CLINICAL MATERNAL–FETAL MEDICINE

CLINICAL MATERNAL–FETAL MEDICINE

Edited by

Hung N. Winn, MD

Professor of Obstetrics and Gynecology
Director, Division of Maternal–Fetal Medicine
Department of Obstetrics, Gynecology & Women's Health
Saint Louis University School of Medicine, and
Chief of Obstetrics, St. Mary's Health Center, St Louis, Missouri, USA

and

John C. Hobbins, MD

Professor of Obstetrics and Gynecology
Chief of Obstetrics
Department of Obstetrics and Gynecology
University of Colorado Health Sciences Center, Denver, Colorado, USA

The Parthenon Publishing Group
International Publishers in Medicine, Science & Technology

NEW YORK   LONDON

Library of Congress Cataloging-in-Publication Data

Data available on request

Published in the UK and Europe by
The Parthenon Publishing Group Limited
Casterton Hall, Carnforth
Lancs., LA6 2LA, UK

Published in the USA by
The Parthenon Publishing Group Inc.
One Blue Hill Plaza
PO Box 1564, Pearl River
NY 10965, USA

British Library Cataloguing in Publication Data
Clinical maternal–fetal medicine
1. Pregnancy - Complications 2. Perinatology
3. Obstetrics 4. Fetus - Diseases
I. Winn, Hung N. II. Hobbins, John C.
618.3

ISBN 1850707987

Copyright © 2000 Parthenon Publishing Group

Typesetting by Siva Math Setters, Chennai, India
Printed by Bookcraft (Bath) Ltd., Midsomer Norton, UK

Contents

List of principal contributors

A. Al-Malt
Fetal Diagnostic Center of Orlando
2905 McRae Avenue, Suite 2
Orlando, FL 32803
USA

G.A. Albright
Bellevue – The Woman's Hospital
Mohawk Anesthesia Associates, P.C.
2210 Troy Road
Niskayuna, NY 12309-4797
USA

S.R. Allen
Section of Maternal–Fetal Medicine
Department of Obstetrics and Gynecology
Texas A & M University College of Medicine
Scott and White Memorial Hospital and Clinic
2401 South 31st Street
Temple, TX 76508
USA

E. Amon
Division of Maternal–Fetal Medicine
Department of Obstetrics and Gynecology
Saint Louis University
6420 Clayton Road, Suite 559
St. Louis, MO 63117
USA

M. Artal
Department of Psychiatry
Saint Louis University
1221 South Grand Boulevard
St. Louis, MO 63104
USA

R. Artal
Division of Maternal–Fetal Medicine
Department of Obstetrics and Gynecology
Saint Louis University
6420 Clayton Road, Suite 559
St. Louis, MO 63117
USA

J.A. Bartelsmeyer
Division of Maternal–Fetal Medicine
Department of Obstetrics and Gynecology
Washington University School of Medicine
3015 North Ballas Road, Ground Floor
St. Louis, MO 63131
USA

M.A. Blinder
Divisions of Hematology and Laboratory Medicine
Departments of Internal Medicine and Pathology
Washington University School of Medicine
660 South Euclid Avenue
St. Louis, MO 63110
USA

B.K. Burton
Division of Genetics and Metabolism
Department of Pediatrics
University of Illinois College of Medicine
840 South Wood Street
Chicago, IL 60612-7324
USA

F.A. Chervenak
Department of Obstetrics and Gynecology
The New York Hospital – Cornell Medical Center
525 East 68th Street – M713
New York, NY 10025
USA

D.B. Clifford
Department of Neurology
Washington University School of Medicine
660 South Euclid Avenue
St. Louis, MO 63110
USA

W.E. Clutter
Division of Endocrinology
Department of Internal Medicine
Washington University School of Medicine
660 South Euclid Avenue, Campus Box 8121
St. Louis, MO 63110
USA

P. Cole
The Heart Health Center
641 North New Ballas Road
St. Louis, MO 63141
USA

C.B. Coulam
Reproductive Immunology
The Center for Human Reproduction
750 N. Orleans Street
Chicago, IL 60610
USA

D.R. Coustan
Department of Obstetrics and Gynecology
Brown University School of Medicine
Women and Infants Hospital of RI
101 Dudley Street
Providence, RI 02905
USA

F. Daffos
Department de Diagnostic
Prenatal et de Medicine Foetale
Institut de Puericulture de Paris
26 Boulevard Brune, 75014 Paris
France

J.G. Dawson
Department of Pediatrics
Washington University School of Medicine
1 Children's Place
St. Louis, MO 63110
USA

J.E. Deaver
Sinai Hospital of Baltimore
Institute for Maternal and Fetal Health
Hoffberger Building Suite 15
2435 West Belvedere Avenue
Baltimore, MD 21215
USA

J.M. Dicke
Department of Obstetrics and Gynecology
Washington University School of Medicine
4911 Barnes-Jewish Hospital Plaza
St. Louis, MO 63110–1094
USA

M.Y. Divon
Department of Obstetrics and Gynecology
Lennox Hill Hospital
100 East 77th Street
New York, NY 10021
USA

M.L. Druzin
Department of Obstetrics and Gynecology
Stanford University School of Medicine
300 Pasteur Drive, Room H-306
Stanford, CA 94306
USA

P. Duff
Division of Maternal–Fetal Medicine
Department of Obstetrics and Gynecology
University of Florida College of Medicine
1600 S.W. Archer Road
Gainesville, FL 32610
USA

C.C. Egley
Division of Maternal–Fetal Medicine
Department of Obstetrics and Gynecology
Methodist Medical Center of Illinois
221 North East Glen Oak Avenue
Peoria, IL 61636
USA

S.A. Gall
Department of Obstetrics and Gynecology
University of Louisville School of Medicine
550 South Jackson Street
Louisville, KY 40202
USA

M.L. Gimovsky
Department of Obstetrics and Gynecology
The Brookdale University Hospital
  and Medical Center
One Brookdale Plaza
Brooklyn, NY 11212–3198
USA

D.K. Grange
Division of Medical Genetics
Department of Pediatrics
Saint Louis University School of Medicine
SSM Cardinal Glennon Children's Hospital
1465 South Grand Boulevard
St. Louis, MO 63104-1095
USA

G.D.V. Hankins
Division of Maternal–Fetal Medicine
Department of Obstetrics and Gynecology
University of Texas Medical Branch
301 University Boulevard
3.4 John Sealy Annex
Galveston, TX 77555-0587
USA

R. Hayashi
Division of Maternal–Fetal Medicine
University of Michigan-Medical Center
Women's Hospital L3208-0264
1500 E. Medical Center Drive
Ann Arbor, MI 48109-0264
USA

T.J. Herzog
Department of Obstetrics and Gynecology
Washington University School of Medicine
4911 Barnes-Jewish Hospital Plaza
St. Louis, MO 63110-1094
USA

W.L. Holcomb, Jr
Division of Maternal–Fetal Medicine
Department of Obstetrics and Gynecology
Saint Louis University
6420 Clayton Road, Suite 559
St. Louis, MO 63117
USA

F. Horvath
Department of Nephrology
University of Illinois College of Medicine at Peoria
515 N.E. Glen Oak, Suite 108
Peoria, IL 61603
USA

J.C. Howitt
Department of Obstetrics and Gynecology
University of Rochester School of Medicine
  and Dentistry
Strong Memorial Hospital
1283 Portland Avenue
Rochester, NY 14621
USA

W.J. Keenan
Department of Pediatrics
Saint Louis University School of Medicine
SSM Cardinal Glennon Children's Hospital
1465 South Grand Boulevard
St. Louis, MO 63104–1095
USA

A.I. Kivikoski
Department of Obstetrics and Gynecology
Washington University School of Medicine
4911 Barnes-Jewish Hospital Plaza
St. Louis, MO 63110-1094
USA

A.B. Levine
Division of Maternal–Fetal Medicine
Department of Obstetrics and Gynecology
Jefferson Medical College
834 Chestnut Street
Philadelphia, PA 19107-5083
USA

A.G. Martin
Division of Dermatology
Washington University School of Medicine
660 South Euclid Avenue, Campus Box 8035
St. Louis, MO 63110
USA

C.M. Martin
Perinatal Laboratory
St. Luke's Hospital
226 S. Woods Mill Road, Suite 62W
Chesterfield, MO 63017-1602
USA

A.T. Masi
Department of Medicine
University of Illinois College of Medicine at Peoria
  (UICOM-P)
1 Illini Drive
Peoria, IL 61605
USA

D. Maulik
Department of Obstetrics and Gynecology
Winthrop-University Hospital
259 First Street
Mineola, NY 11501
USA

J.A. McGregor
Department of Obstetrics and Gynecology
Denver Health Medical Center
777 Bannock Street, Mail Code 0660
Denver, CO 80204
USA

G.R.G. Monif
Department of Obstetrics and Gynecology
Creighton University School of Medicine
Department of Obstetrics and Gynecology
601 N. 30th Street, Suite 4700
Omaha, NB 68131
USA

J.C. Morrison
Division of Maternal–Fetal Medicine
Department of Obstetrics and Gynecology
University of Mississippi Medical Center
2500 North State Street
Jackson, MS 39216-4505
USA

D.J. Mostello
Division of Maternal-Fetal Medicine
Department of Obstetrics and Gynecology
Saint Louis University
6420 Clayton Road, Suite 559
St. Louis, MO 63117
USA

E.R. Newton
Department of Obstetrics and Gynecology
East Carolina University School of Medicine
Room 162 PCMH Teaching Annex
Greenville, NC 27858-4354
USA

M.G. Peters
Division of Gastroenterology
University of California
514 Parnassus Avenue, Room S-357
San Francisco, CA 94143
USA

M. Pietrantoni
Division of Maternal–Fetal Medicine
Department of Obstetrics and Gynecology
University of Louisville School of Medicine
550 South Jackson Street
Louisville, KY 40292
USA

G. Pilu
Clinica Ostetrica e Ginecologia e
    Fisiopatologia Prenatale
Universita degli Studi di Bologna
Policlinico S. Orsola, Via Massarenti, 13
40138 Bologna
Italy

J.M. Piper
Division of Maternal–Fetal Medicine
Department of Obstetrics and Gynecology
The University of Texas Health Science
    Center at San Antonio
7703 Floyd Curl Drive
San Antonio, TX 78284-7836
USA

J. Pratt Rossiter
Division of Maternal–Fetal Medicine
Department of Obstetrics and Gynecology,
    Phipps 228
Johns Hopkins University School of Medicine
600 North Wolfe Street
Baltimore, MD 21287-1228
USA

P.N. Rauk
Department of Obstetrics and Gynecology
    and Reproductive Sciences
University of Pittsburgh School of Medicine
Magee-Womens Hospital
300 Halket Street
Pittsburgh, PA 15213-3180
USA

W.F. Rayburn
Department of Obstetrics and Gynecology
The University of New Mexico
    Health Sciences Center
2211 Lomas Bvd., NE
Albuquerque, NM 87131-5286
USA

R. Romero
Department of Obstetrics and Gynecology
Perinatal Research Branch, NICHD
Wayne State University School of Medicine
Hutzel Hospital
4707 St. Antoine Boulevard
Detroit, MI 48201
USA

D.C. Rubin
Division of Gastroenterology
Washington University School of Medicine
660 South Euclid Avenue, Campus Box 8124
St. Louis, MO 63110
USA

E.P. Schneider
Department of Obstetrics and Gynecology
Cornell University School of Medicine
Northshore Community Hospital
300 Community Drive
Manhasset, NY 11030
USA

D. Schuller
Division of Pulmonary Medicine
    and Critical Care
Washington University School of Medicine
660 South Euclid Avenue, Campus Box 8052
St. Louis, MO 63110-1093
USA

J.B. Shumway
Division of Maternal–Fetal Medicine
Department of Obstetrics and Gynecology
Saint Louis University
6420 Clayton Road, Suite 559
St. Louis, MO 63117
USA

J.M. Shyken
Division of Maternal–Fetal Medicine
Department of Obstetrics and Gynecology
Saint Louis University
6420 Clayton Road, Suite 559
St. Louis, MO 63117
USA

B.M. Sibai
Division of Maternal–Fetal Medicine
Department of Obstetrics and Gynecology
University of Tennessee–Memphis
853 Jefferson, Suite E102
Memphis, TN 38103
USA

J.S. Smeltzer
Wellstar Physicians Group
Wellstar Kennestone Hospital
Marietta, GA 30360
USA

J.L. Swingler
University of Illinois College of Medicine at Peoria
7501 North University, Suite 109
Peoria, IL 61614
USA

P. Tropper
Department of Obstetrics and Gynecology
St. Luke's-Roosevelt Hospital Center
1000 Tenth Avenue
New York, NY 10019
USA

A.M. Vintzileos
Division of Maternal–Fetal Medicine
University of Medicine and Dentistry
  of New Jersey
Robert Wood Johnson Medical School
St. Peter's Medical Center
254 Easton Avenue, MOB 4th Floor
New Brunswick, NJ 08903
USA

R.R. Viscarello
Division of Maternal–Fetal Medicine
Department of Obstetrics and Gynecology
Yale University
Stamford Hospital
1275 Summer Street, Suite 306
Stamford, CT 06905
USA

H.N. Winn
Division of Maternal–Fetal Medicine
Department of Obstetrics and Gynecology
Saint Louis University
6420 Clayton Road, Suite 559
St. Louis, MO 63117
USA

F.R. Witter
Division of Maternal–Fetal Medicine
Department of Obstetrics and Gynecology,
  Phipps 228
Johns Hopkins University School of Medicine
600 North Wolfe Street
Baltimore, MD 21287-1228
USA

Dedication

This textbook is dedicated to Roy H. Petrie, MD, ScD (1940–1995) — an excellent clinician, dedicated teacher, accomplished clinical scientist, and one of the greatest academic leaders of our time. Friends and colleagues around the globe fondly remember his hard work, dedication, ingenuity, honesty, good sense of humor and, most importantly, his genuine concern for his fellow man.

Dr Petrie's innovative research has made a major impact on our obstetrical practices in such important areas as fetal heart rate monitoring, induction of labor, and tocolysis of preterm labor with magnesium sulfate. In addition to authoring numerous articles, he was the editor of several textbooks and co-founded the *Journal of Maternal–Fetal Medicine*. He was instrumental in establishing the Society of Perinatal Obstetricians, now known as the Society of Maternal–Fetal Medicine, the national organization for Maternal–Fetal Medicine physicians. He served as the Society's president in 1984. At the time of his death, he was Professor and Chairman of the Department of Obstetrics and Gynecology at St Louis University School of Medicine.

Dr Petrie is probably best remembered as a great leader in the truest sense of the word. One of the quotes which Roy posted in his office characterized the type of leadership which Roy fostered: "The final test of a leader is that he leaves behind him in other men the conviction and the will to carry on". Roy has left behind, in all of us, the conviction and the will to carry on the mission of progressive education, innovative research, dedication to patient care, and a genuine concern for our fellow man, thus making our society a better place in which to work and to live.

Hung N. Winn and
John C. Hobbins

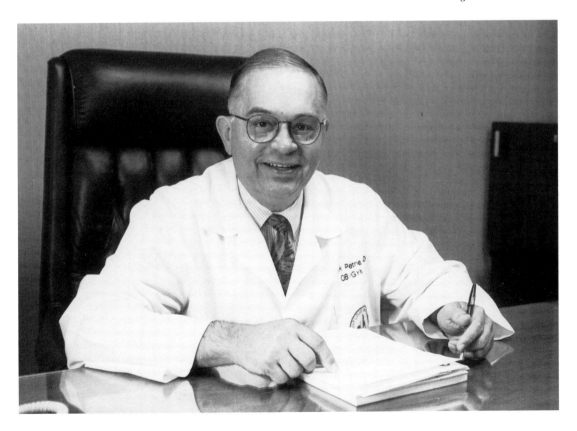

Acknowledgements

To Susan, for her love, support, and her unique perspective.

John C. Hobbins

To my wife, Lee, my children, John, Jessica, and Justin, and my parents –
with love and gratitude. They have made my life meaningful.

Hung N. Winn

Preface

Maternal–fetal medicine has evolved over the last three decades to become a well-established discipline. Its existence is the direct result of the advancements in medicine and medical technology. Its principles and practices derive from the integration of a wide range of disciplines such as critical care, internal medicine, surgery, endoscopic surgery, human genetics, ultrasonography, molecular biology, and toxicology. The current understanding of maternal physiology and pathophysiology has allowed us to obtain more accurate diagnoses and to provide more effective treatments of medical, surgical, and obstetrical maternal complications. More importantly, the fetus has become a distinct individual whose *in utero* environment has become much more accessible to study, diagnosis and treatment.

This textbook is a treatise on the clinical practice of maternal–fetal medicine. It addresses the pathophysiology, diagnosis and treatment of common medical and obstetrical maternal complications and fetal complications. It has been designed to provide a concise and timely review of clinically relevant topics in this discipline. The textbook should serve as a convenient reference for the clinicians and students who have the privilege of caring for a unique symbiotic relationship between a mother and her fetus. It is hoped that our ever-expanding medical knowledge and deep-seated dedication to our patients, and to our profession, will allow all of us to evolve into a healthier and gentler mankind.

Hung N. Winn
and
John C. Hobbins

Section I

Obstetric complications

1

Breech presentation

M.L. Gimovsky, J.P. O'Grady and C. McIlhargie

Breech presentation is a significant obstetric event associated with dramatic increases in perinatal morbidity and mortality[1,2]. The three areas of greatest risk for these infants are the often overlapping problems of preterm delivery, congenital anomalies and birth trauma. More than one-quarter of breech-presenting fetuses are premature. Concomitantly, severe or lethal anomalies further complicate up to 20% of such preterm deliveries and fully 6–7% of term breech deliveries (a relative risk of three- to five-fold), depending on gestational age. In the evaluation of a specific pregnancy with a breech presentation, certain clinical data are important in establishing overall risk. These factors include: the estimated fetal weight, the specific type of breech presentation, the status of the fetal membranes, the size and structure of the maternal bony pelvis, the experience of the operator and the availability of neonatal intensive care. However, with these divergent variables, the central area of concern for clinicians in breech management revolves around the particularly difficult issue of the potential for birth trauma.

Any consideration of breech management involving either a trial of labor or Cesarean delivery is bedevilled by issues of birth injury and medicolegal risk. In the mid-1970s and throughout the 1980s, the response to the perceived risk of physical injury during vaginal breech birth was a dramatic increase in the resort to operative or Cesarean delivery. In addition, external cephalic version was championed as a means of avoiding the issue by converting breech into cephalic presentations. Unfortunately, the results of these major, uncontrolled clinical experiments have not resulted in the substantial reductions in fetal/neonatal injuries that were originally confidently predicted. Utilizing perinatal mortality as an endpoint, a review of the obstetric literature from the 1930s to the 1960s demonstrates a rough linear relationship – i.e. the perinatal death rate for term-sized neonates was reduced as the Cesarean delivery rate increased from 3% to 30% or more (Figure 1). Fetal/neonatal injuries still occur at Cesarean delivery to a surprising degree[2]. In 1981, Green and co-workers[3] reported that, in a relatively controlled setting, i.e. one department over a period of time, increasing the use of Cesarean delivery for breech from 22% to 94% did not eliminate preventable trauma. Therefore, a critical reconsideration

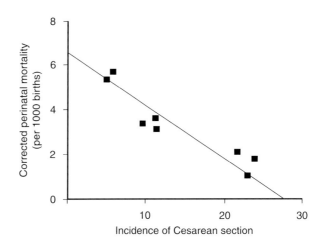

Figure 1 Correlation between Cesarean delivery rates and decreased perinatal mortality in term breech infants in the 1940s and 1950s

of the ideas underlying the assumptions leading to a near-universal resort to Cesarean section for breech presentation is appropriate.

The contribution of delivery route to outcome is hard to measure. It is difficult for even an active and liberal practitioner to develop extensive experience with various management alternatives. Despite inherent limitations, retrospective data are helpful in guiding clinical choices, as individual physicians face a low incidence of such clinical problems.

The intent in this chapter is to consider the current management of breech presentation, the costs and benefits of various management schemes and the documentation and considerations required when clinical choices are made. Our purpose is not necessarily to suggest that the current widespread use of Cesarean section in breech delivery is either excessive or suboptimal, but to emphasize that the data demand a reconsideration of popular practice. Universal Cesarean delivery for breech presentation is far from the whole answer when critically reviewed in the light of present experience. Further, in the long term, universal Cesarean delivery progressively reduces the store of clinical expertise in more traditional obstetric manipulations. The widespread use of Cesarean section does not lessen the need for expertise in performing breech delivery. The problem for the profession is to define which maneuvers can and should be taught, how to maintain a high level of competence in these and how to present the options fairly to our patients.

SPECIAL ISSUES

External cephalic version

A potential technique for reducing the incidence of breech presentation is external cephalic version. External cephalic version performed at 37 weeks to term has decreased the rate of intrapartum breech presentation from 3–4% to 1–2%[4–8]. Earlier groups of investigators had attempted version at 28 to 32 weeks[6] or 30 to 32 weeks[7], but failed to effect any change in the intrapartum rate of breech presentation. These failures erroneously led clinicians to believe that the only versions that succeeded were those that would have occurred spontaneously. These 'early' versions were probably unsuccessful because of the relatively large amount of amniotic fluid relative to the fetus, which therefore reverted to breech after the original procedure. Also, anesthesia and analgesia were employed. This allowed for more forceful procedures, leading to occasional transplacental hemorrhage and isoimmunization, a substantial risk in the era prior to the availability of rhesus immune globulin.

Even in modern practice, version is not without risk, albeit small. Both umbilical cord complications and placental abruption have been described in conjunction with external version[9]. The most common problem associated with version is failure to alter the fetal lie, despite manipulation. Currently, external cephalic version performed under tocolysis (terbutaline, ritodrine or intravenous magnesium sulfate) has a reasonable success rate (50–80%). Also, the concomitant use of non-stress testing, real-time ultrasound and the avoidance of analgesia/anesthesia have contributed to the overall safety of the procedure. An exception to the rule of no analgesia/anesthesia is the occasional use of epidural anesthesia for intrapartum version, a special application for selected cases[10].

There is a place for external cephalic version even in early labor. Depending on the stage of labor at which the patient is admitted and the time when breech presentation is diagnosed, immediate β-mimetic tocolysis is often successful in permitting manipulations. However, after rupture of the membranes and the onset of true labor, any attempt at version becomes both difficult and inherently dangerous, owing to the descent of the presenting part and the potential risk of cord prolapse.

Continued efforts at refinement of external cephalic version have revolved around the issues of tocolysis and anesthesia. Robertson and co-workers[11] found that use of tocolytics for adjunctive treatment after a trial of external cephalic version without tocolytics did not improve success rates. Samuels[12] has described the successful use of regional anesthesia instead of tocolysis for version. No difficulty with sequelae of excessive force was described in his original report. Despite these interesting reports, brief treatment with tocolytics prior to attempting manipulations remains popular, because of the inherent safety, minimal expense and ease of administration of these drugs and their perceived utility. Most clinicians have found that the use of a tocolytic before version (usually 0.125 or 0.250 mg of terbutaline administered subcutaneously) reduces patient discomfort as well as the external force required for the procedure.

CLINICAL ISSUES

The undiagnosed breech

In reaching a decision concerning optimal breech management, it is useful to review data from various breech management protocols. Flanagan and co-workers[13] studied 716 cases of singleton breech presentation at term. Labor and vaginal delivery occurred in 72% of selected patients. Although antepartum external cephalic version was helpful in reducing the overall incidence of breech presentation, nearly 40% of term breeches were not identified until the onset of labor. These data emphasize an important point. Management protocols must be activated at the time of hospital admission to select candidates for a trial of labor as opposed to those for Cesarean section.

Management not according to protocol is a serious clinical issue in breech management. In a prospective study of term breech presentations (all types of breech presentations) involving data collected from two large teaching services, Gimovsky and Petrie[14] reported a 64% success rate for selective trial of labor. Outcomes measured in this study included perinatal mortality and morbidity assessed by low Apgar scores and bony and peripheral nerve injuries. Protocol-managed infants, regardless of delivery mode, had outcomes similar to those of infants undergoing elective Cesarean delivery. As in earlier studies, these authors reported that patients whose vaginal breech deliveries were managed outside the protocol incurred the most severe infant injuries[15] (Table 1).

Based on a literature review from 1974 to 1987, Brigham and Lilford[16] applied a paradigm to estimate the benefits of a selective trial of labor approach vs. elective Cesarean delivery for breech presentations at term. Decision analysis utilizes general assumptions regarding outcome, but faces limitations regarding specific circumstances. Unfortunately, the authors employed data from 25 retrospective studies and had only two prospective studies to form the basis of probability estimates regarding the benefits of a selective trial of labor approach vs. elective Cesarean delivery for breech presentations at term. These studies were from a variety of institutions over a time span in which

Table 1 Perinatal outcome vs. management strategy. Data from reference 14, with permission

	Non-protocol	*Protocol*		
	Elective Cesarean section (protocol bypass)	*Imminent delivery (vaginal delivery)*	*Selective Cesarean section*	*Selective trial of labor (vaginal delivery)*
Number of patients	463	39	72	132
Corrected perinatal mortality	0.002 (2/1000)	0.025 (25/1000)	0.013 (13/1000)	0.007 (7/1000)
Apgar score < 7 at 5 min	0.015 (1.5%)	0.179 (17.9%)	0.041 (4.1%)	0.038 (3.8%)
Brachial plexus injury	(1) moderate Erb's palsy (2/1000)	(1) severe Erb's palsy (25/1000) (2) moderate Erb's palsies (51/1000)	(1) mild Erb's palsy (13/1000)	(2) mild Erb's injury (15/1000)
Bony fractures	(0)	(1) fractured clavicle	(0)	(0)
Other injuries diagnosed at delivery	(1) moderate lacerations	(0)	(2) minor lacerations	(1) minor vulvar hemorrhage
Total minor neonatal injuries	(0)	(0)	(3)	(3)
Total moderate and severe neonatal injuries	(2) moderate	(3) moderate (1) severe		

Symptoms present at discharge, moderate injury; symptoms present at 6 months of life, severe lacerations; minor, no suturing; moderate, requiring sutures

the approach to this clinical problem was undergoing dramatic change. This analysis is also limited by the sizeable percentage of breech presentations that were not identified prior to the onset of labor. A significant proportion of cases were unavailable for elective Cesarean section, or for a trial of prophylactic external cephalic version.

Despite a decision to submit all breeches to Cesarean delivery, some instances of vaginal breech delivery cannot be avoided, owing to unforeseen events such as undiagnosed breech presentation or breech presentation diagnosed too late in labor. Regardless of their view towards vaginal trials or Cesarean delivery, it is vital for all clinicians to develop experience in the management of both breech extraction at Cesarean section and vaginal breech delivery. The routine resort to Cesarean delivery does not guarantee a perfect infant nor obviate the clinician's need for great care and substantial skill as an accoucheur in the operating room. Not surprisingly, measurable rates of the entire range of birth injuries occur in Cesarean sections, although the incidence is low. The occurrence of these injuries at Cesarean section underscores the need for full understanding of the manual maneuvers utilized for breech delivery. In the performance of safe Cesarean section for breech presentation, the surgeon must possess facility with total breech extraction. Even with the exposure possible at laparotomy, breech extraction remains an inherently more dangerous procedure than the assisted breech delivery performed in the majority of vaginal breech births[17]. Such procedures require thoughtful and judicious application of force. Commensurate with the increased use of abdominal operative delivery, maternal morbidity, both immediate and remote, is also greatly increased, although the majority of these complications prove to be of trivial clinical consequence[18].

Selective trial of labor

Protocols for vaginal delivery of breech infants need critical review. An important consideration in determining best management is the type of breech presentation. The largest group of breech fetuses at term are in frank breech position. The best data reflect management protocols for these most favorable cases. Collea and co-workers[18] conducted a prospective randomized study that compared elective Cesarean section with protocol-managed labor for fetuses with frank breech presentation at term. They reported significant maternal morbidity among patients delivered by Cesarean section, without any dramatic improvement in neonatal outcome. Among 60 infants delivered vaginally, there were two instances of brachial plexus injury. O'Leary[19] performed a similar study at the University of South Alabama. Among term frank breech presentations screened by a protocol similar to that described by Collea and co-workers, O'Leary described one injury in 81 vaginal deliveries, and this occurred during a breech extraction performed for fetal distress. In this study the comparison group was a cohort of breech deliveries managed without the specific requirements of protocol. In this same group a similar number of infants were stillborn; however, one infant died of trauma, eight had low Apgar scores and four experienced birth injuries. The author concluded that the use of the protocol had significantly improved the outcome for the breech infants in the study.

In a study of all types of breech presentation (including non-frank or complete, incomplete and footling breeches) at the Sloane Hospital for Women in New York, a protocol similar to that of O'Leary was followed by Gimovsky and co-workers[15]. The authors found that selective management by protocol of term breech fetuses, even those non-frank in presentation, gave acceptable immediate neonatal performance in comparison to elective Cesarean section (Table 2). The outcome for protocol-managed breech fetuses delivered vaginally was essentially identical to that of all patients delivered by elective Cesarean section. The protocol in use at Columbia has since been revised[20]. In 1983, Gimovsky and co-workers[21] reported preliminary results of the new protocol that confirmed a similar outcome between patients with elective Cesarean section and selected protocol-managed patients. In that prospective study of non-frank breech presentations at term, a rigorous protocol was employed for intrapartum management (Figure 2). One fetus in the study group of 105 patients died during the intrapartum period, owing to an unusual complication that emphasized the complex problems of clinical medicine. This occurred when a woman became hysterical during a trial of vaginal delivery. Efforts to place her under anesthesia to effect safe vaginal delivery were prolonged and the infant eventually delivered could not be resuscitated, despite intensive efforts.

Informed consent

In an area such as management of breech presentation which is rife with controversy, informed patient consent for any clinical approach is not only prudent, it is mandatory. The mother (and her spouse) must be advised of the facts necessary to make an informed, independent choice of either undergoing a trial of labor or of proceeding with Cesarean delivery. This explanation needs to be simple, factual, balanced and complete. Despite the complexities that attend such assessment and obstetric decision making, the obstetrician has an obligation to make the essential and pivotal factors that are central to a clinical choice understandable to the patient. Ideally, the actual decision should be made by the patient and not simply surrendered to the obstetrician. To do otherwise invites the risk that a patient who experiences a sad or untoward result will respond with blame and feelings of betrayal.

The focus of the obstetrician's explanation should emphasize a detailed comparison of risks attendant on the alternatives: specifically trial of labor vs. prompt Cesarean delivery once labor begins or term has been reached. The issue of possible version should also be carefully discussed. The nature, purpose and risks (to both mother and infant) should be outlined for both approaches. The obstetrician must explain and discuss the following.

(1) The nature of breech presentation. In this review the clinician explains how breech differs from cephalic presentation and factors that influence perinatal morbidity and mortality in breech delivery.

(2) A comparison of the mechanics of Cesarean section with vaginal delivery after a trial of labor, with emphasis on the increased risk of fetal injuries secondary to the dynamics of the delivery process. This explanation should include the observations that, with cephalic presentation, the largest and most unyielding part comes first and then the softer, more malleable parts follow. With breech presentation, the softer more malleable parts are received first, followed by the relatively larger and unyielding head. If the head proves

Table 2 Results by delivery type, presentation and outcome. Data from reference 15, with permission

	Protocol group	*Non-protocol group*	*Control group 1*	*Control group 2*
Type of delivery	vaginal	vaginal	spontaneous vaginal	elective Cesarean section
Presentation	breech	breech	vertex	vertex (95%), breech (5%)
Mean birth weight (g)	3125	3025	3170	2980
range	2001–4080	2000–4210	2470–4010	2350–4100
Number of deliveries	130	78	130	130
Ward/private ratio	59/41	62/38	60/40	58/42
Mean 5-min Apgar score	8.6	8.1	8.7	8.6
Neonatal morbidity	4/130	12/78	3/130	2/130
		($p < 0.001$)	($p < 0.50$)	($p < 0.34$)
Intrapartum mortality	0	1	0	0
Perinatal mortality*	0	12.8	0	0

* A comparison of the results obtained with a selective management protocol for the management of the term breech fetus, including all types of specific breech presentation

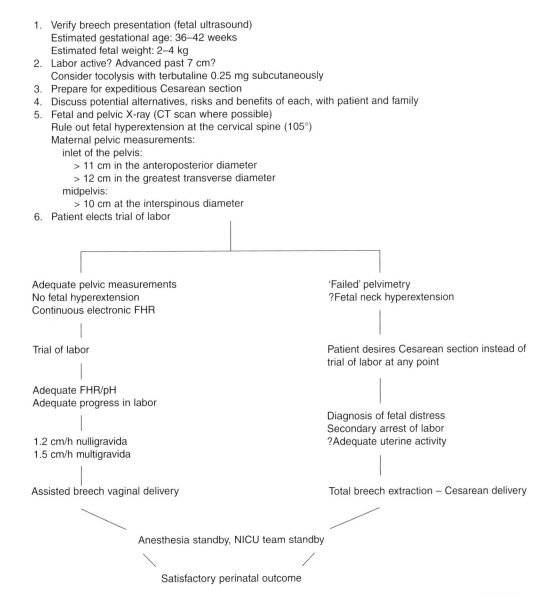

1. Verify breech presentation (fetal ultrasound)
   Estimated gestational age: 36–42 weeks
   Estimated fetal weight: 2–4 kg
2. Labor active? Advanced past 7 cm?
   Consider tocolysis with terbutaline 0.25 mg subcutaneously
3. Prepare for expeditious Cesarean section
4. Discuss potential alternatives, risks and benefits of each, with patient and family
5. Fetal and pelvic X-ray (CT scan where possible)
   Rule out fetal hyperextension at the cervical spine (105°)
   Maternal pelvic measurements:
        inlet of the pelvis:
             > 11 cm in the anteroposterior diameter
             > 12 cm in the greatest transverse diameter
        midpelvis:
             > 10 cm at the interspinous diameter
6. Patient elects trial of labor

Adequate pelvic measurements
No fetal hyperextension
Continuous electronic FHR

Trial of labor

Adequate FHR/pH
Adequate progress in labor

1.2 cm/h nulligravida
1.5 cm/h multigravida

Assisted breech vaginal delivery

'Failed' pelvimetry
?Fetal neck hyperextension

Patient desires Cesarean section instead of
trial of labor at any point

Diagnosis of fetal distress
Secondary arrest of labor
?Adequate uterine activity

Total breech extraction – Cesarean delivery

Anesthesia standby, NICU team standby

Satisfactory perinatal outcome

Figure 2   Selective management protocol for intrapartum breech management. FHR, fetal heart rate; NICU, neonatal intensive care unit. From reference 14, with permission

too big for the pelvic outlet, and the rest of the baby is already delivered, there is a substantially increased risk for significant injury to the infant.

(3) The nature of specific risks of Cesarean section to the mother from hemorrhage, infection or unanticipated lacerations vs. the potential for genital tract lacerations and hemorrhage associated with breech delivery with or without the use of forceps.

(4) Data on potential fetal injury, including the risks to the infants of intracranial hemorrhage and significant long-term neurological injury, either by Cesarean section or by vaginal incidental to breech delivery.

(5) The limitations of current diagnostic techniques (both clinical and radiographic). This discussion explains why these procedures cannot absolutely exclude fetopelvic disproportion.

(6) The basis for recommending a trial of labor or Cesarean delivery. This includes the basis for the obstetrician's judgement as to the risks and benefits in a manner tailored to the specific factors of this patient's clinical presentation.

(7) The protocol for surveillance and availability of emergency Cesarean section if a trial of vaginal delivery is elected. The obstetrician should emphasize the dynamics of ongoing evaluation and the potential for abandoning a trial of labor and proceeding immediately to emergency Cesarean section when there is failed progress of labor or evidence of fetal distress. In this context, consent

to a Cesarean section based upon the physician's clinical judgement must be obtained in advance of undertaking a trial of labor.

(8) The limits of prediction. The clinician needs to emphasize that, although this protocol of surveillance relies on meticulous monitoring, which is reasonably calculated to limit risk of injury to the infant, risks are never completely eliminated. Therefore, there is no guarantee of an outcome free from complications or injuries, regardless of the route of delivery.

(9) The role of version. This discussion critically reviews the advantages vs. the risks of external cephalic version and why this procedure should or should not be attempted in the patient's specific case.

Because there is controversy surrounding the decision to recommend a trial of labor with breech presentation, as opposed to proceeding immediately to Cesarean section, the obstetrician is well advised to make a balanced presentation of both views. The clinician must be prepared to explain that those who favor Cesarean delivery in all cases may rely on statistics which suggest that three times as many fetal injuries occur with vaginal/breech delivery as compared to Cesarean section. Those advocating trial of labor with a breech presentation will want to explain how a meticulously implemented protocol of surveillance can render the statistical difference between these procedures negligible. In making such explanations, the obstetrician should resist favoring the decision he/she wants by either exaggerating or underrating the risks of one management plan over another. The use of dramatic overstatement or florid language will undoubtedly be long remembered by an apprehensive mother or an expectant father. If the decision is to be truly that of the patient, based upon information, the facts and just the facts should be presented in a logical and unemotional manner, as free from bias as possible. At the end of this discussion, an obstetrician is well advised to invite any questions the patient might have and make every effort to ensure that both she and her partner are satisfied with the explanation given.

In cases in which the breech presentation has been recognized prior to the onset of labor, such discussions will be likely to have occurred outside the hospital. It is prudent to review the same date briefly with the woman/family following admission for labor/delivery. These in-hospital conversations are best conducted in the presence of a nurse, who can then independently document in the medical record that the pertinent consent discussions have taken place.

Pelvic measurement and fetal evaluation

When selecting patients as candidates for a trial of labor, careful, objective evaluation of the fetopelvic size is

mandatory. Radiographs can provide this information and also document that the fetal skull is normal in both general appearance and attitude. Ultrasound scanning has also been extensively employed in describing fetal size, structural normality and head attitude and is useful in acute evaluation of the baby[22,23].

Ultrasound or radiographic studies are particularly useful in the diagnosis of hyperextension of the fetal head, a condition that occurs when an angle of more than 105° exists between the fetal mandible and the main axis of the cervical spine. This is an absolute contraindication to an attempt at vaginal delivery[24]. Even at Cesarean delivery with an adequate incision, meticulous attention to minimal force is required for safe delivery of a breech infant with cranial hyperextension. Experience suggests that up to 5% of term breech infants have this additional risk. Early diagnosis is important, as prolonged labor with hyperextended head may also result in cervical spine injury, even when delivery is ultimately accomplished by Cesarean section[25].

The additional purpose of radiographic assessment of the mother is to diagnose women with moderate degrees of pelvic disproportion prior to attempting delivery of the aftercoming head. Entrapment of the fetal head and/or difficult delivery may be largely avoided if such cases are taken to Cesarean section without a trial of labor. Radiography can define patients with potential borderline pelves; however, these studies are not guarantors of perfect safety, nor do they substitute for clinical expertise.

Radiographic pelvimetry first appeared in Europe in the late 19th century following Roentgen's discovery of the X-ray. Over its long history, the popularity of radiographic pelvimetry has waxed and waned, owing, in part, to its risks and to questions regarding its accuracy. Recently, there has been a shift to pelvic measurement by computerized tomography (CT). A pilot study in 1985 indicated the applicability of such management[26]. In 1986 Kopelman and co-workers[27] assessed the reliability of this method in a breech protocol and reported favorable results. Standard pelvimetry techniques in use up to that time, with the radiation exposure to maternal and fetal gonads, were compared with the equally useful single CT scan[28]. CT generates more accurate and more reproducible data than other techniques[26] (Figure 3).

Taken alone, the measurement of pelvic diameters is not capable of reliably directing management, especially for women in labor. Experience has shown that minimal pelvic inlet measurements of 11 cm in the anteroposterior diameter and 12 cm at the transverse of the inlet, coupled with 10 cm at the mid-pelvic plane of the intraspinous diameter, are consistent with a normal bony pelvis (10, 11, 12 rule)[15,20,21,29]. These recommended measurements should be used as a starting point in considering the labor of an average-sized fetus at term. A clinical consideration of fetal size is obviously a major issue in deciding upon the

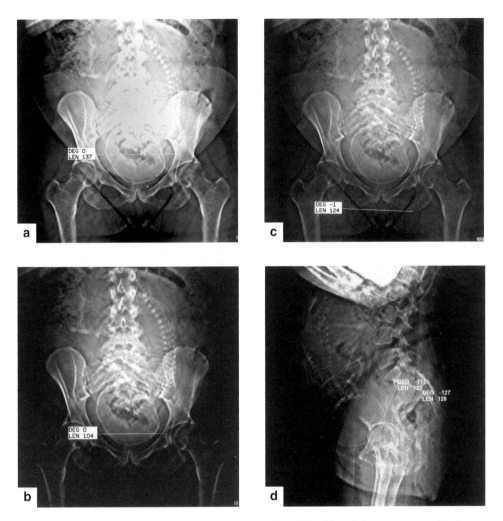

Figure 3 Computer topography of the maternal pelvis and the flexed fetal head demonstrates: (a) the transverse diameter of the pelvic inlet from an anterior-posterior view; (b) transverse diameter of the mid-pelvic from an anterior-posterior view; (c) the transverse diameter of the pelvic outlet from an anterior-posterior view; and (d) the anterior-posterior diameters of the pelvic inlet (123) and mid-pelvis (128) from a lateral view.

appropriateness of a labor trial. It may be helpful for the attending obstetrician to review the pelvimetry directly. At present, we are evaluating the use of the fetal head circumference obtained by ultrasonography in addition to the CT-derived pelvic inlet measurements as a more definitive guide to fetopelvic disproportion[30].

As maternal position during labor affects pelvic diameters, careful maternal placement and positioning during delivery is important. Thorough evaluation of the fetus for structural abnormalities and position by real-time scanning is also critical prior to making decisions regarding management. The use of a β-mimetic (such as terbutaline 0.250 mg subcutaneously) is a useful adjunct to slow down uterine contractions, to permit sufficient time for ultrasonic studies and maternal pelvic measurements. When circumstances dictate an expeditious delivery by Cesarean section, brief tocolysis lessens both operative and anesthetic risks by relaxing the uterus and permitting sufficient time for a proper

discussion of informed consent[10]. It should be noted that clinical pelvic examination is still important. Soft tissue resistance, which can create a significant problem for vaginal delivery, is not directly measurable but can be assessed by an experienced attendant. Although it is difficult to quantify, the slope of the pelvic sidewalls and the position of the sacrum also play a role in the estimated pelvic capacity and the likelihood of an uncomplicated vaginal delivery.

Fetal surveillance

Continuous fetal surveillance is essential in intrapartum management of breech labor, as umbilical cord prolapse is a potential hazard in all breech presentations. Cord complications are most likely to occur in the second stage of labor, which should be conducted in the delivery room. In 1963, in the pre-electronic fetal monitoring era, Rovinsky and co-wokers[31] showed that vertex fetuses had the same risk of intrapartum demise from overt cord prolapse as did frank breeches. It is of interest that both these presentations subject the fetus to a greater risk for compromise from cord accidents than do footling and complete breech presentations, probably because of the close clinical attention paid to the non-frank breech labor.

The usual criteria for interpreting intrapartum electronic fetal monitoring apply, regardless of fetal position. Nishijima and colleagues[32] compared nulliparas' and multiparas' fetal heart rate patterns in labor for breech and vertex presentations and found no essential difference.

Wheeler and Greene[33] have suggested that periodic fetal heart rate accelerations are more common in breech babies, presumably because of a difference in vaginal stimulation. Our experience, based upon umbilical cord gas studies at birth, confirm that the fetal acid–base status is normal when fetal heart rate patterns are normal during labor.

Vaginal breech delivery results in cord respiratory blood gas values and Apgar scores at birth that are similar to those observed at Cesarean delivery. These data are consistent with the previously described findings concerning the similarity between both fetal heart rate monitoring patterns and capillary pH in breech-presenting fetuses, independent of the mode of delivery[32,33].

Anesthesia

Skilled anesthetic support is essential for safe breech management. In the past, practitioners commonly used pudendal nerve blocks in trials of labor, with a general anesthetic supplement in about 10% of cases, if required[2]. Epidural anesthesia, when available, offers further advantages and is the current first choice for many clinicians[34]. For the small breech fetus or the footling breech presentation, adequate anesthesia helps to dampen maternal bearing-down efforts, retarding spontaneous membrane rupture and involuntary pushing. This also decreases the risk of umbilical cord or fetal body prolapse through an incompletely dilated cervix[34]. The absence of such involuntary bearing-down efforts is also desirable when the clinician's intent is to deliver a markedly premature fetus in caul.

The anesthesiologist should be immediately available. Adequate anesthesia for either emergency Cesarean section, should it be necessary, or vaginal manipulations, is essential to a successful and safe trial of labor. Neonatal support is also important for a good outcome. Regardless of the delivery route, the breech presentation is a high-risk situation and neonatal resuscitation, when required, must be prompt, proper and expeditious.

Dynamics of labor

Parity plays little or no role in the outcome of trials of labor. In fact, despite the beliefs of many clinicians, there may actually be an increase in perinatal morbidity among multiparas undergoing vaginal breech delivery[15]. In multiparas, the aftercoming fetal head can deliver so quickly that acute and unpredictable fluctuations occur in fetal intracranial pressure which presumably lowers Apgar scores.

The judicious use of oxytocin in selected cases is permissible and does not prejudice outcome[1,15,18,21]. In their experience at Moffitt Hospital, Flanagan and co-workers[13] reported no difference in the perinatal outcome seen among patients with breech presentation given a trial of labor with or without the administration of oxytocin. In this study almost 20% of the patients received oxytocin, primarily for labor induction.

Therefore, if the breech is engaged, the fetus is of normal size, the fetal head is flexed and the radiographic measurements show the pelvis to be adequate, induction of labor by oxytocin is acceptable[29]. However, oxytocin augmentation of breech labor is rarely indicated, given both the potential risks and the current medicolegal atmosphere. The experience at Los Angeles County-University of Southern California Medical Center indicates that oxytocin augmentation rarely achieves safe vaginal delivery of a breech infant if a secondary arrest of active-phase labor has occurred[2]. Therefore, great care is needed if normal progression in labor does not occur. These data tend to confirm an earlier observation of Friedman[35], that feto-pelvic disproportion is a frequent cause of secondary arrest in breech labor. There is also an association between larger infants and abnormalities in labor. Approximately three-fourths of women who deliver breech infants weighing more than 3500 g develop a dysfunctional labor pattern. An abnormal labor pattern is therefore a critical clue that a decision for vaginal trial should be carefully reasoned and that Cesarean delivery may be indicated.

The authors consider that 3500–4000 g is the upper limit considered as a safe fetal size for vaginal breech delivery. Therefore, the practitioner must be careful to avoid 'forcing' a trial of labor in the presence of a known or suspected large breech fetus. Both ultrasound and clinical weight estimates should be combined in judging fetal size. The lower limits of safe progress in labor are ≥ 1.2 cm per hour for nulliparas and ≥ 1.5 cm per hour for multiparas. In the presence of normal uterine activity, women failing to dilate at this rate should be taken to Cesarean section without an attempt at oxytocin augmentation of labor.

Accouchement

If a vaginal trial is elected, the second stage of labor should be carried out in the delivery room with continuous fetal monitoring. Perhaps more than in any other obstetric setting, vaginal delivery of a breech fetus requires both watchful waiting and gentle manipulation. An experienced, gowned and gloved assistant and a scrub nurse should be present for the delivery.

A safe assisted breech delivery requires that the accoucher understands the judicious application of force. An 80-kg obstetrician can easily overpower a 3000-g neonate. However, excessive force alone is not necessarily the major cause of injury. Acute rotation of the fetal body for delivery of the arms or head exceeding 90° may compromise the vertebral blood supply to the central nervous system. In addition, maintaining flexion of the aftercoming head during the actual birth process is crucial. Gentle but firm and continuous suprapubic force needs to be judiciously applied by an assistant to the aftercoming head as the delivery proceeds. The accoucher must also be prepared either to apply forceps or to reach for the face of the aftercoming fetal head during delivery. It is well to recall that Piper forceps were designed to act as a lever and not as a tractor in aiding the delivery of the head. Good results with forceps to the aftercoming head have been described by Milner[36] (Table 3). If forceps are not applied, the Mariceau–Smellie–Veit (MSV) maneuver is the procedure of choice in completing the breech delivery. The purpose of the suprapubic pressure is not to effect delivery by *accouchement forcé* but simply to maintain cranial flexion during descent, thus facilitating the entry of the fetal skull into the pelvis by continuously presenting the smallest diameter. If the clinician fails to 'follow' the fetal head by exerting gentle but continuous transabdominal pressure on the uterus, cranial extension can occur, resulting in a difficult delivery as a larger diameter of the cranium is presented to the maternal pelvis. Haste is dangerous in the management of breech delivery and almost always unnecessary. Slow, gentle manipulations are always best. Normal cord gases are seen even after a 6-min delay from emergence of the umbilicus to final delivery.

A comparison of duration between the vaginal route of delivery and Cesarean section is illuminating. We have found that, in two-thirds of cases, the duration of time during vaginal delivery is shorter than the incision-to-delivery time at Cesarean section[37].

Table 3 Vaginal breech delivery: impact of forceps to aftercoming head. Data from reference 36

Birth weight (g)	Neonatal deaths (%)	
	No forceps	*Forceps*
1500–1999	22.3	11.0
2000–2499	7.8	0.0
2500–2999	3.5	0.5

Documentation

Complete and accurate records are essential in the conduct of breech management, regardless of the mode of delivery chosen. Within the progress notes, the obstetrician should detail the discussions which are the foundation of patient informed consent. As has already been discussed, the obstetrician is well advised to have a knowledgeable labor and delivery nurse present at the time of these interactions who can, in his/her own nursing notes, confirm the nature and extent of the discussions.

The obstetrician should record in the progress notes the basis for the clinical judgements made in support of the decision to conduct a trial of labor or Cesarean section. This note should stress the clinical and diagnostic factors which favor the choice that was made. If a trial of labor is planned, the note should make a statement of the specifics of the protocol to be followed, with emphasis on the elements of meticulous observation during the progress of labor, ongoing assessment of adequacy of descent, continuous fetal monitoring and preparedness for immediate emergency Cesarean delivery. The progress note recorded during the course of labor itself should set forth in detail the basis for all clinical decisions in response to significant changes in maternal/fetal status. This process may at first appear to be excessive, but it is nothing more than a plan for strict adherence to the usual standards for documentation of high-risk labor.

COMPLICATIONS

Prematurity and low birth weight

The low birth weight breech fetus, between 25 and 36 weeks' gestation, presents a clinical challenge[24,38,39]. These fetuses have up to a one in five chance of having a major congenital malformation[2,38]. Further, such pregnancies are commonly complicated by significant obstetric problems including but not limited to placenta previa, abruptio placentae and multiple gestations[40]. Owing to the relative sizes of head and abdomen, the risk of cord prolapse (or body prolapse) through an incompletely dilated cervix is high.

The limits of ultrasound measurement are also a problem. Underestimation of fetal weight results in fetuses that are essentially dismissed as being too small to survive[41]. Less likely is the overestimation of fetal weight, which can lead to heroic efforts for fetuses with limited chance for survival. A rough summation of the available, complex clinical data suggests improvements in outcome for breech infants with birth weights of 1000–2000 g delivered by Cesarean section[40]. In contrast, above 2000 g, a trial of labor seems reasonable under appropriate select circumstances, particularly for frank and complete breech presentations[42]. There are other more subtle issues as well. The head to

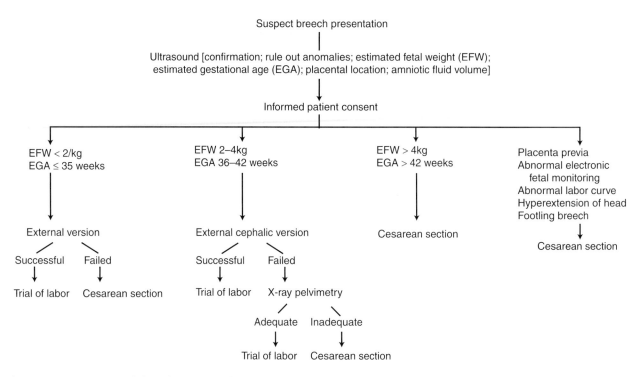

Figure 4   Overview and flow diagram of the management of breech presentation in early labor. From reference 43, with permission

abdomen ratio of 1.0 or less favors a breech delivery of a normally grown 2100-g fetus over a less mature or growth-retarded fetus of the same weight. In the growth-retarded fetus, the abdomen can be significantly smaller than the head and thus more likely to prolapse through a partially dilated cervix, resulting in entrapment of the fetal head.

For the fetus between 34 and 38 weeks' gestation, there may be a crucial difference, based on estimates of gestational age and fetal weight, in the likelihood of success and safety of a trial of labor vs. Cesarean delivery. By insisting on a clinically estimated fetal weight of *more* than 2000 g and gestational age of ≥ 36 weeks, a reasonable margin of error is built into the protocol.

Untoward results

In the event of an untoward result following either a vaginal trial or a Cesarean delivery, the facts of the occurrence must be carefully documented. If the obstetrician has appropriately documented adherence to the originally decided protocol, and clinical decision making throughout the course of the trial of labor or Cesarean delivery has followed this plan, there should be little need for lengthy commentary or explanation in the progress note. Protracted retrospective explanations entered into the medical record with the hope that subsequent medical/legal reviewers will be persuaded to exonerate a physician's conduct seldom prove effective, unless the remainder of the chart

adequately documents a coherent *prospective* plan. In fact, many physicians find themselves compromised by their own 'explanatory remarks', because such hastily formulated notations are frequently either incomplete or poorly articulated.

Initial discussions with the mother concerning the injury or death of her infant ought to be prompt. In these conversations, the clinician should frankly discuss the infant's status and/or prognosis, if it is accurately known. Imparting either falsely hopeful or falsely negative information is more harmful than simply stating that the baby's condition is uncertain or under evaluation. Because an atmosphere of strong emotion often attends this initial communication, it is sometimes wise for the obstetrician to defer detailed discussion of the circumstances which led to the unpleasant result (if they are known) until a later time. Once the mother/family is calm and reasonably receptive to such discussion, the physician should explain what happened. Obstetricians who regularly pride themselves on their skill, knowledge and professional acumen are at that moment met with a singularly demanding challenge: embracing their own human limitations and explaining in plain language why they were powerless to prevent this untoward result. Honest acknowledgment of both human and technical limitations is necessary and appropriate. If done properly this should simply reinforce what the patient should have known before the delivery was ever undertaken. The gift of simple humanity on the part of the physician at this juncture will go a long way towards healing the loss experienced by both the patient and the doctor. It is good practice to have another observer (nurse, colleague, etc.) present during these discussions. Obviously, it is prudent to notify the hospital risk management service of such complications, as it is always uncertain whether formal legal proceedings will result from any complication and the lag time between the event and the legal complaint can be long indeed.

CONCLUSIONS

The results of several recent studies of term breech delivery generally confirm the advice given by earlier generations of obstetricians: a management program consisting of radiological confirmation of pelvic adequacy in conjunction with careful assessment of labor and continuous fetal monitoring produces outcomes in neonates born vaginally that are comparable with those delivered abdominally[15,18–21] (Figure 4).

At the Sloane Hospital for Women[15], such a protocol has resulted in a 55–65% Cesarean section rate for breech presentation at term. This compares favorably with the current national Cesarean section rate of 80–90% for such patients. Nevertheless, all prudent observers recognize that a single numerical expression such as Cesarean section rate is at best an artificial approach to quality of care, especially in optimal management of as complex a problem as breech presentation.

Although liberal use of Cesarean section reduces the potential for trauma and hypoxia in breech delivery, it by no means eliminates it; this would be true even if every breech could be delivered operatively[3]. In establishing any protocol and ultimately in reaching a management plan for any individual patient, it is necessary to balance the risks and benefits for both mother and neonate from Cesarean section and vaginal delivery and to counsel families accordingly. Where facilities allow for expeditious Cesarean section, selected patients may safely be offered a trial of labor. However, to assure maternal and fetal safety, the obstetrician must be committed to thorough evaluation of the maternal pelvis and close attention to the course of labor. Further, the clinician must know the mechanics of safe breech delivery, regardless of the delivery route initially chosen. At Cesarean section, although the infant is being delivered through incisions in the abdominal wall, the mechanism of delivery by extraction has the potential for greatly traumatizing the infant unless extreme care is exercised. Even at Cesarean section, peripheral nerve and bony injuries to the fetus are not only possible, but seen to occur with regularity[14]. The obstetrician can minimize the risk of trauma to the breech fetus born by Cesarean section or vaginally after a labor trial by close attention to detail with the application of the standard obstetric techniques for assisted delivery. The same approaches to delivery apply to both Cesarean section and vaginal delivery: minimal force, careful pressure to the aftercoming head to prevent the loss of flexion and judicious use of the MSV maneuver and/or Piper forceps for cranial extraction.

Based on the cumulative experience of many clinicians on multiple obstetric services, traumatic birth injuries to both the parturient and her fetus can often be avoided and always be minimized in the management of breech presentation. A program of antepartum external cepahlic version offers the advantage of decreasing the incidence of breech presentation in labor, thus avoiding these dilemmas for the clinician. Although Cesarean section will be used to deliver many breech infants, a selective trial of labor employing strict protocol adherence can be satisfying to both physician and parturient and result in an equally good outcome.

REFERENCES

1. Kauppila D. The perinatal mortality in breech deliveries and observation of affecting factors. *Acta Obstet Gynecol Scand* (Suppl) 1975;39:1–145

2. Gimovsky ML, Paul RH. Singleton breech presentation in labor – experience in 1980. *Am J Obstet Gynecol* 1982; 143:733–80

3. Green JE, McLean F, Smtth LP, *et al.* Has an increased Cesarean section rate for term breech delivery reduced the incidence of birth asphyxia, trauma and deaths? *Am J Obstet Gynecol* 1981;142:643–8

4. Van Dorsten JP, Schifrin BS, Wallace R. Randomized controlled trial of external cephalic version with tocolysis in late pregnancy. *Am J Obstet Gynecol* 1981;141: 417–21

5. Hotmyer GJ. Effect of external cephalic version in late pregnancy on breech presentation and Cesarean section rate: a controlled trial. *Br J Obstet Gynaecol* 1983; 90:392–4

6. Brosset A. The value of prophylactic external cephalic version in cases of breech presentation. *Acta Obstet Gynecol Scand* 1956;35:555–7

7. Kasule J, Chimbria T, Brown I. Controlled trial of external cephalic version. *Br J Obstet Gynaecol* 1985;92: 14–17

8. Fortinato S, Mercer L, Guzick D. External cephalic version with tocolysis – factors associated with success. *Obstet Gynecol* 1988;72:59–61

9. Gimovsky ML, O'Grady JO, Keroack E. Immediate neonatal outcome of vaginal breech delivery at term in oxytocin stimulated labor; abstr. *Am J Obstet Gynecol* 1993;168:436

10. Gimovsky ML. Short term tocolysis adjunctive to intrapartum term breech management. *Am J Obstet Gynecol* 1985;153:233

11. Robertson AW, Kopelman JN, Read JA, *et al.* External cephalic version at term – is a tocolytic necessary? *Obstet Gynecol* 1987;70:896–7

12. Samuels P. Epidural facilitates external version. *Obstet Gynecol News* 1990;25:1

13. Flanagan TA, Mulclahey KM, Korenbrot CC, *et al.* Management of term breech presentation. *Am J Obstet Gynecol* 1987;156:1492–9

14. Gimovsky ML, Petrie RH. The intrapartum management of the breech presentation. *Clin Perinatol* 1989;16:975–86

15. Gimovsky ML, Petrie RH, Todd WD. Neonatal performance of the selected term vaginal breech delivery. *Obstet Gynecol* 1980;56:687–91

16. Brigham P, Lilford R. Management of the selected term breech presentation – assessment of the risks of selected vaginal delivery versus Cesarean section for all cases. *Obstet Gynecol* 1987;69:965–9

17. Kerr M. Breech presentation. In Myciscorh P, Mori J, eds. *Munro Kerr's Operative Obstetrics*, 8th edn. Baltimore: Williams & Wilkins, 1971

18. Collea J, Chein C, Quillgean EJ. The randomized management of the term frank breech presentation – a study of 208 cases. *Am J Obstet Gynecol* 1980;137:235–41

19. O'Leary JA. Vaginal delivery of the term breech. *Obstet Gynecol* 1979;53:341–5

20. Todd WD, Steer CM. Term breech: review of 1006 term breech deliveries. *Obstet Gynecol* 1963;22:583–91

21. Gimovsky ML, Wallace RL, Schifrin BS, *et al.* Randomized management of the nonfrank breech presentation at term – a preliminary report. *Am J Obstet Gynecol* 1983;146:34–41

22. Caterini H, Langer A, Sanra JC, *et al.* Fetal risk in hypertension of the fetal head in breech presentation. *Am J Obstet Gynecol* 1975;123:632–5

23. Phelan J, Bethel M, Gimovsky ML, *et al.* Use of ultrasound in breech presentation with hyperextension of the fetal head. *J Ultrasound Med* 1983;2:373–4

24. Myers SA, Glescher N. Breech delivery. Why the dilemmas? *Am J Obstet Gynecol* 1987;156:6–10

25. Queenan JT. Newborn's neck broken during breech delivery. *Contemp Obstet Gynecol* 1991;36:102

26. Gimovsky ML, Willard K, Neglio M, *et al.* X-ray pelvimetry in a breech protocol – a comparison of digital radiography and conventional method. *Am J Obstet Gynecol* 1985;153:887–91

27. Kopelman JN, Duff P, Karl RJ, *et al.* Computed tomographic pelvimetry in the evaluation of breech presentation. *Obstet Gynecol* 1986;68:455–61

28. Federle MP, Cohen HA, Rosenwein MF, *et al.* Pelvimetry by digital radiography – a low dose examination. *Radiology* 1982;143:733–6

29. Gimovsky ML, O'Grady JP, Morris B, *et al.* An assessment of CT pelvimetry within a selective breech management protocol. *J Reprod Med* 1994;39:489–91

30. Gimovsky ML, Petrie RH. Intrapartum ultrasound as an adjunct in the selective management approach to breech presentation. In Transactions of the Tenth Annual Meeting of the Society of Perinatal Obstetricians. *Am J Obstet Gynecol* 1990;163:715–999

31. Rovinsky JJ, Miller JA, Kaplan S. Management of breech presenting at term. *Am J Obstet Gynecol* 1973;115:497–505

32. Nishijima N, Tatsuni H, Amano K, *et al.* Differences of FHR patterns between cephalic and breech presentations at term. *J Perinat Med* (Suppl) 1981;9:129–34

33. Wheeler T, Greene K. FHR monitoring during breech labor. *Br J Obstet Gynaecol* 1975;82:208–14

34. Crawford B. An appraisal of lumbar epidural blockade in patients with singleton fetus presenting by the breech. *J Obstet Gynaecol Br Commonw* 1974;81:867–8

35. Friedman EA (ed). *Clinical Management of Labor*, 2nd edn. New York: Appleton, Century, Crofts, 1978

36. Milner RDG. Neonatal mortality of breech deliveries with and without forceps to the after-coming head. *Br J Obstet Gynaecol* 1975;82:783–5

37. Gimovsky ML, Nishiyama M, Halle J. Fetal respiratory status at birth as reflected by umbilical cord acid–base parameters. Presented at the *9th Annual Meeting of the Society of Perinatal Obstetricians*, San Francisco, CA, February 1989

38. Cruckshank DP, Pitten R. Delivery of the premature breech. *Obstet Gynecol* 1977;50:367–9

39. Ingemarson I, Westgven M, Svennignsen N. Long term follow-up of preterm infants in breech presentation delivered by Cesarean section. *Lancet* 1978;2:172–4

40. Kauppila O, Gronross M, Aro P, *et al.* Management of low birth weight breech delivery. Should Cesarean section be routine? *Obstet Gynecol* 1981;57:289–93

41. Paul RH, Koh KS, Monfared AH. Obstetric factors influencing the outcome in infants weighing from 1000 to 1500 grams. *Am J Obstet Gynecol* 1979;133:503

42. Gimovsky ML, Petrie RH. The intrapartum and neonatal performance of the low birth weight vaginal breech delivery. *J Reprod Med* 1988;8:141–9

43. Gimovsky ML. Diagnostic difficulty after failed external cephalic version under tocolysis. *J Perinatol* 1985;4:59

2

Cesarean section and vaginal birth after Cesarean section

E.P. Schneider, G. Farmakides and H.N. Winn

INTRODUCTION

In the United States, about 23% of approximately 4 million infants born in 1993 were delivered by Cesarean section. The rates of Cesarean section increased dramatically from an annual rate of 5.5% in 1970 to 24.1% in 1986, but have since stabilized. About one-third of the rise in Cesarean section rates results from repeat Cesarean section[1]. Although the USA has reported the largest increase in Cesarean birth rate, other countries have also demonstrated this trend[2].

Cragin's dictum 'once a Cesarean, always a Cesarean' dates back to 1916, when he suggested that uterine rupture following vaginal delivery after previous Cesarean birth was so catastrophic an event that a repeat Cesarean should be done prior to the onset of labor[3]. This opinion was then cited in the fourth edition of *Williams' Obstetrics*[4] and the attitudes favoring repeat Cesarean sections began to prevail. All this dates back to a pre-antibiotic, pre-transfusion era when Cesarean section involved a classical uterine incision. During the past 75 years this wisdom has been challenged by many reports, which were generally ignored by the general obstetric community[5]. In 1980, the National Institutes of Health (NIH) Consensus Development Conference pointed out that repeat Cesarean was one of the major reasons for the rising Cesarean rate. The literature was reviewed and the Consensus Development Task Force on Cesarean Childbirth concurred that labor following a low transverse uterine incision was associated with lower maternal morbidity and mortality, with equivalent infant outcomes. They concluded that vaginal birth after Cesarean (VBAC) was an appropriate option[6]. On the other hand, a recent study from Nova Scotia demonstrated a 1.3% rate of major maternal complications such as uterine rupture, hysterectomy and operative injury in patients undergoing a trial of labor. This rate represents a two-fold increase compared to that of patients undergoing an elective repeat Cesarean section. The rates of perinatal morbidity and mortality were similar between the two groups[7]. However, The American College of Obstetricians and Gynecologists has recommended a trial of labor after a previous Cesarean section, because the studies in the USA have demonstrated its safety[8]. The overall success rates of VBAC ranged from 54% to 89% in an earlier study[9] and range from 75% to 81% in more recent studies[10,11]. The indications for the primary Cesarean sections such as cephalopelvic disproportion or failure to progress, breech presentation, fetal distress and genital herpes infection do not appear to influence the high success rate of VBAC delivery[9-11].

RISKS OF UTERINE RUPTURES

Oxytocin use

Many studies have demonstrated the safety of using oxytocin for induction of labor or augmentation of labor in patients undergoing VBAC. The risk of uterine rupture is not increased if uterine pressure is carefully monitored, preferably with an intrauterine pressure catheter[12]. However, overuse of oxytocin to augment labor for prolonged latent phase in patients undergoing trial of labor has been associated with a risk of uterine rupture 2.7 times that of a control group[13]. The success rate of VBAC in patients who receive intravenous oxytocin for induction or augmentation of labor is about 70% without increased maternal or perinatal morbidity or mortality[9,10,14]. It is unclear whether the success rates of VBAC differ between induction of labor and augmentation of labor with oxytocin[15].

Prostaglandin use

Although uterine rupture has been reported following prostaglandin administration in the absence of previous surgery, MacKenzie and colleagues, in 1984, reported on the use of prostaglandins for induction of labor in women with a surgically scarred uterus[16]. In this series of 143 women, there was a 76% vaginal delivery rate with no maternal or fetal complications reported. Limited data suggest that cervical ripening with prostaglandin (PGE_2) gel appears to be safe, without increased risk of uterine rupture or increased incidence of maternal or perinatal morbidity or mortality in patients undergoing VBAC[17,18]. Careful monitoring of uterine contraction and fetal heart rates is strongly recommended. The safety of induction of labor with PGE_2 gel for fetal demise in patients with a previous Cesarean section remains to be determined.

Epidural anesthesia

The initial concern of epidural anesthesia during labor in masking the symptoms and signs of uterine rupture such as pain or hypotension in patients undergoing a trial of labor has not been supported by clinical data. Epidural anesthesia is not associated with an increased risk of uterine rupture in patients undergoing VBAC[13]. The use of epidural anesthesia allows adequate pain relief during labor and ready access to safe anesthesia when Cesarean section is required.

Fetal macrosomia

Fetal macrosomia is defined as a fetus having an estimated weight of ≥ 4000 g[19]. Trial of labor in patients with fetal macrosomia is not associated with an increased risk of uterine rupture and perinatal or maternal morbidity or mortality[13,20]. It is uncertain whether fetal macrosomia affects the success rates of VBAC. One study showed VBAC success rates of 78% with infants' birth weights of < 4000 g, 58% with birth weights between 4000 g and 4499 g and 26% with birth weights of > 4500 g[21]. Another study showed comparable VBAC success rates of 73–76%[20]. Trial of labor should not be discouraged because of fetal macrosomia, in view of its safety and the inaccuracy of predicting fetal weight in macrosomic fetuses.

Breech presentation

The safety and success rates of VBAC in patients with breech-presenting fetuses remain to be determined. A few small studies have shown that patients with breech-presenting fetuses are least likely to undergo trial of labor, and have VBAC success rates ranging from 46% to 89%[5,22]. External version can be safely performed in patients with a previous Cesarean section, followed by a trial of labor and vaginal delivery. Success rates of 82% for external cephalic version and 65% for subsequent vaginal delivery have been reported[23].

Twins

As with the breech, the management of patients with multiple gestation remains a topic of debate. There are inadequate data on the management of patients with previous Cesarean sections who have multiple gestations. Gilbert and co-workers[24] described 15 women with multiple gestations who underwent a trial of labor and delivered vaginally. The report of Strong and associates[25] involved 25 women with twins and previous Cesarean sections who underwent a trial of labor. Seventy-two per cent ultimately delivered both twins vaginally. There was one dehiscence among the mothers but no neonatal complications due to mode of delivery. Multiple gestation theoretically increases the risk for uterine dehiscence, because of its association with increased uterine size and distension. These retrospective studies show that twin pregnancy with a low transverse uterine segment scar may not increase the risk of uterine rupture. One reason for electing Cesarean section for the multiple gestation is malpresentation of one or both twins.

Amnioinfusion

Amnioinfusion has been performed for indications such as oligohydramnios, meconium-stained amniotic fluid and variable fetal heart rate (FHR) decelerations in patients with previous Cesarean sections. The success rates of VBAC range from 58% to 83% without a significant increase in the incidences of uterine rupture or maternal perinatal morbidity or maternal mortality[26,27]. The incidence of uterine rupture is 0.8%[27]. Amnioinfusion does not appear to be a contraindication for trial of labor in patients with previous Cesarean sections.

Prior uterine incisions

Multiple previous Cesarean sections

Patients undergoing a trial of labor after having more than one previous Cesarean section had VBAC success rates ranging from 64% to 77%[9,10,28–30]. Uterine wound separation appeared to be increased, even though not statistically significantly, in patients with multiple previous Cesarean sections compared to those with a single previous Cesarean section[30]. There was no increased perinatal morbidity or mortality that could be attributed to uterine separation or rupture[9,30]. The American College of Obstetricians and Gynecologists recommend that trial of labor should not be discouraged in patients who had more than one previous low transverse cervical Cesarean section.

A previous low uterine vertical Cesarean section

Patients who undergo a trial of labor after a previous low uterine vertical Cesarean section have VBAC success rates ranging from 83% to 85%, risks of uterine rupture ranging from 1.1% to 1.3% and no maternal deaths reported. There is no significantly increased incidence of perinatal morbidity or mortality due to uterine rupture[31,32]. Therefore, a trial of labor could be attempted in patients who had a previous low vertical uterine Cesarean section with close maternal and FHR monitoring.

Unknown uterine scar

Documentation of the uterine incision in the previous Cesarean section is one of the main criteria for undergoing a trial of labor. A dilemma occurs when the type of uterine incision is unknown. Limited data reveal that the rate of uterine rupture is 2.2% without a significant increase in maternal or perinatal mortality or morbidity[33]. Augmentation of labor during the latent phase with intravenous oxytocin increased the incidence of uterine separation compared to that of patients who were managed expectantly without oxytocin[34].

In 1984 Beall and co-workers[35] reported on 451 women with unknown types of uterine scar. Ninety-seven labored with an 87% vaginal delivery rate. There was 1% scar dehiscence rate in the women who labored and this did not significantly differ from the rate in women with unknown scar who did not labor. Perinatal mortality was similar in both groups.

CONCLUSION

The risk of uterine rupture in patients undergoing a trial of labor after previous Cesarean sections varies with the type of previous uterine incision, and the number of previous Cesarean sections. The risks of uterine rupture range from 0.6% to 0.8% with one previous low transverse uterine incision[11-13,36-39], from 1.1% to 1.3% with more than one previous transverse uterine incision[31, 32] and about 12% with previous classical uterine incision[33]. Other predisposing factors include excessive amount of intravenous oxytocin for augmentation or induction of labor, and dysfunctional labor. Fetal macrosomia and epidural anesthesia do not appear to increase the risk of uterine rupture[13]. Signs of uterine rupture include abnormal FHR patterns indicating fetal distress, such as sudden onset of prolonged fetal bradycardia, abdominal pain, vaginal bleeding and abnormal labor[10,40]. Trial of labor in patients with previous Cesarean sections does not increase maternal mortality compared to those undergoing elective Cesarean section[33]. There has been no maternal death related to uterine rupture reported.

Despite the reassuring data, VBAC has not been readily adopted as the accepted obstetric management for women with a prior Cesarean section. Both obstetricians' and patients' undue concern about the potential maternal and fetal complications associated with uterine rupture and the convenience of scheduled Cesarean section have contributed to the low rate of trial of labor. Patients with a previous low transverse cervical Cesarean section should be encouraged to undergo a trial of labor. In addition to the low risk of uterine rupture, patients who undergo VBAC have shorter hospital stays, fewer blood transfusions and less fever in the postpartum period[11]. Trial of labor may be offered to patients who have more than one

previous low transverse cervical Cesarean section. Patients with a low vertical uterine Cesarean section or unknown uterine scar should not be discouraged from a trial of labor after being informed of the slightly higher risk of uterine ruptures (up to 2%) and potential associated maternal or perinatal complications. Fetal macrosomia is not a contraindication for a trial of labor. Epidural anesthesia for pain control may be offered to patients who undergo VBAC. Fetal heart rate and maternal labor and medical condition should be closely monitored during labor. The institution's resources and the medical staff should be able to respond to peripartum emergencies promptly.

REFERENCES

1. Clarke SC, Taffel S. Changes in Cesarean delivery in the United States, 1988 and 1993. *Birth* 1995;22:63–7
2. Notzen F, Placec P, Taffel S. Comparisons of national Cesarean section rates. *N Engl J Med* 1987;316:386–9
3. Cragin EB. Conservatism in obstetrics. *NY Med J* 1916;104:1–3
4. Williams JM. *Williams' Obstetrics*. New York: S Appleton, 1917
5. Ophir E, Yagoda A, Rojansky N, Oettinger M. Trial of labor following Cesarean section: dilemma. *Obstet Gynecol Surv* 1988;44:19–24
6. The National Institutes of Health, The Cesarean Birth Task Force. National Institutes of Health consensus development statement on Cesarean childbirth. *Obstet Gynecol* 1981;57:537–45
7. McMahon MJ, Luther ER, Bowes WA, Olshan AF. Comparison of a trial of labor with an elective second Cesarean section. *N Engl J Med* 1996;335:689–95
8. The American College of Obstetricians and Gynecologists. *Vaginal Delivery after Previous Cesarean Birth*. ACOG Practice Pattern 1. Washington, DC: ACOG, 1995
9. Rosen MG, Dickinson JC. Vaginal birth after Cesarean: a meta-analysis of indicators for success. *Obstet Gynecol* 1990;76:865–9
10. Cowan RK, Kinch RAH, Ellis B, Anderson R. Trial of labor following Cesarean delivery. *Obstet Gynecol* 1994;83:933–6
11. Flamm BL, Goings JR, Liu Y, Wolde-Tsadik G. Elective Repeat Cesarean delivery versus trial of labor. A prospective multicenter study. *Obstet Gynecol* 1994;83:927–32
12. Rosen MG, Dickinson JC, Westhoff CL. Vaginal birth after Cesarean: a meta-analysis of morbidity and mortality. *Obstet Gynecol* 1991;77:465–70
13. Leung AS, Farmer RM, Leung EK, *et al.* Risk factors associated with uterine rupture during trial of labor after Cesarean delivery: a case–control study. *Am J Obstet Gynecol* 1993;168:1358–63
14. Chelmow D, Laros RK. Maternal and neonatal outcomes after oxytocin augmentation in patients undergoing a trial of labor after prior Cesarean delivery. *Obstet Gynecol* 1992;80:966–71
15. Sakala EP, Kaye S, Murray RD, Munson LJ. Oxytocin use after previous Cesarean: why a higher rate of failed labor trial? *Obstet Gynecol* 1990;75:356–9

16. MacKenzie L, Bradley S, Embrey MP. Vaginal prostaglandins and labor induction for patients previously delivered by Cesarean section. *Br J Obstet Gynaecol* 1984;91:7–10

17. Norman M, Ekman G. Preinductive cervical ripening with prostaglandin E$_2$ in women with one previous Cesarean section. *Am J Obstet Gynecol* 1991;165:996–1001

18. Blanco JD, Collins M, Willis D, Prien S. Prostaglandin E$_2$ gel induction of patients with a prior low transverse Cesarean section. *Am J Perinatol* 1992;9:80–3

19. The American College of Obstetricians and Gynecologists. *Fetal Macrosomia*. ACOG Technical Bulletin 159. Washington, DC: ACOG, 1991

20. Nguyen TV, Dinh TV, Suresh MS, *et al*. Vaginal birth after Cesarean section at the University of Texas. *J Reprod Med* 1992;37:880–2

21. Flamm BL, Goings JR. Vaginal birth after Cesarean section: is suspected fetal macrosomia a contraindication? *Obstet Gynecol* 1989;74:694–7

22. Ophir E, Oettinger M, Yagoda A, *et al*. Breech presentation after Cesarean section: always a section? *Am J Obstet Gynecol* 1989;161:25–8

23. Flamm BL, Fried MW, Lonky NM, Giles WS. External cephalic version after previous Cesarean section. *Am J Obstet Gynecol* 1991;165:370–2

24. Gilbert L, Saunders N, Sharp F. The management of multiple pregnancy in women with a lower-segment Caesarean scar. Is a repeat Caesarean section the 'safe' option? *Br J Obstet Gynaecol* 1989;161:29–32

25. Strong TH, Phelan JP, Ahn MO, Sarno AP. Vaginal birth after Cesarean delivery in the twin gestation. *Am J Obstet Gynecol* 1989;161:29–32

26. Strong TH, Vega JS, O'Shaughnessy MJ, *et al*. Amnioinfusion among women attempting vaginal birth after Cesarean delivery. *Obstet Gynecol* 1992;79:673–4

27. Ouzounian JG, Miller DA, Paul RH. Amnioinfusion in women with previous Cesarean births: a preliminary report. *Am J Obstet Gynecol* 1996;174:783–6

28. Farmakides G, Duvivier R, Schulman H, *et al*. Vaginal birth after two or more previous Cesarean sections. *Am J Obstet Gynecol* 1987;156:565–6

29. Phelan JP, Ahn MO, Diaz F, *et al*. Twice a Cesarean, always a Cesarean? *Obstet Gynecol* 1989;73:161–5

30. Asakura H, Myers SA. More than one previous Cesarean delivery: a 5-year experience with 435 patients. *Obstet Gynecol* 1995;85:924–9

31. Naef RW, Ray MA, Chaunan SP, *et al*. Trial of labor after Cesarean delivery with a lower-segment, vertical uterine incision: is it safe? *Am J Obstet Gynecol* 1995;172:1666–74

32. Adair CD, Sanchez-Ramos L, Whitaker D, *et al*. Trial of labor in patients with a previous lower uterine vertical Cesarean section. *Am J Obstet Gynecol* 1996;174:966–70

33. Rosen MG, Dickenson JC, Westhoff CL. Vaginal birth after Cesarean: a meta-analysis of morbidity and mortality. *Obstet Gynecol* 1991;77:465–70

34. Grubb DK, Kjos SL, Paul RH. Latent labor with an unknown uterine scar. *Obstet Gynecol* 1996;88:351–5

35. Beall M, Eglinton GS, Clark SL, Phelan JP. Vaginal delivery after Cesarean section in women with unknown types of uterine scar. *J Reprod Med* 1984;29:31–5

36. Lavin J, Stephens R, Miodovnik M, Barden T. Vaginal delivery in patients with a prior Cesarean section. *Obstet Gynecol* 1982;59:135–48

37. Nielsen TF, Ljungblad U, Hagberg H. Rupture and dehiscence of Cesarean section scar during pregnancy and delivery. *Am J Obstet Gynecol* 1989;160:569–73

38. Horowitz B, Edelstein S, Lippman L. Once a Cesarean, always a Cesarean. *Obstet Gynecol Surv* 1981;36:592–8

39. Farmer R, Kirschbaum T, Potter D, *et al*. Uterine rupture during trial of labor after previous Cesarean section. *Am J Obstet Gynecol* 1991;1651:996–1001

40. Scott JR. Mandatory trial of labor after Cesarean delivery: an alternative viewpoint. *Obstet Gynecol* 1991;77:811–14

3

Gestational hypertension/pre-eclampsia

B.M. Sibai and A.D. Khoury

Hypertensive disorders are the most common medical complications of pregnancy. Approximately 7–10% of all pregnancies are complicated by hypertension. The two most common forms of hypertension are pregnancy-associated hypertensive disease, which accounts for 70% of hypertension during pregnancy, and pre-existing chronic hypertension, which is responsible for the remaining cases[1]. Hypertensive disorders are associated with increased maternal and perinatal mortality and present as a wide spectrum of disorders, ranging from minimal elevation of blood pressure alone, to severe hypertension with multiple organ dysfunction.

CLASSIFICATIONS

Multiple classifications have been proposed for the hypertensive disorders of pregnancy. In 1972, the Committee on Terminology of the American College of Obstetricians and Gynecologists[2] suggested five categories:

(1) Gestational hypertension, defined as hypertension appearing in the second half of pregnancy or in the first 24 h postpartum without edema or proteinuria, and with a return to normotension within 10 days after delivery. The hypertension should be a level of at least 140 mmHg systolic or 90 mmHg diastolic on at least two occasions 6 h apart.

(2) Pre-eclampsia, defined as hypertension together with abnormal edema or proteinuria.

(3) Eclampsia, defined as the development of convulsions or coma in patients with signs and symptoms of pre-eclampsia in the absence of other causes of convulsions.

(4) Chronic hypertensive disease, defined as chronic hypertension of any cause. This group includes patients with pre-existing hypertension, patients with pre-existing elevation of blood pressure to at least 140/90 mmHg on two occasions before 20 weeks, and patients with hypertension that persists for more than 42 days postpartum.

(5) Superimposed pre-eclampsia or eclampsia, defined as the development of pre-eclampsia or eclampsia in patients with diagnosed chronic hypertension. About 15–30% of chronically hypertensive women will develop pre-eclampsia.

Pre-eclampsia also is classified as either mild or severe. Severe pre-eclampsia is diagnosed when any of the criteria listed in Table 1 is present[2]. These criteria for severe pre-eclampsia do not include other findings that also indicate severe disease, such as marked abnormality in hepatic function, low level of platelets and severe fetal growth retardation.

The classifications and definitions of the hypertension disorders of pregnancy are confusing. It is frequently difficult to differentiate between pre-eclampsia, chronic hypertension and chronic hypertension with superimposed pre-eclampsia. The normal midtrimester fall in blood pressure may conceal the presence of underlying chronic hypertension; therefore, unless the patient presents in the first trimester or has a well documented history of chronic hypertension, accurate classification is impossible.

PRE-ECLAMPSIA

Pre-eclampsia is a disorder peculiar to human pregnancy. Reported incidences rage from 2% to 10% depending on the diagnostic criteria used and the population studied. It is principally a disease of young primigravidas. The incidence is about 6–7% of all nulliparous pregnancies in the USA[3].

Although geographic and racial differences in incidence have been reported, several risk factors have been identified as predisposing to the development of pre-eclampsia in different populations[4–11] (Table 2). On the other hand, the incidence is reportedly reduced in

Table 1 Criteria for the diagnosis of severe pre-eclampsia

Blood pressure ≥ 160 mmHg systolic or ≥ 110 mmHg diastolic on two occasions at least 6 h apart with the patient at bed rest
Proteinuria ≥ 5 g in a 24-h urine collection
Oliguria (≤ 400 ml in 24 h)
Severe and persistent epigastric pain
Pulmonary edema or cyanosis
Thrombocytopenia (platelet count < 100 000/mm[3])

19

Table 2 Risk factors for pre-eclampsia

Nulliparity
Multiple gestation
Family history of pre-eclampsia–eclampsia
Pre-existing hypertension/renal disease
Previous pre-eclampsia–eclampsia
Diabetes (class B to F)
Non-immune hydrops fetalis
Molar pregnancy
Obesity

Table 3 Prevention of pre-eclampsia

Dietary manipulation
Low-calorie diet
High-protein diet
Low-salt diet
Nutritional supplementation
    calcium, magnesium, zinc
    fish oil and evening primrose oil

Pharmacological manipulation
Diuretics
Antihypertensives
β–sympathomimetics
Antithrombic agents
    low-dose aspirin
    dipyridamole
    dazoxiben
    heparin
    vitamin E

Personal habit changes
Frequent prenatal care
Daily rest in lateral position
Keeping the same partner
Avoiding or reducing coffee

women who smoke during pregnancy[12,13], and in those who have had previous abortions or miscarriages[14–16].

DIAGNOSIS

Pre-eclampsia traditionally has been described as a triad of edema, proteinuria and hypertension. However, a spectrum of clinical signs and symptoms, presenting either alone or in combination, makes the diagnosis of pre-eclampsia a subject of great controversy. A finding of abnormal blood pressure is subject to many errors; several variants may influence the readings: faulty equipment, race, obesity, smoking, position, patient anxiety, or duration of the resting period[17].

The diagnosis of pre-eclampsia requires the presence of elevated blood pressure with proteinuria, edema, or both. The presence of proteinuria is usually determined by the use of dipsticks or the sulfosalicylic acid test on random urine samples. The concentration of urinary protein is highly variable. It is influenced by several factors, including contamination with vaginal secretions, blood or bacteria, urine specific gravity and pH, exercise and posture. In addition, urinary protein-to-creatinine excretion is highly variable in patients with pre-eclampsia[18]. Moreover, three recent studies found that urinary dipstick determinations correlate very poorly with the amount of proteinuria found in 24-h urine determinations in hypertensive pregnancies[19–21]. Therefore, the definitive test for diagnosing proteinuria should be quantitative measurement of total protein excretion over a 24-h period. Significant proteinuria should be defined as > 300 mg per 24-h urine sample. For making the diagnosis of severe pre-eclampsia based on proteinuria only, it is recommended that a 24-h urine excretion of protein of > 5 g be documented. Dipstick measurements in urine samples (≥ 3) are not adequate for the diagnosis of severe pre-eclampsia[19].

PREVENTION OF PRE-ECLAMPSIA

There are numerous reports and clinical trials describing the use of various methods to prevent or reduce the incidence of pre-eclampsia. Since the etiology of the disease is unknown, these methods were used to correct the pathophysiological abnormalities in the hopes of ameliorating the course of, or preventing, the disease. Some of the methods used are summarized in Table 3. To date, none of these methods have been shown conclusively to be effective in preventing the disease.

Diets low in salt and high in protein, as well as restricted caloric intake, have been suggested to prevent pre-eclampsia. In addition, the use of diuretics has been recommended to prevent pre-eclampsia[22]. However, the efficacy of these measures has never been proven. Several epidemiological studies and a few clinical supplementation trials have suggested a relationship between calcium, magnesium and zinc intake and pregnancy-induced hypertension. The relationship between dietary calcium intake and hypertension has been the subject of several experimental and observational studies[23]. It has been shown that there is an inverse association between calcium intake and maternal blood pressure and the incidences of pre-eclampsia and eclampsia in epidemiological studies[24]. The blood pressure-lowering effect of calcium was thought to be mediated by alterations in plasma renin activity and parathyroid hormone. In addition, calcium supplementation during pregnancy was shown to reduce angiotensin II vascular sensitivities in such pregnancies[25,26].

There are nine clinical studies that have compared the use of calcium vs. no treatment or placebo in pregnancy[25–33]. The findings of these studies were reviewed in two recent meta-analyses[34,35]. These trials differed regarding the population studied (low-risk or high-risk

Table 4 Pregnancy outcome in healthy nulliparous women receiving aspirin or placebo, in two trials

	Hauth et al.[41]		*Sibai et al.*[42]	
	Aspirin (n = 302)	*Placebo* (n = 302)	*Aspirin* (n = 1485)	*Placebo* (n = 1500)
Pre-eclampsia (%)	1.7	5.6	4.6	6.3
Gestational hypertension (%)	6.3	5.6	6.7	5.9
Mean birth weight (g)	3249	3169	3188	3189
< 10th centile (%)	5.6	6.3	4.6	5.8
Mean delivery gestational				
age (week)	39.1	38.9	38.6	38.7
< 37 weeks (%)	6.7	8.0	10.6	9.8

for hypertensive disorders of pregnancy), study design (randomization, double-blind, or use of a placebo), gestational age at enrolment (20–32 weeks' gestation), sample size in each group (range 22–588), dose of elemental calcium used (156–2000 mg/day). In addition, these studies differed regarding the definition of the hypertensive disorders of pregnancy. The findings suggest that calcium supplementation reduces the overall incidence of hypertensive disorders of pregnancy, with a trend towards reducing the incidence of pre-eclampsia. A critical analysis of the design of eight of these studies was recently reported by Levine and associates[36].

A large multicenter trial to evaluate the benefits and side-effects of calcium supplementation to prevent pre-eclampsia has recently been completed at five medical centers in the USA. This trial randomized over 4500 healthy nulliparous women who were enrolled prior to 20 weeks' gestation. The results of this trial demonstrated no difference between calcium- and placebo-supplemented women in the incidence of either pre-eclampsia or gestational hypertension. In addition, calcium supplementation had no effect on maternal blood pressure throughout gestation[37].

ASPIRIN

Pre-eclampsia is associated with vasospasm and an activation of the coagulation–hemostasis system. Enhanced platelet activation plays a central role in the above process with resultant abnormality in the thromboxane/prostacyclin balance. Several authors have used pharmacological manipulation to alter the above ratio in an attempt to prevent or ameliorate the course of pre-eclampsia.

Aspirin inhibits the synthesis of prostaglandins by irreversibly acetylating and inactivating cyclo-oxygenase. *In vitro*, platelet cyclo-oxygenase is more sensitive to inhibition by very low doses of aspirin (< 80 mg) than vascular endothelial cyclo-oxygenase. Therefore, treatment with low doses of aspirin could alter the balance between prostacyclin and thromboxane[38]. This biochemical selectivity of low-dose

aspirin appears to be related to its unusual kinetics that result in presystemic acetylation of platelets exposed to higher concentrations of aspirin in the portal circulation. Sibai and colleagues[39] found that effective inhibition of thromboxane generation by platelets (98% decrease from baseline) was achieved after 1 week of therapy with 80 mg of daily aspirin during pregnancy. In addition, they found that a 60-mg dose resulted in 60% decrease in platelet thromboxane generation after 1 week and 97% decrease after 2 weeks of therapy.

There are some studies describing the effects of low-dose aspirin (60–81 mg/day) on angiotensin II sensitivity during pregnancy. The results of these studies were reviewed by Dekker and Sibai[40]. Findings from these studies suggest that enhanced vascular responsiveness to angiotensin II infusions may be mediated by an imbalance in thromboxane/prostacyclin production that may be corrected in some women by the use of low-dose aspirin. In addition, several prospective studies have been published which suggest that administration of aspirin in women at high risk for pre-eclampsia might reduce the incidence of hypertensive disorders of pregnancy, fetal growth retardation and preterm delivery. These studies included a limited number of patients who were identified to be at high risk for pre-eclampsia on the basis of a poor obstetric history, chronic hypertension, positive rollover test, increased sensitivity to angiotensin II infusions, or abnormal Doppler studies of the uterine vessels. In general, the findings of these studies suggested that low-dose aspirin was highly effective in the prevention of pre-eclampsia and fetal growth retardation in women considered to be at risk for these complications[40].

Recently, several multicenter randomized prospective studies were reported from various countries. Some of these studies were conducted in healthy nulliparous women[41,42], whereas others included patients with various obstetric and medical complications[43–47].

In general, about 75% of all pre-eclampsia cases occur in nulliparous women. Therefore, prevention of pre-eclampsia in these women has major clinical implications. There are two randomized placebo-controlled trials describing the use of 60 mg/day of aspirin in healthy nulliparous women (Table 4). Hauth and co-workers[41] studied 604 healthy nulliparous women who were randomized at 24 weeks' gestation: 302 women received 60 mg/day of aspirin and 302 women received a matching placebo. The incidence of pre-eclampsia was significantly lower in the aspirin-treated women; however, there were no differences between the two groups regarding gestational age at delivery, neonatal birth weight, or frequency of fetal growth retardation or preterm delivery.

Sibai and associates[42] reported a multicenter study in 2985 healthy nulliparous women who were randomized at 13–26 weeks' gestation: 1485 women received 60 mg/day of aspirin and 1500 women received a matching placebo. The women were enrolled at seven medical centers in the USA, and the study was sponsored by the National Institute of Child Health and Human Development. The incidence of pre-eclampsia was reduced by only 26% in the aspirin-treated women; however, there were no differences in mean gestational age at delivery, birth weight or the frequency of fetal growth retardation or preterm delivery. It is important to note that, despite a reduction in the incidence of pre-eclampsia with aspirin in both trials, perinatal outcome was not improved with such therapy. In addition, the mean gestational age at delivery in women who developed pre-eclampsia and who received aspirin was similar to that of the respective group who received placebo (both trials). Moreover, the trial by Sibai and associates found a significantly higher incidence of abruptio placentae in women receiving aspirin (0.7%) compared to those receiving placebo (0.1%)[42].

Viinikka and colleagues[43] studied 197 women with pre-existing chronic hypertension or a history of severe pre-eclampsia in their previous pregnancies who were randomized at 15 weeks' gestation: 97 received 50 mg/day of aspirin and 100 received a matching placebo. The incidences of exacerbation of hypertension as well as pre-eclampsia were similar in the two groups. In addition, the two groups had similar mean gestational age at delivery. However, patients receiving low-dose aspirin had a higher mean birth weight and lower frequency of fetal growth retardation.

The Italian multicenter trial evaluated the use of 50 mg/day of aspirin compared to no treatment in a large group of pregnant women considered at risk for pre-eclampsia[44]. Eligible women were randomly assigned to treatment with 50 mg aspirin daily until delivery ($n = 583$) or no treatment ($n = 523$); 18 and 46 women, respectively, were lost to follow-up. There were no differences between the two groups regarding the incidences of hypertension only, pre-eclampsia, fetal growth retardation, preterm delivery, abruptio placentae, or perinatal death.

The CLASP (Collaborative Low-Dose Aspirin Study in Pregnancy) is a multinational randomized trial of low-dose aspirin for the prevention and treatment of pre-eclampsia and fetal growth retardation[45]. In this trial, 9364 women were randomly assigned to 60 mg aspirin daily or matching placebo. Seventy-four per cent were entered for prophylaxis of pre-eclampsia, 12% for prophylaxis of fetal growth retardation, 12% for treatment of pre-eclampsia and 3% for treatment of fetal growth retardation. Twenty-eight per cent were primigravid, 20% had chronic hypertension, 5% had renal disease and 3% had diabetes. Outcome data were available for 4659 aspirin-allocated women and 4650 placebo-allocated women. There were no differences between the two study groups regarding the incidences of pre-eclampsia, fetal growth retardation, abruptio placentae, or perinatal deaths. However, the aspirin-treated group had a lower incidence of preterm delivery. In addition, there was a significant trend ($p = 0.004$) towards progressively greater reductions in pre-eclampsia (more in preterm delivery). The study group suggested that low-dose aspirin administration may be justified in women judged to be at risk for early-onset pre-eclampsia. In such women, the study group recommended that low-dose aspirin be started early during the second trimester.

The ECPPA trial had a similar design to the CLASP trial and evaluated the outcome in 476 women receiving low-dose aspirin and 494 assigned to a placebo[47]. A large percentage of randomized women had chronic hypertension. There were no differences between the study groups regarding pre-eclampsia, fetal growth retardation, or preterm births.

Recently, a large multicenter clinical trial has been completed in which pregnant women with high-risk characteristics (previous pre-eclampsia–eclampsia, chronic hypertension, class B to F diabetes, or multifetal gestation) were randomized to either aspirin 60 mg/day or matching placebo. This trial was conducted at 11 centers in the USA and was sponsored by the National Institute of Child Health and Human Development. The results of this trial demonstrated minimal to no benefit from the use of low-dose aspirin in such women[48].

MANAGEMENT OF MILD HYPERTENSION–PRE-ECLAMPSIA

The optimal management of mild pre-eclampsia remote from term is very controversial. In general, there is considerable disagreement regarding the need for hospitalization vs. ambulatory management.

Historically, admission to a hospital was an accepted practice worldwide and its rationale was to reduce eclampsia[49] and improve perinatal outcome[50]. In some centers in the USA, management of these patients has included relative bed rest in the hospital for the duration of pregnancy. This approach has been reported to diminish the frequency of progression to severe disease and to enhance fetal survival[15,50]. In fact, several studies (Table 5) noted the benefits of prolonged hospitalization for patients with mild gestational hypertension remote from term.

Hospital vs. home management

Management of gestational hypertension–pre-eclampsia by hospitalization was based largely on clinical experience rather than being the result of controlled randomized trials. In theory, hospital admission for bed rest could delay or prevent progression to severe hypertension[50,51].

This practice was challenged by Matthews and associates[52], who found no differences in perinatal mortality in women with gestational hypertension between those who were hospitalized for the duration and those who were managed as outpatients. Later on, Matthews and colleagues[53] studied 135 patients with gestational hypertension in a randomized trial. They showed that complete bed rest appeared to have no advantage over 'ambulation as desired' in controlling the severity of maternal disease. Similarly, Crowther and co-workers[54] conducted a randomized controlled trial on 218 patients with gestational hypertension. They showed that bed rest in pregnancies complicated by gestational

hypertension was not associated with an overall improvement in fetal growth or reduced neonatal morbidity. Instead, the recording of fetal kick count at home and continued outpatient antenatal care provided a safe alternative to hospital admission. The results of these two randomized trials are summarized in Table 6.

Management alternatives

Obstetricians are increasingly utilizing outpatient management of gestational hypertension, especially with the increasing pressure to decrease medical expenses and use outpatient therapy. Outpatient management was addressed by the American College of Obstetricians and Gynecologists Technical Bulletin[2], which noted that 'Ambulatory management is acceptable for patients who are compliant, who can have frequent office visits and who can perform some form of adequate blood pressure monitoring at home. Hospitalization should be required for noncompliant patients and those who show unsatisfactory progress as outpatients.' In addition, ambulatory management was recommended for a select group of patients (nulliparous women without proteinuria and with blood pressure of < 140/90 mmHg) in a recent issue of *Williams' Obstetrics*[55].

Recent randomized trials assessing the value of admission to hospital for bed rest found no benefits over outpatient management in women with mild gestational hypertension[56,57]. With the introduction of outpatient management alternatives, evaluation of maternal and fetal status was similar to inpatient therapy. In fact, the incidence of both eclampsia and placental abruption and the perinatal mortality rates were almost the same in both hospitalized and non-hospitalized patients[56,57].

Home-care programs

In an attempt to provide a safe and less expensive alternative to hospital care for women with pre-eclampsia, some home-care programs were initiated in the mid-1980s. Helewa and associates[58] reported their experience with one such program. Patients eligible

Table 5 Traditional hospital management of patients with gestational hypertension and mild pre-eclampsia in three studies

	Gilstrap et al.[50] (1977)	Sibai et al.[51] (1987)	Sibai et al.[56] (1992)
Patients (*n*)	576	200	200
Mean hospitalization (days)	24	21	12
Pregnancy prolongation (days)	24	21	22
Preterm delivery at < 37 weeks (%)	23	—	41–49
Perinatal deaths	9/100	5/1000	0/1000
Abruptio placentae (%)	0.9	1.7	

Table 6 Randomized trials of hospitalization and ambulatory management

Management	No. of patients	Delivery			
		Gestational age (weeks)	37 weeks (%)	< 10th centile (%)	Perinatal deaths (%)
Matthews et al.[53]					
Hospital	71	N/A	2.8	20	2.8
Ambulatory	64	N/A	1.6	16	1.6
Crowther et al.[54]					
Hospital	110	38.3	11.8	14	1.8
Ambulatory	108	38.2	22.8	14	0.9

N/A, not available

for home-care management included those with blood pressure of < 150/100 mmHg, protein level of < 0.6 g in a 24-h collection of urine, absence of symptoms of severe pre-eclampsia, platelet count of > 120 000/mm³ and liver enzymes of < 50 U/l. Enrolled patients were visited at home by a trained nurse. The nurse measured the blood pressure and fetal heart rate, reviewed fetal movement counts, tested for the presence and amount of protein in the urine and checked for signs and symptoms of pre-eclampsia. An assessment of the fetal biophysical profile and biochemical profile and a visit to the attending physician were carried out on a weekly basis. The program nurse contacted the physician if clinical deterioration was noted. Labor was induced electively at term when the patient had a favorable cervix or at any gestational age if the pre-eclampsia became severe or there were signs of fetal distress. In this study, 321 patients met the criteria and were enrolled in the home-care program. A total of 141 patients (44%) were admitted to the antepartum unit for inpatient monitoring: nine had severe pre-eclampsia. The average length of enrolment in the home-care program was 11.5 days (1–42 days). Hospital stay was reduced from 5.7 days to 3.7 days, and cost was reduced by 74%.

Day-care programs

Similarly, and in an attempt to decrease hospital bed occupancy, a fetal-surveillance unit or day-care unit established within the hospital was described by some authors[59–62]. The unit was established within the hospital and run by a nurse-midwife and staffed by an attending physician. Every visit included monitoring of maternal blood pressure, urine testing, assessment of fetal heart rate, biophysical profile and uteroplacental circulation, as needed. The patient remained under the care of the referring physician unless there was need for immediate intervention. Soothill and co-workers[59] reported a decrease in the rate of antenatal bed occupancy by 22% with no significant change in the stillbirth rate. Similarly, Tuffnell and associates[60] reported an 80% reduction in hospital inpatient stay, and a reduction in the number of medical interventions. In addition, Dawson and colleagues[61] showed that telephonic monitoring of the fetal heart rate in such women was also associated with fewer hospital admissions and a smaller percentage of time spent in hospital.

Perinatal outpatient monitoring service

This service depends on a device designed specifically to monitor and record information associated with the major signs of obstetric hypertensive disease (blood pressure determination, weight, sleep/rest documentation, fetal movement count and urinalysis)[57]. Outpatient evaluation includes four times daily automated blood pressure and pulse measurement and daily assessment of weight, fetal kick counts, duration of rest/sleep periods and proteinuria. Each data element is dated and time-coded. Objective and subjective data are then transmitted by phone to a perinatal center daily or immediately, if elevated blood pressure or decreased fetal movements are observed. Patients receive twice weekly antenatal evaluation with non-stress testing and frequent amniotic fluid assessment. Barton and colleagues[57] evaluated the perinatal and maternal outcomes of this outpatient monitoring service in 592 patients with mild gestational hypertension at 24–36 weeks' gestation. The mean pregnancy prolongation was 27.4 ± 3.3 days, whereas the mean antepartum hospitalization for management of similar patients was only 1.7 days. Maternal and perinatal outcome were similar to those reported by investigators using hospitalization for management of similar patients. In a subsequent report, Barton and associates[63] found that a similar program was safe and effective, even in young teenage patients with mild gestational hypertension remote from term.

Management protocol

The success rate of outpatient management depends mostly on maternal status (presence or absence of proteinuria, diastolic blood pressure and gestational age) at time of enrolment. Pregnancies complicated by gestational hypertension with proteinuria are associated with a lower gestational age at delivery, shorter pregnancy prolongation and an increased requirement for antepartum hospitalization as compared to pregnancies with gestational hypertension but absent proteinuria[56,57]. In addition, our observation was that patients with a diastolic blood pressure of < 100 mmHg and absent proteinuria had a longer duration of pregnancy than those with a diastolic blood pressure of > 100 mmHg and significant proteinuria. In our experience, women who develop gestational hypertension–pre-eclampsia at an earlier gestational age tend to have earlier gestational age at delivery and a worsening of the disease status and more unfavorable fetal outcome than those who develop the disease at term.

Our management plan for patients with gestational hypertension is dependent on gestational age as well as maternal and fetal findings. Patients with gestational age beyond 37 weeks are managed on the basis of their cervical Bishop score. Only those with a favorable cervix undergo induction of labor. Those who do not have a favorable Bishop score are either admitted to the hospital for cervical ripening and eventual delivery or managed as outpatients (but not beyond 40 weeks). Patients at < 37 weeks' gestation are assigned to either ambulatory or inpatient management, depending on several criteria. Those who are unreliable, or have a diastolic blood pressure of > 100 mmHg, proteinuria of > 500 mg, abnormal laboratory tests, abnormal fetal testing, preterm labor or bleeding are usually hospitalized. They are allowed to eat regular hospital diet without salt restriction, and their activity is not restricted to complete bed rest. Initially, antihypertensive drugs are not prescribed. If the blood pressure remains below 100 mmHg in the absence of significant proteinuria ($<$ 500 mg/24 h or $< 2+ = < 100$ mg/dl) or there is any evidence of fetal jeopardy, outpatient management may be considered in compliant and motivated patients. These patients should be instructed to have daily urine dipstick measurements of proteinuria, blood pressure monitoring, daily checking of weight gain and daily recording of fetal kick count, and they should be educated to report any symptoms of impending eclampsia (Table 7). The patient is then evaluated in the antepartum testing area for maternal and fetal well-being at least twice per week for patients with proteinuria ($> 1+ = > 30$ mg/dl) and once a week for those with absent proteinuria (0 or trace). If there is any evidence of disease progression and if acute severe hypertension develops, then hospitalization is indicated. During expectant management, these women should have laboratory evaluation of platelet count and liver enzymes (1–2 times per week), serial ultrasound examinations for estimated fetal growth (every 3 weeks), and fetal antenatal testing with the non-stress test (once per week).

In summary, management of women with mild gestational hypertension–pre-eclampsia must always put safety of the mother first and then aim at the delivery of a live, mature newborn that will not require intensive and prolonged neonatal care. Therefore, requirements for outpatient management must include well motivated patients, a perinatal outpatient monitoring service or other management alternative for close maternal and fetal evaluation, and guidelines for contacting the health care provider (Table 8).

Antihypertensive drugs in mild gestational hypertension–pre-eclampsia

There are several retrospective and prospective studies that have described the use of various antihypertensive drugs in women with mild gestational hypertension–pre-eclampsia[51,56,64–72]. Drugs used in these studies included hydralazine, methyldopa, nifedipine, prazosin, diuretics and β-blockers. These studies included women with gestational hypertension (proteinuria absent) and mild pre-eclampsia (proteinuria present). The purpose of using antihypertensive drugs in this group of women was not to improve blood pressure, but rather to improve perinatal outcome by prolonging the pregnancy in those who were remote from term. Some of these studies found that labetalol had some beneficial effects on the disease process (progression to severe hypertension, development of proteinuria)[64,67], whereas other studies reported detrimental effects

Table 7 Home monitoring

Daily visit at home by a nurse (optional)
Daily assessment of blood pressure and urine protein
Daily fetal kick count
Daily checking for excessive weight gain
Education about symptoms of impending eclampsia
   persistent epigastric/right upper quadrant pain
   persistent severe headaches
   persistent visual symptoms
   nausea and/or vomiting

Table 8 Outpatient management requirements

Well motivated patients
Well trained nurses
Perinatal outpatient monitoring service or other
   management alternative
Close maternal and fetal evaluation
Guidelines for contacting health care provider
   labor or rupture of membranes
   vaginal bleeding
   decreased fetal movement
   symptoms of impending eclampsia

(higher frequency of fetal growth retardation) in the treated group[51,70]. In general, none of these studies have reported a better perinatal outcome than those reported in studies using hospitalization only.

In summary, there are currently few data to support the use of antihypertensive drugs in the management of mild gestational hypertension–pre-eclampsia remote from term[73].

MANAGEMENT OF SEVERE PRE-ECLAMPSIA

Pre-eclampsia affects two patients – the mother and the fetus. Traditionally, women with severe pre-eclampsia have been delivered without delay, regardless of fetal considerations. Although delivery is appropriate therapy for the mother, aggressive management with immediate delivery of a fetus remote from term leads to high neonatal mortality and morbidity resulting from prematurity. Recent studies have demonstrated favorable neonatal outcomes after conservative management of severe pre-eclampsia. Candidates for conservative management should be carefully selected and managed with intensive maternal and fetal monitoring at a tertiary perinatal center.

The timing of delivery in women with severe pre-eclampsia in the second trimester is a difficult decision to make for mother and obstetrician. Aggressive management with immediate delivery will result in extremely high neonatal mortality and morbidity resulting from prematurity. Consequently, hospitalization in a neonatal intensive care unit is prolonged, and some surviving infants may have long-term disabilities[74]. Attempts to prolong pregnancy may improve fetal outcome, but may expose the mother to potential morbidity[75].

Therefore, concerning expectant management, one must weigh risks and benefits to the mother and fetus. Fetal gestational age, fetal condition and maternal condition will play an important role in reaching such a decision[74].

Maternal indications

Because the pathophysiology of pre-eclampsia involves diffuse endothelial injury, patients may present with multiple-system involvement and differing degrees of severity. Some women with severe disease have marked improvement in blood pressure, protein excretion and urine output shortly after hospitalization. However, others require immediate delivery because of signs of deterioration. Careful selection of patients with severe disease is advocated[75]. Patients judged suitable for this type of management have one or more of the following clinical findings: controlled hypertension (< 160 mmHg systolic and < 110 mmHg diastolic), proteinuria of > 5 g/day, oliguria that resolves with routine fluid or food intake, elevated liver enzymes (aspartate aminotransferase or alanine aminotransferase) without epigastric pain, or right upper quadrant tenderness (Table 9)[75]. Only 67% of patients with severe pre-eclampsia remote from term would be eligible for conservative management based on these criteria. When the risks of delay outweigh the benefits, delivery within 72 h of admission is the only alternative.

Table 9 Maternal guidelines for expedited delivery or conservative management of severe pre-eclampsia remote from term. Modified from reference 75

Expedited delivery (within 72 h)
One or more of the following:
    uncontrolled severe hypertension
    eclampsia
    thrombocytopenia
    pulmonary edema
    elevated liver enzymes with epigastric pain or right
      upper quadrant tenderness
    persistent severe headache or visual changes
    obstetric complications: premature rupture of
      membranes, bleeding, labor

Conservative management
One or more of the following:
    controlled hypertension
    urinary protein > 5 g/24 h
    oliguria (< 0.5 ml/kg/h) that resolves with routine
      fluid or food intake
    elevated liver enzymes only

Recently, Visser and Wallenburg[76] rejected the general recommendation of prompt termination of pregnancy in pre-eclamptic patients with hemolysis, elevated liver enzymes and low platelets (HELLP syndrome) in the late second or early third trimester. In their study, 128 pre-eclamptic patients with HELLP were matched for gestational age with 128 pre-eclamptic patients without HELLP. Both groups were treated conservatively with volume expansion and pharmacological vasodilatation with the aim of prolonging gestation and enhancing fetal maturity. Complete reversal of HELLP occurred in around 43% of patients. Perinatal mortality was 14.1% in HELLP patients and 14.8% in patients without HELLP. Similarly, Magann and co-workers[77] demonstrated significant improvement in the laboratory and clinical parameters associated with the HELLP syndrome in women who received high-dose antenatal corticosteroids (10 mg intravenously every 12 h).

Fetal indications

Severe pre-eclampsia may affect the fetus in a negative way. Inadequate trophoblastic invasion causing abnormal placentation is one of the main features of pre-eclampsia. This can lead to decreased uteroplacental perfusion with a resulting increased incidence of intrauterine growth retardation, fetal hypoxia and perinatal death. Therefore, careful selection and intensive monitoring of the fetus is essential. Patients judged suitable for conservative management have one or more of the following: biophysical profile > 4, largest vertical amniotic fluid pocket of > 2, ultrasound-estimated fetal weight above the 5th centile.

It is commonly believed that maternal pre-eclampsia has a protective effect on neonatal outcome after delivery before 34 weeks' gestation. This protective effect is thought to be caused by the fact that fetuses of pre-eclamptic mothers are subjected to stress *in utero* and therefore have accelerated maturation and consequently a better prognosis than other preterm infants. This belief has motivated physicians to proceed with delivery of early gestations because of presumed accelerated lung maturity. In a well designed retrospective study. Schiff and colleagues[78] studied fetal lung maturity by amniocentesis in 127 pre-eclamptic patients and a matched control group of women with preterm labor. They found no significant difference in the incidence of an immature result between pre-eclamptic patients and their matched controls (39.4% vs. 38.6%). Surprisingly, the incidence of respiratory distress syndrome in 69 of the matched pairs was slightly, but not significantly, higher in the pre-eclamptic group. In addition, Friedman and associates[79] found no beneficial effect from pre-eclampsia on the postnatal course of infants born at 24–35 weeks' gestation.

The poor perinatal outcome associated with severe pre-eclampsia is believed to be related mainly to prematurity. However, severe pre-eclampsia has been associated with increased vascular resistance and a decreased uteroplacental perfusion leading to an increased incidence of intrauterine growth retardation, fetal hypoxia and perinatal death. Studies have demonstrated the efficacy of umbilical artery velocimetry in identifying fetal acidosis. Doppler ultrasound scanning is now common in the management of pregnancies complicated by hypertension and has become an indirect tool to assess fetal well-being. The absence of end-diastolic velocity has proved to be highly predictive of low birth weight or fetal death[80,81]. Torres and co-workers[81] retrospectively investigated the relationship between abnormal umbilical artery velocimetry and fetal outcome in 172 hypertensive pregnant women. In their study, the absence of end-diastolic velocity predicted low birth weight in 100% of pregnancies and fetal death in 66.6%. All stillbirths in this study had absence of end-diastolic velocity (sensitivity 100%). However, the value of abnormal umbilical artery Doppler results (reversed or absent end-diastolic flow) in predicting poor fetal outcome in hypertensive pregnancies has been studied in only a small number of patients.

Management according to gestational age

In general, management of severe pre-eclampsia is dependent on gestational age. Patients with fetuses at a gestational age older than 34 weeks are delivered within 24 h of admission. Patients at 33–34 weeks' gestation with immature fluid receive steroids to accelerate fetal lung maturity and are delivered 24 h after the last dose of steroids in the presence of any change in maternal or fetal conditions. However, patients found eligible for conservative management should be counseled about the fact that gaining 2 more weeks could make the difference between having an infant admitted to the neonatal intensive care unit or having an infant admitted to the well-baby nursery[74].

Patients at 28–32 weeks' gestation are managed according to their clinical response during the observation period. Recently, Sibai and colleagues[74] published data from a randomized and well controlled study comparing aggressive management (46 patients) vs. expectant management (49 patients) in patients with severe pre-eclampsia between 28 and 32 weeks' gestation. In this study, it was possible to prolong pregnancy by an average of 15.4 days in women assigned to expectant management without a significant increase in maternal morbidity. Additionally, the expectant management group had a lower incidence of admissions to the neonatal intensive care unit (76% vs. 100%), lower average number of days spent in that unit (20.2 vs. 36.6 days), reduced incidence of respiratory

distress syndrome (22.4% vs. 50.0%) and a reduced incidence of necrotizing enterocolitis (0% vs. 10.9%). Similar findings were observed by Odendaal and co-workers[82] and by Fenakel and colleagues[83] (Table 10).

Patients with severe pre-eclampsia at a gestational age of < 27 weeks should receive extensive counseling regarding the risks and benefits of expectant management[84]. Sibai and co-workers[84] reported a perinatal survival rate in conservative management of severe pre-eclampsia between 25 and 27 weeks' gestation of 76% compared with 35.5% in the group that had immediate delivery. In addition, the infants in the conservative management group had a lower incidence of intraventricular hemorrhage (41% vs. 71%) and a lower number of days in a neonatal intensive care unit (70 vs. 115). In the same study, a perinatal survival rate of 6.7% and a 27% incidence of maternal morbidity were reported in conservative management of severe pre-eclampsia at ≤ 24 weeks' gestation. Therefore, expectant management of patients between 25 and 27 weeks' gestation had a significantly higher perinatal survival and a lower acute and long-term neonatal morbidity compared to aggressive management. Maternal complications were infrequent in both groups. Findings concerning patients at ≤ 24 weeks' gestation were different. Perinatal survival was low, morbidity was high and maternal complications were also elevated. Therefore, for patients between 24 and 25 weeks' gestation, a gain of 1 or 2 weeks will markedly improve perinatal survival and reduce neonatal morbidity.

Any deterioration in the status of either the mother or the fetus necessitates urgent delivery. Early detection of maternal or fetal complications or deterioration in their clinical status and immediate therapy and delivery are probably responsible for infrequent maternal complications. This supports our beliefs that such management with frequent and daily monitoring of maternal and fetal status is essential and should be practiced only at a tertiary care center. Chari and colleagues[85] studied 68 women with severe pre-eclampsia remote from term who underwent expectant management with daily fetal testing until delivery. In this study, patients who had non-reassuring testing were delivered. Because neither stillbirths nor fetal compromise at birth occurred in patients undergoing daily antenatal testing, the authors recommended daily testing in patients with severe pre-eclampsia managed

Table 10 Randomized studies of conservative management

Authors	Number of women	Gestational age (weeks)	Prolongation (days)
Sibai et al.[74]	49	28–32	15.4 (nifedipine)
Odendaal et al.[82]	20	28–34	7.1 (prazosin)
Fenakel et al.[83]	49	26–36	15.5 (nifedipine) 9.5 (hydralazine)

expectantly. Odendaal and associates[82] recommended performing the non-stress test at least three times daily in this group of patients. However, such evaluation appears to be excessive, except in a select group of patients.

Intrapartum management

Once a decision for delivery is made, vaginal delivery is preferable if possible, and a trial of induction within a limited time is warranted.

It is generally accepted that pre-eclamptic women are at increased risk for convulsions during labor, compared with normotensive pregnant women. The risk for convulsions depends on the severity of the pre-eclamptic process. Women with gestational hypertension (absent proteinuria) are at a lower risk than those with proteinuric hypertension. The highest risk is usually in women with severe pre-eclampsia, particularly those remote from term, those with cerebral manifestations and those with the HELLP syndrome. The use of magnesium sulfate in patients with pre-eclampsia has been questioned for a long time. The incidence of eclampsia in pre-eclamptic women receiving magnesium sulfate is 0.15–0.3% vs. 1.2% in pre-eclamptic women not receiving magnesium sulfate[86]. As a result, all women who are diagnosed to have pre-eclampsia should receive parenteral magnesium sulfate during labor. Magnesium sulfate has been the drug of choice for the prophylaxis of eclamptic seizures in the USA. Other agents (diazepam, clomethiazole, barbiturates and phenytoin) or no agent at all have been used for the same purpose in Europe and Australia. The most commonly used regimens of magnesium sulfate administration are the standard intramuscular regimen of Pritchard and the intravenous regimens of Zuspan and Sibai (Table 11). Phenytoin, on the other hand, has proved to be an effective anticonvulsant in the setting of pre-eclampsia and eclampsia, and was considered by some to be a desirable alternative to magnesium sulfate, especially because phenytoin possesses certain advantages (more rapid cervical dilatation and a smaller drop in hematocrit) and fewer side-effects[87]. Recently, Lucas and colleagues[88] conducted a randomized study comparing the use of magnesium sulfate to phenytoin in the prevention of eclampsia. They found that magnesium sulfate was clearly superior to phenytoin when given prophylactically for eclamptic seizures to women with peripartum hypertension. In fact, ten of the 1089 women randomly assigned to the phenytoin regimen had eclamptic convulsions, compared with none of 1049 women assigned to magnesium sulfate.

Patients should receive close monitoring during labor and delivery and postpartum, with special attention to fluid intake and output. Patients with severe disease and those with the HELLP syndrome are at an increased risk for the development of pulmonary edema from fluid overload and from acute renal failure from blood loss during delivery or from hemolysis, or from a combination of both. Urinary output needs to be monitored every hour, and fluid administration should not exceed 150 ml/h. If the patient develops oliguria (< 100 ml/4 h), both the rate of fluid administered and the dose of magnesium sulfate need to be adjusted.

Antihypertensive drugs in severe pre-eclampsia

Empirically, antihypertensive therapy is recommended for systolic blood pressure exceeding 160 mmHg and diastolic blood pressure of ≥ 110 mmHg in order to protect the patient from the complications of severe hypertension, especially stroke. The aim of therapy is to maintain the blood pressure within the range of 140–150 mmHg systolic and 90–100 mmHg diastolic or to reduce mean arterial blood pressure by no more than 20% from baseline values. Diuretics are not needed, except in the presence of pulmonary edema. Irrespective of the antihypertensive drug used, care must be taken not to lower blood pressure excessively, as this may exacerbate maternal cerebral ischemia, decrease renal function, or jeopardize fetal well-being by decreasing cerebral, renal and placental blood flow. Attempts should be made to reduce the blood pressure to a safe range within 4 h of diagnosis. The antihypertensive drugs that we currently use in the acute treatment of severe pre-eclampsia are described in Table 12. The doses are usually titrated to blood pressure response. Comparative trials between hydralazine, nifedipine and labetalol have not shown one agent to be superior in the acute management of severe hypertension in pregnancy[89,90].

Hydralazine is given in intravenous boluses of 5–10 mg at intervals of 15–20 min until a satisfactory response is achieved. Hydralazine causes a direct relaxation of arterial smooth muscle, resulting in stimulation of the sympathetic nervous system and causing an increased heart rate and contractility. Maternal side-effects include flushing, headache, palpitations, nausea and vomiting. Uteroplacental perfusion may decrease following parenteral administration leading to fetal distress. The onset of the effect of therapy may be 20–30 min, reaching a peak at 60 min from administration. Therefore, the drug may accumulate after continuous intravenous infusion, resulting in hypotension. In a randomized clinical trial, Fenakel and colleagues[83] compared the effects of nifedipine to hydralazine in patients with severe pre-eclampsia. Nifedipine produced a more predictable reduction in blood pressure without being associated with sudden or excessive falls in blood pressure. This characteristic is an important factor in the avoidance of acute fetal distress from sudden hypotension in pre-eclamptic

Table 11 Recommended regimens of magnesium sulfate

Pritchard's intramuscular regimen
   loading dose: 4 g intravenously + 10 g intramuscularly
   maintenance dose: 5 g intramuscularly every 4 h
Zuspan's regimen
   loading dose: 4 g intravenously
   maintenance dose: 1–2 g intravenously per hour
Sibai's intravenous regimen
   loading dose: 6 g intravenously
   maintenance dose: 2–3 g intravenously per hour

Table 12 Drugs for the acute treatment of severe hypertension

Class	Drug	Onset (min)	Peak (min)	Dose
Arterial dilator	hydralazine	10–20	60	5–10 mg intravenously every 15–30 min
Calcium channel blocker	nifedipine	10	60	10–20 mg orally every 30 min
Alpha/ beta-blocker	labetalol	5	60	20–40–80 mg intravenously every 10–20 min up to 300 mg
Arterial/ venous dilator	sodium nitroprusside	0.5–5	5	0.2–5.0 µg/kg/min

patients who frequently have compromised uteroplacental blood flow. Only one of the 24 nifedipine subjects developed acute fetal distress, as opposed to 11 of the 25 hydralazine patients.

Labetalol is administered in repeated bolus intravenous injections. The starting dose is 20 mg, and if no improvement in blood pressure is noted, repeated doses of 40 mg and then 80 mg can be given every 10–20 min to a maximum total dose of 300 mg. When compared to hydralazine, labetalol has fewer side effects, quicker onset of action and smoother reduction in blood pressure[89].

Nifedipine is started at an initial oral dose of 10–20 mg. It is then repeated in 30 min if necessary. The total dose of nifedipine should not exceed 120 mg over a 24-h period. Large controlled trials using this drug in pregnancy are lacking.

Sodium nitroprusside is a potent arterial and venous dilator. It is given in a continuous intravenous infusion beginning at a rate of 0.2 µg/kg/min. It has a rapid action, with short duration. Because of the potent hypotensive properties of the drug, invasive arterial pressure monitoring is recommended. It should be used only in extreme emergencies in pregnancy, because of

the potential risks of fetal cyanide poisoning and metabolic acidosis[91].

Anesthesia

There is controversy about the use of epidural analgesia–anesthesia in women with pre-eclampsia. Some authors believe that the administration of epidural anesthesia in women with severe pre-eclampsia is detrimental to both the mother and the fetus, owing to possible profound hypotension. Other studies have demonstrated, however, that administration of epidural anesthesia in women with pre-eclampsia has a favorable effect on maternal hemodynamics, decreases catecholamine levels and improves intervillous as well as umbilical blood flow[92–95]. Ramanathan and colleagues[95] prospectively compared the effects of lumbar epidural (n = 11) and general (n = 10) anesthesia on the hemodynamic and neuroendocrine stress response to Cesarean delivery in 21 women with severe pre-eclampsia. The authors found that, in the epidural group, there was a decrease in mean arterial pressure, and the concentrations of adrenocorticotropic hormone, β-endorphin and catecholamine decreased or remained unchanged during the procedure. In contrast, patients receiving general anesthesia demonstrated a significant increase in both mean blood pressure and the concentration of the various hormones studied. In addition, neonatal outcomes were similar in both groups. It is our opinion that the epidural is the anesthetic of choice in women with pre-eclampsia. However, its use is contraindicated in patients with coagulopathy and/or acute fetal distress. For patients with the HELLP syndrome, the use of pudendal block is contraindicated.

Postpartum management

Following delivery, the patient should continue to be monitored in the recovery room for 12–24 h, during which time maternal vital signs including reflexes, and intake and output, should be monitored hourly. Twenty-five per cent of cases of eclampsia are reported to occur postpartum; therefore, close observation is mandatory. Salt restriction and diuretics are not needed. Most patients will show evidence of resolution of the disease process within 24 h. Some, however, mainly those with severe disease in the mid-trimester, and those with the HELLP syndrome, require intensive monitoring for 2–4 days. In such patients, magnesium sulfate may be needed for more than 24 h. In addition, these patients are at increased risk for development of pulmonary edema from fluid overload, fluid mobilization and compromised renal function[96].

If the patient develops severe hypertension during this time, the blood pressure may be controlled with oral nifedipine. In a double-blind study, Barton and co-workers[97] evaluated the effect of nifedipine in postpartum patients with severe pre-eclampsia before delivery. They found oral nifedipine to be effective in the control of blood pressure as well as improving urine output during the 24 h after delivery. In a subsequent report, Barton and co-workers[98] studied the pharmacokinetic and pharmacodynamic parameters of oral nifedipine use in the immediate postpartum period. Again, they found the drug to be efficacious in controlling hypertension associated with pre-eclampsia and they suggested that dosing should be every 3–4 h. Most patients will be normotensive at the time of discharge from the hospital. In these patients, birth control pills may be prescribed without problems. A few patients may continue to have severe hypertension, and this can be controlled with either methyldopa or labetalol. Prophylactic anticonvulsive drugs such as phenobarbital are not needed. The patient is then seen at weekly intervals until her blood pressure is in the normal range without the use of medication. If this change does not occur by 6 weeks, a work-up to assess hypertension should be performed.

In addition to the use of nifedipine, postpartum curettage has been used by some obstetricians as another alternative to enhance postpartum recovery from pre-eclampsia[99]. Gentle postpartum curettage with the banjo curette was described to be as effective as nifedipine use[100]. A recent study comparing the use of these two modalities showed that no statistical difference exists between these two approaches relative to the decrease in mean arterial pressure or the increase in urinary output following either treatment. However, uterine curettage was associated with a more rapid resolution of thrombocytopenia[100]. It is important to note that both these studies had problems with design and sample size. At present, there is no indication to use such management in women with severe pre-eclampsia.

REFERENCES

1. Sibai BM, Usta IM. Chronic hypertension in pregnancy. In Sciarra JJ, ed. *Gynecology and Obstetrics. Service 60.* Philadelphia: JB Lippincott, 1995:1–19
2. American College of Obstetricians and Gynecologists. *Management of Severe Preeclampsia.* Technical Bulletin no. 91. Washington, DC: American College of Obstetricians and Gynecologists, 1986
3. Sibai BM. Hypertension in pregnancy. Chapter 28. In Gabbe SG, Niebyl JR, Simpson JL, eds. *Obstetrics: Normal and Problem Pregnancies*, 3rd edn. New York: Churchill Livingstone, 1996:935–6
4. Long P, Oats J. Preeclampsia in twin pregnancy–severity and pathogenesis. *Aust NZ J Obstet Gynaecol* 1987;27:1–5
5. Coonrod DV, Hickok D, Zhu K, *et al.* Risk factors for preeclampsia in twin pregnancies: a population-based cohort study. *Obstet Gynecol* 1995;85:645–50
6. Sutherland A, Cooper DW, Howie PW, *et al.* The incidence of severe preeclampsia among mothers and mothers-in-law of preeclamptics and controls. *Br J Obstet Gynaecol* 1981;88:785–91
7. Sibai BM, El-Nazer A, Gonzalez-Ruiz A. Severe preeclampsia–eclampsia in young primigravidas: subsequent pregnancy outcome and remote prognosis. *Am J Obstet Gynecol* 1986;1555:1011–16
8. Sibai BM. Preeclampsia–eclampsia. *Curr Prob Obstet Gynecol Fertil* 1990;13:1–45
9. Chesley LC. History and epidemiology of preeclampsia–eclampsia. *Clin Obstet Gynecol* 1984;27:801–20
10. Eskenazi B, Fenster L, Sidney S. A multivariate analysis of risk factors of preeclampsia *J Am Med Assoc* 1991;266:237–41
11. Easterling TR, Benedetti TJ, Schmucker BC, Millard SP. Maternal hemodynamics in normal and preeclamptic pregnancies: a longitudinal study. *Obstet Gynecol* 1990;76:1061–9
12. Sibai BM, Gordon T, Thom E, *et al.* and the National Institute of Child Health and Human Development Network of Maternal–Fetal Medicine Units. Risk factors for preeclampsia in healthy nulliparous women: a prospective multicenter study. *Am J Obstet Gynecol* 1995;172:642–8
13. Marcoux S, Brisson J, Fabia J. The effect of cigarette smoking on the risk of preeclampsia and gestational hypertension. *Am J Epidemiol* 1989;130:950–7
14. Seidman DS, Ever-Hadani P, Stevenson DK, Gale R. The effect of abortion on the incidence of preeclampsia. *Eur J Obstet Gynecol Reprod Biol* 1989;33:109–14
15. Campbell DM, MacGillivray I. Preeclampsia in second pregnancy. *Br J Obstet Gynaecol* 1985;92:131–40
16. Strickland DM, Guzick DS, Cox K, *et al.* The relationship between abortion in the first pregnancy and development of pregnancy-induced hypertension in the subsequent pregnancy. *Am J Obstet Gynecol* 1986;154:146–8
17. Sibai BM. Pitfalls in the diagnosis and management of preeclampsia. *Am J Obstet Gynecol* 1988;159:1–5
18. Lindow SW, Davey DA. The variability of urinary protein and creatinine excretion in patients with gestational proteinuric hypertension. *Br J Obstet Gynaecol* 1992;99:869–73
19. Meyer NL, Mercer BM, Friedman SA, Sibai BM. Urinary dipstick protein: a poor predictor of absent or severe proteinuria. *Am J Obstet Gynecol* 1994;170:137–41
20. Kuo VS, Koumantakis G, Gallery EDM. Proteinuria and its assessment in normal and hypertensive pregnancy. *Am J Obstet Gynecol* 1992;167:723–8
21. Brown MA, Buddle ML. Inadequacy of dipstick proteinuria in hypertensive pregnancy. *Aust NZ J Obstet Gynaecol* 1995;35:366–9
22. Collins R, Yusuf S, Peto R. Overview of randomized trials of diuretics in pregnancy. *Br Med J* 1985;190:17–23
23. Hatton DC, McCarron DA. Dietary calcium and blood pressure in experimental models of hypertension: a review. *Hypertension* 1994;23:513–30
24. Belizan JM, Villar J, Repke J. The relationship between calcium intake and pregnancy-induced hypertension: up-to-date evidence. *Am J Obstet Gynecol* 1988;158:898–902
25. Kawasaki N, Matsui K, Nakamura T, *et al.* Effect of calcium supplementation on the vascular sensitivity to

angiotensin II in pregnant women. *Am J Obstet Gynecol* 1985;153:576–82

26. Sanchez-Ramos L, Briones DK, Kaunitz AM, *et al*. Prevention of pregnancy-induced hypertension by calcium supplementation in angiotensin-II sensitive patients. *Obstet Gynecol* 1994;84:349–53

27. Marya RK, Rathee S, Manrow M. Effect of calcium and vitamin D supplementation on toxaemia of pregnancy. *Gynecol Obstet Invest* 1987;24:38–42

28. Villar J, Repke J, Belizan JM, *et al*. Calcium supplementation reduces blood pressure during pregnancy: results from a randomized clinical trial. *Obstet Gynecol* 1987;70:317–22

29. Lopez-Jaramillo P, Narvaez M, Weigel RM, *et al*. Calcium supplementation reduces the risk of pregnancy-induced hypertension in an Andes population. *Br J Obstet Gynaecol* 1987;96:648–55

30. Villar J, Repke JT. Calcium supplementation during pregnancy may reduce preterm delivery in high-risk populations. *Am J Obstet Gynecol* 1990;163:124–31

31. Montanaro D, Boscutti G, Mioni G, *et al*. Calcium supplementation decreases the incidence of pregnancy-induced hypertension (PIH) and preeclampsia. *Proceedings of the VIIth World Congress of Hypertension in Pregnancy*, Perugia, Italy, October 1990;abstr.91

32. Belizan JM, Villar J, Gonzalez L, *et al*. Calcium supplementation to prevent hypertensive disorders of pregnancy. *N Engl J Med* 1991;325:1399–405

33. Lopez-Jaramillo P, Narvaez M, Felix C, Lopez A. Dietary calcium supplementation and prevention of pregnancy hypertension, letter. *Lancet* 1990;335:293

34. Carroli G, Duley L, Belizan JM, Villar J. Calcium supplementation during pregnancy: a systemic review of randomized controlled trials. *Br J Obstet Gynaecol* 1994;101:753–8

35. Bucher HC, Guyatt GH, Cook RJ, *et al*. Effect of calcium supplementation on pregnancy-induced hypertension and preeclampsia. A meta-analysis of randomized controlled trials. *J Am Med Assoc* 1996;275:1113–17

36. Levine RJ, Raymon E, Der Simonian R, Clemens JD. Preeclampsia prevention with calcium supplementation. *Clin Appl Nutr* 1992;2:30

37. National Institute of Health/Maternal–Fetal Medicine Units Network (Sibai BM). The trial of calcium for preeclampsia prevention (CPEP): rationale, design, and methods. *Controlled Clin Trials* 1996;17:442–69

38. Spitz B, Magness RR, Cox SM, *et al*. Low-dose aspirin. I. Effect on angiotensin II pressor responses and blood prostaglandin concentration in pregnant women sensitive to angiotensin II. *Am J Obstet Gynecol* 1988;159:1035–43

39. Sibai BM, Mirro R, Chesney CM, Leffer C. Low dose aspirin in pregnancy. *Obstet Gynecol* 1989;74:551–7

40. Dekker GA, Sibai BM. Low-dose aspirin: the prevention of preeclampsia and fetal growth retardation: rationale, mechanisms, and clinical trials. *Am J Obstet Gynecol* 1993;168:214–17

41. Hauth JC, Goldenberg RL, Parker R Jr, *et al*. Low-dose aspirin therapy to prevent preeclampsia. *Am J Obstet Gynecol* 1993;168:1083–93

42. Sibai BM, Caritis SN, Thom E, *et al*. and the National Institute of Child Health and Human Development Network of Maternal–Fetal Medicine Units. Prevention of preeclampsia with low-dose aspirin in healthy, nulliparous pregnant women. *N Engl J Med* 1993;329:1213–18

43. Viinikka L, Hartikainen-Sorri A-L, Lumme R, *et al*. Low dose aspirin in hypertensive pregnant women: effect on pregnancy outcome and prostacyclin–thromboxane balance in mother and newborn. *Br J Obstet Gynaecol* 1993;100:809–15

44. Italian Study of Aspirin in Pregnancy. Low-dose aspirin in prevention and treatment of intrauterine growth retardation and pregnancy-induced hypertension. *Lancet* 1993;341:396–400

45. CLASP. A randomized trial of low-dose aspirin for the prevention and treatment of preeclampsia among 9364 pregnant women. *Lancet* 1992;343:619–29

46. Hamid R, Robson M, Pearch JM. Low-dose aspirin in women with raised maternal serum alpha-fetoprotein and abnormal Doppler waveform patterns from the uteroplacental circulation. *Br J Obstet Gynaecol* 1994;101:481–4

47. Estudo Colaborativo para Prevencao da Pre-eclampsia com Aspirina (ECPPA). ECPPA: randomised trial of low dose aspirin for the prevention of maternal and fetal complications in high risk pregnant women. *Br J Obstet Gynaecol* 1996;103:39–47

48. Caritis S for the NICHD MFMU Network (Sibai BM). Low dose aspirin does not prevent preeclampsia in high risk women. *Annual Meeting of the Society of Perinatal Obstetricians*, Anaheim, CA, January 20–25, 1997. *Am J Obstet Gynecol* 1997;1:53

49. Hamlin RHJ. The prevention of eclampsia and preeclampsia. *Lancet* 1952;1:64–8

50. Gilstrap LC, Cunningham GF, Whalley PJ. Management of pregnancy induced hypertension in the nulliparous patient remote from term. *Semin Perinatol* 1978;2:73–81

51. Sibai BM, Gonzalez AR, Mabie WC, *et al*. A comparison of labetalol versus hospitalization alone in the management of preeclampsia remote from term. *Obstet Gynecol* 1987;70:323–7

52. Matthews DD, Patel IR, Sengupta SM. Outpatient management of toxaemia. *J Obstet Gynaecol Br Commonw* 1971;78:610–19

53. Matthews DD, Agarwal V, Shuttleworth TP. The effect of rest and ambulation on plasma urea levels in pregnant women with proteinuric hypertension. *Br J Obstet Gynaecol* 1980;87:1095–8

54. Crowther CA, Bouwmeester AM, Ashurst HM. Does admission to hospital for bed rest prevent disease progression or improve fetal outcome in pregnancy complicated by non-proteinuric hypertension? *Br J Obstet Gynaecol* 1992;99:13–17

55. Cunningham FG, MacDonald PC, Gant NF, *et al*. *Williams' Obstetrics*, 19th edn. Norwalk, CT: Appleton & Lange, 1993:785

56. Sibai BM, Barton JR, Akl S, *et al*. A randomized prospective comparison of nifedipine and bed rest versus bed rest alone in the management of preeclampsia remote from term. *Am J Obstet Gynecol* 1992;167:879–84

57. Barton JR, Stanziano GJ, Sibai BM. Monitored outpatient management of mild gestational hypertension

remote from term. *Am J Obstet Gynecol* 1994;170: 765–9

58. Helewa M, Heaman M, Robinson MA, Thompson L. Community based home-care program for the management of pre-eclampsia: an alternative. *Can Med Assoc J* 1993;149:829–34

59. Soothill PW, Campbell S, Gibbs J, *et al.* Effect of a fetal surveillance unit on admission of antenatal patients to hospital. *Br Med J* 1991;303:269–71

60. Tuffnell DJ, Lilford RJ, Buchan PC, *et al.* Randomized controlled trial of daycare for hypertension in pregnancy. *Lancet* 1992;339:224–7

61. Dawson AJ, Middlemiss C, Coles EC, *et al.* A randomized study of a domiciliary antenatal care scheme: the effect on hospital admissions. *Br J Obstet Gynaecol* 1989;96:1319–22

62. Twaddle S, Harper V. An economic evaluation of day care in the management of hypertension in pregnancy. *Br J Obstet Gynaecol* 1992;99:459–63

63. Barton JR, Stanziano GJ, Jacques DL, *et al.* Monitored outpatient management of mild gestational hypertension remote from term in teenage pregnancies. *Am J Obstet Gynecol* 1995;73:1865–8

64. Rubin PC, Clark DM, Summer DJ, *et al.* Placebo-controlled trial of atenolol in the treatment of pregnancy associated hypertension. *Lancet* 1983;1:431–4

65. Wichman K, Ryden G, Karlberg BE. A placebo controlled trial of metoprolol in the treatment of hypertension in pregnancy. *Scand J Clin Lab Invest* 1984;44: 90–5

66. Plouin PF, Breart GL, Maillard F, *et al.* Comparison of antihypertensive efficacy and perinatal safety of labetalol and methyldopa in the treatment of hypertension in pregnancy: a randomized controlled trial. *Br J Obstet Gynaecol* 1988;95:868–76

67. Pickles CJ, Symonds EM, Broughton-Pipkin F. The fetal outcome in a randomized double-blind controlled trial of labetalol versus placebo in pregnancy-induced hypertension. *Br J Obstet Gynaecol* 1989;96:38–43

68. Plouin F, Beart G, Llado J, *et al.* A randomized comparison of early with conservative use of antihypertensive drugs in the management of pregnancy-induced hypertension. *Br J Obstet Gynaecol* 1990;97:134–41

69. Phippard AF, Fisher WE, Horvath JS, *et al.* Early blood pressure control improves pregnancy outcome in primigravid women with mild hypertension. *Med J Aust* 1991;154:378–82

70. Cruikshank DJ, Robertson AA, Campbell DM, MacGillivray I. Does labetalol influence the development of proteinuria in pregnancy hypertension? A randomized controlled study. *Eur J Obstet Gynecol Reprod Biol* 1992;45:47–51

71. Pickles CJ, Broughton-Pipkin F, Symonds EM. A randomized placebo controlled trial of labetalol in the treatment of mild to moderate pregnancy induced hypertension. *Br J Obstet Gynaecol* 1992;99:964–8

72. Jannet D, Carbonne B, Sebban E, Milliez J. Nicardipine versus metoprolol in the treatment of hypertension during pregnancy: a randomized controlled trial. *Obstet Gynecol* 1994;84:354–9

73. Sibai BM. Treatment of hypertension in pregnant women. *N Engl J Med* 1996;335:257–65

74. Sibai BM, Mercer BM, Schiff E, Friedman SA. Aggressive versus expectant management of severe pre-eclampsia at 28 to 32 weeks' gestation: a randomized controlled trial. *Am J Obstet Gynecol* 1994;171: 818–22

75. Schiff E, Friedman SA, Sibai BM. Conservative management of severe preeclampsia remote from term. *Obstet Gynecol* 1994;84:626–30

76. Visser W, Wallenburg H. Temporizing management of severe preeclampsia with and without the HELLP syndrome. *Br J Obstet Gynaecol* 1995;102:111–17

77. Magann EF, Bass D, Chauhan SP, *et al.* Antepartum corticosteroids: disease stabilization in patients with the syndrome of hemolysis, elevated liver enzymes, and low platelets (HELLP). *Am J Obstet Gynecol* 1994; 171:1148–53

78. Schiff E, Friedman SA, Mercer BM, Sibai BM. Fetal lung maturity is not accelerated in preeclamptic patients. *Am J Obstet Gynecol* 1993;169:1096–101

79. Friedman SA, Schiff E, Kao L, Sibai BM. Neonatal outcome after preterm delivery for preeclampsia. *Am J Obstet Gynecol* 1995;172:1785–92

80. Yoon BH, Lee CM, Kim SW. An abnormal umbilical artery waveform: a strong and independent predictor of adverse perinatal outcome in patients with preeclampsia. *Am J Obstet Gynecol* 1994;171:713–21

81. Torres PJ, Gratacos E, Alonso PL. Umbilical artery Doppler ultrasound predicts low birthweight and fetal death in hypertensive pregnancies. *Acta Obstet Gynecol Scand* 1995;74:352–5

82. Odendaal HJ, Pattison RC, Bam R, *et al.* Aggressive or expectant management for patients with severe pre-eclampsia between 28–34 weeks' gestation: a randomized controlled trial. *Obstet Gynecol* 1990;76:1070–5

83. Fenakel K, Fenakel G, Appelman Z, *et al.* Nifedipine in the treatment of severe preeclampsia. *Obstet Gynecol* 1991;77:331–7

84. Sibai BM, Akl S, Fairlie F, Moretti M. A protocol for managing severe preeclampsia in the second trimester. *Am J Obstet Gynecol* 1990;163:733–8

85. Chari RS, Friedman SA, O'Brien JM, Sibai BM. Daily antenatal testing in women with severe preeclampsia. *Am J Obstet Gynecol* 1995;173:1207–10

86. Sibai BM, Ramanathan J. The case for magnesium sulfate in preeclampsia–eclampsia. *Int J Obstet Anesth* 1992;1:167–75

87. Friedman SA, Lim K, Baker CA, Repke J. Phenytoin versus magnesium sulfate in preeclampsia: a pilot study. *Am J Perinatol* 1993;10:233–8

88. Lucas MJ, Leveno KJ, Cunningham FG. A comparison of magnesium sulfate with phenytoin for the prevention of eclampsia. *N Engl J Med* 1995;333:201–5

89. Mabie WC, Gonzales AR, Sibai BM, Amon E. A comparative trial of labetalol and hydralazine in the acute management of severe hypertension complicating pregnancy. *Obstet Gynecol* 1987;70:328–33

90. Ashe RE, Moodley J, Richards AM, Philpott RH. Comparison of labetalol and dihydralazine in hypertensive emergencies of pregnancy. *S Afr Med J* 1987; 71:354–6

91. Shoemaker CT, Meyers M. Sodium nitroprusside for control of severe hypertensive disease of pregnancy: a

case report and discussion of potential toxicity. *Am J Obstet Gynecol* 1984;149:171–3

92. Abboud T, Artal R, Sarkis F, *et al.* Sympathoadrenal activity, maternal, fetal and neonatal responses after epidural anesthesia in the preeclamptic patient. *Am J Obstet Gynecol* 1982;144:915–18

93. Jouppila P, Jouppila R, Hollmen A, *et al.* Lumbar epidural analgesia to improve intervillous blood flow during labor in severe preeclampsia. *Obstet Gynecol* 1982;59:158–61

94. Miles GJ, Dempster J, Patel NB, Taylor DJ. Epidural analgesia and its effect on umbilical artery flow velocity waveform patterns in uncomplicated labour and labour complicated by pregnancy-induced hypertension. *Eur J Obstet Gynecol Reprod Biol* 1990;36:35–41

95. Ramanathan J, Coleman P, Sibai BM. Anesthetic modification of hemodynamic and neuroendocrine stress responses to cesarean delivery in women with severe preeclampsia. *Anesth Analg* 1991;73:772–9

96. Sibai BM, Mabie BC, Harvey CJ, Gonzalez AR. Pulmonary edema in severe preeclampsia–eclampsia: analysis of 37 consecutive cases. *Am J Obstet Gynecol* 1987;156:1174–9

97. Barton JR, Hiett AK, Conover WC. The use of nifedipine during the postpartum period in patients with severe preeclampsia. *Am J Obstet Gynecol* 1990;162:788–92

98. Barton JR, Prevost RR, Wilson DA, *et al.* Nifedipine pharmacokinetics and pharmacodynamics during the immediate postpartum period in patients with preeclampsia. *Am J Obstet Gynecol* 1991;165:91–4

99. Magann EF, Martin JN Jr, Isaacs JD, *et al.* Immediate postpartum curettage: accelerated recovery from severe preeclampsia. *Obstet Gynecol* 1993;81:502–6

100. Magann EF, Bass JD, Chauhan SP, *et al.* Accelerated recovery from severe preeclampsia: uterine curettage versus nifedipine. *J Soc Gynecol Invest* 1995;1:210–14

4

Incompetent cervix

A.I. Kivikoski

EPIDEMIOLOGY

Uterine cervical incompetence is the inability of the cervix to support the pregnancy to term. Although the incompetent cervix has been discussed in the literature for more than 100 years, information pertaining to the diagnosis is still controversial. The classical presentation is painless cervical dilatation in the second trimester, followed by rupture of membranes, or protrusion of membranes often including fetal parts into the vagina, leading to second-trimester pregnancy loss. The incidence of incompetent cervix in relation to the number of normal deliveries has not been established, with a wide variation in the literature from 0.1% to 1.8%[1].

It is estimated that cervical incompetence is responsible for more than 16% of second-trimester abortions[2]. This variation arises from the lack of standard criteria for the diagnosis of cervical incompetence and possible overdiagnosis.

THE CERVIX

Anatomically, the cervix has two entities: a predominantly fibrous cervix and a more muscular isthmus. The mean proportions of smooth muscle are 6.4%, 18% and 29% in the lower, middle and upper thirds of the cervix, respectively[3]. The transition area from the cervix to the isthmus varies in the non-pregnant uterus from very narrow up to 10 mm[4]. It appears that the amount of cervical muscle tissue is higher in patients with clinical cervical incompetence than in normal patients immediately following regular labor at term[5]. Anatomically and functionally, the isthmus is part of the corpus uteri.

Starting at about the 3rd month of pregnancy, the isthmus dilates and elongates, and beyond the 5th month it represents the lowest part of the uterine cavity[6]. Biochemical changes can be detected in the cervical tissue before labor onset. In one study, the amount of intact collagen chains found antepartum and intrapartum was small, compared to the amount found during the proliferative phase and early pregnancy, and the hydroxyproline : total protein ratio was lower intrapartum[7]. The incompetent cervix has a decreased amount of elastin fibers[8].

ETIOLOGICAL FACTORS

In spite of numerous studies in the literature, there is no generally accepted etiology of cervical incompetence. The most commonly associated factors are cervical trauma, congenital anomaly and structural changes.

Cervical trauma

Cervical trauma may originate from previous pregnancies and is usually mentioned as the most common cause of cervical incompetence. It may follow spontaneous or induced precipitate labor, as well as obstetric operative procedures. Gynecological procedures, such as mechanical cervical dilatation preceding diagnostic procedures or termination of pregnancy, and conization of the cervix are also implicated. It appears that younger patients (17 years or less) are at an increased risk for cervical injury from therapeutic abortions because of small, immature cervices[9]. Interestingly, one study reported that 68% of women with cervical incompetence had a history of cervical dilatation and curettage, and 93% had a history of one or more second-trimester abortions[1].

First-trimester termination of pregnancy is not a risk factor if performed by an experienced operator with the use of *Laminaria*[9]. To minimize cervical trauma, cervical dilatation should be done slowly, as during normal uterine activity.

Cervical conization procedures, especially those which are large and high in the cervix, could contribute to cervical incompetence[10,11].

Congenital anomaly

The most often mentioned anomalies are those associated with intrauterine exposure to diethylstilbestrol (DES). In the late 1970s, when cervical incompetence among DES-exposed women was initially published, poor perinatal outcomes secondary to preterm deliveries and increased perinatal mortality were reported[6]. In a prospective study, as many as 40% of DES-exposed patients with grossly normal cervices on the initial examination demonstrated silent cervical effacement and dilatation in the second trimester requiring intervention[12].

DIAGNOSIS

A history of repeated second-trimester abortions without uterine contractions resulting in delivery of living or non-macerated products of conception is suggestive. Patients with a history of incompetent cervix should be evaluated to rule out other causes of cervical dilatation, such as uterine activity, immunological disorders or infection. Patients may occasionally complain of pelvic pressure, increased vaginal discharge, spotting or urinary urgency. It is also advisable to examine and evaluate nulliparous patients during the second trimester who are at risk for cervical incompetence. A common method of diagnosing cervical incompetence during pregnancy is vaginal examination to document cervical shortening, internal os dilatation, or membranes bulging through the cervical canal.

It should be noted that mild cervical dilatation may normally occur in the second half of pregnancy. Internal os dilatation of a finger's breadth between 21 and 36 weeks' gestation has been reported. When the duration of pregnancy increased, the internal os dilated more often[13,14]. Cervical incompetence is usually operatively treated between 14 and 18 weeks, thus before this 'physiological' opening occurs.

Ultrasonography provides an objective means to evaluate the cervix during pregnancy[15]. Changes in cervical length[16–20] or width of the internal os[18,21,22], and presence of membranes bulging into the cervical canal[18,23,24], have been described as signs of cervical incompetence. Mean normal cervical lengths were reported at 2.0–4.2 cm and 4.09 cm by abdominal and vaginal ultrasound examinations, respectively. Furthermore, the correlation between digital and vaginal ultrasound measurements of cervical length was weak[25], only 0.49[26]. In a study conducted by the National Institute of Child Health and Human Development (NICHD), 2915 women at approximately 24 weeks and 2531 women at approximately 28 weeks were screened by vaginal ultrasonography to predict spontaneous premature delivery. The risk of preterm delivery was increased in women who were found to have a short cervix[20]. Concerning cervical width, the internal os was higher in patients admitted for cerclage than in normal patients. A cervical width of 0.9 cm or more was considered to be diagnostic of cervical incompetence[21].

After insertion of cerclage, membrane protrusion decreased[19]. Appreciation of transfundal pressure during transvaginal ultrasound evaluation increases the detection of the asymptomatic incompetent cervix[27].

The incompetent cervix opens as a result of enlargement of the internal os, followed by the lower part of the cervical canal.

DIAGNOSTIC TESTS IN THE NON-PREGNANT CONDITION

Mechanical tests have been used to measure cervical resistance, assuming that an incompetent cervix would have less resistance. The Hegar test uses a no. 8 dilator passed through the cervix. In the traction test, a Foley catheter is pulled through the cervix with the balloon filled with 1 ml of water. During these tests, the cervix may not function as it does during pregnancy, demonstrating a potential test flaw. In addition, test uniformity is difficult to achieve.

Hysterography has been used to assess cervical canals. In one study of 212 patients with histories of spontaneous second-trimester abortions or early preterm births, a significantly higher proportion of patients (58%) showed wider cervical canals compared to controls[28].

Magnetic resonance imaging (MRI) has also been used to demonstrate cervical changes such as shorter cervical length, wider internal os, or abnormal signal intensity in cervical stroma, suggestive of an incompetent cervix[29].

TREATMENT

The pregnant patient with incompetent cervix, assessed either by a classical history or by cervical change during the second trimester, may benefit from cervical cerclage. This is best done between 14 and 18 weeks, when the isthmus is forming part of the uterine cavity and the risk of spontaneous abortion is substantially reduced. In addition, genetic amniocentesis could be carried out prior to the cerclage. The most common procedures are the Shirodkar[30] and McDonald[31] operations. Ultrasound examination is recommended before the operation to demonstrate the viability of the fetus and to exclude major fetal anomalies. Some obstetricians use tocolysis such as oral terbutaline or indomethacin for 24 h during the preoperative period.

The Shirodkar cerclage is a submucosal band around the cervix. First, the cervical mucosa is opened anteriorly and posteriorly. Second, the bladder is elevated and the cerclage is placed close to the internal os with the use of a mersilene band which is available with its own atraumatic needles. Third, the cerclage is anchored in place to prevent sliding with 4–0 permanent sutures anteriorly and posteriorly. Finally, the mucosa is closed.

The McDonald purse-string procedure (Figure 1) is simpler, involving four or five bites deep into the cervical matrix, underrunning the blood vessels. The suture is placed as high as possible near the internal os without injuring the bladder, with the knot tied in the anterior aspect of the cervix. There are variations on the original technique, e.g. the use of two sutures 1 cm

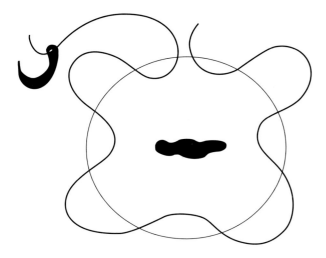

Figure 1 McDonald purse string suture

apart. Permanent no. 1 suture is preferable. These sutures are removed before labor at 37 weeks. The sutures can be removed earlier, in the case of ruptured membranes or uterine contractions unresponsive to tocolysis.

Late cerclage operations, usually emergent procedures done between 18 and 24 weeks of gestation following a significant cervical dilatation, have lower fetal survival rates.

If the cervix is already dilated, Hefner[32] sutures may be used. These are simple or mattress sutures to close the external os. It is important to be sure that there are no contractions before undertaking the operation.

If membranes are already bulging through the cervix, they tend to rupture intraoperatively. It has been helpful to use 6–10 stay sutures at the edges of the cervix. Under traction these sutures help to lift the membranes and close the cervix below the membranes[33]. To minimize rupture of the membranes, one of the following methods can be used. First, a Foley catheter with a 30-ml balloon can be inserted into the cervix to keep the membranes above the cervix. Once the cerclage is in place, the balloon is deflated and the catheter is removed[34]. Another method to displace prolapsed membranes upwards is to fill the bladder with 1000 ml of saline solution while the patient is in the Trendelenburg position. After the membranes are seen to be lifted above the cervix, the cerclage is placed and the bladder is then emptied[35]. Lombardi and colleagues[36] utilized a McDonald cerclage combined with adjunctive medical therapy of antibiotics and tocolysis. The following intravenous antibiotic regimen is administered preoperatively: loading dose of 120 mg gentamycin followed by 80 mg every 8 h; 900 mg of clindamycin every 8 h; and 2 g of ampicillin every 6 h. Indomethacin can be used for tocolysis with a loading dose of 50 mg rectally, followed by 25 mg every 6 h. Surgically a McDonald cerclage is inserted

by the Foley catheter technique with 5 mm Mersilene tape. Postoperative antibiotics are administered with the same regimen listed above for a minimum course of 48 h and a maximum course of 5 days, depending on the risk of infection. Indomethacin is continued postoperatively as 25 mg every 6 h for an average duration of 48 h, a minimum course of 24 h and a maximum course of 72 h[36].

In rare cases when the cervix is amputated, deeply lacerated, or scarred, an abdominal cerclage may be carried out.

RESULTS

When a cerclage is done prophylactically, the rate of live births is 80–100%[1,23,37]. If the procedure is done when there is already significant cervical change, the rate of live births ranges from 12% to 50%[1,36,38]. The type of cerclage procedure used depends on personal preference and has no impact on fetal survival rates[39].

COMPLICATIONS

The most common complication is continued cervical dilatation in spite of the procedure. This may occur soon after the procedure, because of myometrial activity, which necessitates removal of the suture. This complication is less likely to happen if the procedure is carried out prophylactically before cervical dilatation. Displacement of cervical sutures, usually in the posterior cervix, can occur, especially in the presence of myometrial activity. Replacement of the cerclage is usually associated with a much lower success rate. Rupture of membranes may occur perioperatively, more so with emergency cerclage when the cervix is quite dilated and the membranes are bulging into the vagina. Rare complications include uterine rupture associated with active labor with a cerclage in place and infection, such as abscesses along the rupture line, chorioamnionitis and sepsis. Infection appears to occur more frequently following the Shirodkar, as opposed to the McDonald, suture[1].

REFERENCES

1. McDonald IA. Cervical cerclage. *Clin Obstet Gynecol* 1980; 7:461–79
2. Stromme BW, Hayva EW. Intrauterine fetal death in the second trimester. *Am J Obstet Gynecol* 1963;85:223
3. Rorie PK, Newton M. Histological and chemical studies of the smooth muscle in human cervix and uterus. *Am J Obstet Gynecol* 1967;99:466
4. Danforth DN. The fibrous nature of the human cervix and its relation to the isthmic segment in gravid and nongravid uteri. *Am J Obstet Gynecol* 1947;53:541
5. Buckingham JC, Buethe RA, Danforth DN. Collagen–muscle ratio in clinically normal and clinically incompetent cervices. *Am J Obstet Gynecol* 1965;91:232

6. Cousins L. Cervical incompetence, 1980: a time for reappraisal, *Clin Obstet Gynecol* 1980;23:967

7. Kleissl HP, Van Der Rest M, Naftolin G, *et al.* Collagen changes in the human uterine cervix at parturition. *Am J Obstet Gynecol* 1978;130:748

8. Leppert PC, Yu SY, Keller S, *et al.* Decreased elastic fibers and desmosine content in incompetent cervix. *Am J Obstet Gynecol* 1987;157:1134

9. Schulz KF, Grimes DK, Cates W. Measures to prevent cervical injury during suction curettage abortion. *Lancet* 1983;1:1182

10. Leiman G, Harrison NA, Rubin A. Pregnancy following conization of the cervix: complications related to cone size. *Am J Obstet Gynecol* 1980;136:14

11. Larsson G, Grundsell H, Gullberg B, Svennerud S. Outcome of pregnancy after conization. *Acta Obstet Gynecol Scand* 1982;61:461

12. Ludmir J, Landon MB, Gabbe SG, *et al.* Management of the DES-exposed pregnant patient: a prospective study. *Am J Obstet Gynecol* 1987;3:665

13. Parikh MN, Mehta AC. Internal cervical os during the second half of pregnancy. *J Obstet Gynaecol Br Commonw* 1061;68:818

14. Schaffner F, Schanzer SN: Cervical dilatation in the early third trimester. *Obstet Gynecol* 1966;27:130

15. Ludmir J. Sonographic detection of cervical incompetence. *Clin Obstet Gynecol* 1988;31:101.

16. Vaalamo P, Kivikoski A. The length of cervix uteri during pregnancy measured by ultrasound. *XX Nordic Congress of Obstetrics and Gynecology*, Bergen, 1978

17. Zemlyn S. The length of the uterine cervix and its significance. *J Clin Ultrasound* 1981;9:267

18. Varma TR, Patel RH, Pillai V. Ultrasonic assessment of cervix in normal pregnancy. *Acta Obstet Gynecol Scand* 1986;65:229

19. Michaels WH, Montgomery G Karo J, *et al.* Ultrasound differentiation of the competent from the incompetent cervix: prevention of preterm delivery. *Am J Obstet Gynecol* 1986;154:537

20. Iams JD, Goldenberg RL, Meis J, *et al.* The length of the cervix and the risk of spontaneous premature delivery. *N Engl J Med* 1996;334:567

21. Brook I, Feingold M, Schwartz A, Zakut H. Ultrasonography in the diagnosis of cervical incompetence in pregnancy. *Br J Obstet Gynaecol* 1981;88:640

22. Mahran M. The role of ultrasound in the diagnosis and management of the incompetent cervix. In Kurjak A, ed. *Recent Advances in Ultrasound Diagnosis 2*. Amsterdam, Oxford, Princeton: Excerpta Medica, 1980:505–14

23. Vaalamo P, Kivikoski A: The incompetent cervix during pregnancy diagnosed by ultrasound. *Acta Obstet Gynecol Scand* 1983;62:19

24. Sarti DA, Sample WF, Hobel CJ, Staisch KJ. Ultrasonic visualization of a dilated cervix during pregnancy. *Radiology* 1979;130:417

25. Andersen HF, Nugent CE, Wanty SD, Hayashi RH. Prediction of risk for preterm delivery by ultrasonographic measurement of cervical length. *Am J Obstet Gynecol* 1990;163:859

26. Sonek JD, Iams JD, Blumenfeld M, *et al.* Measurement of cervical length in pregnancy: comparison between vaginal ultrasonography and digital examination. *Obstet Gynecol* 1990;76:172

27. Guzman ER, Rosenberg JC, Houlihan JI, *et al.* A new method using vaginal ultrasound and transfundal pressure to evaluate the asymptomatic incompetent cervix. *Obstet Gynecol* 1994;83:248

28. Zlatnik FJ, Burmeister LF, Feddersen PA, Brown RC. Radiologic appearance of the upper cervical canal in women with a history of premature delivery. II. Relationship to clinical presentation and to tests of cervical compliance. *J Reprod Med* 1989;34:525

29. Hricak H, Chang YCF, Cann LE, Parer JT. Cervical incompetence: preliminary evaluation with MR imaging. *Radiology* 1990;174:821

30. Shirodkar UN. A new method of operative treatment for habitual abortion in the second trimester of pregnancy. *Antiseptic* 1955;52:299

31. McDonald IA: Suture of the cervix for inevitable miscarriage. *J Obstet Gynaecol Emp* 1957;63:346

32. Käser O, Iklé FA, Hirsch HA, eds. *Atlas of Gynecological Surgery*. Stuttgart, New York: Georg Thieme Verlag, 1985:13.1

33. Olatunbosun OA, Dyck F. Cervical cerclage operation for a dilated cervix. *Obstet Gynecol* 1981;57:166

34. Holman MR. An aid for cervical cerclage. *Obstet Gynecol* 1973;42:478

35. Schearer LJ, Lam F, Katz M. *A New Technique for Cervical Cerclage in the Presence of Prolapsed Fetal Membranes*. Orlando: Society for Perinatal Obstetricians, 1987

36. Lombardi SJ, Fedrizzi RP, Rosemond RL, Boehm FH. Advanced cervical dilatation: the role of cervical cerclage. *J Matern Fetal Med* 1993;2:48

37. Fieden FJ, Ordonca SA, Hoskins IA, Young BK. The Shirodkar operation: a reappraisal. *Am J Obstet Gynecol* 1990;163:830

38. Whitehead KD, Wise RB, Dunnihoo DR, Otterson WN. Retrospective analysis of cervical cerclage procedures at the Louisiana State University. *South Med J* 1990;83:159

39. Harger JH. Cervical cerclage, patient selection, morbidity and success rate. *Clin Perinatol* 1983;10:321

5
Multiple gestation

H.N. Winn and W.R. Gerber

INCIDENCE

There are two types of twinning: monozygotic twinning (MZ) and dizygotic twinning (DZ). Monozygotic twinning (MZ) occurs when a single egg is fertilized by a single spermatozoon, and the fertilized egg then splits into two genetically identical units. Dizygotic twinning (DZ), or 'fraternal twins', results from the ovulation of two discrete eggs, each of which is fertilized by a different spermatozoon. The ratio of MZ to DZ is about 1 : 2.

Superfecundation refers to a conception of dizygotic twins, each by a different father. This occurs when a woman ovulates two ova in one cycle and has intercourse with two different men, such that each egg is fertilized by a different man. Superfetation refers to the fertilization of two ova, each in a different ovulatory cycle. This would imply that a woman who is pregnant with a singleton then ovulates and conceives again, an unlikely occurrence since pregnancy suppresses ovulation.

The overall incidence of twins at delivery is approximately one in 89 births[1]. The incidence of twinning in the first trimester is much higher, with a rate of 3.29% having been reported[2]. Fetal wastage is much higher in multiple gestations than in singletons. Serial ultrasounds have demonstrated that some pregnancies begin as twins but undergo the silent resorption of one twin, leading to the delivery of an apparent singleton at term. This phenomenon has been referred to as the 'vanishing twin'. The incidences of vanishing of at least one twin of a set range from 21–63%[2–4]. If fetal demise occurs during the second trimester, the dead fetus may be compressed to become a fetus papyraceus which can be observed after delivery.

The rate of MZ twinning is relatively constant, at three to five per 1000 births around the world[5,6]. The incidence of DZ twinning, however, is affected by many factors, such as race, hereditary, maternal age, weight, nutritious status, parity, and *in vitro* fertilization. The DZ twinning rate is increased by a maternal history of twinning, advanced maternal age (peaking at about 30–40 years), maternal obesity, increased parity and *in vitro* fertilization, and is decreased among malnourished mothers[1,7–9]. The rates of MZ and DZ twins in different countries are summarized in Table 1. The pathogenesis of twinning remains unclear, but increased maternal serum levels of follicle stimulating hormone (FSH) have been implicated.

The incidence of higher-order multiple gestations can be estimated by using a mathematical relationship referred to as Hellin's Law[7]. According to this law, if the rate of twins in a given population is x, then the incidence of triplets, quadruplets, and so on, will be x^2, x^3, etc., respectively. This relationship has matched reported incidences until recently, when there have been increased rates of multiple gestations due to fertility drugs and assisted reproductive technology.

Table 1 Incidence of twinning: twinning rates per 1000 births in different countries

	Monozygotic	*Dizygotic*	*Total*
Nigeria	5	49	54
USA			
Black	4.7	11.1	15.8
White	4.2	7.1	11.3
England and Wales	3.5	8.8	12.3
India (Calcutta)	3.3	8.1	11.4
Japan	3.0	1.3	4.3

With permission from reference 1

PLACENTAL CHORIONICITY

There are two major types of placentas in twin gestations, monochorionic and dichorionic, depending on the histological compositions of the dividing membranes. The dividing membranes of dichorionic placentas contain four layers: amnion–chorion–chorion–amnion, while those of monochorionic placentas contain only two layers: amnion–amnion[10–12]. If the dividing membranes are absent, monoamniotic monochorionic twin gestations exist. Dichorionic placentas are found in about 80% of twins and are associated with either MZ or DZ twins. Monochorionic placentation, which may be either monoamniotic or diamniotic, accounts for about 20% of twin gestations and is present only in MZ twins. Dichorionic diamniotic placentas that are fused may appear grossly similar to monochorionic diamniotic placentas, the distinguishing characteristic being the thickness of the partition separating the fetuses.

The special case of monochorionic monoamniotic placentation accounts for about 1% of all twin gestations and carries serious risks from cord entanglement in addition to other complications of monochorionic twins. Therefore, fetal wastage can be as high as 50% or more[13–15]. Furthermore, conjoined twins occur in monochorionic monoamniotic gestations.

Perinatal morbidity and mortality in twin gestations are significantly affected by the status of the placental chorion and amnion. Complications such as preterm labor are increased for monozygotic compared to dizygotic twins and increased for monochorionic compared to dichorionic placentas[9,16]. Since monochorionic placentas almost always have vascular anastomoses between the two fetal circulations, the identification of placental chorion is very useful in the management of twin pregnancies, especially when it is complicated by growth discrepancy, fetal hydrops and demise. While the identification of different fetal genders or two separate placentas indicates dichorionic twinning, differentiation between monochorionic and dichorionic placentas must rely on other parameters when only one placenta and similar fetal genders exist.

Ultrasonography has been extensively used recently for the prenatal diagnosis of placental chorion status. Different proposed sonographic criteria for the dividing membranes include the quality evaluation of the membranous thickness by 'eye-balling', and the number of constituting membranes. Using a membrane thickness of 2 mm as a cut-off point, the accuracy of predicting monochorionic or dichorionic twin gestations is 85% and 92.3%, respectively[17]. Another ultrasonographic sign, the 'twin peak' sign, appears to be reliable evidence of dichorionic placentation. This sign is a triangular projection of placental tissue from the chorionic surface to the area between the two amnions[18].

At the time of delivery, monochorionic or dichorionic membranes can be determined by gross and microscopic examination of the placenta. The information is useful in determining zygosity of the twins.

CHANGES IN MATERNAL PHYSIOLOGY IN MULTIPLE GESTATION

In general, the physiological changes in multiple gestation are exaggerations of the changes in a singleton pregnancy.

Cardiovascular

A 70-kg non-pregnant woman has a circulating blood volume of about 5 l. This increases by 40% and 45%, to approximately 7 l and 7.5 l in singleton and twin pregnancies, respectively. Plasma volume is about 4 l in a singleton pregnancy and 4.7 l in a twin gestation.

Red-cell mass is approximately 1.8 l in a singleton and about 2.3 l in a twin gestation in the third trimester[19]. Compared to the non-pregnant condition, the cardiac output, cardiac index and left ventricular work index increase during pregnancy, starting at about 21 weeks of gestation. The increments in these measurements are higher in twin pregnancies than in singleton pregnancies. In a singleton pregnancy, the mean increment of cardiac index peaks at a value of 44.2% above that of the non-pregnant condition at 25–28 weeks of gestation, then decreases significantly towards the non-pregnant value. In twin pregnancies, the mean increment of cardiac index peaks at a value of 48% higher than that of the non-pregnant condition and persists from 21 weeks of gestation to 32 weeks of gestation, then decreases progressively to about 15.6% above the non-gravid level at term. The changes in left ventricular work parallel those of cardiac index. The cardiac changes are summarized in Table 2[20].

Pulmonary

In general, the pulmonary changes in pregnancy involve decreases in lung volumes (lung capacity, functional reserve capacity, expiratory reserve volume, and residual volume) and increases in ventilation, tidal volume, respiratory rate and oxygen consumption. These changes are somewhat exaggerated with higher gestational numbers[19].

Other systems

Increased relaxation of smooth muscle from increased production of progesterone results in increased incidences of cholestasis, constipation and hydro-ureter[19]. Compared to a singleton pregnancy, a twin gestation:

(1) Is at a higher risk for urinary obstruction and urinary infection due to urinary stasis from mechanical compression of the ureter by the larger uterus;

(2) Has an average weight gain of approximately 1.5 times higher;

(3) Produces a maternal perception of increased fetal movement and more awkwardness, the latter due to a greater change in the center of gravity.

Uterine size of a twin gestation from a pelvic examination is about the same as that of a singleton pregnancy until 13 weeks of gestation when the twin-containing uterus begins to grow at an accelerated rate.

COMPLICATIONS IN MULTIPLE GESTATION

The physiological changes in multiple gestation predispose the mother and her fetuses to many maternal and fetal complications. Maternal complications

Table 2 Mean cardiac output and cardiac index during pregnancy

Category (weeks)	Cardiac output (l/min)	Cardiac index (l/min/m²)	Left ventricular work index (kg m/min/m²)
Controls	5.87	3.46	4.25
Single pregnancies			
21–24	8.10	4.80	6.14
25–28	8.56	4.99	6.39
29–32	7.71	4.65	5.77
33–36	6.52	4.10	4.99
37–40	5.94	3.54	4.47
Twin pregnancies			
21–24	9.01	5.02	6.29
25–28	8.52	5.14	6.49
29–32	7.97	4.99	6.49
33–36	7.83	4.50	5.74
37–40	6.93	4.00	5.51

Modified with permission from reference 20

include preterm labor, premature rupture of membranes, pregnancy-induced hypertension, postpartum hemorrhage, anemia, urinary tract infections and fluid overload, the latter being more common in such situations as maternal severe cardiac diseases and parenteral tocolysis[21,22]. According to a population-based study, the risk of pre-eclampsia is four-fold higher in twins than in singleton pregnancies and 14 times higher in a nulliparous twin pregnancy than in a parous singleton pregnancy[23]. Fetal complications include prematurity, congenital anomalies, twin–twin transfusion, cord accidents, fetal growth retardation and intrauterine fetal demise[22]. The average perinatal mortality of twin gestations has decreased from approximately 100 per 1000 to a range of 20–132 per 1000 in the past decade[24,25]. These rates are two to five times those for singleton pregnancies. Deaths are due mainly to prematurity, followed by congenital abnormalities, fetal growth restriction, and twin–twin transfusion[24,25].

The increased risk of postpartum hemorrhage from uterine atony as a result of uterine overdistension requires careful observation of the patient in the first few postpartum hours. Increasing uterine tone by uterine massage, intravenous oxytocin, intramuscular Methergine and intramyometrial prostaglandin $F_{2\alpha}$ may be effective in controlling the bleeding. Surgical intervention may be necessary in selected situations.

Congenital anomalies

In general, the incidence of congenital anomalies is higher among twins than singletons and increased in MZ twins compared to DZ twins. Twin pregnancies have unique anomalies such as acardia and conjoined twins in addition to those seen among singletons. Single umbilical artery and neural tube defects appear to be more frequent in twin gestations than in singletons. The excess of neural tube defects was attributed mainly to anencephalus and encephalocele[26–29]. Interestingly, there is a very high discordance rate for development and genetic abnormalities in dizygotic twins. Understandably, MZ twins have an almost 100% concordance rate for genetic anomalies. This information may be helpful to the patients who contemplate undergoing the various modalities of prenatal diagnosis.

The maternal serum α-fetoprotein is normally elevated in twin pregnancies compared to singletons. A maternal serum α-fetoprotein > 2.5 multiples of the median (MOM) is seen in 20–40% of twin gestations. A maternal serum α-fetoprotein level of greater than 4 MOM in twin gestations is associated with fetal anomalies, perinatal deaths and premature deliveries[30,31]. The nomograms for amniotic fluid α-fetoprotein in twins are comparable to those of singletons. The reliability of the amniotic fluid α-fetoprotein in predicting fetal anomalies in one twin if the other twin has a fetal anomaly depends on the placental chorionicity. The amniotic fluid α-fetoprotein may be falsely elevated in the normal twin if the other twin has anomalies in the case of monochorionic placentation[32].

Acardia

This is a very rare anomaly which occurs exclusively in multiple gestations with monochorionic placentation. Its incidence is about one in 30 000 to one in 35 000 births[33]. The pathogenesis of acardia remains to be determined. The possibilities of primary cardiac maldevelopment or twin-reversed arterial perfusion have been proposed; the latter occurs in the setting of arterial–arterial or venous–venous anastomosis[34]. The acardiac twin has an umbilical cord containing one artery and one vein and usually does not have a heart or brain[34]. The normal twin coexisting with the acardiac twin is at an increased risk of intrauterine fetal demise and preterm delivery. Cesarean section delivery of an acardiac twin may be necessary if dystocia occurs.

Conjoined twins

Conjoined twins are also very rare, with incidences ranging from one in 25 000 to one in 80 000 births[35]. Conjoined twins arise if the division of the MZ twins occurs within the interval of 13–16 post-ovulatory days[14,36]. Conjoined twins can be diagnosed by ultrasonography as early as 12 weeks of gestation[37]. Different types of conjoined twins are classified according to the most prominent sites of conjunction. The prognosis is generally poor and depends on the classification and the shared organs. About 25% of conjoined twins survive the first 24 h of life and 40% may be stillborn[38]. Cesarean section delivery is necessary if the prognosis is not lethal. Even though postnatal surgical separations are possible, these neonates still suffer significant mortality and morbidity.

Preterm labor and delivery

Preterm labor complicates 20–50% of twin pregnancies, and preterm delivery is the single largest contributor to fetal wastage[39,40]. The average lengths of normal twin, triplet and quadruplet gestations are 35 weeks, 33 weeks and 29 weeks, respectively[41]. A variety of prophylactic measures, such as bedrest and cervical cerclage, have been tried without significant impact. A combination of bedrest at home and oral β-mimetics appears to be a promising prophylaxis[42]. Coital activity is permitted unless preterm labor has occurred, since it does not appear to initiate preterm labor in twin gestations[43]. In general, there is a synchronous fetal lung maturation with a high degree of correlation of lecithin/sphingomyelin (L/S) ratios in a twin pair. Furthermore, when the L/S ratios of a twin pair are discordant, a mature L/S ratio in one twin is likely to predict fetal lung maturity in both twins, even though the other twin may have an immature L/S ratio[44]. However, a twin pregnancy *per se* does not accelerate fetal lung maturity[45].

Fetal growth restriction

Intrauterine growth restriction, defined as growth below the 10th centile for a given gestational age, occurs in at least 25% of twin gestations[46]. Ultrasonography plays an important role in the assessment of fetal growth in twin gestations. The frequency of serial ultrasound examinations ranges from 2–8 weeks, depending on the gestational age, twin chorionicity, severity of existing twin discordance and signs of fetal hydrops. Since the estimated fetal weight can have an error of more than 10% of the birth weight, the discordance of estimated fetal weights should be more than 20% to be clinically significant. The difference in estimated fetal weights could be due to:

(1) Different genders, with male fetuses being larger than female ones;

(2) One twin having normal growth while the other one has abnormal growth;

(3) Twin transfusion syndrome.

To assess fetal growth in twin gestations, nomograms for twin estimated fetal weight should be used instead of those of singletons, because twins normally tend to be smaller than singletons at a given gestational age during the last trimester. The growth of the biparietal diameter does not seem to be affected by twinning[47]. Table 3 provides the nomograms for fetal growth by estimated fetal weight in twins.

Correctable conditions such as diet, smoking, drug use and anemia should be addressed. Plenty of bedrest in the lateral position may facilitate growth of both fetuses.

Table 3 Nomogram of estimated fetal weight in twin gestations. From reference 47

Gestational age (weeks)	Centile				
	5th	25th	50th	75th	95th
16	132	141	154	189	207
17	173	194	215	239	249
18	214	248	276	289	291
19	223	253	300	333	412
20	232	259	324	378	534
21	275	355	432	482	705
22	319	452	540	586	876
23	347	497	598	684	880
24	376	543	656	783	885
25	549	677	793	916	1118
26	722	812	931	1049	1352
27	755	978	1087	1193	1563
28	789	1145	1244	1337	1774
29	900	1266	1395	1509	1883
30	1011	1387	1546	1682	1992
31	1198	1532	1693	1875	2392
32	1385	1677	1840	2068	2793
33	1491	1771	2032	2334	3000
34	1597	1866	2224	2601	3208
35	1703	2093	2427	2716	3336
36	1809	2321	2631	2832	3465
37	2239	2540	2824	3035	3679
38	2669	2760	3017	3239	3894

Twin–twin transfusion

Twin–twin transfusion syndrome represents a severe form of discordant growth occurring almost exclusively in monochorionic placentas where there is a vascular anastomosis (usually arteriovenous) between the placental vessels of the two fetuses[48]. It affects 4% of all twin pregnancies. The differential flow leads to anemia in one twin and polycythemia in the other. Polyhydramnios and oligohydramnios often occur in the amniotic sacs of the larger twin and smaller twin, respectively. Perinatal mortality can be as high as 66%. The diagnosis should be strongly considered when ultrasound examinations reveal differential fetal growth and signs of fetal hydrops[49,50]. Rarely, the twin–twin transfusion occurs in dichorionic placentas without the development of oligohydramnios or polyhydramnios[51]. The diagnosis of twin–twin transfusion is supported by a difference in hemoglobin of more than 1.8 g/dl, with the larger twin having the higher hemoglobin concentration[52]. Fetal hemoglobin can be determined by funicentesis. Doppler umbilical artery blood flow is not better than estimated fetal weight alone in detecting twin–twin transfusion syndrome[53]. Management depends on the severity, gestational age, fetal well-being and fetal lung maturity. After delivery, the diagnosis can be confirmed by injecting milk into the vessels of one placenta and observing the extension of milk into the vessels of the other placenta[54].

Intrauterine demise of one twin

Preterm intrauterine fetal demise of one twin presents an obstetric dilemma between a high neonatal mortality and morbidity from premature delivery of the surviving twin versus potential maternal disseminated intravascular coagulation (DIC) from prolongation of the pregnancy. If expectant management is attempted, close surveillance of maternal homeostasis and fetal well-being is essential. Baseline coagulation profile, which includes platelet count, prothrombin time, activated partial thromboplastin time and fibrinogen split products, is obtained initially, then platelet count and fibrinogen split products are measured weekly. Elevated fibrinogen split products and thrombocytopenia appear to be the most sensitive markers of coagulopathy associated with intrauterine fetal demise. Reversal of consumptive coagulopathy has been demonstrated with the administration of heparin[55,56]. This treatment modality provides an alternative to the transfusion of blood products in the treatment of DIC resulting from intrauterine fetal demise. Caution should be exercised when heparinization is attempted in this clinical setting. Fortunately, maternal coagulopathy in this setting is quite uncommon[57].

The surviving twin, especially of monochorionic twinning, is at risk of having DIC, and also thromboembolism, presumably because the thromboplastic materials from the dead twin can reach the surviving one through the shared circulation. Ultrasonography can be very useful in evaluating fetal growth, well-being and structural abnormalities.

Antepartum management

The diagnosis of twinning should be made as soon as possible, preferably during the first trimester to determine the expected date of delivery. An ultrasound examination provides the best method of diagnosing twin gestations and is recommended in pregnancies with risks for twins or higher-order multiple gestations, such as advanced maternal age, maternal history of twinning, elevated maternal serum α-fetoprotein, larger-than-expected fundal height and assisted reproductive technology. Once the diagnosis is established, the patient should be advised about the need for increased nutritional and vitamin requirements, the adverse effects of illicit drugs on fetal growth, and signs and symptoms of preterm labor or premature rupture of membranes. The patient should be closely observed for the development of anemia, urinary tract infection, preterm labor, pre-eclampsia and fetal growth discordance. Folic acid 1 mg daily and iron sulfate 320 mg two or three times daily, in addition to regular multiple vitamins, may be necessary to prevent anemia.

Titrated activity level and scheduled resting in the lateral decubitus position for 2 h a day, in addition to 8–10 h of sleep at night, may be beneficial in optimizing fetal growth and forestalling preterm labor[58]. Prompt detection and treatment of preterm labor is important to prevent preterm delivery.

Indications and dosages for the administration of betamethasone to induce fetal lung maturity are similar to those for singleton pregnancies when there is a significant risk of preterm delivery such as preterm labor, severe pre-eclampsia or severe discordant growth.

Close monitoring of fetal well-being is recommended when the fetal condition may be compromised in such situations as growth discordance, intrauterine fetal demise of one twin, twin–twin transfusion syndrome, severe pre-eclampsia and fetal anomalies. Nonstress tests, biophysical profiles and Doppler blood flow studies of selected fetal vasculature are available modalities for this purpose.

Intrapartum management

Labor

The labor and delivery of twins should be managed in a hospital where the following supporting services are readily available:

(1) Screen or typing of maternal blood because of the increased risk of peripartum hemorrhage;

(2) Availability of anesthesia and pediatric personnel;

(3) Capability of monitoring of the fetal heart rates of the two fetuses;

(4) Availability of an assistant to assist during the delivery;

(5) Availability of an ultrasound machine to determine the presentation of the second twin after delivery of the first;

(6) Capability of emergency Cesarean section;

(7) Availability of oxytocin, Methergine, prostaglandin E_2 suppositories and prostaglandin $F_{2\alpha}$ injection for controlling postpartum hemorrhage.

Since the twin gestation patient is at risk for uterine rupture from an overdistended uterus, intrauterine pressure should be closely monitored, preferably with an intrauterine pressure catheter, during induction or augmentation of labor.

Mode of delivery

The mode of delivery for twin gestations depends on the presentations of the twins. During the intrapartum period, the possible presentations of twin A (presenting twin)/twin B are vertex/vertex, vertex/non-vertex and non-vertex/vertex and occur in about 42%, 38% and 20% of twin gestations, respectively[59]. It is generally agreed that the vaginal route and Cesarean section are appropriate in the cases of vertex/vertex and non-vertex/vertex presentations, respectively.

The mode of delivery for a vertex/non-vertex presentation remains controversial. Acceptable alternatives include:

(1) Elective Cesarean section of both twins;

(2) Vaginal delivery of twin A followed by vaginal breech extraction of twin B;

(3) Vaginal delivery of twin A, external cephalic version of twin B, followed by vaginal delivery of twin B.

In selected situations, a safe vaginal delivery of both twins could be accomplished.

After delivery of twin A, an ultrasound examination of twin B is carried out to determine its presentation. If the second twin presents as vertex, amniotomy can be performed to allow engagement of the fetal head into the maternal pelvis and application of a direct fetal heart-rate monitor. If the second twin presents as transverse or breech, external cephalic version under ultrasound guidance may be attempted. A success rate of 73% for intrapartum external cephalic version has been reported[60]. Relaxation of the abdominal wall muscles with epidural anesthesia appears to facilitate the external cephalic version. Retrospective studies revealed that vaginal breech delivery of the second twin with birth weight below 1500 g was associated with increased neonatal death or intraventricular hemorrhage[60,61]. Since there is an error of about 10% in estimating fetal weight by ultrasonography, Cesarean section delivery of a non-vertex twin B with an estimated fetal weight of less than 1800 g is acceptable if external cephalic version is unsuccessful. In infants with birth weights above 1500 g, there was no statistically significant difference between vaginal vertex delivery and vaginal breech delivery of the second twin when comparing 5-min Apgar scores, lengths of neonatal hospital stay, neonatal intensive care unit admissions, neonatal deaths or intraventricular hemorrhages[61,62]. A randomized study of 60 twin pregnancies at 35–41 weeks of gestation demonstrated no significance difference in the incidences of 1-min Apgar scores, 5-min Apgar scores, neonatal hypoglycemia, secondary apnea and hyperbilirubinemia between vaginal delivery and Cesarean section of the second twin[63]. Until data from a prospective, randomized study of the optimal modes of delivery of non-vertex second twins are available, vaginal breech extraction by an experienced operator of the second twin, preferably having an estimated fetal weight of more than 1800 g but less than that of the first twin, is an acceptable alternative.

Monochorionic monoamniotic twins

Monoamniotic monochorionic twins have a high perinatal mortality from cord entanglement in addition to other complications of monochorionic twins.

Intense monitoring of fetal growth and well-being is recommended and may necessitate hospitalization as early as 28–30 weeks of gestation. Amniocentesis could be performed starting at 32–34 weeks of gestation and Cesarean section delivery is carried out when fetal lung maturity is documented. This approach is supported by the findings that the survival rates of mono-amniotic twins do not decrease by prolonging the pregnancy beyond 30–32 weeks of gestation[14,15] and that good perinatal outcomes are obtained when delivery is delayed until 33–34 weeks after fetal lung maturity is documented[13].

Locked twins

Twin locking denotes the condition where the inferior aspect of each twin's chin is opposed to each other in a vertical axis. This occurs during vaginal delivery when the co-twins lie vertically with the first twin presenting as a breech and the second twin presenting as vertex. The incidence of twin locking is approximately one in 800 twin gestations or about one in 90 of twin gestations presenting as breech/vertex, based on data from the Obstetrical Statistical Co-operative conducted between 1950 and 1960[64]. It rarely happens in current obstetric practice, since the presentation of both twins can be readily determined by ultrasound examinations and Cesarean section is routinely performed if the presenting twin is in a breech position. The interlocking may occur, first, above the pelvic inlet, resulting in failure of descent of the presenting twin, or, second, at or below the inlet if the presenting twin has been partially delivered. In either case, an acute emergency arises due to mechanical difficulty in accomplishing vaginal delivery. The perinatal mortality of the interlocking twins is about 50%, with the presenting twin accounting for 80% of the perinatal deaths. Decapitation and asphyxia are the major causes of perinatal mortality[64]. If a patient presents with interlocking twins in advanced labor, prompt Cesarean section delivery is recommended to reduce perinatal mortality and morbidity.

MULTIPLE GESTATIONS GREATER THAN TWINS

Pregnancies with a greater number of fetuses than twins are generally rare. For example, triplets occur at a rate of one in 8000 deliveries in the USA. However, the incidence has recently increased, owing to ovulation induction. Complications of higher-numbered fetal gestations are simply an exaggeration of those for twin gestations. The risk of prematurity increases with a higher number of fetuses. Most obstetricians would deliver triplets and higher-numbered fetal pregnancies by elective Cesarean section. It is unclear whether the reduction of triplets to twins would improve perinatal outcomes such as premature deliveries and intrauterine growth restriction[65,66]. The incidence of fetal growth retardation remains higher in reduced multiple gestations than in non-reduced twins and restriction increases with the number of fetuses before reduction[67]. Ethical consideration plays an important role in the patient's decision of selective reduction of a higher-order multiple gestation to twin gestation.

REFERENCES

1. MacGillivray I. Epidemiology of twin pregnancy. *Semin Perinatol* 1986;10:4–8

2. Landy HJ, Weiner S, Corson SL, *et al*. The 'vanishing twin': ultrasonographic assessment of fetal disappearance in the first trimester. *Am J Obstet Gynecol* 1986; 155:14–19

3. Varma TR. Ultrasound evidence of early pregnancy failure in patients with multiple conceptions. *Br J Obstet Gynaecol* 1979;86:290–2

4. Parisi P, Gatti M, Prinzi G. Familial incidence of twinning. *Nature (London)* 1983;304:626–8

5. Marivate M, Norman RJ. Twins. *Clin Obstet Gynaecol* 1982;9:723–43

6. Bulmer, MG. The familial incidence of twinning. *Ann Hum Genet* 1960;24:1–3

7. Benirschke K, Kim CK. Multiple pregnancy. *N Engl J Med* 1973;288:1276–84

8. Nylander PPS. Biosocial aspects of multiple births. *J Biosoc Sci* 1971;3(Suppl):29–38

9. Kovacs B, Shabahrami B, Platt LD. Molecular genetic prenatal determination of twin zygosity. *Obstet Gynecol* 1988;72:954–6

10. Hertzberg BS, Kurtz AB, Choi HY, *et al*. Significance of membrane thickness in the sonographic evaluation of twin gestations. *Am J Radiol* 1987;148:151–3

11. Barss VA, Benacerraf BR, Frigoletto FD. Ultrasonographic determination of chorion type in twin gestation. *Obstet Gynecol* 1985;66:779–83

12. Mahony RS, Filly RA, Callen PW. Amnionicity and chorionicity in twin pregnancies: prediction using ultrasound. *Radiology* 1985;155:205–9

13. Rodis JF, Vintzileos AM, Campbell WA, *et al*. Antenatal diagnosis and management of monoamniotic twins. *Am J Obstet Gynecol* 1987;157:1255–7

14. Tessen JA, Zlatnik FJ. Monoamniotic twins: a retrospective controlled study. *Obstet Gynecol* 1991;77:832–4

15. Carr SR, Aronson MP, Coustan DR. Survival rates of monoamniotic twins do not decrease after 30 weeks' gestation. *Am J Obstet Gynecol* 1990;163:719–22

16. Pridjian G, Nugent CE, Barr M. Twin gestation: influence of placentation on fetal growth. *Am J Obstet Gynecol* 1991;165:1394–401

17. Winn HN, Gabrielli S, Reece EA, *et al*. Ultrasonographic criteria for the prenatal diagnosis of placental chorionicity in twin gestations. *Am J Obstet Gynecol* 1989;161:1540–2

18. Finberg HJ. The 'twin peak' sign: reliable evidence of dichorionic twinning. *J Ultrasound Med* 1992;11: 571–7

19. Parsons M. Effects of twins: maternal, fetal, and labor. *Clin Perinatol* 1988;15:41–53

20. Rovinsky JJ, Jaffin H. Cardiac output and left ventricular work in multiple pregnancy. *Am J Obstet Gynecol* 1966;95:781–6

21. Spellacy WN, Handler A, Ferre CD. A case–control study of 1253 twin pregnancies from a 1982–1987 perinatal data base. *Obstet Gynecol* 1990;75:168–71

22. Naeye RL, Tafari N, Judge D, *et al*. Twins: causes of perinatal death in 12 United States cities and one African city. *Am J Obstet Gynecol* 1978;131:267–72

23. Coonrod DV, Hickok DE, Zhu K, *et al*. Risk factors for preeclampsia in twin pregnancies: a population-based cohort study. *Obstet Gynecol* 1995;85:645–50

24. Farooqui MO, Grossman JR, Shannon RA. A review of twin pregnancy and perinatal mortality. *Obstet Gynecol Surv* 1973;28(Suppl):144–53

25. Hawrylyshyn PA, Barkin M, Berstein A, *et al*. Twin pregnancies – a continuing perinatal challenge. *Obstet Gynecol* 1982;59:463–6

26. Layde PM, Erickson JD, Falek A, *et al*. Congenital malformations in twins. *Am J Hum Genet* 1980;32:69–78

27. Windham GC, Sever LE. Neural tube defects among twin births. *Am J Hum Genet* 1982;34:988–98

28. Windham GC, Bjepkedal T, Sever LE. The association of twinning and birth defects: studies in Los Angeles, California and Norway. *Acta Genet Med* 1982; 31:165–72

29. Heijetz SA. Single umbilical artery, a statistical analysis of 237 autopsy cases and review of the literature. *Perspect Pediatr Pathol* 1984;8:345–78

30. Redford DHA, Whitfield CR. Maternal serum alpha fetoprotein in twin pregnancies uncomplicated by neural tube defect. *Am J Obstet Gynecol* 1985; 152:550–3

31. Johnson JM, Harman CR, Evans JA, *et al*. Maternal serum alpha fetoprotein in twin pregnancy. *Am J Obstet Gynecol* 1990;162:1020–5

32. Stiller RJ, Lockwood CJ, Belanger K, *et al*. Amniotic fluid α-fetoprotein concentration in twin gestations: dependence on placental membrane anatomy. *Am J Obstet Gynecol* 1988;158:1088–92

33. Napolitani FD, Schreiber I. The acardiac monster: a review of the world literature and presentation of two cases. *Am J Obstet Gynecol* 1960;80:582–89

34. Benirschke K, Harper VDR. The acardiac anomaly. *Teratology* 1977;15:311–16

35. Freedman HL, Tafeen CH, Harris H. Conjoined thoracopagus twins. *Am J Obstet Gynecol* 1962;84: 1904–7, discussion 1908–9

36. Benirschke K, Temple WW, Bloor C. Conjoined twins: nosology and congenital malformations. *Birth Defects* 1978;14:179–92

37. Schmidt W, Heberling D, Kubli F. Antepartum ultrasonographic diagnosis of conjoined twins in early pregnancy. *Am J Obstet Gynecol* 1985;139:961–3

38. Edmonds LD, Layde PM. Conjoined twins in the United States, 1970–1977. *Teratology* 1982;25:301–8

39. Medearis AL, Jonas HS, Stockbauer JW, *et al*. Perinatal death in twin pregnancies. A five-year analysis of statewide statistics in Missouri. *Am J Obstet Gynecol* 1979;134:413–21

40. Watson P, Campbell DM. Preterm deliveries in twin pregnancies in Oxford. *Acta Genet Med Gemellol (Roma)* 1986;35:193–9

41. Caspi E, Ronen J, Schreyer P, Goldberg MD. The outcome of pregnancy after gonadotrophin therapy. *Br J Obstet Gynaecol* 1976;83:967–73

42. O'Leary TA. Prophylactic tocolysis of twins. *Am J Obstet Gynecol* 1986;154:904–5

43. Neilson JP, Mutambira M. Coitus: twin pregnancy, and preterm labor. *Am J Obstet Gynecol* 1989;160:416–18

44. Leveno KJ, Quirk JG, Whalley PJ, *et al*. Fetal lung maturation in twin gestation. *Am J Obstet Gynecol* 1984; 148:405–11

45. Winn HN, Romero R, Roberts A, *et al*. Comparison of fetal lung maturation in preterm singleton and twin pregnancies. *Am J Perinatol* 1992;9:326–8

46. Houlton M, Marivate M, Philpott R. The prediction of fetal growth retardation in twin pregnancy. *Br J Obstet Gynaecol* 1981;88:264–73

47. Yarkoni S, Reece EA, Holford T, *et al*. Estimated fetal weight in the evaluation of growth in twin gestations: a prospective longitudinal study. *Obstet Gynecol* 1987; 69:636–9

48. Tan KL, Tan R, Tan SH, Tan AM. The twin transfusion syndrome. Clinical observations on 35 affected pairs. *Clin Pediatr* 1979;18:111–14

49. Danskin FH, Neilson JP. Twin-to-twin transfusion syndrome: what are appropriate diagnostic criteria? *Am J Obstet Gynecol* 1989;161:365–9

50. Brown DL, Benson CB, Driscoll SG, *et al*. Twin–twin transfusion syndrome: sonographic findings. *Radiology* 1989;170:161–3

51. King AD, Soothill PW, Montemagno R, *et al*. Twin-to-twin blood transfusion in a dichorionic pregnancy without the oligohydramnios–polyhydramnios sequence. *Br J Obstet Gynaecol* 1995;102:334–5

52. Okamura K, Murotsuki J, Koauge S, *et al*. Diagnostic use of cordocentesis in twin pregnancy. *Fetal Diagn Ther* 1994;9:385–90

53. Divon M, Girz B, Sklar A, *et al*. Discordant twins – a prospective study of the diagnostic value of real-time ultrasonography combined with umbilical artery velocimetry. *Am J Obstet Gynecol* 1989;161:757–60

54. Bebbington MW, Wittmann BK. Fetal transfusion syndrome: antenatal factors predicting outcome. *Am J Obstet Gynecol* 1989;160:913–15

55. Phillips LL, Sciara JJ. Hypofibrinogenemia with a dead fetus treated with intravenous heparin. *Am J Obstet Gynecol* 1965;92:1161–2

56. Romero R, Duffy TP, Berkowitz RL, *et al*. Prolongation of a preterm pregnancy complicated by death of a single twin *in utero* and disseminated intravascular coagulation: effects of treatment with heparin. *N Engl J Med* 1984;310:772–4

57. Santema JG, Swaak AM, Wallenburg HC. Expectant management of twin pregnancy with single fetal death. *Br J Obstet Gynaecol* 1995;102:26–30

58. Komaromy B, Lampe L. The value of bedrest in twin pregnancies. *Int J Obstet Gynaecol* 1977;15:262–6

59. Chervenak FA, Johnson RE, Youcha S, *et al*. Intrapartum management of twin gestation. *Obstet Gynecol* 1985;65:119–24

60. Chervenak F, Johnson RE, Berkowitz RL, *et al*. Is routine Cesarean section necessary for vertex-breech and vertex-transverse twin gestations? *Am J Obstet Gynecol* 1984;148:1–5

61. Adam C, Allen AC, Baskett TF. Twin delivery: influence of the presentation and method of delivery on the second twin. *Am J Obstet Gynecol* 1991;165:23–7

62. Ellings JM, Newman RB, Hulsey TC, *et al*. Vaginal delivery of the nonvertex second twin. *Am J Obstet Gynecol* 1993;168:861–4

63. Rabinovici J, Barkai G, Reichman B, *et al*. Randomized management of the second nonvertex twin: vaginal delivery or Cesarean section. *Am J Obstet Gynecol* 1987; 156:52–6

64. Cohen M, Kohl SG, Rosenthal AH. Fetal interlocking complicating twin gestation. *Am J Obstet Gynecol* 1965; 91:407–12

65. Lipitz S, Uval J, Achiron R, *et al*. Outcome of twin pregnancies reduced from triplets compared with nonreduced twin gestations. *Obstet Gynecol* 1996;87:511–14

66. Smith-Levitin M, Kowalik A, Birnholz J, *et al*. Selective reduction of multifetal pregnancies to twins improves outcome over nonreduced triplet gestations. *Am J Obstet Gynecol* 1996;175:878–82

67. Depp R, Macones GA, Rosenn MF. Multifetal pregnancy reduction: evaluation of fetal growth in the remaining twins. *Am J Obstet Gynecol* 1996;174:1233–8

6

Abruptio placentae and placenta previa

C.C. Egley

Hemorrhage may be a serious threat to the life of the pregnant woman and her fetus. Although maternal coagulopathy or neoplasm may occasionally be the cause, the most frequent and hazardous etiologies are abruptio placentae, placenta previa and (less commonly) vasa previa.

ABRUPTIO PLACENTAE

Definition and pathological mechanism

The overall incidence of abruptio placentae ranges from 0.4 to 0.9% with a recurrent risk after a previous abruptio placentae of 10–15%[1]. Abruptio placentae occurs when the normally implanted placenta separates before delivery of the fetus. The initial event in abruptio placentae is probably vasospasm leading to necrosis of the decidua basalis. Release of the vasospasm then causes arteriolar rupture and further decidual necrosis[2,3]. Since the fetus and amniotic fluid continue to distend the uterus at this time, the myometrium cannot sufficiently contract to effect hemostasis. Further bleeding will then result in decidual hematoma formation. The blood escaping into the decidua will then seek any of four tracts. It may (1) infiltrate the myometrium, causing uterine contractions and causing the uterus to adopt a blue color ('Couvelaire uterus'); (2) burrow under the membranes (a large volume of blood can be concealed here, but continued burrowing will eventually lead to vaginal bleeding); (3) seep through the membranes (causing the bloody amniotic fluid often seen in cases of abruptio placentae); and (4) continue to dissect the decidua basalis until the placenta becomes completely separated from the uterus. The infiltration of blood into the myometrium leads to tetanic contractions that may lead to fetal hypoxia and acidosis. The increase in amniotic fluid pressure from the tetanic contractions may further compromise fetal oxygenation.

The decidua basalis is very rich in thromboplastin. At the time of placental separation, this thromboplastin may be released into the maternal circulation, causing disseminated intravascular coagulation[4].

Etiology

The etiology of most cases of abruptio placentae is obscure and may relate to poor initial placentation much earlier in pregnancy. We have found, for example, that in one-third of cases of abruptio the maternal serum α-fetoprotein (AFP) level had been inexplicably elevated earlier in pregnancy. It may be that poor placentation allows for leakage of AFP across the placenta and later leads to abruptio[5].

Cigarette smoking appears to be an important etiological factor in abruptio placentae. Smoking has a vasoconstrictive effect on the uteroplacental circulation. Decidual necrosis at the margin of the placenta is common among cigarette smokers[6]. Women who smoke have a six-fold increase in the incidence of abruptio placentae compared to women who do not, and this effect of smoking is independent of maternal age[2,7]. Women who stop smoking early in pregnancy have a lower incidence of abruptio placentae than those who continue to smoke[6].

There is a strong association between cocaine use during pregnancy and abruptio placenta, with as many as 14% of cocaine users suffering this complication. Cocaine is known to decrease uterine blood flow[8].

Sudden uterine decompression at the time of rupture of the membranes in cases of hydramnios may lead to abruptio placentae[9,10]. Abruptio may occur secondary to external trauma such as automobile accidents, with or without the use of lap seat belts[11]. External cephalic versions have been reported occasionally to be etiological[10].

It is known both from experimental animal studies and from human studies (compression of the inferior vena cava just before opening the uterus at Cesarean delivery) that inferior vena caval compression can cause abruptio placentae[12]. Its clinical significance is unclear. Patients have successfully completed pregnancy after surgical inferior vena caval ligation for pulmonary emboli[9]. Also, angiographic studies in humans have shown that the inferior vena cava is often completely occluded when women are in the supine position during late pregnancy[13].

Evidence regarding the relationship between maternal age and abruptio placentae is conflicting, but there is a clearer relationship between high parity and abruptio, especially if parity is more than four[9,10,14,15]. Patients with chronic hypertension or prolonged rupture of membranes have an approximately three-fold increased risk of abruptio placentae compared to patients without either complication[1].

Most recent studies have not confirmed a relationship between folate deficiency and the development of abruptio placentae[6,9]. Furthermore, attempts to prevent abruptio by folate supplementation have not been successful[15].

Signs and symptoms

The onset of abruptio placentae is usually abrupt and without warning, although about 10% of patients will have had at least some vaginal bleeding over the previous 2 months. The onset can occur at any point during the second half of pregnancy, with a peak at 36 to 37 weeks' gestation. The classic onset is that of sudden vaginal bleeding, tetanic uterine contractions, abdominal pain, uterine tenderness and maternal shock that is out of proportion to the amount of visible maternal blood loss.

Some degree of vaginal bleeding is present in nearly all cases[16], but since there may be a large volume of blood concealed behind the fetal membranes, there is a poor relationship between the amount of *visible* bleeding and the total amount of maternal blood loss, the degree of placental separation and the degree of hypofibrinogenemia. In fact, there may be minimal visible bleeding even though maternal shock and disseminated intravascular coagulation are present, the fetus is dead and complete abruptio is present.

Abdominal pain is present in about one-third of cases. The pain is probably caused by myometrial intravasation of blood. The pain usually has an acute onset and is constant. When posterior placentation is present, the abruptio may be 'silent' even though severe, and the only complaint may be that of persistent lower back pain.

On physical examination, the uterus is nearly always tender. Although uterine hypertonia may only be present in 17% of cases, the uterus is usually irritable in that contractions can be elicited by uterine palpation[16].

In severe cases, maternal shock and disseminated intravascular coagulation may be present. Intense vasospasm often ensues, so that the mother may be normotensive or hypertensive in spite of marked blood loss and shock.

Diagnosis

When a patient presents during the second half of pregnancy with vaginal bleeding, uterine tenderness and uterine hypertonia, the diagnosis is straightforward. If she presents with only bleeding, than the diagnosis is difficult. Maternal shock out of proportion to the amount of vaginal bleeding points towards abruptio placentae, as does laboratory evidence of a maternal coagulopathy.

It is now standard to perform ultrasonography on all patients who present with bleeding during the second half of pregnancy. If ultrasound reveals no placenta previa, the physician should be highly suspicious of abruptio placentae, even in the absence of maternal pain or uterine tenderness. Although the diagnosis of abruptio placentae is still a clinical diagnosis, occasional cases can be diagnosed with ultrasound. A retroplacental hematoma may be seen as an anechoic collection between the uterine wall and the placenta. Its echogenicity will then increase as the hematoma becomes organized. Ultrasound, however, is neither a sensitive nor a specific tool for making the diagnosis of abruptio placentae[5].

Finally, we have occasionally confirmed the diagnosis of abruptio placentae by finding bloody amniotic fluid at the time of amniocentesis.

Complications

The major maternal complications of abruptio placentae include disseminated intravascular coagulation, renal failure, acute hypertension and postpartum hemorrhage. Hypofibrinogenemia with fibrinogen levels less than 100 mg/dl occurs in 4–10% of all abruptio cases[17,18], but occurs in 30% of cases severe enough to kill the fetus[4]. After hypofibrinogenemia develops, thrombocytopenia often follows, while levels of factors VII and VIII (normally elevated in pregnancy) fall into the low normal range[4].

When disseminated intravascular coagulation accompanies abruptio placentae, both the perinatal and maternal mortality rates markedly increase[18], and this nearly always occurs within 8 h of clinical onset of the abruptio. Conversely, if the disseminated intravascular coagulation has not occurred within 8 h of the clinical onset of abruptio, it is unlikely to occur at all, even if delivery is delayed for several hours[4].

If the diagnosis of abruptio placentae is entertained, evidence for disseminated intravascular coagulation must be sought. The diagnosis is often suspected clinically when the patient has prolonged bleeding from venipuncture sites. The diagnosis is supported by a serum fibrinogen level of < 100 mg/dl or fibrin split products of > 10 μg/ml. A rapid, easy method of patient evaluation for disseminated intravascular coagulation involves observing her freshly drawn blood in a test tube. If the blood fails to clot within 8 min, it is likely that hypofibrinogenemia is present. Failure of the clot to retract from the sides of the tube within 1 h indicates thrombocytopenia[4].

Renal failure is a leading cause of maternal mortality in cases of abruptio placentae. At autopsy, most of these women are found to have bilateral cortical necrosis and many are found to have lower nephron necrosis. The cause of the renal failure includes maternal hypovolemia and intense systemic vasospasm. The renal failure can be prevented only by sufficient fluid replacement, central monitoring and recognizing that the degree of hypovolemia may be masked by the amount of concealed hemorrhage and the degree of vasospasm[19].

Hypertension accompanies more than half of all abruptio placentae cases. When hypertension occurs, it is often severe, with diastolic blood pressure exceeding 110 mmHg in one-third of cases. There is some debate over whether the hypertension occurs first (and predisposes to abruptio placentae) or whether the hypertension results from the abruptio[10,14].

Postpartum hemorrhage develops in one-third of patients with the combination of abruptio placentae and disseminated intravascular coagulation[20]. However, the hemorrhage is not related to the degree of hypofibrinogenemia but seems to be closely related to the presence of early fibrinolytic products (fragments X or Y). *In vitro* studies of human myometrium have shown that contractility is inhibited when exposed to these fragments.

Treatment

Once the diagnosis of abruptio placentae has been made, the goals of treatment include restoration of an effective maternal circulation, delivery of a well oxygenated neonate and continual surveillance of the maternal coagulation status.

There is a tendency among clinicians to underestimate the degree of maternal hemorrhage and to undertransfuse. Much of the hemorrhage is concealed and the intense vasospasm associated with abruptio placentae may cause the mother to be normotensive or hypertensive in spite of massive hypovolemia. Tachycardia and pallor often do not manifest until 40–50% of the maternal blood volume has been lost[21].

A large-bore (16-g) intravenous line must be secured. A Foley catheter should be placed for accurate monitoring of urine output. At least 4 units of blood should be typed and cross-matched. Fresh blood should be made available if possible. Blood and crystalloid solution should be infused at rates sufficient to keep the hematocrit above 30% and the urine output above 30 ml/h. If the urine output drops below this rate, then a central venous pressure or pulmonary artery catheter should be used to guide further volume replacement. Overtransfusion in this situation is rare, whereas undertransfusion is common. The amount of blood transfused tends to be more adequate if central monitoring is used than if it is not. The hematocrit should be repeated every 2–3 h.

Blood should be drawn for assessment of PT, PTT, fibrinogen, fibrin degradation products and platelet count. If there is evidence of disseminated intravascular coagulation, trauma to the genital tract should be avoided through spontaneous vaginal delivery. If an episiotomy is needed, it should be in the midline and should be carefully repaired. Although hypofibrinogenemia rarely corrects spontaneously until after delivery, treatment of the coagulopathy with blood products is usually unnecessary. If transfusion is required, however, it is best to administer fresh whole blood. Delivery is the treatment of choice for the disseminated intravascular coagulation that accompanies abruptio placentae. After delivery, the fibrinogen concentration will increase by about 100 mg/dl over the next 12–16 h[4]. Other coagulation factors will similarly increase, although the platelet count may require several days to return to normal. After delivery, myometrial contractility augments hemostasis more than the coagulation mechanism. Oxytocin administration, uterine massage and occasionally intramuscular synthetic 15-methyl $F_{2\alpha}$ become important. If postpartum bleeding persists, cryoprecipitate therapy may be indicated. Ten units of cryoprecipitate will increase the fibrinogen concentration by about 100 mg/dl and will similarly increase the concentration of other coagulation factors, although fresh frozen plasma may occasionally be required to replace factor V. If a Cesarean section becomes necessary in the face of disseminated intravascular coagulation, enough cryoprecipitate should be given preoperatively to increase the fibrinogen concentration to 100–150 mg/dl.

If the fetus is alive on admission, vaginal delivery should be hastened. It is essential, however, that internal monitoring of the fetal heart be performed along with liberal use of fetal scalp blood sampling, while recognizing that up to 60% of fetuses will exhibit signs of intrapartum fetal distress. Amniotomy should be performed as early as possible, (1) to allow a fetal scalp electrode to be placed; (2) to decrease the intervillous space pressure, to improve fetal oxygenation; (3) to expedite delivery; and (4) to prevent the escape of thromboplastin into the maternal circulation. Intravenous oxytocin should be used to induce labor.

Prevention

The physician may be able to decrease the incidence of abruptio placentae significantly in two groups of patients: those who smoke cigarettes and those who use cocaine.

Naeye[6] found that, among women who smoked during pregnancy, those who later gave up smoking had a 23% lower incidence of abruption than those who continued smoking, and that these patients had half the number of fetal and neonatal deaths experienced by those who continued smoking. If the mother is able to stop smoking by the time of her first prenatal visit, the risk of perinatal mortality secondary to abruption is nearly identical to that of the patient who never smoked.

Cocaine use has increasingly become a risk factor for abruptio placentae. Since there appears to be a temporal relationship between cocaine use and the onset of abruption[8], it is likely that ceasing cocaine use would lessen the likelihood of abruptio placentae.

If the patient with chronic hypertension has had an abruption in a previous pregnancy, consideration should be given to using antihypertensive agents in the present pregnancy.

PLACENTA PREVIA

Definition and classification

The presence of placental tissue at or over the internal cervical os defines placenta previa. Placenta previa is classified as marginal when the placental edge reaches but does not cross the internal os; partial when the placenta covers part of the internal os; and central or complete when the placenta entirely covers the os. The term low-lying placenta is used to describe the condition in which part of the placenta is implanted over the lower uterine segment but does not reach the edge of the internal os. A low-lying placenta is not a genuine placenta previa.

This classification is important in predicting outcome. The complete placenta previa is less likely to 'migrate' (described below). Complete placenta previa is associated with a higher maternal blood loss before delivery, increased need for maternal transfusion and an increased risk of maternal infection after delivery[22]. Some studies have found that central placenta previa is associated with lower gestational age and lower birth weight at delivery[23], but others have not[22]. Marginal placenta previa, on the other hand, is more commonly associated with preterm contractions necessitating tocolytic therapy. Central previa accounts for about half the cases of placenta previa, and marginal and partial previa account equally for the remainder[22,23].

The relationship between the placental location and position of the internal cervical os may change during pregnancy[24,25]. The incidence of placenta previa in the mid-trimester is as high as 45%[12], with well over 90% of these converting to a fundal implantation site by term. It is not clear how the placenta 'migrates' to its fundal location from the lower uterine segment. Perhaps, as the lower uterine segment forms, it draws the placenta in a cephalad direction. Alternatively, placentation may be a dynamic process with trophoblastic regression occurring in the lower uterine segment along with growth of new trophoblastic tissue towards the fundus.

Incidence and impact

The incidence of placenta previa beyond 24 weeks' gestation is 0.3–0.6%[22,26]. Since Cesarean section is an important risk factor for placenta previa in subsequent pregnancies, the recent increase in the Cesarean rate may increase the incidence of placenta previa over the next decade. The maternal mortality rate in cases of placenta previa has markedly decreased over the past 50 years[27]. Several recent series[22,23,26,28] contain a combined total of 453 cases of placenta previa with no maternal mortalities.

Similarly, the perinatal mortality and morbidity have steadily decreased since the institution of conservative management of placenta previa in 1945[22,29], although the perinatal mortality rate is still 12.6%[22] with the perinatal deaths evenly divided between neonatal and antenatal deaths. If the first bleeding episode occurs before the third trimester, the fetal prognosis is worse[23]. The improved perinatal mortality is largely due to liberal use of maternal transfusion, availability of ultrasound for placental localization and gestational age assignment, availability of biochemical tests of fetal pulmonary maturity, improved neonatal care, improved antenatal fetal surveillance and improved anesthesia[26]. Inpatient management of placenta previa may also improve fetal prognosis[28]. Neonatal complications (respiratory distress syndrome, anemia, jaundice) are mainly secondary to prematurity, although the neonatal anemia may be secondary to fetal bleeding.

Risk factors

Major risk factors for placenta previa include previous Cesarean delivery[23,30], cigarette smoking[31], previous curettage for spontaneous abortion (but not for therapeutic abortion)[23], maternal age and parity, and presence of a male fetus[22,27]. Recurrence rates as high as 8% have been reported[32,33].

Signs and symptoms

The onset of painless, bright red, vaginal bleeding during the third trimester is the hallmark symptom (and sign) of placenta previa. The mean gestational age at onset varies between 29 weeks and 32 weeks[23,26]. The first episode of bleeding is almost never life-threatening to either the mother or the fetus. It has been the author's experience that careful questioning of the patient will reveal that there had been episodes of spotting during the second trimester. Subsequent bleeding episodes are usually more severe and the episodes occur with increasing frequency as pregnancy advances. With the onset of labor, the bleeding again becomes intensified.

The amount of external bleeding associated with previa is nearly always reflected in the patient's vital signs and hematocrit; there is no concealed hemorrhage, as is seen with abruptio placentae. Uterine contractions accompany the first episode of bleeding in 15% to 20% of cases of placenta previa[22,26].

As many as 7% of cases of placenta previa have been diagnosed as 'incidental findings' at the time of ultrasonography done for gestational age assignment[22]. It is anticipated that, as ultrasonography becomes more routine, this will occur more frequently.

If a pelvic examination is performed in the presence of placenta previa, there is a high likelihood of opening thrombosed sinuses and aggravating the bleeding.

Any patient experiencing painless vaginal bleeding during the second half of pregnancy has a placenta previa until proven otherwise. A pelvic examination must never be performed in the presence of vaginal bleeding during the second half of pregnancy except (1) under double set-up conditions; or (2) after expertly performed ultrasonography, unequivocally proving that placenta previa is absent.

Diagnosis

Three tools are extremely valuable to the clinician in making the diagnosis of placenta previa: ultrasound, double set-up examination and magnetic resonance imaging (MRI).

Abdominal ultrasound has an accuracy of more than 90% in diagnosing placenta previa, with false-negative and false-positive rates of 5–10%[25,34]. The echogenic placental tissue can usually be seen overlying the cervical os. The cord insertion onto the chorionic plate should be visualized at the time of examination. If the cord inserts peripherally and the umbilical vessels splay at the placenta, velamentous insertion of the cord is likely. The lower border of a posterior placenta previa is sometimes difficult to visualize because of acoustic shadowing from the overlying fetal calvarium. Transabdominal, manual elevation of the fetal head at the time of the examination may permit adequate visualization in this circumstance. The relationship between the posterior fetal calvarium and the sacrum may also be helpful in ruling out a posterior placenta previa. Careful transvaginal sonography is also helpful in this situation. Although transabdominal sonography should be performed with a full maternal bladder, an overly distended maternal bladder may push an anterior, low-lying placenta against the posterior wall of the uterus, thus giving the appearance of a complete placenta previa. It is therefore important to obtain a confirmatory post-void scan.

An MRI scan more precisely defines the degree of placenta previa. MRI is also more reliable in diagnosing a posterior placenta previa, because the fetal calvarium does not obscure the image[35].

Double set-up examination is reserved for the case in which the diagnosis remains uncertain. A double set-up examination is performed in the operating room after the patient, nurses, obstetricians and anesthesiologist have been completely prepared for a Cesarean delivery. A speculum examination is first performed to visualize placental tissue through the cervical os. If none is visualized, an examining finger is gently placed against the vaginal fornices. The finger is then gently inserted into the cervical canal to palpate for placenta. We stress that the double set-up examination is not performed electively to make a diagnosis. It is performed at a time when the obstetrician feels that delivery is necessary and is performed only to define the route of delivery.

Complications

Several fetal and neonatal complications were addressed earlier in this chapter. It must be emphasized that the chief cause of perinatal mortality is preterm delivery and not fetal anemia or hypoxia[22,23]. It appears, also, that these infants have a high incidence of respiratory distress syndrome for their gestational age[23]. There is a two-fold increase in the incidence of congenital malformations[22,27]. Malpresentation is present in about 30% of cases[22,23]. Most recent studies have shown no higher incidence of growth retardation[23,27].

A major maternal complication is placenta accreta, which occurs in 3–5% of patients with placenta previa. In patients who have had a previous Cesarean delivery and now have a placenta previa, the incidence of placenta accreta increases to 25%. The incidence of accreta is further increased in patients with two or more previous Cesarean deliveries[36]. It has been observed that ultrasonographic visualization of laminar and turbulent blood flow in large placental lakes of placenta previae is predictive of placenta previa accreta[37].

Management

The goal of therapy is to prolong the pregnancy as long as possible, anticipating planned delivery at term or when fetal pulmonary maturity can be documented by amniocentesis[22]. Earlier delivery should be carried out in the face of severe maternal hemorrhage, fetal distress, or unstoppable preterm labor[23]. Even if the initial maternal hemorrhage exceeds 500 ml, the pregnancy can usually be significantly prolonged[22]. We emphasize that this conservative goal applies only to the patient who is hemodynamically stable and in whom the bleeding stops within a reasonable period of time.

The patient should be hospitalized if she has an episode of bleeding after 24 weeks. Although outpatient management can be allowed under certain strict conditions for patients who are reliable, there is evidence[28] that, with inpatient management: (1) the gestational age at birth will be more advanced; (2) the birth weight will be greater; (3) the neonatal mortality will be lower; and (4) neonatal hospitalization will be of shorter duration. In the long run, hospitalization of the mother may be less expensive than outpatient treatment. Stool softeners and a diet high in fiber should be prescribed. Oral iron therapy should be started. Weekly or twice-weekly biophysical profile tests should be undertaken to assure fetal well-being.

Two to four units of red cells must be continuously available for transfusion. If active bleeding subsides and the maternal hematocrit remains greater than 34%, then she is a candidate for autologous blood transfusion, which has been shown to be very safe for both the mother and the fetus[38]. In the face of active bleeding or if the hematocrit drops to less than 30%, red cell transfusions should be administered.

Glucocorticoids should be administered at least once between 28 and 32 weeks' gestation[23]. The rationale for administration is that (1) infants of mothers with previa tend to have delayed pulmonary maturation[23]; (2) glucocorticoids need at least 12–24 h to be effective; and (3) the obstetrician has no way of predicting when emergency delivery may become necessary.

Preterm contractions are not uncommon among patients with previa, particularly with marginal and partial placenta previa[39]. Although controversy surrounds the use of tocolytic agents in this situation, tocolytic therapy may prevent further shearing of the placenta from the lower uterine segment and prolong gestation.

After 36 weeks' gestation, an amniocentesis should be performed every 7–10 days until fetal pulmonary maturity is proven.

If fetal lung maturity can be documented, delivery should be carried out electively within 24 h. At 39 weeks or more, delivery can be carried out without amniocentesis. Emergency delivery should be carried out in the face of (1) excessive maternal hemorrhage; (2) fetal distress; or (3) uterine contractions unresponsive to tocolytic therapy. If central placenta previa is diagnosed, delivery must be by Cesarean. If there is a question of a marginal placenta previa, a double set-up examination should be performed in the Cesarean room before delivery. Occasionally, the obstetrician is surprised to find that no placenta can be palpated through the cervix, in which case the membranes may be ruptured and labor induced in anticipation of a vaginal delivery.

Because of the association between placenta previa and placenta accreta, it has been our policy to obtain written permission for hysterectomy at the time the permission for Cesarean section is obtained.

Finally, an alternative method of management of symptomatic placenta previa before 30 weeks' gestation may be placement of a cervical cerclage. Arias[40] found in a prospective, randomized study that placing a cerclage between 24 and 30 weeks' gestation in these patients decreased the number of maternal bleeding episodes and decreased the total hospital cost. We feel that this method of treatment needs further investigation at the present time, before it can be recommended.

Vasa previa

The term velamentous insertion is used when the umbilical vessels insert onto the membranes instead of onto the body of the placenta. When these vessels cross the lower uterine segment ahead of the fetal presenting part, the term vasa previa is applied. Although vasa previa is present in only about 1 in 5000 pregnancies, it occurs more commonly in association with placenta previa and with multiple gestation[41]. When the fetal umbilical vessels are in this precarious position, they are likely to burst at the time of rupture of the membranes, and they may burst spontaneously or become compressed with descent of the fetal presenting part. With rupture of the membranes, a perinatal loss rate as high as 75% may occur. There may also be an increase in the incidence of fetal anomalies associated with vasa previa.

If vaginal bleeding occurs at the time of rupture of the membranes, vasa previa must be suspected. Concomitant fetal heart rate abnormalities should heighten the suspicion. Since the blood is entirely fetal blood, the diagnosis may be confirmed with an Apt test or with Wright's staining of the blood, looking for nucleated (fetal) red blood cells. If the diagnosis is confirmed, this represents a fetal emergency and a prompt Cesarean delivery should be performed.

REFERENCES

1. Ananth CV, Savitz DA, Williams MA. Placental abruption and its association with hypertension and prolonged rupture of membranes: a methodologic review and meta-analysis. *Obstet Gynecol* 1996;88:309–18
2. Naeye RL, Harkness WL, Utts J. Abruptio placentae and perinatal death: a prospective study. *Am J Obstet Gynecol* 1977;128:740–6
3. Knab DR. Abruptio placentae. *Obstet Gynecol* 1978; 52:625–9
4. Pritchard JA. Treatment of the defibrination syndromes of pregnancy. *Mod Treat* 1968;5:401–18
5. Egley CC, Cefalo RC. Abruptio placentae. In Studd J, ed. *Progress in Obstetrics and Gynecology*. New York: Churchill Livingstone, 1985:108–20
6. Naeye RL. Abruptio placentae and placenta previa. frequency, perinatal mortality, and cigarette smoking. *Obstet Gynecol* 1980;55:701–4
7. Goujard J, Rumeau C, Schwartz D. Smoking during pregnancy, stillbirth and abruptio placentae. *Biomedicine* 1975;23:20–2
8. Townsend RR, Laing FC, Jeffrey RB. Placental abruption associated with cocaine abuse. *Am J Roentgenol* 1988;150:1339–40
9. Pritchard JA, Mason R, Corley M, *et al*. Genesis of severe placental abruption. *Am J Obstet Gynecol* 1970;108:22–7
10. Hibbard BM, Hibbard ED. Aetiological factors in abruptio placentae. *Br Med J* 1963;2:1430–6
11. Crosby WM, Costiloe JP. Safety of lap belt restraint for pregnant victims of automobile collisions. *N Engl J Med* 1971;284:632–6
12. Mengert WF. Observations on the pathogenesis of premature separation of the normally implanted placenta. *Am J Obstet Gynecol* 1953;66:1104–10
13. Kerr MG. The mechanical effects of the gravid uterus in late pregnancy. *J Obstet Gynaecol Br Commonw* 1965; 72:513–19
14. Paintin DB. The epidemiology of ante-partum haemorrhage. *J Obstet Gynecol* 1962;69:614–24
15. Golditch IM, Boyce NE. Management of abruptio placentae. *J Am Med Assoc* 1970;212:288–93

16. Hurd WW, Miodovnik M, Hertzberg V, *et al*. Selective management of abruptio placentae: a prospective study. *Obstet Gynecol* 1983;61:467–73

17. Porter J. Conservative treatment of abruptio placentae. *Obstet Gynecol* 1960;15:690–7

18. Sher G. Pathogenesis and management of uterine inertia complicating abruptio placentae with consumption coagulopathy. *Am J Obstet Gynecol* 1977;129:164–70

19. Nilsen PA. Premature separation of the normally implanted placenta. *Acta Obstet Gynecol Scand* 1958;37:195–260

20. Basu HK. Fibrinolysis and abruptio placentae. *J Obstet Gynaecol BR Commonw* 1969;76:481–96

21. Barry A. Accidental haemorrhage or abruptio placentae clinical features. *J Obstet Gynaecol Br Commonw* 1963;70:708–10

22. Cotton DB, Read JA, Paul RH, *et al*. The conservative aggressive management of placenta previa. *Am J Obstet Gynecol* 1980;137:687–95

23. McShane PM, Heyl PS, Epstein MF. Maternal and perinatal morbidity resulting from placenta previa. *Obstet Gynecol* 1985;65:176–82

24. Wexler P, Gottesfeld KR. Second trimester placenta previa. An apparently normal placentation. *Obstet Gynecol* 1977;50:706–9

25. Comeau J, Shaw L, Marcell CC, *et al*. Early placenta previa and delivery outcome. *Obstet Gynecol* 1983;61:577–80

26. Silver R, Depp R, Sabbagha RE, *et al*. Placenta previa: aggressive expectant management. *Am J Obstet Gynecol* 1984;150:15–22

27. Brenner WE, Edelman DA, Hendricks CH. Characteristics of patients with placenta previa and results of 'expectant management'. *Am J Obstet Gynecol* 1978;132:180–91

28. D'Angelo LJ, Irwin LF. Conservative management of placenta previa: a cost–benefit analysis. *Am J Obstet Gynecol* 1984;149:320–6

29. Lockwood CJ. Placenta previa and related disorders. *Contemp Obstet Gynecol* 1990;26:47–68

30. Singh PM, Rodrigues C, Gupta AN. Placenta previa and previous Cesarean section. *Acta Obstet Gynecol Scand* 1981;60:367–8

31. Rose GL, Chapman MG. Aetiological factors in placenta previa – a case–controlled study. *Br J Obstet Gynaecol* 1986;93:586–8

32. Read JA, Cotton DB, Miller FC. Placenta accreta: changing clinical aspects and outcome. *Obstet Gynecol* 1980;56:31–4

33. Iffy L. Contribution to the etiology of placenta previa. *Am J Obstet Gynecol* 1962;83:969–75

34. Bowie JD, Rochester D, Cadkin AV, *et al*. Accuracy of placental localization by ultrasound. *Radiology* 1978;128:177–80

35. Powell MC, Buckley J, Price H, *et al*. Magnetic resonance imaging and placenta previa. *Am J Obstet Gynecol* 1986;154:565–9

36. Clark SL, Koonings PP, Phelan JP. Placenta previa/accreta and prior cesarean section. *Obstet Gynecol* 1985;66:89–91

37. Guy GP, Peisner DB, Timor-Tritsch IE. Ultrasonographic evaluation of uteroplacental blood flow patterns of abnormally located and adherent placentas. *Am J Obstet Gynecol* 1990;163:723–7

38. Herbert WN, Owen HG, Collins ML. Autologous blood storage in obstetrics. *Obstet Gynecol* 1988;72:166–70

39. Tomich PG. Prolonged use of tocolytic agents in the expectant management of placenta previa. *J Reprod Med* 1985;30:745–8

40. Arias F. Cervical cerclage for the temporary treatment of patients with placenta previa. *Obstet Gynecol* 1988;71:545–8

41. VanDrie DM, Kammeraad LA. Vasa previa: case report, review and presentation of a new diagnostic method. *J Reprod Med* 1981;26:577–80

7

Post-term pregnancy

H.N. Winn

INTRODUCTION

Post-term pregnancy is defined as a gestation of more than 42 weeks or 294 days from the onset of the last normal menstrual cycle which was followed by conception 2 weeks later. Postmaturity syndrome or dysmaturity refers to a constellation of neonatal physical findings reflecting wasting subcutaneous fat, as initially described by Clifford[1]. At birth, infants with dysmaturity have one or a combination of the following features: wrinkled, dry, cracked and desquamated skin, thin extremities, meconium-stained nails and skin, and a very alert look. Although dysmaturity occurs more frequently in post-term pregnancies, it is evident in pregnancies complicated by severe intrauterine growth retardation (IUGR) at other gestational ages as well.

The etiology of post-term gestation remains unknown. The placenta and fetal pituitary and adrenal glands appear to play a role in the onset of spontaneous labor. Gestation has been prolonged in pregnancies complicated by placental sulfatase insufficiency, fetal anencephaly, or fetal adrenal hypoplasia or aplasia[2]. Whether the underproduction of estrogens (estradiol and estriol) in these clinical situations is the culprit remains to be clarified. Interestingly, labor has been initiated in post-term pregnancies with the intraamniotic injection of cortisol[3]. It appears that there is a delicate inter-relationship between fetal steroid production, placental metabolism and prostaglandin production which brings about the onset of labor in normal gestation. More work is needed to shed light on this important issue.

Post-term gestation occurs in about 10% of pregnancies and is associated with significant perinatal morbidity[4,5] mainly from an increased incidence of macrosomia, dysmaturity and intrapartum fetal distress. In addition, compared to normal term pregnancy, the fetal mortality rate doubles and quadruples at 43 and 44 completed weeks of gestation, respectively[6]. Although the high-risk nature of post-term pregnancy has been recognized since the beginning of the century, the best management approach remains unsettled.

Determination of gestational age is the most important initial step in the post-term pregnancy management. Interestingly, one study demonstrated that all of the pregnancies which had been diagnosed as post-term on the basis of certain last menstrual periods actually were found to be term pregnancies when basal body temperature was used to ascertain ovulation[7]. The traditional methods of gestational dating – such as uterine size, the timing of the audible fetal heart sounds by either the fetoscope or the doptone, and the onset of fetal movement perceived by the mother – are not accurate enough in most instances to be clinically useful. Ultrasound examinations, obtained at the appropriate time, can be used to predict gestational age with a high degree of accuracy. The crown–rump length (CRL) can predict the gestational age within 2.7 days from the 7th to 14th weeks when the average of three independent measurements is used[8]. The biparietal diameter (BPD) and femur length (FL) are two useful parameters in estimating gestational age during the second trimester. The accuracy of BPD or FL in gestational dating is about 1 week with 95% confidence limits until about 26 weeks[9-11]. It should be noted that, to use the BPD for gestational dating, the cephalic index, which is the ratio of the BPD to the occipitofrontal diameter, has to be in the normal range of 74–83%[12]. The cerebellum is located in the posterior fossa of the cranium and its transverse diameter can be easily measured. During the second trimester, the linear relationship of the transverse diameter in millimeters with the gestational age in weeks permits the convenient estimation of gestational age with a high degree of accuracy[13]. Since the transverse diameter is not affected by the head shape, it can replace the BPD in dating the pregnancy when the cephalic indices fall outside the normal range. The above ultrasonographic parameters are not reliable for gestational dating, with an error of up to 3 weeks, during the third trimester. The extremity ossification centers, which appear as echodense structures, can be useful for gestational dating during this stage of gestation. The presence of a distal femoral epiphysis, proximal tibial epiphysis and proximal humeral epiphysis generally indicates gestational ages of at least 32 weeks, 34 weeks and 36 weeks of gestation, respectively[14-17]. It should be noted that the timing of the appearance of the epiphyses is affected by the fetal gender, with earlier occurrence in female fetuses[18,19]. If routine ultrasound examination ever becomes a reality, one ultrasound examination at 18–19 weeks of gestation may be sufficient to accomplish both screening for fetal anomalies and determination of gestational age.

ASSESSMENT OF FETAL WELL-BEING

The controversy in the management of post-term pregnancies arises when the cervix is non-inducible. In this clinical setting, the increased risk of perinatal mortality and morbidity associated with expectant management has to be balanced against the increased maternal morbidity and mortality associated with a higher incidence of Cesarean section due to failed induction. It becomes apparent that expectant management of post-term pregnancies is possible only if fetal well-being can be assured.

The contraction stress test

The contraction stress test (CST) was one of the earliest tests to use fetal heart rate (FHR) monitoring to assess fetal well-being in post-term pregnancies on a large scale. The uterine contractions can be spontaneous or elicited by either intravenous oxytocin or manual nipple stimulation. The current CST protocol as developed by Ray and Freeman[20,21] requires the presence of three uterine contractions, each lasting 40–60 s in a 10-min window, to be adequate. The CST is defined as negative or positive depending on whether late decelerations are absent or persistently present with uterine contractions, respectively. The CST is equivocal if the late decelerations of FHR associated with uterine contractions are not persistent.

Since the CST was designed to test the placental reserve of nutritional support to the growing fetus, it appears to be an ideal test of fetal well-being in post-term pregnancies where placental insufficiency is a concern. In fact, a negative CST predicts fetal survival for 1 week with at least 99.5% accuracy in pregnancies at risk for placental insufficiency such as hypertension, IUGR, diabetes and being post-term[20,22]. Interestingly, no perinatal mortality was reported within 1 week of a negative CST in a prospective study of 679 post-term patients which utilized the CST as the sole means of fetal surveillance[23]. In addition, the incidence of intrapartum fetal distress increased in patients with equivocal or positive tests.

The main disadvantages of the CST are the inconvenience of intravenous oxytocin administration and a high incidence of equivocal tests; the latter requires repetitive testing and may prompt unnecessary intervention. The presence of variable decelerations should be noted and requires further evaluation with an ultrasound examination to rule out oligohydramnios, which can cause cord compression. Currently, the CST has been almost replaced by the biophysical profile as the second test of fetal well-being when the non-stress test (NST) is non-reactive.

The non-stress test

The NST has been extensively used for the evaluation of fetal well-being in postdate pregnancies since its introduction. Its popularity rests on its ease of use and interpretation. The current protocol for the NST as developed by Evertson and Paul[24] includes observing the FHR pattern for a period of 10–40 min. A reactive NST is defined as having two accelerations of the FHR, with at least 15 beats/min above the baseline FHR and lasting at least 15 s for each acceleration, during a 20-min observational window. The NST is non-reactive if there are no such FHR accelerations during the 40-min observational period. Although the NST does not directly address the placental insufficiency problem, it monitors the essential endpoint of the pregnancy itself, the fetus. Generally, a reactive NST is reassuring and indicates a non-hypoxic fetus. The incidence of stillbirth within a week of a reactive NST among post-term pregnancies ranges from 2.8/1000 to 24/1000[22,25,26]. Since stillbirth can occur within 2–5 days after a reactive NST[25–27], the NST should be administered at least semiweekly, if it is the only test used to assess fetal well-being in post-term pregnancies. A non-reactive NST does not necessarily mean fetal distress and requires further evaluation with either a CST or an ultrasound examination.

The biophysical profile

The biophysical profile, as introduced by Manning and colleagues[28], consists of an ultrasound evaluation of the amniotic fluid, fetal biophysical characteristics such as breathing movement, body movement and tone, in addition to a standard NST. Each of the five variables is assigned a score of 0 or 2, depending on whether it is abnormal or normal. The biophysical profile was developed on the assumption that the presence of normal fetal breathing movements, body movements and tone reflects a non-depressed fetal central nervous system. In the original study of 216 high-risk patients with 40% of patients being post-term, no perinatal mortality was noted within a week of a normal fetal biophysical profile, regardless of the result of the NST. On the other hand, a poor biophysical profile (a total score of 4/10 or less), which presumably reflected fetal hypoxemia, was associated with a significantly increased perinatal mortality and morbidity. In this study the NST rather than the biophysical profile was used for fetal assessment[28]. Subsequently, the biophysical profile was used in the clinical management of 12 620 high-risk pregnancies complicated by being post-term, with suspected IUGR, hypertension, diabetes and other conditions, with a patient distribution of 11.6%, 20.8%, 17.5%, 9.2% and 40.9%, respectively. The false-negative rate of the biophysical profile, i.e. stillbirth occurring within a week of a normal biophysical profile with a total score of at least 8/10, was 0.634/1000. One of the stillbirths occurred in a post-term pregnancy within 5 days of a normal biophysical profile[28]. Similar to the NST and CST, a poor biophysical profile does not necessarily mean impending fetal distress, because of the inherent cyclicity of the fetal biophysical characteristics during a 24-h period. In fact, one study showed that the accuracy of an abnormal profile in predicting poor neonatal outcome in post-term gestation was only 14%[29].

The biophysical profile appears to be an excellent modality for assessing fetal well-being in post-term pregnancies. First of all, being non-invasive and easily applied, the biophysical profile can be performed in an outpatient setting. Secondly, the biophysical profile has a very low false-negative rate that is comparable to that of the CST. No perinatal mortality was observed when a semiweekly biophysical profile was solely used for fetal assessment in the management of post-term pregnancies. Furthermore, excellent perinatal outcomes with a reduction of Cesarean section rate were observed when expectant management was carried out in the presence of a normal biophysical profile[30]. Thirdly, compared to the NST or CST, the biophysical profile is associated with a much lower percentage of equivocal or abnormal tests[31]. Thus, the expense of time, labor and patients' anxiety associated with false testing is reduced. Fourthly, until routine ultrasound examination of the fetus in early pregnancy becomes a reality, the biophysical profile provides the opportunity to evaluate fetal anatomy. Finally, it permits the detection of oligohydramnios, which has an ominous prognosis in post-term pregnancy.

Even though oligohydramnios is an important clinical finding, its definition remains unsettled. Proposed definitions include: (1) the average of the two diameters measured in two perpendicular planes of the largest cord-free pocket of amniotic fluid less than 1 cm[31]; and (2) amniotic fluid index of less than 5 cm; this is obtained by adding the vertical diameters of the largest cord-free pocket of amniotic fluid, one from each quadrant[32,33]. When the average of the two diameters is 1–2 cm, the amniotic fluid index is considered to be marginal[34]. The pathogenesis of oligohydramnios probably involves increased fetal size, placental insufficiency and reduced fetal urine production[35]. It remains to be determined whether oligohydramnios in post-term pregnancies is due to reduced renal blood flow. Although the change in the amniotic fluid volume appears to correlate with the left cardiac function as reflected by the changes in the aortic peak velocity and the aortic outflow[36], Doppler blood flow studies of the fetal renal arteries in post-term pregnancies reveal inconsistent results. Both an elevated ratio of systolic

frequency shift to diastolic frequency shift (S/D ratio) in patients with oligohydramnios[37] and no change in resistance index[38] have been reported when comparing a group with oligohydramnios to a group with normal amniotic volume. It should be noted that, even though the reduction in amniotic volume is usually a gradual process, oligohydramnios can occasionally develop acutely over a 24-h period[39].

Cord compression secondary to oligohydramnios rather than uteroplacental insufficiency is a major cause of intrapartum fetal distress, as revealed by FHR monitoring in post-term gestation[40,41]. In addition, one fetal death occurred 2 days after a biophysical profile score of 8/10 with the only abnormal variable being oligohydramnios[42]. It appears that the biophysical profile should be done twice-weekly if it is the only prenatal testing used for fetal assessment, and that termination of the expectant management may be considered if oligohydramnios is detected.

The Doppler blood flow study

Doppler ultrasound has been used to measure the relative blood flow velocity in various parts of the human body for quite some time, and its utility in obstetrics is currently being investigated. Its major potential application involves predicting fetal distress and elucidating one of the mechanisms of intrauterine growth retardation: fetoplacental blood flow insufficiency. The relative blood flow is measured by different indices obtained from the Doppler flow velocity waveform (Figure 1) such as: (1) the S/D ratio of the peak systolic frequency shift (S) to peak end-diastolic frequency shift (D); (2) the pulsatility index (PI) [$PI = (S - D)/M$, where M represents the mean frequency shift]; and (3) the resistance index (RI) [$RI = (S - D)/S$]. These indices are related to the vascular resistance beyond the point of measurement. Another Doppler velocimetry parameter, the time-averaged mean velocity, has also been studied in post-term pregnancies[43,44]. In uncomplicated pregnancies, blood flow in the uterine, umbilical, fetal middle cerebral, fetal descending thoracic or renal arteries as reflected by these indices does not significantly change as gestational age advances beyond 40 weeks of gestation[43–47].

Therefore, it does not appear that there is a significant increase in placental resistance to blood flow in post-term pregnancy, as was once thought. In a comparison of post-term pregnancies with and without perinatal complications such as oligohydramnios, intrapartum fetal distress or low 5-min Apgar score, the change in the S/D ratios of uterine arteries has not been found to be significantly different, while that of the umbilical artery has not been consistently reported[44,47–49]. Among these Doppler blood flow indices, the absence of the end-diastolic frequency shift (D) from the umbilical artery waveform appears

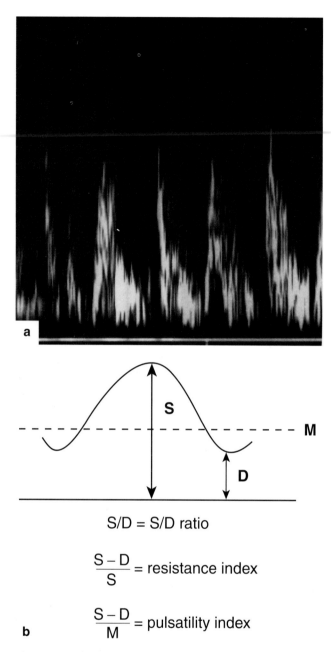

$$S/D = S/D \text{ ratio}$$

$$\frac{S-D}{S} = \text{resistance index}$$

$$\frac{S-D}{M} = \text{pulsatility index}$$

Figure 1   (a) Doppler waveform of the umbilical artery and (b) analysis of the waveform. S, peak systolic frequency shift; D, end-diastolic frequency shift; M, mean frequency shift

to be a useful marker in predicting fetal distress. In a study of 534 patients[46], absent end-diastolic frequency shift had a positive predictive value of 91% for fetal distress during the first stage of labor.

Another promising direct parameter of fetal blood flow, the time-averaged mean velocity in the fetal descending thoracic aorta, has been found to be significantly decreased in post-term pregnancies complicated by oligohydramnios, meconium-stained amniotic fluid, abnormal NST or fetal distress. The latter may necessitate Cesarean section delivery[44].

Similarly, an elevated S/D ratio of the fetal internal carotid artery[49], or a ratio of middle cerebral artery S/D to umbilical artery S/D of less than 1.05[50] is present in complicated post-term pregnancies. At present, there are insufficient data to determine whether Doppler blood flow will offer a better method of identifying fetuses at risk for poor perinatal outcomes in the expectant management of post-term gestation. Doppler blood flow velocimetry could play a role in identifying a subset of post-term patients with abnormal prenatal testing, such as reduced amniotic fluid volume or non-reactive NST, who have an increased risk of fetal compromise during the peripartum period.

PRENATAL MANAGEMENT

Once the diagnosis of post-term pregnancy is made, a plan of management with the goal of optimal maternal and perinatal outcomes should be discussed with the patient and carried out in a timely manner. Unfortunately, the best approach to the management of post-term pregnancy remains to be determined. The main concern with elective induction of labor of all pregnancies at 41 weeks of gestation or greater, regardless of cervical status, is increased maternal morbidity from a higher rate of Cesarean section due to failed induction[51]. However, this concern has not been supported by many randomized clinical trials[52–54]. In addition, intracervical insertion of 0.5 mg of prostaglandin E_2 (PGE_2) 12 h prior to induction of labor with intravenous oxytocin is not more effective than placebo in cervical ripening[52].

If active management of patients with post-term pregnancy and unripe cervix is pursued, cervical ripening with intravaginal PGE_2 can be safely done as an outpatient procedure, provided close fetal monitoring is carried out. One approach involves placing a 2.5-mg PGE_2 suppository in the posterior vaginal fornix, closely monitoring uterine contractions and FHR for the next 2 h on an outpatient basis, and then initiating induction of labor with intravenous oxytocin 12 h later[53]. Other approaches entail the self-administration of 2 mg of intravaginal PGE_2 suppositories daily either for 5 days[55] or until the cervix becomes inducible or fetal well-being is not reassuring[56]. Outpatient cervical ripening with intravaginal suppositories of PGE_2 appears to be cost-effective by inducing labor, thus reducing the cost of antenatal testing, without the increased maternal and perinatal morbidity or mortality.

If expectant management is pursued, fetal evaluation should be started no later than 41 weeks of gestation, since the incidences of fetal macrosomia and perinatal morbidity and mortality rise significantly afterwards[57–60]. The initial step involves assessing fetal weight and amniotic fluid volume by an ultrasound examination. Evaluation of fetal well-being with a combination of semi-weekly NST and weekly evaluation of amniotic volume is adequate and can be conveniently carried out on an outpatient basis. If both tests are normal, the patient can be allowed to await spontaneous labor or ripening of her cervix. Weekly cervical examination should be done. The presence of abnormal fetal testing, such as variable decelerations, oligohydramnios, non-reactive NST, positive CST, or biophysical profile of less than 6/10, indicates that termination of the pregnancy should be considered. In addition, induction of labor is advisable whenever the cervix is inducible. The question of how long expectant management should continue remains debatable. Elective termination of the pregnancy at 44 completed weeks of gestation is not unreasonable, in view of a very high risk of perinatal mortality beyond this gestational age.

INTRAPARTUM MANAGEMENT

The perinatal morbidity of post-term pregnancies does not stop once the decision of induction of labor is made. The post-term fetus is at an increased risk of perinatal hypoxia, severe birth injury from shoulder dystocia and meconium aspiration.

Meconium aspiration

The frequency of meconium-stained amniotic fluid in post-term pregnancies ranges from 22% at 42 weeks to 44% at a later gestation[61] compared to 11.3% in term high-risk pregnancies[62]. Advanced gastrointestinal maturation may play a major role, since passage of meconium is infrequently observed before 32 weeks. Although meconium may pass in response to fetal distress, the presence of meconium-stained amniotic fluid *per se* without concomitant biochemical or biophysical abnormalities does not necessarily mean impending fetal distress[61,63]. Therefore, post-term pregnancies with meconium-stained amniotic fluid and negative CST can be expectantly managed without increased perinatal morbidity and mortality[61]. Meconium tends to be thick in the case of post-term gestation, because of the frequent concomitant oligohydramnios. The merit of peripartum detection of thick meconium lies in the timely initiation of preventive measures to reduce the morbidity associated with meconium aspiration syndrome. Suction of the meconium from the infant's nasopharynx and posterior oropharynx before delivery of the chest and endotracheal suction of the meconium below the infant's vocal cords immediately after delivery has been shown to be effective in reducing the morbidity of the meconium aspiration syndrome. Recently, amnioinfusion has been advocated to reduce the neonatal morbidity associated with meconium aspiration syndrome, probably by diluting the meconium in the amniotic fluid. Intrapartum amnioinfusion has been shown significantly to reduce the incidences of meconium below the vocal cords, neonatal acidemia and the need for positive-pressure ventilation resuscitation during the neonatal period[64].

Perinatal hypoxia

The post-term fetuses are at risk of distress during labor from either cord compression due to oligohydramnios or placental insufficiency. Abnormal FHR patterns during labor or neonatal hypoxia have been observed in 12–30% of post-term pregnancies with normal antenatal testings[23,26,65]. As a result, these fetuses should be closely monitored during labor so that timely and appropriate intervention can be carried out. Amnioinfusion has also been used to relieve repetitive variable decelerations and prolonged decelerations commonly caused by cord compression presumably by restoring the cushioning effect of the amniotic fluid[66–68]. One prospective study shows that, in the presence of oligohydramnios secondary to premature rupture of membranes, patients who receive prophylactic amnioinfusion have significantly higher umbilical arterial and venous pH values than those who do not receive amnioinfusion. Fortunately, the mean umbilical arterial and venous pH values for both groups are within normal limits[69]. The value of prophylactic intrapartum amnioinfusion in parturients with oligohydramnios from either post-term or premature rupture of membranes in improving perinatal outcomes remains to be determined.

Shoulder dystocia

Since the fetus may continue to grow during the post-term period, macrosomia may ensue[70]. The incidence of fetal macrosomia in post-term pregnancies is about 25% compared with 10.2% in term pregnancies[23,57,58,71,72]. Since the risk of shoulder dystocia increases with higher birth weight, shoulder dystocia is a potential problem. Fetal weight should be estimated by ultrasound examination if a large fetus is clinically suspected, recognizing that the error in predicting fetal weight by ultrasound is about 10–15%. It is not unreasonable to perform elective Cesarean section if the fetal weight is estimated to be about 5000 g, because dysfunctional labor and/or shoulder dystocia are the likely outcomes in this clinical setting. Besides macrosomia, other risk factors for shoulder dystocia, such as prolonged second stage of labor, operative vaginal delivery and diabetes[73], should also be recognized. Ultrasonography has also been utilized to predict shoulder dystocia in addition to estimating fetal weight. For example, a difference between the fetal chest circumference and the biparietal diameter of more than 14 mm has been associated with a 3–13% risk of shoulder dystocia in pregnant diabetic patients[74]. Unfortunately, the accuracy of predicting shoulder dystocia with ultrasonography has so far remained limited.

To minimize the perinatal morbidity and mortality associated with shoulder dystocia, those who manage post-term pregnancies should have a high index of suspicion for this condition and be prepared for skilful performance of those maneuvers affecting the delivery before permanent damage has occurred.

In summary, the post-term gestation represents a high-risk clinical situation with potentially significant obstetric mortality and morbidity. Although the ideal management of this clinical entity remains to be determined, any expectant management plan should include the following: (1) determination of the date of confinement early in the gestation, and ultrasound examination for dating if necessary; (2) close monitoring of the fetus, and consideration of delivery if fetal well-being cannot be assured; and (3) being well prepared for potential perinatal complications, such as perinatal asphyxia, meconium aspiration and shoulder dystocia. With a well designed plan of management and the patient's co-operation, excellent perinatal outcomes can be obtained without unnecessarily increased maternal morbidity and mortality. It is somewhat reassuring to know that post-term gestation *per se* without perinatal hypoxia does not appear adversely to affect the offsprings' mental and physical development, as measured by intelligent quotient and physical milestones, respectively[75].

REFERENCES

1. Clifford SH. Postmaturity with placental dysfunction. *J Pediatr* 1954;44:1–13
2. Naeye RL. Causes of perinatal mortality: excess of prolonged gestations. *Am J Epidemiol* 1978;108:429–33
3. Nwosu VC, Wallach EE, Bolognese RJ. Initiation of labor by intraamniotic cortisol instillation in prolonged human pregnancy. *Am J Obstet Gynecol* 1966;96:901
4. Fleischer A, Schulman H, Farmakides G, *et al*. Antepartum nonstress test and the postmature pregnancy. *Obstet Gynecol* 1985;66:80–3
5. Vorherr H. Placental insufficiency in relation to post-term pregnancy and fetal postmaturity. *Am J Obstet Gynecol* 1975;123:67–103
6. McClure-Browne JC. Postmaturity. *Am J Obstet Gynecol* 1963;85:573–82
7. Saito M, Yazawa K, Hashiguchi A, *et al*. Time of ovulation and prolonged pregnancy. *Am J Obstet Gynecol* 1972;112:31–38
8. Robinson HP, Fleming JE. A critical evaluation of sonar 'crown–rump length' measurements. *Br J Obstet Gynaecol* 1975;82:702–10
9. Campbell S. The prediction of fetal maturity by ultrasonic measurement of the biparietal diameter. *J Obstet Gynaecol Br Commonw* 1969;76:603–9
10. O'Brien GD, Queenan JT, Campbell S. Assessment of gestational age in the second trimester by real-time ultrasound measurement of the femur length. *Am J Obstet Gynecol* 1981;139:540–5

11. Sabbagha RE, Barton BA, Barton FB, *et al*. Sonar biparietal diameter. I. Analysis of percentile growth differences in two normal populations using same methodology. *Am J Obstet Gynecol* 1976;126:479–84
12. Hadlock FP, Deter RL, Carpenter RJ, *et al*. Estimating fetal age: effect of head shape on BPD. *AJR Am J Roentgenol* 1981;137:83–5
13. Goldstein I, Reece EA, Pilu G, *et al*. Cerebellar measurements with ultrasonography in the evaluation of fetal growth and development. *Am J Obstet Gynecol* 1987;156:1065–9
14. Chinn DH, Bolding DB, Callen PW, *et al*. The lateral cerebral ventricle in early second trimester. *Radiology* 1983;148:529–31
15. Goldstein I, Lockwood C, Belanger K, *et al*. Ultrasonographic assessment of gestational age with the distal femoral and proximal tibial ossification centers in the third trimester. *Am J Obstet Gynecol* 1988;158:127–30
16. Mahony BS, Bowie JD, Killam AP, *et al*. Epiphyseal ossification centers in the assessment of fetal maturity: sonographic correlation with the amniocentesis lung profile. *Radiology* 1986;159:521–4
17. Tabsh RMA. Correlation of ultrasonic epiphyseal centers and the lecithin/sphingomyelin ratio. *Obstet Gynecol* 1984;64:92–6
18. Kuhns LR, Finnstrom O. New standards of ossification of the newborn. *Radiology* 1976;119:655–60
19. Mahony BS, Callen PW, Filly RA. The distal femoral epiphyseal ossification center in the assessment of third-trimester menstrual age: sonographic identification and measurement. *Radiology* 1985;155:201–4
20. Freeman RK. The use of the oxytocin challenge test for antepartum clinical evaluation of uteroplacental respiratory function. *Am J Obstet Gynecol* 1975;121:481–9
21. Ray M, Freeman R, Pine S, *et al*. Clinical experience with the oxytocin challenge test. *Am J Obstet Gynecol* 1972;114:1–9
22. Khouzami VA, Johnson JWC, Daikoku NH, *et al*. Comparison of urinary estrogens, contraction stress tests and nonstress tests in the management of post-term pregnancy. *J Reprod Med* 1983;28:189–94
23. Freeman RK, Garite TJ, Modanlou H, *et al*. Postdate pregnancy: utilization of contraction stress testing for primary fetal surveillance. *Am J Obstet Gynecol* 1981;140:128–35
24. Evertson LR, Paul RH. Antepartum fetal heart rate testing: the nonstress test. *Am J Obstet Gynecol* 1978;132:895–900
25. Barss VA, Frigoletto FD, Diamond F, *et al*. Stillbirth after nonstress testing. *Obstet Gynecol* 1985;65:541
26. Miyazaki FS, Miyazaki BA. False reactive nonstress tests in postterm pregnancies. *Am J Obstet Gynecol* 1981;140:269–76
27. Eden RD, Gergely RZ, Schifrin BS, *et al*. Comparison of antepartum testing schemes for the management of the postdate pregnancy. *Am J Obstet Gynecol* 1982;144:683–92
28. Manning FA, Platt LD, Sipos L, *et al*. Antepartum fetal evaluation: development of a fetal biophysical profile. *Am J Obstet Gynecol* 1980;136:787–95
29. Hann L, McArdle C, Sachs B. Sonographic biophysical profile in the postdate pregnancy. *J Ultrasound Med* 1987;6:191–5

30. Johnson JM, Harman CR, Lange IR, *et al*. Biophysical profile scoring in the management of the postterm pregnancy: an analysis of 307 patients. *Am J Obstet Gynecol* 1986;154:269–73

31. Manning FA, Morrison I, Lang IR, *et al*. Fetal assessment based on fetal biophysical profile scoring: experience in 12,620 referred high-risk pregnancies. *Am J Obstet Gynecol* 1985;151:343–50

32. Phelan JP, Platt LD, Yeh SY, *et al*. The role of ultrasound assessment of amniotic fluid volume in the management of the post-date pregnancy. *Am J Obstet Gynecol* 1985;151:304–8

33. Phelan JP, Smith CV, Broussard P, *et al*. Amniotic fluid volume assessment with the four-quadrant technique at 36–42 weeks' gestation. *J Reprod Med* 1987;32:540–2

34. Chamberlain PF, Manning FA, Morrison I, *et al*. Ultrasound evaluation of amniotic fluid volume. *Am J Obstet Gynecol* 1984;150:245–9

35. Trimmer KJ, Leveno KJ, Peters MT, Kelly MA. Observations on the cause of oligohydramnios in prolonged pregnancy. *Am J Obstet Gynecol* 1990;163:1900–3

36. Weiner Z, Farmakides G, Barnhard Y, *et al*. Doppler study of the fetal cardiac function in prolonged pregnancies. *Obstet Gynecol* 1996;88:200–2

37. Veille JC, Penry M, Mueller-Heubach E. Fetal renal pulsed Doppler waveform in prolonged pregnancies. *Am J Obstet Gynecol* 1993;169:882–4

38. Bar-Hava I, Divon MY, Sardo M, Barnhard Y. Is oligohydramnios in postterm pregnancy associated with redistribution of fetal blood flow? *Am J Obstet Gynecol* 1995;173:519–22

39. Clement D, Schifrin BS, Kates RB. Acute oligohydramnios in postdate pregnancy. *Am J Obstet Gynecol* 1987;157:884

40. Bochner CJ, Medearis AL, Davis J, *et al*. Antepartum predictors of fetal distress in postterm pregnancy. *Am J Obstet Gynecol* 1987;157:353

41. Leveno KJ, Quirk JG, Cunningham FG, *et al*. Prolonged pregnancy I. Observations concerning the causes of fetal distress. *Am J Obstet Gynecol* 1984;150:465–73

42. Phelan JP, Platt LD, Yeh SY, *et al*. The role of ultrasound assessment of amniotic fluid volume in the management of the postdate pregnancy. *Am J Obstet Gynecol* 1985;151:304–8

43. Rightmire DA, Campbell S. Fetal and maternal Doppler blood flow parameters in postterm pregnancies. *Obstet Gynecol* 1987;69:891–4

44. Battaglia C, Larocca E, Lanzani A, *et al*. Doppler velocimetry in prolonged pregnancy. *Obstet Gynecol* 1991;77:213–6

45. Arduini D, Rizzo G. Fetal renal artery velocity waveforms and amniotic fluid volume in growth-retarded and post-term fetuses. *Obstet Gynecol* 1991;77:370–3

46. Pearce JM, McParland PJ. A comparison of Doppler flow velocity waveforms, amniotic fluid columns, and the nonstress test as a means of monitoring post-dates pregnancies. *Obstet Gynecol* 1991;77:204–8

47. Guidetti DA, Divon MY, Cavalieri RL, *et al*. Fetal umbilical artery flow velocimetry in postdate pregnancies. *Am J Obstet Gynecol* 1987;157:1521–3

48. Fischer RL, Kuhlman KA, Depp R, Wapner RJ. Doppler evaluation of umbilical and uterine-arcuate arteries in the postdates pregnancy. *Obstet Gynecol* 1991;78:363–8

49. Brar HS, Horenstein J, Medearis AL, *et al*. Cerebral, umbilical, and uterine resistance using Doppler velocimetry in postterm pregnancy. *J Ultrasound Med* 1989;8:187–91

50. Devine PA, Bracero LA, Lysikiewicz A, *et al*. Middle cerebral to umbilical artery Doppler ration in post-date pregnancies. *Obstet Gynecol* 1994;84:856–60

51. Gibb DMF, Cardozo LD, Studd JWW, *et al*. Prolonged pregnancy: is induction of labor indicated? A prospective study. *Br J Obstet Gynaecol* 1982;89:292–5

52. The National Institute of Child Health and Human Development Network of Maternal–Fetal Medicine Units. A clinical trial of induction of labor versus expectant management in postterm pregnancy. *Am J Obstet Gynecol* 1995;170:716–23

53. Rayburn W, Gosen R, Ramadei C, *et al*. Outpatient cervical ripening with prostaglandin E$_2$ gel in uncomplicated postdate pregnancies. *Am J Obstet Gynecol* 1988;158:1417–23

54. Dyson DC, Miller PD, Armstrong MA. Management of prolonged pregnancy: induction of labor versus antepartum fetal testing. *Am J Obstet Gynecol* 1987;156:928–34

55. O'Brien JM, Mercer BM, Cleary NT, Sibai BM. Efficacy of outpatient induction with low-dose intravaginal prostaglandin E$_2$: a randomized, double-blind, placebo-controlled trial. *Am J Obstet Gynecol* 1995;173:1855–9

56. Sawai SK, O'Brien WF, Mastrogiannis DS, *et al*. Patient-administered outpatient intravaginal prostaglandin E$_2$ suppositories in post-date pregnancies: a double-blind, randomized, placebo-controlled study. *Obstet Gynecol* 1994;84:807–10

57. Arias F. Predictability of complications associated with prolongation of pregnancy. *Obstet Gynecol* 1987;70:101–6

58. Chervenak JL, Divon MY, Hirsch J, *et al*. Macrosomia in the postdate pregnancy: is routine ultrasonographic screening indicated? *Am J Obstet Gynecol* 1989;161:753–6

59. Guidetti DA, Divon MY, Langer O. Postdate fetal surveillance: is 41 weeks too early? *Am J Obstet Gynecol* 1989;161:91–3

60. Bochner CJ, Williams J, Castro L, *et al*. The efficacy of starting postterm antenatal testing at 41 weeks as compared with 42 weeks of gestational age. *Am J Obstet Gynecol* 1988;159:550–4

61. Knox EG, Huddleston JF, Flowers CE Jr, *et al*. Management of prolonged pregnancy: results of a prospective randomized trial. *Am J Obstet Gynecol* 1979;134:376–384

62. Mandelbaum B. Gestational meconium in the high-risk pregnancy. *Obstet Gynecol* 1973;42:87–92

63. Miller FC, Sacks DA, Yeh SY, *et al*. Significance of meconium during labor. *Am J Obstet Gynecol* 1975;122:573–80

64. Sadovsky Y, Amon E, Bade ME, Petrie RH. Prophylactic amnioinfusion during labor complicated by meconium: a preliminary report. *Am J Obstet Gynecol* 1989;161:613–17

65. Rochard F, Schifrin BS, Goupil F, *et al*. Nonstressed fetal heart rate monitoring in the antepartum period. *Am J Obstet Gynecol* 1976;126:699–706

66. Miyazaki FS, Taylor NA. Saline amnioinfusion for relief of variable or prolonged decelerations. *Am J Obstet Gynecol* 1983;146:670–8

67. Owen J, Henson BV, Hauth JC. A prospective randomized study of saline solution amnioinfusion. *Am J Obstet Gynecol* 1990;162:1146–9
68. Schrimmer DB, Macri CJ, Paul RH. Prophylactic amnioinfusion as a treatment for oligohydramnios in laboring patients: a prospective, randomized trial. *Am J Obstet Gynecol* 1991;165:972–5
69. Nageotte MP, Freeman RK, Garite TJ, Dorchester W. Prophylactic intrapartum amnioinfusion in patients with preterm premature rupture of membranes. *Am J Obstet Gynecol* 1985;153:557–62
70. McLean FH, Boyd ME, Usher RH, Kramer MS. Postterm infants: too big or too small? *Am J Obstet Gynecol* 1991;164:619–24
71. Boyd ME, Usher RH, McLean FH. Fetal macrosomia: prediction, risks, proposed management. *Obstet Gynecol* 1983;61:715–22
72. Golditch IM, Kirkman K. The large fetus. Management and outcome. *Obstet Gynecol* 1978;52:26–30
73. Benedetti TJ, Gabbe SG. Shoulder dystocia: a complication of fetal macrosomia and prolonged second stage of labor with mid-pelvic delivery. *Obstet Gynecol* 1978;52:526–9
74. Elliott JP, Garite TJ, Freeman RK, *et al*. Ultrasonic prediction of fetal macrosomia in diabetic patients. *Obstet Gynecol* 1982;60:159–62
75. Shime J, Librach CL, Gare DJ, Cook CJ. The influence of prolonged pregnancy on infant development at one and two years of age: a prospective controlled study. *Am J Obstet Gynecol* 1986;154:341–5

8
Premature labor

E. Amon

EPIDEMIOLOGY AND DEMOGRAPHY

Preterm birth in this chapter is any birth, regardless of birth weight, that occurs after 20.0 and before 37.0 weeks' gestation based on the best obstetric criteria.

Prior to 20 weeks' gestation, the proper use of clinical terminology depends on whether a spontaneous birth results in a fetus that is liveborn or stillborn. If the fetus is stillborn it is referred to as an abortus, but if the fetus is a spontaneous liveborn, then this is referred to as a live birth. If gestational age is unknown, then a birth weight criterion of 350 g is used to determine the legal status of a dead fetus (stillbirth vs. abortus).

One should refrain from referring to liveborn fetuses as abortuses, because they are indeed liveborn infants. If this terminology departs from the traditional understanding of older obstetric definitions, it is for good reason. Medical terminology relying on gestational age or birth weight to determine the status of a liveborn infant here serves no useful purpose except to propagate tradition. Clearly, a live birth is a live birth, regardless of gestational age. Although this extremely previable newborn will succumb shortly after a birth, clinical concerns about patient-centered emotional care and etiology of death will require acknowledgement that it was a live birth. This information is critical for accurately reporting vital statistics and appropriate epidemiology studies.

Unfortunately, neither the traditional obstetric definitions[1] nor the legal statutory definitions (e.g. Missouri revised statutes, Section 193.165) are based on clinical utility (i.e. the neonate's ability to survive). Although neonatal survival has been reported at 22–23 weeks' gestation, the break-even or 50% survival rate does not commonly occur in most medical centers until at least 24–25 weeks' gestation, or 600–700 g[2,3].

The current classification of low birth weight (LBW) is summarized in Table 1. Many mildly preterm infants have high birth weights of 2500 g or more; conversely, many moderately LBW infants (1500–2499 g) are actually full-term. In some series nearly half of LBW infants were considered term[4].

Preterm birth is one of the most important unsolved problems in reproductive medicine. It is directly responsible for 75–90% of all neonatal deaths not due to lethal congenital malformations[5,6]. Preterm birth

Table 1 Low birth weight classification

Category	Weight (g)
Low birth weight (LBW)	< 2500
Very low birth weight (VLBW)	< 1500
Extremely low birth weight (ELBW) or very very low birth weight (VVLBW)	≤ 1000
Incredibly low birth weight (ILBW)	< 750

also accounts for a large proportion of perinatal mortality and short- and long-term neonatal morbidity, not to mention significant grief, anxiety and financial costs[7].

The major diseases of the preterm infant are due to organ immaturity; therefore, their incidence is inversely related to gestational age. These conditions include respiratory distress syndrome, bronchopulmonary dysplasia, patent ductus arteriosus, necrotizing enterocolitis, hyperbilirubinemia, apnea of prematurity, intraventricular hemorrhage, retinopathy of prematurity and neonatal sepsis. In the past, if preterm infants survived at all, they faced a high risk of significant handicap (blindness, deafness, cerebral palsy, or mental retardation). Today, only 7.5% of very LBW (VLBW) infants (< 1500 g) have a major long-term handicapping condition; the smallest of these surviving infants (450–800 g) have a rate of about 25%[8].

Survival should reach 99% by 32 weeks' gestation. Although surfactant-deficient respiratory distress occurs after 32 weeks, most of these infants are effectively treated. Furthermore, severe grades of intraventricular/periventricular hemorrhage are rare after 32 weeks. Therefore, significant long-term neurological deficit in these older infants should be uncommon.

LBW is a surrogate measure for the health of any society, because it is the leading indicator of infant mortality and morbidity. Its incidence is therefore closely monitored. Most recent improvements in neonatal survival at the lower limits of viability are due to major medical advances in neonatal and perinatal medicine. Further decreases in neonatal mortality will most probably not be achieved unless the focus is shifted to decreasing the incidence of second-trimester preterm birth. There appear to be technical limits to what modern medicine can achieve. Accordingly, non-medical interventions now appear necessary and will be discussed later.

The rates of moderately LBW and VLBW differ substantially between whites and blacks. The relative risk in blacks for moderately LBW is 2.2 and for VLBW is 2.9[9]. The rate of VLBW among whites is 1% and blacks is 3%. In 1997, the incidence of preterm birth (< 37 weeks) was 17.5% in blacks (decreased from 18.5% in 1993) and 10.2% in whites (increased from 9.1% in 1992)[10]. The reasons for these demographic differences are complex and relate to both socioeconomic and biological differences between the races. For instance, pregnant black women are more often poor and unmarried and are more likely to receive inadequate prenatal care, and the adolescent pregnancy rate is higher in blacks. Undoubtedly, such socioeconomic disadvantages are primarily responsible for the substantial differences in rates, but after controlling for some confounding socioeconomic variables, recent investigators found that the two-fold increase in relative risk for LBW remained[10]. In fact, low-risk black women had a rate of VLBW 1.7 times higher than that of high-risk white women. The persistence of these effects needs further investigation. Perhaps improvements in socioeconomic status require more than one generation to result in similar rates of VLBW infants among blacks and whites.

Because up to 30% of gestational assignments are inaccurate, many clinical epidemiologists have come to rely on a more accurate figure: birth weight. The reader should note well that data for the USA for 1997 indicate that the rate of LBW for all races was 7.5% (increased from 6.7% in 1984), the highest level reported since 1976, and the rate of preterm birth is 11.4% (increased from 11.0% in 1993)[10]. Preterm birth and LBW differ in their pathogenesis but share many predisposing factors (Table 2)[11].

It is disheartening that, despite the technical and theoretical advances in reproductive medicine, these rates have not significantly decreased in the last three to four decades. In, fact, the rates have increased. The advances in health-care delivery include risk scoring techniques, liberal use of tocolytic agents, preterm birth prevention programs, regionalized health care and the development of a corporate industry dedicated to the early detection of preterm labor through home uterine activity monitoring programs. Unfortunately, advances in financing of perinatal health care have not kept pace with increases in the rates of preterm delivery.

Many demographic and epidemiological risk factors are not etiological *per se*, but instead are simply markers identifying patients at increased risk. For example, advanced maternal age above 35 years in a primigravida and teenage pregnancy regardless of parity are associated with preterm birth. To illustrate, 23% of mothers < 15 years old gave birth to preterm

Table 2 Categories of risk for low birth weight/preterm birth

Economic
Poverty
Unemployment
Maternal father's poor socioeconomic status
Uninsured, underinsured
Poor access to prenatal care
Poor access to food

Cultural–Behavioral
Low educational status
Poor health-care attitudes
No or inadequate prenatal care
Cigarette, alcohol, drug abuse
Age < 16 or > 35 years
Unmarried
Short interprepregnancy interval
Lack of support group (husband, family, religious institution)
Stress (physical, psychological)
Poor weight gain during pregnancy
Black race

Biological–genetic–medical
Previous low birth weight infant/preterm birth
Low maternal weight at her birth
Black race
Low weight for height
Short stature
Poor nutrition
Chronic medical illnesses
Inbreeding (autosomal recessive?)
Intergenerational effects

Reproductive
Multiple gestation
Premature rupture of membranes
Infections (systemic, amniotic, extra-amniotic, cervical)
Pre-eclampsia/eclampsia
Uterine bleeding (abruptio placentae, placenta previa)
Parity (0 or > 5)
Uterine–cervical anomalies
Fetal demise
Anemia or high hemoglobin
Idiopathic premature labor
Iatrogenic prematurity

infants compared with 10% of women in their twenties, and 13% of women ≥ 40 years old[10].

Table 3 lists the identifiable factors most proximate to preterm birth. Recent studies have shown that clinically evident membrane rupture, medical or obstetric maternal complications or fetal complications account for about 70% of preterm births[6,12,13]. Most patients with preterm labor with intact membranes do not belong to the idiopathic category; only after known or suspected causes are eliminated should patients be diagnosed with idiopathic preterm labor. Although some studies suggest that almost 50% of patients

Table 3 Proximate factors/causes associated with preterm birth

Iatrogenic preterm delivery
Physician error

Maternal causes
Significant systemic medical illness
Significant non-obstetric abdominal pathology
Drug abuse
Severe pre-eclampsia/eclampsia
Trauma

Uterine causes
Malformation
Acute overdistension
Large myomata, degenerating myomata
Deciduitis
Idiopathic uterine activity

Placental causes
Abruptio placentae
Placenta previa
Marginal placental bleeding
Large chorioangioma

Amniotic fluid causes
Oligohydramnios with intact membranes
Preterm rupture of chorioamniotic membranes
Polyhydramnios
Subclinical intra-amniotic infection
Clinical chorioamnionitis

Fetal causes
Fetal malformation
Multifetal gestation
Fetal hydrops
Fetal growth retardation
Fetal distress
Fetal demise

Cervical causes
Cervical incompetence
Cervical foreshortening
Acute cervicitis/vaginitis

giving birth to infants below 2500 g were diagnosed with idiopathic preterm labor[14], this number is a vast overestimate. For example, many infants at highest risk for poor outcome (≤ 1000 g) are born from preterm births that are currently not idiopathic and not necessarily preventable[6]. Many investigators question whether idiopathic preterm labor actually exists. The accuracy of the diagnosis depends on the thoroughness of the assessment. Clearly, subclinical infection or accelerated fetal pulmonary maturation remains undiagnosed unless the diagnostic assessment includes amniocentesis[15]. Histological evaluation of the placenta by knowledgeable pathologists supports the notion that idiopathic preterm labor is quite uncommon[16]. If amniocentesis and placental pathology were commonly performed, the true incidence of unexplained preterm labor would be much lower than the commonly quoted figure of about 30–50%, perhaps accounting for only 5% of cases.

The remainder of this chapter focuses on spontaneous preterm labor with intact membranes.

CLINICAL USE OF RISK FACTORS

Many risk factors antedate the diagnosis of preterm labor, but unfortunately these factors are not very specific. This lack of specificity is further compounded by the inability to diagnose true preterm labor accurately, with implications for progression and delivery, especially if not treated in its early stages. The overlap with false preterm labor is considerable.

Various risk scoring systems have been developed to identify women at above-average risk for preterm birth. These scores subject empirically collected data to various statistical analyses. However, these scores often do not make clear to what extent the predicted preterm birth relates to a treatable entity. Assuming that spontaneous preterm labor with intact membranes is treatable with tocolytic agents, there are many other proximate causes of preterm birth (see Table 3) for which tocolysis is absolutely contraindicated (e.g. antepartum stillbirth, significant maternal hemorrhage, chorioamnionitis, lethal congenital abnormalities, eclampsia).

Further, these scores are limited to empirically derived risk factors. Few if any of these are truly etiological for the predicted outcome. Many risk factors cannot be modified. Some statistical evaluations include only risk 'increasing' factors. Other evaluations additionally include risk 'decreasing' factors.

In the USA, Creasy and colleagues were first to popularize a scoring system of risk factors to predict spontaneous preterm birth[17]. More than 30 items are divided into four categories: socioeconomic, prior medical history, daily habits and current pregnancy problems. Screening is done at the initial prenatal visit and repeated near the end of the second trimester. Patients with a score of 10 points or more are considered to be at high risk.

Holbrook and associates[18] reduced the number of items in their scoring system for the prediction of preterm labor (not preterm birth) from 37 to 18 without any significant statistical loss of identification prevalence, senstitivity, or positive predictive value (Table 4). Fourteen per cent of their prenatal patients were classified as high risk; the sensitivity was 41% and the positive predictive value 25%. This modified risk assessment system is recommended since it is straightforward and does not require the calculation of a risk score. Twelve factors are defined as major (any one indicating high risk) and six as minor (two or more indicating high risk).

The recurrence risk of preterm birth varies from 15% to 40% after one prior preterm birth[19-22]. The risk

Table 4 Major and minor risk factors of the modified scoring system for spontaneous preterm labor. High risk is indicated by one or more of the major factors, or two or more of the minor factors. From reference 18, with permission

Major factors
Multiple gestation
Previous preterm delivery
Previous preterm labor, term delivery
Abdominal surgery during pregnancy
Diethylstilbestrol exposure
Hydramnios
Uterine anomaly
History of cone biopsy
Uterine irritability (admission to rule out preterm labor)
More than one second-trimester abortion
Cervical dilatation (> 1 cm) at 32 weeks
Cervical effacement (< 1 cm) at 32 weeks

Minor factors
Febrile illness during pregnancy
Bleeding after 12 weeks
History of pyelonephritis
Cigarette smoking (> 10 per day)
One second-trimester abortion
More than two first-trimester abortions

significantly increases with two or more prior preterm births. The tendency to repeat preterm birth at the same gestational age as previous preterm births should be noted well. The more preterm the delivery, the less likely the subsequent pregnancy is to deliver at term[21]. For example, a patient with a late second-trimester birth has only 60% likelihood of delivering at term or later in the subsequent pregnancy, whereas a patient with a very mild preterm delivery has a 71% likelihood of delivering at term or later[22]. As a caveat, it should be noted that indicated preterm delivery was not excluded in some of these studies[21,22].

A second-trimester abortion is associated with an increased risk of preterm labor (14%), but one or two first-trimester abortions are not[18]. Three first-trimester abortions are associated with an increased risk of preterm labor (12%)[18].

Twenty per cent of the population-based risk for preterm birth is attributed to cigarette smoking. The incidence of cigarette smoking varies but may be as frequent as 33% in lower socioeconomic groups. This one factor is potentially modifiable and smoking cessation should be pursued.

It is difficult to assess the value of formal risk scoring, since it is never used alone but is combined with many antenatal management modalities. Many scores have been introduced, with claims of success based on historical controls. The most powerful tests of effectiveness and safety are randomized controlled trials, but these have not been carried out to the satisfaction of most. Randomized trials by Main and colleagues[13] and Mueller-Heubach and co-workers[23] have shown no

direct benefit of risk scoring to the patients enrolled, but the use of scoring does appear to make providers and patients more aware of the need for preterm birth prevention.

While risk scoring systems may identify a subset of patients at increased risk for preterm birth, most patients who actually deliver preterm cannot be identified by these methods. Furthermore, the false-positive rate is very high in those identified as being at high risk. As a rule, the positive predictive value of a high-risk score is less than 30%[24]. These concerns are important because most women so identified (70%) will nonetheless deliver at term, regardless of treatment. Accordingly, needless treatments and interventions may cause unnecessary anxiety and stress. There are significant costs and problems associated with initiating and maintaining surveillance and therapy in identified high-risk patients. Furthermore, limited resources may be allocated to populations where they are needed the least. If uterine activity *per se* becomes a significant risk factor for initiating therapy, then in some series up to 50% of all pregnancies would be subject to tocolytic therapy[25].

Despite the limitations of risk scoring for preterm birth and preterm labor, it is an inexpensive index that can be used to identify a group of patients that are at increased risk. Once identified, these women deserve a more intense work-up, ongoing medical supervision and individualized care. The simple act of telling a pregnant woman that she is 'at high risk' can operate as a preventive intervention. After being informed, such a woman may actually change her behavior (e.g. stop smoking, stop cocaine use) and thus decrease her risk status.

There is now a shift towards counselling all pregnant women regarding prevention of preterm labor by emphasizing preterm labor education and signs and symptoms at all prenatal visits.

What can be done to prevent preterm labor?

A number of additional approaches have been proposed to screen for preterm labor. These include evaluation of biochemical markers, clinical assessments of cervical status and monitoring of uterine activity.

Most biochemical markers including progesterone/ estrogen ratios, placental peptides such as corticotropin releasing hormone and mediators of inflammation such as cytokines. Metabolites from prostaglandin synthesis have no clinical utility in day-to-day practice. They are either not predictive of preterm labor or occur too late in the preterm labor state to initiate effective intervention.

Recent interest has centered on cervical vaginal secretions of fetal fibronectin as a predictor of preterm labor. In one study a positive test had a 46% predictive value for preterm birth, with a sensitivity of 93%. A negative test had a 94% predictive value of a term delivery[26]. The assay appears to be promising but its proper role in prenatal care has been neither clearly defined nor agreed upon.

HOME UTERINE ACTIVITY MONITORING

Obstetricians have long sought a way to diagnose preterm labor in its earliest stages, in the belief that early treatment is critically important. With the use of newly developed non-invasive sensing devices and computer technology, uterine activity in the second trimester and beyond can now be detected at home. It is hoped that such detection will decrease the frequency of preterm birth. The critical link here is the appropriateness of treatment interventions; specifically, the choice of intervention, route, timing, duration, efficacy, safety and cost.

Fundamental to the concept of home monitoring is provider-initiated contact, in addition to the standard approach of patient-initiated contact. The patient at risk is physically monitored at home with external tocodynamometers. The data are transmitted via telephone to a central viewing station, where the pattern of uterine activity is assessed by a nursing service. The service contacts the patient once or twice daily and prepares a detailed history on the patient's current status. If the service detects abnormalities, the physician is notified immediately. Further management depends on the circumstances.

The frequency of uterine activity is the principal variable monitored. Studies have shown that the mean frequency of uterine activity per hour rises with increasing gestation[27]. There is a further increase in frequency 24–48 h before the onset of true labor. The mean contraction frequency for women destined to have preterm labor is higher than for those who are not, but the overlap between these two groups is high, limiting its positive predictive value.

Some of these monitoring devices are extremely sensitive and cannot distinguish normal Braxton Hicks contractions from those of early labor. In one study only 10% of women correctly perceived their contractions more than half the time[28].

A few randomized and non-randomized trials have indicated that twice-daily monitoring of high-risk women, along with daily nursing support and high-quality obstetric care, may prevent preterm birth[26,27,29–31]. These studies do not clarify whether the effect is due to monitoring, to daily provider-initiated support, to the extended rest periods required for uterine activity monitoring, or to some combination thereof. Investigator bias may exist, since these studies cannot be blinded. Further, many patients who were enrolled but failed to use the service were often

Table 5 Chief symptoms of preterm labor

Abdominal pain
Back pain
Pelvic pain
'Gas pains'
Menstruation-like cramps
Vaginal bleeding
Pinkish staining
Increased vaginal discharge
Pelvic pressure
Urinary frequency
Diarrhea

excluded from evaluation[32]. Other studies have found no significant benefit[33].

Substantial controversy exists over whether there is sufficient evidence to warrant the routine use of home uterine activity monitoring in high-risk patients. Whereas early detection of cervical change is probable, serious flaws in research study design suggest that home monitoring lacks efficacy in preterm birth prevention. Delay in delivery rather than prevention of preterm birth as a benefit of home monitoring is closer to the truth.

Will these outpatient services for home monitoring of uterine activity become the new standard for high-risk obstetric care? The costs of these intensive services and the potential of inappropriate medical tocolysis and related complications must be weighed against the costs of current standards of care that include conscientious education programs by the physician's office and 24-h access to care. Although these services may be useful in a few circumstances, to date they are not considered to be the standard of care and are not fully endorsed by the American College of Obstetricians and Gynecologists.

CHIEF COMPLAINTS

A host of complaints may herald preterm labor (Table 5). Many of these symptoms are common in normal pregnancy and, unfortunately, are often dismissed by many prenatal care providers. Patients with preterm labor complained of both painful and painless contractions, backache, change in vaginal discharge, pelvic pressure and menstruation-like cramps, each independently in 40–50% of cases[34]. Normal women complained of the same individual symptoms as the preterm labor patient in 10–30% of cases.

In a study of outpatients at increased risk for preterm labor, Iams and co-workers[35] studied 51 patients who subsequently developed preterm labor. Only 67% were symptomatic. The initial evidence of preterm labor was symptoms without monitored contractions in 24%, monitored uterine activity without patient symptoms in 24%, both symptoms and monitored contractions in 43%, and 9% who were asymptomatic were discovered only when advanced cervical dilatation was found during routine cervical examination. The numbers in this study were small, and further research in this area is needed.

Vague constitutional symptoms may also presage preterm labor. A not uncommon set of complaints relates to painless uterine activity, described as 'balling up' or tightening of the uterus. Some complaints are misinterpreted and consequently incorrectly reported by the patient, thus misleading both physician and patient. These include gas pains, constipation and an increase in fetal movements, and may represent undiagnosed increases in rhythmic uterine activity. It is generally good practice to instruct patients, especially those at increased risk, about the importance of vague signs and symptoms of preterm labor. Patients experiencing these should be encouraged to contact the physician as soon as possible. This is especially true since the 'window of opportunity' for early initiation of tocolysis does not extend beyond 12–24 h before actual preterm labor[36].

CERVICAL DILATATION

Asymptomatic cervical dilatation may represent silent preterm labor, cervical incompetence, or a normal anatomical variation. In a general obstetric population, the frequency of preterm asymptomatic cervical dilatation increases as gestation advances. The frequency was evaluated in a large study by Papiernik and associates[37] (Table 6). Cervical dilatation also has been studied by others as a predictor for subsequent preterm birth[38–40]. In these studies the relative risk for developing preterm birth from cervical dilatation compared to an undilated cervix ranged from two- to four-fold, and the positive predictive value was < 30%.

Conversely, at least three previous reports emphasized that such dilatation is a normal anatomical variant, particularly in the multipara[41–43]. These studies showed no significant increase in the rate of preterm birth.

Some investigators have argued that some change in management is useful when a pregnant patient is found to have asymptomatic cervical dilatation at cervical examination. These options include monitoring uterine activity, performing more frequent surveillance, restricting activity, administering tocolytic agents and obtaining endocervical cultures.

Nonetheless, the results of a recently published large randomized controlled trial argue against the usefulness of routine cervical examination during prenatal care in a general obstetric population. These multinational investigators found no significant impact on the incidence of preterm birth, low birth weight, premature rupture of membranes, or perinatal mortality[44]. Notwithstanding the fact that data are sparse regarding its effectiveness, routine cervical examination and associated intervention options appear more reasonable if the patient has been previously identified as at high risk for preterm labor or cervical incompetence.

DIAGNOSIS

Accurately diagnosing preterm labor is difficult unless labor has obviously advanced beyond the point of successful long-term tocolysis. With this caveat in mind, preterm labor can be classified as threatened or actual. The basis for such a classification is the difference in prognosis. Approximately 85% of patients with threatened preterm labor will deliver at term, whereas 50% of patients in actual preterm labor will deliver at term.

The hallmark of threatened preterm labor is uterine activity. The diagnosis of threatened preterm labor is applied to the patient with uterine activity but no evidence of cervical changes. About 85% of patients with threatened preterm labor will deliver at term. In the past, many of these patients may have been diagnosed as having painful or painless Braxton Hicks contractions. The change in terminology is clinically important for placing the clinician 'on guard'. The recurrence rate of threatened preterm labor in the current pregnancy is about 30%; of these women, about half will deliver preterm[45].

Most often, patients with threatened preterm labor respond to simple conservative measures (bed rest, hydration, sedation, or limited doses of subcutaneous terbutaline). Less commonly, continuous infusion of a tocolytic agent may be required for unrelenting, significant uterine activity. The prognosis for a term delivery appears to be improved if preterm labor begins in the third trimester rather than in the second trimester.

During actual preterm labor (as diagnosed by Ingemarsson's criteria) about 20% (3/15) of placebo-treated patients delivered at term, compared to 80% (12/15) of terbutaline-treated patients[46]. These criteria were:

(1) Gestation of 28–36 weeks;
(2) Painful, regular uterine contractions, occurring at intervals of less than 10 min, for at least 30 min, by external tocography;

Table 6 Percentage of general obstetric patients with cervical dilatation of the internal os of > 1 cm

Gestation (weeks)	%	n	% Preterm birth
19–24	2.4	2124	17.3
25–28	4.4	2415	23.4
29–31	10.6	1750	21.6
32–34	12.4	2967	17.4
35–36	22.5	1921	11.1
37–38	32.8	2693	—

(3) Intact membranes; and

(4) Cervix effaced or almost effaced, dilated between 1 and 4 cm.

Patients with bleeding, uterine malformations, fever, multiple gestation and other known etiologies of preterm labor were excluded. All patients were given 10 mg of diazepam intramuscularly; if this had no obvious effect on contractions, treatment was continued with either terbutaline or placebo.

Creasy[47] modified the Ingemarsson criteria as follows:

(1) Gestation of 20 to 37 weeks;

(2) Documented uterine contractions (four in 20 min or eight in 60 min);

(3) Documented cervical change or cervical effacement of 80% or cervical dilatation of 2 cm; and

(4) Intact membranes.

These diagnostic criteria are well accepted for the nulliparous patient. There is general agreement that the same diagnostic criteria can be used for the multipara, but their prognostic values may be lessened.

Documenting cervical change requires serial documentation of cervical status, ideally by the same examiner. One method of determining cervical change is by noting changes in the Bishop score[48]. Dilatation of the internal cervical os and effacement of cervical length are most significant; other measures of change, such as consistency and position, seem to be inadequate for accurate diagnosis.

Fetal station, although not part of the diagnostic criteria for preterm labor, has prognostic value: the lower the station, the greater the risk of spontaneous preterm delivery. A patient who experiences a lower frequency of documented uterine contractions and who is known to have a high degree of cervical compliance based on the Bishop scoring criteria (e.g. Bishop score > 6) is at increased risk for premature delivery.

Many practitioners believe that, for tocolytic therapy to be most successful, it should be started before serial cervical change is documented. Therefore, many practitioners initiate tocolytic therapy as early as possible. However, a recent report by Utter and colleagues[49] disputes these beliefs. The authors compared the preterm delivery rates in 98 patients without serial cervical change before tocolysis (Group 1) and 75 patients with serial cervical change before tocolysis (Group 2). In comparing both groups, the outcome was not statistically different, with 40–50% of patients delivering at term. The authors concluded that, even with significant cervical dilatation, but of < 3 cm, observation was a reasonable alternative until subsequent uterine activity and cervical change could be determined. Thereafter, ritodrine tocolysis could be given without affecting its success rate.

Although these findings are interesting and highlight the problem of making an accurate diagnosis even at dilatations of 2 cm, it seems prudent to await confirmation from other centers before managing patients with preterm labor in such a manner, i.e. waiting for cervical change.

MANAGING PRETERM LABOR

Once the diagnosis of actual preterm labor is made, appropriate evaluations and initial management plans are instituted. The diagnostic evaluation has two major parts. In the first, the need for tocolytic therapy is assessed with attention focused on the specific nature of the agents to be used. The second part is an etiological diagnostic work-up.

During evaluation, the physician seeks contraindications to active prolonging of pregnancy. Absolute contraindications include fetal demise, lethal fetal anomaly, severe pre-eclampsia/eclampsia, severe hemorrhage and chorioamnionitis. Relative contraindications include abnormalities on fetal heart-rate monitoring, fetal growth retardation, mild pre-eclampsia, relatively stable late second-trimester and third-trimester bleeding, progressive structural but non-lethal fetal anomalies, significant maternal medical disease and cervical dilatation of 5 cm or more.

The lower limit for initiating tocolysis in a favorable candidate is about 17–20 weeks' gestation. As for the upper limits of fetal age and weight, differing opinions exist for appropriate tocolytic therapy. In 'uncomplicated' patients, some physicians initiate tocolytic therapy at 36 weeks' gestation and continue oral treatment until 37–38 weeks[50]. However, based on changes in the vascular intracranial anatomy and nursery performance for cardiovascular, pulmonary and gastrointestinal systems, there are few data to support an over aggressive tocolytic approach beyond the 34th week or an estimated fetal weight of 2000 g, particularly if fetal lung maturity is present.

Ideally, tocolysis should be withheld from patients with threatened preterm labor who resolve their uterine activity with conservative therapy. In these patients cervical evaluation for fetal fibronectin, and subtle anatomical changes found on digital and sonographic examinations may help exclude patients from the need for tocolysis. Conversely, tocolysis should be withheld from those in whom the choice of early delivery is clearly outweighed by the risk and lack of efficacy of tocolytic treatment. The fundamental issue is whether the risk of delivery outweighs the risk of prolonging the pregnancy by medical interventions.

During the initial evaluation period, some authors recommend performing microbiological cultures, urine toxicology and baseline maternal cardiac, hematological and electrolyte evaluations. While these test results are pending and both the maternal and fetal vital signs are deemed stable, a thorough ultrasound examination is performed to complete the evaluation.

Factors to be assessed are listed in Table 7. Many of these factors have a tremendous influence on clinical management. Accordingly, these sonographic findings will be discussed in greater detail (see below).

Once the necessity for therapy is determined, the choice of tocolytic agent is the next major decision. The physician must consider the mother's adrenergic and neuromuscular state, and the presence of comorbid conditions such as diabetes mellitus, heart disease, hypertension, renal disease, neuromuscular disease, or gastrointestinal disease. The physician should also consider the amniotic fluid status, fetal age and fetal structural status. These factors are discussed in greater detail later under the specific tocolytic agents. The physician must seek contraindications to β-sympathomimetic agents, including situations in which β-receptor stimulation is undesirable (i.e. New York Heart Association functional class 2 or higher cardiac disease, cardiac arrhythmias, severe hypertension, thyrotoxicosis, asymmetric septal hypertrophy, uncontrolled diabetes mellitus, neurological thromboembolic phenomenon). Contraindications to magnesium sulfate include myasthenia gravis, some cardiac rhythm disturbances, myocardial damage and severe renal disease. Contraindications to indomethacin include maternal peptic ulcer disease, maternal platelet dysfunction, fetal genitourinary disease, fetal

Table 7   Fetal and maternal assessment via sonography

Fetal evaluation
Fetal age, weight and growth status
Fetal life and fetal number
Fetal lie, presentation, position
Fetal well-being
Fetal behavior
Fetal anatomy and gender
Fetal blood sampling (funicentesis) for rapid karyotype, blood gases, disease-specific hematological profiles

Amniotic fluid evaluation
Polyhydramnios
Oligohydramnios
Amniocentesis for infection, fetal pulmonary maturation, fetal hemolysis

Placental and funic evaluation
Previa
Abruption
Marginal bleed with membrane separation
Location, internal anatomy, contour, thickness and grade
Umbilical cord insertion sites
Funic presentation

Uterine and cervical evaluation
Defective uterine scar
Uterine septum
Weak lower uterine segment
Cervical length
Cervical dilatation
Myomatous uterus

structural heart disease and fetal gestational age beyond 32–34 weeks.

Fetal age, weight and growth status

One of the most important determinations that must be made is that of gestational age. This usually has already been determined earlier during prenatal care. Of course, gestational age is not one true number but rather a range of numbers based on the best obstetric estimate. Sonography is often used to confirm optimal menstrual age or to be consistent with suboptimal menstrual age within a given number of days. At best, sonographic fetal age based on biometry is an estimate determined by the mean for a population of normally grown and uncomplicated fetuses. Dating by sonography alone in the third trimester is much less accurate, owing to increasing variation in fetal growth. Requirements for impeccability in timing of conception include basal body temperature, single or infrequent coitus, artificial insemination and *in vitro* fertilization. Most women who present in preterm labor, particularly at the lower limits of viability, do not have such a precisely timed gestational age. In this setting of borderline viability assessments (22–24 weeks), the acceptable range of error for sonographic imaging (10 days) encompasses the range from life to death, which in turn depends both on the biological status and on the willingness of the clinician to intervene on behalf of the fetus/neonate. Furthermore, some of these patients have had inadequate prenatal care, and therefore the gestational age has yet been assigned.

Routine fetal biometric measurements should be taken, including the biparietal diameter, head circumference, cephalic index, abdominal circumference and femur length. After the gestational age is determined or confirmed, fetal weight should be estimated. For practical purposes, at the bedside I recommend using fetal weight tables based on calculations from the formulae of Shepard or Hadlock[51,52].

Determination of weight also becomes a very important issue at the lower limits of viability. As in gestational age, estimating fetal weight by sonography carries with it inherent error. A 10% error in predicting birth weight is usually less than 75 g at the lower limits of viability. This is equivalent to ± 5 days of average fetal growth. Thus the fetal weight error is much less than the ± 10-day error of ultrasound-determined age. Furthermore, unlike gestational age, post-delivery birth weight is a reproducible number without a significant range of error; birth weight has significant prognostic value particularly for infants of < 1000 g[53]. Determining fetal weight is useful for predelivery counselling regarding prognosis, and at times may be superior to standard determinations of gestational age with regard to predictive value for survival.

The shape of the fetal head influences the accuracy of the biparietal diameter prediction of fetal age or weight. With dolichocephaly, age and weight are underestimated; with brachycephaly, overestimation may occur. Doubilet and Greenes[54] significantly improved their prediction of gestational age by using a formula to correct for the shape of the fetal head. Understanding these influences is especially critical to making management decisions near the lower limits of fetal viability (i.e. 22–24 weeks).

After age and weight are determined, intrauterine growth status should be assessed. Several investigators have suggested that fetal growth retardation is more common than expected in the setting of preterm labor[55,56]. The fetal length/abdominal circumference (FL/AC) ratio of $22 \pm 2\%$ between 21 and 42 weeks' gestation is constant and independent of gestational age[57,58]. Westgren and co-workers[59] found that 41% of infants who were delivered prematurely after failed tocolysis had an FL/AC ratio above 23.5 (indicating asymmetric growth restriction) compared to 5% of patients in preterm labor who responded well to tocolytic therapy.

The clinical relevance of finding fetal growth retardation is again of great importance to management at the lower limits of fetal viability (i.e. 22–26 weeks). In these situations sonographic measurements may erroneously underestimate fetal age secondary to suboptimal growth, and the infant may be erroneously declared previable. At the other end of the prematurity spectrum (32–36 weeks), it is not uncommon to find fetal pulmonary maturity when performing transabdominal amniocentesis. One explanation for the presumably 'accelerated' pulmonary phospholipid determinations may be that suboptimal fetal growth manifests as preterm labor.

Fetal demise

In patients with inadequate prenatal care, fetal demise and multiple gestation not uncommonly present as preterm labor. These entities are reliably verified with the use of ultrasound. Tocolytic therapy is contraindicated in fetal demise; labor is either allowed to proceed or augmented.

Fetal number

Multiple gestation results in preterm labor at least 12 times more often than in singleton pregnancies[60]. Moreover, patients with multiple gestations have higher rates of many other maternal and fetal complications that strongly influence decision making regarding preterm labor and delivery. Not uncommonly, multiple gestation is complicated by fetal malformation, polyhydramnios, or non-immune hydrops. The overall likelihood that a multiple gestation will be delivered before 37 weeks is about 40%[61].

In patients with multiple gestation, extreme care must be used when administering parenteral tocolytic therapy. When using either β-agonists or magnesium sulfate combined with fluid therapy, the risk of pulmonary edema is higher in multiple gestation than in singleton pregnancies. To prevent pulmonary edema, total fluid intake should be restricted to 2500 ml per 24 h of salt-poor (i.e. hypotonic) solutions.

Malpresentation

Fetal malpresentation is common in patients with preterm labor and delivery. The incidence of malpresentation is inversely related to gestational age. It is possible with sonography to detect not only fetal malpresentation but also associated uterine malformation, placental abnormality, polyhydramnios, oligohydramnios, or fetal abnormality. The index of suspicion for a fetal malformation or genetic syndrome must be raised because there is a higher incidence of fetal malformation in the preterm breech infant[62,63].

When faced with preterm delivery between 28 and 34 weeks of a singleton breech-presenting fetus in the absence of other clinically pertinent maternal or fetal complications, most maternal–fetal medicine subspecialists in the USA usually perform a Cesarean section, despite the fact that there is little scientific proof to justify this approach[64]. This is also true for the UK[65]. Cesarean section is recommended for breech-presenting fetuses estimated to weigh 750–1500 g with a gestational age of 26–32 weeks. Above 1500 g, there is little information demonstrating any significant advantage of Cesarean section for these infants. Below 750 g or less than 25 weeks' gestation, inherent fetal biology is thought to be a better predictor of survival than the delivery mode. Nonetheless, entrapment of the after-coming head by the incompletely dilated cervix does occur, and it is more likely to occur in infants born vaginally during the second trimester. Thus, individualization is necessary regarding delivery mode of the extremely preterm breech.

External cephalic version under ultrasound guidance should be considered in preparation for preterm delivery of the malpresenting infant to decrease the rate of Cesarean delivery. This technique is well described for the term or near-term infant and can be modified when preterm delivery of a malpresenting fetus is inevitable[66].

Fetal well-being

Fetal well-being in the course of preterm labor is most commonly assessed with the non-stress test. A classically reactive test is most widely defined as at least two accelerations of fetal heart rate of 15 beats per minute for 15 s during a 20-min monitoring period. If the criteria for activity are not met, the test is considered non-reactive; this is usually due to fetal sleep cycles, medication, or prematurity, especially less than 32 weeks' gestation. Once sleep cycles or drugs are eliminated, then further assessment of well-being is indicated.

Since the contraction stress test is contraindicated in the presence of preterm labor, the test of choice for further fetal evaluation is the biophysical profile. Fetal tone, movement, amniotic fluid volume and fetal breathing movements (FBM) all become normally manifest weeks before classical fetal heart reactivity[67]. In fact, all four of these sonographic parameters should be present by 20 weeks' gestation. Fetal oxygenation is sufficient if these four parameters are present, according to the criteria of Manning and co-workers[68], regardless of the absence of classical fetal heart rate reactivity.

Modifications of the classical criteria of a reactive non-stress test for the preterm fetus have been detailed by Castillo and colleagues[69]. With reactivity defined as three accelerations of 10 beats per minute, all fetuses tested at 26 weeks were reactive at the end of 60 min, and about 90% of the 24-week fetuses were reactive. If non-invasive data are contradictory with regard to fetal oxygenation status, particularly in fetuses at high risk for acidosis yet remote from term, funicentesis (percutaneous umbilical cord sampling) may be helpful in the optimal management of preterm labor and timing of delivery[70].

Fetal breathing movements

There seems to be a significant decrease in FBM during true labor. Several investigators have observed that absence of FBM may distinguish the patient in preterm labor destined to deliver within 2–7 days of diagnosis[71,72]. This prediction is most accurate in uncomplicated preterm labor without membrane rupture, antepartum hemorrhage, or multiple gestation, and without prior tocolytic therapy. The use of indomethacin for tocolysis has been associated with an increase in FBM, whereas magnesium sulfate has been associated with a decrease in FBM. How FBM can be applied to the management of preterm labor remains unclear, but in combination with other tests, FBM may help to distinguish true labor from false labor.

Fetal malformation

There is an increased incidence of fetal malformation in patients with preterm labor[73]. Often these patients have advanced preterm labor, spontaneous rupture of membranes, or vaginal bleeding. The rate of central nervous system malformation in patients born preterm is as high as 8/1000. Overall the relative risk of preterm birth in a pregnancy complicated with fetal malformation is two-fold. Rodeck[74] provided a succinct review of fetal abnormality in relation to preterm labor.

It is important to perform a complete fetal malformation screen in preterm labor and delivery. If sonographic evidence suggests a strong possibility of aneuploidy, then a fetal karyotype may be useful for optimal medical and obstetric management of labor, mode of delivery, place of delivery and neonatal resuscitation[75].

The rapidity of a karyotypic determination depends on the clinical exigencies; time is one factor influencing the decision for amniocentesis vs. funicentesis. Blood karyotype results can be obtained within 48 h, whereas with amniotic fluid karyotype results may require 7–10 days. Trisomy 18, trisomy 13 and triploidy are considered lethal chromosomal abnormalities in which heroic medical interventions are not warranted. Cesarean section for fetal indication in these aneuploid fetuses is considered unwarranted. Accordingly, if a virtually lethal chromosomal constitution is discovered, then management should focus on the mother's safety. Tocolytic therapy should be discontinued. Non-aggressive management of the fetus/neonate that is consistent with ethical guidelines for a given institution should be considered.

Polyhydramnios

Polyhydramnios is an uncommon but important cause of preterm labor owing to uterine overdistension. The classical diagnosis is suspected when uterine enlargement is greater than expected for gestational age. Clinically, there is usually difficulty in palpating fetal parts. Occasionally, the uterine wall is exceedingly tense and tender. Maternal respiratory compromise and maternal postrenal obstruction may result from massive uterine overdistension. As much as 40% of patients with clinically evident polyhydramnios experience preterm labor and delivery[76]. Sonography is used to confirm the diagnosis, to help determine the proximate cause and to guide therapeutic mechanical relief via reduction amniocentesis. Sonographic confirmation of the diagnosis is best made subjectively by an experienced observer. Unfortunately, there is a significant number of sonographers who make incidental diagnoses of polyhydramnios based on measured criteria, such as amniotic fluid index. This population has a much milder form of the amniotic fluid abnormality. Accordingly, in these milder cases, the incidence of preterm labor and delivery will approximate 19% of patients. Furthermore, the incidence of structural fetal abnormalities will also be decreased[77].

The proximate cause is then determined; causes may be maternal, fetal, placental, or a combination of these. In some series about 60% of cases are idiopathic[78]. Maternal causes include diabetes mellitus and red cell alloimmunization (anti-D, anti-Kell, etc.). These entities are readily excluded by laboratory tests.

Fetal etiologies include complicated multiple gestation, non-immune hydrops and structural congenital malformation. Up to 75% of singleton pregnancies with non-immune hydrops have associated polyhydramnios.

Fetal congenital malformations occur in up to 50% of cases with polyhydramnios. Fetal malformations were found in 75% of cases with severe polyhydramnios, compared to a 29% rate of fetal abnormality in mild cases[78].

Central nervous system defects account for about 45–50% of all fetal malformations. Upper gastrointestinal defects represent about 30% of associated malformations. The latter category of defects present later in gestation than do central nervous system defects. Circulatory abnormalities, accounting for about 7% of fetal abnormalities, include coarctation of the aorta, interruption of the fetal aorta, cardiac arrhythmias (primarily supraventricular tachyarrhythmias) and myocardial disorders. Miscellaneous disorders, which may account for 18% of malformations, include congenital chylothorax, pancreatic cysts, asphyxiating thoracic dystrophy, thanatophoric dwarfism, other short-limb dwarfisms, trisomies 18 and 21, cystic hygroma and sacrococcygeal, cervical, or mediastinal teratomas.

One placental cause of polyhydramnios is a large chorioangioma, a benign vascular malformation that acts like an arteriovenous shunt. Tumors large enough to produce polyhydramnios and preterm labor are rare. They are usually circumscribed, solid or complex masses protruding from the fetal surface of the placenta and are larger than 5 cm when associated with fetal hydrops[79].

Oligohydramnios

Oligohydramnios is diagnosed easily with ultrasound as a significant reduction in amniotic fluid volume. In the setting of preterm labor this may be due to premature rupture of the membranes, severe intrauterine growth retardation, or a genitourinary malformation in which fetal urination into the amniotic cavity is absent. Serial sonography and invasive procedures allow for differentiation among the etiologies.

The diagnosis of lethal renal diseases is important, since many of these cases may present with fetal distress or malpresentation during preterm labor. About 60% of patients with Potter's syndrome develop preterm labor, and 40–60% are in the breech presentation[80]. In these situations, tocolysis and Cesarean section for fetal indication are not warranted.

Fetal gender

Fetal gender has important prognostic and practical significance. Although not 100% accurate, this parameter is easily determined in most instances with ultrasound. Female fetuses have been found to benefit from the use of antenatal dexamethasone to reduce the incidence of respiratory distress syndrome[81]. This view has been recently questioned on the basis of meta-analysis of data from multiple studies. By regression analysis,

Fleisher and co-workers[82] found that the lecithin/sphingomyelin (L/S) ratio in females reached 2 : 1 at 33.7 weeks, 1.4 weeks earlier than in males. Phosphatidylglycerol first appeared at 34 weeks for females and at 35 weeks for males. The female infant has a significant survival advantage, particularly if her birth weight is 1000 g or more[53].

When funicentesis is done to assist in fetal diagnosis, knowing that the fetus is male allows the laboratory to distinguish fetal cells from maternal cells when there is maternal contamination. This is especially important when a rapid karyotype is indicated or a 100% pure fetal sample is required.

Amniocentesis and neonatal outcome

Amniocentesis in experienced hands carries minimal risk in the late second trimester or third trimester. Leigh and Garite[83] used amniocentesis during idiopathic preterm labor to detect subclinical infection and fetal pulmonary maturity and found that 12% had positive cultures. These colonized patients presented at earlier gestational ages and were more likely to rupture membranes and to deliver within 48 h of admission than those with negative cultures. One-third of the patients at 31–32 weeks and 50% of those at 33 weeks or more had mature L/S ratios.

In review of 11 studies of transabdominal amniocentesis in patients with preterm labor and intact membranes, Romero and Mazor[15] found a positive culture rate of 16%. In the patients with positive cultures, clinical chorioamnionitis occurred in 58%, refractoriness to tocolysis in 65% and membrane rupture in 40%. The respective rates of these complications for the patients with negative cultures were 7%, 16% and 4%. Although a large percentage of the microbes recovered were anaerobic, neonates rarely developed significant anaerobic infections.

The appropriate management of patients with positive intra-amniotic cultures remains controversial. Some regimens include antibiotics and immediate delivery, but in other regimens the fetus is delivered only when there is frank clinical evidence of infection, particularly if the fetus is 28 weeks or younger. If there is no evidence of intra-amniotic infection, there is documented significant immaturity (i.e. L/S ratio of < 1.5) and there is a significant risk of delivery between 24 h and 1 week, then it is reasonable to give a course of betamethasone 12 mg intramuscularly twice, 24 h apart. In these situations aggressive tocolytic therapy is reasonable if the fetus is less than 35 weeks' gestation. In contrast, if the L/S ratio is 2:1 or higher, phosphatidylglycerol is present, or there is a positive shake test, some authors are not as aggressive, because the benefit of tocolysis does not seem to outweigh the risk.

We recently analyzed neonatal morbidity in infants born with mature amniotic fluid tests[84] (Table 8). The mothers presented with spontaneous preterm labor and were potential candidates for tocolytic therapy. In view of the pulmonary maturity, tocolytic agents were discontinued in many patients. Entry criteria were singleton gestation, transabdominal amniocentesis, uncontaminated amniotic fluid, delivery within 72 h of amniocentesis and absence of antenatal steroids, diabetes mellitus and significant malformations. We found that despite 'pulmonary maturity', respiratory distress and other morbidities still occurred as an inverse function of gestational age. Hence, prolongation of pregnancy should still be attempted even in the presence of mature amniotic fluid indices. It should be noted that none of the infants had significant respiratory distress at 34 weeks or more. Wigton and colleagues[85] confirmed our findings regarding the high false mature rate of pulmonary maturity tests in preterm gestations. They also demonstrated that neonatal morbidity is inversely related to gestational age despite pulmonary maturity test results.

A somewhat similar study of neonatal morbidity by Konte and colleagues[86], but excluding amniocentesis data, found a similar inverse relationship between neonatal morbidity and gestational age (Table 9). It should be noted that 23% of the patients at 34 weeks' gestation had significant respiratory distress; this is consistent with the fact that pulmonary maturity was not present and emphasizes the usefulness and predictive value of amniocentesis at this gestational age.

Therefore, one need not be over aggressive in the treatment of preterm labor at 34 weeks if the L/S ratio is mature; nor should one be over aggressive with tocolytic agents at 35–36 weeks when the L/S ratio is unknown.

Uterine malformation

Premature labor occurs in about 25% of pregnancies complicated by structural uterine malformations[87]. The patients with complete bicornuate uteri had the highest incidence of preterm labor (66%), but the number of such patients studied was small (n = 6). Didelphis and all varieties of bicornuate uteri were associated with an incidence of preterm labor that was above 20%. Preterm labor occurred in 10.3–37.5% of patients with unicornuate uteri[88]. Patients with the complete septate uterus had the best fetal survival rate (86%); those with the complete bicornuate uterus (50%) and unicornuate uterus (40%) had the worst.

Unfortunately, uterine anomalies are often not recognized until patients have obstetric or gynecological problems. In cases of uterine anomalies, associated cervical incompetence, malpresentation and preterm labor are not uncommon; therefore, uterine malformation may be suspected when associated obstetric problems arise. We recommend intrauterine exploration after delivery, whether vaginal or Cesarean, to

Table 8 Neonatal morbidity in infants born with mature amniotic fluid tests. From reference 84, with permission

	Gestation (weeks)			
	< 33 (n = 15)	*33 (n = 13)*	*34 (n = 19)*	*35–36 (n = 35)*
Respiratory distress	7 (47%)	2 (15%)	0	0
Air leak	2 (13%)	1 (8%)	0	0
Necrotizing enterocolitis	1 (7%)	3 (23%)	0	0
Intraventricular hemorrhage	4 (27%)	1 (8%)	2 (11%)	0
Sepsis	7 (47%)	2 (15%)	0	0
Blood transfusion	8 (53%)	4 (31%)	2 (11%)	1 (3%)
Total parenteral nutrition	8 (53%)	5 (39%)	1 (5%)	1 (3%)
Mean (± SD) birth weight (g)	1563 ± 489	1925 ± 283	2177 ± 259	2442 ± 333

Table 9 Neonatal morbidity rates by gestational age at birth. Percentages (in parentheses) are rounded to the nearest per cent. From reference 86, with permission

	Gestational age (weeks)					
Complication	*26–27 (n = 16)*	*28–29 (n = 32)*	*30–31 (n = 33)*	*32–33 (n = 44)*	*34 (n = 40)*	*35 (n = 36)*
Intensive care nursery	16 (100)	32 (100)	31 (94)	40 (91)	29 (73)	8 (22)
Respiratory distress syndrome	13 (81)	19 (59)	10 (30)	13 (30)	9 (23)	1 (3)
Patent ductus arteriosus	8 (50)	16 (50)	7 (21)	6 (14)	5 (13)	—
Sepsis	5 (31)	8 (25)	5 (15)	3 (7)	2 (5)	2 (6)
Intraventricular hemorrhage	5 (31)	4 (13)	1 (3)	—	—	—
Necrotizing enterocolitis	4 (29)	2 (6)	2 (6)	1 (2)	—	—

Table 10 Hospital survival of extremely low birth weight infants (survivors/live births). Percentages shown in parentheses

Reference (see reference 89 for specific citation)	Year of birth	Gestation (weeks) 23	24	25	26
Milligan *et al.*	1979–82	1/7 (14)	9/23 (39)	28/44 (64)	34/45 (76)
Kitchen *et al.*	1977–82	—	2/27 (7)	11/54 (20)	36/80 (45)
Yu *et al.*	1977–84	2/28 (7)	13/40 (33)	11/44 (25)	36/62 (58)
Amon *et al.*	1981–85	5/73 (7)*	7/63 (11)	31/66 (47)	32/88 (36)
Dillon and Egan	1977–80	—	4/11 (36)	6/16 (38)	11/18 (61)
Herschel *et al.*	1977–80	—	2/7 (29)	3/28 (11)	17/38 (45)
†Amon *et al.*	1986–92	17/59 (29)	20/43 (47)	14/29 (48)	18/25 (72)
†Hack *et al.*	1989–90	(15)	(54)	(59)	(71)

* All infants thought to be 22 or 23 weeks' gestation are combined
† Modified from reference 89, by adding data from references 2 and 3

exclude any palpable intrauterine malformations. Likewise, in cases of known uterine anomalies or exposure to maternal diethylstilbestrol, there must be a high index of suspicion for the future development of associated problems.

Management decisions at the lower end of viability

Managing preterm delivery at the lower limits of viability – currently 22–24 weeks' gestation – is a vexing problem. The *a priori* determination of viability for a severely preterm yet normally formed fetus requiring delivery remains a statistical, not an absolute, concept. Biological and clinical variables associated with obstetric and neonatal management that favorably influence neonatal outcome have been reviewed[6,53,89–92]. It is optimal in such cases for delivery to occur in immediate proximity to a neonatal intensive-care center[93]. When conditions permit, decisions regarding delivery of a severely preterm fetus (i.e. 22–26 weeks' gestation by best obstetric estimate) are ideally made after the mother is transported to a tertiary-care center with experienced pediatric and obstetric specialists[89]. At these gestational ages, opinions about management differ among obstetric specialists and among neonatologists[94–96]. Therefore, co-ordinated predelivery family counselling by obstetricians and neonatal physicians is recommended to discuss the prognosis and to plan the management, thereby minimizing anxiety, confusion and fear[89].

A highly individualized, thoughtful, thorough and compassionate approach to the patient is required. Survival rates as a function of gestational age and birth weight are shown in Tables 10 and 11[2,3]. Literature reviews have found that subsequent serious handicap rates in severely preterm survivors are about 20–30%[6,8,94,97]. Conversely, of all extremely LBW non-survivors, 70–80% die in the first week of postnatal life, most in the first few days[89,98]. Cesarean section for fetal distress is performed by about 40% of

maternal–fetal medicine specialists, beginning at 24 weeks' gestation[95].

Due to inherent inaccuracies in estimating fetal age and weight, thoughtful consideration on behalf of the fetus should begin between 22 and 23 weeks' gestation and 450–500 g. Since the likelihood for survival in these instances is dismal (i.e. < 5% to 10%), Cesarean section for fetal indications is best avoided. Survival, if it occurs, will generally occur regardless of the delivery mode. To protect the mother from undue risk of Cesarean section for little potential benefit for the newborn, everything short of major surgery (i.e. Cesarean section) should be offered to the mother. These measures include transfer to a tertiary-care center, family counselling, standard hydration, fetal monitoring, maternal positioning, maternal oxygenation, controlled sterile delivery and the presence of a neonatologist at delivery. Newer measures include transcervical amnioinfusion and acute tocolysis for uterine relaxation[99–101]. These therapies are based on the view that mortality and significant handicap rates will increase without optimal therapy.

Table 11 Survival rates* (%) of incredibly low birth weight infants (inborn deliveries only), including those with birth defects. Survival = discharge home alive

Birth weight (g)	Amon *et al.* St Louis University 1986–1992 (reference 2) (n = 156)	Hack *et al.* Multicenter NIH Neonatal network 1989–1990 (reference 3) (n = 329)*
500–750	69/156 (44%)	(39%)
500–599	14/55 (25%)	(20%)
600–699	33/64 (52%)	(41%)
700–750	22/37 (59%)	
701–800		(65%)

* These 329 patients are those with birth weights of 500–750 g only. Data should be compared to those of Amon (reference 89) to note how survival has improved over the past decade

Tocolytic agents

In the last four decades, a host of drugs has been used in the attempt to inhibit preterm labor, including relaxing β-sympathomimetic agents, ethanol, prostaglandin synthetase inhibitors, organic calcium-channel blockers, magnesium sulfate, diazoxide, aminophylline, progestagens and most recently oxytocin analogs that block oxytocin receptors. Many of these agents showed high success rates initially, but subsequently reports showed reduced, somewhat limited efficacy.

Several fundamental issues must be addressed in a discussion of tocolytic treatment for preterm labor. First, can actual preterm labor be accurately diagnosed and distinguished from threatened preterm labor? Second, although uterine activity may be abolished or minimized by treatment, does this really prolong pregnancy, and is this treatment successful? Different studies have defined success rates differently.

Third, and most importantly, what effect does successful tocolytic treatment have on perinatal outcome? Substantive improvement in perinatal outcome should be defined as real reductions in mortality, morbidity and cost of care; unfortunately, the success of most agents is defined in terms of pregnancy prolongation rather than on substantive reduction of morbidity and mortality. Neonatal mortality beyond 32 weeks' gestation in the normally formed infant is minimal and hence is no longer a significant issue. Nonetheless, morbidity remains a significant issue at all preterm gestational ages. The mortality focus now centers on late second-trimester and early third-trimester pregnancies. Although pregnancy may be prolonged to some extent in most studies, actual substantive effects on improved perinatal outcome are lacking.

The final question is whether the mother and fetus should be exposed to potentially significant side-effects, and if so, to what extent? Tocolytic agents are commonly used without a universal acclamation that they should be used. Psychologically, it is very difficult for the practitioner not to treat the patient, and it is difficult for the patient to go to a practitioner who does not treat her.

β-Sympathomimetic agents

β$_1$-Receptors predominate in the heart, small intestine and adipose tissue; β$_2$-receptors predominate in the uterus, blood vessels, bronchioles and liver. Some agents (e.g. ritodrine) have been publicized as having selective β$_2$ activity[102]. β$_2$-selective sympathomimetic amines are structurally related to catecholamines and stimulate all β-receptors throughout the entire body. With continued use, tachyphylaxis is noted[103].

The side-effects of these agents represent an exaggeration of their physiological effects. In the cardiovascular system, there is a decrease in diastolic blood pressure and tachycardia, an increase in cardiac output and a tendency towards arrhythmogenesis[104]. Chest pain not uncommonly occurs with parenteral administration. These drugs increase oxygen demand and decrease coronary artery perfusion. They may cause myocardial ischemia. There may be transient ST segment depression that resolves with discontinuation of drug therapy. These clinical and electrocardiogram findings may relate directly to drug therapy or indirectly to electrolyte disturbance *per se* rather than to ischemia[105].

Pulmonary edema may occur in a small percentage of patients treated with parenteral β-sympathomimetic agents[104]. This life-threatening complication has several predisposing factors: multiple gestation, a positive fluid balance, blood transfusion, anemia, infection, associated hypertension, polyhydramnios and underlying cardiac disease. Ritodrine causes the retention of salt and water at the level of the kidney[106]. Plasma volume expands and the hematocrit drops by 10–15%[107]. Considering that most side-effects contribute to increases in cardiac output, it is surprising that more patients do not develop pulmonary edema. These findings highlight the importance of refraining from the use of isotonic fluids throughout ritodrine therapy. In the past, antenatal steroids, such as betamethasone, were implicated in the genesis of pulmonary edema, but since betamethasone and dexamethasone are almost devoid of mineralocorticoid activity, they are most probably innocent bystanders.

Maternal mortality has been reported with the use of these agents[108]. From an anonymous survey of American obstetricians, it appears that the maternal mortality related to tocolytic agents has been under-reported[109].

Metabolic complications, such as hypokalemia due to increases in glucose and insulin, hyperglycemia due to glucagon stimulation and glycogenolysis, and an increase in free fatty acids due to lipolysis, are common with intravenous therapy. Less common are lactic acidosis and ketosis[110]. Occasionally there have been cases of diabetic ketoacidosis[111]. Once the patient is switched to oral therapy, it appears that ritodrine has less effect on glucose intolerance than does oral terbutaline[112].

The effects on uteroplacental profusion are controversial: some studies show an increase, others a decrease[113,114]. The primary effects on the neonate have been limited to hypoglycemia[115]. Apgar scores have not been significantly affected. Long-term follow-up studies have revealed no significant problems in child development[116].

Ritodrine

Initial favorable reports in 1980 by Barden, Merkatz and Peter[117,118] promulgated the clinical use of ritodrine in the USA. Ritodrine became the first drug approved in the USA by the Food and Drug Administration (FDA) for the inhibition of preterm labor. It was reported to have similar efficacy but fewer side-effects than previously used tocolytic agents. Generally, the side-effects were thought to be acceptable. There was evidence that it prolonged pregnancy. More importantly, when compared with controls, there was a significant reduction in the incidence of neonatal death and respiratory distress syndrome[118].

A subsequent meta-analysis of ritodrine efficacy was performed on 890 women who participated in 16 scientifically acceptable controlled trials[119]. There were significantly fewer deliveries in the β-mimetic group during the first 24 and 48 h of therapy. There was a slight reduction in the percentage of preterm delivery in the group receiving β-mimetic therapy. However, there was no significant reduction in the incidence of LBW infants, respiratory distress morbidity, or perinatal mortality. The lack of any suggestion of effect on substantive outcome challenges the previous claims that had favored such drug therapy. It has been suggested that the increased cost of intensive tocolysis beyond 34 weeks' gestation is offset by the decreased cost of neonatal intensive care[120].

Furthermore, a more recent large, randomized, placebo-controlled, multicenter trial demonstrated that ritodrine was associated with a significant reduction in the proportion of women delivering within 48 h of treatment. This study, however, failed to find any significant beneficial effect on perinatal mortality, frequency of preterm delivery, or birth weight[121].

If ritodrine infusions are used, they should be given according to the guidelines in the manufacturer's package insert, or based on Caritis's method[117,122]. Attention should be paid to contraindications, maternal tachycardia, diabetic status and fluid balance. Some physicians give ritodrine intramuscularly[123]. It is thought that there are fewer side-effects when ritodrine is infused according to the method of Caritis or given intramuscularly, as opposed to the 'Barden protocol' approved by the FDA. Additional precautions to reduce risk include exclusion of congenital heart disease, use of small volumes of fluid, reduction of dosages once uterine activity is controlled, regular monitoring of all vital signs, intake and output, electrolytes, glucose and an electrocardiogram.

To date, β-sympathomimetic agents have not been shown to be effective when given as a prophylactic treatment. They may have some beneficial effect when administered as maintenance after the apparent successful treatment of preterm labor, reducing the number of recurrences. However, there is no evidence that they will affect the incidence of preterm birth. In fact, the lack of efficacy of oral terbutaline has been confirmed, even in dosages sufficient to maintain maternal heart rate above 100 beats per min[124].

Terbutaline

Terbutaline is commonly used in the initial management of preterm labor. At first, its efficacy was thought to be quite significant, but subsequent studies have found that it has only limited efficacy[46,125,126]. Terbutaline has significant, potentially life-threatening side-effects similar to those of ritodrine, especially when given intravenously[127].

An alternative route is subcutaneous administration: the drug effect is rapid and apparently has fewer side-effects[128]. The ease of administration and the avoidance of intravenous hydration makes subcutaneous use a reasonable alternative. In a commonly used regimen, 0.25 mg is given subcutaneously every 20–60 min until contractions have subsided. Close attention is paid to the maternal heart rate and symptoms, to prevent serious complications. Oral administration of terbutaline results in widely varying serum concentrations. The common daily dose ranges from 10 to 30 mg; the maximum daily dose is about 40 mg.

A recent development in terbutaline administration is the use of the continuous subcutaneous infusion pump. Although significant efficacy is claimed, this type of home therapy is very expensive. More data are required before this therapy can be unequivocally advocated.

In general, there seems to be no significant difference in efficacy or safety between terbutaline and ritodrine. Oral terbutaline does cause significant alterations in maternal glucose tolerance, compared to oral ritodrine administration. However, terbutaline is much less expensive[112].

FDA approval   There is confusion among many clinicians regarding the meaning of FDA approval of a drug. The FDA does not and cannot dictate specific medical practice regarding the use of a drug. The FDA approves drugs to be marketed in the USA by pharmaceutical companies for very specific and labelled medical indications. Without this approval, the medication cannot be commercially available to the practitioner. However, once a medication is approved to be marketed and labelled for specific indications, it becomes readily available for general clinical use.

The exact clinical use of a medication must then be determined by the prescribing physician. In fact, the FDA acknowledges that it is appropriate and rational to use a drug for unlabelled indications when such drug therapy has been extensively reported in the literature[129]. For example, the safe and effective use of terbutaline and magnesium sulfate as tocolytic agents has been reported in such a manner.

Since there is a significant database and clinical experience with the use of terbutaline, FDA approval of the specific indication of tocolysis is unnecessary for its continued use in the medical community in the USA.

Prostaglandin synthetase inhibitors

Prostaglandin synthetase inhibitors are among the most effective drugs known for inhibiting preterm labor. They are easily administered and well tolerated by the mother. However, the limiting factor is fetal safety[130].

Maternal side-effects are minimal and include primarily gastrointestinal upset, which may require the use of Maalox®. Indomethacin is contraindicated in patients with hematological dysfunction, peptic ulcer disease and known allergy. Indomethacin does not significantly affect uteroplacental perfusion or Apgar scores.

The most significant potential complications in the fetus are the premature closure of the ductus arteriosus, right-sided heart failure and fetal death[131,132]. Prostaglandin E series allow for the ductus arteriosus to remain patent, but indomethacin in the early third trimester tends to constrict the fetal ductus transiently[133]. It is more likely to close the ductus irreversibly when it is given at a later gestational age, closer to the time of physiological closure.

In the neonate the most feared complication is persistent pulmonary hypertension[131,132]. Fetal and neonatal oliguria is not uncommon[134–136]; in fact, idiopathic polyhydramnios may be treated effectively with indomethacin[137]. Sonographic surveillance for oligohydramnios is indicated when indomethacin is used for 48 h. There are case reports of bowel perforation[138]. Recent analyses have found that very preterm infants delivered after recent exposure to indomethacin experienced significantly more intracranial hemorrhage and necrotizing enterocolitis when compared to gestational age-matched controls. Hyperbilirubinemia may occur, because indomethacin may displace bilirubin from the binding sites of albumin.

Since there is potential for substantial side-effects to the preterm fetus or neonate, the benefits and risks of treatment should be carefully evaluated. Prostaglandin synthetase inhibitors are effective, easily administered and well tolerated by the mother. Many patients respond to 100 mg administered rectally followed by 25 mg orally every 6 h. The daily dose ranges from 100 to 200 mg. Nonetheless, these agents must be used only with proper precautions to minimize fetal and neonatal effects. These include very short courses of therapy (24–48 h) in patients of less than 34 weeks' gestation.

Since there is a significant database and clinical experience with indomethacin, FDA approval is unnecessary for its use in the USA. Its use must be carefully supervised to minimize life-threatening perinatal complications; this may require consultation with maternal–fetal medicine subspecialists and serial sonographic evaluation of the fetus.

Magnesium sulfate

Magnesium sulfate is a commonly prescribed parenteral agent in the USA for tocolytic therapy. Recent evidence and clinical experience favor magnesium over β-sympathomimetics with regard to safety without compromising tocolytic efficacy[139].

The clinical use of magnesium sulfate has several advantages. American obstetricians have extensive experience with it in patients with pre-eclampsia/eclampsia. Properly used, magnesium sulfate is safe for both tocolysis and seizure prophylaxis. Most clinicians monitor reflexes, respiration, urine output and intermittent serum magnesium levels to prevent serious complications of hypermagnesemia. A diminished glomerular filtration rate decreases the excretion of magnesium and continued administration of parenteral magnesium sulfate may result in toxicity as serum levels rise. Fortunately, an antidote is available. Intravenous injection of calcium gluconate or chloride rapidly antagonizes the actions of excessive magnesium.

Pharmacology Oral magnesium is absorbed in the upper small bowel by an active process. Only 30% of normal daily intake is absorbed. The recommended dietary allowance of magnesium by the National Research Council for pregnant women is 450 mg daily. Dietary sources of magnesium are meat, milk, dark-green vegetables, seafood and chocolate. Oral preparations readily available in the USA and currently used in pregnant women are the gluconate and oxide salts of magnesium, although other varieties exist. The kidney is the major regulator of the serum magnesium concentration, since magnesium is almost totally excreted in the urine[140].

The mechanism by which hypermagnesemia exerts its relaxant effects on smooth muscle differs from that of skeletal muscle. Smooth muscle undergoes pharmacomechanical coupling mediated by various agonists rather than the electromechanical coupling characteristic of skeletal muscle. Excess magnesium depresses the peripheral neuromuscular system in three ways: the inhibition of acetylcholine release, the reduction of sensitivity of the motor endplate and the reduction of the amplitude of the motor endplate potential. Acetylcholine is unnecessary for spontaneous contractility of smooth muscle.

The exact mechanism by which magnesium diminishes or abolishes uterine activity remains unclear. Experimental data support the view that the extracellular magnesium ion concentration affects the uptake, binding and distribution of intermolecular calcium in vascular smooth muscle. Similar mechanisms may operate in gravid uterine smooth muscle.

It has been noted that magnesium sulfate in an extracellular concentration of 9.6–12.0 mg/dl (1.0 mEq/l = 1.2 mg/dl) almost completely inhibits spontaneous uterine contractility in muscle strips excised from pregnant women[141]. This inhibition is dose-related. The duration of labor is longer in pre-eclamptic patients receiving high doses of parenteral magnesium sulfate compared to those receiving low doses.

In general, drug-induced maternal hypermagnesemia is associated with increased urinary excretion of both magnesium and calcium. Three-quarters of the elemental magnesium infused is excreted during the infusion and 90% by 24 h after the end of the infusion[142]. The urinary excretion of calcium is increased three-fold. The mean total maternal serum calcium decreased by 12% and the mean serum ionized calcium decreased by 25%. Acutely, phosphate and calcitonin levels did not change significantly, but the mean parathyroid hormone level increased by about 25% from baseline to the end of the infusion. However, there are observed increases in maternal serum phosphate with longer-term (> 1 week) chronic intravenous magnesium sulfate therapy for tocolysis.

Maternal side-effects   Table 12 summarizes the major maternal clinical side-effects of maternal hypermagnesemia. The loss of patellar reflexes has been reported

Table 12   Potential maternal effects of hypermagnesemia

Common side-effects
Loss of deep tendon reflexes
Warmth during infusion
Mild central hypothermic effects
Increase in skin temperature
Cutaneous vasodilatation
Nausea, possible emesis

Not uncommon side-effects (seen with moderately elevated serum levels)
Somnolence, lethargy, lightheadedness
Visual blurring, diplopia
Dysarthria
Nystagmus
Constipation and dyspepsia

Uncommon side-effects
Potentiation of other neuromuscular blockers
Lengthening of the P-R and QRS interval
Controversial effect on the T wave
Chest pain
Pulmonary edema

Effects seen at very high serum concentrations
Respiratory depression
Cardiac arrest
Profound muscular paralysis
Amnesia
Decreased rate of impulse formation of the S-A node

Rare side-effects
Profound hypotension
Maternal tetany
Hypersensitivity urticarial reaction
Paralytic ileus

at magnesium concentrations of 8.4–12.0 mg/dl (7–10 mEq/l) and respiratory depression begins at levels of 12–14.4 mg/dl (10–12 mEq/l)[143]. Clinically, respiratory depression from hypermagnesemia does not occur before the disappearance of the deep tendon reflexes. The absence of the reflex arc should serve as a warning sign of impending magnesium toxicity, but this sign is of no value in those few patients who inadvertently receive high doses of magnesium intravenously over a short period (usually as the result of a dosing mistake). The initial clinical presentation may be respiratory or cardiac arrest[144].

Somnolence, drowsiness, lightheadedness and visual blurring occasionally occur at therapeutic concentrations during the usual period (12–72 h) of standard tocolytic therapy. Signs and symptoms of 'apparent' depression of the central nervous system and respiratory effort may be potentiated by the use of other depressant agents, particularly at high magnesium concentrations.

Various side-effects – primarily neuromuscular or gastrointestinal – have been observed during clinical trials of magnesium sulfate as a tocolytic agent[145,146]. During prolonged therapy, psychological effects secondary to prolonged hospitalization may become prominent[147].

During initial magnesium sulfate infusion of 4–6 g over 20–30 min, the acute effects in patients with preterm labor are similar to those observed in patients receiving an intravenous loading dose for pre-eclampsia. Early in the intravenous infusion, perspiration and flushing are observed and the patient feels warm; this finding continues more or less throughout the infusion. The face, neck and hands are particularly affected, and a rise in skin temperature is easily demonstrated. These manifestations occur in both hypertensive and normotensive patients. The intensity of the effect is in part rate-related. Excessive magnesium causes vasodilatation by direct action on blood vessels and ganglionic blockade. Nausea and possibly emesis may occur.

During maintenance therapy, lethargy, somnolence, diplopia, dysarthria, blurred vision, dry mouth, dizziness and nystagmus may occur. These effects generally occur at a dose of more than 2 g/h (2.5–4.0 g/h). Reducing the rate in half-gram increments is generally all that is needed; discontinuation of therapy for side-effects is rarely needed. If necessary, intravenous injection of 1 g calcium gluconate will result in rapid symptomatic relief. During long-term magnesium sulfate infusion therapy which includes bed rest, constipation and dyspepsia may occur and can be symptomatically treated.

One of the most important side-effects encountered during standard tocolytic therapy with magnesium sulfate is chest pain, possibly due to myocardial ischemia. This rarely occurs due to magnesium sulfate therapy alone; more often there are additional factors, such as concomitant ritodrine use.

The other potentially lethal side-effect encountered during magnesium sulfate tocolytic therapy is pulmonary edema. Its incidence is about 1%, compared to 5% in patients receiving β-sympathomimetics[146]. Generally, these cases are complicated by other factors associated with pulmonary edema: multiple gestation, polyhydramnios, pre-eclampsia, anemia, blood transfusion, chorioamnionitis, positive fluid balance, operative delivery, dual-agent therapy and prolonged therapy[148]. With proper patient selection, judicious use of therapy and close monitoring, the risk of pulmonary edema can be minimized and it can easily be treated with diuretics.

Perinatal side-effects Neonatal and fetal effects are summarized in Table 13. None of the neonatal effects appear to be due to magnesium alone. They may be related to confounding variables such as maternal illness, fetal growth retardation and prematurity. Some infants develop proximal humeral radiographic abnormalities consisting of transverse radiolucent or sclerotic bands after exposure to long-term magnesium sulfate (> 7 days)[149]. The clinical significance of these findings is unknown. More studies are required to address this concern, particularly with a control group of pregnant women receiving prolonged bed rest for the same interval.

Efficacy and relative safety In 1966, Rusu and colleagues[150] performed the first therapeutic trials of magnesium as a tocolytic agent. In 1977, Steer and Petrie[151] were the first investigators to publish (in English) a clinical trial evaluating such therapy. They demonstrated both safety and efficacy when treating patients with preterm labor and intact membranes who had a painful, identifiable contraction pattern with a frequency of 5 min or less.

In 1983, Elliott[146] reported on 355 patients with and without intact membranes who were treated with magnesium sulfate as the primary tocolytic agent. Only 5% (14/309) of all patients treated with intact membranes had no apparent reason for failure; if only patients

Table 13 Potential fetal/neonatal effects of hypermagnesemia

Controversial effects on fetal heart rate variability
Lack of significant effect on fetal umbilical
  Doppler studies
Fetal breathing movements decrease
Mean baseline fetal heart rate decreases
Flaccidity, hyporeflexia
Need for assisted ventilation
Weak or absent cry
Transient decreased active tone of neck extensors
Possible transient radiographic bony changes

with cervical dilatations of 2 cm or less were included, 2% (5/309) had unexplained failure. Failures were often due to chorioamnionitis, advanced cervical dilatation and abruptio placentae. Seven per cent of patients experienced some side-effects, but only 2% required discontinuation of medication for this reason. There was a 1% incidence of pulmonary edema (each of these patients had predisposing factors); this compared favorably to the 5% rate for β-sympathomimetic agents. Side-effects were found to be less serious and also fewer in number than the known effects of intravenous ritodrine.

In 1987, Hollander and co-workers[139] performed an excellent prospective randomized study analyzing the efficacy and safety of magnesium sulfate vs. ritodrine. All patients had preterm labor with intact membranes and associated cervical changes. Successful tocolysis was defined as cessation of uterine activity and delay in delivery for 72 h or more from the onset of tocolysis. The success rate of ritodrine and magnesium sulfate as primary agents were 83% (30/36) and 91% (31/34), respectively. When administered as either a primary or a secondary agent, the success rate of ritodrine was 79% (31/39) and magnesium sulfate was 88% (35/40). The mean rate of ritodrine required to achieve tocolysis was 210 µg/min. The mean serum level of magnesium required to achieve tocolysis was 6.6 mg/100 ml. Although the side-effects differed in type and severity, the proportion of patients with a side-effect was comparable in both groups. Two patients in the ritodrine group required discontinuation of therapy due to chest pains and tachycardia. No patient receiving magnesium required discontinuation because of side-effects, but two patients did require a downward adjustment in dosage for lethargy with diplopia as its major symptom. The authors concluded that magnesium sulfate was easy to administer and clinically efficacious and that the side-effects were less alarming than in the ritodrine group. They recommended that magnesium sulfate should be used as the first line of tocolytic therapy, with ritodrine to be used as back-up.

Cox and co-workers performed a recent randomized trial comparing magnesium sulfate to no tocolytic therapy in 156 women thought to be in preterm labor[152]. They found no significant pregnancy prolongation in the group receiving magnesium and concluded that magnesium sulfate is ineffective in preventing preterm birth. This study has potential bias because the clinicians were not blinded to the patient groups. Also, only 28% of the control group delivered within 24 h. Almost two-thirds of the control patients had a delay in delivery of at least 1 week, and most of them had pregnancy that continued more than 28 days. There appears to be a major flaw in the diagnosis of 'true preterm labor' in the control group. This renders the study conclusions suspect and speculative, at best. It serves as a reminder of the difficulty in making a true diagnosis of actual preterm labor. This difficulty is compounded in a very busy indigent-care obstetric service.

A report by Madden and colleagues[153] found no threshold relationship of specific serum magnesium concentrations and tocolytic efficacy. This is in contrast to the reports of Elliot[146] and Hollander[139] and their colleagues, who recommended that levels should be at least 5.0–5.7 mg% for efficacy. The desired effect of magnesium sulfate is best achieved when titrated between the clinical findings of toxicity and uterine responsiveness.

In summary, as a single agent, magnesium sulfate is as effective as intravenous β-sympathomimetic agents and is safer than β-mimetic agents.

Dual-agent therapy In 1984, Ferguson and associates[154] performed the first trial of dual-agent primary therapy of magnesium sulfate and intravenous ritodrine vs. intravenous ritodrine, and noted serious maternal side-effects. Ten patients had chest pain, and seven of these had electrocardiogram changes consistent with myocardial ischemia; one additional patient had adult respiratory distress syndrome. Most of these patients subsequently did well on magnesium sulfate alone.

Other studies also showed the potential for complications. In summary, dual-agent intravenous therapy with magnesium sulfate and a β-sympathomimetic agent carries with it the potential for extremely serious effects compared to single-agent therapy and thus cannot be recommended. These effects may be due to the infusion of both drugs, the increased duration of therapy common in patients requiring a second agent, the extensive concurrent use of isotonic crystalloids, patient selection, or some combination of factors. Other drug combinations containing magnesium sulfate have been empirically used quite successfully and safely in our hands (e.g. magnesium sulfate and intermittent oral or subcutaneous terbutaline); studies of these regimens are needed.

Long-term therapy In 1986, Wilkins and colleagues[147] reported a normal outcome in two patients in preterm labor who had been treated continuously for 6–13 weeks with intravenous magnesium sulfate for tocolysis. In each case, conventional therapy with intravenous and oral ritodrine failed to abate uterine contractions and attempts to wean magnesium sulfate were unsuccessful. In 1989, Dudley and colleagues[145] added 51 patients to the database, successfully supporting long-term magnesium sulfate therapy. In fact, they concluded that there need be no time limit and that magnesium sulfate tocolysis may be continued as clinically indicated. In contrast, some reports seem to implicate long-term continuous infusion of magnesium sulfate for tocolysis in the genesis of transient neonatal radiographic bony lesions[149,154].

The most important problem arising from prolonged therapy appears to be emotional depression and anxiety of the patient and family due to prolonged bed rest and hospitalization.

Oral magnesium as prophylaxis for preterm delivery Serum magnesium levels are usually lower in pregnancy than in the non-pregnant state, and during preterm labor levels appear to drop still further[155,156]. Some investigators have suggested an etiological relationship between low magnesium concentration and preterm delivery.

Oral tocolysis with magnesium oxide and gluconate may be used. The mean serum concentration of magnesium may increase from 1.44 ± 0.22 mg/100 ml before therapy to 2.16 ± 0.32 mg/100 ml after oral therapy[157].

In 1988, Martin and colleagues studied 50 successfully tocolyzed patients with preterm labor[158]. The authors concluded that both oral magnesium and oral ritodrine were equally effective in prolonging pregnancy to term, although the ritodrine patients had more side-effects. It is difficult to understand how oral magnesium, which raises magnesium levels only slightly, could be effective in maintaining uterine quiescence and preventing preterm delivery. Since this study was not randomized, selection bias could have influenced the results. Furthermore, since there was no placebo control group, it could be argued that neither agent was effective.

A randomized trial comparing oral terbutaline and magnesium oxide for maintenance of tocolysis revealed no significant difference in efficacy[159]. Again, there were fewer side-effects and a significant cost advantage with the magnesium therapy.

Of greater interest is a recent study that compared oral ritodrine, oral magnesium and no oral maintenance therapy. The investigators were unable to demonstrate any benefits of either oral drug therapy in terms of five different measures of pregnancy prolongation[160].

In a double-blind randomized controlled study of 400 primigravid young normotensive patients, prophylactic oral daily administration of 365 mg of magnesium aspartate hydrochloride was compared to an aspartic acid placebo[161]. No significant differences were found in the incidence of preterm labor, preterm delivery, abruptio placentae, fetal growth retardation, pre-eclampsia or admission to the neonatal intensive-care unit. They concluded that magnesium supplements had no demonstrable benefit. Even with a sample size ten times larger, no decrease in preterm labor would be detected in the magnesium group.

Recommended clinical protocol A review of the literature and extensive clinical experience in managing patients with active preterm labor leave little doubt that intravenous magnesium sulfate is an important drug of choice for most patients in preterm labor. The signs and symptoms of hypermagnesemia seen in patients with preterm labor are not generally encountered in patients with pre-eclampsia. This may be related to the higher serum magnesium level required in some patients to achieve tocolysis and to a longer average duration of therapy in patients with preterm labor. Unlike the adverse side-effects seen with hypermagne-semia, the beta-adrenergic side-effects of ritodrine do not appear to be dose-related and hence may be less predictable.

Most reports in the literature have used a loading dose of 4 g intravenous magnesium sulfate followed by 2 g/h, but Sibai and co-workers, Petrie and Elliott have advocated 6-g loading doses[162–163]. The clinical protocol in Table 14 allows for fine-tuning of infusion rates

Table 14   A clinical recipe for administration of magnesium sulfate

(1)   100 ml of a 50% solution of magnesium sulfate is easily obtained from readily available products. This volume contains 50 g magnesium sulfate.

(2)   100 ml is removed with sterile technique from a 500-ml bag of 5% dextrose in water. 50 g magnesium sulfate is injected into the remaining 400 ml of fluid for intravenous infusion. It should be noted that 10 ml of this final solution equals 1 g magnesium sulfate.

(3)   A loading dose of 6 g is infused over 30 min. Perspiration and flushing are observed and occur with a feeling of warmth due to vasodilatation. These findings are usually noted early during the intravenous infusion and continue to a greater or lesser degree throughout the infusion. The face, neck and hands are particularly affected. Nausea and emesis may occur.

(4)   The initial continuous maintenance rate is 2–3 g/h for 30–60 min. One or two doses of subcutaneous terbutaline 0.25 mg per dose may be used during this interval if there are no contraindications and rapid diminution in uterine activity is desired.

(5)   Complete and rapid uterine quiescence is unnecessary.

(6)   The infusion rate is increased in increments of 0.5 g/h every 30 min until uterine activity begins to decrease or signs and symptoms of toxicity occur. These findings include lethargy, somnolence, diplopia, dysarthria, blurred vision, dry mouth, dizziness and nystagmus. These effects generally occur at a dose greater than 2 g/h (2.5–4.0 g/h). Downward adjustments in the rate by half-gram increments are generally all that is needed; discontinuation of therapy for side-effects is rarely needed. If necessary, intravenous injection of 1 g calcium gluconate can be used in the symptomatic patient; this will be followed by rapid symptomatic relief.

(7)   The infusion is continued at the lowest effective rate or 2 g/h, whichever is greater, for at least 12 h of relative uterine quiescence.

(8)   The infusion rate is decreased at 0.5 g/h and oral β-sympathomimetic therapy is administered. Should uterine activity begin to increase during this weaning interval, the rate of magnesium sulfate infusion should be increased to the effective rate.

(9)   If the patient cannot be successfully weaned from intravenous magnesium therapy, continuous short-term therapy (24–72 h) may be safely administered, usually at rates of 2–3 g/h. During this interval, another attempt at weaning, albeit at a slower rate, may be attempted.

(10)   If uterine activity recurs coincident with a decrease in the rate of magnesium sulfate infusion, the dosage rate should again be increased to an effective level. Attempts to use other tocolytic agents may be instituted.

(11)   Should these fail to decrease uterine activity, continuous intermediate-term to long-term therapy with magnesium sulfate may be given. In general, cervical dilatation will not change significantly during these therapeutic maneuvers. During long-term magnesium sulfate infusion therapy, constipation and dyspepsia may occur; these can be symptomatically treated. The health-care team should be ready to provide emotional and moral support for patients requiring long-term hospitalization.

(12)   Most true failures of magnesium sulfate therapy and progressive preterm labor are due to cervical dilatation of > 4 cm, abruptio placentae or chorioamnionitis.

(13)   The occasional patient continues to have increased uterine activity, yet has no associated cervical changes while on magnesium sulfate therapy. Other tocolytic agents may be tried in these cases in an attempt to quieten the uterus.

(14)   Patients who are refractory to treatment for preterm labor are likely to have an identifiable pathophysiological process, most notably amniotic infection or abruptio placentae. An amniocentesis for studies of infection is indicated.

(15)   Dual-agent combination therapy with intravenous magnesium sulfate and intravenous β-sympathomimetic agents is not recommended, owing to a significantly increased risk of side-effects. However, dual therapy combining magnesium with oral subcutaneous ß-sympathomimetics is reasonable. Combined use of magnesium with nifedipine, indomethacin, or oxytocin analogs needs further study.

(16)   In the severely preterm gestation with inevitable delivery because of advanced cervical dilatation (4–8 cm), aggressive magnesium tocolysis alone or in combination may be extremely useful in delaying delivery for 24–48 h, to improve the neonatal survival advantage by giving antenatal betamethasone during tocolysis[164].

without the potential for fluid overload, and is well tolerated by most patients. Of course, this assumes that contraindications to magnesium therapy are respected (myasthenia gravis, heart block, recent myocardial infarction and severe renal disease). Paying careful attention to fluid intake and output diminishes the risk of pulmonary edema and magnesium toxicity. Although solutions containing some salt are used, continuous isotonic crystalloid infusion is restricted to patients undergoing the final labor and delivery process.

Nifedipine

The calcium-channel blockers are better called 'calcium antagonists', since they do not completely block calcium influx into the cell; such an action would be incompatible with life. Rather, calcium antagonists are used to normalize excessive transmembrane calcium influx, thus controlling excessive pathological muscle contractility and pacemaker activity at the cardiac, vascular and uterine tissue and organ level[165]. Calcium antagonists are divided into three classes: phenylalkylamines, 1,4-dihydropyridines and benzothiazepines. The respective prototypes are verapamil, nifedipine and diltiazem.

Nifedipine inhibits uterine activity but has less of an effect on the cardiac conduction system than verapamil. Therefore, nifedipine may be used to inhibit uterine activity in acceptable doses, but verapamil's tocolytic effect is limited by its cardiac effects.

The mechanism of action of nifedipine appears limited to the inhibition of the slow voltage-dependent channels regulating calcium influx. Adverse pharmacological effects include vasodilation, negative inotropism and sinoatrial or atrioventricular node conduction disturbances. Because it is a potent vasodilator, nifedipine may cause dizziness, lightheadedness, flushing, headache and peripheral edema. While the overall incidence of side-effects is 17%, severe effects necessitating discontinuation of therapy occur in 2–5% of patients[166]. The negative inotropic and dromotropic (affecting cardiac nodal conduction) effects of nifedipine are minimal. This is due in large part to the heart's baroreflex response to peripheral vasodilatation. Idiosyncratic reactions to nifedipine are rare.

Nifedipine is rapidly and almost completely absorbed from the gastrointestinal tract. Absorption after sublingual administration is rapid but less complete, with levels being measurable in the plasma within 5 min. The rate of absorption of oral and sublingual capsules varies widely among patients. Ferguson and colleagues[167] have shown the mean elimination half-life to be 81 ± 26 min (range 49–137 min) in patients with preterm labor treated with sublingual nifedipine (bitten and held between molars). The mean ratio of fetal cord to maternal serum concentrations of nifedipine was 0.93 ± 0.2, whereas the mean amniotic fluid concentration was $53 \pm 15\%$ of simultaneously obtained maternal vein samples[168].

Clinical experience   In the 1980s, the use of nifedipine for tocolysis came into the clinical arena[169–171]. The results were favorable.

In a randomized study on 58 women in preterm labor who received either oral nifedipine or intravenous ritodrine, the authors found that nifedipine was as effective as ritodrine with significantly fewer side-effects[172].

Ferguson and colleagues[173] studied 66 women randomized to receive tocolysis with either nifedipine or intravenous ritodrine. Maternal side-effects were more serious and more common in the ritodrine group (47%) than in the nifedipine group (13%); perinatal outcome was similar in both groups.

Nifedipine was not associated with alterations in serum electrolytes or dramatic hyperglycemia. The systolic pressure did not significantly change, but the diastolic pressure dropped from 68.5 ± 8.7 mmHg to 64.5 ± 8.3 mmHg 10 min after the initial sublingual dose. The maximum mean pulse was 98 beats/min, which occurred 1 h after the last sublingual dose. Maximal change in blood pressure and pulse were of the same magnitude as those measured during sublingual administration[174].

More recent prospective randomized studies have also supported nifedipine as an equally effective tocolytic agent to more commonly used agents. Kupferminc and colleagues[175] found that nifedipine had equal efficacy to intravenous ritodrine, but caused less nausea, chest pain, palpitations and tachycardia. Nifedipine caused a statistical decrement in blood pressure but one that was of unlikely physiological importance and it was significantly less than the decrease associated with ritodrine. Nifedipine was, however, associated with more flushing. In this study the regimen was a 30 mg oral loading dose and if uterine activity persisted after 90 min an additional dose followed with 20 mg orally. In successfully tocolyzed patients, a maintenance dose of 20 mg every 8 h was employed thereafter.

In a study comparing nifedipine to magnesium sulfate as a first-line tocolytic agent, Glock and Morales[176] found that both treatment regimens were equally effective in the treatment of uncomplicated preterm labor. Both regimens were associated with a similar frequency of side-effects. However, patients in the magnesium group experienced chest pain and need for discontinuation of drug therapy more often. Patients in the nifedipine group experienced more episodes of transient hypotension, but none of these episodes were clinically significant. The authors stressed that the associated decrements in blood pressure indicate the need for adequate hydration prior to initiation of the nifedipine regimen.

Glock and Morales initiated nifedipine tocolysis with a 10-mg capsule given sublingually. If uterine activity persisted, this dose was repeated every 20 min up to an initial maximum of 40 mg during the first hour of treatment. If tocolysis was then successful, oral therapy with 20 mg of nifedipine was initiated 4 h after the last sublingual dose. This dose was repeated every 4 h for 48 h. The patients were then maintained on a regimen of oral nifedipine l0 mg every 8 h. Intravenous ritodrine was added if the initial regimen failed. It is unclear from the report whether side-effects were more common in patients receiving dual agent tocolysis. It should be noted however, that the nifedipine regimen used was relatively aggressive in that the usual maximum dose of nifedipine is 120 mg per day.

Circulatory effects   Because of concerns about potentially untoward effects on uteroplacental blood flow in animals, clinical applications of nifedipine during human pregnancy were limited[177]. However, Doppler velocity waveform analysis revealed the lack of significant effect of nifedipine on various measures of fetal and uteroplacental circulation[178].

Clinical implications   Although drug-induced maternal hypotension, particularly in the hypertensive patient, can cause fetal distress, the literature on untoward fetal effects of nifedipine has been limited to animal models. No human studies to date have documented significant adverse effects on the fetus, owing to careful administration of nifedipine. Nifedipine is a potentially valuable therapeutic agent during pregnancy. Owing to recent safety and efficacy studies in the clinical arena, more clinicians are re-evaluating their initial trepidations and are moving towards the clinical use of nifedipine as a tocolytic agent.

Progestational agents

Progestational agents have been widely used to prolong pregnancy in women who are judged to be at increased risk of miscarriage or preterm birth. The most commonly used agent is 17α-hydroxyprogesterone caproate. Keirse analyzed seven relevant published reports of controlled trials using 17α-hydroxyprogesterone caproate and found no significant difference in the miscarriage rate; however, there was a significant difference in the preterm labor and preterm birth rates in favor of drug therapy[179]. Similar to the results of the β-mimetic studies, there was no significant impact on neonatal morbidity or mortality. This drug was primarily given weekly in doses of 250–1000 mg. Therapy was often started at the initiation of prenatal care or in the third trimester. There are questions regarding efficacy of this drug. If this drug is at all efficacious, it seems to be more useful for prophylaxis than for inhibiting active preterm labor.

Oxytocin receptor blockade

The concentration of oxytocin receptors in uterine tissues increases dramatically just before and during labor. Augmented uterine sensitivity to constant serum levels of oxytocin may result in increases in uterine activity. Oxytocin receptors are also noted in decidua. Stimulation at this level appears to increase the production of prostaglandins. Therefore, oxytocin antagonists may have pharmacological actions at a dual level. Recent reports have focused on the development of oxytocin antagonists as new tocolytic agents; theoretically, they may offer greater specificity with fewer side-effects than agents in current use[180]. Clinical trials are under way. Early results appear to be promising and information from larger controlled trials is awaited.

Nitroglycerin

Glyceryl trinitrate, also known as nitroglycerin, has been the subject of recent reports regarding acute uterine relaxation in the setting of uterine inversion, breech extraction and external cephalic version. Nitroglycerin patches have also been used in a small case series as a tocolytic agent for the treatment of preterm labor. These new uses for an older drug seems to warrant further clinical research regarding its proper role in obstetrics.

Antenatal glucocorticoids

The initial report by Liggins and Howie in 1972[181] revealed a significant decrease in respiratory distress syndrome and neonatal death in patients receiving two 12-mg doses of betamethasone 24 h apart. Several subsequent trials have found similar results. The optimal glucocorticoid preparation and the ideal dose are unknown. Most studies have used betamethasone or dexamethasone. These two agents are quite similar, although a methyl group is in the beta position in the betamethasone molecule rather than the alpha position. Neither agent has significant mineralocorticoid activity (as opposed to hydrocortisone or methylprednisolone).

Concern about the harmful effects of corticosteroids has limited the widespread application of this therapy[182]. Animal data have suggested alterations in immune response, neurological development and fetal growth. These harmful effects seem to be limited to studies in which large pharmacological doses of steroids were used in early gestation. They have not been replicated to any significant degree in the human.

Data from 12 controlled trials involving over 3000 participants demonstrated that corticosteroids reduced the incidence of respiratory distress syndrome in each subgroup examined[183]. Reductions in respiratory morbidity were also associated with reductions in intraventricular hemorrhage, necrotizing enterocolitis and neonatal death. Fortunately, these beneficial effects occurred in the absence of strong evidence for adverse effects of corticosteroids. In this meta-analysis, patients with premature rupture of membranes were included. Overall, neonatal respiratory morbidity was decreased by 40–60% in the group receiving antenatal steroids. Most patients in these studies were between 30 and 34 weeks' gestation. The beneficial effects were noted during any of these gestational ages. The effects were also noted regardless of whether there was premature rupture of membranes. The most dramatic effects were noted in infants born after 24 h but within 7 days of the dose of steroids. In this meta-analysis both male and female infants benefited. It should be noted that pulmonary maturity testing was not used as a basis for the administration of corticosteroids; as a result, the basis for administration was gestational age and not demonstrated pulmonary maturity.

Non-randomized trials have supported the use of corticosteroids in very preterm gestations[184]. A survey of maternal–fetal specialists has shown that this therapy, even at 24 weeks' gestation, is not unreasonable[95]. There are also data indicating that the combination of postnatal surfactant treatment and antenatal glucocorticoid therapy is more beneficial than either therapy alone.

Finally, a consensus statement from a National Institute of Health (NIH) consensus conference concluded that all women at risk for preterm delivery between 24 and 34 weeks are potential candidates for antenatal glucocorticoid therapy, including those with preterm membrane rupture prior to 30–32 weeks[185]. Lest, in the setting of preterm birth, steroids become used as frequently as water, some important caveats are suggested. Thoughtful consideration must be exercised in diabetic pregnant women, in women in whom gestational diabetic screening has not yet been performed, in those with active viral infections, in those with active peptic ulcer disease, in those with active tuberculosis and in those with known or suspected chorioamnionitis.

Adjunctive therapy

Administering thyrotropin releasing hormone and antenatal steroids to prevent respiratory distress syndrome, chronic lung disease and ventilator days in the intensive care nursery has been promising. Nonetheless, a recent large Australian trial has cast doubt on the benefit/risk ratio of thyrotropin administration[186].

Preventing intraventricular hemorrhage by medical therapies such as the antenatal administration of phenobarbital and vitamin K, although apparently useful in initial studies, still requires further confirmation before these can be acceptable as clinically useful adjunctive therapy.

Administering antenatal antibiotics, as a general rule, to prolong 'subclinically' infected pregnancies and to prevent neonatal sepsis[187,188] is somewhat controversial and not an established practice. In the American NIH randomized, double-blinded placebo-controlled study, treatment with ampicillin and erythromycin during preterm labor with intact membranes was ineffective in prolonging pregnancy or decreasing neonatal morbidity[188,189]. In contrast, a much smaller randomized but non-blinded, non-placebo-controlled trial of ampicillin and metronidazole treatment in preterm labor demonstrated greater pregnancy prolongation and decreased neonatal morbidity in the treatment group[190].

Outpatient prenatal treatment of women colonized with group B streptococci with erythromycin was ineffective at decreasing preterm birth[191]. However, in patients with a history of prematurity in the preceding pregnancy, treatment of bacterial vaginosis during pregnancy was effective in reducing preterm births[192].

Operative intervention such as prophylactic forceps use and prophylactic Cesarean section have not been proven to be successful at preventing intraventricular hemorrhage[193,194].

With the exceptions of standard therapy for group B streptococci in labor, antenatal treatment for bacterial vaginosis and operative delivery for standard obstetric indications, none of these adjunctive therapies for the prevention of specific prematurity-related complications have gained widespread acceptance. Further research regarding their safety and efficacy is warranted before their use can be recommended outside a research protocol.

PREVENTING PRETERM BIRTH

Preventing preterm birth is a major undertaking. Success would lead to a major improvement in health and welfare. It is difficult to imagine, though, how such a multifaceted problem could be solved by simple interventions, especially when we lack an essential understanding of the mechanisms that give rise to the multitudinous proximate causes of preterm birth (Table 3).

Numerous investigators have attempted to prevent indicated preterm deliveries with some modicum of success. Interventions have included low-dose aspirin and calcium for the prevention of pre-eclampsia, eclampsia and intrauterine growth retardation. In most cases, fetal hemolytic disease is well understood and preventable.

Most preterm births appear to be due to spontaneous but not idiopathic labor. We must be able to predict these events accurately before we can prevent them. Predictions based on risk-scoring systems, biochemical markers and cervical examination are of limited value; prophylaxis with bed rest, cerclage, tocolytic agents and progestational agents are also of limited value. Commercial programs for the early detection of preterm labor are being developed and fostered as representative of the forefront of outpatient modern perinatal medicine. These programs are based on the maternal diagnosis of vague symptomatology, high-risk patient scoring, cervical evaluation and assessment of uterine activity.

Since there is no single treatable factor that can prevent all preterm births, many investigators have developed comprehensive preterm birth prevention programs. Papiernik and colleagues were among the first to institute such a program[195]. Its fundamental components include 'universal' preterm birth and preterm labor education of patients, families, staff and payor sources. Critical to the program's success is 24-h access to care and a continued commitment to the program. Results are not achieved overnight and in fact may take years to develop. Although most preterm birth prevention programs seem to be ineffective in indigent populations, a model program from the West Los Angeles Preterm Birth Prevention Project has promising results which appear to demonstrate cost effectiveness in the prevention of prematurity[196].

Regardless of the medical component of these programs, it is clear that socioeconomic variables, such as educational status, income, nutrition, housing, child care and sociological and psychological stress, place a substantial burden on those experiencing preterm delivery, before and after the fact. Many investigators believe that the greatest potential impact will not come from the medical component *per se*; rather, reduction of preterm delivery will come from preventive social, educational and economic changes. That is not to say that medical advancements cannot affect prematurity to a limited extent: Iams and colleagues[197] have emphasized that the obstetrician's attitude with regard to preterm birth prevention is of critical importance. Thorough attention to detail, early therapy and modification of behavioral risk factors throughout prenatal care is advocated as a useful antidote to preterm birth[197].

A study by Miller and Merritt[198] is a prime example of the potential impact of behavior modification on prematurity. They studied six modifiable behavioral risk factors that are significantly related to LBW: low maternal weight for height, low maternal weight gain, lack of prenatal care, age less than 17 or more than 35 years at delivery, cigarette smoking and the use of drugs or alcohol. Among white women, if three of these variables were present, the risk of LBW was 29%, with two variables 10%, with one variable 6.7% and with none of these variables 1%.

Nevertheless, there is no clearly proven method to prevent the onset of preterm labor. Policy-makers must address several issues. Should existing healthcare resources be reallocated to the beginning of life? To what extent is this the responsibility of the medical profession, and to what extent is this the responsibility of society at large (e.g. legislators, business executives, agency directors, judges, foundations, non-governmental organizations, hospital directors, labor negotiators, insurance companies, churches and schools)? It appears that only when there is a critical mass of concern and commitment will there be a comprehensive frontal attack on all aspects of preterm birth rather than just on the medical front alone.

Finally, a simple truth may lie in the notion of universal education to all pregnant patients, not just those who are identifiable as being at high risk. The 'grandfather of preterm birth prevention', Emile Papiernik, cogently argues that prevention programs are unlikely to work when the risk is very high. Conversely, prevention programs for preterm birth in France have been applied to 20 million pregnant women since the early 1970s. The greatest benefit of these programs were in patients at 'low risk'. In the USA, most prematurity derives from unrecognizable risk factors in low-risk pregnant women; therefore, we have much to learn from the French experience with low-risk pregnant women[199].

REFERENCES

1. Pritchard JA, MacDonald PC, Gant NF, eds. Preterm and post-term pregnancies and fetal growth retardation. In *Williams' Obstetrics*, 17th edn. Connecticut: Appleton-Century-Crofts, 1985:745

2. Amon E, Steigerwald J, Winn H. Obstetric factors associated with surival of the borderline viable liveborn infant (500–750 grams). *Am J Obstet Gynecol* 1995; 172:418

3. Hack M, Wright LL, Shankaran S, *et al*. Very-low-birth-weight outcomes of the National Institute of Child Health and Human Development Neonatal Network, November 1989 to October 1990. *Am J Obstet Gynecol* 1995;172:457–64

4. Fedrick J, Anderson ABM. Factors associated with spontaneous preterm birth. *Br J Obstet Gynaecol* 1976; 83:342–50

5. Rush RW, Keirse MJ, Houlat P, *et al*. Contribution of preterm delivery to perinatal mortality. *Br Med J* 1976;2:965–8

6. Amon E, Anderson GD, Sibai BM, *et al*. Factors responsible for a preterm delivery of the immature newborn infant (≤ 1000 gm.). *Am J Obstet Gynecol* 1987;156:1143–8

7. Center for the Future of Children. *The Future of Children: Low Birth Weight*, vol 5. Los Angeles, California: The David and Lucille Packard Foundation, 1995

8. Ehrenhaft PM, Wagner JL, Herdman RC. Changing prognosis for very low birth weight infants. *Obstet Gynecol* 1989;74:528

9. Trends in fertility and infant and maternal health – United States, 1980–1988. *Morbid Mortal Weekly Rep* 1991;40:381

10. Ventura SJ, Martin JA, Curtin SC, *et al*. Births: Final data for 1997. *National Vital Statistics Reports*, vol 47, no 18. Hyattsville, Maryland: National Center for Health Statistics, 1988

11. Kliegman RM, Rottman CJ, Behrman RE. Strategies for the prevention of low birth weight. *Am J Obstet Gynecol* 1990;162:1073

12. Arias F, Tomich P. Etiology and outcome of low birth weight and preterm infants. *Obstet Gynecol* 1982; 60:277–81

13. Main DM, Gabbe SG, Richardson D. Can preterm deliveries be prevented? *Am J Obstet Gynecol* 1985; 151:892–8

14. Meis PJ, Ernest JM, Moore ML. Causes of low birth weight births in public and private patients. *Am J Obstet Gynecol* 1987;156:1165–8

15. Romero R, Mazor M. Infection and preterm labor. *Clin Obstet Gynecol* 1988;31:533–84

16. Lettieri L, Vintzileos AM, Rodis JF, *et al.* Does 'idiopathic' preterm labor resulting in preterm birth exist? *Am J Obstet Gynecol* 1993;168:1480–5

17. Creasy RK, Gummer BA, Liggins GC. System for predicting spontaneous preterm birth. *Obstet Gynecol* 1980;55:692–5

18. Holbrook RH, Laros RK, Creasy RK. Evaluation of a risk-scoring system for prediction of preterm labor. *Am J Perinatol* 1989:6:62–8

19. Carr-Hill RA, Hall MH. The repetition of spontaneous preterm labour. *Br J Obstet Gynaecol* 1985; 92:921–8

20. Keirse M, Rush R, Anderson A, Turnbull A. Risk of preterm delivery in patients with previous preterm delivery and/or abortion. *Br J Obstet Gynaecol* 1978;85:81–5

21. Bakketeig LS, Hoffman HJ, Harley EE. The tendency to repeat gestational age and birth weight in successive births. *Am J Obstet Gynecol* 1979;135:1086–103

22. Hoffman HJ, Bakketeig LS. Risk factors associated with the occurrence of preterm birth. *Clin Obstet Gynecol* 1984;27:539–52

23. Mueller-Heubach E, Reddick D, Barnett B, Bente R. Preterm birth prevention: evaluation of a prospective controlled randomized trial. *Am J Obstet Gynecol* 1989; 160:1172–8

24. Keirse MJNC, Phil D. An evaluation of formal risk scoring for preterm birth. *Am J Perinatol* 1989; 6:226–33

25. Breart G, Goujard J, Blondel B, *et al.* A comparison of two policies of antenatal supervision for the prevention of prematurity. *Int J Epidemiol* 1981;10:241–4

26. Lockwood CJ, Senyei AE, Dische MR, *et al.* Fetal fibronectin in cervical and vaginal secretions as a predictor of preterm delivery. *N Engl J Med* 1991;325: 669–74

27. Katz M, Gill PJ, Newman RB. Detection of preterm labor by ambulatory monitoring of uterine activity: a preliminary report. *Obstet Gynecol* 1986;68:773–8

28. Newman RB, Gill PJ, Wittreich P, Katz M. Maternal perception of prelabor uterine activity. *Obstet Gynecol* 1986;68:765–9

29. Morrison JC, Martin JN Jr, Martin RW, *et al.* Prevention of preterm birth by ambulatory assessment of uterine activity: a randomized study. *Am J Obstet Gynecol* 1987;156:536–43

30. Hill WC, Fleming AD, Martin RW, *et al.* Home uterine activity monitoring is associated with a reduction in preterm birth. *Obstet Gynecol* 1990;76:13S–18S

31. Knuppel RA, Lake MF, Watson DL, *et al.* Preventing preterm birth in twin gestation: home uterine activity monitoring and perinatal nursing support. *Obstet Gynecol* 1990;76:24S–27S

32. Rhoads GG, McNellis DC, Kessel SS. Home monitoring of uterine contractility. *Am J Obstet Gynecol* 1990; 165:2–6

33. A multicenter randomized control trial of home uterine monitoring (HUAM): active vs. sham device. *Am J Obstet Gynecol* 1995;172:1120–7

34. Iams JD, Stilson R, Johnson FF, *et al.* Symptoms that precede preterm labor and preterm premature rupture of the membranes. *Am J Obstet Gynecol* 1990;162:486–90

35. Iams JD, Johnson FF, Hamer C. Uterine activity and symptoms as predictor of preterm labor. *Obstet Gynecol* 1990;76:42S–46S

36. Iams JD, Johnson FF, Parker M. A prospective evaluation of the signs and symptoms of preterm labor. *Obstet Gynecol* 1994;84:227–30

37. Papiernik E, Bouyer J, Collin D, *et al.* Precocious cervical ripening and preterm labor. *Obstet Gynecol* 1986;67:238–42

38. Wood C, Bannerman RHO, Booth RT, Pinkerton JHM. The prediction of premature labor by observation of the cervix and external tocography. *Am J Obstet Gynecol* 1965;91:396–402

39. Leveno KJ, Cox K, Roark ML. Cervical dilatation and prematurity revisited. *Obstet Gynecol* 1986;68:434–5

40. Stubbs TM, Van Dorsten P, Miller MC. The preterm cervix and preterm labor; relative risks, predictive values, and change over time. *Am J Obstet Gynecol* 1986; 155:829–34

41. Parikh MN, Mehta AC. Internal cervical os during the second half of pregnancy. *J Obstet Gynaecol Br Commonw* 1961;68:818

42. Schaffner F, Schanzer SN. Cervical dilatation in the early third trimester. *Obstet Gynecol* 1966;27:130–3

43. Floyd WS. Cervical dilatation in the mid-trimester of pregnancy. *Obstet Gynecol* 1961;18:380

44. Buekins P, Alexander S, Boutsen M, *et al.* Randomized controlled trial of routine cervical examinations in pregnancy. *Lancet* 1994;344:841–44

45. Valenzuela G, Cline S, Hayashi R. Follow-up of hydration and sedation in the pretherapy of premature labor. *Am J Obstet Gynecol* 1983;147:396–8

46. Ingemarsson I. Effect of terbutaline on premature labor: a double-blind placebo-controlled study. *Am J Obstet Gynecol* 1976;125:520–4

47. Creasy RK. Implications of treatment of preterm labor. In MacDonald PC, Portr J, eds. *Initiation of Parturition: Prevention of Prematurity*. Ohio: Ross Laboratories 1983:73

48. Catalano PM, Ashikaga T, Mann LI. Cervical change and uterine activity as predictors of preterm delivery. *Am J Perinatol* 1989;6:185–90

49. Utter GO, Dooley SL, Tamura RK, Socol ML. Awaiting cervical change for the diagnosis of preterm labor does not compromise the efficacy of ritodrine tocolysis. *Am J Obstet Gynecol* 1990;63:882–6

50. Gonik B, Creasy RK. Preterm labor: its diagnosis and management. *Am J Obstet Gynecol* 1986;154:3–8

51. Shepard MJ, Richards VA, Berkowitz RL, *et al.* An evaluation of two equations for predicting fetal weight by ultrasound. *Am J Obstet Gynecol* 1982;142:47–54

52. Hadlock FP, Harrist RB, Carpenter RJ. Sonographic estimation of fetal weight. *Radiology* 1984;150:535–40

53. Amon E, Sabai BM, Anderson GD, *et al.* Obstetric variables predicting survival of the immature newborn (– 1000 gm.): a five-year experience at a single perinatal center. *Am J Obstet Gynecol* 1987;156:1380–9

54. Doubilet PM, Greenes RA. Improved prediction of gestational age from fetal head measurements. *Am J Roentgenol* 1982;142:47

55. Tamura RK, Sabbagha RE, Depp R, *et al.* Diminished growth in fetuses born preterm after spontaneous labor or rupture of membranes. *Am J Obstet Gynecol* 1984;148:1105–10

56. Weiner CP, Sabbagha RE, Visrub N, *et al.* A hypothetical model suggesting suboptimal intrauterine growth in infants delivered preterm. *Obstet Gynecol* 1985; 65:323–6

57. Hadlock FP, Deter RL, Harrist RB, *et al.* A date-independent predictor of intrauterine growth retardation: femur length/abdominal circumference ratio. *Am J Roentgenol* 1983;141:979–84

58. Ott WJ. Fetal femur length, neonatal crown–heel length, and screening for intrauterine growth retardation. *Obstet Gynecol* 1985;65:460–4

59. Westgren M, Beall M, Divon M, *et al.* Fetal femur length/abdominal circumference ratio in preterm labor patients with and without successful tocolytic therapy. *J Ultrasound Med* 1986;5:243–5

60. Rush RW, Kierse MJNC, Howat P, *et al.* Contribution of preterm delivery to perinatal mortality. *Br Med J* 1976;2:965–8

61. National Center for Health Statistics. *Vital Statistics of the United States, 1985*, DHHS Publication (PHS) 88–1113, Natality. Washington, DC: U.S. Government Printing Office, 1988:1

62. Nisell H, Bistoletti P, Palme C. Preterm breech delivery: early and late complications. *Acta Obstet Gynecol Scand* 1981;60:363–6

63. Braun FHT, Jones KL, Smith DW. Breech presentation as an indicator of fetal abnormality. *J Pediatr* 1975; 86:419–21

64. Amon E, Sibai BM, Anderson GD. How perinatologists manage the problem of the presenting breech fetus. *Am J Perinatol* 1988;5:247–50

65. Penn ZJ, Steer PJ. How obstetricians manage the problem of preterm delivery with special reference to the preterm breech. *Br J Obstet Gynaecol* 1991; 98:531–4

66. Amon E. External cephalic version. In Sabbagha RE, ed. *Diagnostic Ultrasound Applied to Obstetrics and Gynecology*. Philadelphia: JB Lippincott, 1987

67. Vintzileos AM, Campbell WA, Nochimson DJ, *et al.* The use and misuse of the fetal biophysical profile. *Am J Obstet Gynecol* 1987;156:527–33

68. Manning FA, Morrison I, Harman CR, *et al.* Fetal assessment based on fetal biophysical profile scoring: experience in 19,221 referred high risk pregnancies. II. An analysis of false negative results. *Am J Obstet Gynecol* 1987;157:880–4

69. Castillo RA, Devoe LD, Arthur M, *et al.* The preterm nonstress test: effects of gestational age and length of study. *Am J Obstet Gynecol* 1989;160:172–5

70. Amon E, Dacus JV, Mabie BC, *et al.* Ultrasonically guided direct umbilical cord blood sampling. *J Reprod Med* 1987;32:851–4

71. Castle BM, Turnbull AC. The presence or absence of fetal breathing movements predicts the outcome of preterm labour. *Lancet* 1987;2:471–3

72. Besinger RE, Compton AA, Hayashi RH. The presence or absence of fetal breathing movements as a predictor of outcome in preterm labor. *Am J Obstet Gynecol* 1987;153:753–7

73. Stubblefield PG. Causes and prevention of preterm birth: an overview. In Fuchs F, Stubblefield PG, eds. *Preterm Birth: Causes, Prevention, and Management*, 2nd edn. New York: Macmillan, 1993

74. Rodeck CH. Fetal abnormality and preterm labour. In Beard RW, Sharp R, eds. *Preterm Labour and its Consequences*. London: Royal College of Obstetricians and Gynaecologists, 1985

75. Donnenfeld AE, Mennuti MT. Sonographic findings in fetuses with common chromosome abnormalities. *Clin Obstet Gynecol* 1988;31:80–96

76. Kirbinen P, Jouppila P. Polyhydramnios: a clinical study. *Ann Chir Gynaecol* 1978;67:117–22

77. Many A, Hill LM, Lazebnik N, *et al.* The association between polyhydramnios and preterm delivery. *Obstet Gynecol* 1995;86:389–91

78. Barkin SZ, Pretorious DH, Beckett MN, *et al.* Severe polyhydramnios: incidence of anomalies. *Am J Roentgenol* 1987;148:155–9

79. Wallenburg HCS. Chorioangioma of the placenta. *Obstet Gynecol Surv* 1971;26:411–25

80. Ratten GJ, Beischer AN, Fortune DW. Obstetric complications when the fetus has Potter's syndrome. *Am J Obstet Gynecol* 1973;115:890–6

81. Collaborative Group on Antenatal Steroid Therapy. Effect of antenatal dexamethasone administration on the prevention of respiratory distress syndrome. *Am J Obstet Gynecol* 1981;141:276–87

82. Fleisher B, Kulovich MV, Hallman M, *et al.* Lung profile: sex differences in normal pregnancies. *Obstet Gynecol* 1985;66:327–30

83. Leigh J, Garite TJ. Amniocentesis and the management of preterm labor. *Obstet Gynecol* 1986;67:500–6

84. Amon E, Leventhal S, Allen GS, Sibai BM. Neonatal outcome following spontaneous preterm labor after demonstrated lung maturity by amniocentesis. *Society for Gynecologic Investigation 37th Annual Meeting*, St Louis, Missouri, 1990;abstr.l69

85. Wigton TR, Tamura RK, Wickstrom E, *et al.* Neonatal morbidity after preterm delivery in the presence of documented lung maturity. *Am J Obstet Gynecol* 1993; 169:951–5

86. Konte JM, Holbrook RH Jr, Laros RK Jr, Creasy RK. Short-term neonatal morbidity. *Am J Perinatol* 1986; 3:283–8

87. Heinonen PK, Saarikoski S, Pystynen P. Reproductive performance of women with uterine anomalies: an evaluation of 182 cases. *Acta Obstet Gynecol Scand* 1982; 61:157–62

88. Fedele L, Zamberletti D, Vercellini P, *et al.* Reproductive performance of women with unicornuate uterus. *Fertil Steril* 1987;47:416–19

89. Amon E. Limits of fetal viability. *Obstet Gynecol Clin North Am* 1988;15:321–38

90. Yu VYH, Downe L, Astbury J, *et al.* Perinatal factors and adverse outcome in extremely low birthweight infants. *Arch Dis Child* 1986;61:554–8

91. Yu VYH, Loke HI, Bajuk B, *et al.* Prognosis for infants born at 23–28 weeks' gestation. *Br Med J* 1986; 293:1200–3

92. Hack M, Fanaroff AA. How small is too small? Considerations in evaluating the outcome of the tiny infant. *Clin Perinatol* 1988;15:773–88

93. Kitchen W, Ford G, Orgill A, *et al.* Outcome of extremely low birthweight infants in relation to the hospital of birth. *Aust NZ J Obstet Gynaecol* 1984;24:1–5

94. Amon E, Shyken JM, Sibai BM. How small is too small and early is too early? A survey of American obstetricians specializing in high-risk pregnancies. *Am J Perinatol* 1992;9:17–21

95. Amon E, Moyn S. Cesarean section for fetal indications at the limits of fetal viability (1986 to 1991). *Society of Perinatal Obstetricians, Proceedings of the 12th Annual Meeting*, Orlando, Florida, 1991;abstr.4

96. DeGaris C, Kuhse H, Singer P, Yu VYH. Attitudes of Australian neonatal paediatricians to the treatment of extremely preterm infants. *Aust Paediatr J* 1987; 23:223–6

97. Hack M, Fanaroff AA. Changes in the delivery room care of the extremely small infant (– 750 g): effects on morbidity and outcome. *N Engl J Med* 1986;314:660–4

98. Yu VYH, Wong PY, Bajuk B, *et al.* Outcome of extremely low birthweight infants. *Br J Obstet Gynaecol* 1986;93:162–70

99. Miyazaki FS, Taylor NA. Saline amnioinfusion for relief of variable or prolonged decelerations. *Am J Obstet Gynecol* 1983;146:670–8

100. Reece EA, Chervenak FA, Romero R, Hobbins JC. Magnesium sulfate in the management of acute intrapartum fetal distress. *Am J Obstet Gynecol* 1984; 148:104–6

101. Mendez-Bauer C, Shekarloo A, Cook V, Freese U. Treatment of acute intrapartum fetal distress by beta$_2$ sympathomimetics. *Am J Obstet Gynecol* 1987;156:638–42

102. Lipshitz J, Bailie P. Uterine and cardiovascular effects of beta$_2$-selective sympathomimetic drugs administered as an intravenous infusion. *S Afr Med J* 1976;50:1973–7

103. Caritis SN, Chiao JP, Moore JJ, *et al.* Myometrial desensitization after ritodrine infusion. *Am J Physiol* 1987;253:E410–17

104. Benedetti TJ. Maternal complications of parenteral beta-sympathomimetic therapy for preterm labor. *Am J Obstet Gynecol* 1983;145:1–6

105. Hendricks SK, Keroes J, Katz M. Electrocardiographic changes associated with ritodrine-induced maternal tachycardia and hypokalemia. *Am J Obstet Gynecol* 1986;154:921–3

106. Grospietsch G, Kuhn W. Effects of beta-mimetics on maternal physiology. In Fuchs F, Stubblefield PG, eds. *Preterm Birth: Causes, Prevention and Management*, 2nd edn. New York: Macmillan, 1993

107. Philipsen T, Eriksen PS, Lynggaard F. Pulmonary edema following ritodrine–saline infusion in premature labor. *Obstet Gynecol* 1981;58:304–8

108. Milliez S, Blot PH, Sureau C. A case report of maternal death associated with betamimetic and betamethasone administration in premature labor. *Eur J Obstet Gynecol Reprod Biol* 1980;2:95–100

109. Taslimi MM, Sibai BM, Amon E, *et al.* A national survey on preterm labor. *Am J Obstet Gynecol* 1989;160:1352–7

110. Lenz S, Kuhl C, Wang P, *et al.* The effects of ritodrine on carbohydrate and lipid metabolism in normal and diabetic pregnant women. *Acta Endocrinol* 1979; 92:669–79

111. Wager J, Fredholm B, Lunell N, *et al.* Metabolic and circulatory effects of intravenous and oral salbutamol in late pregnancy in diabetic and non-diabetic women. *Acta Obstet Gynecol Scand Suppl* 1982;108:41–6

112. Angel JL, O'Brien WF, Knuppel RA, *et al.* Carbohydrate intolerance in patients receiving oral tocolytics. *Am J Obstet Gynecol* 1988;159:762–6

113. Lippert TH, DeGrandi PB, Fridrich R. Actions of the uterine relaxant, fenoterol, on uteroplacental hemodynamics in human subjects. *Am J Obstet Gynecol* 1976; 125:1093–8

114. Lunell NO, Joelsson I, Lewander R, *et al.* Uteroplacental blood flow and the effect of beta$_2$-adrenoceptor stimulating drugs. *Acta Obstet Gynecol Scand Suppl* 1982;108:25–8

115. Hancock PJ, Setzer ES, Beydoun SN. Physiologic and biochemical effects of ritodrine therapy in the mother and perinate. *Am J Perinatol* 1985;2:1–6

116. Haddengra M, Touwen BCL, Huisjes JH. Longterm follow-up of children prenatally exposed to ritodrine. *Br J Obstet Gynaecol* 1986;93:156–61

117. Barden TP, Peter JB, Merkatz IR. Ritodrine hydrochloride: a betamimetic agent for use in preterm labor. I. Pharmacology, clinical history, administration, side effects, and safety. *Obstet Gynecol* 1980;56:1–6

118. Merkatz IR, Peter JB, Barden TP. Ritodrine hydrochloride: a betamimetic agent for use in preterm labor. II. Evidence of efficacy. *Obstet Gynecol* 1980; 56:7–12

119. King JF, Grand A, Keirse MJN, *et al.* Betamimetics in preterm labour: an overview of randomized controlled trials. *Br J Obstet Gynaecol* 1988;95:211–22

120. Korenbrot CC, Aalto LH, Laros RK. The cost effectiveness of stopping preterm labor with beta-adrenergic treatment. *N Engl J Med* 1984;310:691–6

121. Canadian Preterm Labor Investigators Group. Treatment of preterm labor with the beta-adrenergic agonist ritodrine. *N Engl J Med* 1992;327:308–12

122. Caritis S. A pharmacologic approach to the infusion of ritodrine. *Am J Obstet Gynecol* 1998;158:380–4

123. Gonik B, Benedetti T, Creasy RK, *et al.* Intramuscular versus intravenous ritodrine hydrochloride for preterm labor management. *Am J Obstet Gynecol* 1988; 159:323–8

124. Parilla BV, Dooley SL, Minogue JP, *et al.* The efficacy of oral terbutaline after intravenous tocolysis. *Am J Obstet Gynecol* 1993;169:965–9

125. Howard TE, Killam AP, Penney LL, *et al.* A double blind randomized study of terbutaline in premature labor. *Milit Med* 1982;147:305–7

126. Cotton DB, Strassner HT, Hill LM, *et al.* Comparison of magnesium sulfate, terbutaline and a placebo for inhibition of preterm labor. A randomized study. *J Reprod Med* 1984;29:92–7

127. Caritis SN, Tolg G, Heddinger LA, *et al.* A double-blind study comparing ritodrine and terbutaline in the treatment of preterm labor. *Am J Obstet Gynecol* 1984;150:7–14

128. Stubblefield PG, Heyl PS. Treatment of premature labor with subcutaneous terbutaline. *Obstet Gynecol* 1982;59:457–62

129. Food and Drug Administration. Use of approved drugs for unlabeled medications. *FDA Drug Bull* 1982;12:4

130. Repke JT, Niebyl JR. Role of prostaglandin synthetase inhibitors in the treatment of preterm labor. *Semin Reprod Endocrinol* 1985;3:259

131. Csaba IF, Sulyok E, Ertl T. Relationship of maternal treatment with indomethacin to persistence of fetal circulation syndrome. *J Pediatr* 1978;92:484

132. Itskovitz J, Abramovich H, Brandes JM. Oligohydramnios, meconium and perinatal death concurrent with indomethacin treatment in human pregnancy. *J Reprod Med* 1980;24:137–40

133. Moise KJ, Huhta JC, Dawood S, *et al.* Indomethacin in the treatment of preterm labor: effects on the human fetal ductus arteriosus. *N Engl J Med* 1988; 319:327–31

134. Cantor B, Tyler T, Nelson RM, *et al.* Oligohydramnios and transient neonatal anuria: a possible association with the maternal use of prostaglandin synthetase inhibitors. *J Reprod Med* 1980;24:220–3

135. Kirshon B, Moise KJ, Wasserstrum N, *et al.* Influence of short-term indomethacin therapy on fetal urine output. *Obstet Gynecol* 1988;72:51–3

136. Hickok DE, Hollenbach KA, Reilley SF, *et al.* The association between amniotic fluid volume and treatment with nonsteroidal anti-inflammatory agents for preterm labor. *Am J Obstet Gynecol* 1989;160:1525–30

137. Kirshon B, Mari G, Moise KJ. Indomethacin therapy in the treatment of symptomatic polyhydramnios. *Obstet Gynecol* 1990;75:202–5

138. Vanhaesebrouck P, Thiery M, Leroy JG, *et al.* Oligohydramnios, renal insufficiency, and ileal perforation in preterm infants after intra-uterine exposure to indomethacin. *J Pediatr* 1988;113:738–43

139. Hollander DI, Nagey DA, Pupkin MJ. Magnesium sulfate and ritodrine hydrochloride. *Am J Obstet Gynecol* 1987;156:631–7

140. Gilman AG, Goodman L, Gilman A, eds. *Goodman and Gilman's The Pharmacologic Basis of Therapeutics*, 6th edn. New York: Macmillan, 1980

141. Hall DG, McGaughey HS, Corey EL, *et al.* The effects of magnesium therapy on the duration of labor. *Am J Obstet Gynecol* 1959;78:27–32

142. Cruikshank DP, Pitkin RM, Donnelly E, Reynolds WA. Urinary magnesium, calcium, and phosphate excretion during magnesium sulfate infusion. *Obstet Gynecol* 1981;58:430–4

143. Hoff HE, Smith PK, Winkler AW. Effects of magnesium on nervous system in relation to its concentration in serum. *Am J Physiol* 1940;130:292

144. McCubbin JH, Sibai BM, Abdella TN, Anderson GD. Cardiopulmonary arrest due to acute maternal hypermagnesaemia. *Lancet* 1981;1:1058–9

145. Dudley D, Gagnon D, Varner M. Long-term tocolysis with intravenous magnesium sulfate. *Obstet Gynecol* 1989;73:373–8

146. Elliott JP. Magnesium sulfate as a tocolytic agent. *Am J Obstet Gynecol* 1983;147:277–84

147. Wilkins IA, Goldberg JD, Phillips RN, *et al.* Long-term use of magnesium sulfate as a tocolytic agent. *Obstet Gynecol* 1986;67:38S–40S

148. Elliott JP, O'Keefe DF, Greenberg P, Freeman RK. Pulmonary edema associated with magnesium sulfate and betamethasone administration. *Am J Obstet Gynecol* 1979;134:717–19

149. Holcomb WL, Schackelford GD, Petrie RH. Magnesium tocolysis and neonatal bone abnormalities. *Obstet Gynecol* 1991;78:611–14

150. Rusu O, Lupan C, Baltescu V. Magnezivl serie in sarcina normala la termen si nasterea prematura. Rolvl magneziterapiei in combatera nasterii premature. *Obstet Gynecol* 1966;14:215

151. Steer CM, Petrie RH. A comparison of magnesium sulfate and alcohol for the prevention of premature labor. *Am J Obstet Gynecol* 1977;129:1–4

152. Cox SM, Sherman ML, Leveno KJ. Randomized investigation of magnesium sulfate for prevention of preterm birth. *Am J Obstet Gynecol* 1990;163:767–72

153. Madden C, Owen J, Hauth JC. Magnesium tocolysis: serum levels versus success. *Am J Obstet Gynecol* 1990; 162:1177–80

154. Ferguson JE II, Hensleigh PA, Kredenster D. Adjunctive use of magnesium sulfate with ritodrine for preterm labor tocolysis. *Am J Obstet Gynecol* 1984; 148:166–71

155. Hall DG. Serum magnesium in pregnancy. *Obstet Gynecol* 1957;9:158

156. Martin RW, Martin JN, Pryor JA, *et al.* Comparison of oral ritodrine and magnesium gluconate for ambulatory tocolysis. *Am J Obstet Gynecol* 1988;158:1440–5

157. Martin RW, Gaddy DK, Martin JN, *et al.* Tocolysis with oral magnesium. *Am J Obstet Gynecol* 1987;156:433–9

158. Martin JN, Pryor JA, Gaddy DK, *et al.* Comparison of oral ritodrine and magnesium gluconate for ambulatory tocolysis. *Am J Obstet Gynecol* 1988;158:1440–5

159. Ridgeway LE, Muise K, Wright JW, *et al.* A prospective randomized comparison of oral terbutaline and magnesium oxide for the maintenance of tocolysis. *Am J Obstet Gynecol* 1990;163:879–82

160. Ricci J, Hariharan S, Helfgott A, *et al.* Oral tocolysis with magnesium flouride: a randomized controlled prospective clinical trial. *Am J Obstet Gynecol* 1991;165: 603–10

161. Sibai AM, Villar MA, Bray E. Magnesium supplementation during pregnancy: a double-blind randomized controlled clinical trial. *Am J Obstet Gynecol* 1989; 161:115–19

162. Sibai BM. The use of magnesium sulfate in pre-eclampsia–eclampsia. In Petrie RH, ed. *Perinatal Pharmacology*. Oradell, NJ: Medical Economics, 1989

163. Petrie RH. Tocolysis using magnesium sulfate. *Semin Perinatol* 1981;5:266–73

164. Amon E, Midkiff C, Shumway J, *et al.* Advanced cervical dilation and tocolysis. *Am J Obstet Gynecol* 1999; 180:522

165. Fleckenstein A. History of calcium antagonists. *Circ Res* 1983;52(suppl I):3

166. Talbert RL, Bussey HI. Update on calcium channel blocking agents. *Clin Pharm* 1983;2:403–16

167. Ferguson JE II, Schutz T, Pershe R, *et al.* Nifedipine pharmacokinetics during preterm labor tocolysis. *Am J Obstet Gynecol* 1989;161:1485–90

168. Rogers RC, Akl SA, Sibai BM, Whybrew WD. Oral nifedipine pharmacokinetics in pregnancy induced hypertension. *Proceedings of the 10th Annual Meeting of the Society of Perinatal Obstetricians*, Houston, Texas, 1990;abstr.

169. Ulmsten U, Andersson KE, Wingerup L. Treatment of premature labor with the calcium antagonist nifedipine. *Arch Gynecol* 1980;229:1–5

170. Kaul AF, Osathanondh R, Safon LE, *et al.* The management of preterm labor with the calcium channel blocking agent nifedipine combined with the beta mimetic terbutaline. *Drug Intell Clin Pharm* 1985;5:369–71

171. Read MD, Wellby DE. The use of a calcium antagonist (nifedipine) to suppress preterm labor. *Br J Obstet Gynaecol* 1986;93:933–7

172. Meyer WR, Randall HW, Graves WL. Nifedipine versus ritodrine for suppressing preterm labor. *J Reprod Med* 1990;35:649–53

173. Ferguson JE, Dyson DC, Schutz T, Stevenson DK. A comparison of tocolysis with nifedipine or ritodrine: analysis of efficacy and maternal, fetal, and neonatal outcome. *Am J Obstet Gynecol* 1990;163:105–11

174. Ferguson JE II, Dyson DC, Holbrook RH Jr, *et al.* Cardiovascular and metabolic effects associated with nifedipine and ritodrine tocolysis. *Am J Obstet Gynecol* 1989;161:788–95

175. Kupferminc M, Lessing JB, Yaron Y, *et al.* Nifedipine vs ritodrine for suppression of preterm labour. *Br J Obstet Gynaecol* 1993;100:1090–4

176. Glock JL, Morales WJ. Efficacy and safety of nifedipine vs magnesium sulfate in the management of preterm labor: a randomized study. *Am J Obstet Gynecol* 1993;169:960–4

177. Parisi VM, Salinas J, Stockmar EJ. Fetal vascular responses to maternal nicardipine administration in the hypertensive ewe. *Am J Obstet Gynecol* 1989; 161:1035–9

178. Mari G, Kirshon B, Moise KJ Jr, *et al.* Doppler assessment of the fetal and uteroplacental circulation during nifedipine therapy for preterm labor. *Am J Obstet Gynecol* 1989;161:1514–18

179. Keirse MJNC. Progestogen administration in pregnancy may prevent preterm delivery. *Br J Obstet Gynaecol* 1990;97:149–54

180. Wilson L, Parsons MT, Quano L, Flouret G. A new tocolytic agent: development of an oxytocin antagonist for inhibiting uterine contractions. *Am J Obstet Gynecol* 1990;163:195–202

181. Liggins GC, Howie RN. A controlled trial of antepartum glucocorticoid treatment for prevention of the respiratory distress syndrome in premature infants. *Pediatrics* 1972;50:515–25

182. U.S. Department of Health and Human Services. *Prevention of Respiratory Distress Syndrome. Effect of Antenatal Dexamethasone Administration*, NIH Publication no. 85-2695 Washington, DC: U.S. Government Printing Office, 1985

183. Crowley P, Chalmers I, Keirse MJNC. The effects of corticosteroid administration before preterm delivery: an overview of the evidence from controlled trials. *Br J Obstet Gynaecol* 1990;97:11–25

184. Doyle LW, Kitchen WH, Ford GW, *et al.* Effects of antenatal steroid therapy on mortality and morbidity in very low birth weight infants. *J Pediatr* 1986;108:287–92

185. NIH Consensus Development Conference Statement. Effect of corticosteroids for fetal maturation on perinatal outcomes, February 28–March 2, 1994. *Am J Obstet Gynecol* 1995;173:246–52

186. Anonymous. Australian Collaborative trial of antenatal thyrotropin-releasing hormone (ACTOBAT) for prevention of neonatal respiratory disease. *Lancet* 1995;345:877–82

187. Morales WJ, Angel JF, O'Brien WF, *et al.* A randomized study of antibiotic therapy in idiopathic preterm labor. *Obstet Gynecol* 1988;72:829–33

188. Newton ER, Dinsmoor MJ, Gibbs RS. A randomized blinded, placebo-controlled trial of antibiotics in idiopathic preterm labor. *Obstet Gynecol* 1989;74:562–6

189. Romero R, Sibai B, Caritis S, *et al.* Antibiotic treatment of preterm labor with intact membranes: a multicenter, randomized, double-blinded, placebo-controlled trial. *Am J Obstet Gynecol* 1993;169:764–74

190. Norman K, Pattinson RC, de Souza J, *et al.* Ampicillin and metronidazole treatment in preterm labour: a multicentre, randomized controlled trial. *Br J Obstet Gynaecol* 1994;101:404–8

191. Klebanoff MA, Regan JA, Rao AV, *et al.* Outcome of the vaginal infections and prematurity study: results of a clinical trial of erythromycin among pregnant women colonized with group B streptococci. *Am J Obstet Gynecol* 1995;172:1540–5

192. Morales WJ, Schoor S, Albritton J. Effect of metronidazole in patients with preterm birth in preceding pregnancy and bacterial vaginosis: a placebo controlled, double-blind study. *Am J Obstet Gynecol* 1994;171:345–7

193. Schwartz D, Miodovnik M, Lavin J. Neonatal outcome among low birth weight infants delivered spontaneously or by low forceps. *Obstet Gynecol* 1983;62:283–6

194. Dietl J, Arnold H, Mentzel H, *et al.* Effect of Cesarean section on outcome in high- and low-risk very preterm infants. *Arch Gynecol Obstet* 1989;246:91–6

195. Behrman RE, *et al.* Committee to Study the Prevention of Low Birthweight, Division of Health Promotion and Disease Prevention. *Preventing Low Birthweight*. Washington, DC: Institute of Medicine, National Academy Press, 1985

196. Hobel CJ, Ross MG, Bemis RL, *et al.* The West Los Angeles preterm birth prevention project. I. Program impact on high-risk women. *Am J Obstet Gynecol* 1994;170:54–62

197. Iams JD, Johnson FF, Creasy RK. Prevention of preterm birth. *Clin Obstet Gynecol* 1988;31:599–615

198. Miller HC, Merritt TA. *Fetal Growth in Humans*. Chicago: Yearbook Medical Publishers, 1977

199. Papiernik E, Breart G. Should a prevention program be proposed to high-risk patients or all patients? *Am J Obstet Gynecol* 1994;171:1676–7

9

Premature rupture of the fetal membranes

A. Al-Malt

INTRODUCTION

Premature delivery is the leading cause of neonatal morbidity and mortality. Premature rupture of the membranes (PROM) is the single most identifiable cause of preterm delivery[1,2]. PROM at < 32 weeks is the major contributor to perinatal mortality and morbidity. Chorioamnionitis and postpartum endometritis are the most common maternal complications associated with PROM.

THE HUMAN FETAL CHORIOAMNIOTIC MEMBRANE

The fetal membranes are the amnion and chorion. The term amnion is derived from the Greek word *amnos*, which means 'lamb'. Amnion was also used to describe the bowl in which the blood of sacrificed animals was collected. Synonyms for amnion were given in 1879 by Hyrtl in his work on Arabic and Hebrew contributions to anatomical terminology[3]. The human amnion develops by cavitation of the inner cell mass of the early blastocyst by the 7–8th day of development of the fertilized ovum[4]. It arises as a single sheet of cells dorsal to the embryonic disc. The amniotic vesicle is formed by fluid accumulation and enlarges gradually to form the amniotic sac. The amniotic sac, which initially covers the dorsal surface of the embryo, enlarges gradually to surround it. The chorion develops into the chorion frondosum at the placental site and the chorion laeve that surrounds the rest of the gestational sac (Figure 1). The amniotic sac is initially separated from the chorion laeve by the extracelomic cavity. Gradual distension of the amniotic sac obliterates the extracelomic cavity by the end of the first trimester and brings the amnion into direct contact with the chorion. The amnion and chorion are slightly adherent, but can easily be separated, owing to the spongy layer in between the two[5]. Histologically, the normal amnion consists of a single layer of unciliated cuboidal cells and measures 0.02–0.5 mm in thickness. By the third trimester, the amnion consists of epithelial cells superimposed on a layer of dense connective tissue rich in collagen filaments[6,7]. The combination of the two layers gives the amnion a thickness of 0.05–0.1 mm. No blood vessels, nerve fibers or lymphatic channels can be identified in the amnion[8]. The underlying

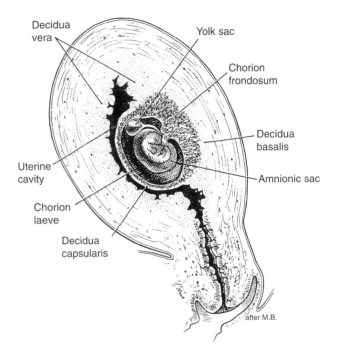

Figure 1 Atrophic chorion laeve and chorion frondosum (chorionic villi) proliferating into the decidua basalis. From reference 179

chorion contains several collagen layers, cellular, reticular and basement membrane, the outermost of which is closely attached and may be indistinguishable from the decidua (Figure 2). The chorion measures 0.04–0.4 mm in thickness[6]. The amnion and chorion form the chorioamniotic membranes, which possess dynamic properties characteristic of viscoelastic material[9]. Normally the preterm chorioamniotic membrane is more resistant to rupture (i.e. has higher bursting pressure) than the term membrane[10].

DEFINITION

Premature rupture of membranes is rupture of the membranes evidenced by leakage of amniotic fluid (amniorrhexis) before the onset of labor. Preterm PROM is rupture of membranes before 37 weeks' gestation. The latency period is the interval between the onset of PROM and the onset of labor. Prolonged

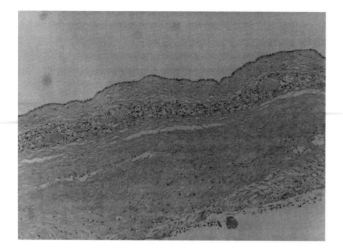

Figure 2 Fetal membranes consist of 4 layers (from top to bottom): amnion, connective tissues, chorion and connective tissues. With permission from reference 180

PROM is PROM with a latency period of more than 24 h[1,10].

INCIDENCE

The incidence of PROM varies with gestational age and diagnostic accuracy. Approximately 10% of all pregnancies (term and preterm) are complicated by PROM. Preterm PROM occurs in 2–4% of gestations, and it is responsible for 30–40% of all preterm deliveries[1,11–14].

The role of amniocentesis, antibiotics and steroids in the management of PROM has been controversial. This chapter discusses the diagnosis, etiology, risk factors, maternal and neonatal morbidity and mortality of preterm PROM as well as management strategies.

DIAGNOSIS OF PREMATURE RUPTURE OF MEMBRANES

The diagnosis of PROM should be considered in pregnant patients with history of watery discharge, a gush of fluid from the vagina, preterm labor or oligohydramnios. Information about the onset, color, consistency and odor of the discharge may be helpful in differentiating PROM from normal leukorrhea of pregnancy, urinary incontinence, vaginal infection and mucoid discharge due to cervical dilatation. The diagnosis should be confirmed by sterile speculum examination and other confirmatory tests. Visualization of the leakage of the amniotic fluid from the cervix confirms the diagnosis. Fluid in the posterior vaginal fornix should be obtained by a sterile swab and smeared on a clean glass slide and on Nitrazine (phenaphthazine paper) (Bristol-Myers Squibb Co)

Microscopically, the amniotic fluid shows 'arborization' or the 'palm leaf pattern' upon drying. This ferning is caused by crystallization of electrolytes, mainly sodium chloride, in the amniotic fluid under the effect of estrogen hormone. False-positive ferning may occur when the sample is contaminated with semen or cervical mucus[15,16]. The overall accuracy of this test in diagnosing PROM is ≥ 95%, with a 5–10% false-negative rate owing to contamination with blood or insufficient drying of the sample[10,17,18]. The value of the fern test in diagnosing PROM has been challenged in a recent survey. The test has high sensitivity and specificity in laboring patients (98% and 88%, respectively), but not in non-laboring patients (51% and 71%, respectively)[19].

The normal vaginal pH in pregnancy is 4.0–4.5, and the pH of the amniotic fluid is 7.0–7.5. The yellow Nitrazine paper turns blue when exposed to the less acidic amniotic fluid. The accuracy of the Nitrazine test is 80–90%, with 10% false-positive and 10% false-negative rates[12]. Contamination with urine, semen, blood and bacteria can cause false-positive results. If amniotic fluid leakage cannot be demonstrated or seen in the posterior fornix, the patient should be re-examined after lying in bed for a few hours. Samples from cervical mucus should be avoided.

A simple two-tablet oral Pyridium (phenazopyridine hydrochloride; Warmer Chilcott Labs) test may be helpful in ruling out urinary incontinence with demonstration of the orange-stained dye on the perineal pad. Although Pyridium crosses the placenta, it does not cause discoloration of the normal amniotic fluid with a pH of 7–7.5[20].

Ultrasound evaluation of amniotic fluid volume can be helpful in the diagnosis of PROM, especially in patients with a previously normal fluid volume. Oligohydramnios can occur with PROM as well as with fetal urinary tract anomalies and intrauterine growth retardation. Amniocentesis and instillation of indigo carmine dye into the amniotic cavity may be necessary to confirm the diagnosis of PROM in the presence of oligohydramnios without evident leakage of amniotic fluid. Staining of a vaginal tampon with the blue indigo carmine dye within a few hours of amniocentesis confirms the diagnosis of PROM. The use of a perineal pad may be preferred to vaginal insertion of a tampon with the theoretical risk of infection. It should be noted that the dye may reach the maternal bladder after many hours of instillation and may stain the pad in the presence of urinary incontinence. Methylene blue is no longer used, because of potential risks of fetal methemoglobinemia and hemolytic crises in patients with glucose 6-phosphate dehydrogenase (G6PD) deficiency[21,22].

Recently, amniotic fluid markers such as α-fetoprotein, diamino-oxidase, fetal fibronectin, prolactin and insulin-like growth factor binding protein-1 in the vaginal secretions have been evaluated for confirming the diagnosis of PROM[23-25]. The sensitivity and specificity are comparable to those of fern and Nitrazine testing.

ETIOLOGY OF PREMATURE RUPTURE OF MEMBRANES

The chorioamniotic membranes have an elastic component which enables them to resist deformation and to recover to their original state[9]. Weakening of the membranes and/or increased intra-amniotic pressure may lead to PROM. Repetitive stretching of the term membranes can cause splitting and breaking down of the compact layer and separation of the amnion from the spongy layer[26]. Acute or chronic stress may cause thinning out of the membranes as a result of breakdown of the non-recoverable elastic component[27]. Membranes that rupture prematurely may have decreased elasticity[28,29].

The quality and/or quantity of collagen in the chorioamniotic membranes may be altered in PROM. The collagen content of the human amniotic membranes was found to be significantly lower in patients with PROM than in patients with intact membranes[30]. More specifically, type III collagen, an interstitial collagen for tissue support, was significantly reduced in the amniotic membranes of patients with PROM[31]. These findings, however, have not been confirmed[32,33]. Others found a higher percentage of soluble collagen despite normal total membrane collagen content[34]. The role of collagen and membrane integrity in PROM remains unresolved. Changes in collagen content, arrangement or degradation may predispose to PROM. These changes, however, may be localized to the site of the rupture only.

Membrane surface energy, bursting pressure and membrane strain may play a role in PROM. Membrane surface energy is maximum at 32 weeks' gestation and then decreases to term, presumably secondary to production of surfactant[35]. High surface energy in early gestation may predispose the new membranes to wear and abrasion, increasing the risk for PROM. Membrane bursting pressure is lower at term, despite there being the same amount of collagen[32]. No difference, however, is found in bursting tension with or without PROM[36-39].

Other studies suggest a role for decreased α_1-antitrypsin activity and increased activity of protease, phospholipase and plasminogen activators in the etiology of PROM. Cytokines associated with infection have recently been implicated in the etiology of PROM. Microbial invasion of the fetal membrane is a source of proteases and phospholipases that could predispose to PROM[40]. Incubation of the membranes with activated neutrophils reduces bursting tension and elasticity of the fetal membranes[41]. Interleukin-1 (IL-1) and tumor necrosis factor (TNF) stimulate collagenase activity[42-44]. Moreover, IL-1 increases chorionic production of hyaluronic acid, which may reduce the tensile strength of the membranes, and tumor necrosis factor can alter multiplication of the amniocytes[42].

RISK FACTORS FOR PREMATURE RUPTURE OF MEMBRANES

The most common risk factors associated with PROM are previous preterm delivery/PROM, vaginal bleeding, placental abruption, smoking and microbial invasion of the amniotic cavity.

History of previous premature rupture of membrane

Previous preterm labor or premature rupture of membrane is the most significant predictor for PROM. The recurrence risk for preterm PROM is 21%[45]. In a case–control study, the demographic features and medical, obstetric, gynecological and sexual histories of the 341 patients with PROM between 20 and 36 weeks were compared to 253 controls[46]. Data were collected by comprehensive questionnaire from six perinatal centers. Multiple logistic regression analysis demonstrated that only previous preterm delivery, vaginal bleeding and cigarette smoking during the index pregnancy were significantly associated with PROM.

In another case–control study of 133 patients and a similar number of controls, smoking and previous PROM were significant predictors for PROM. Patients with a previous history of PROM were 3.5 times more likely to have recurrent PROM (odds ratio 3.6, 90% confidence interval 2–6.8)[47].

Vaginal bleeding

Vaginal bleeding due to placental abruption or placenta previa increases the risk of PROM by two- to three-fold[48]. Vaginal bleeding occurred in 41% of patients with PROM vs. 17% in the control group[46]. The risk for preterm PROM was two-, four- and six-fold if the vaginal bleeding occurred in the first, second or third trimester, respectively. The risk was found to increase to seven-fold if bleeding occurred in more than one trimester. Whether vaginal bleeding is a reflection of cervical changes associated with preterm labor, or a direct causative factor for preterm labor/PROM, is uncertain. Vaginal bleeding may impair nutritional support of the fetal membranes and cause ascending infection and deciduitis, which weaken the fetal membranes. It is noteworthy that PROM can occur in the presence of placenta previa, either by leakage from a high rupture site or by thinning and weakening of the placental part covering the cervical os.

Placental abruption

Placental abruption is positively correlated with PROM[49]. Abruption is five times more frequent in patients with PROM than in the general obstetric population. It is not clear whether abruption is a cause or a consequence of PROM. Placental abruption may increase the intra-amniotic pressure, causing PROM. Patients with abruptio placentae following PROM have a higher incidence of vaginal bleeding before the PROM and during the latency period[50–52]. On the other hand, leakage of amniotic fluid may lead to a disproportion between the placenta surface and uterine wall, favoring placenta separation[53].

Smoking

An older study using data from a United States Perinatal Collaborative Project (1958–66) found no association between smoking and PROM[45]. Recent studies, however, have demonstrated that smoking is a significant risk factor for PROM. A history of previous PROM and smoking more than ten cigarettes a day are significant independent predictors for PROM. Smoking through pregnancy increases the risk of PROM by two- to three-fold and has a dose–response relationship[46,47,54]. The mechanism by which smoking causes PROM is speculative. A significantly decreased level of lymphocytotoxic antibodies was found in pregnant smokers[55]. Smoking may reduce ascorbic acid levels by lowering the overall nutritional status of the patient. It decreases the ability of the immune system to produce protease inhibitors, making the membrane more susceptible to infection. Decidual ischemia as a result of nicotine-induced vasoconstriction is another proposed mechanism.

Infection

Ascending infection from the genital tract may play an important role in the etiology of PROM[56,57]. Organisms linked to prematurity and PROM include *Neisseria gonorrhoeae*, group B streptococcus, *Bacteroides* species, *Gardnerella* and *Trichomonas vaginalis*[56]. Infection increases the production of polymorphonuclear leukocytes and inflammatory cytokines (e.g. IL-1, -6 and -8), which stimulate phospholipase-A$_2$ activity and the production of prostanoids and endothelin. Those substances enhance the production of proteases, which weaken the membranes. This same mechanism is proposed to play a role in initiating preterm labor.

Neisseria gonorrhoeae

One study found no significant increase in prevalence of PROM in patients with positive *N. gonorrhoeae* culture compared to matched controls[58]. Other studies found that PROM and *N. gonorrhoeae* infection were independently associated with preterm labor and delivery[59,60]. A significantly increased incidence of PROM was found in patients with positive *N. gonorrhoeae* cultures than in patients with negative cultures. However, a cause–effect relationship was not demonstrated and the presence of a positive *N. gonorrhoeae* culture may simply identify patients at higher risk for PROM by other mechanisms.

Group B streptococcus

The association of group B streptococcus with preterm labor and PROM has been addressed in many studies. Group B streptococcus has been associated with preterm delivery and PROM[61,62]. A higher frequency of positive genital culture was found on admission in patients with PROM than in those with intact membranes (16% vs. 4%, respectively)[63]. On the other hand, a higher rate of PROM was found in patients with positive genital cervical culture than those with negative culture (42% vs. 19%, respectively)[64]. Currently, there is no evidence that antibiotic prophylaxis for group B streptococcus genital colonization reduces the risk of PROM.

Other bacterial infections

Staphylococcus aureus, *Bacteroides* species, *Enterobacter* and other strains of aerobic and anaerobic bacteria are associated with increased collagenase activity, which may predispose to PROM. The effect of antibiotic treatment on membrane strength was tested *in vitro* with different inhibitory concentrations. Larger doses inhibited bacterial growth, protease release and membrane damage, and smaller doses reduced membrane damage despite bacterial growth[65]. The clinical implications of these findings are not clear.

Bacterial vaginosis

Bacterial vaginosis is characterized by overgrowth of vaginal bacterial flora with anaerobic bacteria such as *Bacteroides* species and peptococci, predominantly. Both *Gardnerella* and *Mycoplasma* are present in high numbers. Bacterial vaginosis may increase vaginal pH by increasing the number of anaerobes, outnumbering the corynebacteria in the vaginal flora. The increased vaginal pH has been implicated as a risk factor for preterm labor and PROM[66]. In recent years, increasing attention has been given to the relationship between altered vaginal bacterial flora and preterm birth. Evidence suggesting that bacterial vaginosis may have a pathological role in preterm labor is gradually accumulating[67–69].

Bacterial vaginosis is a condition of the vagina characterized by overgrowth of anaerobic species, thus outnumbering the normal hydrogen peroxide-degrading *Corynebacterium* species. *Gardnerella vaginalis* is not the only causative organism. Bacterial vaginosis-associated organisms include *Mobiluncus* species, *Mycoplasma hominis*, *Fusobacterium nucleatum*, *Bacteroides ureolyticus*, *Ureaplasma urealyticum*, *Prevotella* species and peptostreptococci.

Bacterial vaginosis and preterm labor Clinical studies have demonstrated a two- to three-fold increased risk of preterm labor and delivery as well as endometritis when bacterial vaginosis is present during pregnancy. This relationship has been demonstrated with bacterial vaginosis diagnosed by clinical or laboratory criteria, and by recovering bacterial vaginosis-associated organisms from the amniotic fluid. The presence of bacterial vaginosis in mid-trimester is significantly and independently related to preterm delivery of infants of low birth weight. A few studies have reported significantly decreased incidences of preterm birth when bacterial vaginosis was treated. The benefit of such treatment is lacking in subsets of patients with a history of previous preterm deliveries. Bacterial vaginosis is more common in African–American unmarried patients with low income. This racial predilection is not fully understood.

Diagnosis of bacterial vaginosis Diagnosis is made when three of the following four criteria are met: (1) vaginal pH greater than 4.5; (2) the presence of amine odor on adding 10% potassium hydroxide to vaginal secretions; (3) detection of 'clue cells' – vaginal epithelial cells heavily coated with bacilli; and (4) the presence of homogeneous vaginal discharge. The specificity and predicting value of the last three criteria alone is approximately 90%. Other diagnostic modalities include vaginal culture for *Gardnerella*, Gram-stain evaluation of lactobacilli, *Gardnerella* and *Mobiluncus*, gas liquid chromatography and proline aminopeptidase tests. The sensitivity of the vaginal culture for diagnosis varies widely. The Gram stain has sensitivity of 60–95%, specificity of 75–95% and positive predictive value of 70–75%. The gas liquid chromatography and proline aminopeptidase tests are used mainly in research.

It is important to recognize that at least 15–20% of all pregnant patients are colonized with bacterial vaginosis. Up to 50% of the colonized patients are asymptomatic. These patients have *Gardnerella* on vaginal culture but do not meet clinical criteria for diagnosis. This type of *Gardnerella* is probably insensitive to hydrogen peroxide produced by the vaginal lactobacilli. A higher frequency of positive rectal isolates for organisms associated with bacterial vaginosis is found in women with bacterial vaginosis than in those without. This suggests that sexual transmission is not the only means of acquiring bacterial vaginosis and urges us to rethink the efficacy of treating the male partners of patients with this infection.

Treatment of bacterial vaginosis Ampicillin was once recommended for treatment but is no longer considered effective. The standard treatment in the non-pregnant population is oral metronidazol, 500 mg twice daily or 250 mg three times a day for 7 days. The immediate cure rate is 98% with a long-term cure rate of 60–95%. Vaginal metranidazol cream can be used twice daily for 5 days. Similar efficacy has been observed with oral clindamycin 300 mg orally twice daily for 7 days, but the side-effects, particularly pseudomembranous colitis, have prevented its widespread use. When 2% clindamycin cream 5 g is used daily for 7 days, vaginal candidiasis occurs in approximately 10% of all patients treated.

Chlamydia trachomatis

The causal relationship between chlamydial genital infection and preterm PROM also remains unclear. While most of the studies showed no significant increase in preterm PROM/preterm delivery of patients with chlamydial infection[70,71], a few[63,67] found a significant association. An increased risk was suggested in a subset of patients with positive IgM antibodies[70]. A higher IgM titer, defined as 1:32, was significantly associated with a higher incidence of preterm delivery and PROM. Although these findings suggest that acute chlamydial infection in the presence of PROM is a risk factor for preterm labor, evidence is lacking for its role in causing PROM.

Mycoplasma infection

Mycoplasma differ from viruses in their ability to grow on cell-free media and differ from bacteria in lacking a cell wall. Only three species have been isolated from the human genital mucosa. *Mycoplasma genitalis* is of uncertain significance. *Ureaplasma urealyticum* alone may be present in 15% of amniotic fluid cultures of PROM of ≤ 34 weeks[72]. A positive genital culture for *U. urealyticum* does not predict preterm labor or PROM[73]. *M. Hominis* and *U. urealyticum* are common isolates of sexually active adults. They become predominant components of the genital flora in the presence of bacterial vaginosis.

In summary, PROM increases the risks of microbial invasion of the amniotic cavity. However, subclinical infection may play a role in preterm PROM by causing membrane inflammation, increasing collagenase activity and altering amniocyte multiplication.

Other factors that may play a role in preterm PROM are connective tissue disorders, incompetent cervix, previous dilatation and curettage (D&C), sexual intercourse and deficiencies of vitamin C and trace elements.

Connective tissue disorders

Fetal membranes are primarily a connective-tissue structure. Type I Ehlers–Danlos syndrome is inherited as an autosomal dominant disorder and has a striking association with PROM, cervical incompetence and preterm labor. Preterm PROM occurred in 72% (13/18), and preterm delivery occurred in 78% (14/18) of patients with Ehlers–Danlos syndrome[74].

Incompetent cervix and cervical cerclage

Cervical incompetence may play a role in the etiology of PROM. Exposure of a large surface area of the fetal membranes to the vaginal flora may predispose the membranes to weakening and rupture. Transudation of amniotic fluid across the exposed fetal membranes is not uncommon in the presence of advanced cervical dilatation (≥ 4 cm) and should not be mistaken for PROM. The role of cervical cerclage in preventing PROM, however, has not been confirmed by large studies. Moreover, there is an increased risk of chorioamnionitis and PROM with cervical cerclage[75]. The risk increases as gestation advances, with 40% incidence of chorioamnionitis associated with late cervical cerclage (> 19 weeks) in the presence of bulging membranes. The role of cervical cerclage in the presence of PROM has been evaluated[76,77]. It is generally advised that the cerclage be removed once the membranes rupture, to decrease the risk of chorioamnionitis.

Dilatation and curettage

Univariant analysis of risk factors for PROM revealed an increased risk of PROM in patients with previous D&C or elective termination of pregnancy[46]. Neither risk factor remained significant when multivariant analysis was used. In another study using step-wise regression analysis, no significant difference in PROM was found between patients with one or more previous abortion and those without abortions[78]. On the other hand, second-trimester termination of pregnancy is considered to be a recognized risk factor for cervical incompetence and subsequent PROM[79].

Ascorbic acid and trace element deficiency

Vitamin C is essential in the formation of collagen. A significant increase in preterm PROM was found in patients with low ascorbic acid levels[47,80]. Low copper concentrations can affect collagen maturation and decrease elastin production. A significantly lower level of serum copper was found in patients with PROM when compared with controls without PROM[81]. No difference in membrane copper content was observed between the two groups. These findings were not confirmed by other investigators[82]. Zinc may play an important role in the antimicrobial activity of amniotic fluid. No significant difference in maternal and umbilical cord zinc serum concentration was found between patients with preterm PROM and patients with preterm delivery without PROM. When a zinc index was calculated from serum, colostrum, scalp and pubic hair zinc, patients with term PROM had a lower index than those without PROM[83]. In summary, there is no conclusive evidence that trace element deficiency plays a significant role in causing PROM.

Coitus

It is believed that coitus temporarily increases the frequency of uterine contractions, either by orgasmic activity or by the high concentration of prostaglandins in the seminal fluid. However, there is no strong evidence to support coitus as an etiological risk factor for PROM. There is no significant difference in coital and orgasmic activity between patients with preterm PROM/preterm labor and patients with term delivery[84]. Coitus during the last month of pregnancy was not found to be associated with preterm labor or PROM[85–87]. A slight increase in preterm PROM was reported when delivery occurred within 9 days of coitus[45]. This increase, however, was not statistically significant. Most recently, only male superior position was found to double the risk of preterm PROM[88].

NEONATAL MORTALITY

Reports on mortality vary, according to the place of delivery, accurate estimation of gestational age, level of the intensive neonatal care resources available and the definition of survival. Neonatal survival is defined as survival at the 28th day of life. Perinatal death rate is the sum of the number of antepartum deaths plus the number of early neonatal deaths (up to 7 days of life) per 1000 births. Most of the data on neonatal survival considered survival as being discharged alive from the hospital. Many reports have excluded antepartum/intrapartum fetal deaths, thus spuriously overestimating the true perinatal survival.

Neonatal survival is approximately 35% at 24 weeks, 55% at 25 weeks, and increases weekly by approximately 10% until 28 weeks. Survival for birth weight of 1250–1500 g at 29 weeks is approximately 90%[89,90]. A recent retrospective study of 142 infants born between 22 and 25 weeks demonstrated a neonatal survival rate of 0% (0/29), 15% (6/40), 56% (19/34) and 79% (31/39) at 22, 23, 24 and 25 weeks, respectively[91]. Only 2% of infants born at 23 weeks' gestation survived without severe abnormalities visualized on cranial ultrasound examination (grade III and IV intraventricular hemorrhage or periventricular leukomalacia) as compared with 21% of those born at 24 weeks and 69% of those born at 25 weeks[91]. In another study, administration of surfactant to the infants with very low birth weight reduced the odds of death in hospital by 30%[92].

NEONATAL MORBIDITY

Morbidity and mortality secondary to preterm PROM are primarily affected by the gestational age at the time of PROM[93,94]. Birth weight is the second most important factor for determining neonatal morbidity and mortality. Short-term complications of preterm PROM include fetal malpresentation, fetal distress due to cord accident or placental abruption, acute respiratory distress and neonatal sepsis. Respiratory distress is the most significant predictor of neonatal morbidity and mortality. A study defining major long-term neonatal morbidity as chronic lung disease, necrotizing enterocolitis and significant intraventricular hemorrhage found 55%, 39% and 26% incidences for neonates with birth weights of ≤ 750 g, 751–1000 g and 1001–1251 g, respectively[89]. The incidence of significant intraventricular hemorrhage (grade III or IV) was 32%, 26% and 12% for the same birth weight ranges, respectively. In a follow-up study, the authors compared 65 school-aged survivors with birth weights of < 750 g to 65 children with birth weights of 750–1499 g, and 61 children born at term. The rates of mental retardation (IQ < 70) in the three groups were 21%, 8% and 2%, respectively, and the rates of cerebral palsy were 9%, 6% and 0%, respectively[95].

PULMONARY HYPOPLASIA

The risk for pulmonary hypoplasia inversely correlates with gestational age at the onset of PROM. The incidence is highest with PROM at ≤ 26 weeks and lowest after 30 weeks[96]. In a review of 100 neonates of mothers with PROM lasting for more than 1 week, a strong relationship was found between PROM at < 26 weeks' gestation and pulmonary hypoplasia[97]. The incidence of pulmonary hypoplasia ranged from 10% to 32% with prolonged PROM at < 26 weeks[93,98,99]. This wide range may be due to inclusion of patients with other causes of oligohydramnios in some studies. The impact of oligohydramnios on obstetric outcome may be related to its onset, duration or severity. Oligohydramnios following mid-trimester PROM is of particular interest, owing to the potential fetal viability and the state of lung development. While gestational age at PROM seems to be the most important predictive factor for the development of pulmonary hypoplasia, the impact

of the latent period and of oligohydramnios is less clear[100–102]. In a recent study of 119 patients with PROM at 18 to 28 weeks gestation, it was found that neonates with oligohydramnios were twice as likely to develop pulmonary hypoplasia (20 vs. 10%), and more likely to experience neonatal death (30 vs. 20%) when compared to those with adequate fluid, even though the difference was not statistically significant[103].

The mechanism of pulmonary hypoplasia associated with PROM is not clearly understood. Animal studies suggest that the effect of gestational age at the time of PROM is more important than the duration of PROM[104]. Chronic drainage of amniotic fluid causing oligohydramnios leads to pulmonary hypoplasia[105,106]. Oligohydramnios causing extrinsic compression of the fetal thorax may impair lung growth either by inhibiting breathing movement or by squeezing out lung fluid. Chronic loss of lung fluid and reduction of intra-amniotic pressure is proposed to increase the pressure gradient of intra-alveolar to amniotic fluid and to alter the laryngeal retentive mechanism leading to pulmonary hypoplasia. The role of low intra-amniotic pressure and low ratio of amniotic fluid to alveolar pressure in causing lung hypoplasia is controversial[107–109]. Alteration of fetal pulmonary arterial flow is also proposed to delay fetal lung growth and maturation[110].

NEONATAL SEPSIS

The risk of acute chorioamnionitis associated with PROM increases after a 24-h latency period[111]. However, this may be affected by other factors, such as the presence of infection at the time of PROM, the number of digital examinations, the volume of amniotic fluid and the population studied. The incidence of acute chorioamnionitis is increased in patients with low socioeconomic status when compared with middle-income patients[112,113]. In PROM at < 34 weeks' gestation, the incidence of neonatal sepsis is positively correlated with the duration of the rupture of the membrane[111,114]. PROM increases the risk of neonatal infection ten- to 15-fold (from 0.1% to 1.4%)[115,116]. The risk increases dramatically to 8% with the presence of chorioamnionitis[117]. Other risk factors for neonatal sepsis are prematurity, genital group B streptococcus colonization and male gender[93,115–119]. In one study, the predominant organisms colonizing the genital tract were found to be *Escherichia coli* (46%), *Bacteroides fragilis* (15%), *Streptococcus faecalis* (11%) and group B streptococcus (10%)[120]. The relative frequencies of such organisms may vary with different populations and different geographical distribution.

MATERNAL MORBIDITY

Maternal complications include chorioamnionitis, postpartum endometritis, increased risk of Cesarean section owing to placental abruption, fetal malpresentation or distress. Septic morbidity and maternal mortality have been significantly reduced with the new era of antibiotics[121,122].

ASSESSMENT OF FETAL WELL-BEING

Biophysical profile

The fetal biophysical profile is designed to evaluate fetal well-being by the non-stress test (NST) and four ultrasonographic parameters during a 30–60-min period. These include fetal movement, fetal tone, fetal breathing and the presence of a 2 × 2 cm pocket of amniotic fluid[123]. A score of 2 is assigned to each of the individual components when it is present and a score of zero when it is absent. A total score of 8 or 10 is reassuring, a score of 6 is equivocal and a score of 4 or less is worrisome. A low biophysical profile may be an early predictor of neonatal sepsis. Modifications of this original score are currently used in clinical practice; the most common is the NST and amniotic fluid volume[124,125].

Non-stress test

The NST alone or as part of the biophysical profile has been the main test for evaluating fetal well-being in the presence of PROM. The oxytocin challenge test and the nipple stimulation test are avoided, for fear of initiating preterm labor in patients with PROM. Preterm PROM has little or no effect on the reactivity of the fetal heart tracing[126,127]. Therefore, the lack of reactivity of the NST in those patients should not be simply ascribed to PROM. Variable decelerations may be observed with PROM, and their frequency has been correlated with the amniotic fluid volume[128]. A non-reactive NST without significant deceleration has a high false-positive rate (50%)[129] and should be repeated within 24 h, or a biophysical profile should be performed. A biophysical profile score of ≥ 8 in the presence of a non-reactive NST is reassuring and further fetal testing can be delayed. A score of 6 is equivocal and should be repeated within 24 h, and a score of ≤ 4 is concerning. The earliest biophysical activities to disappear in response to fetal hypoxia are those that develop later in fetal life. This gradual hypoxic concept is that loss of fetal heart rate reactivity and fetal breathing movements would occur before loss of fetal movement and finally loss of fetal tone. Absence of fetal tone is associated with the highest perinatal death rate (43%), followed by absence of fetal breathing and body movement[130].

Amniotic fluid volume

The volume of amniotic fluid is maintained by a dynamic process, with production by fetal urine and alveolar lung fluid and removal by fetal swallowing and the fetal membrane interface with the maternal uterine wall. Fetal urine first enters the amniotic cavity at 8–11 weeks' gestation. Fetal urine production increases from approximately 5 ml/h in the midtrimester to approximately 50–90 ml/h at term[131,132]. Fetal urine is hypotonic and of low osmolarity. Fetal lungs produce about 200–400 ml of amniotic fluid per day at term. Fetal swallowing accounts for reabsorption of up to 1500 ml/day, and approximately 80 ml/day can be removed by fetal membranes. The fetal membranes play an active role in the production and reabsorption of amniotic fluid. It should be noted that a normal amniotic fluid volume does not exclude preterm PROM and oligohydramnios is not always associated with PROM. Oligohydramnios has been associated with a shorter latency period, variable decelerations and increased incidence of chorioamnionitis[132,133]. However, management decisions should not be based solely on the amount of amniotic fluid.

Fetal breathing movement

PROM is associated with a significant and prolonged reduction of fetal breathing movement[133–135]. The mechanism for this phenomenon is unknown and could be related to the PROM *per se*, increased prostaglandins or preterm labor. Fetal breathing movement decreases with intra-amniotic infection, fetal infection[135,136], preterm labor and increased intra-amniotic prostaglandin E_2 (PGE_2) levels[138,139].

Fetal body movement

Studies have demonstrated that fetal body movement decreases in frequency and duration in patients with preterm PROM and amnionitis confirmed by positive amniotic fluid culture[124,136,137]. Fetal body movement has sensitivity of 32%, specificity of 97%, positive predictive value of 89% and negative predictive value of 69% in diagnosing positive amniotic fluid culture[137]. Others found no correlation between any of the biophysical profile components and clinical chorioamnionitis[140]. It seems logical that fetal body movement may decrease only when there is fetal compromise such as fetal septicemia or hypoxia.

EXPECTANT VS. ACTIVE MANAGEMENT

Fetal growth and maturation continues after PROM[33]. Furthermore, prematurity is the major contributing factor to neonatal morbidity and mortality[141]. Therefore, expectant management is advocated in the absence of evidence of mature fetal lungs. Approximately 40% of patients with PROM at 28–34 weeks' gestation were found to have an lecithin/sphingomyelin (L/S) ratio of

≥ 2:1 for amniotic fluid obtained by amniocentesis[142] and 24% were positive for phosphatidylglycerol. Of those patients with phosphatidylglycerol-negative amniotic fluid, 40% converted to positivity before delivery[143].

Expectant management is favored over active intervention in premature PROM prior to 34 weeks' gestation in the absence of active labor, infection or fetal distress[49,144,145]. The main objectives for management are accurate estimation of gestational age and fetal weight, evaluation of fetal well-being and early detection of preterm labor or infection. A detailed obstetric and gynecological history should be obtained. Since there is a good correlation between speculum and digital examination of the cervix[145–147], digital examination should be avoided unless active labor is established or delivery is imminent. The effect of digital examination on the length of the latency period is controversial, but a higher incidence of chorioamnionitis and endometritis is observed in many studies[148–150]. An increased risk of neonatal infection is reported when the interval from the initial examination to delivery exceeds 24 h[151]. This, however, was not confirmed by other studies. Cervical assessment by perineal ultrasound or vaginal ultrasound using a sterile probe cover can be helpful, although the risk of chorioamnionitis with these techniques remains to be determined. Cervical, vaginal and urinary cultures should be obtained and maternal condition should be evaluated for chorioamnionitis and preterm labor. Prophylactic antibiotics for group B streptococcus such as ampicillin, erythromycin or clindamycin may be initiated pending the result of genital cultures. Ultrasound examination is helpful in evaluating estimated fetal weight, fetal anatomy, fetal presentation and amniotic fluid index. Color flow Doppler ultrasound may be helpful in identifying cord (funic) presentation or cord-free pockets of amniotic fluid, especially in the presence of oligohydramnios.

Amniotic fluid leaking per vagina could be sent for pulmonary maturity studies. Evaluation of results must be cautiously undertaken in the context of other clinical findings. The L/S ratio is altered when amniotic fluid is contaminated with blood or meconium and false-positive phosphatidylglycerol results may occur, owing to bacterial colonization[152].

The use of tocolytic agents, prophylactic antibiotics and corticosteroids in the management of preterm PROM is controversial.

CORTICOSTEROIDS

The effect of premature PROM on fetal lung maturation is controversial. Many individual studies have failed to demonstrate a significant reduction in the incidence of respiratory distress syndrome (RDS) with steroid administration for PROM. However, meta-analyses of randomized trials have shown that steroid administration results in a significant reduction (≥ 50%) in the incidence of RDS (relative risk 0.6, 95% confidence interval 0.5–0.81, $p \leq 0.01$)[153,154]. A recent NIH consensus concluded that corticosteroid therapy is indicated for women at risk of preterm delivery with few exceptions[155]. Corticosteroid administration may be considered in the conservative management of PPROM before 30 to 32 weeks of gestation. This may decrease the risks of severe RDS and/or severe intraventricular hemorrhage. The benefit of multiple courses of corticosteroids in PPROM has not been proven. Administration of corticosteroids with PROM carries a theoretical risk of enhancing maternal and neonatal infection. However, randomized controlled trials failed to demonstrate a significant increase in perinatal infection or puerperal infection as a result of antenatal corticosteroid therapy[156–161].

In summary, antenatal corticosteroid therapy may be considered in premature PROM at 24 to 34 weeks, unless there is evidence of lung maturity, imminent delivery, chorioamnionitis or fetal distress. Different corticosteroids have different rates of placental transfer. A few protocols exist for the administration of different steroids. Betamethasone crosses the placenta more readily than dexamethasone, and prednisone has minimal transfer. Betamethasone is usually given by intramuscular injection in two doses of 12 mg, 24 h apart. The benefit of repeated steroid injection at weekly intervals has not been demonstrated. Evaluation of fetal lung maturity should be considered after 32 weeks' gestation. Recent animal studies have suggested that thyrotropin releasing hormone in combination with corticosteroids can significantly accelerate lung maturation and increase lung compliance in the premature fetus[162]. The clinical utility of this combination therapy remains to be proven. Maternal intravenous administration of thyrotropin releasing hormone has been found to exacerbate hypertension especially in preeclamptic patients[163,164].

TOCOLYTICS

Prophylactic oral tocolytic therapy does not significantly prolong gestation or improve perinatal outcome[165,166]. Three randomized trials evaluated the efficacy of intravenous tocolysis and bed rest in the presence of PROM[167–169]. Only one used a double-blind placebo design[167]. Tocolytics appeared to prolong gestation in two of the trials[167,168]. Intravenous tocolysis significantly prolonged gestation before 28 weeks[168] and decreased the proportion of women delivering within 24 h after PROM when compared to bed rest[167]. There were no significant differences in maternal or neonatal outcomes. Meta-analysis of the two trials that provided adequate information revealed that tocolysis did not result in prolongation of pregnancy for more than 48 h[168,169]. The benefit of tocolytic use in prolonging gestation in patients with preterm PROM remains to be proven. Mercer and Lewis have proposed that PPROM may be the optimal situation for aggressive short-term tocolysis to allow time for the benefit of corticosteroid therapy[170].

ANTIBIOTICS

Preterm infants are at an increased risk for GBS sepsis, particularly with prolonged PPROM. Prophylaxis is recommended with intravenous penicillin for 24 hours pending GBS culture results. Clindamycin or erythromycin can be used if the patient is allergic to penicillin; however, clindamycin may have a better transplacental crossing than erythromycin. The duration of prophylactic therapy for GBS carriers is controversial. Penicillin offers the narrow spectrum coverage but has not been shown to prolong gestation.

The effect of prophylactic antibiotics and the incidence of chorioamnionitis, neonatal sepsis and intraventricular hemorrhage is controversial[171–173]. Prolonged use of prophylactic ampicillin and amoxicillin is reported to be associated with resistant enterobacteriaceae chorioamnionitis and adverse perinatal outcomes[174].

Two recent meta-analyses of randomized prospective trials of adjunctive broad-spectrum antibiotics with expectant management of PPROM have demonstrated significant pregnancy prolongation at one week (38.5% vs. 24.1%)[175,176]. There was no evidence of decrease in RDS or perinatal mortality. The NICHD multi-center trial antibiotics with PPROM at 24 to 32 weeks gestation has demonstrated a significant reduction in perinatal morbidity including RDS[177]. In these trials, the combination of ampicillin and erythromycin, was given intravenously for 48 h, followed by oral administration for an additional 5 days.

In summary, the role of antibiotic administration in the presence of PPROM is controversial. It may be limited to treating culture-proven sepsis and to a short-term prophylaxis for group B streptococcus. The benefit of prophylactic antibiotic therapy should be weighed against the risk of overgrowth of resistant bacteria. A course of broad spectrum antibiotics for 1 week may be helpful to prolong gestation in the absence of infection.

AMNIOCENTESIS

Amniocentesis has been used in the management of preterm PROM. The success and complication rates of obtaining fluid by transabdominal amniocentesis vary widely with the experience of the operator and the amount of the amniotic fluid. Amniocentesis is an invasive procedure that carries risks of, for instance, chorioamnionitis, preterm labor and injury to the placental vessels, umbilical cord, or the fetus. Amniotic fluid obtained by amniocentesis can be assessed for fetal lung maturity and microbial colonization of the amniotic cavity. When the diagnosis of PROM is uncertain, amniocentesis with dye instillation is helpful. The value of amniocentesis in diagnosing intra-amniotic infection is limited by the low sensitivity and the specificity of diagnostic tests for chorioamnionitis. Although amniotic fluid culture remains the gold standard for detection of infection, the results may take 2–3 days. Gram staining of the amniotic fluid has a low sensitivity of 50% for detecting infection[178]. In summary, amniocentesis in experienced hands is useful to confirm the diagnosis of PROM, document lung maturity and exclude colonization of the amniotic cavity. This invasive procedure carries risks to the mother and her fetus, and should be offered only to selected cases after careful evaluation.

CONCLUSION

PROM complicates 10% of all gestations and 2–4% of preterm pregnancies. Our success in preventing preterm PROM and preterm birth is hampered by our limited knowledge of its etiology. Previous PROM/preterm labor is the major risk factor for recurrent PROM. Other risk factors include vaginal bleeding, smoking during pregnancy, cervical incompetence and bacterial colonization of the genital tract. While a great deal of controversy surrounds the management of PROM, emphasis should be applied to preventive measures. Perhaps avoidance of smoking, early detection and management of cervical incompetence, early treatment of vaginal infection and an improvement of overall maternal nutrition can be beneficial in reducing the risk of PROM in certain subsets of patients. The objectives of managing patients with preterm PROM are accurate assessment of gestational age and fetal weight, evaluation of fetal well-being and early detection of infection or preterm labor. Expectant management is recommended for PROM at < 32–34 weeks in absence of evidence of lung maturity, active labor, fetal infection or fetal distress. Corticosteroid therapy should be considered in these circumstances. Currently there is insufficient evidence to recommend routine use of tocolytic agents or amniocentesis for management of preterm PROM. Antibiotic prophylaxis for genital group B streptococcus colonization should be considered until culture results are available. Antibiotic therapy should be initiated in all cases with group B streptococcus culture-positive results. A repeat culture is recommended if the latency period is prolonged and conservative management is expected. PROM remains the single most identifiable cause of preterm delivery and the major contributor to perinatal morbidity and mortality. Its clinical management continues to be controversial. While the role of antibiotics and tocolytics remains to be determined by large prospective trials, recent data support the value of antepartum steroid administration for accelerating lung maturity in the presence of PROM. Future research is warranted to clarify the etiology of PROM and enhance our efforts in its prevention and treatment.

REFERENCES

1. Johnson JW, Daikoku NY, Niebyl JR, *et al*. Premature rupture of the membranes and prolonged pregnancy. Obstet Gynecol 1981;57:547–56
2. Gibbs RS. Premature rupture of the membranes. *Obstet Gynecol* 1982;60:671–9
3. Boyd JD, Hamilton WJ. *The Human Placenta*. Cambridge: Heffer, 1970
4. Hoyes AD. Fine structure of human amniotic epithelium in early pregnancy. *Br J Obstet Gynaecol* 1968;75:949
5. Wynn RM, Davies J. Comparative electron microscopy of the hemochorial villous placenta. *Am J Obstet* 1965;91:533
6. Wynn RM. Fetomaternal cellular relations in the human basal plate: an ultrastructural study of the placenta. *Am J Obstet Gynecol* 1967;97:832–50
7. Bourne GL. The microscopic anatomy of the human amnion and chorion. *Am J Obstet Gynecol* 1960;74:1070
8. Bourne GL. *The Human Amnion and Chorion*. Chicago: Yearbook, 1962
9. Lavery JP, Miller CE. The viscoelastic nature of chorioamniotic membranes. *Obstet Gynecol* 1977;50:467–72
10. Verber IG, Pearce JM, New LC, *et al*. Prolonged rupture of the fetal membranes and neonatal outcome. *J Perinat Med* 1989;17:469–76
11. Lebherz TB, Hellman LB, Madding R, *et al*. Double-blind study of premature rupture of the membranes. *Am J Obstet Gynecol* 1963;87:218
12. Gunn CS, Mishell DR, Morton DG. Premature rupture of the fetal membranes. *Am J Obstet Gynecol* 1970; 106:469–83
13. Sachs M, Baker TH. Spontaneous premature rupture of the membranes. *Am J Obstet Gynecol* 1967;97:888–93
14. Fayez JA, Hasan AA, Jonas HS, Miller GL. Management of premature rupture of the membranes. *Obstet Gynecol* 1978;52:17–21
15. Friedman ML, McElin TW. Diagnosis of ruptured fetal membranes: clinical study and review of literature. *Am J Obstet Gynecol* 1969;104:544–50
16. Lodeiro JG, Hsieh KA, Byers JH, Feinstein SJ. The fingerprint, a false-positive fern test. *Obstet Gynecol* 1989;73:873–4
17. Reece EA, Chervenak FA, Moya FR, Hobbins JC. Amniotic fluid arborization: effect of blood, meconium, and pH alterations. *Obstet Gynecol* 1984;64:248–50
18. Rosemond RL, Lombardi SJ, Boehm FH. Ferning of amniotic fluid contaminated with blood. *Obstet Gynecol* 1990;75:338–40
19. de Haan HH, Offermans PM, Smits F, *et al*. Value of the fern test to confirm or reject the diagnosis of ruptured membranes is modest in nonlaboring women presenting with nonspecific vaginal fluid loss. *Am J Perinatol* 1994;11:46–50
20. Meyer BA, Gonik B, Creasy RK. Evaluation of phenazopyridine hydrochloride as a tool in the diagnosis of premature rupture of the membranes. *Am J Perinatol* 1991;8:297–9
21. Cowett RM, Hakanson DO, Kocon RW, Oh W. Untoward neonatal effect of intra-amniotic administration of methylene blue. *Obstet Gynecol* 1976; 48:74s–5
22. Troche BI. The methylene blue baby. *N Engl J Med* 1989;320:1756–7
23. Gaucherand P, Guibaud S, Rudigoz RC, Wong A. Diagnosis of premature rupture of the membranes by the identification of alpha feto-protein in vaginal secretions. *Acta Obstet Gynecol Scand* 1994;73:456–9
24. Lockwoood CJ, Wein R, Chien D, *et al*. Fetal membrane rupture is associated with the presence of insulin-like growth factor-binding protein-1 in vaginal secretions. *Am J Obstet Gynecol* 1994;171:146–50
25. Gaucherand P, Guibaud JS, Awada A, Rudigoz RC. Comparative study of three amniotic fluid markers in premature rupture of membranes: fetal fibronectin, alpha feto-protein, diamino-oxydase. *Acta Obstet Gynecol Scand* 1995;74:118–21
26. Toppozada M, Sallam N, Gaafar A, *et al*. Role of repeated stretching in the mechanism of timely rupture of the membranes. *Am J Obstet Gynecol* 1970; 108:243–9
27. Lavery J, Miller C. Deformation and creep in the human chorioamniotic sac. *Am J Obstet Gynecol* 1979; 134:366–75
28. Artal R, Sokol RJ, Neuman M, *et al*. The mechanical properties of prematurely and non-prematurely ruptured membranes. *Am J Obstet Gynecol* 1976; 125:655–9
29. Parry-Jones E, Priya S. A study of the elasticity and tension of fetal membranes and of the relation of the area of the gestational sac to the area of the uterine cavity. *Br J Obstet Gynaecol* 1976;83:205–12
30. Skinner S, Campos G, Higgins G. Collagen content of human amniotic membranes: effect of gestational length and premature rupture. *Obstet Gynecol* 1981; 57:487s
31. Kanayama N, Terao T, Kawashima Y. Collagen types in normal prematurely ruptured amniotic membranes. *Am J Obstet Gynecol* 1985;153:899–903
32. Al-Zaid NS, Bou-Resli MN, Goldspink G. Bursting pressure and collagen content of fetal membranes and their relation to premature rupture of the membranes. *Br J Obstet Gynaecol* 1980;87:227–9
33. Evaldson GR, Larsson B, Jiborn H. Is the collagen content reduced when the fetal membranes rupture? A clinical study of term and prematurely ruptured membranes. *Gynecol Obstet Invest* 1987;24:92–4
34. Vadillo-Ortega F, Gonzalex-Avila G, Karchmer S, *et al*. Collagen metabolism in premature rupture of amniotic membranes. *Obstet Gynecol* 1990;75:84–8
35. Hills B, Cotton D. Premature rupture of membranes and surface energy: possible role of surfactant. *Am J Obstet Gynecol* 1984;149:896–902
36. Danforth DN, McElin TW, States MN. Studies on fetal membranes. I. Bursting tension. *Am J Obstet Gynecol* 1953;65:480

37. MacLachlan TB. A method for the investigation of the strength of the fetal membranes. *Am J Obstet Gynecol* 1965;91:309

38. Meudt R, Meudt E. Rupture of the fetal membranes: an experimental, clinical, and histologic study. *Am J Obstet Gynecol* 1967;99:562–8

39. Polishuk WZ, Kohane S, Hadar A. Fetal weight and membrane tensile strength. *Am J Obstet Gynecol* 1964; 88:247

40. McGregor JA, Lawellin D, Franco-Buff A, *et al*. Protease production by microorganisms associated with reproductive tract infection. *Am J Obstet Gynecol* 1986;154:109–14

41. McGregor JA, French JL, Lawelin D, *et al*. Bacterial protease-induced reduction of chorioamniotic membrane strength and elasticity. *Obstet Gynecol* 1987; 69:167–74

42. Casey ML, Cox SM, Beutler B, *et al*. Cachectin/tumor necrosis factor-alpha formation in human decidua: potential role of cytokines in infection-induced preterm labor. *J Clin Invest* 1989;83:430–6

43. Dayer J-M, Beutler B, Cerami A. Brief definitive report: cachectin/tumor necrosis factor stimulates collagenase and prostaglandin E$_2$ production by human synovial cells and dermal fibroblasts. *J Exp Med* 1985;162: 2163–8

44. Katsura M, Ito A, Hirakawa S, Mori Y. Human recombinant interleukin-1-alpha increases biosynthesis of collagenase and hyaluronic acid in cultured human chorionic cells. *FEBS Lett* 1989;244:315–8

45. Naeye RL. Factors that predispose to premature rupture of the fetal membranes. *Obstet Gynecol* 1982; 60:93–8

46. Harger JH, Hsing A, Tuomola R, *et al*. Risk factors for preterm premature rupture of fetal membranes: a multicenter case-controlled study. *Am J Obstet Gynecol* 1990;163:130–7

47. Hadley C, Main D, Gabbe S. Risk factors for preterm premature rupture of the fetal membranes. *Am J Perinatol* 1990;7:374

48. Alger L, Pupkin M. Etiology of preterm premature rupture of the membranes. *Clin J Obstet Gynecol* 1986; 29:758

49. Major CA, de Veciana M, Lewis DF, Morgan MA. Preterm premature rupture of membranes and abruptio placentae: is there an association between these pregnancy complications? *Am J Obstet Gynecol* 1995; 172:672–3

50. Vintzileos AM, Campbell WA, Nochimson DJ, Weinbaum PJ. Preterm premature rupture of the membranes: a risk factor for the development of abruptio placentae. *Am J Obstet Gynecol* 1987;156:1235–8

51. Gonen R, Hannah ME, Milligan JE. Does prolonged preterm premature rupture of the membranes predispose to abruptio placentae? *Obstet Gynecol* 1989; 74:347–50

52. Major CA, Nageotte MP, Lewis DF, *et al*. Preterm premature rupture of membranes and placental abruption: is there an association between these pregnancy complications? *Am J Obstet Gynecol* 1991;164:381

53. Nelson DM, Stempel LE, Zuspan FP. Association of prolonged, preterm premature rupture of the membranes and abruptio placentae. *J Reprod Med* 1986;21:429–53

54. Meyer MB, Tonascia JA. Maternal smoking, pregnancy complications, and perinatal mortality. *Am J Obstet Gynecol* 1987;128:494–502

55. Nymand G. Maternal smoking and immunity. *Lancet* 1974;2:1379–80

56. Ledger WJ. Premature rupture of membranes and maternal–fetal infection. *Clin Obstet Gynecol* 1979; 22:329–37

57. Lockwood J. Recent advances in elucidating the pathogenesis of preterm delivery, the detection of patients at risk and preventative therapies. *Curr Opin Obstet Gynecol* 1994;6:7–18

58. Edwards LE, Barrada MI, Hamann AA, *et al*. Gonorrhea in pregnancy. *Am J Obstet Gynecol* 1978; 132:637–41

59. Elliott B, Brumham R, Laga M, *et al*. Maternal gonococcal infection as a preventable risk factor for low birth weight. *J Infect Dis* 1990;161:531–6

60. Amstey MS, Steadman KT. Asymptomatic gonorrhea and pregnancy. *J Am Ven Dis Assoc* 1976;33:14

61. Regan J, Chao S, James L. Premature rupture of membranes, preterm delivery, and group B streptococcal colonization of mothers. *Am J Obstet Gynecol* 1981;141:184–6

62. Thomsen A, Morup L, Hansen K. Antibiotic elimination of group-B streptococci in urine in prevention of preterm labour. *Lancet* 1987;1:591–3

63. Alger LS, Lovchik JC, Hebel JR, *et al*. The association of *Chlamydia trachomatis*, *Niesseria gonorrhoeae*, and group B streptococci with preterm rupture of the membranes and pregnancy outcome. *Am J Obstet Gynecol* 1988;159:397–404

64. Matorras R, Perea AG, Usandizaga JA, *et al*. Group B streptococcus and premature rupture of membranes and preterm delivery. *Gynecol Obstet Invest* 1989;27:14–18

65. McGregor J, Schoonmaker J, Hunt D. Antibiotic inhibition of bacterially induced fetal membrane weakening. *Obstet Gynecol* 1990;76:124–8

66. Riedewald S, Krentzman I, Heinze T, *et al*. Vaginal and cervical pH in normal pregnancy and pregnancy complicated labor. *J Perinat Med* 1990;18:181–6

67. Hauth JC, Goldenberg RL, Andrews WM, *et al*. Reduced incidence of preterm delivery with metronidazole and erythromycin in women with bacterial vaginosis. *N Engl J Med* 1995;333:1732–6

68. McGregor JA, French JI, Parker R, *et al*. Prevention of premature birth by screening and treatment for common genital tract infections: results of a prospective controlled evaluation. *Am J Obstet Gynecol* 1995; 173:157–67

69. Meis PJ, Goldenberg RL, Mercer B, *et al*. The preterm prediction study: significance of vaginal infections. *Am J Obstet Gynecol* 1995;173:1231–5

70. Cohen I, Tenenbaum E, Fejgin M, *et al*. Serum-specific antibodies for *Chlamydia trachomatis* in preterm premature rupture of the membranes. *Gynecol Obstet Invest* 1990;30:155–8

71. Sweet RL, Landers DV, Walker C, Schacter J. *Chlamydia trachomatis* infection and pregnancy outcome. *Am J Obstet Gynecol* 1987;156:824–33

72. Gauthier DW, Meyer WJ, Bieniarz A. Expectant management of premature rupture of membranes with amniotic fluid cultures postive for *Ureaplasma urealyticum* alone. *Am J Obstet Gynecol* 1994;170:587–90

73. Carey JC, Blackwelder WC, Nugent RP, *et al*. Antepartum cultures for *Ureaplasma urealyticum* are not useful in predicting pregnancy outcome. The Vaginal Infections and Prematurity Study Group 1991;164:728–33

74. Barabas AP. Ehlers–Danlos syndrome associated with prematurity and premature rupture of foetal membranes; possible increase in incidence. *Br Med J* 1966;2:682–4

75. Charles D, Edwards W. Infectious complications of cervical cerclage. *Am J Obstet Gynecol* 1981;141:1065–71

76. Yeast J, Garite T. The role of cervical cerclage in the management of preterm premature rupture of membranes. *Am J Obstet Gynecol* 1988;158:106–10

77. Ludmir J, Bader T, Chen L, *et al*. Poor perinatal outcome associated with retained cerclage in patients with premature rupture of membranes. *Obstet Gynecol* 1984;84:828

78. Harlap S, Davies AM. Late sequelae of induced abortion: complications and outcome of pregnancy and labor. *Am J Epidemiol* 1975;102:217–24

79. Holbrook RH Jr, Laros RK Jr, Creasy RK. Evaluation of a risk-scoring system for prediction of preterm labor. *Am J Perinatol* 1989;6:62

80. Wideman G, Baird A, Bolding D. Ascorbic acid deficiency and premature rupture of fetal membranes. *Am J Obstet Gynecol* 1964;88:592

81. Artal R, Burgeson R, Fernandez F, *et al*. Fetal and maternal copper levels in patients at term with and without premature rupture of membranes. *Obstet Gynecol* 1976;53:608–10

82. Kiiholma P, Gronroos M, Erkkola R, *et al*. The role of calcium, copper, iron and zinc in preterm delivery and premature rupture of fetal membranes. *Gynecol Obstet Invest* 1984;17:194–201

83. Sikorski R, Juszkiewicz T, Paszkowski T. Zinc status in women with premature rupture of membranes at term. *Obstet Gynecol* 1990,76:675

84. Georgakopoulos PA, Dodos D, Mechleris D. Sexuality in pregnancy and premature labour. *Br J Obstet Gynaecol* 1984;91:891–3

85. Mills JL, Harlap S, Harley EE. Should coitus late in pregnancy be discouraged? *Lancet* 1981;1:136

86. Perkins RP. Sexual behavior and response in relation to complications of pregnancy. *Am J Obstet Gynecol* 1979;134:498–505

87. Rayburn WF, Wilson EA. Coital activity and premature delivery. *Am J Obstet Gynecol* 1980;137:972–4

88. Ekwo EE, Gosselink CA, Woolson R, *et al*. Coitus late in pregnancy: risk of preterm rupture of amniotic sac membranes. *Am J Obstet Gynecol* 1993;168:22–31

89. Hack M, Horbar JD, Malloy MH, *et al*. Very low birth weight outcomes of the National Institute of Child Health and Human Development Neonatal Network. *Pediatrics* 1991;87:587

90. Phelps DL, Brown DR, Tung B, *et al*. 28-day survival rates of 6676 neonates with birth weights of 1250 grams or less. *Pediatrics* 1991;87:7

91. Allen MC, Donohue PK, Dusman AE. The limit of viability – neonatal outcome of infants born at 22 to 25 weeks' gestation. *N Engl J Med* 1993;329:1597

92. Schwartz RM, Luby AM, Scanlon JW, Kellogg RJ. Effect of surfactant on morbidity, mortality and resource use in newborn infants weighing 500 to 1500 g. *N Engl J Med* 1994;330:1476

93. Taylor J, Garite TJ. Premature rupture of membranes before fetal viability. *Obstet Gynecol* 1984;64:615

94. Veille JC. Management of preterm premature rupture of membranes. *Clin Perinatol* 1988;15:851

95. Hack M, Taylor HG, Klein N, *et al*. School-age outcomes in children with birthweights under 750 g. *N Engl J Med* 1994;331:753

96. Blackmon LR, Alger LS, Crenshaw C. Fetal and neonatal outcomes associated with premature rupture of the membranes. *Clin Obstet Gynecol* 1986;29:779–815

97. Nimrod C, Varela-Gittings F, Machin G, *et al*. The effect of very prolonged membrane rupture on fetal development. *Am J Obstet Gynecol* 1984;148:540

98. Blott M, Greenough A. Neonatal outcome after prolonged rupture of the membranes starting in the second trimester. *Arch Dis Child* 1988;63:1146–50

99. Taylor J, Garite TH. Premature rupture of membranes before fetal viability. *Obstet Gynecol* 1984;64:615–20

100. Thibeault DW, Beatty EC, Hall RT, *et al*. Neonatal pulmonary hypoplasia with premature rupture of fetal membranes and oligohydramnios. *J Pediatr* 1985;107:273

101. Vintzileos AM, Campbell WA, Nochimson DJ, *et al*. Degree of oligohydramnios and pregnancy outcome in patients with premature rupture of the membranes. *Obstet Gynecol* 1985;66:162

102. Rotschild A, Ling EW, Puterman ML, Farquharson D. Neonatal outcome after prolonged preterm rupture of the membranes. *Am J Obstet Gynecol* 1990;162:46–52

103. Shumway JB, Al-Malt A, Amon E, *et al*. Impact of oligohydramnios on maternal and perinatal outcomes of spontaneous premature rupture of the membranes at 18 to 28 weeks. *J Matern Fetal Med* 1999;8:20–3

104. Vergani P, Ghidini A, Locatelli A, *et al*. Risk factors for pulmonary hypoplasia in second trimester premature rupture of membranes. *Am J Obstet Gynecol* 1994;170:1359–64

105. Moessinger AC, Collins MH, Blanc WA, *et al*. Oligohydramnios-induced lung hypoplasia: the influence of timing and duration in gestation. *Pediatr Res* 1986;20:951

106. Adzick NS, Harrison MR, Glick PL, *et al*. Experimental pulmonary hypoplasia and oligohydramnios: relative contributions of lung fluid and fetal breathing movements. *J Pediatr Surg* 1984;19:658

107. Fewell JE, Hislop AA, Kitterman JA, Johnson P. Effect of tracheostomy on lung development in fetal lambs. *J Appl Physiol* 1983;55:1103

108. Nicolini U, Fisk NM, Rodeck CH, *et al*. Low amniotic pressure in oligohydramnios: is this the cause of pulmonary hypoplasia? *Am J Obstet Gynecol* 1989;161:1098–101

109. Fisk NM, Parker MJ, Moore PJ, *et al*. Mimicking low amniotic pressure by chronic pharyngeal drainage

does not impair lung development in fetal sheep. *Am J Obstet Gynecol* 1992;166:991–6

110. Wallen LD, Perry SF, Alton JT, Maloney JE. Fetal lung growth. Influence of pulmonary arterial flow and surgery in sheep. *Am J Resp Crit Care Med* 1994; 149:1005–11

111. Evaldson G, Lagrelius A, Winiarski J. Premature rupture of the membranes. *Acta Obstet Gynecol Scand* 1980; 59:385

112. Schreiber J, Benedetti T. Conservative management of preterm premature rupture of the fetal membranes in a low socioeconomic population. *Am J Obstet Gynecol* 1980;136:92–6

113. Spinnato JA, Shaver DC, Bray EM, *et al*. Preterm premature rupture of the membranes with fetal pulmonary maturity present: a prospective study. *Obstet Gynecol* 1987;69:196

114. Johnston M, Sanchez-Ramos L, Benrubi GI. Premature rupture of membranes prior to 34 weeks gestational age. One year experience at a tertiary center. *J Fla Med Assoc* 1989;76:767

115. Siegel JD, McCracken GH Jr. Sepsis neonatorum. *N Engl J Med* 1981;304:642

116. St Geme JW Jr, Murray DL, Carter J, *et al*. Perinatal bacterial infection after prolonged rupture of amniotic membranes: an analysis of risk and management. *J Pediatr* 1984;104:608

117. Levine CD. Premature rupture of the membranes and sepsis in preterm neonates. *Nurs Res* 1991;40:36

118. Boyer KM, Gotoff SP. Antimicrobial prophylaxis of neonatal group B streptococcal sepsis. *Clin Perinatol* 1988;15:831

119. Gerdes JS. Clinicopathologic approach to the diagnosis of neonatal sepsis. *Clin Perinatol* 1991;18:563

120. Simon C, Schroder H, Weisner D, *et al*. Bacteriologic finding after PROM. *Arch Gynecol Obstet* 1989;244:69

121. Daikoku NH, Kaltreider DF, Khouzami VA, *et al*. Premature rupture of membranes and spontaneous labor: maternal endometritis risks. *Obstet Gynecol* 1982;59:13

122. Christensen KK, Christensen P, Ingemarsson I, *et al*. A study in complications in preterm deliveries after prolonged premature rupture of the membranes. *Obstet Gynecol* 1976;48:670

123. Manning FA, Morrison I, Lange IR, *et al*. Fetal assessment based on fetal biophysical profile scoring: experience in 12,620 referred high-risk pregnancies. *Am J Obstet Gynecol* 1985;151:343–50

124. Vintzileos AM, Campbell WA, Nochimson DJ, *et al*. The fetal biophysical profile in patients with premature rupture of the membranes – an early predictor of fetal infection. *Am J Obstet Gynecol* 1985;152:510–16

125. Vintzileos AM, Feinstein SJ, Lodeiro JG, *et al*. Fetal biophysical profile and the effect of premature rupture of the membranes. *Obstet Gynecol* 1986;67:818

126. Vintzileos AM, Campbell WA, Nochimson DJ, Weinbaum PJ. The use of nonstress test in patients with premature rupture of the membranes. *Am J Obstet Gynecol* 1986;155:149–53

127. Zeevi D, Sadovsky E, Younis J, *et al*. Antepartum fetal heart rate characteristics in cases of premature rupture of membranes. *Am J Perinatol* 1988;5:260

128. Smith CV, Greenspoon J, Phelan JP, Platt LD. Clinical utility of the nonstress test in the conservative management of women with preterm spontaneous premature rupture of the membranes. *J Reprod Med* 1987;32:1

129. Thacker SB, Berkelman RL. Assessing the diagnostic accuracy and efficacy of selected antepartum fetal surveillance techniques. *Obstet Gynecol Surv* 1986;41:121

130. Vintzileos AM, Campbell WA, Ingardia CJ, *et al*. The fetal biophysical profile and its predictive value. *Obstet Gynecol* 1983;62:271

131. Rabinowitz R, Peters MT, Vyas S, *et al*. Measurement of fetal urine production in normal pregnancy by real-time sonography. *Am J Obstet Gynecol* 1989;161:1246–6

132. Groome LJ, Owen J, Neely CL, Hauth JC. Oligohydramnios: antepartum fetal urine production and intrapartum fetal distress. *Am J Obstet Gynecol* 1991; 165:1077–80

133. Gonick B, Bottoms SF, Cotton DB. Amniotic fluid volume as a risk factor in preterm premature rupture of the membranes. *Obstet Gynecol* 1985;65:456

134. Kivikoski AL, Amon E, Vaalamo PO, *et al*. Effect of third-trimester premature rupture of membranes on fetal breathing movements: a prospective case–control study. *Am J Obstet Gynecol* 1988;159:1474–7

135. Roberts AB, Goldstein I, Romero R, Hobbins JC. Fetal breathing movements after preterm premature rupture of membranes. *Am J Obstet Gynecol* 1991;164: 821–5

136. Vintzileos AM, Campbell WA, Nochimson DJ, Weinbaum PJ. Fetal breathing as a predictor of infection in premature rupture of the membranes. *Obstet Gynecol* 1986;67:813

137. Goldstein I, Romero R, Merrill S, *et al*. Fetal body and breathing movements as predictors of intra-amniotic infection in preterm premature rupture of membranes. *Am J Obstet Gynecol* 1988;159:363–8

138. Koos BJ. Central effects on breathing in fetal sheep of sodium meclofenamate. *J Physiol* 1982;330:50

139. Amon E, Rossick K, Sibai BM. The biophysical profile in patients undergoing cervical ripening by PGE₂ prior to induction of labor. *Am J Obstet Gynecol* 1991; 164(suppl 1):243

140. Miller JM Jr, Kho MS, Brown HL, *et al*. Clinical chorioamnionitis is not predicted by an ultrasonic biophysical profile in patients with premature rupture of membranes. *Obstet Gynecol* 1990;76:1031

141. Cox SM, Williams ML, Leveno KJ. The natural history of preterm ruptured membranes. What to expect of expectant management. *Obstet Gynecol* 1988;71:588

142. Garite TJ, Freeman RK, Linzey EM, *et al*. Prospective randomized study of corticosteroids in the management of premature rupture of the membranes and the premature gestation. *Am J Obstet Gynecol* 1981;141:508–15

143. Stedman CM, Crawford S, Staten E, *et al*. Management of preterm premature rupture of membranes: assessing amniotic fluid in the vagina for phosphatidyl-glycerol. *Am J Obstet Gynecol* 1981;140:34–8

144. Druzin ML, Toth M, Ledger WJ. Nonintervention in premature rupture of the amniotic membrane. *Surg Gynecol Obstet* 1986;163:5

145. Moretti M, Sibai BM. Maternal and perinatal outcome of expectant management of premature rupture of

membranes in the mid-trimester. *Am J Obstet Gynecol* 1988;159:390–6

146. Munson LA, Graham A, Koos BJ, Valenzuela GJ. Is there a need for digital examination in patients with spontaneous rupture of the membranes? *Am J Obstet Gynecol* 1985;153:562–3

147. Brown CL, Ludwiczak MH, Blanco JD, Hirsch CE. Cervical dilation: accuracy of visual and digital examinations. *Obstet Gynecol* 1993;81:215–6

148. Sukcharoen N, Vasuratna A. Effects of digital cervical examinations of duration of latency period, maternal and neonatal outcome in preterm premature rupture of membranes. *J Med Assoc Tailand* 1993;76:203–9

149. Lewis DF, Towers CV, Asrat T, *et al*. Effects of digital vaginal examinations on latency period in preterm premature rupture of membranes. *Obstet Gynecol* 1992; 80:630–4

150. Adoni A, Ben Chetrit A, Zacut D, *et al*. Prolongation of the latent period in patients with premature rupture of the membranes by avoiding digital examination. *Int J Gynaecol Obstet* 1990;32:19–21

151. Schutte MF, Treffers PE, Kloosterman GJ, *et al*. Management of premature rupture of membranes: the risk of vaginal examination to the infant. *Am J Obstet Gynecol* 1983;146:395–400

152. Schumacher RE, Parisi VM, Steady HM, Tsao FHC. Bacteria causing false-positive test for phosphatidyl-glycerol in amniotic fluid. *Am J Obstet Gynecol* 1985; 151:1067–8

153. Ohlsson A. Treatments of preterm premature rupture of the membranes: a meta-analysis. *Am J Obstet Gynecol* 1989;160:890–906

154. Crowley PA. Corticosteroids after preterm premature rupture of membranes. *Obstet Gynecol Clin* 1992; 19-2:317

155. NIH Consensus Conference. Effect of corticosteroids for fetal maturation on perinatal outcomes. Corticosteroids for fetal maturation. *J Am Med Assoc* 1995; 273:413–18

156. Collaborative Group on Antenatal Steroid Therapy. Effect of antenatal steroid administration on prevention of respiratory distress syndrome. *Am J Obstet Gynecol* 1981;141:276

157. Doran TA, Swyer P, MacMurray B, *et al*. Results of a double-blind controlled study on the use of betamethasone in the prevention of respiratory distress syndrome. *Am J Obstet Gynecol* 1980;136:313

158. Gamsu HR, Mullinger BM, Donnai P, *et al*. Antenatal administration of betamethasone to prevent respiratory distress syndrome in preterm infants. Report of a UK multicentre trial. *Br J Obstet Gynaecol* 1989;96:401–10

159. Morales WJ, Diebel ND, Lazar AJ, *et al*. The effect of antenatal dexamethasone on the prevention of respiratory distress syndrome in preterm gestation with premature rupture of membranes. *Am J Obstet Gynecol* 1986;154:59

160. Papageorgiou AN, Desgranges MF, Masson M, *et al*. The antenatal use of betamethasone in the prevention of respiratory distress syndrome. A controlled double-blind study. *Pediatrics* 1979;63:73

161. Schmidt PL, Sums ME, Strassner HT, *et al*. Effect of antepartum glucocorticoid administration upon neonatal respiratory distress syndrome and perinatal infection. *Am J Obstet Gynecol* 1984;148:178

162. Moraga FA, Riquelme RA, Lopez AA, *et al*. Maternal administration of glucocorticoid and thyrotropin releasing hormone enhances fetal lung maturation in undisturbed preterm lambs. *Am J Obstet Gynecol* 1994; 171:729–34

163. Tan AS, Hsu CD, Marder S, *et al*. Is maternal thyrotropin releasing hormone administration safe in the pregnant woman with preeclampsia? *Am J Perinatol* 1997;14:5–6

164. Peek MJ, Bajoria R, Shennan AH, *et al*. Hypertensive effect of antenatal thyrotropin-releasing hormone in pre-eclampsia. *Lancet* 1995;345:793

165. Levy DL, Warsof SL. Oral ritodrine and preterm premature rupture of membranes. *Obstet Gynecol* 1985; 66:621

166. Dunlop PDM, Crowley PA, Lamont RF, Hawkins DF. Preterm ruptured membranes, no contractions. *J Obstet Gynaecol* 1986;7:92

167. Christensen KK, Ingemarsson I, Liedeman T, *et al*. Effect of ritodrine on labor after premature rupture of the membranes. *Obstet Gynecol* 1980;55:187

168. Weiner CP, Renk K, Klugman M. The therapeutic efficacy and cost-effectiveness of aggressive tocolysis for premature labor associated with premature rupture of the membranes. *Am J Obstet Gynecol* 1988;159:216

169. Garite TJ, Keegan KA, Freeman RK, Nageotte MP. A randomized trial of ritodrine tocolysis versus expectant management in patients with premature rupture of membranes at 25 to 30 weeks of gestation. *Am J Obstet Gynecol* 1987;157:388

170. Mercer BM, Lewis R. Preterm labor and preterm premature rupture of the membranes. Diagnosis and management. *Infect Dis Clin North Am* 1997;11:177–201

171. Amon E, Lewis SV, Sibai BM, *et al*. Ampicillin prophylaxis in preterm premature rupture of the membranes: a prospective randomized study. *Am J Obstet Gynecol* 1988;159:539

172. Morales WJ, Angel JL, O'Brien WF, Knuppel RA. Use of ampicillin and corticosteroids in premature rupture of membranes: a randomized study. *Obstet Gynecol* 1989;73:721

173. Johnston MM, Sanchez-Ramos L, Vaughn AJ, *et al*. Antibiotic therapy in preterm premature rupture of membranes: a randomized, prospective, double-blind trial. *Am J Obstet Gynecol* 1990;163:743

174. McDuffie RS Jr, McGregor JA, Gibbs RS. Adverse perinatal outcome and resistant Enterobacteriaceae after antibiotic use for premature rupture of the membranes and GBS carriage. *Obstet Gynecol* 1993;82:487–9

175. Mercer BM, Arheart KL. Antimicrobial therapy in expectant management of preterm premature rupture of the membranes. *Lancet* 1995;346;1271–9

176. Egarter C, Leitich H, Karas H, *et al*. Antibiotic treatment in preterm premature rupture of membranes and neonatal morbidity: a metaanalysis. *Am J Obstet Gynecol* 1996;174:589–97

177. Mercer BM, Miodovnik M, Thurnau GR, *et al*. Antibiotic therapy for reduction of infant morbidity after preterm premature rupture of the membranes. A randomized controlled trial. National Institute of

Child Health and Human Development Maternal-Fetal Medicine Units Network. *J Am Med Assoc* 1997;278:989–95

178. Romero R, Emamian M, Quintero R, *et al.* The value and limitations of the Gram stain examination in the diagnosis of intraamniotic infection. *Am J Obstet Gynecol* 1988;159:114

179. Cunningham FG, MacDonald PC, Gant NF, *et al.* The endometrium and decidua: menstruation and pregnancy. *In Williams Obstetrics*, 20th ed. Stamford, Connecticut: Appleton & Lange, 1997:89

180. Fuchs, Stubblefield. *Preterm Birth*, 2nd edn. 1993:407

10
Recurrent pregnancy losses

C.B. Coulam

The inability of a couple to achieve desired family size affects an estimated 3 million married couples in the USA[1]. Reproductive life table analysis indicates that the majority of reproductive failure results from postfertilization failures occurring before or after implantation. Childlessness as a consequence of repeated postimplantation losses has been described as a syndrome[2] and has been termed recurrent spontaneous abortion. Primary recurrent spontaneous abortion occurs in women who have experienced three or more consecutive abortions and have had no pregnancies beyond 20 weeks of gestation. Secondary recurrent spontaneous abortions are defined as three or more consecutive abortions after a viable pregnancy or a stillbirth.

While recurrent spontaneous abortion has been defined as three or more consecutive spontaneous abortions, a number of studies describing etiological factors include women with two spontaneous abortions. The greatest change in risk of losing a subsequent pregnancy comes after two consecutive spontaneous abortions[3] (Table 1). No differences in the prevalence of etiological factors exist between couples with up to two compared with three or more abortions[4] (Table 2). These two observations along with the emotional frustration of two pregnancy losses are the prime factors motivating and providing rationale for evaluation of couples after experiencing two spontaneous abortions.

EPIDEMIOLOGY

Recurrent spontaneous abortion occurs in approximately 2–5% of reproductive aged women each year[3,5]. Risk factors for recurrence of pregnancy loss are listed in Table 3 and include the number of previous miscarriages[6–9], a history of other adverse pregnancy outcomes[9–11] and a history of subfertility[10–13]. Maternal age as a risk factor for recurrence of pregnancy wastage has been reported[7,14] and refuted[6,9].

Number of previous abortions

A number of studies have demonstrated that the risk for recurrent spontaneous abortion rises in proportion to the number of prior miscarriages (Table 1)[6–9,11]. In predicting the success of the next pregnancy, the odds ratio for number of miscarriages was 0.36, i.e. each

Table 1 Prevalence of pregnancy loss as a function of pregnancy order. From reference 3

Pregnancy order	No. of patients	Pregnancy loss	
		n	*%*
1	2836	357	12.6
2	295	49	16.6
3	40	15	37.5

Table 2 Prevalence of various causes of recurrent spontaneous abortion among 214 couples experiencing two or more abortions and 179 couples with three or more abortions

	Recurrent spontaneous abortions			
	≥ 2		≥ 3	
Etiology	*n*	*%*	*n*	*%*
Chromosomal	13	6	11	6
Anatomic	3	1	2	1
Hormonal	11	5	9	5
Immunological	139	65	117	66
Unexplained	48	23	40	22
Total	214	100	179	100

Table 3 Risk factors for recurrence of pregnancy loss

Number of previous abortions
History of other adverse pregnancy outcome
History of infertility
Maternal age

additional miscarriage after three more than doubled the risk of loss for the next pregnancy[9]. The observed frequency of recurrent abortion is higher than that expected by chance, implying an underlying cause or causes contributing to the recurrent loss[11].

Other adverse reproductive outcomes

An association has been reported between recurrent spontaneous abortion and other reproductive failures, including ectopic pregnancy[11,15–17], hydatidiform mole[11,18,19], preterm births[11,20–23], stillbirths[11], small-for-gestation-age (SGA) infants[11,23,24], congenital anomalies[25] and increased prenatal mortality[20]. Women with a history of recurrent spontaneous abortion have a higher frequency of other types of pregnancy wastage than the general population. Table 4 summarizes the outcomes of 1968 pregnancies occurring in 455 women with recurrent spontaneous abortion[11]. When these pregnancy outcomes were compared with the expected proportions of each in the general population[26–28], the observed/expected ratios were 2–3 times increased for ectopic pregnancies and preterm births; 7 times increased for hydatidiform mole; and 16 times increased for stillbirths (Table 4). A history of a single late pregnancy loss in a series of at least three reproductive failures decreased the chance for successful pregnancy with an odds ratio of 0.18[9]. No association between gravidity and observed/expected ratios were noted for any of the pregnancy outcomes (Table 5), suggesting that these adverse pregnancy outcomes are not risk factors for recurrent abortion, nor vice versa. A common etiology for recurrent spontaneous abortion and ectopic and molar pregnancies has been proposed[16–19]. However, a common mechanism is not obvious. Current understanding of the etiology of hydatidiform mole suggests that the determining event occurs at fertilization[29]. Therefore, whatever the common event that links the different clinical manifestations of reproductive wastage, it could occur at the time of fertilization.

Table 4 Outcome of 1968 pregnancies experienced by 455 women with a history of recurrent spontaneous abortion compared with the expected outcome in the general population

Outcome	Observed	Expected	Ratio	95% CI
Term birth	184	1547	0.1	0.10–0.14
Preterm birth	30	18[*]	1.6	1.11–2.34
Stillbirth	16	1[*]	16.0	8.0–22.65
Molar pregnancy	6	0.8[†]	7.5	2.62–15.57
Ectopic pregnancy	63	24[†]	2.6	2.60–3.33
Spontaneous abortion	1669	252[†]	6.6	6.30–9.94

[*]per 1000 livebirths; [†]per 1000 pregnancies

Table 5 Ratio of observed/expected pregnancy outcome by pregnancy order reported by 455 women with recurrent spontaneous abortion

Gravida	Preterm birth[*]	Stillbirth[*]	Molar[†]	Ectopic[†]
1	1.1	5.3	10	2.7
2	2.3	0.5	5	2.7
3	2.3	1.2	5	2.0
4	2.5	2.3	7.7	3.5
5+	2.8	0.6	5	2.1

[*]per 1000 livebirths; [†]per 1000 pregnancies

Subfertility

That subfertility should be included in the spectrum of reproductive disorders associated with recurrent spontaneous abortion has been suggested by data showing an increased frequency of infertility among couples with recurrent spontaneous abortion and by data indicating that the best predictor of successful pregnancy after immunotherapy for recurrent spontaneous abortion is the time interval between immunization and pregnancy[9,11,30,31]. In addition to an increased frequency of infertility among women with recurrent spontaneous abortions[10], infertile women have an increased risk for miscarriage[12].

Table 6 summarizes the results of a study of the reproductive histories of 175 women with recurrent spontaneous abortion[11]. The occurrence of subfertility among these 175 women was evaluated in three ways. A diagnosis of infertility was made if the couple had not been able to achieve desired pregnancy for 1 or more years of unprotected intercourse. The second indicator of subfertility was the determination of the mean number of pregnancies achieved by each couple per year. This figure was calculated as the total number of pregnancies divided by the number of years over which they occurred. Thirdly, to estimate fecundability, the time interval from diagnosis of recurrent spontaneous abortion to conception of subsequent pregnancy was studied. The women with recurrent spontaneous abortion had a two-fold increase in the frequency of infertility when compared with the general population ($p < 0.05$)[1]. There were 35 couples who complained of infertility, and 69 couples who experienced less than one pregnancy per year (observed/expected ratio of 4.1; $p < 0.05$). The 175 women with recurrent spontaneous abortion had a total of 797 pregnancies over 890 years for a mean of 0.9 pregnancies per year. The outcome of the first pregnancy after evaluation was recorded in 54 pregnancies: 30 terminated in pregnancy loss and 24 resulted in viable births. When the time interval from diagnosis of recurrent pregnancy losses to conception was 30 weeks or more, the risk of spontaneous abortion was significantly higher than conception

Table 6 Observed/expected ratios of subfertility indices among 175 women with recurrent spontaneous abortion

	Observed	Expected	Ratio	p Value
History of infertility	35	17	2.0	< 0.05
<1 pregnancy/year	69	17	4.1	< 0.05
Conception ≤ 6 months after diagnosis of recurrent spontaneous abortion	54	140	0.4	< 0.05

occurring before 30 weeks ($p < 0.05$) (Figure 1). Therefore, couples with a history of recurrent spontaneous abortion experiencing infertility or subfertility and taking longer than 30 weeks to conceive are more

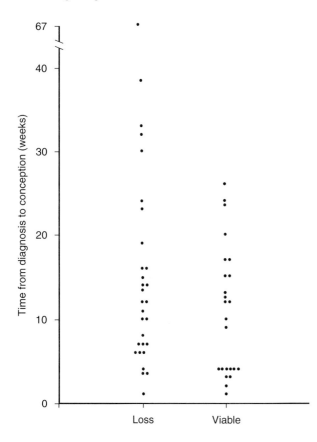

Figure 1 Reproductive outcome based on time interval to time of conception. Pregnancy loss, $n = 30$; viable pregnancy, $n = 24$

likely to have a miscarriage. Subfertility should be included in the spectrum of reproductive disorders associated with recurrent spontaneous abortion. It has been estimated that only 50% of fertilized eggs actually implant in the endometrium[30] and 43% of those that do implant are lost before clinical pregnancy is recognized[31]. Therefore, 85% of all reproductive wastage occurs prior to clinical awareness[32]. Those individuals who are experiencing recurrent pregnancy loss prior to perception of pregnancy would present with the complaint of unexplained infertility rather than recurrent spontaneous abortion. Figure 2 depicts the possible fates of a fertilized oocyte. The common event that links all of the adverse reproductive outcomes is fertilization. Therefore, understanding the factors involved at fertilization that predispose to adverse reproductive outcomes would provide insight into the mechanisms of reproductive wastage.

ETIOLOGY

The etiologies of recurrent spontaneous abortion have been reported as being due to anatomic, hormonal, chromosomal and immunological causes[33]. The prevalence rates for causes of recurrent spontaneous abortion vary in the studies reported[33–36] and are compared in Table 7. Recently, the roles of anatomic defects[33,37] and hormonal deficiencies[37,38] have been questioned.

Anatomic defects

Müllerian duct anomalies have been thought to be causal in recurrent spontaneous abortion[33–37]. Although reports have shown a marked improvement in fetal salvage rates after metroplasty among women with

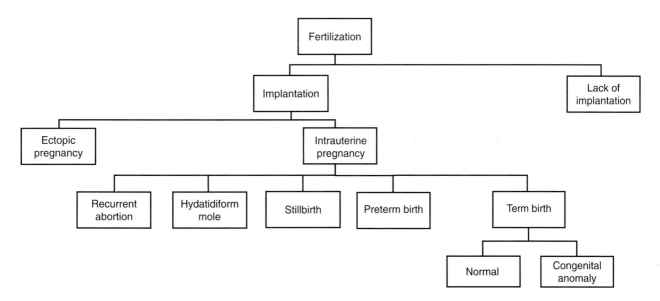

Figure 2 Association between fertilization and other possible reproductive outcomes

Table 7 Comparison of prevalence (%) of diagnosis in couples with recurrent spontaneous abortion from various centers

Diagnosis	MCH[34]	MWH[35]	Norway[36]	Mayo[33]	Indianapolis[4]	Virginia[37,46]
Chromosomal	12	8	3	6	6	58
Anatomic	15	27	28	10	1	1
Hormonal	23	—	5	29	5	1
Immunological	—	8	—	40	65	30
Other	—	20	20	—	—	—
Unexplained	50	37	44	15	23	10

MCH, Medical College of Georgia; MWH, Magee Women's Hospital

Müllerian duct defects and a history of recurrent spontaneous abortion, live birth rates were the same when the women with the same uterine anomaly who did not have surgery were followed for the same period of time[33,37].

Hormonal deficiencies

The role of luteal phase deficiency as a cause of recurrent spontaneous abortion has also been questioned. Reasons for the queries have accumulated in three areas. (1) Studies purporting to correct luteal phase defects using exogenous progesterone administration in women with recurrent spontaneous abortion did not have control groups, whereas other studies showed no difference in pregnancy outcome between hormone-treated and placebo-treated groups[39,40]; (2) the existence of a luteal phase defect has been a subject of considerable debate, because of the inconsistencies in diagnosis based upon the endometrial biopsy[41]; and (3) fertile control women have a higher prevalence of diagnosis of luteal phase defect than do women with a history of recurrent spontaneous abortion[41,42].

Chromosomal abnormalities

Although sporadic spontaneous abortions are assumed to be the result of identifiable karyotypic abnormalities[43], the frequency of abnormal chromosomal analyses among recurrent spontaneous abortions has been thought to be low[4,33–36]. Only about 6% of recurrent spontaneous abortuses (range 3–12%) had been reported to display abnormal chromosomes[4,33]; More recent studies indicate that 58% of all abortuses from women experiencing recurrent abortion are chromosomally abnormal[37] (Table 7). The prevalences of chromosomal abnormalities or at least 50% of all first-trimester abortions contrast with chromosomal abnormalities observed among stillbirths (5%) and livebirths (0.5%)[44]. The most plausible explanation for the large number of chromosomal abnormalities among lost pregnancies is that most chromosomal abnormalities result in disordered development incompatible with prolonged intrauterine survival. The frequency of disordered development may be

increased in pregnancies from a subset of women experiencing recurrent pregnancy loss compared to a control group; aneuploid conceptions occur more frequently in couples experiencing recurrent spontaneous abortion (0.3% vs. 1.6%)[45].

Immunological causes

A body of literature is accumulating which suggests that immunological mechanisms provide an explanation for a large proportion of recurrent spontaneous abortions which were heretofore unexplained. It is not surprising that a large proportion of unexplained recurrent pregnancy loss could result from immunological maladaptation to the pregnancy, since the conceptus is both an autograft and an allograft to its host mother. If the maternal immunological response to the conceptus is not appropriate and the problem involves a maternally derived target antigen, an auto-immune cause of recurrent spontaneous abortion is diagnosed. Alternatively, if an inappropriate response to a paternally derived antigen is found, an alloimmune cause of recurrent spontaneous abortion is diagnosed. Laboratory tests used to identify auto-immune causes of recurrent pregnancy loss have included the following autoantibodies: antiphospholipid, antinuclear and antithyroid antibodies[46]. Laboratory tests used to identify autoimmune causes include quantitation of circulating natural killer (NK) or CD56+ cells and detection of circulating embryotoxins[46]. The conclusions that autoimmune and alloimmune mechanisms are causes of recurrent pregnancy loss are supported by basic laboratory studies as well as results of clinical trials using various forms of immunotherapy for treatment. The association of autoantibodies and recurrent pregnancy loss has been known for over a decade[47,48]. A number of clinical trials have shown that women with circulating autoantibodies respond to treatment with low-dose aspirin and heparin or prednisone[49,50].

Mononuclear cells that express CD56, present in early pregnancy decidua, have been associated with successful pregnancy outcome[51]. A deficiency of these CD56+ cells has been observed in placentae from women with incipient miscarriage[51]. Animal studies have demonstrated a role of CD56+ cells in the prevention of abortion[52].

In the mouse, the success of the fetal allograft is, in part, the result of local suppression at the level of the decidua by factors secreted by NK cells[53]. Other studies have proposed that the systemic regulation of antitrophoblast lymphokine-activated killer (LAK) cells determines reproductive success[54]. Peripheral NK cells from women with recurrent spontaneous abortion have cytotoxic actions to autologous placental extracts[55]. A study of peripheral circulating NK cells in women with recurrent spontaneous abortion has reported the levels of these to be significantly elevated as compared to the levels in normal fertile controls[56], and the concentrations of circulating NK cells have been shown to be correlated with pregnancy outcome in pregnant women carrying a singleton gestation and in women with an obstetric history of recurrent pregnancy loss[57].

Immunotherapy in the forms of intravenous immunoglobulin (IVIG) and leukocyte immunization have been shown by level I evidence (randomized, blinded, placebo-controlled trials or meta-analysis of sufficient power to avoid type II errors) to be effective treatment for recurrent pregnancy loss[58–60].

PATHOPHYSIOLOGY

The mechanisms by which pregnancies are lost are not known; however, they involve either the processes of abnormal implantation or interference with placental blood flow once normal implantation has occurred. For better appreciation of the pathophysiology of recurrent pregnancy loss, normal implantation will be reviewed. The events which occur during normal gestations will then be compared with those associated with recurrent pregnancy loss.

Normal implantation

The process of implantation involves adhesion of the trophectoderm to the uterine epithelium and subsequent penetration, proliferation, protection from immunological attack and metastasis of the trophoblast.

Adhesion

Recognition signals for adhesion of the trophoblast to the uterine epithelium remain elusive. It is well established that preimplantation embryos synthesize and secrete human chorionic gonadotropin (hCG)[61], interleukin-1 (IL-1)[62] and platelet activating factor (PAF)[63]. Receptors for hCG[64], IL-1[62] and PAF[65] have been found in the endometrium. These observations suggest that hCG, IL-1 and PAF made by trophoblast may directly regulate the functions of the endometrium and allow normal implantation.

Penetration

Implantation is initiated at day 6 or 7 after fertilization, approximately 3 weeks from the onset of the last menstrual period (LMP). The process of penetration of the endometrium by the blastocyst ensues. The mechanisms of trophoblastic invasion into the endometrium is analogous to the processes involved in cancer invasion and occurs in three steps[66]: first, adherence of the invading cell to the extracellular matrix and basement membrane; second, local proteolysis associated with breakdown of extracellular matrix and basement membrane components; and third, migration and locomotion of the invading cell through the defect in the extracellular matrix and basement membrane. The laminin receptor, a cell-surface protein that binds the laminin component of the extracellular matrix, has been postulated to play a role in the first step of adhesion[67]. Type IV collagenase, a metalloprotease that specifically degrades type IV collagen of the extracellular matrix, may be important for the second step of local proteolysis[68]. A new class of cytokines – autocrine motility factors – have been suggested to play a role in stimulating locomotion through the permeabilized extracellular matrix and basement membrane in the third step of migration[69].

Proliferation

As the trophoblastic cells penetrate the endometrium, they proliferate. Stimuli for trophoblastic proliferation include a number of growth factors present in the placental bed such as granulocyte–macrophage colony stimulating factor (GM-CSF), granulocyte colony stimulating factor (G-CSF or CSF-1), interleukin-3 (IL-3), interleukin-4 (IL-4), epidermal growth factor (EGF), insulin-like growth factor (IGF) and basic fibroblast growth factor. All of these growth factors are present in the decidua and are known to play important roles in the stimulation and regulation of all growth, including that of the cells participating in angiogenesis[70,71]. The trophoblastic surface is rich in receptors for a number of growth factors including GM-CSF, G-CSF, IGF-I, IGF-II, EGF, which also binds transforming growth factor alpha (TGFα) and platelet-derived growth factor (PDGF)[72–78]. The findings of growth factors in the decidua and their receptors on trophoblastic cells suggest that these growth factors may directly regulate trophoblastic proliferation and facilitate normal implantation. A number of other cytokines are present in uteroplacental tissues, including TGFβ, tumor necrosis factor alpha (TNFα) and interferon gamma (IFNγ)[79]. Human placentae also express receptor activity for IFNγ and TNFα[77,78]. TNFα and INFγ have both been shown to be toxic to the growth and development of trophoblasts[80,81].

An immunotrophic hypothesis has been proposed which holds that, at the implantation site, maternal

T cells, NK-type cells (large endometrial granular lymphocytes) and macrophages recognize antigens on trophoblastic surfaces and release cytokines[82]. Cytokines such as GM-CSF, CSF-1 and IL-3 stimulate placental growth and hence fetal growth[83]. The TNFα product of activated macrophages seems to serve as a stop signal for invasion[78,79]. A 34-kDa protein produced by CD8+ cells with progesterone receptors and the TGFβ cytokines appears to account for some of the suppressive activity for NK cell function[79,84], thus protecting the trophoblast from the 'normal' maternal immunological response to the allograft. The source of TGFβ suppressor activity is a small, granulated, Fc receptor-negative, non-T, non-B lymphocyte which appears in the endometrium after progesterone exposure and releases TGFβ in response to trophoblastic signals[79]. One trophoblastic signal appears to be mediated by antibody binding to a trophoblastic cell-surface antigen. Whether this antibody is the same as the previously reported 'blocking antibody', which has been postulated to prevent maternal cytotoxic cells from attacking the trophoblast[85], is not clear. However, a concept is emerging that the production of blocking or protective antibodies occurs in response to an antigen present on the trophoblast that has a molecular weight of 80 kDa. This antigen, R80K, is a non-HLA placental antigen to which the mother makes an immune response[86]. A maternal immune response has been demonstrated by eluting the IgG from term placental syncytiotrophoblast (on villi in contact with blood) bound to Fc receptors mediating the transport of maternal IgG into the fetus. The remaining IgG is bound to an 80-kDa molecule[87]. The specificity of the antigen does vary between individual placentae, and appears to be determined by the father's (and his father's) genes[88,89]. The antigen is also expressed on the father's (and his father's) lymphocytes, and immunization of antibody-negative women using husband's lymphocytes results in antigenic generation[88]. The placentae of all successful pregnancies at term have antibody bound to R80K, and women with recurrent miscarriage who lack antibody in their blood, when immunized, and at the end of a successful pregnancy, do have the antibody to R80K on their placentae[89].

IL-1 is released by activated macrophages and is present in uteroplacental tissues very early in pregnancy. Around the time of implantation the source of IL-1 is both the maternal macrophages and the trophoblastic cells. As pregnancy progresses, fetal macrophages can be identified in early and term chorionic villous mesenchyme. Some but not all placental macrophages express HLA DR and hence are interpreted as being activated. Activated macrophages produce significant quantities of IL-1. IL-1 up-regulates the expression of tissue factor (TF)[90,91]. The placenta is abundant in TF, which can form a complex with coagulation factor VII and thus initiate hemostasis that results in fibrin formation[91]. It has long been known that fibrin deposition is common in human placenta[92], and a controlled expression of this process seems to be essential for the development of normal pregnancy[91,92].

Protection from immunological attack

By day 14 after fertilization, 4 weeks from LMP (i.e. the date of the expected next menstrual period), the blastocyst is completely embedded in the maternal decidua and covered by endometrial epithelium[93]. Thus, throughout normal pregnancy, maternal and fetal cells lie side by side with no apparent detrimental effect on each other. The ability of maternal and fetal cells to coexist as a successful allograft has been attributed to the lack of classical major histocompatibility antigens expression on the cell surface of the trophoblast and protection of the pregnancy from maternal immunological attack. Protection of the pregnancy from maternal immunosurveillance has been attributed to five mechanisms. (1) Lack of classical human leukocyte antigen (HLA) class I antigen expression by trophoblast protects against cytotoxic T cell recognition and attack[94]. (2) Expression of the non-classical HLA-G antigen protects against NK cell attack[95]. (3) Local decidual suppressor factors suppress IL-2 and IL-2 receptor expression by maternal T cells and NK cells in the decidua[79]. Most of the suppressive activity appears to belong to the TGFβ family of molecules[79]. However, PAF secreted by the fertilized egg stimulates the secretion of early pregnancy factor (EPF)[96,97]. When EPF binds to lymphocytes, two soluble suppressor factors are released[98]. The relationship of these suppressor factors to TGFβ is unknown. (4) Block-ing anitbodies have been postulated to prevent maternal cells from attacking the conceptus[85]. (5) Trophoblastic membrane cofactor protein (MCP or CD46) inactivates the complement cascade and negates complement-mediated damage[99].

Metastasis

At the time at which the blastocyst is completely embedded in the decidua, chorionic villi are evident. Concurrent with the formation of the villous placenta, a number of non-villous trophoblastic cells invade the maternal decidua further and metastasize to spiral arteries[100]. The metastatic phenotype is analogous to that described for invasion and proliferation and is the result of a balance between production and response to adhesion receptors, growth factors, proteases, protesase inhibitors and autocrine motility factors[66]. Trophoblastic migration into spiral arteries appears to begin at about 6 weeks of gestation[100]. The endovascular trophoblast migrates up spiral arteries, replaces maternal endothelium and reaches terminal segments of the radial arteries by 16–20 weeks of gestation[100]. As a result of endovascular trophoblast metastasis, the muscular and elastic tissue in the arterial wall is replaced by a fibroid material, thereby converting the arteries into flaccid distended tubes. These changes, termed physiological changes, result in a ten-fold increase in blood flow through the uteroplacental arteries and into the placental intervillous space[101]. These physiological changes occur temporally to coincide with the metastasis of endovascular trophoblasts[102]. Physiological changes occur in decidual segments of spiral arteries from 6–12 weeks' gestation and in myometrial segments from about 16 weeks' gestation[100–102]. By about 24 weeks' gestation these structural changes are completed; in normal pregnancy all spiral arteries in the placental bed show these physiological changes[101].

Abnormal implantation

Mechanisms by which defective implantation leads to recurrent pregnancy loss can involve any of the processes necessary for normal implantation. Abnormalities which could occur during implantation are summarized in Table 8. These abnormalities can result from defective trophoblast functioning, or inappropriate maternal response to the blastocyst at either the local (endometrial) or systemic level.

Abnormal trophoblastic function

At the time of implantation, trophoblastic cells communicate with endometrial and lymphoid cells. Communication is mediated by cytokines and cell-surface proteins. HLA-G, a protein expressed on the cell surface of the trophoblast[103], is recognized by a CD8+ lymphocyte. The CD8+ lymphocyte secretes cytokines that promote trophoblastic cell growth and differentiation[104]. As the trophoblastic cells proliferate and invade the endometrium, they differentiate into an inner cytoblastic and an outer syncytiocytoblastic layer. Any agent that interferes with differentiation of cytotrophoblast to syncytiotrophoblast can inhibit the normal development of a pregnancy. Antiphospholipid antibodies (APA) have been shown to inhibit the differentiation of cytotrophoblast to syncytiotrophoblast[105] and their presence in sera of women have been associated with adverse pregnancy outcome[106].

Abnormal endometrial immunological response

At the time of implantation, the endometrium contains maternal immune cells including macrophages, CD8 (suppressor) T cells and CD56+ CD16– NK cells. Trophoblastic cells are resistant to lysis by cytotoxic T lymphocytes and NK cells, but they are susceptible to activated NK cells or LAK cells[107]. Suppression of

Table 8   Proposed mechanisms of abnormalities occurring during implantation which results in reproductive failure

Implantation event	Time of event (days from LMP)	Molecule affecting event	Abnormality	Clinical presentation
Adhesion	21	hCG, PAF hCG-R, IL-1, IL-1R, IL-1Ra	defective blastocyst non-responsive endometrium	infertility
Penetration	22	laminin-R collagenase autocrine motility factors growth factors growth factor receptor	defective blastocyst non-responsive endometrium defective blastocyst	infertility
Allograft acceptance	22–280	HLA-G, MCP suppressor factors blocking antibodies	defective blastocyst non-responsive endometrium inappropriate maternal immune response	infertility RSA RPL
Metastasis	40–140	laminin receptor collagenase autocrine motility factors serpines	defective blastocyst non-responsive endometrium defective blastocyst	RSA RPL

RSA, recurrent spontaneous abortion; RPL, recurrent pregnancy loss activation of NK to LAK cells is necessary for successful pregnancy to occur. A number of cytokines have been shown to prevent LAK cell activation and abortion in mice. These cytokines include IL-3, GM-CSF, TGFβ$_2$[51,108] and a 34-kDa protein produced by CD8+ cells with progesterone receptors[84]. TGFβ$_2$ is produced by decidual cells that have a CD56+ CD16– phenotype[53]. A subpopulation of patients with recurrent pregnancy loss that lacks these TGFβ$_2$ CD56+ CD16– cells has been identified[52,109]. Further, an infiltrate of CD56+ CD16+ LAK cells has been noted in placental bed biopsies in incipiently aborting patients with a history of recurrent spontaneous abortion[53].

In addition to NK and T cell production of suppressive factors, activated decidual mononuclear cells including macrophages release IL-1. IL-1 down-regulates endothelial thrombomodulin and makes TF available on endothelial plasma membranes[90,92]. Human placentae contain substantial amounts of TF[91], which is potentially able to trigger or activate the extrinsic pathway of coagulation and results in fibrin deposition. Since fibrin is necessary for successful implantation, inappropriate allogeneic stimulation or recognition of the implanting blastocyst would lead to insufficient fibrin formation to secure the implantation site[92].

Abnormal fibrin depositions are associated with abnormal pregnancies[91,92]. A possible mechanism for the increased fibrin deposition is the production of cytokines or antibodies which recognize antigens on the endothelial cell surface and activate the endothelial cell to convert from thromboresistant to thrombogenic surfaces[92]. Evidence in support of this mechanism is available from studies describing the placental bed in women with the antiphospholipid syndrome; placental vessel thrombosis, infarction and placental insufficiency have been demonstrated[110].

In other abnormal pregnancies including cases of pre-eclampsia and a proportion of normotensive pregnancies complicated by fetal growth retardation, physiological changes in spiral arteries occurring as a result of metastasis of endovascular trophoblasts are absent in the myometrial segments of spiral arteries. Further, physiological changes have been noted also to be absent from decidual segments in these pregnancy disorders, indicating that there is not only a reduction in depth of physiological changes in the spiral arteries that are partially transformed but also a reduction in the number of uteroplacental arteries that are actually formed[110]. In those vessels that have not undergone physiological changes, an arteriopathy characterized by fibrinoid necrosis of smooth muscle, perivascular mononuclear inflammatory infiltrate and intramural and intraluminal lipophages is seen[111]. Immunohistochemical and clinical studies suggest that immunological mechanisms are important in the pathogenesis of this lesion[112].

Abnormal systemic immunological response

Local production of these cytokines at the fetodecidual interface has been studied, but there is also evidence of systemic activity. These factors can be measured systemically as circulating embryotoxins in an embryotoxicity assay[113–119]. Circulating NK (CD56+) cells can be measured, and identification of elevated percentages of circulating CD56+ cells has been associated with early loss of karyotypically normal pregnancies[57]. Thus, identification of circulating elevated concentrations of antiphospholipids (and other autoantibodies including antithyroid and antinuclear antibodies) and elevated percentages of CD56+ cells and embryotoxins has been used to identify women at risk for immunological components contributing to pregnancy wastage.

DIAGNOSIS AND MANAGEMENT

Diagnostic investigation of couples experiencing two or more consecutive pregnancy losses includes chromosome analysis of previous products of conception as well as of both partners, hysterosonography, hysterosalpingography or hysteroscopy, luteal phase evaluation with measurement of uterine receptivity and immunological tests (Table 9). Understanding the mechanisms involved in the pathophysiology of recurrent pregnancy loss allows a more focused approach to applying these tools to identify risk factors that can be corrected.

Management of couples suffering from recurrent pregnancy loss should be directed towards the cause of the reproductive wastage.

Anatomic defects

Metroplasty has been advocated for treatment of Müllerian duct anomalies in women with recurrent pregnancy loss. However, when 140 women with uterine abnormalities were studied for subsequent pregnancy outcome, the live birth rate was the same in women undergoing metroplasty and those not

Table 9   Evaluation of couples experiencing recurrent pregnancy loss

---

Chromosomal analysis
Parents, Products of conception

Examination of uterine cavity
Hysteroscopy, Hysterosalpingography
Hysterosonography

Evaluation of endometrial receptivity
Serum progesterone, Endometrial biopsy,
Integrins, Ultrasonography

Immunological tests
Autoantibodies, CD56+ cells,
Embryotoxicity assay, Leukocyte
antibody detection assay

---

having surgery[120]. In this study 21 women underwent metroplasty and 119 did not. Seventeen of the non-surgical patients were matched with the surgical patients by age, chief complaint at the time of diagnosis, gravidity and type of anomaly, and these women served as matched controls. The remaining 102 non-surgical patients did not have significant clinical problems and served as additional controls. Follow-up data were available after the diagnosis of uterine anomaly for 20 of the surgical patients, 17 of the non-surgical matched controls and 52 of the other controls. The percentages of patients with living children after the diagnosis of uterine anomaly were 71% and 80% for each of the non-surgical groups, compared with 70% for those who underwent metroplasty. Although fetal salvage rates improved markedly after metroplasty, outcome was similar to that of the controls for whom surgery was deferred. Moreover, the frequency of congenital uterine anomalies was similar among normal parous women and women experiencing recurrent spontaneous abortion[121,122].

Observations with the hysteroscope have provided evidence that uterine adhesions represent an effect rather than a cause of multiple pregnancy losses[123]. Just as the efficacy of metroplasty in the treatment of multiple pregnancy loss is being questioned, so too is the role of these anatomic defects as a cause.

Two additional anatomic defects deserve mention. A small, T-shaped uterus identified by hysterosalpingogram suggests *in utero* exposure to diethylstilbestrol. The hypoplastic uterine corpus is associated with recurrent spontaneous abortions and premature labor. No treatment exists for these problems. A history of recurrent second-trimester pregnancy losses preceded by painless cervical effacement and dilatation is a typical history of an incompetent cervix. Treatment involves placing a McDonald or Shirodkar cervical cerclage during the second trimester of the subsequent pregnancy.

Hormonal deficiencies

The role of progesterone deficiency in recurrent spontaneous abortion has been investigated in two areas. The first was an attempt to implicate low pregnanediol levels in pregnancy. Results in women who were treated with exogenous progesterone were no different from those in patients who received placebo[39,40]. The second approach was to diagnose the insufficient effect of progesterone on the endometrium during the luteal phase of the menstrual cycle, and to initiate treatment with exogenous hormones a few days after ovulation. To date, these studies have not been controlled to determine whether correcting the luteal phase defect prior to the missed menstrual period is of value in recurrent spontaneous aborters who are diagnosed as having an inadequate luteal phase.

Genetic causes

Chromosomal abnormalities have been found in 60% of karyotyped products of conception and 6% of parental leukocytes among women who experience recurrent spontaneous abortion[37]. Trisomies and monosomy for the X chromosome are the most frequent chromosomal abnormalities in first-trimester abortions[43], and Robertsonian translocations usually are seen in members of couples who experience recurrent abortions[124].

At the time of the initial visit, pedigree analysis and chromosomal studies of peripheral blood in both parents will identify known genetic factors. At present there is no available treatment either for a detected parent chromosomal translocation, or for a multifactorial genetic disorder that is operative in the production of abortions, with or without fetal malformations. Therapeutically, the chance of a full-term living child is in the range of 20–30% depending on the specific translocation or genetic disorder. Cytogenetic studies of chorionic villi and amniotic fluid, ultrasonography, and α-fetoprotein levels are indicated in future pregnancies for these women. Use of donor gametes is a treatment option, and high successful pregnancy rates have been reported.

Immunological causes

Various forms of immunotherapy have been introduced to treat couples experiencing recurrent spontaneous abortion. Understanding the mechanisms involved in recurrent spontaneous abortion allows a more focused approach to specific treatment. Tests available to help direct the approach to treatment include measurement of antiphospholipid antibodies and antinuclear antibodies, quantitation of circulating CD56+ cells and assays for the detection of embryotoxicity and lymphocyte antibodies.

Immunotherapy for recurrent spontaneous abortion associated with antiphospholipid antibodies

Treatments involving aspirin, heparin, glucocorticoids, intravenous immunoglobulin, all four or a combination of two or three of these have been used.

Aspirin

Low-dose aspirin alone has been advocated in the treatment of recurrent spontaneous abortion associated with antiphospholipid antibodies. Sbracia and colleagues[125] reported a successful pregnancy outcome of 85% in the treatment arm (ASA 50 mg/day) and 53% in the placebo arm of a clinical trial ($p < 0.02$). However, results of other clinical trials have shown aspirin alone to be half as effective as other treatments including prednisone and heparin[49]. In a recent prospective controlled trial of 50 women receiving aspirin alone or heparin plus aspirin for treatment of recurrent spontaneous abortion associated with antiphospholipid antibodies, heparin plus aspirin provided a significantly better outcome than aspirin alone (livebirth rate of 80% vs. 44%, $p < 0.01$)[49]. A rationale for the use of low-dose aspirin therapy during pregnancy for women with antiphospholipid antibodies is provided by the observation that IgG from women with antiphospholipid antibodies has been shown to increase the concentration of placental thromboxane[126]. Platelets also produce thromboxane, resulting in vasoconstriction and platelet aggregation. Thromboxane production leads to thrombosis. In fact, 85% of placentae from antiphospholipid-positive women have evidence of thrombosis[110,127]. Low-dose aspirin has been shown to be a thromboxane inhibitor[128].

Heparin and aspirin

Heparin has also been used in conjunction with aspirin to prevent placental thrombosis[49,129,130]. The rationale for heparin use has been that the anticoagulant activity overrides the thrombotic events caused by antiphospholipid binding to phospholipid[126]. Plasma from women with antiphospholipid antibodies has been shown to inhibit endothelial cell production of prostacyclin[126]. Prostacyclin is a potent vasodilator and inhibitor of platelet aggregation. Decreased production of prostacyclin facilitates the thromboxane-dominant milieu that leads to thrombosis. A recent study has shown that the addition of heparin to antiphospholipid-positive serum from women with recurrent pregnancy loss caused a dose-dependent decrease in IgG binding to cardiolipin and phosphatidylserine in an enzyme-linked immunosorbent assay (ELISA)[131]. Heparin may have multiple mechanisms of action in the antiphospholipid antibody syndrome.

Various treatment regimens of heparin have been used. Heparin has been used with aspirin with or without prednisone. With prednisone, live birth rates after heparin and aspirin treatment were 74%[132], and without prednisone were 80%[49]. Thus, no enhancement of live birth rates has been noted when prednisone is added to heparin and aspirin therapy for recurrent spontaneous abortion. A prospective controlled trial compared live birth rates in 50 women with antiphospholipid antibodies and recurrent spontaneous abortion after treatment with either heparin and aspirin or aspirin alone[49]. A greater number of women in the group with heparin and aspirin (80%) delivered viable infants than did women in the aspirin-alone group (44%) ($p < 0.05$). There were no significant differences between the low-dose aspirin and the heparin plus low-dose aspirin groups with respect to gestational age at delivery, number of Cesarean sections, or complications. The investigators concluded that heparin plus low-dose aspirin provided a significantly better pregnancy outcome than did low-dose aspirin alone for antiphospholipid antibody-associated recurrent pregnancy loss[49]. The randomized controlled clinical trial of Cowchock and associates[130] that compared heparin and aspirin with prednisone and aspirin for treatment of recurrent spontaneous abortion associated with antiphospholipid antibodies had live birth rates of 75% in both groups. However, both maternal morbidity and the frequency of preterm delivery with premature rupture of membranes and pre-eclampsia were significantly higher in pregnant women treated with prednisone and aspirin. Therefore, the current recommendations for 'first attempt' treatment for recurrent spontaneous abortion associated with antiphospholipid antibodies is heparin and aspirin. Heparin is usually administered at a dose of 5000–10 000 units subcutaneously twice a day along with aspirin 80 mg each day instituted prior to pregnancy. The possible side-effects of low-dose heparin therapy include prolonged coagulation times, thrombocytopenia and osteoporosis[133,134].

Prednisone and aspirin

The majority of reported cases of recurrent spontaneous abortion have been treated with combinations of prednisone and aspirin. Prednisone is usually given as a daily dose of 40–80 mg beginning at the diagnosis of pregnancy. A daily dose of 80 mg aspirin is usually started preconceptually. The rationale for prednisone therapy is suppression of autoantibodies such as antiphospholipid and antinuclear antibodies.

Hasegawa and co-workers[50] published a randomized controlled trial that evaluated the efficacy of prednisone and aspirin for treatment of recurrent spontaneous abortion associated with antiphospholipid antibodies. In this study, women treated with prednisone and aspirin had a live birth rate of 77% compared with non-treated control women who had a live birth rate of 8%. In the trial of Silber and colleagues[135], 39 women were randomized to receive either prednisone plus aspirin or aspirin alone. All 34 pregnancies included in the analysis ended in live birth, but the aspirin with prednisone group demonstrated a greater incidence of preterm delivery. Others have reported a high frequency of premature rupture of membranes and associated preterm delivery with the administration of prednisone[130,136]. Non-obstetric risks associated with high doses of prednisone include iatrogenic Cushing's syndrome, severe acne, increased risk of gestational diabetes, osteopenia, posterior capsular cataract, listeriosis, pneumonia and even maternal death from miliary tuberculosis[130,136,137]. Collectively, these studies suggest that glucocorticoid therapy is probably best reserved for heparin and aspirin treatment failures or for women with antiphospholipid antibodies and active autoimmune diseases such as systemic lupus erythematosus[138].

Intravenous immunoglobulin therapy

Intravenous immunoglobulin (IVIG) therapy has been used as treatment for recurrent spontaneous abortion associated with antiphospholipid antibodies. Originally, IVIG therapy was used to treat women who had not been successful in pregnancies previously treated with aspirin and prednisone or aspirin alone. The rationale for use of IVIG therapy in the original studies was the suppression of the lupus anticoagulant in a woman being treated for severe thrombocytopenia[139]. Intravenous immunoglobulin was often given with prednisone or heparin plus aspirin. The estimated total success rate of 71% for women at very high risk for failure with a history of previous treatment failures suggested that the IVIG treatment was effective[129]. More recently, IVIG therapy alone has been used successfully to treat women with antiphospholipid antibodies[140]. This series, along with a previous report of successful treatment with IVIG in a woman who had lost 12 previous pregnancies while being treated with aspirin and heparin or prednisone[141], suggested that IVIG therapy alone is successful in treating women with recurrent spontaneous abortion associated with antiphospholipid antibodies. IVIG has been used successfully to treat women who became refractory to conventional autoimmune treatment and experienced obstetric complications[142,143].

Immunotherapy for recurrent spontaneous abortion not associated with antiphospholipid antibodies

Management of unexplained recurrent spontaneous abortion has been controversial. Results of meta-analyses and randomized clinical trials have provided evidence for successful treatment of recurrent spontaneous abortion by immunotherapy in the forms of immunization with allogeneic monocytes[60,144,145] or IVIG[58,146,147].

Allogeneic mononuclear cell immunotherapy for recurrent spontaneous abortion

Clinical trials evaluating allogeneic monocyte immunization have both supported[60,144,145] and challenged[148,149] the efficacy of immunotherapy for the treatment of recurrent spontaneous abortion. To address the uncertainties caused by these conflicting results, a worldwide collaborative observational study and meta-analysis was performed[60]. Fifteen collaborating centers participated in the study. Nine randomized trials (seven double-blinded) were evaluated independently by two data analysis teams to assure that conclusions were robust.

Although the independent analyses used different definitions and statistical methods, the results were similar. The per cent live birth ratios (ratio of live births in treatment and control groups, respectively) with 95% confidence intervals were 1.16 (range 1.01–1.34; $p = 0.03$) and 1.21 (range 1.04–1.37; $p = 0.02$). The absolute differences in live birth rates between treatment and control groups were 8% and 10%. These results were based on a data set that included couples in whom the female partner had autoimmune abnormalities (positive antinuclear antibodies and/or positive anticardiolipin antibodies), for which treatment reduced the probability of a live birth; or pre-existing antipaternal lymphocyte antibodies; or one prior successful pregnancy with their partner, when the probability of success without treatment was high[60]. Logistic regression analysis indicated negative prognostic variables of abnormal autoimmunity and increasing numbers of losses with partner, and positive prognostic variables of presence of pretreatment paternal antibody. A supplementary analysis of primary recurrent aborters (no prior live births), excluding those with autoimmunity and pre-existing antipaternal antibodies, has subsequently been published[150]. By selecting patients most likely to benefit from immunotherapy, the outcome may be improved by at least 50%. When the analysis was restricted to patients who became pregnant after intervention, similar results were obtained[150].

The original rationale for treating recurrent spontaneous abortion with allogeneic leukocyte immunization was to present an allogeneic stimulus to the maternal immune system that would evoke an appropriate response to antigens on the fetal trophoblastic cells needed to protect the pregnancy from failure[151]. Fetal trophoblastic cells have been considered to have little immunogenicity even though they do express HLA-C and HLA-G[152,153]. Recently, an 80-kDa antigen (R80K) has been found on human syncytiotrophoblasts that can be recognized immunologically by the mother[86]. The R80K antibody obtained from placenta or maternal serum reacts with an antigen on her partner's B lymphocytes and monocytes and with her partner's father's B cells and monocytes[88,89]. The genetic basis for this unusual pattern of transmission is consistent with selective expression of the paternal genome in trophoblast. The antibody response to R80K is T-cell dependent, but conventional T cells do not appear to be able to recognize or react to trophoblast[154].

In humans, there is evidence that CD8+ T cells may recognize trophoblast. These particular CDs and T cells carry the γδ type receptor rather than the conventional αβ T-cell receptor that recognizes HLA A, B and C[155]. In successful pregnancy or after T-cell activation, as occurs with immunization, CD8+ cells are activated, express progesterone receptors and secrete a factor that inhibits activation of NK cells[84,156,157]. Other cytokines may also be produced by activated CD8+ T cells, and it is hypothesized that some of these may enhance antibody responses (IL-4), inhibit macrophages (IL-10) and facilitate activation of CD56+, CD16– bone marrow-derived TGFβ-producing suppressor cells (IL-3, GM-CSF) found in decidua[158,159]. Women with recurrent miscarriage show a lack of activation of their CD8+ cells in early pregnancy[160]. Whether allogeneic mononuclear cell immunization enhances activation of CD8+ cells is not known. In fact, the mechanism by which allogeneic leukocyte immunization enhances live birth rates is not known. The fact that the treatment effect of allogeneic mononuclear cell immunization is small (11 patients have to be immunized to achieve one additional live birth)[60] suggests that it is either incomplete treatment for some, or complete treatment for a smaller proportion of couples experiencing recurrent spontaneous abortion.

Intravenous immunoglobulin therapy for treatment of recurrent spontaneous abortion

Because of the low treatment effect of allogeneic mononuclear cell immunization[60], other treatments for recurrent spontaneous abortion were sought. Further understanding of the mechanisms involved in recurrent spontaneous abortion helped in selecting potential alternative treatments. Recent research has indicated that the basis for failure of early pregnancy is NK cells. NK cells have been shown to recognize trophoblastic cells[161]. NK cells cannot kill trophoblastic cells *in vitro*, but NK cells activated by cytokines (LAK cells) such as IL-2 may kill trophoblastic cells *in vitro*[162]. Decidual bed biopsies from women experiencing recurrent spontaneous abortion reveal an increase in LAK cells (CD56+, CD16+ NK cells)[52]. Peripheral blood CD56+, CD16+ NK cells were significantly elevated in women with recurrent spontaneous abortions as compared with normal control women[163]. Quantitation of CD56+ NK cells in the peripheral blood of patients with recurrent spontaneous abortion with a failing pregnancy has shown a significant elevation associated with spontaneous abortion of a conceptus of normal karyotype, and a normal level associated with loss of embryos that are karyotypically abnormal[157]. Furthermore, high blood NK levels in non-pregnant women are predictive of recurrent spontaneous abortion[164]. Thus, NK cells and failure to suppress NK-cell activation play an important role in immunologically preventable spontaneous abortion.

Intravenous immunoglobulin has been shown to down-regulate NK cell killing activity[165] and to regulate CD8+ cells. Both of these events may be necessary for successful pregnancy to occur[154]. Provided there is adequate quality control, commercially available IVIG should be virus-free[166], theoretically decreasing the risk of viral transmission of disease compared to mononuclear cell immunization[167]. Three randomized controlled trials of IVIG for treatment of recurrent spontaneous abortion have been published[58,146,147]. A Europe-based study showed a positive trend but did not achieve statistical significance, owing to too few patients for adequate statistical power, given the magnitude of the effect[146]. However, a second USA-based trial did show a significant benefit[58]. This prospective, randomized, placebo-controlled trial showed the difference in live birth rates between women receiving IVIG (62%) and those receiving placebo (34%) ($p = 0.04$)[58]. As the USA-based trial did not have larger numbers than the Europe-based trial, the positive result was due to an effect of greater magnitude. From the magnitude of the effect in the USA-based trial, it is concluded that one needs to treat four women to achieve one additional live birth, making IVIG therapy more effective than mononuclear cell immunization in the treatment of recurrent spontaneous abortion[168]. The greater magnitude of effect in the USA-based study compared to the Europe-based trial could have arisen by the use of a different study design. One of the potentially significant differences in study design between the two trials was timely initiation of treatment. Patients began IVIG treatment prior to conception in the USA-based trial[58], but after implantation in the Europe-based trial[146]. By waiting until 5–8 weeks of gestation (for diagnosis of pregnancy), women with NK cell-related pathology occurring earlier would be excluded and pregnancies with the best prognosis would be included, providing an opportunity for selection bias. Studies using other forms of immunotherapy have shown a significant increase in live birth rates when treatment was begun preconceptually compared to postconceptually[132]. A third study[147] treated only patients with secondary recurrent spontaneous abortion, a group that showed no significant benefit to treatment using leukocyte immunization[60]. A non-controlled study by the same investigators using IVIG to treat 11 women who had 4–8 unexplained pregnancy losses reported a live birth rate of 85%[169]. A meta-analysis of the randomized controlled studies using IVIG for treatment of recurrent spontaneous abortion[59] revealed an overall relative risk of 1.38 (95% confidence interval of 1.04–1.84; $p = 0.02$). These results show IVIG to be effective in the treatment of recurrent spontaneous abortion, but it is still not clear what is the ideal dosage, or how frequently and how long IVIG therapy should be given.

Immunotherapy for recurrent spontaneous abortion associated with elevated concentrations of circulating CD56+ cells

Recent data suggest that IVIG therapy is useful in maintaining pregnancies in women with a history of recurrent spontaneous abortion who lose karyotypically normal embryos after detection of embryonic cardiac activity on ultrasonographic examination and who demonstrate elevated levels of NK (CD56+) cells in maternal blood[57]. Viable pregnancies were found in a significantly higher proportion of women with CD56+ cell levels of >12% who received IVIG than those who did not receive IVIG ($p = 0.0002$)[57].

Peripheral NK cell activities were studied in women experiencing recurrent spontaneous abortion before and after immunotherapy with partner's mononuclear cell immunization[54]. All women in whom NK activity decreased following immunotherapy became pregnant and had healthy babies. In contrast, women in whom NK activity greatly increased following immunotherapy failed to become pregnant more than 12 months after treatment[55].

However, more recent studies have documented decreases in NK activity *in vivo* in women with a history of recurrent spontaneous abortion previously treated with mononuclear cell immunization after IVIG administration[56,170].

Immunotherapy for recurrent spontaneous abortion associated with circulating embryotoxins

Hill and colleagues[113] reported that embryotoxic factors were produced by activated leukocyte cultures from 90% of 180 women with recurrent spontaneous abortion. Other studies have identified embryotoxic factors in 24–60% of women experiencing recurrent spontaneous abortion[114–118]. Successful pregnancies have been observed in these women following IVIG therapy or progesterone supplementation[57,117]. However, none of these studies reported control results. Randomized controlled clinical trials of immunotherapy for the treatment of recurrent spontaneous abortions associated with circulating embryotoxins are required to determine efficacy.

SUMMARY

Recurrent pregnancy loss is a health care concern. Safe and effective treatments are necessary. Because women who experience recurrent pregnancy loss are a heterogeneous population, specific markers are necessary to identify those who will respond to various treatments. The presence of antiphospholipid antibodies helps identify women with recurrent pregnancy loss who are most likely to respond to heparin and aspirin treatment. An elevated concentration of NK cells in maternal blood and a loss of karyotypically normal embryos after detection of cardiac activity at ultrasonographic examination helps identify women who are most likely to respond to IVIG treatment. An obstetric history of recurrent primary abortion with an absence of maternal antipaternal lymphocytotoxic antibodies and antiphospholipid antibodies is used to predict the women who are most likely to respond to allogeneic leukocyte immunization. However, the treatment effect is low, with a live birth rate of 60%, representing an enhancement over no treatment in the range of 8–10%. The difference in live birth rates between women receiving IVIG therapy and women receiving placebo was 28%. Women experiencing recurrent spontaneous abortion who have high, as opposed to low, levels of leukocyte antibody do not respond to leukocyte immunization therapy. They do, however, respond to treatment with IVIG, the overall success rate of IVIG being 70%.

It is important to be able to identify women likely to respond to various forms of immunotherapy. Chromosomal abnormalities are evident in 60% of recurrent abortions. Women who experience recurrent aneuploidy in their abortuses would not be expected to respond to immunotherapy. At present, the only way to identify such women is to have the results of chromosome analysis of previous pregnancy losses available. Having access to this information will require a change in current obstetric practice in obtaining karyotyping of all pregnancy losses. The cost effectiveness of chromosomal studies of abortuses is apparent when the costs of evaluation and treatment are considered.

REFERENCES

1. Mosher WD. Infertility trends among U.S. couples, 1965–1976. *Fam Plann Perspect* 1982;14:22
2. Strobino BR, Kuni J, Shrout P, *et al.* Recurrent spontaneous abortion: definition of a syndrome. In Porter IH, Hook EB, eds. *Human Embryonic and Fetal Death.* London: Academic Press, 1980:315–29
3. Roman E. Fetal loss rates and their relation to pregnancy order. *J Epidemiol Commun Health* 1984;38:29
4. Coulam CB. Epidemiology of recurrent spontaneous abortion. *Am J Reprod Immunol* 1991;26:23
5. Mills JE, Simpson JL, Driscoll SG, *et al.* Incidence of spontaneous abortion among normal women and insulin-dependent diabetic women whose pregnancies were identified within 21 days of conception. *N Engl J Med* 1988;319:1617
6. Parazzini F, Acaia B, Ricciardeiello O, *et al.* Short-term reproductive prognosis when no cause can be found for recurrent miscarriage. *Br J Obstet Gynaecol* 1988;95:654–8
7. Risch HA, Weiss NS, Clarke EA, Miller AB. Risk factors for spontaneous abortion and its recurrence. *Am J Epidemiol* 1988;128:420
8. Poland BJ, Miller JR, Jones DC, Trimble BK. Reproductive counseling in patients who have had a spontaneous abortion. *Am J Obstet Gynecol* 1977; 127:685–91

9. Cowchock FS, Smith JB, David S, *et al.* Paternal mononuclear cell immunization therapy for repeated miscarriage: predictive variables for pregnancy success. *Am J Reprod Immunol* 1990;22:12

10. Strobino B, Fox HD, Kline J, *et al.* Characteristics of women with recurrent spontaneous abortions and women with favorable reproductive histories. *Am J Public Health* 1986;76:986

11. Regan L. Recurrent miscarriage. *Br Med J* 1991; 302:543

12. Jansen RPS. Spontaneous abortion incidence in the treatment of infertility. *Am J Obstet Gynecol* 1982; 143:451

13. Peters A, Coulam CB, Critser ES. Association between recurrent spontaneous abortion and subfertility. *Am J Reprod Immunol* 1990;22:87

14. Regan L. A prospective study of spontaneous abortion. In Beard RW, Sharp F, eds. *Early Pregnancy Loss: Mechanisms and Treatment.* London: RCOG, 1988:23

15. Honore LH. A significant association between spontaneous abortion and tubal ectopic pregnancy. *Fertil Steril* 1979;32:401

16. Fedele L, Acaia B, Parazzini F, *et al.* Ectopic pregnancy and recurrent spontaneous abortion: two associated reproductive failures. *Obstet Gynecol* 1989;73:206–8

17. Coulam CB, Johnson PM, Ramaden GH, *et al.* Occurrence of ectopic pregnancy among women with recurrent spontaneous abortion. *Am J Reprod Immunol* 1989;21:105

18. Masserli ML, Lillienfeld MD, Parmley T, *et al.* Risk factors for gestational trophoblastic neoplasia. *Am J Obstet Gynecol* 1985;153:294

19. Parazzini F, LaVecchia C, Pampallona S, Franceschi S. Reproductive patterns and the risk of gestational trophoblastic disease. *Am J Obstet Gynecol* 1985;152:866

20. Reginald PW, Beard RW, Chapple J, *et al.* Outcome of pregnancies progressing beyond 28 weeks gestation in women with a history of recurrent miscarriage. *Br J Obstet Gynaecol* 1987;94:643

21. Branch DW, Blackwell J, Dudley DJ, Scott JR. Antiphospholipid antibody syndrome (APAS): treated pregnancy outcome and medical follow up. Presented at the *37th Annual Meeting of the Society for Gynecologic Investigation*, St Louis, Missouri, March 21–24, 1990; abstr. 377

22. Funderburk SJ, Guthrie D, Meldrum D, Suboptimal pregnancy with prior abortions and premature births. *Am J Obstet Gynecol* 1976;126:55

23. Schoenbaum SC, Monson RR, Subblefield PG, *et al.* Outome of the delivery following induced and spontaneous delivery. *Am J Obstet Gynecol* 1980;136:19

24. Alberman E, Roman E, Pharoah POD, Chamberlain C. Birthweights before and after spontaneous abortions. *Br J Obstet Gynaecol* 1980;87:275

25. Coulam CB, Smith JB, Branch DW. Report of Workshop on Unification of Immunotherapy Protocols. *Am J Reprod Immunol* 1991;25:1

26. Miller JF, Williamson E, Glue J, *et al.* Fetal loss after implantation. A prospective study. *Lancet* 1980; 2:554

27. Rubin GL, Peterson HB, Dorfman SF, *et al.* Ectopic pregnancy in the United States: 1970 through 1978. *J Am Med Assoc* 1983;249:1725

28. Cunningham FG, MacDonald PC, Gant NF, eds. In *Preterm and Post-term Pregnancy and Inappropriate Fetal Growth*, 18th ed. Norwalk CT, San Mateo CA: Appleton and Lange, 1989:741

29. Kaji T, Okama K. Androgenic origin of hydatidiform mole. *Nature (London)* 1977;268:633

30. Poland BJ, Miller JR, Harris M, Livingston J. Spontaneous abortion. A study of 1961 women and their conceptuses. *Acta Obstet Gynecol Scand* (suppl) 1981;102:1

31. Miller JF, Williamson E, Glue J, *et al.* Fetal loss after implantation. A prospective study. *Lancet* 1980;2:554

32. Leridan H. *Human Fertility: the Basic Components.* Chicago: University of Chicago, 1977

33. Coulam CB. Unexplained recurrent pregnancy loss: epilogue. *Clin Obstet Gynecol* 1986;29:999

34. Tho PT, Byrd JR, McDonough PG. Etiologies and subsequent reproductive performance of 100 couples with recurrent abortion. *Fertil Steril* 1979;32:389

35. Harger JH, Archer DF, Marchese SG, *et al.* Etiology of recurrent pregnancy losses and outcome of subsequent pregnancies. *Obstet Gynecol* 1983;62:574

36. Stray-Pedersen B, Stray-Pedersen S. Etiologic factors and subsequent reproductive performance among 195 couples with a prior history of habitual abortion. *Am J Obstet Gynecol* 1984;148:140

37. Stern JJ, Dorfmann A, Gutierez-Najar AJ, *et al.* Frequency of abnormal karyotypes among abortuses from women with and without a history of recurrent spontaneous abortion. *Fertil Steril* 1996;65:250

38. Lloyd R, Coulam CB. Recurrent spontaneous abortion: frequency of diagnosis of luteal phase defects. *Am J Reprod Immunol Microbiol* 1988;16:103

39. Goldzieher JW. Double-blind trial for a progestin in habitual abortion. *J Am Med Assoc* 1964;188:651

40. Klopper A, Macnaughton MC. Hormones in recurrent abortion. *Br J Obstet Gynaecol* 1965;72:1022

41. Lloyd R, Coulam CB. Role of endometrial biopsy in diagnosing luteal phase defect. *Fertil Steril* Suppl 1988:S57

42. Peters AJ, Lloyd RP, Coulam CB. Prevalence of out of phase endometrial biopsy specimens. *Am J Obstet Gynecol* 1992;166:1738

43. Hassold T, Chen N, Funkhouse J, *et al.* A cytogenetic study of 1000 spontaneous abortions. *Ann Hum Genet* 1980;44:151

44. Boklage CE. Survival of human conceptions from fertilization to term. *Int J Fertil* 1991;35:189–94

45. Drugan A, Koppitch FC, Williams JC, *et al.* Prenatal genetic diagnosis following recurrent early pregnancy loss. *Obstet Gynecol* 1990;75:381–4

46. Roussev RG, Kaider BD, Price DE, Coulam CB. Laboratory evaluation of women experiencing reproductive failure. *Am J Reprod Immunol* 1996;35:415–20

47. Lubbe WF, Liggins GC. Lupus anticoagulant and pregnancy. *Am J Obstet Gynecol* 1985;153:322

48. Branch DW, Scott JR, Kochenour NR, Hershgold E. Obstetrical complications associated with the lupus anticoagulant. *N Engl J Med* 1985;313:1322

49. Kutteh WH. Antiphospholipid antibody-associated recurrent pregnancy loss: treatment with heparain and low-dose aspirin is superior to low-dose aspirin alone. *Am J Obstet Gynecol* 1996;174:1–6

50. Hasegawa I, Takakiwa K, Goto S, *et al.* Effectiveness of prednisone/aspirin therapy for recurrent aborters

with antiphospholipid antibody. *Hum Reprod* 1992; 7:203–7

51. Clark DA, Lea RG, Flanders KC, *et al*. Role of a unique species of transforming growth factor beta in preventing rejection of the conceptus during pregnancy. In Gergeley L, ed. *Progress in Immunology*. New York: Springer-Verlag, 1992:841–7

52. Lea RG, Underwood J, Flanders KC, *et al*. A subset of patients with recurrent spontaneous abortion is deficient in transforming growth factor beta 2-producing suppressor cells in decidua near the placental attachment site. *Am J Reprod Immunol* 1995;34:52–64

53. Clark DA, Lea RG, Podor T, *et al*. Cytokines determining the success or failure of pregnancy. *Ann NY Acad Sci* 1991;626:524–44

54. Makida R, Minami M, Takamizawa M, *et al*. Natural killer cell activity and immunotherapy for recurrent spontaneous abortion. *Lancet* 1991;2:579–80

55. Yokoyama M, Sano M, Sonoda K, *et al*. Cytotoxic cells directed against placental cells detected in human habitual abortions by an *in vitro* terminal labeling assay. *Am J Reprod Immunol* 1994;31:197–204

56. Kwak FM-Y, Kwak JYH, Beer AE. Peripheral blood natural killer cells are effectively suppressed by immunoglobulin G infusions in women with recurrent spontaneous abortions. *Am J Reprod Immunol* 1995;33:466

57. Coulam CB, Goodman C, Roussev RG, *et al*. Systemic CD56+ cells can predict pregnancy outcome. *Am J Reprod Immunol* 1995;33:40–6

58. Coulam CB, Krysa L, Stern JJ, Bustillo M. Intravenous immunoglobulin for treatment of recurrent pregnancy loss. *Am J Reprod Immunol* 1995;34:333–8

59. Clark DA. Alloimmunity and pregnancy loss. In Gleicher *et al*. eds. *Principles and Practice of Medical Therapy in Pregnancy*, 3rd ed. New York: Plenum Press, 1996

60. Coulam CB, Clark DA, Collins JA, *et al*. (The Recurrent Miscarriage Immunotherapy Trialist Group). World-wide collaborative observational study and meta-analysis on allogeneic leukocyte immunotherapy for recurrent spontaneous abortion. *Am J Reprod Immunol* 1994;32:55–72

61. Hay DL, Lopata A. Chorionic gonadotropin secretion by human embryos *in vitro*. *J Clin Endocrinol Metab* 1988;67:1322

62. Simon C, Pellicer A, Polan ML. Interleukin-1 system crosstalk in embryonic implantation. *Hum Reprod* 1995;10:43–54

63. O'Neill C. Partial characterization of the embryo-derived platelet activating factor in mice. *J Reprod Fertil* 1985;75:375–80

64. Reshep F, Lei ZM, Rao CV, *et al*. The presence of gonadotropin receptors in nonpregnant human uterus, human placenta, fetal membranes and decidua. *J Clin Endocrinol Metab* 1990;70:421

65. Harper MJK. Platelet activating factor: a paracrine factor in implantation stages of reproduction? *Bine Reprod* 1984;40:917–13

66. Liotta LA. Cancer invasion and metastasis. *J Am Med Assoc* 1990;263:1123

67. Rao CN, Margulies IMK, Tralka S, *et al*. Isolation of a subunit of laminin and its role in molecular structure and tumor cell attachment. *J Biol Chem* 1982;257:9740

68. Liotta LA, Tryggvason K, Garbisa S, *et al*. Metastatic potential correlates with enzymatic degradation of basement membrane collagen. *Nature (London)* 1980; 284:67

69. Liotta LA, Mandler R, Murano G, *et al*. Tumor cell autocrine motility factor. *Proc Natl Acad Sci USA* 1986; 83:3302

70. Chaouat G, Menu E, Szelares-Bartho J, *et al*. Lymphokines, steroids, placental factors and trophoblast intrinsic resistance to immune cell-mediated lysis are involved in pregnancy success or immunologically-mediated pregnancy failure. In Wegmann TG, Gill TJ, eds. *Molecular Biology of the Feto-maternal Interface*. New York: Oxford University Press, 1989

71. Bensaid M, Tauber MT, Malecaze F, *et al*. Effect of basic and acidic FGF and TBG-β in controlling the proliferation of retinal capillary endothelial cells. *Acta Paediatr Scand* (suppl) 1988;343:230

72. Richards RC, Beardmore JM, Brown PJ, *et al*. Epidermal growth factor receptors on isolated human placental syncytiotrophoblast plasma membrane. *Placenta* 1983;4:133

73. Hagid M, Manney LB, Stoscheck CM, King LE Jr. Epidermal growth factor binding and receptor distribution in term human placenta. *Placenta* 1985;6:519

74. Jonas HA, Cox AJ, Harrison LC. Delineation of atypical insulin receptors from classical insulin and type I insulin-like growth factor receptors in human placenta. *Biochem J* 1989;257:101

75. Muller R, Tremblay JM, Adamson ED, Verma IM. Tissue and cell type-specific expression of two human c-*onc* genes. *Nature (London)* 1983;304:1062

76. Gouston AS, Betsholtz C, Pfeiffer-Ohlsson S, *et al*. Coexpression of the *sis* and *myc* proto-oncogenes in developing human placenta suggests autocrine control of trophoblast growth. *Cell* 1985;41:301

77. Calderon J, Sheehan KCF, Chance C, *et al*. Purification and characterization of the human interferon-γ receptor from placenta. *Proc Natl Acad Sci USA* 1988; 85:4837

78. Eades DK, Cornelium P, Pekala PH. Characterization of the tumor necrosis factor receptor in human placenta. *Placenta* 1988;9:247

79. Clark DA, Chaouat G. What do we know about spontaneous abortion mechanism? *Am J Reprod Immunol* 1989;19:28

80. Hill JA, Haimovici F, Anderson DJ. Products of activated lymphocytes and macrophages inhibit mouse embryo development *in vitro*. *J Immunol* 1987;139:2250

81. Berkowitz RS, Hill JA, Kurtz CB, Anderson DJ. Effects of the products of activated leukocytes (lymphokines and monokines) on the growth of malignant trophoblast cells *in vitro*. *Am J Obstet Gynecol* 1988;158:199

82. Wegmann TG. Placental immunotropism. Maternal T cells enhance placental growth and function. *Am J Reprod Immunol Microbiol* 1987;15:67

83. Wegmann TG. Maternal T cells promote placental growth and prevent spontaneous abortion. *Immunol Lett* 1988;17:297

84. Szekeres-Bartho J, Kinsky R, Chaouat G. The effect of progesterone-induced immunologic blocking factor on NK-mediated resorption. *Am J Reprod Immunol* 1990;24:105–7

85. Rocklin RE, Ktizmiller JL, Carpenter CB, *et al.* Maternal–fetal relation. Absence of an immunologic blocking factor from the serum of women with chronic abortions. *N Engl J Med* 1976;295:1209

86. Jalali G, Rezai A, Underwood JL, *et al.* An 80 kDa syncytiotrophoblast alloantigen bound to maternal alloantibody in term placenta. *Am J Reprod Immunol* 1995;33:213–20

87. Jalali GR, Underwood JL, Mowbray JF. IgG on normal human placenta is bound both to antigen and Fc receptor. *Transplant Proc* 1989;21:572–4

88. Underwood JL, Rezai A, Jalali GR, *et al.* Transmission ratio distortion of a paternally derived syncytiotrophoblast antigen. *Am J Reprod Immunol* 1995;33:474–9

89. Rezai A, Underwood JL, Jalali GR, *et al.* Anomalous inheritance of a paternally derived trophoblast antigen. *Am J Reprod Immunol* 1996;35:245–51

90. Helin H, Edgington TS. A distinct 'slow' cellular pathway involving soluble mediators for the T cell-instructed induction of monocyte tissue factor activity in an allogeneic immune response. *J Immunol* 1984;132:2457

91. Nemerson Y. Tissue factor and hemostasis. *Blood* 1988;71:1

92. Faulk WP. Placental fibrin. *Am J Reprod Immunol* 1989; 19:132

93. Moore, KL. *The Developing Human*, 2nd edn. Philadelphia: W.B. Saunders, 1977:40

94. Faulk WP, McIntyre JA. Trophoblast survival. *Transplantation* 1981;32:1

95. Lolce VW, King A. Immunology of human implantation: an evolutionary perspective. *Hum Reprod* 1996; 11:283–6

96. Sueoka K, Dharmarajan AM, Miyazaki T, *et al.* Platelet activating factor (PAF)-induced early pregnancy factor (EPF) activity from the perfused rabbit ovary and oviduct. *Am J Obstet Gynecol* 1988;159:1580

97. Cavanagh AC, Morton H, Rolfe BE, Gidley-Baid AA. Ovum factor: a first signal of pregnancy. *Am J Reprod Immunol* 1982;2:97

98. Rolfe BE, Cavanagh AC, Quinn KA, Morton H. Identification of two suppressor factors induced by early pregnancy factor. *Clin Exp Immunol* 1988; 73:219

99. Ballard LL, Bora NS, Yu GH, Atkinson JP. Biochemical characterization of membrane cofactor protein of the complement system. *J Immunol* 1988; 141:3923

100. Pijnenborg R, Dixon G, Robertson WB, Brosens I. Trophoblastic invasion of human decidua from 8 to 18 weeks of pregnancy. *Placenta* 1980;1:3

101. Brosens I, Robertson WB, Dixon HG. The physiological response of the vessels of the placental bed to normal pregnancy. *J Pathol Bacteriol* 1967;93:569

102. Bronsons I, Dixon HG. Anatomy of the maternal side of the placenta. *J Obstet Gynaecol Br Commonw* 1966; 73:357

103. Wei X, Orr HT. Differential expression of HLAE, HLAF and HLAG transcripts in human tissue. *Hum Immunol* 1990;29:131

104. Chaouat G, Menu E, Athanassakis I, Wegmann TG. Maternal T cells regulate placental size and fetal survival. *Reg Immunol* 1988;1:143

105. Rote NS. Antiphospholipid antibodies: lobsters or red herrings? *Am J Reprod Immunol* 1992;28:31

106. Cowchock S. The role of antiphospholipid antibodies in obstetric medicine. *Curr Obstet Med* 1991;1:229

107. King A, Loke YW. Human trophoblast and JEG choriocarcinoma cells are sensitive to lysis by IL-2-stimulated decidual NK cells. *Cell Immunol* 1990; 129:435

108. Clark DA, Vinci G, Flanders KC, *et al.* CD56+ lymphocytic cells in human first trimester decidua as a source of novel TGF beta 2 related immunosuppressive factors. *Hum Reprod* 1994;9:2270–7

109. Michel M, Underwood J, Clark DA, *et al.* Histologic and immunologic study of uterine biopsy tissue of incipiently aborting women. *Am J Obstet Gynecol* 1989; 161:409–14

110. DeWolf F, Carreras LO, Moermann P, *et al.* Decided vasculopathy and extensive placental infarction in a patient with repeated thromboembolic accidents, recurrent fetal loss, and a lupus anticoagulant. *Am J Obstet Gynecol* 1982;142:829

111. Yee KT, DeWolf F, Robertson WB, Bronson I. Inadequate maternal vascular response to placentation in pregnancies complicated by pre-eclampsia and small for gestational age infants. *Br J Obstet Gynaecol* 1986;93:1049

112. Yee KT. Pathology of intrauterine growth retardation. *Am J Reprod Immunol* 1989;21:132

113. Hill JA, Polgar K, Harlow BL, Anderson DJ. Evidence of embryo and trophoblast-toxic cellular immune response(s) in women with recurrent spontaneous abortion. *Am J Obstet Gynecol* 1992;166:1044–52

114. Chavez DJ, McIntyre JA. Sera from women with histories of repeated pregnancy losses cause abnormalities in mouse peri-implantation blastocyst. *J Reprod Immunol* 1984;6:273–81

115. Oksenberg JR, Brautbar C. *In vitro* suppression of murine blastocysts growth by sera from women with reproductive disorders. *Am J Reprod Immunol* 1986;11: 118–24.

116. Zigril M, Fein A, Carp H, Toder V. Immuno-potentiation reverses the embryotoxic effect of serum from women with pregnancy loss. *Fertil Steril* 1991;56:653–9

117. Eckler JL, Laufer MR, Hill JA. Measurement of embryotoxic factors is predictive of pregnancy outcome in women with a history of recurrent abortion. *Obstet Gynecol* 1993;81:84–7

118. Roussev RG, Stern JJ, Thorsell L, *et al.* Validation of an embryotoxicity assay. *Am J Reprod Immunol* 1994;32:1–5

119. Thomason EG, Roussev RG, Stern JJ, Coulam CB. Prevalence of embryotoxic factor in sera from women with unexplained recurrent abortion. *Am J Reprod Immunol* 1995;33:333

120. Kirk EP, Chuong CJ, Coulam CB, Williams TJ. Pregnancy after metroplasty for uterine anomalies. *Fertil Steril* 1993;59:1164–8

121. Simon C, Martinez L, Pardo F, *et al.* Mullerian defects in women with normal reproductive outcome. *Fertil Steril* 1991;56:1192–3

122. Clifford K, Rai R, Watson H, Regan L. An informative protocol for the investigation of recurrent miscarriage:

preliminary experience of 500 consecutive cases. *Hum Reprod* 1994;9:1328–32

123. Bennett MJ. Congenital abnormalities of the fundus. In Bennett MJ, Edmonds DK, eds. *Spontaneous and Recurrent Abortion*. Oxford: Blackwell Scientific Publications, 1987:109–29

124. Dewald GW, Michels VV. Recurrent miscarriages: cytogenetic causes and genetic counseling of affected families. *Clin Obstet Gynecol* 1986;29:865

125. Sbracia M, Grasso JA, Scarpillini F. A prospective controlled trial of aspirin versus placebo for treatment of women with recurrent spontaneous abortion associated with antiphospholipid antibodies. *Am J Reprod Immunol* 1994;31:242

126. Rote NS. Pregnancy associated immunologic disorders. *Curr Opin Immunol* 1989;1:1165–72

127. Out HJ, Kooijman CD, Bruinse HW, Derksen RHWM. Histopathological findings from patients with intrauterine fetal death and antiphospholipid antibodies. *Eur J Obstet Gynecol* 1991;41:179–86

128. Dekker GA, Sibai BM. Low-dose aspirin in the prevention of pre-eclampsia and fetal growth retardation: rationale, mechanisms, and clinical trials. *Am J Obstet Gynecol* 1993;168:214–17

129. Coulam CB. Immunotherapy for recurrent spontaneous abortion. *Early Preg Biol Med* 1995;1:13–26

130. Cowchock FS, Reece EA, Balaban D, *et al.* Repeated fetal losses associated with antiphospholipid antibodies: a colloborative randomized trial comparing prednisone with low-dose heparin treatment. *Am J Obstet Gynecol* 1992;155:1318–23

131. McIntyre JA, Taylor CG, Torry DS, *et al.* Heparin and pregnancy in women with a history of repeated miscarriages. *Hemostasis* 1993;23:202–11

132. Kwak JYH, Gilman-Sachs A, Beaman KD, Beer AE. Reproductive outcome in women with recurrent spontaneous abortions of alloimmune and autoimmune causes: preconception versus postconception treatment. *Am J Obstet Gynecol* 1992;166:1787–95

133. Babcock RB, Dumper CW, Scharfman WB. Heparin-induced immunothrombocytopenia. *Engl J Med* 1976; 295:237–41

134. Dahlman T, Sjoberg HE, Ringertz H. Bone mineral density during long-term prophylaxis with heparin in pregnancy. *Am J Obstet Gynecol* 1994;170:1315–20

135. Silber RK, MacGregar SN, Small JS, *et al.* Comparative trial of prednisone plus aspirin versus aspirin alone in the treatment of anticardiolipin-antibody positive obstetric patients. *Am J Obstet Gynecol* 1993; 169:1411–17

136. Ramsdon CF, Farquharson RG. A woman with twelve first trimester losses in whom lupus anticoagulant was detected and treated with steroids, sandoglobulin and heparin. *Clin Exp Rheumatol* 1990;8:221–2

137. Branch DW, Scott JR, Kochenaur NK, Hershgold E. Obstetric complications associated with lupus anticoagulant. *N Engl J Med* 1985;313:1322–6

138. Rubbert A, Pirner K, Wildt L, *et al.* Pregnancy course and complications in patients with systemic lupus erythematosus. *Am J Reprod Immunol* 1992;28: 205–7

139. Wapner RJ, Cowchock FS, Shapiro SS. Successful treatment in two women with antiphospholipid antibodies and refractory pregnancy losses with intravenous immunoglobulin infusions. *Am J Obstet Gynecol* 1989;161:1271–2

140. Christiansen OB, Mathiesen O, Lauristen JG, Grunnet N. Intravenous immunoglobulin treatment of women with multiple miscarriages. *Hum Reprod* 1992;7:718–22

141. Bernstein RM, Crawford RJ. Intravenous IgG therapy for anticardiolipin syndrome: a case report. *Clin Exp Rheumatol* 1988;6:198–9

142. Scott JR, Branch W, Kochenour NK, Ward K. Intravenous immunoglobulin treatment of pregnant patients with recurrent pregnancy loss caused by antiphospholipid antibodies and Rh immunization. *Am J Obstet Gynecol* 1988;159:1055–6

143. Kwak JYH, Quilty EA, Gilman-Sachs A, *et al.* Intravenous immunoglobulin G infusion therapy in women with recurrent spontaneous abortions of immune etiologies. *J Reprod Immunol* 1995;28:175–88

144. Mowbray JF, Liddel H, Underwood JL, *et al.* Controlled trial of treatment of recurrent spontaneous abortion by immunization with paternal cells. *Lancet* 1985;1:941–9

145. Gatenby PA, Cameron K, Simes RJ, *et al.* Treatment of recurrent spontaneous abortion by immunization with paternal lymphocytes: results of a controlled trial. *Am J Reprod Immunol* 1993;29:88–94

146. Mueller-Eckhardt G, Mohr-Pennert A, Heine O, *et al.* Controlled trial on intravenous immunoglobulin treatment for prevention of recurrent spontaneous bortion. *Br J Obstet Gynaecol* 1994;101:1072–7

147. Christiansen OB, Mathiesen O, Husth M, *et al.* Placebo-controlled trial for treatment of unexplained secondary recurrent abortions and recurrent late spontaneous abortions with i.v. immunoglobulin. *Hum Reprod* 1995;10:2690–4

148. Ho HN, Gill TJ, Hsieh HJ, *et al.* Immunotherapy for recurrent spontaneous abortion in a Chinese population. *Am J Reprod Immunol* 1991;25:10–15

149. Cauchi MN, Lim D, Young DE, *et al.* Treatment of recurrent aborters by immunization with paternal cells – controlled trial. *Am J Reprod Immunol* 1991; 25:16–17

150. Daya S, Gunby J (The Recurrent Miscarriage Immunotherapy Trialist Group). The effectiveness of allogeneic leukocyte immunization in unexplained primary recurrent spontaneous abortion. *Am J Reprod Immunol* 1994;32:294–302

151. Faulk WP, McIntyre JA. Trophoblast survival. *Transplantation* 1981;32:1–5

152. Stern PL, de Wit TFR. The role of MHC class expression in developmental tumors. *Sem Cancer Biol* 1991; 2:11–15

153. Parkam P. Review: antigen presentation by class I major histocompatability complex molecules: a context for thinking about HLA G. *Am J Reprod Immunol* 1995;34:10–15

154. Clark DA. Controversies in reproductive immunology. *Cit Rev Immunol* 1991;11:215–47

155. Heyborne K, Fu Y-X, Nelson A, *et al.* Recognition of trophoblasts by gamma-delta T cells. *J Immunol* 1994;153:2918–26

156. Szekeres-Bartho J, Autran B, Debre P, *et al.* Immuno-regulatory effects of suppressor factor from healthy pregnant women's lymphocytes after progesterone induction. *Cell Immunol* 1989;122:281–94

157. Szekeres-Bartho J, Szekeres G, Debre P, *et al.* Reactivity of lymphocytes to a progesterone receptor-specific monoclonal antibody. *Cell Immunol* 1990;125:273–83

158. Erard F, Garcia-Sanz JA, Le Gros G. Switch of CD8 T cells of noncytolytic CD8– CD4– cells that make TH2 cytokines and help B cells. *Science* 1993;260:1802–5

159. Moore SC, Soderberg LSF. Mouse bone marrow natural suppresser cells: induction and activity. *FASEB J* 1990;4:435–9

160. Szekeres-Bartho J, Reznikoff-Etievant MF, Varga P, *et al.* Lymphocytic progesterone receptors in normal and pathological human pregnancy. *J Reprod Immunol* 1989;16:239–47

161. Wegmann T, Waters CA, Drill DW, *et al.* Pregnant mice are not primed but can be primed to fetal alloantigens. *Proc Natl Acad Sci* USA 1979;76:2410–14

162. Head JR. Can trophoblasts be killed by cytotoxic cells? *In vitro* evidence and *in vivo* possibilities. *Am J Reprod Immunol* 1989;20:100–5

163. Kwak JYH, Biaman KD, Gilman-Sachs A, *et al.* Upregulated expression of CD56+, CD56+16+ and CD19+ cells in peripheral blood lymphocytes in women with recurrent pregnancy losses. *Am J Reprod Immunol* 1995;34:93–9

164. Aoki KI, Kajiura S, Matsumoto Y, *et al.* Preconceptual natural killer cell activity as a predictor of miscarriage. *Lancet* 1995;345:1340–2

165. Ruiz JE, Kwak JYH, Baum L, *et al.* Intravenous immunoglobulin inhibits natural killer cell activity *in vivo* in women with recurrent spontaneous abortion. *Am J Reprod Immunol* 1996;35:370–5

166. Kempf C, Jentsch P, Poirier B, *et al.* Virus inactivation during production of intravenous immunoglobulin. *Transfusion* 1991;31:423–7

167. Soto B, Garcia-Bengrechea M, Reistra S, *et al.* Heterosexual transmission of hepatitis C virus and the possible role of coexistent human immunodeficiency virus infection in the index case. A multicenter study of 423 pairings. *J Intern Med* 1994;236:515–19

168. Coulam CB, Stephenson M, Stern JJ, Clark DA. Immunotherapy for recurrent pregnancy loss: analysis of results from clinical trials. *Am J Reprod Immunol* 1996;35:352–9

169. Christiansen OB, Mathiesen O, Lauristen JG, Grunnet N. Intravenous immunoglobulin treatment of women with multiple miscarriages. *Hum Reprod* 1992;7:718–22

170. Aoki K, Higuchi K, Yagami Y. Suppression of natural killer cell activity by monocytes following immuno-therapy for habitual aborters. *Am J Reprod Immunol* 1995;33:465

Section II

Obstetrical emergencies

11
Amniotic fluid embolism

H.N. Winn and R.H. Petrie

Amniotic fluid embolism is a life-threatening complication characterized by a sudden onset of respiratory distress, cyanosis, cardiovascular collapse and coma. Although the entry of amniotic fluid into the maternal circulation was first reported in the Brazilian literature in 1926[1] and in the English-language literature in relation to studies on the etiology of pre-eclampsia[2], the status of amniotic fluid embolism as a clinical entity was not accepted until 1941, when Steiner and Lushbaugh reported clinical and experimental findings in the *Journal of the American Medical Association*[3]. These investigators described the clinical and pathological course of eight women who suddenly expired during labor or in the immediate postpartum interval following major disturbances in cardiorespiratory function; autopsies revealed amniotic particulate matter in the lungs. It was not until 1947–50 that cases involving a significant bleeding, either immediate or delayed, were reported[4,5]. Subsequently, a number of papers were published that clearly demonstrated that a consumptive coagulopathy may accompany this disorder[6–9].

MATERNAL AND PERINATAL MORBIDITY AND MORTALITY

The medical literature offers a wide range of incidences for amniotic fluid embolism, but the best data probably came out of England and Wales, where the incidence is about 1 in 80 0000 deliveries[10]. In the USA, the incidences range from 1 in 3700 deliveries to 1 in 45 000 deliveries[11,12]. Although pre-eclampsia, hemorrhage and infection still head the list of primary causes of maternal mortality, the number of deaths from these has been decreasing. As a result, other potentially life-threatening conditions such as amniotic fluid embolism are now being given greater attention. It is estimated that between 10% and 15% of all maternal deaths in the USA are due to amniotic fluid embolism[13]. These figures include not only patients at term but also patients in early pregnancy. In 1979, Morgan[8] reviewed 272 cases of amniotic fluid embolism that had been reported in the English-language literature; he could find only 39 survivors with a mortality rate of 86%. Death occurred between 10 min and 32 h after the embolus; one-quarter of the fatalities occurred within 1 h of the initial symptom. In the same year, Wasser and co-workers[14] found only 25 instances in which a patient had survived a probable amniotic fluid embolism. Since that time, there appears to have been an increase in the number of reports of probable or proven cases of amniotic fluid embolism in which the patients survived[15–18]. A maternal mortality of 61% was more recently reported[9]. Interestingly, surviving patients may have subsequent uncomplicated gestations[8,19].

In the setting of amniotic fluid embolism, the overall rate of neonatal survival is 79%. However, the overall rate of neonatal survival with intact neurological status is only 39%. Although the neonatal mortality increases with the duration of time from the onset of cardiac arrest to delivery, neonatal survival is possible even if delivery is delayed for as long as 35 min from the onset of cardiac arrest[9].

ETIOLOGY

Earlier, many investigators believed that the mother had to be in labor for amniotic fluid embolism to occur. They reasoned that some contractile stress during labor could bring about a rent or tear between the amniotic fluid compartment and the maternal venous system, allowing the egress of amniotic fluid from the fetal compartment into the vascular aspect of the maternal compartment. It was thought that such conditions only exist in active labor or in the immediate postpartum period. A number of papers have subsequently demonstrated that amniotic fluid embolism may occur spontaneously under circumstances other than labor, such as during the second trimester[18], termination of pregnancy[20–22], amniocentesis[23], abruption due to cord entanglement[24] and/or saline amnioinfusion[25].

For a number of years it was felt that the diagnosis of amniotic fluid embolism, without such demonstrable particulate matter as lanugo hair, vernix, mucin, fetal squamous cells, or meconium in the maternal circulation, was highly suspect[26]. Many authorities would discount cases reported without these findings. Although many of the investigators believed that some amniotic fluid probably reached the maternal circulation with each delivery, a number of them were unable to demonstrate this using reasonably sophisticated investigative efforts[27,28].

With the emergence of such subspecialty areas within obstetrics and gynecology as maternal–fetal medicine, a growing number of obstetricians have developed skills in critical care medicine. This includes the use of Swan–Ganz catheters for hemodynamic observations and measurements, important to the management of patients with obstetric catastrophes such as amniotic fluid embolism. Accordingly, a number of investigators have sampled maternal pulmonary artery blood from these catheters in patients with amniotic fluid embolism and demonstrated the presence of such debris as fetal mucin, squamous cells, fat cells, meconium and lanugo hair – all particulate matter of amniotic fluid[8,15,16,29]. However, squamous and trophoblastic cells are also found in the pulmonary artery in patients undergoing invasive hemodynamic monitoring for medical conditions without amniotic fluid embolism[30–32]. One potential error would be the contamination of maternal skin squamous cells during the insertion of the Swan–Ganz catheters. It appears that varying amounts of amniotic fluid may escape from the fetal compartment far more frequently than was believed.

CLINICAL PRESENTATION

Amniotic fluid typically presents with a sudden onset of dyspnea, cyanosis, seizures, cardiovascular collapse, respiratory arrest and coma[8,9]. Cardiac dysrhythmia includes electromechanical dissociation, bradycardia, ventricular tachycardia or fibrillation and asystole[9]. Probably as a result of cerebral hypoxia[8,9], 10–48% of patients manifest tonic–clonic seizures. Fetal distress manifested by fetal bradycardia or prolonged fetal heart rate decelerations often develops within minutes of maternal symptoms[8,9,33].

In an excellent clinical review of the subject, Morgan evaluated 272 cases of amniotic fluid embolism demographically[8]. In more than half the patients, respiratory distress and cyanosis were the initial presenting symptoms. In approximately one-quarter, the first sign was hypotension out of proportion to the amount of blood loss. Although labor was associated with amniotic fluid embolism in 90% of cases, tumultuous labor or usage of intravenous oxytocin was present in less than 30% of the cases.

In 1982, Barrows[33] reported a case in which the first sign involved the fetus. The mother showed no symptoms of impending difficulty, but there was long deceleration of the fetal heart rate. However, during the Cesarean section performed for fetal distress, the mother began to exhibit signs pointing to amniotic fluid embolism.

Almost all patients with amniotic fluid embolism develop coagulopathy[8,9]. Morgan found that 12% of the patients had a bleeding tendency from the start as one of their primary problems. After the first hour, almost all survivors demonstrated laboratory evidence of a consumptive coagulopathy; approximately half of these also demonstrated significant bleeding. The bleeding may have come from various sites in the skin that had been broken or from the reproductive tract itself[8].

Pulmonary edema or adult respiratory distress syndrome developed in approximately 24% to 93% of patients[8,9]. This may have occurred as a result of fluid overload from vigorous attempts at resuscitation or left heart failure. Survivors did not have long-term pulmonary problems[8].

The symptoms that occur with amniotic fluid embolism are common to a number of other catastrophic as well as less severe disorders[34]. The diagnosis of amniotic fluid embolism should be considered in any patient presenting with a sudden onset of cardiovascular collapse, respiratory distress, or severe coagulopathy. Documentation of squamous cells or other components of amniotic fluid in the maternal pulmonary artery circulation is neither required nor pathognomonic for the diagnosis of amniotic fluid embolism. Differential diagnoses include eclampsia, severe abruptio placentae, a ruptured uterus, aspiration pneumonia, septic shock and myocardial infarction.

PATHOGENESIS

Although a large amount of autopsy and experimental animal data have been collected, the exact pathogenesis of amniotic fluid embolism is still open to debate. At autopsy, the pathologist is usually able to find a site of entry of the amniotic fluid into the maternal circulation[3]. The major sites of entry include the endocervical vein, traumatic uterine lacerations or the placental site itself. What happens after the entry of the fluid remains unknown; animal studies have not provided the answers. If unfiltered amniotic fluid is injected into the maternal vascular compartment of a sheep, for example, a disorder very similar to that seen in the human will be produced. Filtered amniotic fluid does not have this effect[35]. Furthermore, injection of a large amount of autologous amniotic fluid appears to be innocuous in monkeys[36,37]. Overall, the results differ depending on the species of animal involved – dog, monkey, or cat – and the exact variables being examined[36,38]. The animal data appear to add more confusion than clarity to the issue.

It is tempting to suggest that amniotic fluid particulate matter produces the obstruction of the pulmonary circulation. However, Macmillan[39] showed that there were approximately 560 cells/ml of human amniotic fluid; extrapolating from animal data, he estimated that it would take about 7 l of amniotic fluid to block pulmonary vessels sufficiently to cause death, if this were the basic pathophysiological mechanism.

A number of investigators have implicated the metabolites of arachidonic acid, particularly prostaglandin

(PG)F$_{2\alpha}$ and leukotriene, in the pathogenesis of amniotic fluid embolism[40–43]. PGF$_{2\alpha}$ can cause pulmonary hypertension. Leukotriene inhibitor can modify the hemodynamic responses to infusion of amniotic fluid in rats[43]. Again, different animals respond differently to different prostaglandins, and the prostaglandin content of their amniotic fluid varies at different stages of labor. At present, the roles of arachidonic acid metabolites in the etiology of this syndrome are uncertain.

The mechanism for the bleeding disorder that is common with amniotic fluid embolism is likewise not clearly understood. The amniotic fluid contains factors IIa, VIIa and Xa which can evoke intravascular clotting[44,45]. However, the very low concentrations of these coagulant factors may be insufficient to cause major clotting disorders in the human[45,46]. A marked activation of the fibrinolytic system in amniotic fluid embolism could contribute to the bleeding problem[47]. In addition, the substantial tissue factor-specific procoagulant activity of the amniotic fluid may play a major role in the development of coagulopathy in amniotic fluid embolism[45].

Hemodynamic data from patients with amniotic fluid embolism have been evaluated. In humans, the hemodynamic evidence suggests that the primary problem is left heart failure without pulmonary hypertension[48–51]. Pulmonary edema from left heart failure causes maternal hypoxia, which leads to cyanosis, tachypnea, restlessness, mental function alterations, convulsions and/or coma. The traditional concept of pulmonary hypertension and cor pulmonale is based mainly on animal model data[48,51].

It appears that the causes of amniotic fluid embolism may be cumulative and divergent in origin – or perhaps we have overlooked the major problem altogether. Steiner and Lushbaugh[3] believed that the effects of amniotic fluid embolism could be due to an anaphylactic shock-like syndrome secondary to the fetal elements found in the lung. Other authors have supported this consideration. Meigs[52], for example, described intense phagocytic activity that he thought was directed at the granular material in the meconium in a fatal case of amniotic fluid embolism. He felt that an anaphylactoid reaction might also be the cause of the blood clotting problem. Clark and colleagues[9] suggested that the term 'amniotic fluid embolism' be replaced by 'anaphylactoid syndrome of pregnancy' to emphasize the anaphylactic nature of this condition.

MANAGEMENT

Although more that 40 years have elapsed since amniotic fluid embolism was first described, the management of the disorder remains supportive. Correction of hypoxia and coagulopathy and maintenance of the cardiovascular system are essential. The following management protocol for the acute management of amniotic fluid embolism is suggested:

(1) Initiate advanced cardiopulmonary life support as indicated;

(2) Intubate the patient and ventilate the patient with a high concentration of oxygen (90–100%), and positive end-expiratory pressure to maintain pO$_2$ at > 60 mmHg. The setting of the ventilator is further guided with arterial blood gases and or pulse oximetry;

(3) Establish intravenous access with a large-bore needle to allow transfusion of fluid, blood products and medications;

(4) Insert a Swan–Ganz catheter for central hemodynamic monitoring as soon as possible to guide further fluid administration and response to medications;

(5) Maintain systolic blood pressure above 90 mmHg by rapid infusion of saline solution to provide adequate preload; administer pressor agents such as dobutamine, and inotropic agents such as digoxin;

(6) Correct coagulopathy with infusion of fresh frozen plasma and platelets. The amount, frequency and type of blood products depend on the laboratory data and clinical responses;

(7) Monitor fetal heart rate if fetal viability is reached. Perimortem Cesarean section should be considered;

(8) Consultation with a medical intensivist or other appropriate medical subspecialist is recommended.

Many steps are usually carried out simultaneously. Cardiopulmonary bypass and pulmonary artery thrombolectomy has been attempted in the treatment of amniotic fluid embolism resulting in patient survival[53].

SUMMARY

Entry of amniotic fluid into the maternal circulation may trigger a maternal anaphylactic reaction causing respiratory distress, cardiovascular collapse, convulsions and death in the majority of affected women. There are no known steps for prevention, no warning signs or symptoms and no known therapeutic modalities other than supportive therapy.

It is interesting to consider that the recent increase in the number of reports of patients who have survived amniotic fluid embolism may be due to a higher index of suspicion for the disorder, immediate institution of hemodynamic monitoring and effective management of respiratory and cardiovascular collapse and coagulopathy. Hopefully, once the underlying mechanism of this condition is understood, specific therapy can be aimed at the causative insult. Meanwhile, it can be expected that this sudden catastrophic disorder will continue to be highly lethal, with less than 15% of affected patients surviving with intact neurological status.

REFERENCES

1. Meyer JR. Embolia pulmonaramniocaseosa. *Brazil Med* 1926;2:301–3
2. Warden MR. Amniotic fluid as a possible factor in the etiology of eclampsia. *Am J Obstet Gynecol* 1927;14: 292–300
3. Steiner PE, Lushbaugh CC. Maternal pulmonary embolism by amniotic fluid as a cause of obstetric shock and unexpected deaths in obstetrics. *J Am Med Assoc* 1941;117:1245,1340
4. Hemmings CT. Maternal pulmonary embolism by contents of the amniotic fluid. *Am J Obstet Gynecol* 1947; 53:303–6
5. Weiner AE, Reid DE. The pathogenesis of amniotic fluid embolism. III. Coagulant activity of amniotic fluid. *N Engl J Med* 1950;243:597–8
6. Reid DE, Weiner AE, Roby CC. Intravascular clotting and afibrinogenemia. The presumptive lethal factors in the syndrome of amniotic fluid embolism. *Am J Obstet Gynecol* 1953;66:465–74
7. Ratnoff OD, Vosburgh GJ. Observations on the clotting defect in amniotic fluid embolism. *N Engl J Med* 1952; 247:970–3
8. Morgan M. Amniotic fluid embolism. *Anaesthesia* 1979;34:20–32
9. Clark SL, Hankins GDV, Dudley DA, *et al*. Amniotic fluid embolism: analysis of the national registry. *Am J Obstet Gynecol* 1995;172:1158–69
10. Lewis TLT. *Progress in Clinical Obstetrics and Gynaecology*, 2nd edn. London: Churchill, 1964:48
11. McLeod AGW. Fatal amniotic fluid embolism in Dade County: an unusual incidence. *Am J Obstet Gynecol* 1972; 113:1103–7
12. Martin RW. Amniotic fluid embolism. *Clin Obstet Gynecol* 1996;39:101–6
13. Duff P, Engelsgjerd B, Zingery LW, *et al*. Hemodynamic observations in a patient with intrapartum amniotic fluid embolism. *Am J Obstet Gynecol* 1983;146:112–5
14. Wasser WG, Tessier S, Kamath CP, *et al*. Nonfatal amniotic fluid embolism: a case report of postpartum respiratory distress with histopathologic studies. *Mt Sinai J Med (NY)* 1979;46:388–91
15. Resnik R, Swartz WH, Plumer MH, *et al*. Amniotic fluid embolism with survival. *Obstet Gynecol* 1976;47: 295–8
16. Masson RG, Ruggieri J, Siddigui MM. Amniotic fluid embolism: definitive diagnosis in a survivor. *Am Rev Respir Dis* 1979;120:187–92
17. Dolyniuk M, Orfei E, Vania H, *et al*. Rapid diagnosis of amniotic fluid embolism. *Obstet Gynecol* 1983;61: 28S–30S
18. Meier PR, Bowes WA Jr. Amniotic fluid embolus-like syndrome presenting in the second trimester of pregnancy. *Obstet Gynecol* 1983;61:31S–34S
19. Clark SL. Successful pregnancy outcomes after amniotic fluid embolism. *Am J Obstet Gynecol* 1992;167:511–12
20. Guidotti RJ, Grimes DA, Cates W Jr. Amniotic-fluid embolism and abortion. *Lancet* 1979;2:911–12
21. Cates W Jr, Boyd C, Halvorson-Boyd G, *et al*. Death from amniotic fluid embolism and disseminated intravascular coagulation after a curettage abortion. *Am J Obstet Gynecol* 1981;141:346–8
22. Guidotti RJ, Grimes DA, Cates W Jr. Fatal amniotic fluid embolism during legally induced abortion, United States, 1972 to 1978. *Am J Obstet Gynecol* 1981;141: 257–61
23. Hassart TH, Essed GG. Amniotic fluid embolism after transabdominal amniocentesis. *Eur J Obstet Gynecol Reprod Biol* 1983;16:25–30
24. Corridan M, Kendall ED, Begg JD. Cord entanglement causing premature placental separation and amniotic fluid embolism. Case report. *Br J Obstet Gynaecol* 1980; 87:935–40
25. Maher JE, Wenstrom KD, Hauth JC, Meis PJ. Amniotic fluid embolism after saline amnioinfusion: two cases and review of the literature. *Obstet Gynecol* 1994;83:851–4
26. Garland IWC, Thompson WD. Diagnosis of amniotic fluid embolism using an antiserum to human keratin. *J Clin Pathol* 1983;36:625–7
27. Roche WD, Norris HJ. Detection and significance of maternal pulmonary amniotic fluid embolism. *Obstet Gynecol* 1974;43:729–31
28. Sparr RA, Pritchard JA. Studies to detect the escape of amniotic fluid into the maternal circulation during parturition. *Surg Gynecol Obstet* 1958;107:560
29. Duff P, Engelsgjerd B, Zingery LW, *et al*. Hemodynamic observations in a patient with intrapartum amniotic fluid embolism. *Am J Obstet Gynecol* 1983;146:112–5
30. Plauche WC. Amniotic fluid embolism. *Am J Obstet Gynecol* 1983;147:982–3
31. Clark SL, Pavlova A, Horenstein J, *et al*. Squamous cells in the maternal pulmonary circulation. *Am J Obstet Gynecol* 1986;154:104–6
32. Lee W, Ginsburg KA, Cotton DB, *et al*. Squamous cells in the maternal pulmonary circulation. *Am J Obstet Gynecol* 1986;155:999–1001
33. Barrows JJ. A documented case of amniotic fluid embolism presenting as acute fetal distress. *Am J Obstet Gynecol* 1982;143:599–600
34. Peterson EP, Taylor HB. Amniotic fluid embolism. *Obstet Gynecol* 1970;35:787–93
35. Halmagyi DFJ, Starzecki B, Shearman RP. Experimental amniotic fluid embolism: mechanism and treatment. *Am J Obstet Gynecol* 1962;84:251–6
36. Adamsons K, Mueller-Heubach E, Myer RE. The innocuousness of amniotic fluid infusion in the pregnant rhesus monkey. *Am J Obstet Gynecol* 1971;109: 977–84
37. Stolte K, van Kessel H, Seelen J, *et al*. Failure to produce the syndrome of amniotic fluid embolism by infusion of amniotic fluid and meconium into monkeys. *Am J Obstet Gynecol* 1967;98:694–7
38. Attwood HD, Downing SE. Experimental amniotic fluid and meconium embolism. *Surg Gynecol Obstet* 1965;120:255–62
39. MacMillan D. Experimental amniotic fluid infusion. *J Obstet Gynaecol Br Commonw* 1968;75:849–52
40. Kitzmiller JL, Lucas WE. Studies on a model of amniotic fluid embolism. *Abstr. Obstet Gynecol* 1972;39:626–7
41. Reeves JT, Daoud FS, Estridge M, *et al*. Pulmonary pressor effects of small amounts of bovine amniotic fluid. *Respir Physiol* 1974;20:231–7
42. Clark SL. Arachidonic acid metabolites and the pathophysiology of amniotic fluid embolism. *Semin Reprod Endocrinol* 1985;3:253

43. Azegami M, Mori N. Amniotic fluid embolism and leukotrienes. *Am J Obstet Gynecol* 1986;155:1119–24

44. Courtney LD, Allington LM. Effect of amniotic fluid on blood coagulation. *Br J Haematol* 1972;22:353–5

45. Lockwood CJ, Bach R, Guha A, *et al*. Amniotic fluid contains tissue factor, a potent initiator of coagulation. *Am J Obstet Gynecol* 1991;165:1335–41

46. Phillips LL, Davidson EC Jr. Procoagulant properties of amniotic fluid. *Am J Obstet Gynecol* 1972;113:911–19

47. Beller FK, Douglas GW, Debrovner CH, *et al*. The fibrinolytic system in the amniotic fluid embolism. *Am J Obstet Gynecol* 1963;87:48–55

48. Clark SL, Montz FJ, Phelan JP. Hemodynamic alterations associated with fluid embolism: a reappraisal. *Am J Obstet Gynecol* 1985;151:617–21

49. Girard P, Mal H, Laine JF, *et al*. Left heart failure in amniotic fluid embolism. *Anesthesiology* 1986;64:262–5

50. Vanmaele L, Noppen M, Vincken W, *et al*. Transient left heart failure in amniotic fluid embolism. *Intensive Care Med* 1990;16:269–71

51. Clark SL, Cotton DB, Gonik B, *et al*. Central hemodynamic alterations in amniotic fluid embolism. *Am J Obstet Gynecol* 1988;158;1124–6

52. Meigs LC. Amniotic fluid embolism. Pulmonary histopathologic findings in a rapidly fatal occurrence of amniotic fluid embolism. *Am J Obstet Gynecol* 1971;111:1069–74

53. Esposito RA, Grossi EA, Coppa G, *et al*. Successful treatment of postpartum shock caused by amniotic fluid embolism with cardiopulmonary bypass and pulmonary artery thromboembolectomy. *Am J Obstet Gynecol* 1990;163:572–4

12

Coagulopathies in obstetrics

H.N. Winn and R. Romero

CHANGES IN THE HEMOSTATIC SYSTEM DURING PREGNANCY

During pregnancy, blood vessels become more prominent, probably owing to the combination of increased blood volume and vasodilatation normally observed during gestation. A specialized regional circulation (the placental vascular bed) develops to ensure an adequate supply of maternal blood to the conceptus.

The platelet count tends to decrease with advancing gestational age. This has been attributed to hemodilution and placental trapping. Nevertheless, the platelet count during pregnancy remains within the limits of the normal adult range (150 000 to 350 000/μl). The lifespan of platelets during pregnancy is similar to that in non-pregnant women[1–4].

As pregnancy progresses, there is activation of the coagulation components of the hemostatic system, as evidenced by the increased concentrations of fibrinopeptide A[5] and high-molecular-weight fibrinogen complexes[6]. This hypercoagulable state seems to be related to the participation of the hemostatic system in the modelling of the placental bed and spiral arteries in response to maternal preparation for the eventual separation of the placenta.

Fibrin is deposited in the placental bed as pregnancy progresses and it can be found in the floor of the placenta (Nitabuch's layer), lining the intervillous space and on the surface of the villi[7]. The spiral arteries undergo important morphological changes during pregnancy, including the replacement of the elastic lamina and the smooth muscle of the vascular wall by a matrix containing fibrin. Physiological consequences of these changes include[8]:

(1) Non-responsive vessels known as uteroplacental arteries, which are able to accommodate the increased blood flow to the conceptus as pregnancy progresses. Removal of the elastic lamina also reduces the variation in pressure in the blood flowing to the placenta.

(2) Fibrin replacement of the tunica media also facilitates the severance of the terminal part of the spiral arteries at the time of separation of the placenta and their occlusion by the action of myometrial contractions.

McKay[7] has proposed that normal pregnancy is a state of chronic intravascular coagulation localized to the placental bed. This state would result in a compensatory increase in the synthesis of coagulation factors and a decrease in the platelet count.

The activity of all coagulation factors, except factors XI and XIII, is increased[9–17]. The decreased level in factor XIII is, however, consistent with the increased deposition of fibrin at the end of pregnancy, since recent evidence suggests that the concentration of factor XIII decreases during the acute phase of thromboembolism.

The activity of coagulation inhibitors has been the subject of contradictory reports, but it does not seem to be substantially altered with pregnancy. The traditional concept has been that fibrinolysis is depressed during pregnancy[8,18,19]. Evidence to support this view includes the detection during gestation of the following[20–24]:

(1) Falling levels of plasminogen activator;

(2) Decreased fibrinolytic activity of plasma;

(3) Decreased fibrinolytic capacity in response to venous occlusion;

(4) The presence of an inhibitor of urokinase-induced fibrinolysis;

(5) Increased concentration of plasmin inhibitors, such as macroglobulin and antiplasmin, with no change in inhibitors of plasminogen activator.

Several investigators, using studies of fibrinogen catabolism, have challenged this concept of fibrinolysis depression during pregnancy[25]. They have proposed that there is an appropriate fibrinolytic response, but that the levels of plasminogen activator are depressed because of its sequestration in sites of fibrin deposition.

Indications for hemostatic testing in the obstetric patient

Screening tests are indicated whenever there is a significant risk of hemostatic failure. The most frequent reasons for testing in the obstetric patient are:

(1) To evaluate the relative contributions of the different components of the hemostatic system causing excessive spontaneous or surgical hemorrhage.

(2) To look for subclinical activation of the hemostatic system in patients with obstetric complications that may be associated with disseminated intravascular coagulation (e.g. pre-eclampsia, fetal death, abruptio placentae). Detection of significant activation of the hemostatic system could change clinical management in these conditions.

(3) Laboratory monitoring of the progress of hemostatic therapy in cases of coagulation failure or of anticoagulation in patients with thromboembolic disease.

(4) Antepartum or preoperative hemostatic testing of the patient with a history suggestive of a bleeding diathesis or a medical disorder associated with hemostatic problems.

Abnormalities in any of the four components of the hemostatic system may cause an increased bleeding tendency. Screening tests should include evaluation of vascular integrity, platelet number and function, the different pathways of the coagulation cascade, and fibrinolytic activity. Specific tests of hemostatic competence include:

(1) Tests of vascular integrity;
(2) Platelet count;
(3) Bleeding time;
(4) Prothrombin time,
(5) Partial thromboplastin time;
(6) Fibrinogen concentration;
(7) Fibrinogen degradation products.

BLOOD REPLACEMENT THERAPY IN COAGULATION FAILURE

The most common indications for transfusion therapy in the obstetric patient are hypovolemia, anemia and the need to replace hemostatic components. The optimal use of blood component therapy for hemostatic replacement requires familiarity with the composition of the different available preparations. The causes of transfusion-associated deaths include the following: acute hemolysis from ABO incompatibility (51%), acute pulmonary injury (15%), bacterial contamination of blood products (10%), delayed hemolysis (10%), damaged blood products (3%) and graft-versus-host disease (0.4%)[26].

Whole stored blood

When a unit of blood is drawn, it can be kept as whole blood or separated into its individual components. In general, deterioration of the hemostatic function of whole blood begins 6 h after collection and this, along with volume considerations, limits the usefulness of stored whole blood for replacement of hemostatic components.

Whole stored blood, or the combination of red blood cells and crystalloid solution, is appropriate therapy for replacement of volume and oxygen-carrying capacity in the acutely hemorrhaging obstetric patient without a coagulopathy. However, when the amount transfused within a 24-h period exceeds the patient's circulating blood volume, a bleeding disorder, in part caused by the loss and dilution of platelets and plasma coagulation factors, can occur[27,28]. Because of this possibility, some authors have suggested that, during massive transfusions, one-third of the blood administered should be fresh. A more practical alternative is the administration of fresh-frozen plasma and/or platelet concentrates.

Fresh whole blood

The term 'fresh blood' is generally used to designate blood that has been collected less than 24 h prior to administration. This preparation has an acceptably minimal loss of hemostatic factors, it is less expensive than blood component therapy, and its use is not associated with the problems of microaggregates of platelets, white blood cells and fibrin formed during the storage of whole blood. The major disadvantages of using fresh blood are the risk of hepatitis, since there may be insufficient time to complete hepatitis screening, and the risk of circulatory overload if fresh blood is administered to replace coagulation factors in a patient who is not actively bleeding. At present, the use of fresh whole blood is being actively discouraged by blood-bank services in the USA. Insufficient time for hepatitis screening, limited availability of donors and more efficient utilization of blood components are the reasons for this policy. The use of fresh blood will probably be limited to those parts of the world where transfusion services are not appropriately developed.

Fresh-frozen plasma

Fresh-frozen plasma is obtained by separation and freezing of the plasma derived during the preparation of red blood cells and platelet concentrates from a unit of whole blood. The plasma must be frozen within 8 h of donation and can be stored at temperatures lower than − 18 °C, preferably at − 30 °C or lower, for a period of 12 months. The product is available in 200–250-ml bags[29].

Fresh-frozen plasma is devoid of platelets, but contains all the other coagulation factors, including factors V and VIII and naturally occurring inhibitors. Its concentration of clotting factors is similar to that found in an equivalent volume of circulating plasma in a normal person (1 ml of fresh-frozen plasma = 1 unit of factor activity)[29]. It carries the same risk of hepatitis as a unit of whole blood. The product should be administered to ABO-compatible recipients.

Fresh-frozen plasma is a good source of coagulation components and is frequently used to administer these factors, along with volume, to the obstetric patient with hemorrhage and disseminated intravascular coagulation. Since none of the factors are concentrated, large volumes of fresh-frozen plasma are usually needed to achieve hemostatic levels of depleted coagulation components. The risk of circulatory overload is, therefore, the most important limiting factor in the use of fresh-frozen plasma for hemostatic replacement. For this reason, most congenital deficiencies of factors are best treated with concentrates of specific factors[29].

Fresh-frozen plasma is indicated for coagulopathy resulting from congenital or acquired deficiency of coagulation factors as documented by:

(1) A prothombin time greater than 1.5 times the mid-point of the normal range, usually > 18 s;

(2) An activated partial thromboplastin time greater than 1.5 times the top of the normal range, usually > 55 s; or

(3) An activity of a specific coagulation factor of < 25% of normal.

Fresh-frozen plasma can be used to stop active bleeding or to prevent excessive bleeding from an operative or invasive procedure. Fresh-frozen plasma should not be used as a volume expander because of its risks and the availability of safer alternatives. Indications for the use of fresh-frozen plasma include[29]:

(1) Massive blood transfusion of more than one blood volume (about 5 l in a 70-kg adult) with evidence of coagulopathy;

(2) Deficiencies of antithrombin III or isolated coagulation factors, such as factors VIII, IX and X, when no safe concentrate is available;

(3) Deficiency of heparin cofactor II, protein C or protein S;

(4) Reversal of warfarin (Coumadin) effect when it is unsafe to wait for the time required for correction by administration of parenteral vitamin K;

(5) Disseminated intravascular coagulation from liver disease, prolonged intrauterine fetal demise and severe pre-eclampsia.

The starting dose is one or two bags of fresh-frozen plasma and further transfusion should be determined by prothrombin time or activated partial thromboplastin time obtained at the end of the transfusion. A transfusion of five or six units of platelets provides the patient with an equivalent of one bag of fresh-frozen plasma. Thus, the dosage should be adjusted accordingly. Since factor VII has a much shorter half-life (5–6 h), activated partial thromboplastin time is a better indicator of the efficacy of the treatment than prothrombin time if the latter is not determined within 1–2 h after transfusion[29].

Cryoprecipitate

Cryoprecipitate is the term used to designate the white gelatinous precipitate produced by the thawing of fresh-frozen plasma at 1–6 °C. A unit of cryoprecipitate has a volume of 15–25 ml and is an excellent source of fibrinogen, von Willebrand factor, factor VIII:C and factor XIII[29–31].

Once prepared, cryoprecipitate can be stored at − 18 °C for up to 1 year. When it is needed for transfusion, cryoprecipitate is thawed at 37 °C. Several units of cryoprecipitate are generally pooled into one bag for ease of administration. Once pooled, cryoprecipitate must be used or discarded within 6 h because of the danger of bacterial contamination. It is preferable to administer this preparation to ABO-compatible recipients[32].

The main indication for administering cryoprecipitate in the obstetric patient is the need to replace fibrinogen. Currently, cryoprecipitate is the only fibrinogen concentrate approved by the Food and Drug Administration. Each unit contains about 250 mg of fibrinogen, so that significant amounts of this protein can be delivered in a relatively small volume. Ten units of cryoprecipitate generally increase the circulating fibrinogen in an average-sized person by 50 mg/dl[30]. A fibrinogen level of l00 mg/dl or higher is considered adequate for hemostasis. Other uses of cryoprecipitate are for replacement of factors VIII and XIII and in the management of bleeding in von Willebrand's disease. A factor VIII concentrate preparation (Humate-P, Armour, Kankakee, IL) is preferable to cryoprecipitate for the treatment of von Willebrand's disease, because the preparation of the former involves inactivation of contaminating viruses[33]. The risk of hepatitis with one unit of cryoprecipitate is the same as with one unit of whole blood[29].

Platelets

Platelets can be administered in fresh whole blood, platelet-rich plasma and platelet concentrate. The use of fresh blood and platelet-rich plasma as a source of platelets should be discouraged, because a large volume is generally necessary to achieve a platelet hemostatic level and circulatory overload is likely to occur before such a level is reached[34].

Platelet-rich plasma is obtained by low-speed centrifugation of one unit of fresh whole blood. Platelets remain in the plasma phase, whereas red blood cells and white blood cells precipitate because of their higher specific gravity. One unit of platelet concentrate is obtained from one unit of platelet-rich plasma by centrifugation at a higher speed to precipitate the platelets. Each unit is suspended in 30–50 ml of donor plasma, and its platelet content is dependent upon the donor's platelet count and the blood volume from which the platelets were extracted. Platelet concentrates are stored at room temperature (22 °C) for a maximum of 2–5 days, depending on the type of bag used. Storage for longer periods of time or at 4 °C results in a shorter platelet lifespan[35–37]. In the case of autologous transfusion, cryopreservation of platelets may be necessary to extend the storage period.

The response to platelet-concentrate transfusions is expressed in terms of the increment in platelet count per square meter (m^2) of body area. This method permits evaluation of the effectiveness of platelet transfusions independently of blood volume and allows comparisons between individuals. One unit of transfused platelets generally raises the platelet count by 5000–10 000/μl per m^2 of body surface[38]. Fever, infection, alloimmunization and drug-induced platelet antibodies can shorten the lifespan of transfused platelets. Platelets are contaminated with red blood cells, and rhesus sensitization can occur after the administration of platelets from rhesus-positive donors to rhesus-negative recipients. Rhesus-negative platelet concentrates should be used for rhesus-negative obstetric patients. If this is not possible, rhesus immunoglobulin or RhoGAM (300 μg) should be administered to prevent the development of isoimmunization when platelets from a rhesus-positive donor are given to a rhesus-negative recipient. Although platelets have ABO antigens, they can be transfused to ABO-incompatible recipients[39] if ABO-compatible platelets are not available. Episodes of mild hemolysis can occur if large amounts of group O platelet concentrates (with anti-A and anti-B plasma) are administered to group A or B recipients. Both shortened and normal lifespans of non-allogenic platelets with respect to the ABO group have been reported, but this does not seem to be a significant clinical problem[40].

Indications for the use of platelet transfusions include prophylaxis against, and treatment of, excessive bleeding caused by thrombocytopenia and platelet dysfunction. The combined use of platelet counts and bleeding times permits assessment of the contribution of platelet abnormalities to hemostatic failure. Platelet concentrate therapy is indicated in the following circumstances:

(1) Prophylaxis of bleeding in surgical patients with a platelet count below 50 000/μl. The risk of bleeding from trauma and surgical procedures is extremely high at platelet counts of less than 5000/μl, high at counts of between 5000/μl and 10 000/μl and variable at counts of between 10 000/μl and 50 000/μl. Bleeding from thrombocytopenia is exceedingly rare with a platelet count of > 50 000/μl[41,42].

(2) Prophylaxis of spontaneous bleeding in patients with platelet counts below 10 000/μl. The risk of spontaneous hemorrhage is increased with a platelet count of between 5000/μl and 10 000/μl, and the risk is very high at a platelet count of less than 5000/μl[41,42]. Prophylactic transfusion of platelets whenever the platelet count is less than 20 000/μl may not be advisable, considering the potential complications of transfusion[43].

(3) Prophylaxis and treatment of excessive bleeding in patients with known platelet dysfunction[29].

(4) Therapy of excessive bleeding in the patient who has been subjected to massive transfusion therapy and has developed severe dilutional thrombocytopenia. Between six and ten units of platelet concentrate are usually administered at any one time. The optimal dose naturally depends on the cause of the thrombocytopenia, the initial platelet count, the level that needs to be reached, the presence of known platelet dysfunction and alloimmunization or other factors that increase platelet dysfunction. The common starting dose is one unit of platelet concentrate per 10 kg of body weight. A platelet count should be obtained 1 h after the transfusion to determine its effectiveness[29].

Platelet concentrates are more effective in treating patients with impaired platelet production than in those with increased destruction. A notable example of the latter is the patient with immune thrombocytopenic purpura, in whom transfused platelets may be destroyed within hours or minutes.

Occasionally, patients receiving frequent transfusions of platelet concentrates may become refractory to random donor platelets. This refractoriness to platelet transfusion may be related to fever, infection, splenomegaly or medications[29]. The most common underlying mechanism for this phenomenon is the development of alloantibodies to platelet-associated human leukocyte antigens. Under these circumstances, human leukocyte antigen-compatible concentrates can be used if platelet transfusions are necessary[44]. A rare complication associated with the administration of platelets is infection. The etiologic agents are similar to those involved in administration of other blood products and include human immunodeficiency virus, hepatitis C virus, cytomegalovirus, hepatitis B virus and bacterial infections.

Plasma fractions (fibrinogen and factor IX complexes)

Plasma obtained from whole blood or plasmapheresis can be used as fresh-frozen plasma, or pooled and fractionated into different components such as fibrinogen, antihemophilic factor (AHF or factor VIII), factor IX complex, gamma globulin or albumin. Pooling of several units of plasma is performed to allow efficient large-scale preparation of the plasma fractions. However, the act of mixing plasma from many donors increases the risk of hepatitis virus. Heat treatment can inactivate the hepatitis virus. This procedure is used in the preparation of albumin and gamma globulin, rendering these products virtually free of risk of hepatitis. Coagulation fractions, however, cannot be heated and, therefore, these pooled preparations are associated with a significant risk of hepatitis transmission. For this reason, fibrinogen concentrates are no longer a licensed product in the USA. Cryoprecipitate is the preparation of choice for efficient fibrinogen replacement[29].

Factor IX complex (Proplex or Konyne) is a stable, dried, purified plasma that contains factors II, VII, IX and X. It is available in vials whose contents are reconstituted with sterile water. The concentration of factors II, VII, IX and X is roughly equivalent to 500 ml of fresh-frozen plasma. Factor IX complex is prepared from large pools of plasma and therefore carries a substantial risk of hepatitis. It is preferable to administer fresh-frozen plasma to replace the factors contained in the factor IX complex and reserve this complex for those cases in which time and volume considerations prevent therapy with vitamin K and/or fresh-frozen plasma. The administration of factor IX complex has been associated with the production of venous thrombosis or disseminated intravascular coagulation in the recipient. These side-effects are possibly attributable to the presence of procoagulant activity in most factor IX preparations[45–48].

The other plasma fraction with hemostatic value is factor VIII concentrate. This preparation is rarely used in the obstetric patient, except in the occasional instance of a specific factor deficiency or a circulating inhibitor.

Autologous blood donation

Autologous transfusion involves collection and reinfusion of the patient's own blood components to reduce or eliminate the transfusion-related reactions or infections. This is accomplished in patients who are very likely to require transfusion of blood products during or after the procedure. Three options for autologous transfusions are preoperative blood donation, perioperative blood salvage and acute normovolemic hemodilution. In pregnant patients, autologous transfusion usually involves preoperative donation of blood when there is a significant risk for peripartum hemorrhage such as placenta previa and placenta accreta. Autologous donation of half a unit (approximately 250 ml) or one unit (approximately 500 ml) of blood at an interval of at least 1 week can be safely done during the third trimester, without increased perinatal morbidity or mortality. It is recommended that the pre-donation hemoglobin be at least 11.0 g/dl and that

the last donation is completed before the anticipated date of delivery to allow the red-cell mass to recover[49]. The overall rate of autologous transfusion after donation ranges from 7.7–11%, with the highest incidence of 83% in patients having placenta previa[49,50]. The Food and Drug Administration recommends that all blood, homologous or autologous, be tested for the presence of hepatitis B virus (HBV), hepatitis C virus (HCV), human immunodeficiency virus (HIV), cytomegalovirus (CMV), and syphilis. Most blood centers also test for antibody to human T-cell lymphotropic virus type I, alanine aminotransferase and antibody to hepatitis B core antigen[51]. Vasovagal reactions, such as light-headedness, occur as a result of transient hypotension and bradycardia in about 2–5% of patients[49,51]. External fetal heart-rate monitoring may be used to monitor the fetal condition when autologous donation is carried out after fetal viability is reached. Fetal heart-rate decelerations may occur if maternal hypotension develops.

DISSEMINATED INTRAVASCULAR COAGULATION

Disseminated intravascular coagulation is a pathological state caused by excessive thrombin activity. It is kinetically and pathologically characterized by increased thrombin generation, increased turnover of platelets and coagulation factors, formation of thrombi in the microcirculation and secondary activation of the fibrinolytic system. These events are manifested clinically by varying degrees of bleeding and ischemic tissue damage.

Disseminated intravascular coagulation is not a specific disease, but rather a sequence of pathological events that can be associated with many different conditions.

Familiarity with the pathophysiology, diagnosis and management of disseminated intravascular coagulation is important, since this condition is the most frequent cause of acquired coagulopathy in the obstetric patient. Inappropriate handling of this pathological process can lead to serious and potentially fatal complications.

Management
General principles

(1) Disseminated intravascular coagulation is always secondary to a disease that causes excessive thrombin generation. The most effective treatment is to eliminate the cause of activation of the hemostatic system. This implies therapy of the primary disease and, in obstetrics, frequently indicates the need for delivery.

(2) The association of disseminated intravascular coagulation with any obstetric entity (e.g. abruptio placentae, chorioamnionitis) transforms a local disorder into a systemic disease and introduces the risk of multiple organ failure. Therefore, the presence of disseminated intravascular coagulation magnifies the severity of the underlying disease.

(3) As a mode of delivery, the vaginal route is preferable to Cesarean section or hysterotomy in a patient with a decompensated coagulopathy. The vaginal approach places less stress on the hemostatic mechanism than an abdominal operation, in which there is a significant risk of bleeding from the uterine and abdominal wall incisions. It would be ideal if an episiotomy or any other obstetric operative intervention could be safely avoided during the course of a vaginal delivery.

(4) The administration of conduction anesthesia (caudal, epidural or spinal) is contraindicated in a patient with hemostatic failure, because of the increased risk of formation of an epidural hematoma and subsequent neurologic damage.

(5) Replacement therapy of the depleted hemostatic components is indicated only in the presence of bleeding or to correct subnormal levels of hemostatic factors prior to surgical intervention or a vaginal delivery. If the fibrinogen level is above 100 mg/dl and the platelet count is more than 50 000/μl, replacement therapy is not generally required.

(6) The rationale for the use of heparin in disseminated intravascular coagulation is to decrease the excessive thrombin generation and activity. This would arrest coagulation factor consumption and fibrin deposition and reduce the risk of consumptive coagulopathy and ischemic damage. Although the most effective treatment for disseminated intravascular coagulation is the elimination of the cause of activation of the hemostatic system, this cannot always be immediately accomplished, particularly when the cause is infection or neoplasia. Heparin has been used with some success under these circumstances to prevent the deleterious consequences of disseminated intravascular coagulation. Heparin therapy, however, is rarely indicated in the obstetric patient, because most episodes are self-limited and because detachment of the placenta at delivery or during abruption creates significant vascular disruption and heparin magnifies the potential for life-threatening hemorrhage. Its use should be limited to those cases in which there is an intact intravascular bed and delivery is not anticipated during the period of anticoagulation. Heparin has a high molecular weight and does not cross the placenta; therefore, it is an ideal anticoagulant for obstetric use[8,52].

Abruptio placentae

Abruptio placentae is the most frequent cause of acute decompensated disseminated intravascular coagulation in the obstetric patient. The incidence of abruptio placentae varies from 0.2 to 2.4% of all pregnancies[53], and disseminated intravascular coagulation with fibrinogen concentrations of less than 100 mg/dl complicates one-third to one-quarter of the cases[54]. The etiology of abruptio placentae is usually unknown. Risk factors include a history of severe abruptio placentae in a previous pregnancy, high parity, hypertensive disease of the mother, cigarette smoking, cocaine use, and external trauma. The role of other proposed causes, such as polyhydramnios, a short umbilical cord, uterine anomalies and folate deficiencies, remains obscure and is not likely to be significant[55,56].

The initial event is likely to be an ischemic lesion of the decidual, leading to decidual necrosis, vascular disruption and bleeding. As hemorrhage occurs, laceration and dissection along a decidual plane and placental separation take place. The latter produces more vascular rhexis, arterial hemorrhage, retroplacental accumulation of blood and further placental separation[57].

Following delivery, control of uterine bleeding is dependent on myometrial contraction, which constricts the severed vessels at the placental implantation site. This mechanism cannot operate efficiently in abruptio placentae because the uterine cavity remains distended by the presence of the fetus. Since the maternal venous sinuses are opened, thromboplastic material can be infused into the maternal circulation. Bleeding stops following delivery of the fetus and placenta or, less frequently, by self-limitation of the precipitating event.

The clinical manifestations of abruptio placentae depend upon the site of placental implantation, the type and degree of separation, the amount of blood loss and the presence of disseminated intravascular coagulation. It has been suggested that abruption of posteriorly implanted placentas tends to be less symptomatic than that occurring with anterior placentas[58]. The site of separation also has clinical importance, as it may determine the intensity of blood loss. Central detachments involve disruption of the spiral arteries and the resulting high-pressure arterial bleeding causes an expanding retroplacental hemorrhage. On the other hand, marginal separations produce bleeding from veins at the edge of the placental disk or from the intervillous space. In either case, the bleeding is not of arterial origin and is therefore less serious than that seen with central separations[59]. Not all central detachments lead to total separation of the placenta and fetal death. If a hematoma can form before the separation and hemorrhage become extensive, the process may stop and only be detected at the time of delivery as an organized thrombus in an area of infarcted placenta.

It must be remembered that the amount of vaginal bleeding is not a reliable indicator of the degree of placental separation. Significant amounts of blood can be concealed within the uterus until delivery. When fetal death occurs, blood loss commonly amounts to 2500 ml and may exceed 5000 ml. Therefore, anemia and hypovolemic shock can be present with little evidence of major vaginal bleeding.

Maternal complications include anemia, hypovolemic shock, acquired consumptive coagulopathy, renal failure, postpartum hemorrhage and the sequelae of ischemic damage to distant organs.

The occurrence of disseminated intravascular coagulation seems to be related to the degree of placental separation and retroplacental bleeding. The greater the separation, the higher the likelihood of significant bleeding and acquired coagulopathy[8].

The fetal mortality rate in abruptio placentae has been reported to be over 50% and a significant number of perinatal deaths occur prior to hospital admission[53]. The fetal complications in this disorder are related to hypoxemia and occasionally to anemia. Hypoxemia results from maternal hypovolemia, anemia and reduction of the available placental interface for fetal–maternal exchange. When fetal anemia occurs, it is probably caused by bleeding from lacerated villi[53,60].

Three main theories have been proposed to explain the fibrinogen depletion and the hemorrhagic diathesis associated with abruptio placentae[21,54,61]:

(1) Release of tissue thromboplastin into the maternal circulation, with the production of disseminated intravascular coagulation[62–68];

(2) Intrauterine consumption of fibrinogen and other coagulation factors during the formation of the retroplacental clot;

(3) Primary fibrinolysis, with digestion of the circulating fibrinogen[69].

The first theory seems to provide the most plausible explanation for the occurrence of a coagulopathy in abruptio placentae. The placenta and decidua are rich in thromboplastic material and disseminated intravascular coagulation has been experimentally induced by injecting placental extracts into animals[64–66]. It has been postulated that thromboplastic material is introduced through the maternal venous sinuses and that activation of the extrinsic mechanism of blood coagulation results in disseminated intravascular coagulation.

It must be stressed that the bleeding diathesis associated with abruptio placentae is due not only to fibrinogen consumption, but also to the depletion of other coagulation factors, such as factors V and VIII, and to the anticoagulant effects of fibrin degradation products[70]. The incidence of postpartum hemorrhage has been better correlated with a high level of circulating fibrin degradation products than with fibrinogen concentration. This underlines the importance of fibrinolysis in the production of clinical manifestations of bleeding in disseminated intravascular coagulation[61,71–73].

The clinical course and laboratory findings of the coagulopathy of abruptio placentae are those of decompensated acute disseminated intravascular coagulation. Fibrinogen and factors V and VIII levels are low, whereas fibrinogen degradation products are elevated. Platelets are either low or normal, and frequently the degree of thrombocytopenia is less than that expected from the hypofibrinogenemia. It has been suggested that a very active fibrinolytic system lyses the clots and avoids excessive traumatic destruction of platelets and red blood cells[54].

A patient with a placental abruption should be cared for in the labor and delivery unit. Women with extensive placental separations usually present with abdominal pain and vaginal bleeding. The uterus is often tetanically contracted and fetal heart tones may be absent. Initial evaluation includes recording of vital signs, assessment of vaginal bleeding, electronic fetal heart-rate monitoring and drawing blood for baseline studies (hematocrit, platelet count, fibrinogen, prothrombin time, partial thromboplastin time, fibrinogen split products and clot observation test). A secure intravenous route for the administration of blood and fluid should be set up by using a 16- or 18-gauge cannula. Since fluid can be administered more rapidly under pressure than by gravity alone, it is preferable to use plastic fluid bags rather than glass bottles. Fluid bags can be compressed by a pressor infusion set to increase the rate of infusion. The infusion should be initiated with a crystalloid solution such as Ringer's lactate. A Foley catheter should be inserted to follow urinary output; 30 ml/h is indicative of adequate renal perfusion.

Tests that can be performed in the labor-floor laboratory include hematocrit, a clot observation test and a peripheral smear for platelet enumeration. The clot observation test is carried out by collecting 5 ml of maternal venous blood in a glass tube and inverting it four or five times. An abnormality should be suspected if a clot fails to form in 6 min. If the clot forms in less then 6 min, the concentration of fibrinogen is likely to be more than 150 mg/dl. If a clot is not formed in 30 min, the fibrinogen concentration is likely to be less than 100 mg/dl. This test is simple and may be performed in every patient suspected of having an abruptio placentae[53]. Rapid clot formation essentially makes the possibility of severe hypofibrinogenemia unlikely and, under these circumstances, surgical intervention can be undertaken for fetal indications. If a clot has not formed in 30 min, however, a serious disruption of the hemostasis mechanism is likely to exist. In institutions where blood components are immediately available upon request, surgery for fetal distress may be started and replacement therapy begun during the procedure. If a delay in obtaining blood products is anticipated, however, it is best to delay surgery until they are available because of the possibility of maternal exsanguination during the operation. A Wright's stain of a peripheral smear can be used to quickly screen for a platelet deficiency. If less than four platelets per high-power field are seen, thrombocytopenia should be strongly suspected.

The management of individual cases of severe abruptio placentae depends on gestational age, fetal status, severity of the abruption, feasibility of vaginal delivery, and the presence of shock and disseminated intravascular coagulation. If the fetus is dead, every effort should be made to accomplish vaginal delivery, because this imposes less severe demands on the hemostatic system than hysterotomy or Cesarean section. If fetal distress is present in a viable infant, delivery should be accomplished in the most expeditious way. If fetal distress is not present and vaginal delivery is anticipated within 6–8 h, vaginal delivery may be attempted, provided means of fetal assessment and access to anesthesia, blood and operating room are continuously available. If these conditions are not present, Cesarean section is likely to improve perinatal salvage, because fetal distress may suddenly occur[74].

Induction of labor should begin with amniotomy if it is feasible. The loss of amniotic fluid decreases intrauterine volume and allows more effective hemostasis at the placental site. Oxytocin administration by intravenous infusion should be started immediately following the amniotomy.

If there are signs of circulatory collapse in association with disseminated intravascular coagulation, rapid volume replacement is necessary in order to prevent acute renal failure. Replacement with Ringer's lactate solution is initiated pending availability of blood. When fetal death has occurred, a deficit of at least 1–2 l of blood can be estimated. A central venous pressure line may be placed to assess the effectiveness of intravascular volume replacement. The average central venous pressure in the third trimester is about 10 cmH$_2$O, which can be used as a guide to follow the progress of fluid replacement.

Packed red cells are indicated if anemia is present. The goal is to maintain the hematocrit at around 30%. Each unit of packed red blood cells can be expected to increase the hemoglobin by 1–1.5 g/dl and the hematocrit by 3%. Fresh-frozen plasma can be used to replace the hemostatic components consumed in disseminated intravascular coagulation, such as fibrinogen, factor V, factor VIII and antithrombin III. Cryoprecipitate is the most volume-efficient form of fibrinogen replacement. Its use is indicated when fibrinogen concentrations are below 100 mg/dl. Each unit of cryoprecipitate contains approximately 250 mg of fibrinogen and raises the fibrinogen concentration by approximately 5 mg/dl.

If the fibrinogen level is above 100 mg/dl, volume replacement therapy can be given as whole blood, packed red cells and fresh-frozen plasma, or packed red cells and crystalloid solutions. The best combination is packed red cells and fresh frozen plasma, because it provides more labile coagulation factors than whole blood and avoids crystalloid-induced dilution of circulating coagulation factors.

Since fibrinolysis in abruptio placentae is a protective mechanism against intravascular coagulation, interfering with its natural course by the use of fibrinolytic inhibitors is potentially dangerous. When uterine inertia is refractory to amniotomy and oxytocin, it may be associated with hyperfibrinolysis and resolved with the administration of the fibrinolytic inhibitor Trasylol. Although the explanation for these observations remains speculative, their confirmation could create an indication for fibrinolytic inhibitors in abruptio placentae complicated by refractory uterine inertia[75].

Occasionally, severe bleeding from the placental site occurs several hours after delivery. Active local fibrinolysis may be responsible for this phenomenon. If a surgical cause for the hemorrhage is excluded and bleeding cannot be controlled by manual or pharmacological stimulation of the myometrium, amniocaproic acid or other inhibitors of fibrinolysis might be used. This should rarely be necessary, however, and consultation with a hematologist is advised prior to starting a patient on these agents.

Prolonged retention of a dead fetus

The association between prolonged retention of a dead fetus and hemostatic failure has been recognized for many years. The coagulopathy seems to be caused by the slow release of tissue thromboplastin from the fetoplacental unit into the maternal circulation. The resultant activation of the extrinsic pathway of blood coagulation leads to excessive generation of thrombin and disseminated intravascular coagulation. This pathologic process is initially low-grade, but the progressively increased and sustained generation of thrombin may eventually transform an early-compensated disseminated intravascular coagulation into a decompensated state[76–80].

The frequency of disseminated intravascular coagulation associated with fetal demise is related to the length of time the fetus has been retained in the uterine cavity and to the laboratory criteria employed to diagnose disseminated intravascular coagulation. Jimenez and Pritchard[78] studied over 100 patients who had retained a dead fetus for more than 1 week and found that none demonstrated a fibrinogen concentration below 150 mg/dl less than 5 weeks after the detection of fetal death. When more than 5 weeks had elapsed, one-third of the patients had fibrinogen concentrations below 150 mg/dl. The factors responsible for the development of hypofibrinogenemia in some patients and not in others are not known.

Active management of the patient with a fetal death has made prolonged retention of a dead fetus a rare cause of coagulopathy in modern obstetrics. The availability of ultrasonography and effective means to induce premature labor has virtually eliminated the delay in uterine evacuation caused by diagnostic uncertainty or fear of induction failure. All patients with a fetal death should be screened with coagulation studies prior to pregnancy termination, because clinical manifestations of disseminated intravascular coagulation are often minimal and the first sign of hemostasis failure may be a dangerously severe postpartum hemorrhage[78,81].

The initial changes in the coagulation profile of a patient with a retained dead fetus are an elevation in the circulating levels of fibrinogen degradation products and a fall in the concentration of fibrinogen. These changes precede the development of abnormalities in the partial thromboplastin time and prothrombin time. The fall in platelet count is less marked than that in fibrinogen levels.

The management of a patient with disseminated intravascular coagulation caused by a retained dead fetus depends on the state of hemostatic compensation and whether or not the patient is in labor. If the disseminated intravascular coagulation is either compensated or overcompensated (elevated fibrinogen degradation products, normal or elevated fibrinogen and platelets), the risk of hemostatic failure is small. The management goal in this setting is to accomplish delivery of the dead infant in order to eliminate the source of thromboplastic material and suppress the excessive generation of thrombin. The duration of pregnancy and the cervical status determine whether intravenous oxytocin, prostaglandin preparations, or misoprostol suppository should be used for induction of labor.

If the patient has decompensated disseminated intravascular coagulation (low fibrinogen or platelets), the management objective should be to decrease the risk of peripartum hemorrhage by restoring hemostatic levels of the consumed coagulation components prior to delivery. This can be accomplished by the administration of heparin if the patient is not in labor or by supplying the consumed factor with blood component therapy if labor is in progress.

When the patient is in labor, potential areas of vascular disruption and injury are likely to develop (e.g. placental implantation site, episiotomy or lacerations). Under these circumstances, the administration of heparin is contraindicated because it may increase the bleeding tendency by reducing the ability to form clots in areas of vascular injury. Management should be directed toward replacing the deficient hemostatic components. Fibrinogen is the most frequently depleted coagulation factor in this setting. Platelet counts and levels of factors V and VIII are frequently within a safe hemostatic range (platelets > 50 000/µl; factor V = 10–20%; and factor VIII = 25–30%). Fibrinogen replacement is best accomplished by administration of cryoprecipitate. Approximately ten units of this product are necessary to increase the circulatory level of plasma fibrinogen by 50 mg/dl. Cryoprecipitate is preferred to fresh-frozen plasma, because the correction of hypofibrinogenemia with the latter product requires the administration of large volumes of colloids, placing the patient at risk for circulatory overload.

If the patient is not in labor, the administration of heparin can arrest the consumption of coagulation factors, permit restoration of hemostatic competence, and obviate the need for blood replacement therapy. Heparin is best administered by continuous intravenous infusion. This reduces the risk of bleeding that may accompany intermittent bolus administration. A recommended program for heparin therapy is to give an initial bolus of 5000 units, then start an infusion at a rate of 1000 units/h. Modification of the maintenance rate may be necessary to avoid bleeding complications and achieve therapeutic goals.

Heparin therapy is monitored with serial fibrinogen levels, platelet counts and partial thromboplastin times. The objective of the therapy is to increase the concentrations of fibrinogen, coagulation factors and circulating platelets above safe hemostatic levels. A reasonable goal is to achieve a fibrinogen concentration between 150 and 300 mg/dl and a platelet count above 50 000/µl. The activated partial thromboplastin time is performed to assess the risk of excessive anticoagulation and should not be prolonged for more than 2.5 times the patient's control value.

Patients should be cautioned to avoid trauma and to report any episode of bleeding during heparin administration. Treatment goals can usually be accomplished in 24–48 h, after which time heparin therapy can be stopped. Induction of labor may begin 5 h after discontinuation of therapy, since the anticoagulant activity of heparin is virtually non-existent 4 h after the infusion has been stopped.

Another indication for heparin therapy is the management of a multiple gestation complicated by decompensated disseminated intravascular coagulation secondary to the death of one fetus during labor[82]. Heparin therapy should be administered in order to achieve safe levels of hemostatic factors. The anticoagulant should then be stopped and labor induced. If the gestation is preterm, however, significant prolongation of the pregnancy can be achieved by anticoagulation of the mother[83]. This can be accomplished initially with intravenous administration of heparin, until the fibrinogen concentration has reverted to acceptable levels, and then by subcutaneous therapy. The dose of subcutaneous heparin used for maintenance therapy is

5000 units every 6 h. Modification of the treatment plan depends on changes in plasma fibrinogen concentration. Platelet counts should be monitored during heparin therapy, because thrombocytopenia can be a side-effect of heparin administration. Heparin therapy should be discontinued prior to elective induction when the living twin has been shown to have achieved pulmonary maturity. Total discontinuation of heparin therapy many weeks prior to delivery without a recurrence of the coagulopathy is possible.

Pregnancy-induced hypertension

Pregnancy-induced hypertension, also known as toxemia of pregnancy, is a common cause of chronic disseminated intravascular coagulation in the pregnant patient. The mechanism of activation of the hemostatic system in pregnancy-induced hypertension is unknown. Several authors have proposed that such an activation occurs prior to the clinical onset of hypertension and is an integral part of the pathophysiology of the disease[84–88]. Evidence for excessive thrombin activity is provided by the increased concentrations of fibrinopeptide A and soluble fibrin complexes in pre-eclamptic patients as compared with normal pregnant women[89–91]. The kinetic consequences of excessive thrombin generation, namely thrombocytopenia, decreased fibrinogen concentrations and a decreased factor VIII activity/VIII antigen ratio, have been well documented in the course of the disease[92,93]. Thrombi in the microcirculation of the liver[94], kidney[95] and placental bed of patients with pregnancy-induced hypertension have been identified and may account for the multi-organ manifestations of the disease.

Elevated levels of fibrinogen degradation products are consistent with secondary activation of the fibrinolytic system. The presence of thrombotic lesions in the microcirculation in pregnancy-induced hypertension, however, may be due to a relative impairment of fibrinolytic activity. Activation of the hemostatic system is important in this disease, because a correlation has been demonstrated between the severity of hypertension and proteinuria and the degree of coagulation abnormality[93].

The most frequent manifestations of disseminated intravascular coagulation in pregnancy-induced hypertension are thrombocytopenia and elevated circulatory levels of fibrin degradation products. Platelet counts of less than 150 000/μl have been reported in as many as 15% of patients with pre-eclampsia and 30% of those with eclampsia[96]. This thrombocytopenia is caused by intravascular consumption of platelets. In pre-eclamptic women with thrombocytopenia, fibrinogen levels are usually normal or may even be elevated. This may be due to a greater degree of compensation afforded by the liver as compared with the bone marrow. Alternatively, it is possible that platelets participate in

the process of initiation of disseminated intravascular coagulation in pregnancy-induced hypertension and, therefore, are consumed to a greater degree than fibrinogen and other coagulation factors[97].

The typical hemostatic profile of a patient with chronic disseminated intravascular coagulation associated with pregnancy-induced hypertension includes thrombocytopenia, normal prothrombin time, normal partial thromboplastin time, normal thrombin time, normal, low or high fibrinogen levels, elevated fibrinogen degradation products and microangiopathic hemolytic changes of the red blood cells. Decreased activities of factors XII, XI, IX and VIII as a result of the activation of the intrinsic pathway have been observed in severe pregnancy-induced hypertension. Bone marrow aspiration typically demonstrates a normal or elevated number of megakaryocytes. Serum levels of lactate dehydrogenase can be elevated, reflecting its release from mechanical destruction of red blood cells. Patients with these laboratory findings frequently present with epigastric pain and elevation of the serum aminotransferases levels. On occasion, the triad of abdominal pain, thrombocytopenia and liver dysfunction may precede the development of hypertension[84,85].

The process of chronic disseminated intravascular coagulation invariably resolves after delivery of the infant. Antepartum resolution of thrombocytopenia and correction of the liver dysfunction have been observed to occur spontaneously or after the administration of corticosteroids[98] and antiplatelet agents such as aspirin and dipyridamole[99]. Spontaneous antepartum resolution of the thrombocytopenia does not mean that the process of disseminated intravascular coagulation has resolved. Frequently, elevated levels of fibrinogen degradation products can still be demonstrated, despite a normal platelet count. This evidence of fibrinolysis is generally accepted to indicate a state of chronic compensated disseminated intravascular coagulation. The consequences of ongoing compensated disseminated intravascular coagulation have not been established, but worsening of the hypertension and delivery of growth-restricted infants have been observed in patients managed conservatively after resolution of their thrombocytopenia.

Although the thrombocytopenia associated with acute pregnancy-induced hypertension can be severe, antepartum bleeding is rare. Frequently, the nadir platelet count is reached during the first postpartum day, with spontaneous resolution occurring 72 h after delivery in most cases[100].

Patients with pregnancy-induced hypertension and thrombocytopenia should be considered to have severe pre-eclampsia, regardless of the degree of systemic hypertension. These women are at risk of multiple organ ischemic involvement and their fetuses are at risk of intrauterine growth restriction. The mechanism responsible for intrauterine growth restriction has been postulated to be suboptimal placental perfusion and poor fetal–maternal exchange because of platelets and fibrin deposits in the uteroplacental microcirculation.

Delivery of the infant is the treatment of choice for patients with pregnancy-induced hypertension and disseminated intravascular coagulation. Platelet transfusions are not indicated unless the platelet count is less than 20 000/µl, there is active bleeding or the patient is being prepared for surgery. A reasonable goal is to raise the platelet count to 50 000/µl prior to any surgical intervention. Fibrinogen replacement with cryoprecipitate is rarely necessary, because serum fibrinogen levels generally exceed 100 mg/dl.

The role of heparin and antiplatelet agents in the treatment of disseminated intravascular coagulation associated with pre-eclampsia has not been definitely established. Their use in patients with severe hypertension is contraindicated because of the risk of cerebral hemorrhage. On the other hand, they may prove to be useful in prolonging an early gestation in patients with mild hypertension but significant activation of the hemostatic system.

PRESENCE OF CLOTTING INHIBITORS: CIRCULATING ANTICOAGULANTS

Circulating anticoagulants are endogenous blood components that inhibit the action of clotting factors. They may be directed against a specific coagulation factor or may interfere with a phase of blood coagulation.

Specific inhibitors

Specific inhibitors can occur in patients with congenital coagulation defects or in individuals with previously normal hemostasis. Most specific inhibitors are thought to be antibodies. Their appearance has been suggested to be the result of an immunological response of the host to a transfused factor (e.g. factor VIII in hemophilia A), although spontaneous inhibitors have also been reported. Among specific inhibitors, the most frequent one is that directed against factor VIII. The inhibitor generally irreversibly inactivates factor VIII by means of a time- and temperature-dependent reaction[101-103]. The clinical manifestations of this condition are similar to those of hemophilia A, except for a lower frequency of hemarthroses and a higher prevalence of ecchymosis, muscle bleeding, hematuria and menorrhagia[104-110]. The inhibitor may appear at any time during pregnancy, but its most frequent occurrence is in the puerperal period. The hemorrhagic diathesis associated with this circulating anticoagulant may be severe and difficult to treat. The diagnosis is usually made by the presence of a prolonged partial thromboplastin time that is not corrected by the addition of normal plasma;

prothrombin time and thrombin time are typically normal. On occasion, demonstration of the inhibitor may require incubation of the mixture of plasmas for 1 h at 37 °C. It is possible to quantitate the activity of the inhibitor, and standardized inhibitor units (Bethesda or Oxford) have been described.

Therapeutic modalities employed in the management of patients with acquired inhibitors to factor VIII include replacement of factor VIII alone (human, porcine or bovine) or in combination with plasmapheresis, exchange transfusions, corticosteroids, antimetabolites, alkylating agents, and/or Autoplex, and anti-inhibitor coagulation complex[109,111]. A promising therapy is a combination of immunosuppression with either azathioprine or cyclophosphamide and methylprednisolone. This therapy causes disappearance of the factor VIII inhibitors, normalization of the coagulation tests and reversal of bleeding tendency within 6 weeks of treatment. During pregnancy, the therapy may include only corticosteroids initially and add immunosuppression if remission does not occur[112]. Another promising therapy involves the suppression of autoantibody production by immunoglobulin G (IgG) intravenous infusion. The recommended course of treatment includes daily infusions of IgG at a dose of 0.5 g/kg body weight for 8 days. Hemostasis with a prolonged concomitant rising serum level of factor VIII and a falling autoantibody titer has been observed[113]. This mode of therapy should be considered when either immunosuppression or corticosteroid fails to control the recurrent bleeding caused by factor VIII inhibitors. Although the traditional approach to the management of the acute crisis has been administration of factor VIII, encouraging results have been reported recently with Autoplex. This preparation contains activated clotting factors and its postulated mechanism of action is to bypass the site of action of factor VIII in the coagulation cascade. The recommended dose is 76 U/kg over 15–20 min. Therapy can be followed by observing the clinical response and by serial partial thromboplastin times. This preparation is very expensive and should not be used without a precise diagnosis. Patients with an acute hemorrhagic diathesis due to a coagulation inhibitor represent serious management problems. They should be treated in conjunction with an expert hematologist and the blood-bank service.

The prognosis for patients with factor VIII inhibitor is good, provided they survive the acute stage of the disease. Most anticoagulants disappear in months or years after detection. A meta-analysis of 51 published cases of postpartum factor VIII inhibitors revealed a 2-year survival rate of 97% and complete remission rate of 100% at 30 months[114]. Complete remission was defined as absence of factor VIII inhibitors and normalization of factor VIII activity. Immunosuppressive therapy with cyclophosphamide, azathioprine or

6-mercaptopurine shortened the interval from onset of the disease to complete recovery[114]. Although most infants born to mothers with circulating anticoagulants have been clinically normal, factor VIII inhibitor can cross the placenta and cause severe intracranial hemorrhage[115]. In a recent review of the hemostatic performance in successive pregnancies of 12 patients with a factor VIII inhibitor, nine were found to have uneventful pregnancies and to be in remission at the time of the subsequent delivery. These subjects included two patients with inhibitors present at the onset of their second pregnancies, but whose antifactor VIII titers continued to decrease and finally disappeared before the second delivery. Bleeding manifestations persisted in three patients in their subsequent pregnancies and in one of them the disease became worse[109,116].

It must be stressed that pregnancy or surgery in a patient with a high titer of a factor VIII inhibitor is a potentially life-threatening condition. It seems wise to follow patients who are known to have this problem with serial inhibitor titers and to advise them to wait until they are in remission before conceiving. If the disease is detected during pregnancy, or if patients become pregnant before remission is achieved, they should be advised as to their risk and followed with serial inhibitor titers. Consideration should be given to the use of steroids in the event of high or rising inhibitor titers.

LUPUS-TYPE INHIBITORS

A lupus-type inhibitor was originally described in patients with systemic lupus erythematosus, but has now been observed in association with other conditions and in patients without any demonstrable disease. The presence of this inhibitor may be the first manifestation of systemic lupus erythematosus[117,118].

The inhibitor is an immunoglobulin of the IgG or IgM type. Its mechanism of action has not been completely established, but most evidence suggests that it interferes with the reaction in which factor Xa, factor V and phospholipid form a complex (prothrombinase) that transforms prothrombin into thrombin. It has been proposed that this inhibitor occupies the binding site of the phospholipid molecule, which is generally available for the coagulation factor[119].

Bleeding is uncommon, despite the significant abnormalities in *in vitro* coagulation. Thrombosis, on the other hand, seems to be a more significant problem in these patients. To explain this paradox, it has been proposed that bleeding does not occur because after saturation of the inhibitor molecule with phospholipid, enough phospholipid is still available to react with the coagulation factors and accomplish effective hemostasis. The mechanism of thrombosis associated with lupus anticoagulant remains unclear, but several hypotheses have been proposed. The anticoagulant, in its antiphospholipid capacity, may damage both platelets and vascular endothelial cells, resulting in increased thromboxane release and reduced prostacyclin production, respectively[118]. These effects predispose to thrombosis. The presence of the circulating anticoagulant is generally discovered by the detection of a prolonged activated partial thromboplastin time that is not corrected by the addition of normal plasma, or an abnormal kaolin clotting time curve. The kaolin clotting time seems to have a higher sensitivity than the activated partial thromboplastin time. Both tests are not specific for the lupus anticoagulant because they can be abnormal in the presence of other anticoagulants. The presence of the lupus anticoagulant can be confirmed by the platelet neutralization procedure, in which the prolonged activated partial thromboplastin time is corrected by the addition of excess platelet phospholipid. The prothrombin time and thrombin time are frequently prolonged. The reasons for the prolongation of the latter are unclear. Thrombocytopenia is occasionally present. Excessive platelet destruction caused by a relative deficiency of prostacyclin or by platelet antibodies could be the mechanism responsible for the low platelet count.

The presence of the lupus anticoagulant is associated with increased fetal loss throughout gestation, in addition to recurrent thromboembolic disorders. Extensive atheromatous, thrombotic lesions and infarction in the placenta associated with the anticoagulant have also been reported[117,118,120]. These observations are important, because they suggest a link between autoimmune mechanisms and reproductive wastage, and provide new possibilities for therapeutic interventions. Prednisone and low-dose aspirin have been shown to improve fetal salvage in patients with anticoagulants. The recommended doses of prednisone and aspirin are 20–80 mg/day and 80 mg/day, respectively. The dosage of prednisone is adjusted to return the coagulation tests, such as activated partial thromboplastin time, to normal. At this low dose, aspirin inhibits thromboxane synthesis without much impact on prostacyclin production and appears to be safe for use in pregnancy. Interestingly, successful pregnancies have been observed in patients with anticoagulants who received neither aspirin nor immunosuppressive medications during pregnancy. A well-designed clinical trial is needed to evaluate the impact of corticosteroids and/or aspirin on the pregnancy outcomes of lupus anticoagulant-positive patients.

IMMUNE THROMBOCYTOPENIC PURPURA

Immune thrombocytopenic purpura (ITP) is defined as a condition characterized by a low platelet count, with otherwise normal complete blood count and peripheral blood smear, and no clinically apparent associated diseases or factors which can cause thrombocytopenia. Conditions which may be associated with thrombocytopenia include viral infection (human immunodeficiency virus), systemic lupus erythematosus, lymphoproliferative disorders, myelodysplasia, drugs, alloimmune thrombocytopenia, congenital thrombocytopenia and pre-eclampsia. Thus, the diagnosis of ITP is a diagnosis of exclusion and involves a comprehensive history, a thorough physical examination, a complete blood count and a blood smear. Other work-up studies are unnecessary, unless indicated by the history and physical examination[121].

In ITP, a shortened platelet lifespan due to increased platelet destruction is the mechanism of thrombocytopenia. A circulating antibody, which is frequently an IgG, is produced against an unidentified platelet-membrane antigen. This antibody coats the platelets, which are then destroyed at an increased rate in the reticuloendothelial system, mainly in the spleen[122]. The severity of the disease correlates with the quantity of platelet-bound IgG and not with serum antiplatelet IgG[123]. The antibody can cross the placenta, coat fetal platelets and enhance their destruction by the fetal reticuloendothelial system[124]. The antibody may be present in women who are in remission; therefore, their fetuses remain at risk for neonatal thrombocytopenia, even though they have normal platelet counts[124–129].

ITP is not uncommon during pregnancy, as the disease predominantly affects young women during their reproductive years. The consequences of this disorder are related solely to thrombocytopenia and to the disruption of the normal hemostatic mechanism that a low platelet count can produce. The ever-present threat of hemorrhage poses special problems for both the mother and her fetus during pregnancy and the aim of management is to minimize that threat. The risks of antepartum, intrapartum and postpartum hemorrhage, present in all obstetric patients, are increased in women with ITP, as is the potential for increased surgical bleeding during Cesarean section. The main risk to the infant is intracranial hemorrhage secondary to transplacental acquired thrombocytopenia.

The signs and symptoms of this disease are directly related to the platelet count and are not specific for ITP. Capillary bleeding generally occurs when the platelet count is less than 20 000/µl and is predominantly dermal or mucosal (e.g. petechiae, ecchymosis, epistaxis, hematuria). Retinal hemorrhages are particularly important to recognize, because they are signs of impending intracranial hemorrhage. With the exception of these findings, the physical examination is usually normal. An enlarged spleen suggests that the thrombocytopenia is secondary to another disorder, such as systemic lupus erythematosus, infectious mononucleosis or a lymphoproliferative disorder.

The clinical course of the disease may be acute (associated with drug reactions or viral infections) or chronic. Chronic ITP usually has an insidious course, with episodes of intermittent exacerbations and remissions. When the diagnosis of ITP is made in a female of reproductive age, family planning and contraception should be discussed. Since medical therapy and spleenectomy during pregnancy are not without risk, patients should be advised to postpone childbearing until a remission of the disease is obtained or steroid or immunosuppressive therapy is not required. Spleenectomy may be necessary to achieve this state. Occasionally, however, this goal may not be accomplished, because some patients require medical therapy even following spleenectomy. If this is the case, patients who desire to become pregnant should be made aware of the potential risks of steroids or immunosuppressants to the fetus. Patients should also be informed that they may need a Cesarean section for fetal indications and that there is an increased risk to both the fetus and the mother with this disease. However, ITP is by no means an absolute contraindication to pregnancy[3]. Regarding contraception, it is not wise to use intrauterine devices because, in addition to the risks of menorrhagia and uterine perforation, there is an increased failure rate of this method in patients taking steroids. There is no specific contraindication to the use of birth-control pills in women with ITP[3].

Once the patient with ITP is pregnant, the management goals are to decrease the risk of antepartum, intrapartum and postpartum maternal hemorrhage and to prevent intracranial hemorrhage in the neonate. Treatment programs for patients with ITP during pregnancy largely reflect personal bias, since most of the management recommendations have not been evaluated in well-designed clinical trials[121].

Management of ITP in pregnancy

The management of ITP is directed toward preventing platelet underproduction, platelet consumption and impairment of platelet function. The mainstays of treatment are glucocorticoids, intravenous immunoglobulin and spleenectomy. Hospitalization is not indicated if the patient has a platelet count of greater than 20 000/µl and is asymptomatic or has only minor purpura. Hospitalization is appropriate if the patient has a platelet count of less than 20 000/µl and substantial mucous membrane bleeding[121].

General measures

Iron, folic acid and vitamin B_{12} deficiencies impair platelet production[3,130]. Therefore, identification of a deficiency, as well as adequate supplementation of the deficient substances during pregnancy, is important.

Myelotoxic agents, such as alcohol, should be avoided. If present, fever and infection should be identified and treated, since they shorten platelet survival[131]. Drugs that impair platelet function or cause thrombocytopenia should be avoided[132].

Steroid therapy

Therapy in patients with ITP always begins with steroids. The immediate effects of steroid administration are inhibition of antibody attachment to platelets and suppression of platelet phagocytosis by the reticuloendothelial system. The long-term effect is inhibition of antibody synthesis[121,125,133,134].

The objective of steroid therapy during pregnancy is not only to increase the platelet count to the level at which spontaneous hemorrhage is unlikely to occur (generally above 20 000/μl), but also to provide an adequate reserve so that hemostatic failure will not occur in the case of an unforeseen maternal hemorrhage. Although the ideal goal is to bring the platelet count to normal levels, this frequently is difficult to achieve or requires prohibitively high doses of steroid therapy. A more reasonable goal is to maintain a platelet count above 50 000/μl, since excessive surgical hemorrhage rarely occurs above this level if platelet function is normal. If platelet dysfunction is identified by a prolonged bleeding time, the goal should be to normalize the bleeding time.

Therapy with steroids usually begins with administration of prednisone at a dose of 0.5–1 mg/kg per day in divided doses. If the patient has severe bleeding, a higher initial dose of intravenous methylprednisolone of up to 1.0 g daily may be given[135]. Because the placental transfer of prednisone is less than that of other glucocorticoids (e.g. betamethasone, dexamethasone), this has been the corticosteroid of choice in the therapy of ITP in pregnancy. Some authors have recently suggested the use of corticosteroids that readily cross the placenta, with the aim of delivering steroids to the fetus in whom they might have the same therapeutic effect as in the mother[135]. A short course of steroids prior to delivery has been proposed for this purpose. The effect of this approach in the prevention of neonatal thrombocytopenia has been inconsistent. Some authors have reported a favorable response and others have not. There is a theoretical risk of acute worsening of fetal thrombocytopenia with this modality of therapy, since corticosteroids could potentially displace the antibodies from the platelets, resulting in an increase in the unbound antiplatelet IgG antibodies in the maternal circulation.

The effect of steroids on the mother is usually noted within the first 24–48 h, but may take as long as 2–3 weeks. The therapeutic plan is to give the shortest course of steroids that will bring the platelet count to a safe level. Once the platelet count is above 50 000/μl,

the steroids should be continued for 1 week and then tapered slowly. If, on the other hand, the platelet count has not reached 50 000/μl in 3 weeks, the dose of prednisone should be increased to 1.5–2 mg/kg of body weight per day. If continued steroid therapy is needed, it should consist of the lowest dose that will maintain the platelet count above 50 000/μl. This parameter must be checked during reduction and after termination of steroid therapy, because a fall in the platelet count is the earliest indication of relapse in asymptomatic patients. Most pregnant women respond to steroids and, therefore, the performance of a spleenectomy can be deferred until the postpartum period.

The potential risks of steroid administration during pregnancy are difficult to assess. However, the risk of maternal hemorrhage outweighs the potential hazards of the judicious use of these drugs. Although animal studies have shown an increased incidence of cleft palate[136], this has not been substantiated by the limited studies done in humans[137]. Other potential complications of steroids that are rarely reported include transient adrenal insufficiency in the neonate, neonatal hypoglycemia and intrauterine growth retardation[138–140].

Estriol production can be decreased if the equivalent of 75 mg of cortisol is administered daily, because, at this level, transplacental steroids can depress the fetal adrenal production of estriol precursors. Prednisone is secreted into the breast milk, but, if the dose is less than 30 mg per day, it is unlikely to cause any problems in the breastfed neonate[141].

Spleenectomy

Removal of the spleen eliminates the major site of platelet destruction and an important site of antibody production. Furthermore, since a significant portion of the platelets are normally sequestered in the spleen, this operation increases the number of platelets available for circulation. Spleenectomy is usually performed in patients with ITP if the platelet counts remain less than 30 000/μl and bleeding exists after 4–6 weeks of medical therapy[121]. During pregnancy, however, spleenectomy is indicated only in those women who have life-threatening hemorrhage and in whom primary therapies with corticosteroids and intravenous immunoglobulin have failed to increase the platelet count and bleeding manifestations continue to occur[121]. The major risks of performing a spleenectomy in an obstetric patient are premature labor and the occurrence of a surgical accident when ligating the splenic pedicle. During pregnancy, all the blood vessels in the abdomen dramatically increase in size. The technical difficulties of operating on these dilated vessels are compounded by the presence of a gravid uterus, which makes access to the splenic pedicle difficult to attain during the second half of pregnancy. Spleenectomy is performed preferably in the second trimester to minimize the risk of preterm labor and the obstruction by an enlarging uterus. In addition, the operation can be performed immediately following a Cesarean section with few additional complications[142]. Preoperative prophylaxis with intravenous immunoglobulin or oral glucocorticoids to raise the platelet count above 20 000/μl is appropriate[121].

Spleenectomy has been reported to produce permanent remission in 60–70% of patients, temporary remission in 20% and no response in 10%[143,144]. At present, the maternal operative risk of elective spleenectomy during pregnancy is probably similar to that for a non-pregnant patient.

Immunosuppressive therapy

Immunosuppressive agents (vinca alkaloids, cyclophosphamide and azathioprine) have been used with some success to treat non-pregnant patients whose disease is refractory to corticosteroids and spleenectomy as evidenced by a persistent platelet count of less than 30 000/μl and active bleeding[121,123,145]. The rationale for their use is to depress the production of antiplatelet antibodies and the host's cellular immunity. Their role in the management of a pregnant patient with ITP has not been established and concern exists about fetal side-effects[3].

Immunoglobulin G infusion

Favorable responses in maternal platelet counts and hemostasis have been reported with the intravenous infusion of IgG as a treatment for ITP. Rising platelet counts usually occur within 24 h. This modality of therapy can be very useful in preparing patients for surgery or delivery and offers an attractive alternative to spleenectomy in refractory cases. The dosage varies from 0.3 to 0.49 mg/kg of body weight given over a period of 4–6 h daily for 5 days. This course of treatment can be repeated weekly as needed. No adverse maternal or fetal effects have been reported. Interference with the phagocytosis of the antibody-coated platelets by blocking the macrophage Fc receptors of the reticuloendothelial system has been proposed as a mechanism of action for the infused IgG. Actually, a decrease in the Fc receptor-mediated clearance of autologous IgG-coated erythrocytes following immunoglobulin infusion has been observed. The impact of this modality of therapy on fetal platelet counts remains to be determined because both normal platelet counts and thrombocytopenia have been observed in neonates whose mothers had received immunoglobulin infusion for refractory ITP.

Platelet transfusions

Platelet transfusions have no place in the maintenance therapy of ITP. Transfused platelets are not only rapidly destroyed, but they also become progressively less effective in raising the platelet count, because the antigenic load they provide induces the production of antiplatelet antibodies. Platelet transfusions are indicated in the face of life-threatening hemorrhage and to maintain hemostasis during surgery. A rule of thumb is to transfuse platelets to maintain a platelet count above 50 000/μl and a normal bleeding time prior to surgery. High-dose corticosteroid therapy (prednisone 2 mg/kg of body weight or an intravenous preparation of equivalent dose) should be administered with platelet transfusions to prolong platelet survival[146].

Mode of delivery

The most serious perinatal problem associated with ITP is fetal thrombocytopenia, which makes the neonate susceptible to hemorrhages and particularly to intracranial bleeding if the platelet count is less than 50 000/μl. It is believed that the trauma associated with delivery is a determining factor in the production of intracranial hemorrhage. Since most trauma to the fetal head occurs during its passage through the birth canal, Cesarean section has been proposed as the method of choice for delivering these infants. Although this is a logical assumption, it must be noted that the protective effect of Cesarean section has not been, and probably will never be, demonstrated in clinical trials. However, adherence to a policy of routine Cesarean section as the mode of delivery for patients with ITP exposes the mothers to the risks of defective intra- and postoperative hemostasis. Since severe fetal thrombocytopenia (< 50 000/μl) occurs in only about 4–20% of patients with ITP[147–150], a significant number of unnecessary Cesarean sections would be performed for putative fetal indications. A more logical approach would be to assess the neonatal risk of thrombocytopenia antenatally. Maternal platelet counts, a history of spleenectomy and the titers of platelet-associated antibodies are poor predictors of fetal thrombocytopenia[151,152]. Similarly, maternal treatment with corticosteroids does not appear to be effective in preventing neonatal thrombocytopenia[153]. On the other hand, the absence of circulating antiplatelet antibody is associated with a much lower risk of fetal thrombocytopenia[150] and neonatal platelet counts of subsequent pregnancies are similar to those of older siblings[154,155]. The risk of intracranial hemorrhage from ITP is much less, probably 1%[156].

A platelet count can be determined from the fetal scalp capillary blood obtained at the beginning of spontaneous or induced labor and the result can be used to select the mode of delivery. The technique of scalp platelet count determination has been validated by its good correlation with umbilical cord and heel capillary platelet counts[157].

The incidence and extent of neonatal bleeding was related to the neonatal platelet count. No bleeding manifestations and only mild cutaneous manifestations occurred in those with counts above 100 000/µl and 50 000/µl, respectively. Serious bleeding requiring treatment was confined to infants with counts of less than 50 000/µl. Therefore, it was proposed that a platelet count of 50 000/µl in a scalp sample be used as a cut-off value for selecting the mode of delivery. Cesarean section would be indicated only for those infants with platelet counts below 50 000/µl[157]. It must be stressed that the possibility exists that some infants with platelet counts above 50 000/µl have had subclinical bleeding. A study including ultrasonographic examination and neurologic follow-up of infants born to mothers with ITP is necessary to assess the prevalence of asymptomatic bleeding and to establish the long-term significance of these findings.

The technique for scalp platelet count is simple, but must be mastered before it is used in a patient with ITP. The scalp platelet count should be performed at the beginning of labor or after elective amniotomy in patients with dilated cervix at term. A plastic cone is placed in the vagina and directly applied to the fetal scalp. A stab wound scalp incision is then created, similar to that used for scalp pH capillary collection. A Unopette test 5855 system (Becton–Dickinson) is used to collect the sample. This is a plastic pipette that fills by capillary action to 0.02 ml. This pipette is held in an Allis' clamp to collect the sample. Once the pipette has been filled, it is emptied into a reservoir containing 1.98 ml of diluent and then mixed. Determination of platelet count is performed by an automated technique or a standard manual hemocytometer method. A critical part of the scalp platelet determination technique is the speed with which the procedure is performed. If the blood is collected slowly, it tends to clot, giving falsely low results. Fetal platelet count could also be determined with a smear of capillary blood. The technique of blood collection for smear preparation is similar to that previously described. Fetal platelet clumping on a smear is considered an indication of adequate platelet count[158]. Heparinized tubes should not be used for sample collection, because heparin can cause platelet clumping and produce abnormally low platelet counts.

Complications with the use of this technique have not yet been reported. Compression of the scalp incision should be maintained until bleeding has stopped completely. The capability of performing an emergency Cesarean section is essential when this technique is used, as continued fetal bleeding could become a problem.

The inability to determine the fetal platelet count prior to the onset of labor has been considered a drawback of the fetal scalp sampling technique. Even though the impact of labor and delivery on the thrombocytopenic fetuses, especially those with platelet counts below 50 000/µl, remains to be determined, it seems desirable not to subject these fetuses to the trauma of labor and/or precipitous delivery. Funicentesis, or percutaneous umbilical cord blood sampling technique to determine fetal platelet counts at term has been utilized to overcome the above problems. There is a good correlation between the fetal platelet count determined by funicentesis and the neonatal platelet count obtained at the time of delivery[147,159]. However, further studies need to be carried out to evaluate the merits of this approach. At present, the management of ITP in pregnancy with regard to the determination of fetal platelet count and the mode of delivery remains to be determined. Some investigators advocate prenatal determination of fetal platelet count by either funicentesis or fetal scalp blood sampling and Cesarean section delivery if the fetal platelet count is less than 50 000/µl [158,159], while others recommend abandonment of prenatal determination of fetal platelet count and Cesarean section only for obstetric indications[156].

THROMBOTIC THROMBOCYTOPENIC PURPURA

Pathophysiology and laboratory findings

Thrombotic thrombocytopenic purpura (TTP) is a syndrome characterized clinically by thrombocytopenia, microangiopathic hemolytic anemia, neurological abnormalities, renal dysfunction and fever, and pathologically by the presence of intravascular hyaline thrombi consisting of platelets and fibrin. Erythrocytes become disrupted into schistocytes as they travel through vessels which are partially occluded by microthrombi. The presence of schistocytes is the prominent feature of this syndrome[160].

The pathophysiology of this disease has not been definitively established. Increasing evidence suggests that TTP is a disorder of the mechanism that regulates the blood vessel wall–platelet interaction. The initial event may be an injury to discontinuous segments of the endothelium of small arteries and capillaries. The nature of the insult has not been determined, but is likely to be diverse and may involve infectious agents and an immunological mechanism.

Thrombotic thrombocytopenic purpura in pregnancy

TTP is an uncommon disorder, but it affects women more frequently than men and is seen predominantly in those between the ages of 10 and 40 years. It occurs in association with pregnancy in 10–25% of the cases and tends to recur in subsequent pregnancies[161]. Eighty-nine per cent of TTP cases in pregnancy develop during the prenatal period and the remainder develop during the postpartum period. Although fetal mortality can be as high as 80%, fetal thrombocytopenia does not seem to occur, suggesting that whatever factor is causing maternal TTP is not able to cross the placenta readily[162]. Maternal mortality ranged from 68 to 93% prior to the development of effective treatments[162,163]. Currently, 70–80% of patients with TTP survive with minimal or no sequelae[161].

The diagnosis of TTP remains clinical, because there are no pathognomonic tests for the condition[160]. When the symptoms or signs of TTP present prior to or during the first half of pregnancy, the diagnosis of TTP should be strongly considered. When the symptoms or signs of TTP take place in the third trimester of pregnancy, the diagnosis is much more difficult because of the striking similarities between eclampsia and TTP. Both diseases may be manifested by thrombocytopenia, microangiopathic hemolytic anemia, renal dysfunction, fever, and coma and/or seizures[164]. It has been suggested recently that gingival biopsies may provide a diagnostic tool to differentiate the two entities[165]. Biopsy specimens of patients with TTP should show microthrombi in small vessels without evidence of vasculitis and peripheral clot lysis, whereas patients with pre-eclampsia have been assumed to have no thrombotic lesions. The problem with this approach is that gingival biopsies have been reported to be negative in as many as 40% of patients with TTP and the experience with gingival biopsies in women with pre-eclampsia is limited[166]. Furthermore, it is possible that pre-eclamptic patients with decompensated disseminated intravascular coagulation have thrombotic fibrin deposits in small vessels similar to those found on light microscopy in cases of TTP. Differentiation between the thrombotic lesions of TTP and disseminated intravascular coagulation currently requires the histochemical identification of plasminogen activator activity. Lesions of disseminated intravascular coagulation have increased fibrinolytic activity, whereas this is absent in TTP lesions. Determination of the plasma levels of the unusually large von Willebrand multimers (vWMs) appears to be promising in the diagnosis and/or follow-up of patients with TTP. The damaged endothelial cells release the unusually large vWMs, which act synergistically with a plasma platelet-agglutinating factor to cause the segmental intravascular deposition of platelets and platelet-derived fibrin. The unusually large vWMs are absent from the plasma of normal subjects, are greatly reduced or even absent during the acute episode of TTP, and recur in the recovery or remission periods[167]. On the other hand, the vWM levels are normal in patients with severe pre-eclampsia[168].

Management of TTP in pregnancy

Therapy for TTP has been empirical and has involved many different regimens, including steroids, spleenectomy, heparin, heparin and urokinase, antiplatelet agents, immunosuppressive agents, hemodialysis and plasma transfusions. Evaluation of the success of different therapeutic modalities is very difficult because they have frequently been used in combination. Furthermore, it is possible that several disorders with different pathophysiological mechanisms have been inappropriately labelled as TTP. This, of course, will result in variable responses to different therapeutic modalities.

The management of TTP in pregnancy depends on the gestational age at the time of presentation. It is important to differentiate between TTP and eclampsia, because the former requires plasmapheresis without necessitating delivery, whereas the latter responds dramatically to delivery. If a patient presents with the typical TTP pentad in the first or early second trimester, the diagnosis can be established with reasonable certainty, because pre-eclampsia is unlikely to occur at this gestational age. Therapy should be directed toward inducing a hematological remission. If the patient presents in the third trimester, however, it is very difficult to distinguish between TTP and eclampsia. Since eclampsia is the more prevalent condition, it should be assumed to be present if clinical and pathological data are not helpful in differentiating between these disorders, and the patient should be delivered. Every effort should be made to accomplish a vaginal delivery, since this imposes less stress on the hemostatic system than a Cesarean section. Patient failure to improve following delivery suggests the diagnosis of TTP, and specific therapy for that disease can be initiated.

Obstetric patients with TTP are best managed in conjunction with the hematology and blood-bank services. The cornerstone therapy for TTP is either infusion of fresh-frozen plasma or exchange transfusion with fresh-frozen plasma or von Willebrand factor-depleted cryosupernatant[160,169,170]. Plasma exchange is preferable to plasma infusion because:

(1) It requires less fresh-frozen plasma;
(2) It is more effective in inducing remission of TTP;
(3) Plasma infusion is potentially associated with volume overload, especially in patients whose heart and kidneys are affected[160].

The rationale for the use of plasma is based on the demonstration that patients with TTP are deficient in a factor that is present in normal plasma and can inhibit platelet aggregation[171–173]. Plasmapheresis with solutions other than plasma or its cryosupernatant is ineffective. The biochemistry of this factor remains to be determined. It may be reasonable to initiate the treatment of TTP using plasma exchange with the cryosupernatant fraction of plasma instead of fresh-frozen plasma, because the former has been effective in patients who are refractory to fresh-frozen plasma[174]. The patient's status should be monitored with serial platelet counts, serum creatinine, lactate dehydrogenase and bilirubin determinations, as well as frequent neurological examinations. Daily plasma transfusions should be instituted until a spontaneous increase in platelet count to near normal values is obtained and neurological manifestations have disappeared. The volume of the transfusion should be sufficient to maintain the lactate dehydrogenase concentration below 300 U/ml. The initial volume for exchange plasmapheresis has been recommended as 35–40 ml/kg of body weight. Glucocorticoid alone or in combination with plasma exchange has also been shown to be useful in the management of TTP. In fact, glucocorticoid should be considered as a part of the initial treatment. Antiplatelet agents, such as aspirin, dipyridamole, indomethacin, ibuprofen and prostacyclin, fail to prevent the *in vitro* platelet aggregation induced by plasma from patients with TTP. This observation supports the poor clinical responses to the antiplatelet agents in patients with TTP. Patients who have failed to respond to the initial therapy can be empirically treated with spleenectomy or immunosuppressive agents with varying degrees of success. The choice of therapy after initial failure is arbitrary and in most cases reflects the personal experience and preference of the physicians managing the case.

REFERENCES

1. Pitkin RM, Witte DL. Platelet and leukocyte counts in pregnancy. *J Am Med Assoc* 1979;242:2696–8
2. Rakoczi I, Tallian F, Bagdany S, Gati I. Platelet lifespan in normal pregnancy and pre-eclampsia as determined by a non-radioisotope technique. *Thromb Res* 1979;15:553
3. Romero R, Duffy TP. Platelet disorders in pregnancy. *Clin Perinatol* 1980;7:327–48
4. Wallenburg HCS, van Kessel PH. Platelet lifespan in normal pregnancy as determined by a nonradioisotopic technique. *Br J Obstet Gynaecol* 1978;85:33–6
5. Fletcher AP, Alkjaersig NK, Burstein R. The influence of pregnancy upon blood coagulation and plasma fibrinolytic enzyme function. *Am J Obstet Gynecol* 1979; 134:743–51
6. Graef H, Kuhn W. Coagulation disorders in obstetrics. In Friedman EA, ed. *Major Problems in Obstetrics and Gynecology*, vol 13. Philadelphia: WB Saunders, 1980
7. McKay DG. The clinical spectrum and management of acquired coagulopathy in pregnancy. In Reid DE, Christian CD, eds. *Controversy in Obstetrics and Gynecology*, vol II. Philadelphia: WB Saunders, 1974:285
8. Bonnar J. Haemostasis and coagulation disorders in pregnancy. In Bloom AL, Thomas DP, eds. *Haemostasis and Thrombosis*. Edinburgh: Churchill Livingstone, 1981:454
9. Biland L, Duckert F. Coagulation factors of the newborn and his mother. *Thromb Diath Haemorrh* 1973; 29:644–51
10. Coopland AT, Alkjaersig N, Fletcher AP. Reduction in plasma factor XIII (fibrin stabilizing factor) concentration during pregnancy. *J Lab Clin Med* 1969;73:144–53
11. Fresh JW, Ferguson JH, Lewis JH. Blood-clotting studies in parturient women and the newborn. *Obstet Gynecol* 1956;7:117
12. Gilabert J, Aznar J, Parrilla JJ, *et al.* Alterations in the coagulation and fibrinolysis system in pregnancy, labour and puerperium, with special reference to a possible transitory state of intravascular coagulation during labour. *Thromb Haemost* 1978;40:387–96
13. Kennan AL, Bell WN. Blood coagulation during normal pregnancy, labor, and the puerperium. *Am J Obstet Gynecol* 1957;73:57
14. Nilsson IM, Kullander S. Coagulation and fibrinolytic studies during pregnancy. *Acta Obstet Gynecol Scand* 1967;46:273–85
15. Nossel HL, Lanzkowsky P, Levy S, *et al.* A study of coagulation factor levels in women during labour and in their newborn infants. *Thromb Diath Haemorrh* 1966; 16:185–97
16. Pechet L, Alexander B. Increased clotting factors in pregnancy. *N Engl J Med* 1961;265:1093
17. Ratnoff OD, Colopy JE, Pritchard JA. The blood-clotting mechanism during normal parturition. *J Lab Clin Med* 1954;44:408
18. Teisner B, Davey MW, Grudzinskas JG. Circulating antithrombins in pregnancy. *Br J Obstet Gynaecol* 1982; 89:62–4
19. Weiner CP, Brandt J. Plasma antithrombin III activity: an aid in the diagnosis of preeclampsia–eclampsia. *Am J Obstet Gynecol* 1982;142:275–81
20. Astedt B. Fibrinolytic activity during labour. *Acta Obstet Gynecol Scand* 1972;51:171–4
21. Bonnar J, McNicol GP, Douglas AS. Coagulation and fibrinolytic mechanisms during and after normal childbirth. *Br Med J* 1970;2:200–3
22. Hedner U, Astedt B. Studies on fibrinolytic inhibitors during pregnancy. *Acta Obstet Gynecol Scand* 1971;50: 99–103
23. Shaper AG, MacIntosh DM, Kyobe J. Fibrinolytic activity in pregnancy, during parturition, and in the puerperium. *Lancet* 1966;2:874–6
24. Sheppard BL, Bonnar J. Fibrinolysis in decidual spiral arteries in late pregnancy. *Thromb Haemost* 1978;39: 751–8
25. Fletcher AP, Alkjaersig N, Sherry S. Pathogenesis of the coagulation defect developing during pathological plasma proteolytic ('fibrinolytic') states. I. The significance of fibrinogen proteolysis and circulating fibrinogen breakdown products. *J Clin Invest* 1962;41:896
26. Sazama K. Reports of 355 transfusion-associated deaths:1976 through 1985. *Transfusion* 1990;30:583–90
27. Krevens JR, Jackson DP. Hemorrhagic disorder following massive whole blood transfusions. *J Am Med Assoc* 1955;159:171
28. Wilson RF, Bassett JS, Alexander JW. Five years of experience with massive blood transfusion. *J Am Med Assoc* 1965;194:851–4
29. Lundberg GD. Practice parameter for the use of fresh-frozen plasma, cryoprecipitate, and platelets. *J Am Med Assoc* 1994;271:777–81

30. Ness PM, Perkins HA. Cryoprecipitate as a reliable source of fibrinogen replacement. *J Am Med Assoc* 1979;241:1690–1

31. Pool JG, Hershgold EJ. High-potency antihaemophilic factor concentrate prepared from cryoglobulin precipitate. *Nature (London)* 1964;203:312

32. Widmann FK, ed. Preparation of blood components. *Technical Manual of the American Association of Blood Banks*, 8th edn. Baltimore: Williams & Wilkins, 19:38

33. Berntorp E, Nilsson IM. Use of a high-purity factor VIII concentrate (Humate-P™ [Hemate-P™]) in von Willebrand's disease. *Vox Sang* 1989;56:212–17

34. Huestis DW, Bove JR, Busch S, eds. Blood components, fractions, and derivatives. In *Practical Blood Transfusion*. Boston: Little, Brown, 1981:285

35. Filip DJ, Aster RH. Relative hemostatic effectiveness of human platelets stored at 4° and 22 °C. *J Lab Clin Med* 1978;91:618–24

36. Murphy S, Gardner FH. Platelet preservation. Effect of storage temperature on maintenance of platelet viability–deleterious effect of refrigerated storage. *N Engl J Med* 1969;280:1094–8

37. Murphy S, Gardner FH. Platelet storage at 22 °C; metabolic, morphologic, and functional studies. *J Clin Invest* 1971;50:370–7

38. Levin RH, Pert JH, Freireich EJ. Response to transfusion of platelets pooled from multiple donors and the effects of various techniques of concentrating platelets. *Blood* 1965;5:54

39. Goldfinger D, McGinniss MH. Rh-incompatible platelet transfusions – risks and consequences of sensitizing immunosuppressed patients. *N Engl J Med* 1971;284:942–4

40. Aster RH. Effect of anticoagulant and ABO incompatibility on recovery of transfused human platelets. *Blood* 1965;26:732

41. National Institutes of Health Consensus Conference. Platelet transfusion therapy. *J Am Med Assoc* 1987;257:1777–80

42. Slichter SJ. Controversies in platelet transfusion therapy. *Ann Rev Med* 1980;31:509–40

43. Beutler E. Platelet transfusion: the 20 000/μl trigger. *Blood* 1993;81:1411–13

44. Klein CA, Blajchman MD. Alloantibodies and platelet destruction. *Semin Thromb Hemost* 1982;8:105–15

45. Blatt PM, Lundbald RL, Kingdon HS, *et al*. Thrombogenic materials in prothrombin complex concentrates. *Ann Intern Med* 1974;81:766–70

46. Cederbaum AI, Blatt PM, Roberts HR. Intravascular coagulation with use of human prothrombin complex concentrates. *Ann Intern Med* 1976;84:683–7

47. Davey RL, Shashaty GG, Rath CE. Acute coagulopathy following infusion of prothrombin complex concentrate. *Am J Med* 1976;60:719–22

48. Iwarson S, Kjellman H, Teger-Nilsson A-C. Incidence of viral hepatitis after administration of factor IX concentrates. *Vox Sang* 1976;31:136–40

49. McVay PA, Hoag RW, Hoag MS, Toy P. Safety and use of autologous blood donation during the third trimester of pregnancy. *Am J Obstet Gynecol* 1989;160:1479–88

50. Kruskall MS, Leonard S, Klapholz H. Autologous blood donation during pregnancy: analysis of safety and blood use. *Obstet Gynecol* 1987;70:938–40

51. NBREP, National Heart, Lung, and Blood Institute. The use of autologous blood. *J Am Med Assoc* 1990;263:414–17

52. Heene DL. Disseminated intravascular coagulation: evaluation of therapeutic approaches. *Semin Thromb Hemost* 1977;3:291

53. Abdul-Karim RW, Chevli RN. Antepartum hemorrhage and shock. *Clin Obstet Gynecol* 1976;19:533–59

54. Pritchard JA, Brekken AL. Clinical and laboratory studies on severe abruptio placentae. *Am J Obstet Gynecol* 1967;97:681–700

55. Pritchard JA. Genesis of severe placental abruption. *Am J Obstet Gynecol* 1970;108:22–7

56. Dahmus MA, Sibai BM. Blunt abdominal trauma: are there any predictive factors for abruptio placentae or maternal–fetal distress? *Am J Obstet Gynecol* 1993;169:1054–9

57. Naeye RL, Harkness WL, Utts J. Abruptio placentae and perinatal death: a prospective study. *Am J Obstet Gynecol* 1977;128:740–6

58. Notelovits M, Bottoms SF, Dase DF, Leichter PJ. Painless abruptio placentae. *Obstet Gynecol* 1979;53:270–2

59. Ferguson JH, Hatton RL. Abruptio placentae and rupture of the marginal sinus of the placenta: some relationships. *Am J Obstet Gynecol* 1959;78:947

60. Myers RE, Brann AW Jr. Abruptio placentae in rhesus monkey causing brain damage to the fetus. *Am J Obstet Gynecol* 1976;126:1048–9

61. Basu HK. Fibrinolysis and abruptio placentae. *J Obstet Gynaecol Br Commonw* 1969;76:481–96

62. Fulton LD, Page EW. Nature of the refractory state following sublethal dose of human placental thromboplastin. *Proc Soc Exp Biol Med* 1948;68:594

63. Schneider CL. The inactivation of placental toxin by human serum. *Am J Physiol* 1945;146:140

64. Schneider CL. The active principle of placental toxin: thromboplastin; its inactivator in blood: antithromboplastin. *Am J Physiol* 1947;149:123

65. Schneider CL. Complications of late pregnancy in rabbits induced by experimental placental trauma. *Surg Gynecol Obstet* 1950;90:613

66. Schneider CL. 'Fibrin embolism' (disseminated intravascular coagulation) with defibrinations as one of the end results during placenta abruptio. *Surg Obstet Gynecol* 1951;92:27

67. Schneider CL. Rupture of the basal (decidual) plate in abruptio placentae: a pathway of autoextraction from the decidua into the maternal circulation. *Am J Obstet Gynecol* 1952;63:1078

68. Schneider CL. Disseminated intravascular coagulation thrombosis versus fibrination, in clinical disease states. *Thromb Diath Haemorrh* 1969;36:1

69. Phillips LL, Skrodelis V, Taylor HC Jr. Hemorrhage due to fibrinolysis in abruptio placentae. *Am J Obstet Gynecol* 1962;84:1447

70. Barbaro C, Hirsh J. Severe post-partum bleeding in abruptio placentae: failure to respond to fibrinogen infusion. *Med J Aust* 1968;2:1182

71. Bonnar J, McNicol GP, Douglas AS. The behaviour of the coagulation and fibrinolytic mechanisms in abruptio placentae. *J Obstet Gynaecol* 1969;76:799

72. Coopland AT, Israels ED, Zipusrky A, Israels LG. The pathogenesis of defective hemostasis in abruptio placentae. *Am J Obstet Gynecol* 1968;100:311

73. Coopland AT, Livingstone RA. Heparin treatment in abruptio placentae. *Can Med Assoc J* 1970;103:377

74. Page EW, King EB, Merrill JA. Abruptio placentae. Dangers of delay in delivery. *Obstet Gynecol* 1954;3:385

75. Sher G. Pathogenesis and management of uterine inertia complicating abruptio placentae with consumption coagulopathy. *Am J Obstet Gynecol* 1977;129:164–70

76. Hafter R, Graeff H. Molecular aspects of defibrination in a reptilase-treated case of 'dead fetus syndrome'. *Thromb Res* 1975;7:391–9

77. Jennison RF, Walker AHC. Fetal death *in utero* with hypofibrinogenaemia managed conservatively. *Lancet* 1956;2:607

78. Jimenez JM, Pritchard JA. Pathogenesis and treatment of coagulation defects resulting from fetal death. *Obstet Gynecol* 1968;32:449–59

79. Pritchard JA, Ratnoff OD. Studies of fibrinogen and other hemostatic factors in women with intrauterine death and delayed delivery. *Surg Gynecol Obstet* 1955;101:467

80. Tricomi V, Kohl SG. Fetal death *in utero*. *Am J Obstet Gynecol* 1957;74:1092

81. Nilsson IM, Astedt B, Hedner U, Berezine D. Intrauterine fetal death and circulating anticoagulant (antithromboplastin). *Acta Med Scand* 1975;197:153–9

82. Skelly H, Marivate M, Norman R, *et al*. Consumptive coagulopathy following fetal death in a triplet pregnancy. *Am J Obstet Gynecol* 1982;142:595–6

83. Romero R, Duffy TP, Berkowitz RL, *et al*. Prolongation of a preterm pregnancy complicated by death of a single twin *in utero* and disseminated intravascular coagulation: effects of treatment with heparin. *N Engl J Med* 1984;310:772–4

84. Goodlin RC. Severe pre-eclampsia: another great imitator. *Am J Obstet Gynecol* 1976;125:747–53

85. Goodlin RC, Holdt D. Impending gestosis. *Obstet Gynecol* 1981;58:743–5

86. Hathaway WE, Bonnar MD. Physiology of coagulation in pregnancy. In *Perinatal Coagulation*. New York: Grune & Statton, 1978:27

87. Imrie AH, Raper CGL. Severe intravascular coagulation preceding severe pre-eclampsia. *Br J Obstet Gynaecol* 1977;84:71–2

88. Redman CWG, Bonnar J, Beilin L. Early platelet consumption in preeclampsia. *Br Med J* 1978;1:467–9

89. Douglas JT, Shah M, Lowe GDO, *et al*. Plasma fibrinopeptide A and β-thromboglobulin in pre-eclampsia and pregnancy hypertension. *Thromb Haemost* 1982;47:54–5

90. Edgar W, McKillop C, Howie PW, Prentice CRM. Composition of soluble fibrin complexes in pre-eclampsia. *Thromb Res* 1977;10:567–74

91. McKillop C, Forbes CD, Howie PW, Prentice CRM. Soluble fibrinogen/fibrin complexes in pre-eclampsia. *Lancet* 1976;1:56–8

92. Howie PW. The haemostatic mechanisms in pre-eclampsia. *Clin Obstet Gynaecol* 1977;4:595–611

93. Howie PW, Begg CB, Purdie DW, Prentice CRM. Use of coagulation tests to predict the clinical progress of pre-eclampsia. *Lancet* 1976;1:323–5

94. Arias F, Mancilla-Jimenez R. Hepatic fibrinogen deposits in pre-eclampsia. *N Engl J Med* 1976;295:578–82

95. Morris RH, Vassalli P, Beller FK, McCluskey RT. Immunofluorescent studies of renal biopsies in the diagnosis of toxemia of pregnancy. *Obstet Gynecol* 1964;24:32

96. Pritchard JA, Cunningham FG, Mason RA. Coagulation changes in eclampsia: their frequency and pathologies. *Am J Obstet Gynecol* 1976;124:855–64

97. Roberts JM, May WJ. Consumptive coagulopathy in severe preeclampsia. *Obstet Gynecol* 1976;48:163–6

98. Magann EF, Bass D, Chauhan S, *et al*. Antepartum corticosteroids: disease stabilization in patients with the syndrome of hemolysis, elevated liver enzymes, and low platelets (HELLP). *Am J Obstet Gynecol* 1994;171:1148–53

99. Jespersen J. Disseminated intravascular coagulation in toxemia of pregnancy. Correction of the decreased platelet counts and raised levels of serum uric acid and fibrinogen degradation products by aspirin. *Thromb Res* 1980;17:743–6

100. Trudinger BJ. Platelets and intrauterine growth retardation in pre-eclampsia. *Br J Obstet Gynaecol* 1976;83:284

101. Biggs R, Austen DEG, Denson KWE, *et al*. The mode of action of antibodies which destroy factor VIII. I. Antibodies which have second-order concentration graphs. *Br J Haematol* 1972;23:125–35

102. Bloom AL, Davies AJ, Res JK. A clinical and laboratory study of a patient with an unusual factor VIII inhibitor. *Thromb Diath Haemorrh* 1966;15:12–28

103. Bruno MS, Brody HS. Hypothromboplastinemia associated with a circulating anticoagulant and hemorrhage diathesis. *Am J Med* 1954;7:756

104. Edgar W, McKillop C, Howie PW, Prentice CRM. Composition of soluble fibrin complexes in pre-eclampsia. *Thromb Res* 1977;10:567–74

105. Frick PG. Hemophilia-like disease following pregnancy with transplacental transfer of an acquired circulating anticoagulant. *Blood* 1953;8:598

106. Greenwood RJ, Rabin SC. Hemophilia-like postpartum bleeding. *Obstet Gynecol* 1967;30:362–6

107. Hewlett JS, Haden RL. Hemophilia-like disease in women. *J Lab Clin Med* 1949;34:151

108. Marengo-Rowe AJ, Murff G, Leveson JE, Cook J. Hemophilia-like disease associated with pregnancy. *Obstet Gynecol* 1972;40:56–64

109. Michiels JJ, Bosch LJ, van der Plas PM, Abels J. Factor VIII inhibitor post-partum. *Scand J Haematol* 1978;26:97–107

110. Voke J, Letsky E. Pregnancy and antibody to factor VIII. *J Clin Pathol* 1977;30:928–32

111. Files JC, Morrison FS, Halbrook J. Post-partum treatment of a patient with a factor VIII inhibitor. *N Engl J Med* 1981;305:1650

112. Sohngen D, Specker C, Bach D, *et al*. Acquired factor VIII inhibitors in nonhemophiliac patients. *Ann Hematol* 1997;74:89–93

113. Hudak CD, Spiridonidis CH, Hart AJ, *et al*. Pregnancy-associated factor VIII inhibitor: treatment with intravenous high-dose immunoglobulin. *Am J Hematol* 1993;43:158

114. Hauser I, Schneider B, Lechner K. Post-partum factor VIII inhibitors. A review of the literature with special reference to the value of steroid and immunosuppressive treatment. *Thromb Haemost* 1995;73:1–5

115. Ries M, Wolfel D, Maier-Brandt B. Severe intracranial hemorrhage in a newborn infant with transplacental transfer of an acquired factor VII:C inhibitor. *J Pediatr* 1995;127:649–50

116. Coller BS, Hultin MB, Hoyer LW, *et al*. Normal pregnancy in a patient with a prior postpartum factor VIII inhibitor: with observations on pathogenesis and prognosis. *Blood* 1981;58:619–24

117. Carreras LO, Machin SJ, Deman R, *et al*. Arterial thrombosis, intrauterine fetal death and lupus anticoagulant detection of immunoglobulin interfering with prostacyclin formation. *Lancet* 1981;1:244–6

118. Carreras LO, Spitz B, Vermylen J, Van Assche A. Lupus anticoagulant and inhibition of prostacyclin formation in patients with repeated abortion, intrauterine growth retardation and intrauterine fetal death. *Br J Obstet Gynaecol* 1981;88:890–4

119. Prentice CRM. In Hoffbrand AV, Lewis SM, eds. *Acquired Disorders of Haemostasis in Postgraduate Haematology*, 2nd edn. Norwalk, CT: Appleton–Century–Crofts, 1981

120. De Wolf F, Carreras LO, Moerman P, *et al*. Decidual vasculopathy and extensive placental infarction in a patient with repeated thromboembolic accidents, recurrent fetal loss, and a lupus anticoagulant. *Am J Obstet Gynecol* 1982;142:829–34

121. The American Society of Hematology Idiopathic Thrombocytopenic Purpura Practice Guideline Panel. Diagnosis and treatment of idiopathic thrombocytopenic purpura: recommendations of the American Society of Hematology. *Ann Intern Med* 1997;126:319–26

122. George JN, El-Harake MA, Raskob GE. Chronic idiopathic thrombocytopenic purpura. *N Engl J Med* 1994;331:1207–11

123. Karpatkin S. Autoimmune thrombocytopenic purpura. *Blood* 1980;56:329–43

124. Kernoff LM, Malan E, Gunstson K. Neonatal thrombocytopenia complicating autoimmune thrombocytopenia in pregnancy. *Ann Intern Med* 1979;90:55–6

125. Cines DB, Schreiber AD. Immune thrombocytopenia. *N Engl J Med* 1979;300:106–11

126. Karpatkin M, Porges RF, Karpatkin S. Platelet counts in infants of women with autoimmune thrombocytopenia. *N Engl J Med* 1981;305:936–9

127. Minchinton RM, Dodd NJ, O'Brien H, *et al*. Autoimmune thrombocytopenia in pregnancy. *Br J Haematol* 1980;44:451–9

128. Van Leeuwen EG, Helmerhorst FM, Engelfriet CP, von dem Borne AEG Jr. Maternal autoimmune thrombocytopenia and the newborn. *Br Med J* 1981;283:104

129. Veenhoven WA, van der Schans GS, Nieweg HO. Platelet antibodies in idiopathic thrombocytopenic purpura. *Clin Exp Immunol* 1980;39:645–51

130. Karpatkin S, Garg SK, Freedman ML. Role of iron as a regulator of thrombopoiesis. *Am J Med* 1974;57:521

131. Higby DJ, Cohen JE, Holland JF, Sinks L. The prophylactic treatment of thrombocytopenic leukemic patients with platelets: a double blind study. *Transfusion* 1974;14:440

132. Hackett T, Kelton JG, Powers P. Drug-induced platelet destruction. *Semin Thromb Hemost* 1982;8:116

133. McMillan R, Longmire RL, Tavassoli M, *et al*. *In vitro* platelet phagocytosis by splenic leukocytes in idiopathic thrombocytopenic purpura, *N Engl J Med* 1974:290;249

134. McMillan R, Longmire R, Yelenosky R. The effect of corticosteroids on human IgG synthesis. *J Immunol* 1976;1216:1592

135. Laros RK Jr, Sweet RL. Management of idiopathic thrombocytopenic purpura during pregnancy. *Am J Obstet Gynecol* 1975;122:182

136. Fainstat T. Cortisone-induced congenital cleft palate in rabbits. *Endocrinology* 1954;55:502

137. Schatz M, Patterson R, Zeitz S, *et al*. Corticosteroid therapy for the pregnant asthmatic patient. *J Am Med Assoc* 1975;233:804

138. Reinisch JM, Simon NG, Karow WG, Gandelman R. Prenatal exposure to prednisone in humans and animals retards intrauterine growth. *Science* 1978;202:436

139. Bongiovanni AM, McPadden AJ. Steroids during pregnancy and possible fetal consequences. *Fertil Steril* 1960;11:181

140. Heys RF. Steroid therapy for idiopathic thrombocytopenic purpura during pregnancy. *Obstet Gynecol* 1966;28:532

141. Katz FH, Duncan BR. Entry of prednisone into human milk. *N Engl J Med* 1975;293:1154

142. Jones WR, Storey B, Norton G, Neische FW Jr. Pregnancy complicated by acute idiopathic thrombocytopenic purpura. A report of two patients treated by simultaneous Cesarean section and spleenectomy. *J Obstet Gynaecol Br Commonw* 1974;81:330

143. Ahn YS, Harrington WJ. Treatment of idiopathic thrombocytopenic purpura (ITP). *Ann Rev Med* 1977;28:299

144. MacPherson AIS, Richmond J. Planned spleenectomy in treatment of idiopathic thrombocytopenic purpura. *Br Med J* 1975;1:64

145. DiFino SM, Lachant NA, Kirschner JJ, Gottlieb AJ. Adult idiopathic thrombocytopenic purpura. Clinical findings and response to therapy. *Am J Med* 1980;69:430

146. Kelton JG, Gibbons S. Autoimmune platelet destruction: idiopathic thrombocytopenic purpura. *Semin Thromb Hemost* 1982;8:83

147. Garmel SH, Craigo SD, Morin LM, *et al*. The role of percutaneous umbilical blood sampling in the management of immune thrombocytopenic purpura. *Prenat Diagn* 1995;15:439–45

148. Hohlfeld P, Forestier F, Kaplan C, *et al*. Fetal thrombocytopenia: a retrospective survey of 5 194 fetal blood samplings. *Blood* 1994;84:1851–6

149. Burrows RF, Kelton JG. Fetal thrombocytopenia and its relation to maternal thrombocytopenia. *N Engl J Med* 1993;329:1463–6

150. Samuels P, Bussel J, Braitman LE, *et al*. Estimation of the risk of thrombocytopenia in the offspring of

pregnant women with presumed immune thrombocytopenic purpura. *N Engl J Med* 1990;323:229–35

151. Scott JR, Rote NS, Cruikshank DP. Antiplatelet antibodies and platelet counts in pregnancies complicated by autoimmune thrombocytopenic purpura. *Am J Obstet Gynecol* 1983;145:932–9

152. Burrows RF, Kelton JG. Low fetal risks in pregnancies associated with idiopathic thrombocytopenic purpura. *Am J Obstet Gynecol* 1990;163:1147–50

153. Christiaens GCML, Nieuwenhuis HK, Von Dem Borne AEGK, *et al*. Idiopathic thrombocytopenic purpura in pregnancy: a randomized trial on the effect of antenatal low dose of corticosteroids on neonatal platelet count. *Br J Obstet Gynaecol* 1990;97:893–8

154. Bussel JB, Christiaens G. Birth platelet counts in sequential newborns of mothers with ITP: do the platelet counts change with subsequent babies? *Blood* 1993;82(Suppl 1):202a

155. Yamada H, Fujimoto S. Perinatal management of idiopathic thrombocytopenic purpura in pregnancy: risk factors for passive immune thrombocytopenia. *Ann Hematol* 1994;68:39–42

156. Silver RM, Branch DW, Scott JR. Maternal thrombocytopenia in pregnancy: time for a reassessment. *Am J Obstet Gynecol* 1995;173:479–82

157. Scott JR, Cruikshank DP, Kochenour NK, *et al*. Fetal platelet counts in the obstetric management of immunologic thrombocytopenic purpura. *Am J Obstet Gynecol* 1980;136:495

158. Skupski DW, Bussel JB. Comments on: Silver RM, Branch DW, Scott JR. Maternal thrombocytopenia in pregnancy: time for a reassessment. *Am J Obstet Gynecol* 1996;174:1944–6

159. Scioscia AL, Grannum PAT, Copel JA, Hobbins JC. The use of percutaneous umbilical blood sampling in immune thrombocytopenic purpura. *Am J Obstet Gynecol* 1988;159:1066–8

160. McCrae KR, Cines DB. Thrombotic microangiopathy during pregnancy. *Semin Hematol* 1997;34:148–58

161. Rose M, Rowe JM, Eldor A. The changing course of thrombotic thrombocytopenic purpura and modern therapy. *Blood Rev* 1993;7:94–103

162. Weiner CP. Thrombotic microangiopathy in pregnancy and the postpartum period. *Semin Hematol* 1987;24:119–29

163. May HV Jr, Harbert GM, Thornton WN Jr. Thrombotic thrombocytopenic purpura associated with pregnancy. *Am J Obstet Gynecol* 1976;126:452

164. Schwartz ML, Brenner WE. The obfuscation of eclampsia by thrombotic thrombocytopenic purpura. *Am J Obstet Gynecol* 1978;131:18

165. Thiagarajah S, Harbert GM Jr, Caudle MR, Sturgill BC. Thrombotic thrombocytopenic purpura in pregnancy: a reappraisal. *Am J Obstet Gynecol* 1981;141:20

166. Berkowitz LR, Daliforf FG, Blatt PM. Thrombotic thrombocytopenic purpura. *J Am Med Assoc* 1979; 241:1709

167. Moake JL, Rudy CK, Troll JH, *et al*. Unusually large plasma factor VIII: von Willebrand factor multimers in chronic relapsing thrombotic purpura. *N Engl J Med* 1982;307:1432–5

168. Thorp JM, White GC, Moake JL, Bowes WA. Von Willebrand factor multimeric levels and patterns in patients with severe preeclampsia. *Obstet Gynecol* 1990;75:163

169. Byrnes JJ, Khurana M. Treatment of thrombotic thrombocytopenic purpura with plasma. *N Engl J Med* 1977;297:1386

170. Hayward CPM, Sutton DMC, Carter WH, *et al*. Treatment outcomes in patients with adult thrombotic thrombocytopenic purpura – hemolytic uremic syndrome. *Arch Intern Med* 1994;154:982–7

171. Bowie EJW, Owens CA Jr. Hemostatic failure in clinical medicine. *Semin Hematol* 1977;14:341

172. Lian E C-Y, Harkness DR, Byrnes JJ, *et al*. Presence of a platelet aggregating factor in the plasma of patients with thrombotic thrombocytopenic purpura (TTP) and its inhibition by normal plasma. *Blood* 1979; 53:333

173. Upshaw JD Jr. Congenital deficiency of a factor in normal plasma that reverses microangiopathic hemolysis and thrombocytopenia. *N Engl J Med* 1978; 298:1350

174. Byrnes JJ, Moake JL, Klug P, Periman P. Effectiveness of the cryosupernatant fraction of plasma in the treatment of refractory thrombotic thrombocytopenic purpura. *Am J Hematol* 1990;34:169–74

13

Invasive hemodynamic monitoring in obstetrics

G.D.V. Hankins

INTRODUCTION

The flow-directed pulmonary artery catheter transformed what had previously been limited to the cardiac catheterization and research laboratories into a clinical instrument available at the woman's bedside for ongoing monitoring of cardiovascular status and function[1]. Information obtained from its use can facilitate diagnosis, management and evaluation of therapeutic decisions. Often, clinical impressions can be reinforced or refuted with accurate hemodynamic measurements in critically ill women. The indications for the use of invasive hemodynamic monitoring are much the same in obstetrics as in any other area of medicine[2] and it is reasonable to expect that similar results can be gained from its use in pregnant women[3]. Moreover, understanding of the pathophysiology of many conditions unique to obstetrics, such as pulmonary edema associated with the use of β-agonists and the hemodynamics of pre-eclampsia/eclampsia, have been significantly advanced by invasive cardiovascular monitoring[4–8].

VENOUS ACCESS

Venous access for invasive monitoring is usually obtained via the internal or external jugular vein or the subclavian vein. The femoral and antecubital veins are used less frequently because of greater difficulty in positioning the catheter. Additionally, use of the inguinal area in obstetrics may limit access to and manipulation of the catheter at critical times such as during delivery. Under certain conditions, however, such as those involving a patient with a coagulopathy, the antecubital approach may be prudent in order to avoid the possibility of an intrathoracic bleed. In such cases venous access may be easier to achieve by venous cut down as opposed to percutaneous cannulation of the vessel.

The majority of the complications of invasive hemodynamic monitoring relate to two factors: (1) gaining venous access; and (2) the experience and skill of the operator. In gaining venous access the Seldinger technique or a modification of this technique is recommended. After an inquiry as to allergies, the site selected is prepared and draped in a sterile fashion.

The operator is gowned and gloved for gaining venous access and for positioning the pulmonary artery catheter. If the internal jugular approach is selected, the patient is positioned and their head tilted below the horizontal and asked to turn their head to the side opposite the vessel selected for cannulation. With the use of 1% xylocaine and a 21 or 22 gauge 2-inch needle the skin is injected and a wheal made over the carotid artery. The needle is then directed into the patient's neck and towards the ipsilateral nipple at a 45° angle, aspirating for blood as a tract towards the vessel is anesthetized (Figure 1). Often the vein walls will be collapsed, one against the other, by the pressure of the needle, and the vessel is completely penetrated

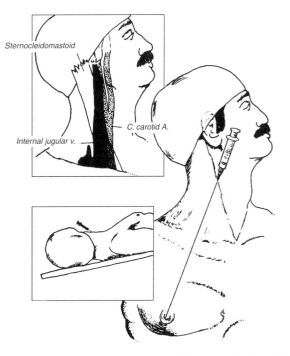

Figure 1 Use of the modified Seldinger technique for vessel cannulation. The technique uses sequentially larger caliber needles for vessel localization, wiring the vessel and finally passing a vein dilator and catheter port over the wire. Emphasis is on avoidance of trauma to the patient or her vessel

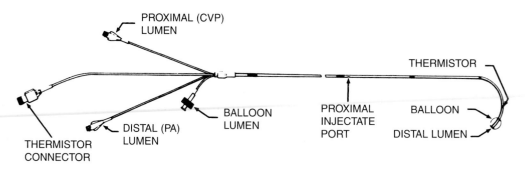

Figure 2   Diagram of a flow-directed pulmonary artery catheter

without blood return. Accordingly, if a tract of the entire length of the needle has been anesthetized and no blood has returned, the operator should slowly withdraw the needle, maintaining a small amount of negative pressure on the syringe. If free-flowing blood returns, the needle should be disconnected from the syringe and left free in the patient's neck to serve as a guide for recannulation of the vessel with a larger bore catheter. Failure to achieve blood return merits repositioning the patient and further attempts – each time redirecting the angle by approximately 5° medial or lateral to the prior attempt. Once the vessel is located, an 18-gauge needle can be used to recannulate it, following which a vascular wire is passed into the vessel. The wire should pass freely and without resistance, and should *never* be withdrawn through the cutting edge of the needle for fear of severing the wire. After the wire is passed into the vessel the needle is withdrawn over the wire. A scalpel is used to make a 3–4 mm cut about the wire, following which the larger 7.5- or 8-F vascular access catheter is passed, with the assistance of a vein dilator, over the wire. The wire and dilator are then withdrawn and ready withdrawal of blood through the catheter introducer should be able to be achieved. If doubt exists as to whether the blood is arterial or venous, blood gas analysis can be performed.

CATHETER ANATOMY

The standard flow-directed thermodilution pulmonary artery catheter (Figure 2) includes a distal lumen at the catheter tip, a proximal lumen 30 cm from the catheter tip, a balloon lumen and a thermistor. The distal lumen provides continuous pulmonary artery pressure measurements when the balloon is deflated, and pulmonary capillary wedge pressures when the balloon is inflated. The proximal port can be used to monitor central venous pressure or to administer fluids or drugs. Both the proximal and the distal lumina of the catheter may be used to withdraw samples of venous blood for laboratory studies. Cardiac output and central core temperature can be measured if the pulmonary artery catheter is used in conjunction with a thermodilution cardiac output computer. Catheters

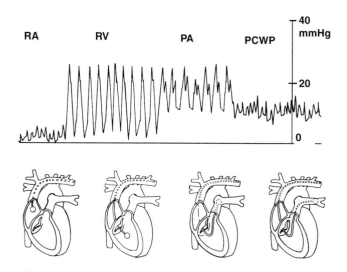

Figure 3 Pressure waveforms observed on an oscilloscope as the pulmonary artery catheter passes through the right atrium (RA), right ventricle (RV) and pulmonary artery (PA), to the pulmonary capillary wedge position (PCWP)

are available with additional ports through which medication can be given. The small size of these ports renders them ineffective for rapid acute infusion of large volumes of fluid or blood. Fiberoptic pulmonary artery catheters are also increasingly used in critically ill patients, in whom, in conjunction with a bedside microprocessor and strip chart recorder, they can provide a continuous reading of the patient's mixed venous oxygen saturation. The standard adult pulmonary artery catheter is 7 FR and will require a 7.5-FR venous introducer, whereas the fiberoptic catheters are 7.5 FR and require an 8.0-FR introducer.

The pulmonary artery catheter is directed into position by venous return to the heart. Its passage is reflected indirectly by pressure waveforms viewed on an oscilloscope that are characteristic of the specific heart chambers (Figure 3). Continuous electrocardiographic monitoring is necessary during catheter positioning to observe for ventricular ectopia and arrhythmias. Prior to catheter insertion the proximal and distal lumina should be flushed and purged of air and the balloon checked for symmetrical inflation, absence of an air leak and ease of spontaneous deflation. The catheter is next advanced through an introducer at the venous access site. The balloon is inflated after insertion of approximately 15 cm of the catheter. If resistance to balloon inflation is encountered, the catheter should be advanced further into the vessel and a repeat attempt made at inflation. This will usually be successful, as the caliber of the vessels increase as the catheter is advanced centrally. As the balloon-tipped catheter is carried along by venous blood flow, the chest cavity is entered, and a low-amplitude pressure tracing is obtained demonstrating respiratory variation, i.e. pressure falls with inspiration and rises with expiration. Continued advancement of the catheter tip into the right ventricle results in a spiking waveform whose baseline is 0 mmHg. Subsequently, as the pulmonary artery is entered, another spiking waveform of lower amplitude is identifiable, measuring diastolic pressures above 0 mmHg. The next waveform obtained, a damped tracing with respiratory variation, is the pulmonary capillary wedge pressure. If the balloon is deflated, a pulmonary artery tracing reappears. A true pulmonary capillary wedge pressure is verified by (1) conversion of a pulmonary artery pressure tracing to a pulmonary capillary wedge pressure tracing when the balloon is inflated; (2) the presence of respiratory variation in the pressure tracing; and (3) a calculated mean pulmonary artery pressure higher than the pulmonary capillary wedge pressure.

The ability to obtain accurate tracings over prolonged periods can be enhanced by the use of two devices which are particularly useful in situations that mandate catheter repositioning. A catheter introducer system containing a one-way valve allows a malfunctioning catheter to be advanced, withdrawn, or changed without loss of the venous access. Additionally, sheaths are available which fit over the catheter itself and attach to the introducer port. The sheaths maintain sterility of a segment of the pulmonary artery catheter, allowing its advancement or withdrawal as necessary to obtain accurate pressure tracings. Routine chest radiography to verify catheter positioning is not necessary if the insertion was uncomplicated and the surgeon is certain the chest cavity was not entered. Verification of proper positioning of the pulmonary artery catheter is dependent upon obtaining a high-quality and appropriate pressure tracing, and not by chest radiograph.

DATA COLLECTION

Continuous central venous and pulmonary artery pressures and intermittent pulmonary capillary wedge pressure measurements are afforded directly by use of the pulmonary artery catheter. Cardiac output can be measured as necessary by the thermodilution technique. Both the heart rate and the rhythm are observed through the use of continuous electrocardiographic monitoring. Systemic arterial pressure can be measured by manual or automatic sphygmomanometer or percutaneous arterial catheterization; the latter also readily provides access for arterial blood sampling and analysis. Mean pressure values are of clinical significance and can be determined for both the pulmonary arterial and the systemic circulations by electronic dampening of the respective tracing, or they can be calculated by the following equation:

$$\text{Mean pressure} = [\text{systolic pressure} + 2(\text{diastolic pressure})]/3$$

The pulmonary capillary wedge pressure, a damped pressure tracing, has a mean value that is the arithmetic average of its maximum and minimum deflections on the oscilloscope. Although oscilloscopic readings are usually adequate for clinical management, strip chart recordings are recommended when dealing with complex waveforms, such as may be encountered with mitral valvular disease, or with data collection for clinical research. If marked respiratory variations exist, these pressures should be read directly from the oscilloscope or the strip chart recorder, since reliance on the digital display will underestimate the wedge pressure if the patient is spontaneously breathing, and overestimate it if positive pressure ventilation is being used.

Various other hemodynamic values that reflect cardiac function and vascular resistance can be calculated or derived (Table 1). Stroke volume is a measure of the

Table 1 Formulas for deriving various hemodynamic parameters

Stroke volume (SV) (ml/beat)

SV = CO/HR

Stroke index (SI) (ml/beat/m²)

SI = SV/BSA

Cardiac index (CI) (l/min/m²)

CI = CO/BSA

Pulmonary vascular resistance (PVR) (dynes × s × cm⁻⁵)

PVR = [(MPAP − PCWP)/CO] × 80

Systemic vascular resistance (SVR) (dynes × s × cm⁻⁵)

SVR = [(MAP − CVP)/CO] × 80

Conversion factor: 1 mmHg/l l/min = 80 dynes × s × cm⁻⁵

BSA, body surface area (m²); CO, cardiac output (l/min); CVP, central venous pressure (mmHg); HR, heart rate (beats/min); MAP, mean systemic arterial pressure (mmHg); MPAP, mean pulmonary artery pressure (mmHg); PCWP, mean pulmonary capillary wedge pressure (mmHg)

Table 2 Central hemodynamic changes

	Non-pregnant	*Pregnant*
Cardiac output (l/min)	4.3 ± 0.9	6.2 ± 1.0
Heart rate (beats/min)	71 ± 10.0	83 ± 10.0
Systemic vascular resistance (dynes × s × cm⁻⁵)	1530 ± 520	1210 ± 266
Pulmonary vascular resistance (dynes × s × cm⁻⁵)	119 ± 47.0	78 ± 22
Colloid oncotic pressure (mmHg)	20.8 ± 1.0	18.0 ± 1.5
Colloid oncotic pressure – pulmonary capillary wedge pressure (mmHg)	14.5 ± 2.5	10.5 ± 2.7
Mean arterial pressure (mmHg)	86.4 ± 7.5	90.3 ± 5.8
Pulmonary capillary wedge pressure (mmHg)	6.3 ± 2.1	7.5 ± 1.8
Central venous pressure (mmHg)	3.7 ± 2.6	3.6 ± 2.5
Left ventricular stroke work index (g × min × m⁻²)	41 ± 8	48 ± 6

amount of blood pumped per contraction by the heart. Both the cardiac output and the stroke volume may be corrected for body size by division of the values by body surface area to obtain cardiac index and stroke index. Resistance to flow can be calculated from right and left ventricles through determinations of the pulmonary vascular resistance and systemic vascular resistance, respectively. Pulmonary shunts and arterial–venous oxygen content differences are calculated by analyses of simultaneously obtained samples of mixed venous blood (drawn from the distal port of the pulmonary artery catheter) and arterial blood. Normal values for healthy non-pregnant and pregnant subjects are given in Table 2[9].

INTERPRETATION OF DATA

Cardiac function

In an assessment of cardiac function, four areas are addressed: preload; afterload; contractile or inotropic state of the myocardium; and heart rate[10–15].

Preload

Preload is determined by intraventricular pressure and volume, thus setting the initial myocardial muscle fiber length. Clinically the right and left ventricular end-diastolic filling pressures are assessed by central venous pressure and pulmonary capillary wedge pressure, respectively. A plotting of cardiac output against central venous pressure or pulmonary capillary wedge pressure gives a cardiac function curve for the right or left ventricle (Figure 4). The ventricular function curve demonstrates that a failing heart requires a higher preload or filling pressure to achieve the same cardiac output as a normally functioning heart (Figure 5). Therapeutic manipulation of the ventricular filling pressures and simultaneous measurement of cardiac output allows calculation of the optimal preload, i.e. the construction of a Starling ventricular function curve at the patient's bedside. The preload can be increased by the administration of crystalloid, colloid,

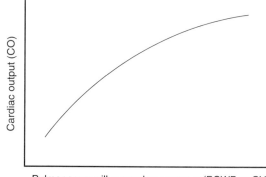

Figure 4 Ventricular function (Starling) curve for the normal heart. Pulmonary capillary wedge pressure (PCWP) or central venous pressure (CVP) represents fiber length, and cardiac output (CO) represents fiber shortening

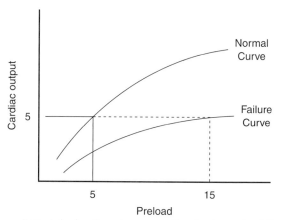

Figure 5 Ventricular function curve for the heart in failure. In order to maintain cardiac output (CO), the failing heart is required to function at higher preloads (pulmonary capillary wedge pressure or central venous pressure)

or blood and can be decreased by the use of a diuretic, a vasodilator, or by phlebotomy.

Afterload

Afterload is defined as the ventricular wall tension during systole and is dependent on the end-diastolic radius of the ventricle, the aortic diastolic pressure and the ventricular wall thickness[16]. The extent to which the right or left intraventricular pressure rises during systole depends primarily on the pulmonary or systemic vascular resistance (Figure 5). In the presence of heart failure, increases in afterload worsen the degree of failure by decreasing both the stroke volume and the cardiac output (Figure 6).

Afterload, like preload, can be increased or decreased therapeutically as mandated by the clinical setting. Increases in afterload are mediated through modulation of the α-adrenergic system; phenylephrine is an agent with almost pure α-agonist effects. Decreases in afterload or systemic vascular resistance can be achieved with numerous agents[17]. Sodium nitroprusside, by continuous intravenous infusion, is used most commonly to decrease afterload in the intensive care setting, while hydralazine is the agent most commonly used in obstetrics. The intermittent intravenous administration of small, incremental doses of hydralazine, without continuous arterial pressure monitoring, has been proved safe for both mother and fetus. Sodium nitroprusside and nitroglycerine infusions should not be used, however, unless intra-arterial blood pressure monitoring has been instituted. Additionally, the potential for fetal cyanide toxicity exists when nitroprusside is used[18,19]. It has been recommended arbitrarily that antepartum use be limited to 30 minutes.

Contractile or inotropic state of the heart

This is defined as the force and velocity of ventricular contractions when preload and afterload are held constant. While cardiac output can be measured directly, its adequacy must be assessed indirectly from acid–base status, arterial–venous oxygen content differences, mixed venous oxygen content or saturation, and urinary output. In low-output cardiac failure both preload and afterload should be optimized through therapeutic manipulation. If this fails to restore the cardiac output to an acceptable level, attention should be directed to improving myocardial contractility. β-Sympathomimetics, such as dopamine and isoproterenol, are effective in improving cardiac output acutely. Depending on the cause of myocardial failure, either short-term or long-term therapy with digitalis may be necessary.

Heart rate

Heart block is rare in pregnant women, but cardiac output can be compromised if the heart rate is too slow. In this circumstance, either treatment with atropine or cardiac pacing is indicated. Conversely, sustained tachycardia can lead to congestive heart failure due to shortened systolic ejection and diastolic filling times or myocardial ischemia, especially in the clinical setting of valvular heart disease. The pathophysiological basis of tachycardia should be determined and corrected (fever, hypovolemia, pain, hyperthyroidism). Treatment with propranolol, digoxin, or a calcium channel blocker such as verapamil is seldom required in obstetric patients; however, when indicated, all can prove effective in limiting heart rate.

Mixed venous blood analysis

Fiberoptic pulmonary artery catheters and bedside microprocessors now make continuous plotting of the mixed venous blood oxygen saturation possible. It has been shown that the mixed venous oxygen content may fall well before any other evidence of hemodynamic instability is manifest, making this potentially useful as an early warning system[20,21].

Traditionally mixed venous blood samples have been analyzed much the same as arterial blood samples: intermittently and often paired with an arterial specimen. As with arterial blood, mixed venous blood can be analyzed for oxygen tension (PvO_2, in millimeters of mercury) and for saturation (SvO_2, in percentage). Ultimately mixed venous blood saturation reflects the balance between oxygen delivery and oxygen utilization. It reflects tissue perfusion, the variation in oxygen requirements of different organs, and the affinity of hemoglobin for acceptance and subsequent release of oxygen. The normal value for PvO_2 is 40 mmHg with an average saturation of 73%, saturations below 60% being abnormally low[21]. Pericapillary interstitial fluid pO_2 is 10–20 mmHg and intracellular pO_2 is estimated to be 6 mmHg. To maintain an adequate intravascular to interstitium to

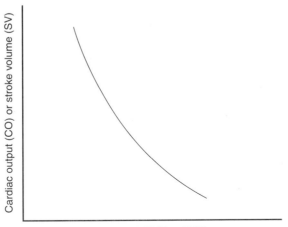

Figure 6 Relationship of afterload (systemic vascular resistance or pulmonary vascular resistance) to cardiac output (CO) or stroke volume (SV) at a constant preload

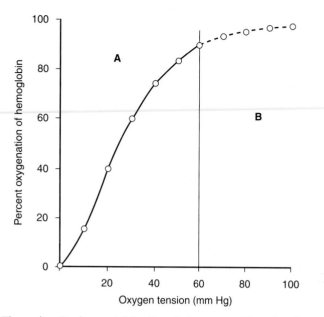

Figure 7   Oxyhemoglobin dissociation curve. Note that the mixed venous oxygen saturations operate on the 'dissociation' or linear phase of the curve and are very sensitive to physiological instability

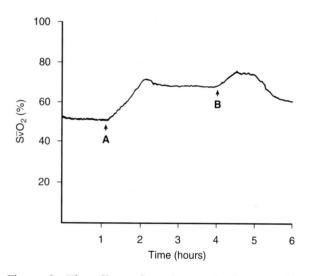

Figure 8   The effects of sepsis on mixed venous blood oxygen saturation (SvO_2). At point A the cardiac output has already increased disproportionately to oxygen utilization even before the patient has clinically apparent infection, resulting in an increase in SvO_2. At point B the patient develops rigors with a further increase in both cardiac output and SvO_2

cellular gradient requires a minimal capillary pO_2 of 30 mmHg. Values below this result in impaired oxygen delivery and anaerobic metabolism. In humans, unconsciousness accompanies a PvO_2 of less than 20 mmHg and irreversible brain damage occurs below 12 mmHg[22,23].

The advantages of continuous monitoring of mixed venous blood saturation, as opposed to arterial blood saturation, are many. First, arterial blood samples will almost always have a saturation of 90% or greater, corresponding to a pO_2 of 60–100 mmHg or greater. Because of the shape of the hemoglobin dissociation curve (Figure 7), fluctuations at these higher levels of oxygen tension are reflected by very small corresponding changes in saturation. Conversely, at the lower levels of oxygen present in venous blood a linear relationship exists between saturation and tension, making it a sensitive test for detection of physiological instability. Second, although an arterial blood analysis provides useful information concerning pulmonary oxygen exchange, ventilation and shunt, it provides little information regarding the overall adequacy of oxygen delivery to peripheral tissues. Because the mixed venous gas reflects the end product of supply and demand, it is superior in this respect. Finally, the addition of a thermodilution cardiac output, in conjunction with a mixed venous gas, can support or refute clinical assumptions made on the basis of the mixed venous oxygen saturation. For example, improvement of mixed venous oxygen saturation with a stable cardiac output is a good prognostic sign and heralds clinical improvement. If however, the same change in the mixed venous oxygen saturation is accompanied by a 100% increase in cardiac output, it may simply be the first sign of sepsis.

Continuous monitoring of SvO_2 has been advocated for titration of vasoactive and inotropic drugs, adjustment of positive end-expiratory pressure, evaluation of fluid therapy, routine patient care and an early warning system for changes in cardiorespiratory status. In Figure 8 the effect of sepsis on SvO_2 is demonstrated. Because the rise in cardiac output exceeds the increase in tissue oxygen demands, SvO_2 increases even before clinical sepsis is apparent (Figure 8, point A). Shortly before and during rigors (Figure 8, point B) a further increase is noted. Another patient care scenario, the titration of 'optimal or best' positive end-expiratory pressure using SvO_2, is demonstrated in Figure 9. Incremental increases in positive end-expiratory pressure at points A and B resulted in airway recruitment, decreased shunt and improved oxygen delivery. At point C, however, more positive end-expiratory pressure resulted in a fall in venous return and a fall in cardiac output with a proportional fall in oxygen delivery, reflected in a declining SvO_2. At point D, the amount of positive end-expiratory pressure is reduced, venous return increases and both cardiac output and SvO_2 improve. Thus, the SvO_2 can be a very simple and efficient method to define best positive end-expiratory pressure.

Pregnancy results in physiological alterations of the mixed venous blood gas. Because the increase in cardiac output exceeds the increase in oxygen utilization,

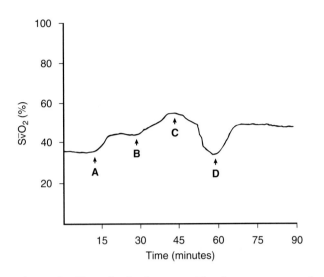

Figure 9 Use of mixed venous blood oxygen saturation (SvO$_2$) to select the best positive end-expiratory pressure

the PvO$_2$ and SvO$_2$ both normally increase[24]. During labor, however, both will be abnormally low if measured during contractions due to the return of desaturated venous blood from the uterus, placenta and lower extremities. Between contractions, however, they will again be abnormally high relative to non-pregnant levels[25].

Few data are available on the use of this relatively new technology in pregnant women. We anticipate, however, that continuous monitoring of mixed venous oxygen saturation may be particularly useful in women who develop the adult respiratory distress syndrome (ARDS) or who have a very prolonged illness and time spent in an intensive care unit.

Pulmonary edema – heart or lung?

The greatest utility of invasive hemodynamic monitoring in obstetrics may lie in differentiation of the pulmonary edema of heart failure (hydrostatic pulmonary edema) from that of lung failure (permeability pulmonary edema)[26], for only after the correct diagnosis has been made can therapy be optimized.

McHugh and colleagues[27] have correlated radiographic findings of pulmonary edema with absolute pulmonary capillary wedge pressure in patients with myocardial infarction. Pulmonary congestion is apparent first at a pressure of 18 mmHg, is mild to moderate at 18–25 mmHg, and is moderate to severe at 20–30 mmHg. Development of frank pulmonary edema at a pulmonary capillary wedge pressure above 30 mmHg was noted. This model represents pure hydrostatic pulmonary edema secondary to left ventricular failure or acute volume overload. In pulmonary edema of this origin, therapy should be directed at improving myocardial contractility and reducing the preload to a high-normal range.

Pulmonary edema can also result from damage to the pulmonary alveolar capillary membrane by any of a host of insults, ranging from sepsis (most common) to hypersensitivity reactions mediated by non-HLA leukoagglutinins at the time of blood transfusion[28–31]. In this model, there is a disturbance of membrane permeability resulting in the flux of both protein and water into the pulmonary interstitium and the alveolus despite normal cardiac function and filling pressures. Unlike the situation in hydrostatic or pressure-induced pulmonary edema, which resolves within a few hours after normal pulmonary capillary wedge pressure is restored, alveolar membrane lesions require days to heal. This process may eventuate in the adult respiratory distress syndrome without eradication of the source of the injury, e.g. a focus of infection leading to septic emboli. The therapeutic goals in pulmonary edema due to permeability defects are (1) to maintain filling pressures in the lower-normal range to minimize transudation of protein and fluid into the lungs; and (2) to eradicate the source of injury.

To illustrate these concepts, let us consider the hypothetical case of a pregnant woman with premature labor who is being treated with intravenous ritodrine. On initial presentation she was treated with bedrest and hydrated with 2 l of normal saline, but had continued contractions. Now, despite high doses of intravenous ritodrine, her contractions are increasing in intensity and frequency and her cervix is progressively dilating. Eighteen hours into ritodrine therapy acute dyspnea develops and physical findings are consistent with pulmonary edema. Concomitantly the patient's temperature is 39°C and now, for the first time, uterine tenderness is elicited. Any of a number of factors could account for this edema: (1) sepsis with alveolar membrane injury; (2) heart failure secondary to the β-agonist ritodrine, i.e. hydrostatic pulmonary edema; or (3) iatrogenic volume overload causing hydrostatic pulmonary edema. The diagnosis and management of patients such as this may be enhanced by invasive hemodynamic monitoring with precise knowledge of myocardial function and filling pressures.

CARDIOVASCULAR MONITORING AND OBSTETRICS

Currently, the flow-directed pulmonary artery catheter is used in obstetrics in (1) the management of critically ill patients or those at risk for sudden cardiovascular decompensation; and (2) clinical investigations that attempt to define the pathophysiology of various disease processes or evaluate therapy of a specific condition.

Obstetric patients with cardiac or pulmonary complications who are critically ill or whose condition is subject to rapid deterioration[2,3,8] are essentially the same patients who would receive invasive cardiovascular monitoring in medical or surgical intensive care units. Management of patients with severe sepsis complicated by hypotension or oliguria[8] and of those with heart failure or pulmonary edema of unclear etiology certainly might be aided by placement of a pulmonary artery catheter[32]. Women with sudden intraoperative cardiovascular decompensation also are candidates for hemodynamic monitoring. For example, the diagnosis of amniotic fluid embolism is facilitated by the demonstration of pulmonary hypertension and a high degree of pulmonary shunting. Additionally, fetal squamous cells or amniotic fluid debris might be obtained in smears of blood aspirated from the pulmonary artery[33]. Similarly, patients with massive blood loss and large transfusion requirements (e.g. with placental abruption or uterine rupture) benefit from invasive monitoring, particularly in the face of oliguria or pulmonary edema.

Another group of high-risk obstetric patients for whom invasive hemodynamic monitoring of labor and delivery affords a margin of safety are those with chronic cardiovascular disease. Patients with significant structural lesions or physiological disturbances of the heart or great vessels, in addition to those with symptoms from compromised cardiac status, are at risk for peripartum decompensation. Included in this group at high risk for cardiac decompensation are all patients with New York Heart Association functional class III or IV. Particularly dangerous structural or physiological disturbances include primary pulmonary hypertension, Eisenmenger's physiology, aortic coarctation and mitral stenosis[33–35]. More precise assessment of their baseline condition, both early in pregnancy to assess the risk of continuing the pregnancy and during labor and delivery, as well as prompt evaluation of complications and subsequent therapeutic decisions, should favorably affect both management and outcome.

Patients with coronary artery disease manifested by angina or a history of myocardial infarction should also be monitored invasively during labor, delivery and the early postpartum period[36]. Similarly, women with a cardiomyopathy should be monitored irrespective of the cause of the cardiac lesion[37]. Additional high-risk patients include those with uncontrolled hyperthyroidism or pheochromocytomas in the predelivery or perioperative period.

SUMMARY

The development of the flow-directed pulmonary artery catheter in the early 1970s moved invasive monitoring from the laboratory to the patient's bedside. Its current use in obstetrics is directed towards definition of certain pathophysiological states unique to pregnancy and towards diagnosis and management of critically ill or potentially critically ill patients.

REFERENCES

1. Swan HJC, Ganz W, Forrester J, *et al*. Catheterization of the heart in man with use of a flow-directed balloon-tipped catheter. *N Engl J Med* 1970;283:447
2. Hankins GDV. *Techniques and Principles of Invasive Hemodynamic Monitoring in Obstetrics and Gynecology*. ACOG Technical Bulletin no.121. Washington DC: American College of Obstetricians and Gynecologists, 1988
3. Clark SL, Horenstein JM, Phelan JP, *et al*. Experience with the pulmonary artery catheter in obstetrics and gynecology. *Am J Obstet Gynecol* 1985;152:374
4. Benedetti TJ, Hargrove JC, Rosene KA. Maternal pulmonary edema during premature labor inhibition. *Obstet Gynecol* 1982;59:335
5. Clark SL, Cotton DB. Clinical Opinion: Clinical indications for pulmonary artery catheterization in the patient with severe pregnancy-induced hypertension. *Am J Obstet Gynecol* 1988;158:453–8
6. Hauth JC, Hankins GDV, Kuehl TJ. Ritodrine hydrochloride infusion in pregnant baboons. I. Biophysical effects. *Am J Obstet Gynecol* 1983;146:916
7. Hankins GDV, Wendel GD, Cunningham FG, Leveno KJ. Longitudinal evaluation of hemodynamic changes in eclampsia. *Am J Obstet Gynecol* 1984;150:506
8. Lee W, Clark SL, Cotton DB, *et al*. Septic shock during pregnancy. *Am J Obstet Gynecol* 1988;159:410–16
9. Clark SL, Cotton DB, Lee W, *et al*. Central hemodynamic assessment of normal term pregnancy. *Am J Obstet Gynecol* 1989;161:1439–42
10. Braunwald E. Regulation of the circulation (Part I). *N Engl J Med* 1974;290:1124
11. Braunwald E. Regulation of the circulation (Part II). *N Engl J Med* 1974;290:1420
12. Mason DT, Spann JF Jr, Zelis R, *et al*. Alterations of hemodynamics and myocardial mechanics in patients with congestive heart failure. Pathophysiologic mechanisms and assessment of cardiac function and ventricular contractility. *Progr Cardiovasc Dis* 1970;12:507
13. Soonenblick EH, Parmley WW, Ursch ICS, *et al*. Ventricular function: evaluation of myocardial contractility in health and disease. *Progr Cardiovasc Dis* 1970;12:449
14. Herman MV, Gorlin RV. Implications of left ventricular asynergy. *Am J Cardiol* 1969;23:538
15. Braunwald E. On the difference between the heart's output and its contractile state (Editorial). *Circulation* 1971;43:171–4
16. Lappas DG, Powell WM, Daggett WM. Cardiac dysfunction in the perioperative period. Pathophysiology, diagnosis and treatment. *Anesthesiology* 1977;47:117
17. Cohn JN, Franciosa JA. Vasodilator therapy of cardiac failure. *N Engl J Med* 1977;297:247
18. Strauss RG, Keefer JR, Burke T, Civetta JM. Hemodynamic monitoring of cardiogenic pulmonary edema complicating toxemia of pregnancy. *Obstet Gynecol* 1980;55:170–4
19. Naulty JS, Cefalo R, Rodkey FL. Placental transfer and fetal toxicity of sodium nitroprusside. Presented at the *Annual Meeting of the American Society of Anesthesiology*, San Francisco, 1976;abstr.543

20. Divertie MG, McMichan JC. Continuous monitoring of mixed venous oxygen saturation. *Chest* 1984;85:423–8

21. Schmidt CR, Frank LP, Estafanous FG. Utility of continuous pulmonary artery oximetry as an early warning monitor in cardiac surgery patients. Presented at the *5th Annual Meeting, Society of Cardiovascular Anesthesiologists*, San Diego, April 1983

22. Gibbs FA, Williams D, Gibbs EL. Modification of the cortical frequency spectrum by changes in CO_2, blood sugar, and O_2. *J Neurophysiol* 1940;3:49–58

23. Thews G. Die sauerstoff diffusion im gehirn. Ein beitrag zur frage sauerstoff diffusion der organe. *Pfluger's Arch Gens Physiol* 1960;271:197–226

24. Kerr MG. Maternal cardiovascular adjustments in pregnancy and labour. In Goodwin JW, Godden JO, Chance GW, eds. *Perinatal Medicine: The Basic Science Underlying Clinical Practice*. Baltimore: Williams & Wilkins, 1976:395–408

25. Ueland K, Hansen JM. Maternal cardiovascular dynamics. II. Posture and uterine contractions. *Am J Obstet Gynecol* 1969;103:1

26. Rinaldo JE, Rogers RM. Adult respiratory distress syndrome. Changing concepts of lung injury and repair. *N Engl J Med* 1982;206:900

27. McHugh TJ, Forrester JS, Alder L, *et al*. Pulmonary vascular congestion in acute myocardial infarction: hemodynamic and radiologic correlations. *Ann Intern Med* 1972;76:29

28. Petty TL. Adult respiratory distress syndrome. *Semin Respir Med* 1982;3:219

29. Anderson RR, Holliday RL, Driedger AA, *et al*. Documentation of pulmonary capillary permeability in the adult respiratory distress syndrome accompanying human sepsis. *Am Rev Respir Dis* 1979;119:869

30. Trambaugh RF, Lewis FR, Christensen JM, *et al*. Lung water changes after thermal injury – the effects of crystalloid resuscitation and sepsis. *Ann Surg* 1980;192:479

31. Thompson JS, Severson CD, Parmely MF. Pulmonary hypersensitivity reactions induced by transfusion of non-HL-A leukoagglutinins. *N Engl J Med* 1971;284:1120

32. Cunningham FG, Lucas MJ, Hankins GDV. Pulmonary injury complicating ante-partum pyelonephritis. *Am J Obstet Gynecol* 1987;156:797

33. Clark SL, Montz FJ, Phelan JP. Hemodynamic alterations in the patient with amniotic fluid embolism: a reappraisal. *Am J Obstet Gynecol* 1985;151:617

34. Clark SL, Phelan JP, Greenspoon J, *et al*. Labor and delivery in the presence of mitral stenosis: central hemodynamic observations. *Am J Obstet Gynecol* 1985;152:984–8

35. Hankins GDV, Brekken AL, Davis LM. Maternal death secondary to a dissecting aneurysm of the pulmonary artery. *Obstet Gynecol* 1985;65:45S

36. Hankins GDV, Wendel GD, Leveno KJ, Stoneham J. Myocardial infarction during pregnancy. A review. *Obstet Gynecol* 1985;65:139

37. Cunningham FG, Pritchard JA, Hankins GDV, *et al*. Peripartum heart failure: a specific pregnancy-induced cardiomyopathy or the consequence of coincidental compounding cardiovascular events? *Obstet Gynecol* 1986;67:157

14

Postpartum hemorrhage

P. Tropper

Postpartum hemorrhage accounts for 4% of all maternal deaths, comprising one-third of maternal deaths due to bleeding[1]. The traditional definition of postpartum hemorrhage is blood loss of more than 500 ml after a vaginal delivery and more than 1000 ml after Cesarean section[2]. Visual estimates of blood loss, which typically underestimate the true amount, are used to determine if bleeding is excessive. The incidence of hemorrhage is approximately 6% after vaginal delivery[3] and 4% after Cesarean section[4], although two-thirds of all obstetric transfusions are given during Cesarean delivery[5]. As uterine blood flow in the peripartum period represents one-fifth of total cardiac output, hemorrhage may be rapid and blood loss massive. Ten per cent of hemorrhages are identified as severe, i.e. associated with hypotension, blood loss of more than 1000 ml or a decrease in hemoglobin of 3 g[6]. One-quarter of these are due to delayed postpartum hemorrhage, i.e. bleeding more than 24 h after delivery. In recent years, the management of postpartum hemorrhage has been dramatically affected by changes in pharmacological treatment, specifically the use of prostaglandin analogs, as well as increasing use of pelvic arterial embolization under fluoroscopic guidance. These management techniques have limited the need for surgical intervention to a very small percentage of cases. Unfortunately, the high overall number of Cesarean sections may be producing a group of obstetric patients who will have an increased incidence of placenta accreta and an increased risk of postpartum hemorrhage.

Normal hemostasis postpartum depends on the ability of the uterus to contract effectively and for normal coagulation mechanisms to occur. Most institutions routinely use oxytocics after delivery, which effectively reduce postpartum blood loss by enhancing uterine contractility[7]. In all cases, following the third stage of labor, the patient should be evaluated for uterine firmness, the presence of cervical or vaginal lacerations and amount of bleeding. When bleeding is greater than normal, identification of excessive blood loss and initiation of appropriate resuscitative measures must be prompt. In all cases of postpartum hemorrhage, attention must be given to volume resuscitation (with the use of two large-bore intravenous lines), monitoring of vital signs and urine output, and blood transfusion as needed. While initial use of crystalloids (3 ml/ml of blood loss) and plasma volume expanders (such as Hespan) are appropriate, reluctance to transfuse should not preclude replacement of blood loss with whole blood or packed cells (preferable) when necessary. With the exception of some experimentally available agents, such as perfluorocarbons, none of the volume expanders can replace blood in terms of its oxygen-carrying capacity. Consideration may be given to the use of autologous donations of blood in the third trimester from patients considered to be at high risk for peripartum hemorrhage. These may be safely obtained during pregnancy. However, the use of autologous donations is limited; less than 2% of patients with identifiable risk criteria subsequently require transfusion and when bleeding does occur, the transfusion of multiple units of blood is often necessary[8]. All bleeding patients should be managed as being at risk for shock, including, in the most severe cases or when transfer of the patient is necessary, the use of a G (MAST) suit inflated to 25–40 mmHg[9] or aortic compression[10] when indicated, until the bleeding can be controlled and the patient stabilized.

UTERINE ATONY

The most common cause of postpartum hemorrhage is uterine atony, accounting for approximately 75% of all cases[11]. Several factors have been identified as predisposing to bleeding from atony, including: delivery of a macrosomic infant, multiple gestation, prolonged first or second stage of labor, antepartum use of magnesium sulfate, use of halogenated anesthetic agents and grand multiparity. The use of oxytocin for labor induction or augmentation is associated with a higher incidence of postpartum hemorrhage but this is probably due to the indications for its use rather than being a primary effect[3,12].

The onset of heavy bleeding after completion of the third stage of labor may be initially managed as uterine atony while further evaluations and resuscitative measures are performed. Bimanual uterine massage and intravenous oxytocin should be initiated. Oxytocin is given in dilute solutions of 40 units per liter of isotonic solution. Infusion of undiluted oxytocin as an intravenous bolus may precipitate acute hypotension even in relatively low doses. Oxytocin may be given directly into the myometrium but there is no evidence that this is more effective than intravenous administration. If the uterus still fails to contract adequately, methergine 0.2 mg intramuscularly should be administered if the patient has no history of hypertension.

If bleeding is not controlled at this point, prior to further intervention, the presumptive diagnosis of uterine atony must be confirmed. First, retained products of conception, uterine rupture and uterine inversion must be ruled out by examination under anesthesia and gentle curettage when necessary. Factors which might predispose to uterine rupture include: traumatic delivery, use of forceps, internal version and presence of a uterine scar. Retained portions of placenta or difficulty removing the placenta may suggest the presence of placenta accreta. Adequate anesthesia and operative assistance are essential to thoroughly examine the cervix and vaginal walls and to rule out lacerations as the primary source of bleeding. Normal coagulation processes may be rapidly ascertained by evaluating puncture sites and by performing a bedside clotting test while more specific coagulation parameters are obtained.

After thorough assessment, if uterine atony is the cause of hemorrhage, prostaglandin $F_{2\alpha}$(Hemabate) is the agent of choice. This may be administered intramuscularly or intramyometrially (directly through the abdominal wall after normal delivery). Although there is no clear advantage to the latter, it has been suggested that onset of action may be more rapid (5 min) with intramyometrial compared to intramuscular injection (45 min)[13]. The dosage is 0.25–0.50 mg in 5 ml normal saline repeated at 30–90-min intervals to a total maximum dose of 15 mg. The overall success rate in controlling hemorrhage is 85% with most patients responding within one or two doses. The majority of failures are attributable to the presence of chorioamnionitis or placenta accreta[6,14]. Complications of prostaglandin $F_{2\alpha}$ include bronchospasm, hypertension, fever, vomiting and oxygen desaturation. Decreases in oxygen saturation by 10% following injection of prostaglandin F have led to the recommendation that all patients receiving prostaglandin should be monitored with pulse oximetry[15].

Prostaglandin E has also been used effectively to increase uterine contractility and decrease hemorrhage, but its vasodilatory effect may result in severe hypotension in these already volume-depleted patients[16]. Intrauterine infusions via Foley catheter of dilute prostaglandin E solutions (1.5 µg/ml in Ringers' lactate) have been effectively used with no serious side-effects[17].

If medical therapy fails, surgical intervention in a timely fashion is necessary. It should not be delayed until the patient is so compromised that resuscitation is not possible. Prior to surgery, the patient is positioned in a semi-dorsolithotomy position so that the effect of intervention on bleeding may be monitored by observing vaginal blood loss. Bilateral uterine artery ligation may be attempted first. The arteries are ligated with chromic suture but not divided. An area of myometrium should be incorporated into the suture to avoid tearing and the suture should be placed high enough to avoid bladder or ureteral injury. Bilateral uterine artery ligation is effective in over 80% of postpartum hemorrhages. Failures are usually associated with placenta previa or accreta or in the presence of coagulation defects[18,19]. Recanalization of the vessels and normal pregnancies have followed bilateral uterine artery ligation. If uterine atony and hemorrhage persist, hysterectomy is probably necessary and should not be delayed in the face of continued significant blood loss. Ligation of the utero-ovarian vessels, bilateral hypogastric artery ligation or uterine packing may be considered prior to hysterectomy but are probably more effective when postpartum hemorrhage is due to other causes. The same applies to pelvic artery embolization which would be limited in the presence of uterine atony as the bleeding is not limited to a specific indentifiable vessel. In addition, unless hemorrhage has been anticipated, there may be a significant delay before invasive radiology techniques are available for any given patient.

PLACENTA ACCRETA

Placenta accreta is usually recognized when a manual attempt is made to remove a retained placenta. Difficulty is encountered in finding a smooth plane between the placenta and the uterus. More and more, ultrasound is helping us in making this diagnosis before delivery. On ultrasound examination, one can identify large vascular spaces, an inability to see an interface between placenta and uterine wall and, occasionally, even blood flow through the aberrant vessels which penetrate the myometrium. (In such cases, preoperative placement of angiography catheters for use in embolizing pelvic vessels to control hemorrhage should be considered.) The incidence of placenta accreta is increasing as the number of patients with previous Cesarean sections increases. This complication, as well as bleeding from the lower uterine segment (associated with placenta previa) is initially managed using uterotonic agents. When this fails, however, other techniques may be attempted. Uterine packing has been used with good results[20]. Uterine packing had lost favor as a technique but recent reports suggest that there is a role for packing in controlling postpartum hemorrhage. Because it is theoretically unphysiological (packing does not allow the uterus to decrease its volume), careful observation is warranted. In addition, while the pack is in place, it may conceal large volumes of blood loss behind the packing. With these reservations in mind, it has, nonetheless, been used in many instances successfully to avoid surgical intervention[21,22] or to decrease blood loss before surgical or other interventions (e.g. radiological embolization) can take place.

If these techniques fail, hysterectomy or an attempt at bilateral uterine artery or hypogastric artery ligation (depending on the extent of placental invasion) are appropriate. If the patient is unstable, hysterectomy may be more rapidly performed to control bleeding. Supracervical hysterectomy has been used to shorten operative time in the very unstable patient.

CERVICAL OR VAGINAL LACERATIONS AND HEMATOMA

Lacerations of the vagina or cervix are less common causes of massive hemorrhage. They can, however, result in large volumes of blood loss which may be underestimated if hematoma are developing and extending into the broad ligament. Vaginal or vulvar hematoma should be evacuated and, if the site of bleeding can be identified, the injury repaired by suture ligation. The vagina may then be packed for further compression of the bleeding site or, if the bleeding is from the perineum, sandbags may be used for compression.

If hemorrhage is massive or if bleeding sites cannot be locally repaired, consideration should be given to techniques of invasive radiology to assist in the management of the hemorrhage. Introduction of a catheter via the femoral vessels and pelvic angiography are likely to identify the source of bleeding as an extravasation of contrast material. Blood loss of 2 ml/min is necessary for angiographic detection. When bleeding can be identified, pelvic embolization may be performed using small pieces (1 mm) of gelatin sponge particles (gelfoam), polyvinyl alcohol or metallic springs[23,24]. The gel particles dissolve in 7–10 days. This technique can be used to occlude the uterine vessels, or if a more specific bleeding site is seen, a particular vessel. It has been used successfully for many types of postpartum hemorrhage[9,25]. As with surgical techniques, unless a specific vessel can be identified as the source of bleeding, embolization must be done bilaterally. This technique is particularly helpful when bleeding occurs after a vaginal delivery. In these instances, embolization may avoid laparotomy in an already compromised patient. Attempting embolization after some of the pelvic vessels have already been ligated makes the technique more difficult to apply. Possible complications of embolization include sciatic and femoral neuropathies and gluteal pain.

If surgery does become necessary, bilateral hypogastric artery ligation should be attempted. Identify and ligate the anterior division of the hypogastric arteries bilaterally. The main purpose of ligation is to decrease pulse pressure and allow normal coagulation to occur. Pulse pressure is decreased 77% if unilateral ligation is performed, and 85% if bilateral ligation is undertaken[26]. Blood flow to injured areas is not totally reduced, owing to the large collateral circulation in the pelvis. Immediate complications of hypogastric artery ligation are injury to the hypogastric vein or ureter. Delayed complications are similar to those identified after pelvic artery embolization of these vessels, as noted above. Normal pregnancies have been reported following bilateral hypogastric artery ligation.

COAGULATION DISORDERS

Bleeding postpartum may be a manifestation of an inherited or acquired coagulation defect. In the evaluation of bleeding, if there is evidence of a coagulopathy (poor bedside clotting test or bleeding from other sites), the patient may be empirically treated with fresh frozen plasma to restore coagulation factors until more specific results can be obtained. The most common inherited coagulation disorder present in pregnant women is Von Willebrand's disease. In over half the pregnancies, primary or secondary (delayed) postpartum hemorrhages are reported. Women who are carriers of hemophilia A or B may also have significant bleeding associated with 10% of their pregnancies. Bleeding may occur despite the normal increase in factor VIII seen during pregnancy and in some cases despite cryoprecipitate treatment[27,28]. In cases in which cryoprecipitate is given, postpartum hemorrhage may be delayed. Desmopressin may be appropriate therapy in the presence of these coagulation disorders.

Acquired coagulation problems are most likely due to the presence of placental abruption, pre-eclampsia/eclampsia, amniotic fluid embolus, retained dead fetus, massive transfusion or idiopathic thrombocytopenic purpura. Coagulation problems which occur as a result of multiple transfusions are more often due to thrombocytopenia than to loss of coagulation factors[29]. Therefore, there is no need to routinely transfer plasma when multiple transfusions have been given. Treatment of disseminated intravascular coagulation in the postpartum period primarily involves resolution of the primary problem and then supportive measures. When necessary, plasma or cryoprecipitate may be used.

DELAYED HEMORRHAGE

Delayed postpartum hemorrhage is defined as bleeding between 24 h and 6 weeks postpartum. Bleeding may be severe and sudden in onset. Causes include subinvolution with resultant uterine atony, retained products of conception, endometritis, dissolution of suture material after operative delivery, and congenital coagulation disorders. Initially the patient should be managed as someone with early postpartum hemorrhage using resuscitation techniques and uterotonic agents. Antibiotics should be administered as well if there is any sign of infection. Patients should undergo curettage only if the above measures fail, since only half of patients with postpartum hemorrhage have retained placental tissue and curettage in the remaining group of patients will only make bleeding worse. Ultrasound is not helpful in discriminating which patients have retained tissue, as clots in the uterine cavity can mimic placental fragments[30].

Effective management of postpartum hemorrhage requires early identification of the problem, appropriate use of anesthesia for thorough evaluation and an awareness of the various pharmacological, surgical and radiological techniques available. Appropriate initial measures and then flexibility in management as the situation evolves are essential to ensure the patient's safety and optimal future health.

REFERENCES

1. Kaunitz AM, Hughes JM, Grimes DA, *et al*. Causes of maternal mortality in the United States. *Obstet Gynecol* 1985;65:605–12

2. Pritchard JA, Baldwin RM, Dickey JC, *et al*. Blood volume changes in pregnancy and puerperium. II. Red blood cell loss and changes in apparent blood volume during and following vaginal delivery, cesarean section, and cesarean section plus total hysterectomy. *Am J Obstet Gynecol* 1962;84:1271–82

3. Combs CA, Murphy EL, Laros RK. Factors associated with postpartum hemorrhage with vaginal birth. *Obstet Gynecol* 1991;77:69–76

4. Combs CA, Murphy EL, Laros RK. Factors associated with hemorrhage in cesarean deliveries. *Obstet Gynecol* 1991;77:77–82

5. Kamani A, McMorland G, Wadsworth L. Utilization of red blood cell transfusion in an obstetric setting. *Am J Obstet Gynecol* 1988;159:1177–83

6. Hayashi RH, Castillo MS, Noah ML. Management of severe postpartum hemorrhage with a prostaglandin F2 alpha analogue. *Obstet Gynecol* 1984;63:806–8

7. Prendiville W, Elbourne D, Chalmers IL. The effects of routine oxytocic administration in the management of the third stage of labour: an overview of the evidence from controlled trials. *Br J Obstet Gynaecol* 1988;95:3–16

8. Andres RL, Piacquadio KM, Resnik R. A reappraisal of the need for autologous blood donation in the obstetric patient. *Am J Obstet Gynecol* 1990;163:1551–3

9. Mud HJ, Schattenkerk E, de Vries JE, *et al*. Nonsurgical treatment of pelvic hemorrhage in obstetric and gynecologic patients. *Crit Care Med* 1987;15:534–5

10. Riley D, Burgess R. External abdominal aortic compression: a study of a resuscitation manoeuvre for postpartum haemorrhage. *Anaesth Intensive Care* 1994;22:571–5

11. Weekes LR, O'Toole DM. Postpartum hemorrhage: a five year study at Queen of Angels Hospital. *Am J Obstet Gynecol* 1956;71:45–50

12. Gilbert L, Porter W, Brown VA. Postpartum haemorrhage – a continuing problem. *Br J Obstet Gynaecol* 1987;94:67–71

13. Bigrigg A, Chui D, Chissell S, *et al*. Use of intramyometrial 15-methyl prostaglandin F2 alpha to control atonic postpartum haemorrhage following vaginal delivery and failure of conventional therapy. *Br J Obstet Gynaecol* 1991;98:734–6

14. Buttino L, Garite TJ. The use of 15 methyl F2 alpha prostaglandin (Prostin 15 M) for the control of postpartum hemorrhage. *Am J Perinatol* 1986;3:241–3

15. Hankins GDV, Berryman GK, Scott RT, *et al*. Maternal arterial desaturation with 15-methyl prostaglandin F2 alpha for uterine atony. *Obstet Gynecol* 1988;72:367–70

16. Kilpatrick AWA, Thorburn J. Severe hypotension due to intramyometrial injection of prostaglandin E2. *Anaesthesia* 1990;43:848–9

17. Peyser MR, Kupferminc MJ. Management of severe postpartum hemorrhage by intrauterine irrigation with prostaglandin E2. *Am J Obstet Gynecol* 1990;162:694–6

18. Fahmy K. Uterine artery ligation to control postpartum hemorrhage. *Int J Gynaecol Obstet* 1987;25:363–7

19. O'Leary JA. Uterine artery ligation in the control of postcesarean hemorrhage. *J Reprod Med* 1995;40:189–93

20. Druzin ML. Packing of lower uterine segment for control of postcesarean bleeding in instances of placenta previa. *Surg Gynecol Obstet* 1989;169:543–5

21. Hester JD. Postpartum hemorrhage and reevaluation of uterine packing. *Obstet Gynecol* 1974;45:501–4

22. Maier RC. Control of postpartum hemorrhage with uterine packing. *Am J Obstet Gynecol* 1993;169:317–23

23. Ito M, Matsui K, Mabe K, *et al*. Transcatheter embolization of pelvic arteries as the safest method for postpartum hemorrhage. *Int J Gynaecol Obstet* 1986;24:373–8

24. Yamashita Y, Takahashi M, Ito M, *et al*. Transcatheter arterial embolization in the management of postpartum hemorrhage due to genital tract injury. *Obstet Gynecol* 1991;77:1603

25. Vedantham S, Goodwin SC, McLucas B, *et al*. Uterine artery embolization: an underused method of controlling pelvic hemorrhage. *Am J Obstet Gynecol* 1997;176:938–48

26. Burchell RC. Internal iliac artery ligation: hemodynamics. *Obstet Gynecol* 1964;24:737–9

27. Greer IA, Lowe GO, Walker JJ, *et al*. Haemorrhagic problems in obstetrics and gynaecology in patients with congenital coagulopathies. *Br J Obstet Gynaecol* 1991;98:909–18

28. Foster PA. The reproductive health of women with von Willebrand disease unresponsive to ddavp: results of an international survey. *Thromb Haemost* 1995;74:784–90

29. Consensus conference. Fresh-frozen plasma. *J Am Med Assoc* 1985;253:552–3

30. Lee CY, Maorazo B, Drukker BH. Ultrasonic evaluation of the postpartum uterus in the management of postpartum bleeding. *Obstet Gynecol* 1981;581:227–32

15
Septic shock

P. Duff and K.M. Davidson

EPIDEMIOLOGY

Shock is a severe derangement of the normal circulatory system characterized by decreased cardiac output, decreased tissue perfusion and cellular dysfunction. The three most common types of shock are hypovolemic or hemorrhagic shock, septic shock and cardiogenic shock. Septic shock has increased in incidence in the past decade. In 1988 it ranked 13th among the leading causes of mortality in the USA, accounting for nearly 21 000 deaths[1].

The incidence of bacteremia in obstetric and gynecological patients varies with the source of underlying infection. Bacteremia has been reported in 8–10% of women with chorioamnionitis[2,3], 5–25% of women with endometritis[4] and up to 7% of women with pyelonephritis[5]. In general, the incidence of bacteremia is 7.5 cases/1000 admissions in an obstetric service[6] and 2–7 cases/1000 admissions in a combined obstetrics–gynecology service[7,8]. In an overall hospital population, septic shock complicates 20–50% of bacteremias due to Gram-negative organisms and 5% of those due to Gram-positive organisms[9]. However, in obstetrics and gynecology, the incidence of shock as a complication of bacteremia appears to be lower[6–8].

The prognosis in septic shock is principally determined by host immunocompetence. The underlying disease is an important determinant of prognosis. The severity of the underlying disease has been classified into three categories. Rapidly fatal disease includes acute leukemia and blastic relapse of chronic leukemia. Diseases believed to be fatal within 5 years such as carcinoma with proved metastasis, aplastic anemia and severe renal or liver failure are classified as ultimately fatal. All other disease states not believed to be fatal within 5 years are characterized as non-fatal underlying disease[10–12]. Patients with rapidly fatal, ultimately fatal or non-fatal underlying diseases display progressively lower mortality rates[10–12].

The majority of obstetric patients who develop septic shock fall into the category of 'non-fatal underlying disease'. Mortality for these patients is about 15–20%[10,11,13]. In contrast, the mortality for non-obstetric patients ranges from 50% to 80% because these individuals are much more likely to have underlying debilitating diseases[10].

MICROBIOLOGY

Any organism capable of infecting a human host can cause septic shock. Genital infections are the most likely source of shock in an obstetrics service and are usually caused by a combination of anaerobic and aerobic bacteria. The most common pathogens that cause septic shock in obstetric patients are the aerobic Gram-negative bacilli. Of these bacteria, *Escherichia coli* is the predominant pathogen. *Klebsiella pneumoniae* and *Proteus* species are less frequent causes of infection. *Pseudomonas* and *Serratia* species are uncommon pathogens except in immunocompromised gynecological oncology patients. Approximately 20% of obstetric patients with sepsis have a polymicrobial bacteremia[14].

PREDISPOSING FACTORS

In obstetric patients, the principal entities that predispose to septic shock are post-Cesarean endomyometritis, infected abortion, acute pyelonephritis and, in rare instances, acute chorioamnionitis[13]. Other causes include instrumentation of the genitourinary tract, such as chorionic villus sampling[15]. In gynecological patients the condition most likely to be associated with septic shock is ruptured tubo-ovarian abscess.

PATHOPHYSIOLOGY

Septic shock is characterized by a complex series of derangements in the cellular and humoral immune systems, coagulation cascade and sympathetic nervous system that, together, lead to multiorgan failure and, ultimately, cardiovascular collapse. The initial stimulus for these pathophysiological alterations is endotoxin, a complex lipopolysaccharide that is present in the cell wall of Gram-negative bacteria. The critical component of endotoxin is a substituent termed lipid A[16]. Upon destruction of the bacterial cell wall, endotoxin is released into the host's circulation. Once in the bloodstream, endotoxin initiates the progression of changes summarized in Figure 1.

Tumor necrosis factor

Cytokines are members of a large family of endogenous proteins or glycoproteins that are released by

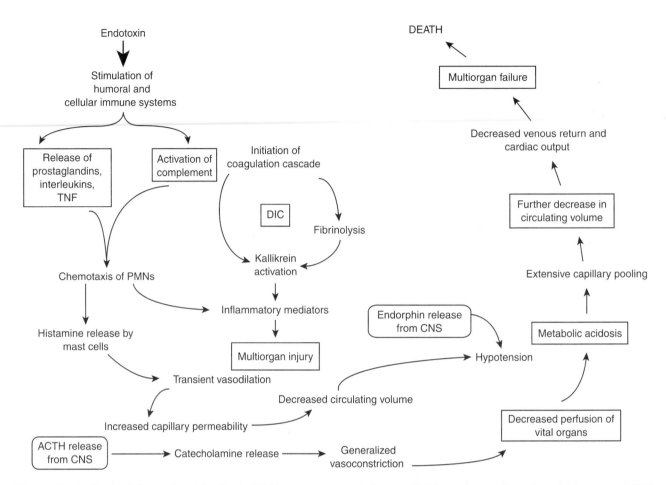

Figure 1   Pathophysiology of septic shock. TNF, tumor necrosis factor; PMNs, polymorphonuclear leukocytes; ACTH, adrenocorticotropic hormone; CNS, central nervous system; DIC, disseminated intravascular coagulation

host cells and mediate the function of diverse target cells. One cytokine that plays a critical role in septic shock is tumor necrosis factor (TNF), also known as cachectin. TNF is a 17-kDa polypeptide that functions as a 'second messenger' for endotoxin. Macrophage stimulation by endotoxin initiates RNA transcription and translation and release of TNF. Through direct feedback on the macrophage, TNF then triggers the release of interleukin 1 (IL-1), an endogenous pyrogen that may be responsible for the fever that often accompanies bacteremia.

Prostaglandin activation

Together, IL-1 and TNF initiate production of eicosanoids through the action of cyclooxygenase on arachidonic acid (Figure 2). Prostacyclin causes vasodilatation and hypotension, and thromboxane A_2 incites platelet aggregation, microthrombus formation and vascular damage. Leukotrienes, which are products of the lipoxygenase pathway, attract and activate polymorphonuclear leukocytes and thereby cause increased vascular permeability.

Activation of the coagulation cascade

One of the other important effects of endotoxin and TNF is activation of Hageman factor (XII), which initiates the intrinsic clotting cascade[17]. Hageman factor also directly activates factor VII, thus stimulating the extrinsic coagulation pathway. Activation of the coagulation system leads to concurrent activation of the fibrinolytic system. Plasmin, the active component of the latter system, then acts on Hageman factor to produce fragments termed prekallikrein activators[18]. These substances convert prekallikrein to kallikrein. Kallikrein causes conversion of plasminogen to plasmin and also directly activates Hageman factor. This sequence of events results in enhanced coagulation and accelerated fibrinolysis and precipitates the phenomenon of disseminated intravascular coagulation (DIC). Another major effect of kallikrein activation is the production of a variety of inflammatory mediators such as hydrogen peroxide, free radicals and bradykinin. These substances cause intense inflammatory injury to vital organs.

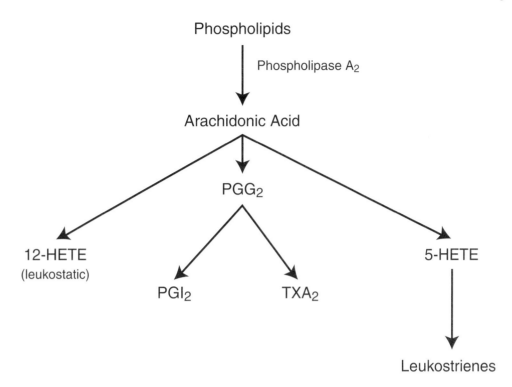

Figure 2 Prostaglandin pathway. 12-HETE, 12-hydroxyeicosatetraenoic acid; 5-HETE, 5-hydroxyeicosatetraenoic acid; PGG_2, prostaglandin G_2; PGI_2, prostacyclin; TXA_2, thromboxane A_2

Activation of the complement system

Endotoxin also activates the complement cascade through the classic and alternate (properdin) pathway and by direct activation of the first component of complement. There are three major effects of complement activation. First, C_{5a} and the $C_{5,6,7}$ complex interact to exert a chemotactic effect, promoting migration of leukocytes into injured tissue. Second, leukocytes release a variety of inflammatory mediators termed leukotrienes[19]. As noted previously, these substances cause vasoconstriction and increased vascular permeability in the postcapillary venules. They also accelerate neutrophil chemotaxis and aggregation, resulting in release of hydrolytic enzymes and superoxides. Progressive vascular injury results in platelet aggregation, release of thrombogenic platelet factors and intensification of the coagulation cascade.

Components C_{3a} and C_{5a} interact to cause degranulation of mast cells and release of histamine. Histamine causes disruption of endothelial integrity, resulting in an increase in capillary permeability, decrease in plasma volume, vasodilatation and hypotension[17]. In response to this initial state of hypotension, the host's heart rate and cardiac output increase and peripheral resistance decreases. In this early stage of sepsis, the patient appears warm, flushed and maximally vasodilated. For this reason septic shock is often referred to as 'warm shock'[20–23].

Activation of the sympathetic nervous system

The initial vasodilatation and decreased peripheral resistance are usually transient. As sepsis evolves, intense activation of the sympathetic nervous system occurs as catecholamines are released from peripheral nerves and the adrenal medulla. This sympathetic discharge causes generalized vasoconstriction in virtually every vascular bed. Vasoconstriction is intensified by the local effects of prostaglandins released from injured endothelial tissue[24].

The most serious effect of generalized vasoconstriction is marked diminution in perfusion of vital organs, resulting in localized tissue hypoxia and acidosis and, ultimately, in systemic metabolic acidosis. As acidosis evolves, there is a marked change in circulatory hemodynamics, characterized by relaxation of smooth muscle in the wall of arterioles and constriction of smooth muscle in the wall of venules. This process leads to extensive pooling in most capillary beds, increased hydrostatic pressure and transudation of intravascular fluid into the extravascular space[17,25–27]. Generalized capillary pooling causes significant decrease in effective circulating blood volume with resultant decrease in venous return to the heart and progressive decrease in cardiac output and systemic blood pressure.

In addition to decreased venous return, at least three other factors contribute to impaired myocardial contractility. First, circulating β–endorphins are significantly increased. These peptides are released from the pituitary gland along with adrenocorticotropic hormone (ACTH) in response to stress. Their principal hemodynamic effects are to lower blood pressure and decrease heart rate[28–30]. Second, endotoxin itself has a direct depressant effect on myocardial contractility. Third, several studies have identified the presence of a specific shock factor, termed myocardial depressant factor (MDF), which apparently is released into the circulation as shock develops. MDF is a glycopeptide with a molecular weight of 500–1000. The most important biological effect of MDF is depression of myocardial contractility. It also enhances vasoconstriction within splanchnic blood vessels, thus accelerating its own production, and directly depresses the phagocytic capacity of the reticuloendothelial system, resulting in impaired clearance of lysosomal enzymes and MDF from the circulation. Other substances that have been implicated as myocardial depressant agents are leucine, cathepsin D and prostaglandins[20,31].

As cardiac output initially begins to fall, local regulatory mechanisms attempt to preserve perfusion of the coronary and cerebral vascular beds. However, if the hemodynamic changes precipitated by septicemia are not corrected, there is progressive diminution in cardiac output and, ultimately, compromise of both coronary and cerebral blood flow. Maintenance of cardiac output correlates directly with ultimate survival[21].

Respiratory failure

Endotoxemia also causes profound derangement in the host's respiratory physiology (Figure 3). Endotoxin directly damages the endothelium of the pulmonary vasculature. As disruption of capillaries occurs, platelets adhere to fragments of exposed collagen. The intrinsic coagulation cascade is activated, resulting in microembolization and stasis of blood flow in the pulmonary microcirculation[17]. Prostaglandins are released from platelets and injured endothelium and cause pulmonary vasoconstriction. The net effect of these processes is profound impairment of pulmonary perfusion, ischemia and progressive injury to the vascular endothelium. Cerebral ischemia resulting from hypotension intensifies pulmonary vasoconstriction.

Endothelial injury also leads to activation of the complement cascade. Increased serum concentration of C_{5a} is a useful predictor of subsequent development of adult respiratory distress syndrome (ARDS)[32]. Complement activation causes damage to the lung by enhancing leukocyte migration into the pulmonary parenchyma. Leukocytes, in turn, release inflammatory mediators that injure the lung. The activity of the proteolytic enzyme elastase is increased in bronchoalveolar lavage obtained from patients with ARDS[33].

Continued inflammation results in increased capillary permeability, transudation of protein-rich fluid into the interstitium and alveolar space, and destruction of surfactant[34]. The functional consequences of these events are extensive atelectasis, perfusion–ventilation imbalance, decreased compliance, interstitial and intra-alveolar edema, severe hypoxemia and, ultimately, respiratory failure.

Other effects of endotoxin

Endotoxin adheres to the cell membrane of circulating leukocytes, causing these cells to be removed from the circulation by reticuloendothelial cells in the spleen. Therefore, the early shock state may be distinguished by neutropenia. As cell-mediated immunological defenses are mobilized, however, rebound leukocytosis usually ensues[17]. This rebound effect, of course, does not occur in immunosuppressed patients, precisely those at greatest risk for developing septic shock.

Endotoxin also exerts a prominent effect on the temperature-regulating center of the hypothalamus. In the early phase of sepsis, the hypothalamic center may be depressed, resulting in hypothermia. As shock evolves, however, the principal effect of endotoxin is activation of the hypothalamic center and elevation of body temperature, an effect mediated by an endogenous pyrogen, probably IL-1, released from host leukocytes.

CLINICAL MANIFESTATIONS

Early recognition and diagnosis of septic shock are essential. Without rapid institution of supportive measures, shock may prove fatal within 36–48 h of onset. Shock may progress through three stages: (1) primary (reversible), early 'warm hypotensive' phase; (2) primary, late 'cold hypotensive' phase; and (3) secondary (irreversible) phase[13].

The initial manifestations of the early phase of primary shock are restlessness, anxiety, disorientation and temperature instability, which may first present as hypothermia and then progress to hyperthermia. A hyperdynamic state is present initially. Cardiac output, myocardial oxygen consumption and oxygen utilization by peripheral tissue are increased, and total peripheral resistance is decreased. Cardiac output is increased at this stage due to compensatory tachycardia, yet loss of contractility and resultant myocardial depression have already begun[20]. The pulse pressure and urinary output remain adequate.

As the patient enters the late phase of primary shock, she may become less apprehensive and alert. Intense generalized vasoconstriction occurs. Hypotension, tachycardia, tachypnea and oliguria ensue, as there is a transition to a hypodynamic cardiac state. Finally, in secondary irreversible shock, cellular hypoxia and a shift to anaerobic metabolism occur, resulting in

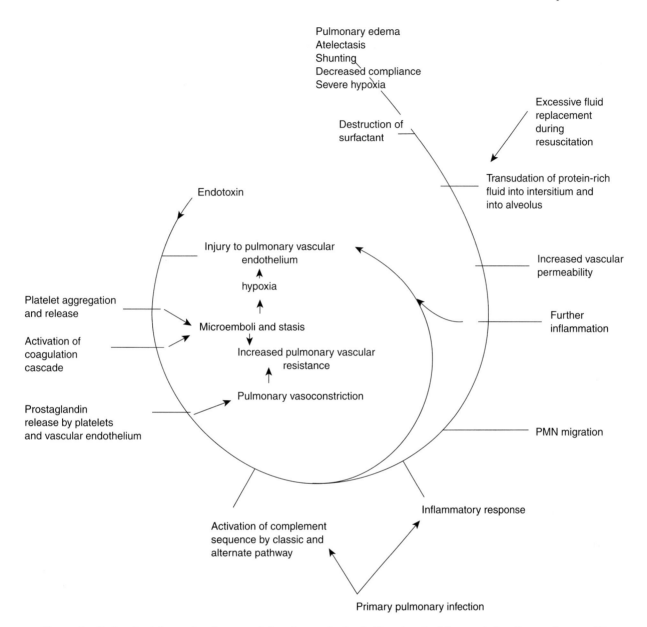

Figure 3 Pathophysiology of pulmonary injury in septic shock. Reprinted with permission from reference 20

an unremitting metabolic acidosis. Myocardial dysfunction is manifested by tachycardia, arrhythmia, myocardial ischemia and, ultimately, biventricular failure and refractory hypotension[13].

ARDS develops in up to 50% of patients with septic shock[35]. The usual clinical signs are tachypnea, dyspnea, stridor and central cyanosis. Examination of the chest demonstrates dullness to percussion, decreased tactile and vocal fremitus, diminished breath sounds and prominent rales throughout both lung fields.

Other clinical manifestations of septic shock may include hematuria, pyuria, oliguria, jaundice, nausea and vomiting. Spontaneous hemorrhage from the gastrointestinal or genitourinary tracts or bleeding from venipuncture sites indicate the presence of a coagulopathy. These prominent clinical findings are summarized in Table 1[36].

DIAGNOSIS

Several important clinical entities must be differentiated from septic shock (Table 2). The diagnosis can be established by thorough history, physical examination, laboratory testing, radiographic examination and hemodynamic monitoring.

Examination of the abdomen and pelvis is important in establishing the primary site of infection and in

Table 1 Target organ effects in septic shock. Adapted from reference 36

Organ system	Clinical and laboratory findings
Brain	confusion, obtundation
Hypothalamus	thermal instability
Cardiovascular	myocardial depression, arrhythmias, tachycardia, hypotension
Lungs	tachypnea, arteriovenous shunting, hypoxia
Gastrointestinal	vomiting, diarrhea
Liver	increase in SGOT, SGPT and bilirubin
Kidney	oliguria, azotemia
Hematopoietic	hemoconcentration, thrombocytopenia, leukopenia, leukocytosis, DIC

SGOT, serum glutamic–oxaloacetic transaminase; SGPT, serum glutamic–pyruvic transaminase DIC, disseminated intravascular coagulation

Table 2 Differential diagnosis of septic shock

Acute adrenal insufficiency
Amniotic fluid embolism
Aortic dissection
Cardiac tamponade
Cardiogenic shock
Diabetic ketoacidosis
Hemorrhagic pancreatitis
Hypovolemic shock
Pulmonary embolism
Thyroid storm

Table 3 Laboratory evaluation of patients with septic shock

Test	Result	Cause
White blood cell count	initially decreased subsequently increased	splenic sequestration granulocytosis
Hematocrit	variable	varies with plasma volume and degree of hemolysis
Platelet count	decreased	DIC
Fibrinogen	decreased	DIC
Fibrin degradation products	increased	DIC
PT, PTT	prolonged	DIC, liver failure
pH	initially increased subsequently decreased	respiratory alkalosis metabolic and respiratory acidosis
Lactic acid	increased	anaerobic metabolism
Arterial pO_2	decreased	respiratory failure
Arterial pCO_2	increased	respiratory failure
HCO_3	decreased	metabolic acidosis
Potassium	increased	acidosis, renal failure

DIC, disseminated intravascular coagulation

identifying other organ systems compromised by the shock state. Physical examination of the upper abdomen should include a careful search for hepatobiliary disease such as cholecystitis or ascending cholangitis, renal parenchymal disorders such as acute pyelonephritis or perinephric abscess and intestinal obstruction. Septicemia may also result from surgical complications such as ureteral injury, wound infection, necrotizing fasciitis and evisceration.

The finding of generalized peritonitis should direct attention to problems such as perforated viscus, appendicitis, diverticulitis, or inflammatory bowel disease. Palpation of enlarged and tender pelvic viscera or a pelvic mass suggests the possibility of disorders such as septic abortion, chorioamnionitis, endomyometritis, ruptured uterus and pelvic abscess.

Many abnormalities in laboratory results are evident early in the course of septic shock (Table 3). Initially, the white blood cell count may be decreased due to sequestration of neutrophils in the spleen. Neutropenia is usually followed by a prominent leukocytosis as demargination of leukocytes from peripheral reserves and release of immature granulocytes from the bone marrow ensues. The hematocrit may be decreased if acute blood loss accompanies sepsis or if DIC has begun. Alternatively, the hematocrit may be increased as a result of decreased circulating plasma volume.

A variety of coagulation abnormalities commonly occur. As DIC develops, the prothrombin and activated partial thromboplastin times become prolonged. Serum fibrinogen often falls, but the size of the decrease depends on the balance between consumption and acute phase synthesis. The serum concentration of fibrin degradation products increases, liver dysfunction worsens and shock progresses. Decreased concentrations of factor XII and antithrombin III contribute to the coagulopathy.

Acid–base abnormalities are prominent in septic shock. Respiratory alkalosis resulting from hyperventilation is often the first change. Metabolic acidosis quickly follows as hypoxia, cellular dysfunction and a shift to anaerobic metabolism occur. Decreased hepatic clearance of lactate accentuates the lactic acidemia. Hyperkalemia may develop as intracellular potassium effluxes from the cell in exchange for hydrogen ions.

Renal function often deteriorates as ischemic injury ensues. Oliguria and azotemia mark the loss of renal function. Hyperkalemia resulting from acidosis worsens as sodium–potassium exchange in the renal tubules fails.

Liver function abnormalities become apparent as multiple organ system failure continues. Serum bilirubin levels rise as a result of hepatocellular dysfunction and hemolysis. Serum transaminases and alkaline phosphatase levels also increase.

Blood cultures are essential to establish the diagnosis of sepsis. At least two aerobic and anaerobic blood cultures should be obtained during the initial evaluation of the patient. Hypertonic blood culture media or culture systems with antibiotic-removal devices can be used to increase the sensitivity of the culture if antibiotics were given prior to obtaining the cultures[37]. In patients receiving parenteral hyperalimentation or immunosuppressive drugs, blood specimens also should be cultured for fungal organisms.

Because blood cultures may be negative in more than 60% of patients diagnosed with septic shock[38], microbiological cultures of operative and local sites must be obtained to identify the primary site of infection and the invading organism. A sample of urine should be obtained from the indwelling catheter for microscopic examination and culture. Sputum culture and Gram stain are indicated in patients who have pneumonia. Transbronchial brush biopsy or open-lung biopsy may be necessary to establish the diagnosis of fungal or *Pneumocystis carinii* pneumonia.

A limited number of radiographic studies are indicated in evaluating the patient with septic shock. A chest radiograph is helpful in detecting the presence of pneumonia, septic pulmonary emboli, pulmonary edema and ARDS (Figure 4). Immediate recognition of the latter disorder is essential, since it so adversely affects the patient's ultimate prognosis.

Radiographs are also helpful in diagnosing intestinal obstruction or perforated viscus. Intravenous pyelography may identify an intraparenchymal or perinephric abscess, ureteral fistula, or ureteral injury. Computerized tomography, magnetic resonance imaging and ultrasonography may aid in delineating a pelvic or abdominal abscess (Figures 5 and 6)[39].

MANAGEMENT

Correction of hemodynamic derangements

Once shock is recognized, treatment with fluid resuscitation and placement of physiological monitors should begin immediately. An arterial line should be inserted to monitor blood pressure and arterial oxygenation, and an indwelling bladder catheter should be placed to measure urine output. Right heart catheterization is required to guide volume replacement and administration of inotropic and vasopressor agents. Central venous monitoring cannot be substituted for right heart catheterization because central venous and pulmonary capillary wedge pressures correlate poorly.

As physiological monitors are being placed, fluid resuscitation should be initiated with an infusion of isotonic crystalloid such as normal saline or lactated

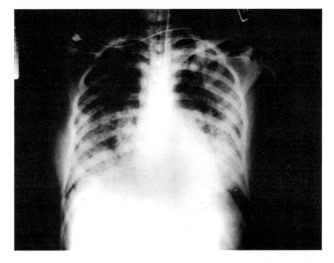

Figure 4   Chest X-ray of a patient with adult respiratory distress syndrome with characteristic bilateral infiltrates reflecting extensive intra-alveolar and interstitial edema. Reprinted with permission from reference 20

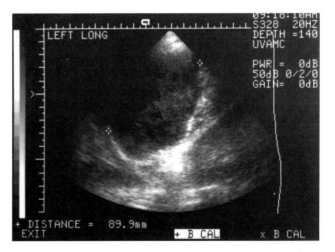

Figure 5   Longitudinal ultrasound scan of left upper quadrant demonstrates subphrenic abscess (A). Photograph courtesy of Patricia Abbitt, MD, Department of Radiology, University of Florida

Ringer's solution. If the patient has experienced acute blood loss, replacement with packed red cells should be given. Initial fluid replacement should be in small increments of 150–200 ml infused over 10 min. Further fluid replacement should be guided by blood pressure, pulse, urine output and myocardial function.

Continued restoration of intravascular volume should be guided by direct measurement of pulmonary capillary wedge pressure. The optimal pulmonary capillary wedge pressure in septic shock is approximately 12 mmHg[40]. Further increases above this level do not result in improved cardiac output and may precipitate or worsen pulmonary edema.

The '7–3' rule is useful for managing fluid replacement in patients with septic shock. Five to 20 ml/min of

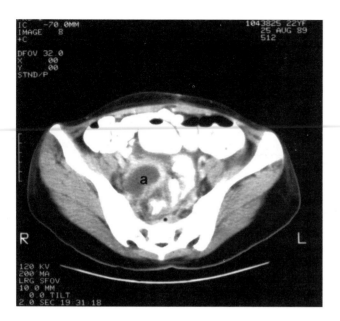

Figure 6 CT scan of pelvis demonstrates well-defined abscess cavity with central lucency (a). Photograph courtesy of Patricia Abbitt, MD, Department of Radiology, University of Florida

fluid is administered for 10 min. If the pulmonary capillary wedge pressure increases more than 7 mmHg above the baseline, the infusion should be discontinued temporarily. If the pulmonary capillary wedge pressure does not increase more than 3 mmHg, the fluid challenge should be repeated and the '7–3' rule applied.

While fluid resuscitation is being initiated, application of a pneumatic antishock garment may result in immediate improvement in cardiac function and tissue perfusion[41]. The antishock garment mobilizes blood that has pooled in the lower portion of the body and returns it to the central circulation. Early use of the garment may decrease the amount of fluid needed for resuscitation, thereby reducing the risk of iatrogenic pulmonary edema. The unit should be deflated gradually as normal perfusion pressure is re-established by intravenous fluid administration.

If tissue hypoperfusion persists after these measures, vasopressor therapy should be initiated to improve myocardial function. Dopamine and dobutamine are the preferred agents in septic shock. These agents increase myocardial contractility and heart rate without causing a disproportionate increase in myocardial oxygen consumption. They may stimulate alpha, beta, or dopaminergic receptors, depending upon the dose (Table 4).

Dopamine is administered by continuous intravenous infusion. Therapy should be initiated at a dose of 2–5 μg/kg/min, and the infusion rate should be increased slowly until the desired hemodynamic response is achieved. At low doses, dopamine stimulates dopaminergic receptors in the renal, mesenteric,

coronary and cerebral circulation to cause vasodilatation. At higher doses, dopamine causes vasoconstriction and decreased tissue perfusion. In doses exceeding 15–20 μg/kg/min, alpha stimulation predominates, leading to a transient increase in cardiac output followed by a sustained decrease in tissue perfusion.

A second inotropic agent, dobutamine, should be added if the desired cardiac function has not been achieved. Dobutamine does not appear to cause the untoward effects associated with dopamine, and it may be a more effective inotropic agent[42]. If a third-line inotropic agent is needed, isoproterenol can be added, but it has the potential side-effects of ventricular ectopy, excessive tachycardia and undesired vasodilatation[43].

Digitalization is indicated in patients with overt congestive heart failure. Initially, a loading dose of digoxin (0.5 mg) should be administered intravenously. Subsequent intravenous doses of 0.25 mg should be given every 4 h until a total dose of 1.0 mg has been administered. A daily maintenance dose in the range of 0.125–0.375 mg/day should then be used to provide a therapeutic serum concentration of 0.5–2.5 ng/ml.

If systemic vascular resistance and cardiac afterload remain low and tissue hypoperfusion persists despite the implementation of the above measures, a vasoconstrictor should be added. Phenylephrine is the agent of choice because it exerts pure α–adrenergic activity. Other vasoconstrictive agents also exert β-mimetic activity, which may cause adverse cardiac effects.

Several experimental modalities have been considered for patients who have refractory hypotension despite volume replacement, inotropic support and vasopressor therapy. Because experimental evidence has shown a role for both β-endorphins and prostaglandins in the pathogenesis of septic shock, treatment with naloxone infusion and prostaglandin synthetase inhibitors has been suggested. There is insufficient evidence at present to recommend routine use of either of these agents in humans. However, in the critically ill patient who has failed vasopressor and inotropic support, naloxone (30 μg/kg initial dose, followed by 30 μg/kg/h by continuous infusion) can be considered[44].

Corticosteroids have also been studied extensively for treatment of severe infections. In several experimental models, pharmacological doses of corticosteroids have been shown to block various steps in the pathogenesis of septic shock. However, several recent clinical trials have demonstrated that steroids do not reduce mortality and may even increase morbidity as a result of superinfection[38,45,46].

Use of intra-aortic balloon counterpulsation has also been reported in gravely ill patients. The principal effects of the aortic balloon are increased diastolic blood pressure, increased coronary blood flow,

Table 4 Pharmacological therapy for septic shock

Drug	Classification	Dose	Receptor	Action
Dopamine	inotrope	2–5 µg/kg/min	dopaminergic	dilatation of renal and mesenteric vasculature
		5–10 µg/kg/min	beta-1	↑ myocardial contractility, stroke volume and cardiac output
		15–20 µg/kg/min	alpha	generalized vasoconstriction
Dobutamine	inotrope	2–10 µg/kg/min	beta-1	↑ cardiac output; mild tachycardia
Isoproterenol	inotrope	1–20 µg/min	beta-1 and -2	↑ contractility ↑ heart rate
Digoxin	cardiac glycoside	0.5 mg loading dose followed by 0.25 mg every 4 h × 2; 0.125–0.375 mg/day to maintain serum digoxin concentration of 0.5–2.5 ng/ml		↑ contractility
Phenylephrine	vasopressor	1–5 µg/kg/min	alpha	vasoconstriction ↑ systemic vascular resistance

decreased afterload, increased cardiac output and increased left ventricular stroke volume index. Therefore, the technique would have greatest application in the hypodynamic phase of septic shock. This therapy remains experimental, however[47,48].

Treatment of infection

Antibiotic therapy should be quickly initiated once cultures have been obtained. Because pelvic infections are polymicrobial, coverage for all potential major pathogens is essential. One acceptable regimen is a combination of penicillin (5 million units every 6 h) or ampicillin (2 g every 6 h), tobramycin or gentamicin (7 mg/kg of ideal body weight every 24 h) and clindamycin (900 mg every 8 h) or metronidazole (500 mg every 12 h). If renal dysfunction is present, aminoglycoside levels should be closely monitored and the dosing interval appropriately adjusted. Alternatively, aztreonam can be used instead of an aminoglycoside.

Imipenem–cilastatin is a bactericidal carbapenem antibiotic which has a wide spectrum of activity. It may be used as a single agent in the treatment of septi shock. The dose is 500 mg every 6 h. An aminoglycoside may be added if *Pseudomonas* infection is suspected. Once cultures identify the invading organism, antibiotic therapy can be more selectively focused.

Adjustments in the antibiotic combinations may be required in certain situations. Immunosuppressed patients who are neutropenic may specifically require coverage for *Pseudomonas* organisms. In such instances, carbenicillin or ticarcillin should be used in conjunction with an aminoglycoside to provide adequate therapy.

If staphylococcal infection is suspected, a semisynthetic penicillin such as nafcillin sodium (2 g every 4–6 h) should be substituted for penicillin. Alternatively, vancomycin (500 mg every 6 h) should be used when infections with methicillin-resistant staphylococci are prevalent. Finally, pentamidine or trimethoprim–sulfamethoxazole may be required to treat *Pneumocystis carinii* infections.

Immunotherapy is a relatively new form of treatment that holds future promise for the treatment of septic shock. Experimental data suggest that passive immunization with antibodies directed against endotoxin or lipopolysaccharide may significantly reduce mortality from septic shock. Ziegler and co-workers[49] have shown that administration of human antiserum to the lipopolysaccharide core significantly reduces mortality in patients with Gram-negative sepsis. However, because this treatment is experimental, routine use cannot be recommended at this time.

In some cases surgical therapy may be required in addition to antibiotic treatment. For example, infected products of conception should be removed by uterine curettage. Devitalized tissue of the abdominal wall or grossly infected pelvic organs also must be resected (Figure 7). Wound abscesses and abdominal and pelvic abscesses must be drained. Indicated surgery should not be delayed even though the patient is unstable, for surgical intervention may be the essential step to stabilize the critically ill patient.

Management of the patient with septic shock due to chorioamnionitis requires special consideration of fetal well-being. Once shock is recognized, cardiovascular support of the mother should be initiated. If the

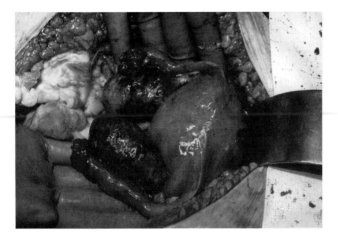

Figure 7   Grossly infected pelvic organs in a patient with Group A streptococcal sepsis. Photograph courtesy of David Soper, MD, Department of Obstetrics and Gynecology, Medical University of South Carolina

parturient's cardiovascular dysfunction does not respond to medical therapy, the fetus should be delivered promptly. If maternal blood pressure, cardiac output and tissue perfusion improve, trial of labor is acceptable provided that the fetus is monitored continuously. Immediate delivery by the most expeditious route is indicated if there is any evidence of deterioration in the condition of the fetus or worsening of maternal cardiovascular function.

Support of the respiratory system

The most common cause of death in septic shock is respiratory failure due to ARDS. Twenty-five to 50% of patients with septic shock develop ARDS, and the mortality rate for this group of patients approaches 90%[35].

A major objective in the management of the critically ill patient is prevention of respiratory failure. Patients with septicemia and shock are, by definition, hypoxic. Therefore, oxygen should be administered by nasal cannula or face mask. Pulse oximetry and periodic sampling of arterial blood gases should be performed to detect early onset of respiratory failure. Excessive fluid replacement should be avoided.

Mechanical ventilation should be initiated at the earliest manifestation of decreased pulmonary compliance to prevent irreversible hypoxic damage to the pulmonary vasculature. A large tidal volume should be used to prevent atelectasis. Forced inspiratory oxygen concentration (FIO_2) should be high enough to maintain a PaO_2 of > 60 mmHg. Initially, 100% oxygen may be required to correct hypoxemia, but, because of the potential oxygen toxicity, the FIO_2 should be reduced to < 50% within 24 h if possible[50]. Positive end-expiratory pressure is also vital in the

treatment of the ARDS, and should be initiated at 3–5 cmH$_2$O and increased only if needed to maintain oxygenation. At optimal pressures, positive end-expiratory pressure increases lung volume, decreases shunting of pulmonary blood flow and decreases oxygen requirements. However, at excessively high pressures, positive end-expiratory pressure can cause a decrease in cardiac output, pneumothorax, pneumomediastinum, fluid retention and increased intracranial pressure[50].

Fetal oxygenation must also be considered in the hypoxemic patient. Fetal pO_2 is maintained until maternal pO_2 falls below 60 mmHg, at which point fetal hemoglobin saturation falls sharply because of the steep slope of the fetal oxygen dissociation curve. Just as small decreases in fetal pO_2 can cause sharp drops in fetal oxygen saturation, small increases in pO_2 that result from improved maternal ventilation may cause a significant increase in fetal oxygen saturation[9,51].

Additional supportive measures

Wide fluctuations in the patient's temperature should be prevented since thermal instability may aggravate cardiovascular dysfunction. Prophylactic administration of antacids or an H$_2$ blocking agent should be considered for the prevention of stress ulceration. Coagulation abnormalities should be identified promptly and corrected by administration of cryoprecipitate, fresh frozen plasma, fresh whole blood, or platelets. Only in rare circumstances should it be necessary to consider use of heparin for management of a consumption coagulopathy. In immunosuppressed neutropenic patients, especially those with infections due to *Pseudomonas* organisms, transfusion of compatible white cells may be indicated.

PREVENTIVE MEASURES

Despite current therapeutic strategies, septic shock is often fatal. Though not all cases can be prevented, attempts can be made to identify and correct predisposing factors and illnesses. During the antepartum period, asymptomatic bacteremia should be identified and treated to prevent progression to pyelonephritis. Upper urinary tract infection should be aggressively treated, and chronic urinary tract infections should be suppressed with antibiotic therapy.

Intrapartum, the number of vaginal examinations should be restricted, especially in patients who have ruptured membranes. Early amniotomy should be performed for clear indications only. Labor abnormalities should be promptly identified and corrected to reduce the risk of prolonged labor. Prophylactic antibiotics should be used at the time of Cesarean delivery to reduce the risk of endometritis. Furthermore, careful surgical technique is of primary importance in reducing the incidence of infection. During the postpartum period, puerperal endometritis should be identified promptly and treated aggressively. While under therapy, infected patients should be observed carefully for early warning signs of impending hemodynamic instability.

REFERENCES

1. National Center for Health Statistics. *Annual Summary of Births, Marriages, Divorces, and Deaths: United States, 1988. Monthly Vital Statistics Report*, vol 37, no 13. Hyattsville, MD: Public Health Service, 1989
2. Gibbs RS, Castillo MS, Rodgers PJ. Management of acute chorioamnionitis. *Am J Obstet Gynecol* 1980;136:709
3. Gibbs RS, Blanco JD, St Clair PJ, Castaneda YS. Quantitative bacteriology of amniotic fluid from women with clinical intraamniotic infection at term. *J Infect Dis* 1982;145:1
4. Swartz WH, Grolle K. The use of prophylactic antibiotics in cesarean section. *J Reprod Med* 1981;26:595
5. Duff P: Pyelonephritis in pregnancy. *Clin Obstet Gynecol* 1984;27:17
6. Blanco JD, Gibbs RS, Castaneda YS. Bacteremia in obstetrics: clinical course. *Obstet Gynecol* 1981;58:621
7. Bryan CS, Reynolds KL, Moore EE. Bacteremia in obstetrics and gynecology. *Obstet Gynecol* 1984;64:155
8. Ledger WJ, Norman M, Gee C, Lewis W. Bacteremia on an obstetric–gynecologic service. *Am J Obstet Gynecol* 1975;121:205
9. Clark SL. Shock in the pregnant patient. *Semin Perinatol* 1990;14:52
10. Freid MA, Vosti KL. The importance of underlying disease in patients with gram-negative bacteremia. *Arch Intern Med* 1968;121:418
11. Kreger BE, Craven DE, Carling PC, McCabe WR. Gram-negative bacteremia. *Am J Med* 1980;68:332
12. Kreger BE, Craven DE, McCabe WR. Gram-negative bacteremia. *Am J Med* 1980;68:344
13. Cavanagh D, Knuppel RA, Shepherd JH, *et al*. Septic shock and the obstetrician/gynecologist. *South Med J* 1982;75:809
14. Monif GRG, Baer H. Polymicrobial bacteremia in obstetric patients. *Obstet Gynecol* 1976;48:167
15. Barela AI, Kleinman GE, Golditch IM, *et al*. Septic shock with renal failure after chorionic villus sampling. *Am J Obstet Gynecol* 1986;154:1100
16. Bernheim HA, Block LH, Atkins E. Fever: pathogenesis, pathophysiology, and purpose. *Ann Intern Med* 1979;91:261
17. Eskridge RA. Septic shock. *Crit Care Q* 1980;2:55
18. Mason JW, Kleeberg U, Dolan P, Colman RW. Plasma kallikrein and Hageman factor in gram-negative bacteremia. *Ann Intern Med* 1970;73:545
19. Samuelsson B. Leukotrienes: mediators of immediate hypersensitivity reactions and inflammation. *Science* 1983;220:568
20. Duff P, Gibbs RS. Maternal sepsis in Benkowitz RL, ed. *Critical Care of the Obstetric Patient*. New York: Churchill-Livingstone, 1983:184–217
21. Weisel RD, Vito L, Dennis RC, *et al*. Myocardial depression during sepsis. *Am J Surg* 1977;133:512
22. Raffa J, Trunkey DD. Myocardial depression in sepsis. *J Trauma* 1978;18:617
23. Pasque MK, Murphy CE, Trigt PV, *et al*. Myocardial adenosine triphosphate levels during early sepsis. *Arch Surg* 1983;118:1437
24. Fletcher JR, Ramwell PW, Herman CM. Prostaglandins and the hemodynamic course of endotoxin shock. *J Surg Res* 1976;20:589
25. Hinshaw LB, Emerson TE, Reins DA. Cardiovascular responses of the primate in endotoxin shock. *J Physiol* 1966;210:335
26. Motsay GJ, Dietzman RH, Ersek RA, Lillehei RC. Hemodynamic alterations and results of treatment in patients with gram-negative septic shock. *Surgery* 1970;67:577
27. Roberts JM, Laros RK. Hemorrhagic and endotoxic shock: a pathophysiologic approach to diagnosis and management. *Am J Obstet Gynecol* 1971;110:1041
28. Guillemin R, Vargo T, Rossier J, *et al*. β-Endorphin and adrenocorticotropin are secreted concomitantly by the pituitary gland. *Science* 1977;197:1367
29. Holaday JW, Faden AI. Naloxone reversal of endotoxin hypotension suggests role of endorphins in shock. *Nature (London)* 1978;275:450
30. Moberg GP. Site of action of endotoxins on hypothalamic–pituitary–adrenal axis. *Am J Physiol* 1971;220:397
31. Lefer AM. Role of a myocardial depressant factor in shock states. *Am Heart Assoc* 1973;17:59
32. Hammerschmidt DE, Weaver LJ, Hudson LD, *et al*. Association of complement activation and elevated plasma-C5a with adult respiratory distress syndrome. *Lancet* 1980;1:947
33. Lee CT, Fein AM, Lippmann M, *et al*. Elastolytic activity in pulmonary lavage fluid from patients with adult respiratory-distress syndrome. *N Engl J Med* 1981;304:192
34. Sibbald WJ, Anderson RR, Reid B, *et al*. Alveolo-capillary permeability in human septic ARDS. *Chest* 1981;79:133
35. Kaplan RL, Sahn SA, Petty TL. Incidence and outcome of the respiratory distress syndrome in gram-negative sepsis. *Arch Intern Med* 1979;139:867
36. American College of Obstetricians and Gynecologists. *Septic Shock. Technical Bulletin No. 75*. Washington DC. 1984
37. Threlkeld MG, Cobbs CG. Gram-negative bacteremia and the sepsis syndrome. In Stein JH, ed. *Internal Medicine*. Boston: Little, Brown, 1990
38. Bone RC, Fisher CJ, Clemmer TP, *et al*. Methylprednisolone Severe Sepsis Study Group. A controlled clinical trial of high-dose methylprednisolone in the treatment of severe sepsis and septic shock. *N Engl J Med* 1987;317:653
39. Knochel JQ, Koehler PR, Lee TG, Welch DM. Diagnosis of abdominal abscesses with computed tomography, ultrasound, and ^{111}In leukocyte scans. *Radiology* 1980;137:425
40. Packman MI, Rackow EC. Optimum left heart filling pressure during fluid resuscitation of patients with hypovolemic and septic shock. *Crit Care Med* 1983;11:165

41. Waeckerle JF. Antishock garments. *Crit Care Q* 1980; 2:15

42. Jardin F, Sportiche M, Bazin M, *et al*. Dobutamine: a hemodynamic evaluation in human septic shock. *Crit Care Med* 1981;9:329

43. Lee W, Clark SL, Cotton DB, *et al*. Septic shock during pregnancy. *Am J Obstet Gynecol* 1988;159:410

44. Roberts DE, Dobson KE, Hall KW, Light RB. Effects of prolonged naloxone infusion in septic shock. *Lancet* 1988;8613:699

45. Sprung CL, Caralis PV, Marcial EH, *et al*. The effects of high-dose corticosteroids in patients with septic shock. *N Engl J Med* 1984;311:1137

46. The Veterans Administration Systemic Sepsis Cooperative Study Group. Effect of high-dose glucocorticoid therapy on mortality in patients with clinical signs of systemic sepsis. *N Engl J Med* 1987;317:659

47. Mercer D, Doris P, Salerno TA. Intra-aortic balloon counterpulsation in septic shock. *Can J Surg* 1981; 24:643

48. Foster ED, Subramanian VA, Vito L, *et al*. Response to intra-aortic balloon pumping. *Am J Surg* 1975;129:464

49. Ziegler EJ, McCutchan JA, Fierer J, *et al*. Treatment of gram-negative bacteremia and shock with human antiserum to a mutant *Escherichia coli*. *N Engl J Med* 1982;307:1225

50. Eriksen NL, Parisi VM. Adult respiratory distress syndrome and pregnancy. *Semin Perinatol* 1990;14:68

51. Yancey MK, Duff P. Acute hypotension related to sepsis in the obstetric patient. *Obstet Gynecol Clin North Am* 1995;22:91–109

16
Shoulder dystocia

J.S. Smeltzer

One of the most frightening experiences in obstetrics is the failure of the shoulders to deliver spontaneously. This sequence, the cardinal sign of its occurrence, and the usual methods and frequently tragic consequences of its inappropriate management were described most vividly by Morris[1]:

Antenatally, a careful observer may have recognized that the child was unusually large, though this is notoriously difficult to judge...it may have been necessary to intervene in the second stage... The hairy scalp slides out with reluctance. When the forehead has appeared it is necessary to press back the perineum to deliver the face. Fat cheeks eventually emerge. A double chin has to be hooked over the vulval commissure, to which it remains tightly opposed [Turtle sign, see Figure 1]... Time passes. The child's face becomes suffused... Abdominal efforts by the mother or by her attendants produce no advance, gentle head traction is equally unavailing. Usually equanimity forsakes the attendants. They push, they pull. Alarm increases. Eventually 'by greater strength of muscle or by some infernal juggle' the difficulty appears to be overcome...

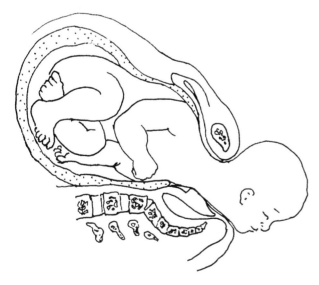

Figure 1 Classic shoulder dystocia. The head is delivered, but retracted by the tension between the chin and the shoulders, which are at the inlet. Further progress for the anterior shoulder or fetus is not safe until the posterior enters the pelvis

It dawns on the attendants that their anxiety was not ill-founded, the baby lies limp and voiceless, and only too often remains so.

Such a disaster and the more common but also tragic result of fetal brachial plexus injury can usually be averted by appropriate management. This management is based on a solid understanding of the biomechanics of normal shoulder delivery and of shoulder dystocia, and the pathophysiology of excessive fetal growth. The steps in this management are prevention of the condition when it can be prevented prenatally, detection of the possibly large infant and avoidance of operative vaginal delivery, preparation for the possible occurrence of shoulder dystocia when a large infant is anticipated, prompt recognition of the dystocia when it occurs and employment of maneuvers with proven effectiveness which are least likely to harm the fetus or mother.

THE MECHANISM OF SHOULDER DYSTOCIA

The mechanism of normal shoulder delivery is not treated in obstetrics texts. The mechanism can be partly verified by pelvic examination of a normal patient after delivery of the fetal head, if there is a generous episiotomy. During delivery of the head, one shoulder has entered the pelvis obliquely and is resting in the sciatic notch, or hollow of the sacrum. This is the posterior shoulder on restitution. The identity of this shoulder, not any 'memory' of previous attitude, determines the direction of 'restitution'[1,2]. This position in the hollow of the sacrum or sacrosciatic notch provides room for the anterior shoulder to slide under the pubis or rotate from the obturator foramen. The turtle sign of fetal head retraction after delivery indicates that the above sequence has not occurred, and that a shoulder dystocia exists.

The position of the shoulders in shoulder dystocia is anterior–posterior. In the more common high dystocia the posterior shoulder is lodged at the inlet on the sacral promontory, and the anterior shoulder is wedged against the pubis[1,3,4] (Figure 1). The turtle sign is produced by traction between the delivered head and the posterior shoulder, and this traction locks the shoulders in an unfavorable position. As observed by Jacquemier[5] and by Woods[6] and demonstrated conclusively by Schwartz and Dixon[3], direct traction and pressure applied to such a 'locked' position are likely both to fail to deliver the infant and to produce injury. This position will not let the posterior shoulder enter the pelvis, will not provide room for the anterior shoulder to slip under the pubis and will stretch the cervical brachial plexus roots of the posterior arm, causing a greater chance of injury to this plexus[7].

This ominous situation occurs because the shoulders do not normally fit through the pelvic inlet together, and the shoulder destined to be the posterior must enter first. This fact is ignored by most writers on the subject, but is ascertainable by episiotomy and pelvic examination before performing maneuvers when the turtle sign is present. Most term infants have a minimum shoulder diameter that is greater than the maximum diameter of the normal maternal pelvic inlet, and cannot traverse it together[8]. The gynecoid pelvis, perfectly adapted to delivery of the fetal head, has a higher relative risk for shoulder dystocia than other types of pelves and maternal pelvic capacity is not a factor in shoulder dystocia and fetal brachial plexus injury[9].

This situation can be made worse by ignorance and panic. The parturient wants to push the baby out, perhaps with 'help' from others by fundal pressure, further wedging the shoulders at the inlet. Attempting to push the anterior shoulder through the inlet with suprapubic pressure would further impact the posterior shoulder. The inclination of the novice accoucheur is to overcome the impaction by force, pulling the fetal head posteriorly, which stretches the brachial plexus of the anterior arm, or inferiorly, which further stretches the plexus of the posterior arm. The fetus is lucky if dystocia is mild or the obstruction is overcome by the

fracture of a clavicle, either spontaneously or by suprapubic pressure. The inclination to use suprapubic pressure is reinforced by many articles and texts on shoulder dystocia. It is usually ineffective in high dystocia[10] and should not be used until it is verified that the posterior shoulder is in the pelvis or in an attempt to fracture the clavicle. Once the posterior shoulder is definitely in the pelvis, suprapubic pressure becomes rational, indicated, and likely to work.

The pelvic inlet, like the walls of Troy, cannot be breached by force without unacceptable loss[5,3,11,12]. The posterior shoulder alone, like the Trojan horse, is small and mobile and can enter easily if permitted to do so. Once the posterior shoulder is in the pelvis, the anterior usually has room to traverse the pubis, or can be persuaded to do so by other means. The mechanism of successful treatment of the normal high shoulder dystocia is to break the tie that occurs at the pelvic inlet and emulate the natural sequence of shoulder delivery. Successful treatments involve the following principles (Table 1):

(1) Relieve the traction that is locking the posterior shoulder in an undeliverable position. This is the opposite of the pushing and pulling that is sometimes employed. Traction is relieved by a large episiotomy, McRoberts maneuver or supine squat[12] and the Hibbard maneuver or partial cephalic replacement[4] or by hands and knees position.

(2) Rotate the posterior shoulder into an oblique diameter. Rock the anterior shoulder abdominally or push the posterior forward from behind (Rubin maneuver)[8], push the distal clavicle back from in front (Woods maneuver)[6] or do this while pushing the anterior shoulder in the opposite

Table 1 Sequence of action when shoulder dystocia is encountered

---

(1) Recognize turtle sign: posterior shoulder is arrested at inlet or high in pelvis. Anterior shoulder is NOT deliverable and do not attempt to deliver it

(2) Obtain help for McRoberts maneuver, neonatal resuscitation and anesthesia, or use hands and knees position

(3) Perform McRoberts maneuver. Insure adequate flexion of hips (knees to shoulders). If it fails, reapply and continue

(4) If turtle sign is released, attempt gentle delivery of anterior shoulder

(5) If turtle sign is not released or anterior does not progress, cut generous episiotomy

(6) Examine patient vaginally:
   where is posterior shoulder?
   is there a fetal tumor obstructing delivery?

(7) Unlock locked shoulders with partial cephalic replacement (Hibbard maneuver)

(8) Rotate posterior shoulder off sacral promontory if this can be done easily

(9) Deliver posterior arm across chest (Jacquemier maneuver) if posterior shoulder not in pelvis. This delivers posterior shoulder into pelvis

(10) Deliver anterior arm (Couder maneuver), or use suprapubic pressure if posterior shoulder is in pelvis and anterior does not deliver easily. This delivers the anterior shoulder under pubis symphysis

(11) If this is not possible, rotate posterior shoulder to anterior (delivered position). Anterior will now be in mid-pelvis and deliverable (Woods maneuver)

(12) Replace head, relax uterus and perform Cesarean section (Zavanelli maneuver) if above measures cannot be performed for some reason or fetus has a tumor obstructing delivery

---

direction from behind above the pubis with the opposite hand (DeLee maneuver). If the shoulders rotate in either direction, the posterior shoulder will enter the pelvis.

(3) If the posterior shoulder cannot be rotated, it will enter the pelvis over the sacral promontory when the posterior arm is delivered (Jacquemier maneuver)[3,5].

(4) When there is insufficient room to deliver the anterior shoulder with the posterior shoulder in the pelvis (either turtle sign absent or after delivery of the posterior shoulder into the pelvis), the anterior arm can be delivered (Couder maneuver), which brings the anterior shoulder out under the pubis. This is my choice[13]. Alternatively, the shoulders can be rotated until the posterior is anterior and delivered under the pubis. This requires the posterior shoulder to be inferior to the ischial spines[2,6]. Once the posterior shoulder is delivered under the pubis, the anterior shoulder is now posterior, is in the pelvis, and can be spontaneously delivered.

(5) If all these fail, replace the head, relax the uterus and perform a Cesarean section (Zavanelli maneuver)[14], or perform a symphysiotomy[15].

(6) If shoulder dystocia should occur during an in-bed delivery, these maneuvers may be difficult or impossible in the supine position. If the McRoberts maneuver cannot be applied, or fails, the hands and knees position[16] should be used. This position gives good access to the posterior shoulder and arm if necessary, gives a favorable angulation of the pelvis, and gravity aids rather than impedes release of the posterior shoulder from the inlet. The hands and knees position has been shown to be safe and very effective for treatment of shoulder dystocia.

PREVENTION

The incidence of shoulder dystocia is 0.2–0.8% and this risk increases directly with birth weight, especially among macrosomic infants. There is no way to predict with any confidence that a shoulder dystocia will occur in a particular delivery, however[13,17–20].

Shoulder dystocia cannot be strictly prevented because normal term fetuses, with shoulders wider than the fetal head, are at some risk for shoulder dystocia, and most infants of mothers without diabetes with shoulder dystocia are not macrosomic[17–21]. The risk is increased by factors that increase the discrepancy between fetal body and shoulder size and head size. About two-thirds of fetuses with shoulder dystocia are male. The risks for macrosomia and shoulder dystocia are increased by a history of prior shoulder dystocia, prior large infant and a large maternal birth weight. The mnemonic DOPE – diabetes, obesity, prolonged pregnancy and excessive fetal size or maternal weight gain – indicates current pregnancy factors that should alert the clinician to an increased risk for shoulder dystocia (Table 2).

PROLONGED PREGNANCY

As body growth continues and head growth diminishes at term, shoulder dystocia risk increases with prolonged pregnancy and is negligible before term. The incidence of shoulder dystocia in pregnancies beyond 41 weeks is 1.5% but the risks of macrosomia (5.2% > 4500 g), birth trauma (0.7%) and shoulder dystocia were not reduced by routine induction of labor at 41 weeks vs. observation and antenatal testing in one randomized study of 3407 pregnancies. However, Cesarean section for fetal distress was reduced by routine induction using prostaglandin gel at 41 weeks[22].

Fetal body and bone growth, unlike brain growth, are sensitive to fetal insulin, which in turn responds to a maternal–fetal glucose load. Maternal conditions such as diabetes, gestational glucose intolerance, excessive weight gain and obesity can cause fetal overnutrition and are associated with an increased risk for macrosomia, operative delivery and shoulder dystocia[17–21].

OBESITY

Maternal obesity is not preventable but is treatable. Past blanket proscriptions against excessive weight

Table 2 Prevention of shoulder dystocia and injury

(1) Offer Cesarean section for high-risk vaginal deliveries:
    extremely large fetuses (over 5 kg)
    very large fetuses (over 4.5 kg) with maternal diabetes
    large fetuses (over 4 kg) with history of shoulder dystocia
    second-stage protraction with large fetus
(2) Identify and treat diabetes mellitus
(3) Be prepared with a plan
(4) Recognize the presence of dystocia before maternal pushing, staff assistance (fundal and suprapubic pressure) and traction have produced or contributed to injury
(5) Note times and get help when shoulder dystocia is recognized. Help includes assistants for McRoberts, obstetric back-up, neonatal resuscitation and anesthesia

gain were obviously misguided. A woman who starts pregnancy 50 kg overweight already has caloric reserves that are the equivalent of 200 days of a normal diet. Her ideal weight gain is in the range of 5–10 kg. Moreover, fat exacerbates the normal gestational resistance to insulin, and thus provides the fetus excess glucose. A balanced diet emphasizing complex carbohydrates, moderate portion size, distribution of calories throughout the day and high fiber intake[23] would seem prudent. These women should know that the objective is not to lose weight, but to limit heavy intake of simple sugars and provide the fetus with appropriate nutrition. The urine should be checked for ketones if weight gain is not adequate, and calories should be increased or distributed more favorably if ketonuria is present.

EXCESSIVE MATERNAL WEIGHT GAIN

Increased maternal weight gain is associated with shoulder dystocia, especially when the mother is already obese. Overall perinatal mortality is generally lower when weight gain during pregnancy is 10–20 kg for normal-weight women or over 20 kg for slim women. Caloric limitations would not be indicated for these women. Increased maternal weight gain and fundal height suggest the possibility of fetal macrosomia, however.

DIABETES

Infants of diabetic mothers have a greater risk for macrosomia and a greater risk of excess shoulder size[24] and shoulder dystocia for a given fetal weight[21,25]. Glucose is the primary energy source for the fetus. It is absorbed by facilitated diffusion, with a rate regulated only by maternal serum glucose concentration. Fetal insulin responds to the fetal absorbed glucose, and it in turn acts as a trophic hormone on fetal liver, bone, muscles and fat. Prevention of fetal overnutrition and macrosomia requires maternal glucose homeostasis.

Tight glucose control, with target fasting glucose of 60–80 mg/dl and preprandial glucose of 60–90 mg/dl is associated with a significant reduction of the risk for macrosomia, shoulder dystocia, operative delivery and, most importantly, perinatal mortality among diabetic women[26]. It is also clear that recognition and control of hyperglycemia prior to 32 weeks is more successful than late control for reducing the risk of macrosomia[27]. Obese women have insulin resistance, high insulin production and delayed insulin secretion, rather than a lack of insulin. Thus, they may require large doses of insulin to achieve euglycemia, but have considerable range between adequate and oversupply of exogenous insulin because the endogenous insulin production moderates their response to exogenous insulin. Excellent glucose control can be readily accomplished with a balanced regular diet high in fiber and complex carbohydrates, with calories and carbohydrates distributed throughout the day.

The problem of hypoglycemia may limit the ability to meet these objectives in Type 1 diabetics who have little endogenous insulin production. For these women, 'tight' control requires close attention to regularization of calories, carbohydrates and exercise; fiber is even more important. Regular insulin administered at abdominal sites has more rapid and predictable absorption, and can be taken before each meal, with small doses of long-acting insulin provided to meet basal needs.

Women with possible gestational glucose intolerance, as evidenced by family history of diabetes, prior large infant, prior shoulder dystocia or stillbirth, should have a preconceptional glucose screen of fasting and 2-h determinations. These women should also have mid-pregnancy screening to exclude the possibility of overt diabetes. The risks of miscarriage and congenital anomalies are increased if maternal glucose is not controlled in the first trimester. In addition, early treatment of maternal hyperglycemia would better reduce the risk of macrosomia. Non-obese patients with non-suggestive history should undergo the regular early third-trimester screening[28].

Untreated women with an abnormal screen but only one abnormal value on glucose tolerance test are at higher risk for macrosomia than women identified and treated as gestational diabetics[29]. These patients should follow the same diet as those with an abnormal glucose tolerance test, and have periodic screening for overt diabetes.

Optimal glycemic control reduces but cannot eliminate the risk of macrosomia. Maintaining maternal serum glucose at normal fasting levels during labor may alleviate fetal asphyxia if a difficult labor or delivery occurs[30,31].

Kjos and colleagues[32] found that induction of labor routinely at 38–39 weeks' gestation in insulin-requiring diabetes reduced the risk for macrosomia and shoulder dystocia vs. conservative management, and did not increase the Cesarean section rate.

DETECTING FETAL MACROSOMIA AND PREDICTING SHOULDER DYSTOCIA

Most fetuses who experience shoulder dystocia but are not macrosomic have non-diabetic mothers, while most macrosomic fetuses with shoulder dystocia have diabetic mothers[18,21,24,25]. Accurate prediction of the fetal weight could identify fetuses at increased risk for shoulder dystocia in this group. Unfortunately, error in predicting birth weight from ultrasonography is 15–20% of the actual birth weight. More babies are born at normal weights as opposed to very large weights; an infant predicted to be over 4000 g is as likely to be less than 4000 g as over 4000 g[20]. With a predicted birth weight over 5000 g, the fetus is likely to be at least over 4000 g. This also means that some large fetuses will be missed.

Elective Cesarean section for prevention of fetal injury has been proposed for macrosomic infants of non-diabetic and diabetic mothers with estimated fetal weights of above 5000 g and above 4500 g or even 4000 g, respectively. As large infants of diabetic mothers have a higher risk for shoulder dystocia and fetal trauma, weight for weight, elective Cesarean section may be indicated if estimated fetal weight could be accurately identified[21]. Our experience was more sanguine in terms of neonatal outcome, and conclusions based on these data are different[33].

Elliott and colleagues[34] described a sonographic finding of abdominal minus biparietal diameter difference of greater than 1.4 cm as predictive of an infant over 4000 g in diabetics, with a sensitivity of 87% and specificity of 72%. Using a similar difference measure for fetuses with an estimated weight of 3800–4200 g also in diabetic mothers, Cohen and associates[35] found that a cut-off value of 2.6 cm identified 20 fetuses with a 30% incidence of shoulder dystocia.

Kitzmiller and co-workers[36] described detection of macrosomia by measurement of shoulder diameter in diabetes by computed tomography scan, with 14.5 cm as the cut-off level for macrosomia. Sensitivity was 100% and specificity was 87% for fetal weight over 4200 g.

The reported incidences of shoulder dystocia with a fetus over 4500 g vary from 2% to 35%, with most studies reporting incidences of 20–40% among infants of diabetic mothers delivering vaginally[21,25,33] and less than half that risk among non-diabetic patients[21,25]. The risk for permanent brachial plexus neurological injury arising from shoulder dystocia varies from 0.6%[19] to 27.5%[37]. The risk for perinatal mortality varies between zero[33] and 28%[21]. There appears to be considerable variation in the ability to diagnose and safely manage shoulder dystocia. The advocacy for elective Cesarean section based on estimated weight by the various authors is directly proportional to their own morbidity and mortality rate.

No rational Cesarean section policy can completely prevent shoulder dystocia[9,11,12,17–21]. Centers with high neonatal morbidity and mortality rates from shoulder dystocia would probably prevent more neonatal morbidity and mortality by meticulous treatment of diabetes in pregnancy and provision of formal training of staff in safe management of shoulder dystocia, rather than expending these resources on performing more elective Cesarean sections.

Four studies have examined methods of treatments of shoulder dystocia and associated neonatal morbidity and mortality[3,11,12,19]. The highest rates of neurological injury and/or death in the first three studies were associated with the 'frontal assault method' of traction and fundal or suprapubic pressure. The last study, which concluded that the method of treatment made no difference in neonatal morbidity and mortality found only one permanent lesion among 33 brachial plexus injuries in 204 cases of shoulder dystocia[19].

The risk for a brachial plexus injury sustained at birth to become permanent is about 5%, based on the collaborative perinatal project data[9].

The recognition of the possibility of a large infant is definitely beneficial for management during labor. Labor disorders of all types are more common in pregnancies destined for shoulder dystocia[9,25,38]. All studies with a significant number of operative vaginal delivery cases clearly indicate that there is a three-to-six-fold increased risk for shoulder dystocia in association with abnormal labor curves. Infants over 4000 g with operative vaginal delivery, especially mid-pelvic delivery, have a several-fold increased risk (23%) for shoulder dystocia[9,38]. Macrosomic infants of diabetic mothers have even a greater risk of shoulder dystocia (50%) and subsequent traumatic injury[25]. It is uncertain whether operative vaginal delivery causes birth of the head when the shoulders are too large too follow, or fails to give the shoulders time to follow the proper mechanism for birth. In any case, non-emergent operative vaginal delivery should be avoided in those patients with anticipated large infants. The mnemonic for the above becomes DODOPE (Disordered labor, Operative vaginal delivery, Diabetes, Obesity, Prolonged pregnancy and Excessive fetal size or maternal weight gain), an association that is becoming extinct. The exceptions are cases of fetal distress and severe maternal disease, in which the actual risks of additional time to delivery or Cesarean section must be weighed against the potential risk of shoulder dystocia individually.

PREPARATION

The delivery team has time physically, mentally and psychologically to prepare themselves and the patient for the possibility of shoulder dystocia when a large infant is suspected. This permits review of maneuvers to be used and effective co-ordination of treatment if the problem is encountered. This physical and mental preparation is the antidote for the panic that can arise in a difficult shoulder delivery. It is helpful to have an anesthetist and a physician experienced in the treatment of shoulder dystocia available, and two people familiar with the McRoberts maneuver in the room. It may also help to have someone experienced in neonatal evaluation and resuscitation. Delivery should be performed without the legs strapped into stirrups.

RECOGNITION

Usually the diagnosis is obvious, when the 'turtle sign' of head retraction after final extension is found. Rarely, shoulder dystocia occurs when the posterior shoulder is in the pelvis and the turtle sign may not be present. These cases will become apparent when the anterior shoulder does not deliver easily with normal effort. Either situation calls for assistance, including all experienced help, anesthesia and neonatal care.

Considerable force is often applied to the fetal head prior to the recognition and appropriate treatment of shoulder dystocia[39]. Traction, neck twisting and lateral head force are not only ineffective, but all stretch the cervical brachial plexus roots and can avulse them.

TREATMENT

The McRoberts maneuver

The McRoberts maneuver should be employed immediately. Assistants should be coached to use and continue the McRoberts maneuver. This accomplishes delivery in most cases and aids in delivery in others[40]. It also provides assistants with a constructive alternative to fundal and downward suprapubic pressure, which only impacts the shoulders further. The McRoberts maneuver or supine squat flexes the lumbar spine and retracts the perineum (Figure 2). The maneuver releases the traction that is locking and depressing the posterior shoulder against the sacral promontory. This spontaneous traction by itself can cause an Erb's palsy, especially if the parturient spontaneously extends rather than flexes the pelvis[13,41]. The McRoberts maneuver also straightens out the lumbosacral lordosis and the sacral promontory and removes the compressive force of the delivery table on the sacrum. In addition, it pushes the anterior shoulder superiorly and places the pelvic inlet perpendicular to the axis of the fetus. These actions together usually place the posterior shoulder of the fetus in the maternal pelvis as the maneuver is being applied; it reduces the force necessary for delivery by 30% and produces less risk for injury of a simulated fetus[42].

As the posterior shoulder enters the pelvis, the baby's neck appears to get longer, usually as the maneuver is being applied. This 'lengthening' should not be confused with the moderate release of tension that occurs with the McRoberts maneuver when the posterior shoulder is still at the inlet. If there is a good regional block and generous episiotomy, this maneuver should be applied with a hand in the pelvis to feel it work. If this succeeds, easy delivery of the anterior shoulder is to be anticipated without further maneuvers. If this fails, the legs can be relaxed somewhat and the maneuver repeated once, in conjunction with pressure on the fetal head towards the sacral promontory to free the shoulders (Hibbard maneuver)[4].

When the McRoberts maneuver is applied correctly, the patient's knees almost or actually touch her shoulders. An excited patient can make the maneuver difficult, as the hamstrings, gluteus and low back muscles of a large patient are quite strong. Maternal pelvic

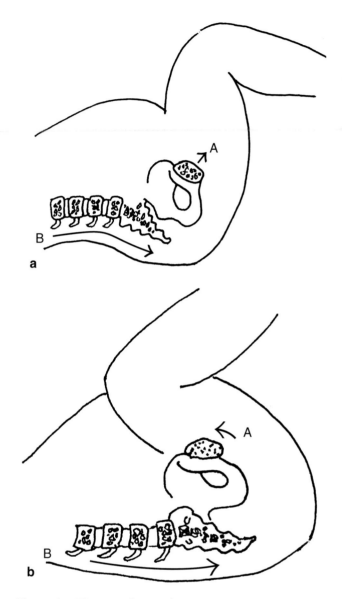

Figure 2   The McRoberts maneuver (a and b) rotates the pelvis cephalad, straightens the lumbosacral lordosis, pushes the anterior shoulder back and lifts the posterior off the sacral promontory. It also relieves the tension between the posterior shoulder and soft tissues by retracting them

extension should be avoided, however, as it can injure the fetus.

An average-sized assistant can effectively apply the maneuver with correct application of force and mass to mechanical advantage in the following fashion: (1) face the patient's head from near the stirrup; (2) place her knee on your inboard shoulder; (3) lock your hands or forearms around the upper thigh and pull the upper thigh snugly against your hip and bend forward, using your mass to flex the hip. The McRoberts maneuver works most of the time if it is used in experienced hands[40], and over 80% of the time at many institutions.

Episiotomy

If the McRoberts maneuver position has not effected release of the posterior shoulder and delivery, it can be continued through the other maneuvers, as it facilitates their action. This position should be relaxed during induction of anesthesia if general anesthesia is required at this time. It is imperative to determine the actual cause of the dystocia and to determine the position of the posterior shoulder and take appropriate action for a safe delivery. It is essential to release the tension between the fetal head and shoulders with minimum impediment and risk for serious fetal injury and extensive maternal vaginal lacerations. Some recommend a large mediolateral episiotomy. Others prefer a complete perineotomy. The simplest way to achieve the latter is a proctoepisiotomy. This is usually not necessary[19]. The proper episiotomy depends on the clinical setting, the size of the fetus and the size of the operator's hand. The only 'wrong' episiotomy is the one that is not sufficient to permit the maneuvers needed to effect delivery without lasting fetal injury.

Examination

The next step is to verify the location of the posterior shoulder and to confirm the absence of dorsal tumors which would make further attempt at vaginal delivery either fruitless or dangerous. This can be accomplished with the hand towards the infant's back after restitution. This leads immediately to the Rubin maneuver.

The Rubin maneuver

In the Rubin maneuver[8] the posterior shoulder is located, usually on the sacral promontory. The shoulder is rotated forward from behind, either by direct pressure or by hooking the scapula. The anterior shoulder can be rocked laterally to free it or rotated in the opposite direction with the heel of the free hand suprapubically. If the posterior shoulder is at the inlet, rotation will permit it to enter the pelvis and rest in the sacrosciatic notch. If it is already in the pelvis while the anterior shoulder is undeliverable, rotation of the posterior shoulder should be continued until it is anterior and can be delivered under the pubis. Rotation using the fetal head has been described, but this may increase stretching of the brachial plexus, similar to direct and lateral traction on the fetal head[1]. If the posterior shoulder does not rotate with moderate pressure, the operator should proceed immediately to the next maneuver.

The Woods maneuver

In the Woods maneuver[6], the hand toward the fetal back is withdrawn, and the opposite hand is placed in the pelvis in front of the fetus. Although anterior fetal tumors are rarer than dorsal ones, if they obstruct further delivery, the operator should proceed to the Zavanelli maneuver. The posterior shoulder is rotated backwards by pressure on the distal clavicle. This may be assisted by pressure with the opposite hand on the anterior shoulder to the front suprapubically (DeLee maneuver). If no rotation occurs with moderate pressure, the operator should proceed immediately to the next maneuver.

Delivery of the posterior arm (Jacquemier maneuver)

The most effective maneuver is delivery of the posterior arm[3,5,9,11,12]. The main risks are vaginal lacerations and fetal humeral fracture. The latter risk can be minimized in the following way (Figure 3): The operator's hand is extended further into the uterus to find the humerus attached to the posterior shoulder. The humerus is brought to the front along the side of the fetus. The elbow is flexed so that the forearm is brought across the body. The forearm is firmly grasped by the operator's entire hand and pulled out in a reverse Pinard sequence. The delivery of the arm causes the posterior shoulder to enter the pelvis. The anterior shoulder should now be easily deliverable under the pubis. Otherwise, an identical maneuver is performed on the anterior arm, except that the traction on the forearm is more towards the mother's posterior[13] (Figure 3c,d). This sequence of advance of the shoulders – the posterior one into the pelvis, the anterior one under the pubis and the posterior one out of the pelvis – is exactly that of a normal delivery. The only difference is that this advance is accomplished by sequential delivery of the arms.

As an alternative, the posterior shoulder can be rotated forward to turn the fetus until it is anterior[6]. The formerly anterior shoulder will be the posterior and in the pelvis. Unlike the sequential arm delivery, this may increase traction on the cervical brachial plexus with manipulation.

Potential problems encountered with arm delivery are: (1) failure to get the operator's hand into the pelvis from inadequate episiotomy; (2) difficulty in getting the operator's hand through the inlet, which can be facilitated by working the flat hand against the chest (which is compressible) and bringing the arm out through the deltopectoral triangle of the opposite shoulder; (3) difficulty finding the posterior arm, which can be corrected by starting at the shoulder; and (4) difficulty in flexing the elbow, which can be corrected by freeing the forearm from the umbilical cord, the knees, etc. Like the Pinard maneuver, it may be necessary to start flexion by pushing the elbow toward the fetal back.

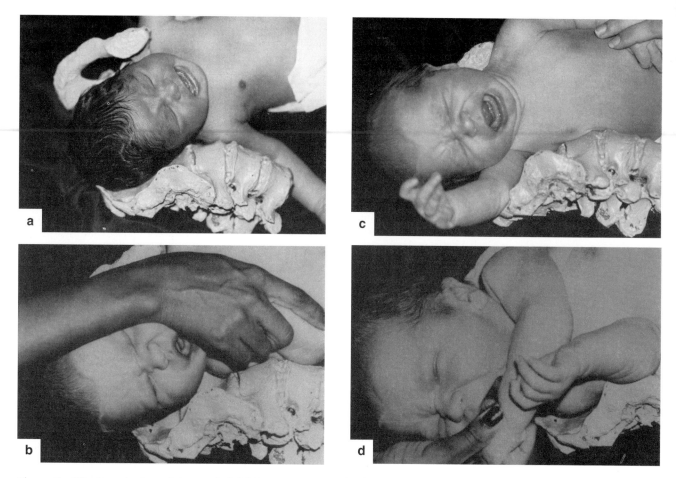

Figure 3   The fetus in the pelvis revealed. (a) Even an average-sized fetus has shoulders too large to enter the pelvis together. (b) Delivery of the posterior arm (Jacquemier maneuver). The posterior forearm has been located and grasped. It will be pulled straight out. With this method, forearm fracture is less likely. (c) The posterior arm delivered. The posterior shoulder has entered the pelvis. There is still not sufficient room to deliver the anterior shoulder, and a low (turtle sign-negative) shoulder dystocia exists. If the baby can be rotated, the posterior shoulder becomes the anterior and is delivered. (d) Delivery of the anterior arm (Couder maneuver) relieves the impaction of the anterior shoulder. This time the pull is more downward

Hands and knees position

This position is difficult in the delivery room, but should be tried immediately during a delivery in bed if the McRoberts maneuver fails, or immediately if the head is delivered with the mother not supine. It can be atraumatic and highly effective[16]. It partially flexes the maternal pelvis, especially if the patient rocks back into a knee–chest position. Gravity aids rather than impedes maneuvers because it brings the fetal body in line with the pelvic inlet and disimpacts the anterior (now dependent) shoulder from the pubis, freeing the posterior from the sacrum. The position provides excellent access for episiotomy, examination and delivery of the posterior arm from a position of comfort, if needed, in bed. The McRoberts maneuver brings the buttocks out of the mattress but requires the operator to assume truly awkward positions to try other maneuvers.

Anesthesia

All of these maneuvers can usually be accomplished within 5 min with no local or regional anesthesia and calm instructions with the patient's co-operation. If things are not in order, then induction of general anesthesia, if immediately available, can provide time to restore calm, relax the patient and get expert assistance.

The Zavanelli maneuver

If the above maneuvers fail or cannot be performed, the fetal head can be replaced in the pelvis, with or without relaxing the uterus (with terbutaline, nitroglycerine, $MgSO_4$ or inhalation anesthetics). Replacement is accomplished by depressing the perineum and reversing the fetal head extension. Delivery can be completed by Cesarean section, at a time indicated by fetal monitoring. This usually results in an intact infant, but possibilities of hypoxic ischemic encephalopathy or stillbirth or permanent brachial plexus injury still exist[14]. The risks may be comparable to those associated with forceful vaginal delivery.

Symphysiotomy and other maneuvers

The reader can find many other maneuvers that have been described for the treatment of shoulder dystocia, and other variations of those presented. The ones presented here have either been observed by the author to be effective without injury or are theoretically likely to be effective biomechanically (hands and knees position) and have been reported to be safe and effective. The other maneuvers that may be safe and effective are: (1) fracture of the clavicle, often the result of sharply applied suprapubic pressure; and (2) symphysiotomy, which is simple, rapid and effective[15].

Prognosis and medicolegal concerns

Stillbirth may occur if delivery is greatly prolonged. Unlike survivors of the Zavanelli maneuver, survivors of shoulder dystocia, even with brachial plexus injury, do not have excessive risk for cognitive deficit when compared to national norms[7] or appropriate controls[9].

Effective delivery with shoulder dystocia is therefore a life-saving treatment for the fetus. The most frequent severe disability for the fetus is Erb's palsy, usually of the posterior arm[7]. This will resolve spontaneously in about 90–95% of cases[9,11,19,43]. There may be some increase in speech dysfunction[7].

Many cases of neonatal brachial plexus injury are not associated with recognized shoulder dystocia, some not even with vaginal delivery[9,11,12,44]. Brachial plexus injury has been observed by myself[13] and others in the absence of any traction to effect delivery. It is likely that the traction between the locked head and posterior shoulder at the pelvic inlet is sufficient at times to harm, even when resolved spontaneously or by McRoberts maneuver.

Malpractice suits have been brought, by parents of children saved by the effective treatment of shoulder dystocia, for the brachial plexus injury sustained during that birth, which may or may not have actually resulted from the treatment. Most shoulder dystocia suits have been successfully defended. Avoiding injury to the extent possible is the most effective prevention.

A fetus without previous compromise has at least 10 min from the time shoulder dystocia occurs until there is any risk of death from asphyxia. Previously compromised infants, or those exposed to high maternal serum glucose levels in the hours prior to delivery, may die or develop cerebral compromise after a shorter period of anoxia[30,31].

The best way to prevent potential lawsuits is a sincere attempt to render the best care possible, applying a learned sequence of effective procedures, such as that described above, honest communication with the family and adequate documentation of exactly what happened.

CONCLUSION

Shoulder dystocia risk increases with increasing fetal body size. There is no effective way to predict with confidence the occurrence of shoulder dystocia, or even macrosomia. The risk for shoulder dystocia may be reduced by early and adequate glucose screening and appropriate diet and insulin therapy.

An estimated weight of over 5 kg in non-diabetics, a bisacromial diameter of 14.5 cm by computed tomography or estimated fetal weight of 4.5 kg in diabetics, or estimated weight of over 4 kg with a history of shoulder dystocia[43] are situations that warrant a discussion of shoulder dystocia and the potential risks and benefits of elective Cesarean section with the mother.

When dystocia is encountered, planned orchestrated action is undertaken to unlock the locked fetal position, and to deliver the fetus with procedures involving minimal invasion and least risk. These should emulate the natural mechanism of shoulder delivery. These are: the McRoberts or hands-and-knees position, generous episiotomy and partial cephalic replacement to unlock the shoulders, delivery of the posterior shoulder into the pelvis by fetal rotation or delivery of the posterior arm, followed if necessary by delivery of the anterior shoulder by delivery of the anterior arm or rotation of the posterior shoulder into the anterior position.

It is important to have a health care provider who is proficient in neonatal resuscitation present in the delivery room. Neurological evaluation of the infant is indicated when fetal injury occurs. The delivery should be clearly and completely documented and discussed with the patient.

REFERENCES

1. Morris W. Shoulder dystocia. *J Obstet Gynaecol Br Emp* 1955;62:302
2. Beer E, Folghera MG. La distocia della spalle: considerazioni su un caso risolto con la manovra di McRoberts. *Arch Obstet Ginecol* 1994;1:3
3. Schwartz BC, Dixon DM. Shoulder dystocia. *Obstet Gynecol* 1958;11:468
4. Hibbard LT. Shoulder dystocia. *Obstet Gynecol* 1969;34:424–9
5. Jacquemier J. Distocie par volume exagere et absence de rotation des epaules. *Gaz Hebd* 1860;7:661–4, 692–775
6. Woods CE. A principle of physics as applicable to shoulder delivery. *Am J Obstet Gynecol* 1962;83:1486–90
7. McCall JO Jr. Shoulder dystocia. A study of aftereffects. *Am J Obstet Gynecol* 1943;45:769–804
8. Rubin A. Management of shoulder dystocia. *J Am Med Assoc* 1964;189:835–7

9. Gordon M, Rich H, Deutschberger J, Green M. The immediate and long-term outcome of obstetric birth trauma 1. Brachial plexus paralysis. *Am J Obstet Gynecol* 1973;51–6

10. Lurie S, Ben-Arie A, Hagay Z. The ABC of shoulder dystocia management. *Asia-Oceana J Obstet Gynecol* 1994;20:195–7

11. Gross SJ, Shime J, Farine D. Shoulder dystocia: predictors and outcome. A five-year review. *Am J Obstet Gynecol* 1987;156:334–6

12. Gonik B, Hollyer VL, Allen R. Shoulder dystocia recognition: differences in neonatal risk for injury. *Am J Perinatol* 1991;8:31–4

13. Smeltzer JS. Prevention and management of shoulder dystocia. *Clin Obstet Gynecol* 1986;29:299–306

14. Sandberg EC. The Zavanelli maneuver extended: progression of a revolutionary concept. *Am J Obstet Gynecol* 1988;158:1347–53

15. Maharry J. Symphysiotomy for shoulder dystocia. *Am J Obstet Gynecol* 1988;158:1352–3

16. Meenan AL, Gaskin IM, Hunt P, Ball CA. A new (old) maneuver for the management of shoulder dystocia. *J Fam Prac* 1991;32:625–9

17. American College of Obstetricians and Gynecologists. *Fetal Macrosomia. ACOG Technical Bulletin 159.* Washington DC: ACOG,1991

18. Gross TL, Sokol RJ, Williams T, Thompsom K. Shoulder dystocia: a fetal–physician risk. *Am J Obstet Gynecol* 1987;156:1408–18

19. Nocon JJ, McKenzie DK, Thomas LJ, Hansell RS. Shoulder dystocia: an analysis of risks and obstetric maneuvers. *Am J Obstet Gynecol* 1993;168:1732–7

20. Sandmire HF. Whither ultrasonic prediction of fetal macrosomia? *Obstet Gynecol* 1993;82:860–2

21. Langer O, Berkus MD, Huff RW, Samueloff A. Shoulder dystocia: should the fetus weighing ≥ 4000 g be delivered by Cesarean section? *Am J Obstet Gynecol* 1991;165:831–7

22. Hannah ME, Hannah WJ, Hellmann J, *et al.* Induction of labor as compared with serial antenatal monitoring in post-term pregnancy. A randomized controlled trial. The Canadian Multicenter Post-term Pregnancy Trial Group. *N Engl J Med* 1992;326:1587–92

23. Fraser RB, Ford FA, Milner RDG. A controlled trial of a high dietary fibre intake in pregnancy – effects on plasma glucose and insulin levels. *Diabetologia* 1983;60:417

24. Modanlou HD, Komatsu G, Dorchester W, *et al.* Large-for-gestational-age neonates: anthropometric reasons for shoulder dystocia. *Obstet Gynecol* 1982;60:417

25. Acker DB, Sachs BP, Friedman EH. Risk factors for shoulder dystocia. *Obstet Gynecol* 1985;66:762–8

26. Langer O, Rodriguez DA, Xenakis EM, *et al.* Intensified versus conventional management of gestational diabetes. *Am J Obstet Gynecol* 1994;170:1036–46

27. Lin C-C, River J, River P, *et al.* Good diabetic control early in pregnancy and favorable fetal outcome. *Obstet Gynecol* 1986;67:51–6

28. Coustan DR, Imarah J. Prophylactic insulin treatment of gestational diabetes reduces the incidence of macrosomia, operative delivery and birth trauma. *Am J Obstet Gynecol* 1984;150:836–42

29. Langer O, Brustman L, Anyaegbunam A, Mazze R. The significance of one abnormal glucose tolerance test value on adverse outcome in pregnancy. *Am J Obstet Gynecol* 1987;157:758–63

30. Myers RE, Wagner KR, deCourten-Myers GM. Brain metabolic and pathologic consequences of asphyxia. *Adv Perinat Med* 1983;3:67

31. Mimouni F, Miodovnik M, Siddiqi TA, *et al.* Perinatal asphyxia in infants of insulin-dependent diabetic mothers. *J Pediatr* 1988;113:345–53

32. Kjos SL, Henry OA, Montoro M, *et al.* Insulin-requiring diabetes in pregnancy: a randomized trial of active induction of labor and expectant management. *Am J Obstet Gynecol* 1993;169:611–5

33. Keller JD, Lopez-Zeno JA, Dooley SL, Socol ML. Shoulder dystocia and birth trauma in gestational diabetes: a five-year experience. *Am J Obstet Gynecol* 1991;165:928–30

34. Elliott JP, Garite TJ, Freeman RK, *et al.* Ultrasonic prediction of fetal macrosomia in diabetic patients. *Obstet Gynecol* 1982;60:159–62

35. Cohen B, Penning S, Major C, *et al.* Sonographic prediction of shoulder dystocia in infants of diabetic mothers. *Obstet Gynecol* 1996;88:10–3

36. Kitzmiller JL, Mall JC, Gin GD, *et al.* Measurement of fetal shoulder width with computed tomography in diabetic women. *Obstet Gynecol* 1987;70:941–5

37. Bahar AM. Risk factors and fetal outcome in cases of shoulder dystocia compared with normal deliveries of a similar birthweight. *Br J Obstet Gynaecol* 1996;103:868–72

38. Benedetti TJ, Gabbe SG. Shoulder dystocia: a complication of fetal macrosomia and prolonged second stage of labor with midpelvic delivery. *Obstet Gynecol* 1978;52:526–9

39. Allen R, Sorab J, Gonik B. Risk factors for shoulder dystocia: an engineering study. *Obstet Gynecol* 1991;77:352–5

40. O'Leary JA, Pollack NB. McRoberts maneuver for shoulder dystocia: a survey. *Int J Gynecol Obstet* 1991;35:129–31

41. Hankins GD, Clark SL. Brachial plexus palsy involving the posterior shoulder at spontaneous vaginal delivery. *Am J Perinatol* 1995;12:44–5

42. Gonik B, Allen R, Sorab J. Objective evaluation of the shoulder dystocia phenomenon: effect of maternal pelvic orientation on force reduction. *Obstet Gynecol* 1989;74:44–8

43. Lewis DF, Raymond RC, Perkins MB, *et al.* Recurrence rate of shoulder dystocia. *Am J Obstet Gynecol* 1995;172:1369–71

44. Jennett RJ, Tarby TJ, Kreinick CJ. Brachial plexus palsy: an old problem revisited. *Am J Obstet Gynecol* 1992;166:1673–6

17
Sickle cell crisis

J.C. Morrison

INTRODUCTION

Hemoglobinopathies complicating pregnancy number in the hundreds, but fortunately most of them are very rare[1]. These inherited disorders usually result from structural abnormalities such as additions, deletions, or substitutions in the amino acids that comprise the two pairs of polypeptide chains common to each hemoglobin molecule (Table 1). These amino acid linkages contain either 141 or 147 amino acids, are responsible for the nomenclature and comprise the common types of hemoglobin such as A, A_2, F, etc[2]. Abnormalities in these globin chains result in hemoglobinopathies such as sickle hemoglobin, in which there is substitution of valine for glutamic acid in the sixth position on the β-globin chain. It is this minor substitution that is responsible for the high incidence of maternal and perinatal adverse effects noted during pregnancy as well as in the non-pregnant state[3].

Sickle cell crisis occurring at any time during gestation is a medical emergency[4]. Vaso-occlusive sickle cell crisis is the most common maternal complication noted in gestations complicated by sickle hemoglobinopathies[3]. Crisis is associated with increased maternal and perinatal morbidity and mortality[5]. The severity as well as frequency of crises among pregnant women are extremely variable, and crises may occur during the prenatal or intrapartum period as well as the puerperium[6]. Improvements in management over the last two decades have resulted in improved outcome for such women and their progeny. Nevertheless, providers who care for these high-risk patients must be prepared to practice preventive medicine, recognize the early signs of crisis and respond rapidly with a well-founded perinatal management plan.

EPIDEMIOLOGY

Sickle hemoglobin is the most common hemoglobinopathy in the USA. Its homozygous state (Hb S-S) complicates one in 625 births of blacks (one per 1875 blacks of reproductive age), while 10% of those with African heritage have sickle cell trait (Hb A-S)[7]. Patients with Hb S-S, as well as the more severe variants, such as hemoglobin S-C (Hb S-C) and hemoglobin S-thalassemia (Hb S-Thal), are said to have sickle cell disease and this is most often responsible for adverse effects on the mother, fetus and newborn[4]. These are also the disorders most likely to be associated with sickle cell crisis. Other sickle hemoglobinopathies such as Hb S-D, Hb A-S and Hb S-E are unlikely to result in sickling episodes.

Table 1 Normal/abnormal hemoglobin

Hemoglobin classification	Globin defect	Chain present	Common name	Hematological destination
Adult hemoglobin*	none	2α 2β	Hb A	$\alpha_2^A \beta_2^A$
Adult hemoglobin*	none	2α 2δ	Hb A_2	$\alpha_2^A \delta_2^A$
Adult fetal hemoglobin*	none	2α 2γ	Hb F	$\alpha_2^A \gamma_2^F$
Sickle hemoglobin†	β-chain substitution	2α 2β	Hb S	$\alpha_2^A \beta_2^S$ (6 glu → val)
C-hemoglobin†	β-chain substitution	2α 2β	Hb C	$\alpha_2^A \beta_2^C$ (6 glu → lys)
Methemoglobin†	α-chain substitution	2α 2β	Hb M Boston	α_2^M(58 his → tyr)β_2^A
β-Thalassemia*	none (decreased synthesis)	2α 2β	Hb B Thal	$\alpha_2^A \beta_2^{Thal}$

*Structurally normal; †structural abnormalities include substitution, inversion or deletions of amino acids in either chain

Patients with Hb S-S or Hb S-C have no hemoglobin A, therefore the predominant hemoglobin is Hb S, 90–95%, with the remainder being Hb F. Patients with this disorder have been shown to have a shorter life span, more common infections and, when pregnant, a higher maternal as well as perinatal mortality/morbidity[1]. The fertility rate does not appear to be decreased unless there are frequent crises and disseminated disease affecting many systems. The spontaneous abortion rate likewise does not appear to be increased.

On the other hand, adverse fetal and neonatal effects are common[2,4,6]. Decreased placental blood flow due to sickling in the tortuous, arcuate vessels of the myometrium have been associated with growth retardation[2]. Premature labor is also increased in 10–55% of those with sickle cell disease. Stillbirths are also common, occurring in 5–13%, and appear to be related to maternal crises[4]. The neonatal mortality rates are not increased in patients with sickle cell disease *per se* but may appear to increase due to preterm deliveries.

Clinical manifestations of sickle cell anemia usually involve the maternal cardiovascular, pulmonary and neurological systems. Although babies are asymptomatic at birth because of a higher concentration of hemoglobin F, the incidence of neonatal mortality increases after about 6 months with 20% of overall deaths from sickle cell disease occurring in the first 2 years, 10% between the ages of 2 and 5 years, and the remainder between 5 and 30 years[8]. During pregnancy, severe anemia is the rule among patients with sickle cell disease and rarely does the packed cell volume rise above 25%. Infections are also common and usually involve the urinary tract, pulmonary system and orthopedic system. In summary, most of the maternal morbidity as well as neonatal problems are related to sickle cell crisis.

Diminished oxygenation in the intravascular compartment in patients with sickle cell disease converts the normal oval red blood cells into the classic sickle-shaped erythrocytes noted in subjects undergoing crisis (Figure 1). These sickle cells lodge in the microvasculature of many organs and result in a decreased life span of red blood cells as well as the maternal and perinatal complications mentioned above. Any event leading to deoxygenation can initiate a sickle cell crisis. For instance, infections from viruses or bacteria, acidosis, dehydration, trauma, blood loss, severe stress, strenuous physical activity, high altitude and hypothermia have been incriminated.

There are several different kinds of sickle cell crisis. The most common is the vaso-occlusive crisis which is most frequently noted in pregnant women and adults. The less common hematological type of crisis is more often seen, but not exclusively so, in children (Table 2). The clinical expressions of the vaso-occlusive crises are extremely variable in their presentation but usually follow a characteristic pattern in each patient. These

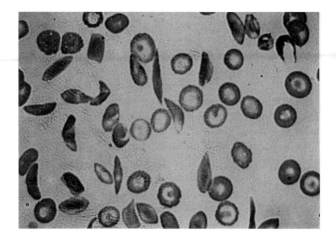

Figure 1   Blood film in patient with sickle cell crisis

Table 2   Sickle cell crisis classification

Vaso-occlusive
Abdominal
Chest
Joints
Central nervous system
Hematological
Aplastic
Hemolytic
Megaloblastic
Splenic sequestration

recurrent and sudden attacks of pain most often involve the abdomen, extremities, central nervous system and chest, although no body area is immune from these attacks[9]. Some patients exhibit generalized pain and malaise, while others have more localized syndromes involving a compromised microcirculation in various areas of the body.

On the other hand, hematological crises are infrequent among pregnant women but, if they occur, aplastic crisis is the most common type. Fortunately, this type of crisis is usually self-limited and most often associated with infection. Hemolytic crises, in contrast, are most commonly related to concomitant spherocytosis or glucose-6-phosphate dehydrogenase deficiency. Megaloblastic crises are usually secondary to folate depletion and are remedial to supplementation. Finally, splenic sequestration crises are usually limited to childhood. As a group, hematological crises are characterized by sudden anemia without icterus, pale conjunctiva, malaise, reticulocytopenia and cardiopulmonary failure.

ETIOLOGY

In a patient with sickle cell disease, the symptom constellation of the chronic, severe anemia and frequent pain lead one to suspect a vaso-occlusive crisis. Most commonly, this event in the pregnant adult is associated with apparent or occult infection (20–33%)[9]. Pneumonia, urinary tract infection and puerperal endomyometritis, as well as osteomyelitis, are the infectious sites commonly encountered with sickle cell crisis. Pneumococcal pneumonia or meningitis is particularly common in adolescent pregnant patients with sickle cell disease[11]. Gram-negative bacteria, such as *Escherichia coli* or *Salmonella* are the most common organisms noted in the third decade[4]. These organisms are particularly likely to attack the renal and gastrointestinal (gallbladder) systems, respectively. During the second decade, *Mycoplasma pneumoniae* is also common.

Factors other than infection have been associated with vaso-occlusive crisis in these patients. Acidosis from dehydration and hypotension have been noted to initiate such crises[1]. Strenuous activity, as well as drug overdose and hypothermia, have likewise been associated with these events[2]. Therefore, when confronted with a suspected vaso-occlusive crisis in a parturient with sickle cell disease, one should suspect infection first but rule out other factors during this intensive assessment.

PATHOPHYSIOLOGY

The variable clinical symptoms with which these patients present is not fully explained. There is evidence, however, to suggest that this variability may be related to the presence of linked and unlinked genes which modify the disease expression[12]. Another theory has been that of incomplete penetrance. The molecular basis for sickle cell crisis can be traced to the single amino acid substitution in the sickle hemoglobin molecule which distinguishes it from hemoglobin A. During deoxygenation or under conditions of acidosis as well as hypoxia the molecules of Hb S aggregate in a process called nucleation.

Hydrophobic bonding occurs between the abnormally substituted valine, owing to the change in electromagnetic charge. These hydrophobic bonds lead to the formation of polymerized hemoglobin strands, which become tactoids and microcables that eventually transform the cell into the half-moon or crescent shape (Figure 1)[13]. This overall process of gelation of the sickle hemoglobin is enhanced by changes in the vascular endothelium. It is reduced by lowering the oxygenation or pH[10].

Repetitive cycles of gelation during the red blood cell life cycle distort the cellular membrane, with resultant potassium and water reduction as well as calcium accumulation and membrane fragmentation[13]. This leads to an increase in the intracellular hemoglobin concentration with a concomitant increase in membrane rigidity to form discocytes or irreversibly sickled cells[15].

The irreversibly sickled cells retain the half-moon shape despite oxygenation. These irreversibly sickled cells constitute up to 50% of the red cell mass in such parturients. This index, however, does not appear to correlate well with vaso-occlusive crisis or its severity, but does have a positive relationship to the degree of anemia.

However, these abnormalities of the red cells themselves do not, alone, explain the pathophysiology of the sickle cell crisis. It is currently felt that there exists a combination of the erythrocyte abnormalities, plasma flow alterations and vessel wall interactions that is associated with sequestration and destruction of abnormal red cells in the microcirculation (Figure 2)[16]. This would explain patient variability noted in the clinical expression of a sickle crisis. Another factor involved in the pathophysiology of sickle cell crisis appears to be the large oscillation in blood flow in the microcirculation[17]. Most recently, with the use of laser-Doppler velocimetry, rather large changes in blood flow in periods of 7–10 s with peak/trough magnitudes measured at 50% of mean flow were found. These findings would suggest that during sickle cell crisis there is periodic flow in the microcirculation with synchronized rhythmic oscillations vs. the continuous even-flow pattern observed in patients with normal hemoglobin.

Therefore, although the environmental factors may stimulate deoxygenation resulting in aggregation, polymerization and subsequent formation of sickled red cells, flow dynamics as well as microcirculation factors are important determinants of the crisis cycle (Figure 2). These factors combine to increase whole blood viscosity and, thus, alter vasomotion in the microcapillaries. This would lead to sludging and destruction of red cells in the microcirculation. This promotes further deoxygenation that leads to vascular injury via ischemic necrosis, which results in pain and the other symptoms expressed during vaso-occlusive crises.

The marked susceptibility of parturients with sickle hemoglobinopathies to infection is related to functional hyposplenism, defective activation of complement fixation, decreased serum IgM, impaired serum opsonizing capacity and defective granulocyte phagocytosis[18]. There does not appear to be any difference in the percentage of helper or suppressor T cells or B cells in subjects in crisis[19]. This finding is compatible with the observation that patients with sickle hemoglobinopathies do not show increased susceptibility to those infections that are normally associated with depressed cell-mediated immunity[20].

DIAGNOSIS

Although some tests for crisis are helpful, the diagnosis is largely a clinical experience and basically one of exclusion. Fortunately, most women with sickle hemoglobinopathies are known prior to pregnancy. For

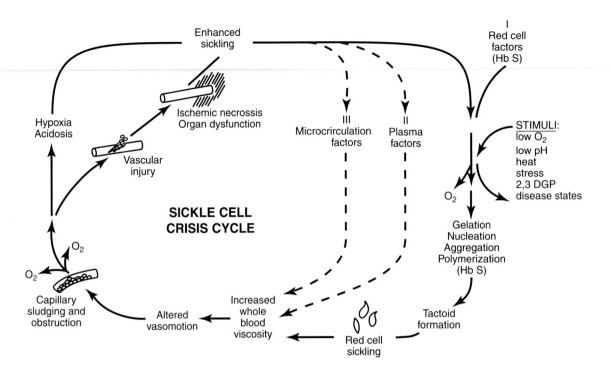

Figure 2   Vicious cycle of sickle cell crisis. Figure by J. Martin

patients with sickle cell disease, the first step is to confirm the diagnosis with hemoglobin electrophoresis. Once the diagnosis is documented, surgical/medical/obstetric conditions associated with a similar symptom complex or even malingering must be ruled out (Table 3). Because a parturient may have any one of many medical, surgical or obstetric complications, pain in a pregnant woman with sickle cell disease does not always result from vaso-occlusive crisis.

Several laboratory tests may be of assistance. Transcranial ultrasonography has been used in those with cerebral symptoms to detect or even predict strokes[21]. Likewise, infection and crises are usually associated with an increase in the total and the segmented neutrophil counts. However, only patients with significant bacterial infection have a consistent increase in the number of non-segmented leukocytes above 1000/mm[3,22]. Serum lactic dehydrogenase activity is also increased in sickle cell crisis. Elevation of isoenzymes 1 and 2 (α-hydroxybutyrate dehydrogenase) are particu-larly predictive[23]. Also, a rise in these isoenzyme levels is usually proportional to the severity of the vaso-occlusive crises.

MANAGEMENT

General

Despite advances during the past 20 years in the appreciation of the molecular basis of sickle cell crisis, there is no specific therapy available. However, an

Table 3   Differential diagnosis of sickle cell anemia

Obstetric factors
Threatened abortion
Preterm labor
Placental abruption
Uterine rupture
Ectopic pregnancy
Degenerating leiomyomata
Ovarian torsion
Pregnancy-induced
   hypertension

Medical factors
Renal/ureteral colic
Cystitis
Pyelonephritis

Other factors
Pneumonia
Pulmonary embolism
Arthritis

Surgical factors
Cholecystitis
Cholelithiasis
Appendicitis
Pancreatitis
Peptic ulcer disease
Perforated viscus
Intestinal obstruction
Volvulus
Ischemic colitis

Malingering
Drug addiction

understanding of the pathophysiology involved in vaso-occlusive crisis allows the provider to address those aspects of this event that can be treated. Such therapeutic regimens generally include: (1) adding fluids to reduce intracellular hemoglobin concentration; (2) correcting acidosis when present; (3) treating infection; and (4) increasing oxygen concentration.

Antepartum

During the prenatal period when the patient in crisis is not in labor and remote from term, hospitalization in a quiet area where bed rest, analgesia and hydration can be carried out is optimal. For mild sedation, phenobarbital can be useful, and analgesics such as meperidine or butorphanol can be helpful. Because of the risk of fetal loss, health assessment via biophysical profile and/or fetal heart rate monitoring is carried out during crisis treatment if gestational age is sufficient to consider intervention for fetal distress. In addition, continuous fetal heart rate monitoring is helpful, because resolution of worrisome signs, such as late decelerations, has been demonstrated during treatment of sickle cell crisis with blood infusion[24].

Vigorous rehydration is useful, particularly in crisis patients who are febrile[4]. In the absence of cardiopulmonary disease, infusion of a liter of Ringer's lactate or isotonic saline during the first 2-h period with continuing replacement at 125 ml/h is undertaken. Careful monitoring of intake and output is essential, but invasive hemodynamic monitoring and urinary catheterization are usually avoided, because of the risk of infection. The administration of alkali during the hydration process has not been found to be helpful[25]. For analgesia, acetaminophen is preferable to acetylsalicylic acid if mild analgesia is needed[4]. For severe pain, meperidine in combination with a sedative or ataractic agent is usually adequate. As soon as the pain begins to regress, non-narcotic agents are recommended.

Although the utility of oxygen therapy is unproven, it is often employed during crisis. Oxygen is administered at 3–6 l/min by tight face mask or nasal cannula. Arterial blood gas assessment is usually recommended if hypoxemia is suspected. Because infection is present in up to one-third of patients with vaso-occlusive crisis and since it is frequently associated with maternal death occurring in sickle cell crisis, attempts to detect occult infection are undertaken immediately. If an infection is suspected, then broad-spectrum antibiotic therapy is begun after appropriate cultures are obtained. Prophylactic antibiotic use, however, is not generally recommended.

Exchange transfusion

Partial exchange transfusion is one of the more important therapeutic agents for the interruption as well as the prevention of vaso-occlusive crises during pregnancy[26–28]. It may be given prophylactically, but some prefer to use this modality on the basis of the severity of the crisis[29]. If hydration, oxygen therapy and mild sedation/analgesia are sufficient, blood is not administered. On the other hand, if the crisis does not respond to conservative therapy, this therapeutic intervention will reduce the Hb S concentration while increasing the oxygen-carrying capacity in the patient[4].

We favor the prophylactic administration of blood in pregnant women with sickle cell disease and administer it by continuous automated erythrocytapheresis using the IBM 2997 cell separator[28]. This is also employed for such parturients during crises. This methodology has largely replaced the manual method of phlebotomy and infusion of packed red cells in most centers. The erythrocytapheresis allows the Hb S-containing cells and irreversibly sickled cells to be removed by extracorporeal, differential centrifugation. It also affords the simultaneous return by venous access in the other arm of the patient's own plasma, leukocytes, platelets and clotting factors along with donor, leukocyte-poor, washed Hb A-containing red cells. In addition, this method maintains isovolemia at all times and allows the provider accurately to monitor the patient's hematological indices such as packed cell volume, etc. It also has the advantage of administration on an outpatient basis. If such a device is not available, the manual 'push–pull' mechanism still works quite well (Table 4)[26].

The goal of the partial exchange transfusion, regardless of how it is accomplished, is to achieve a Hb A concentration of 50–60%[4,27,28]. Generally, six units of donor packed red cells are exchanged by this process and there is rapid resolution of crisis symptomatology and ongoing sickling. In addition to being more isovolemic, automated continuous erythrocytapheresis also requires less transfusion time[28]. About 2 h are usually required compared to 24–36 h by the manual method. Regardless of the methodology, each parturient usually has a Hb A concentration greater than 50% and a hematocrit above 30%. If the packed cell volume is very low (< 16%), a simple transfusion of 1–2 units (packed cells) is administered before the partial exchange transfusion is carried out.

Obviously, most of the complications associated with this approach are related to the risk of the blood

Table 4 Manual partial exchange transfusion

Measure hemoglobin A level and hematocrit
Type and match 6 units packed red blood cells
Start intravenous administration of 1 l normal saline (200–400 ml in the first hour) then 150–250 ml/h
Phlebotomize 500 ml blood from opposite arm over 30 min
Give 2 units leukocyte-poor, washed red cells (under pressure and warmed) over 1–2 h
Repeat procedure after 4 h
If hematocrit ≥ 35% and hemoglobin A ≥ 50%, discharge home
If hemoglobin A < 50%, repeat procedure

products. The use of all volunteer donor blood, screening for infection and washing of the red cells reduces the risk of hepatitis or HIV. Careful cross-matching to minimize minor blood incompatibilities and isoimmunization is critical in avoiding problems later for these patients who may need blood products at various points during their life. The use of blood from family members or friends matched for recipient and donor red cell antigens is clinically helpful in reducing the number of post-transfusion crises. Such episodes, also known as delayed hemolytic reactions, usually occur 2–21 days following transfusion, and are diagnosed by positive direct Coomb's antiglobulin tests[4]. Most often, such patients develop fever, arthritis and a clinical course very similar to that of serum sickness.

Intrapartum

The occurrence of a vaso-occlusive crisis during labor offers additional challenges to the provider. Obviously, with painful uterine contractions the diagnosis of a vaso-occlusive crisis may be more difficult. In addition, while oxygen and hydration therapy can be performed, exchange transfusion may be of limited availability, unless the patient is in a level III center. If delivery is expected within a short time, a simple transfusion of two units of leukocyte-poor, washed red cells can be substituted for the partial exchange transfusion.

During labor, patients should remain in the lateral recumbent position and receive oxygen by tight-fitting face mask. Careful monitoring of maternal and fetal vital signs are essential. Usually, when crisis has been diagnosed during labor and late decelerations appear, infusion of blood products has been associated with resolution of suspected fetal hypoxemia. Maternal blood gas assessment, if necessary, is carried out but invasive hemodynamic monitoring is avoided unless other concomitant disease processes such as pregnancy-induced hypertension, etc., are present. Urinary catheters, as well as intrauterine catheters, are discouraged, because of their association with increased infection.

Intrapartum analgesia and anesthesia for the parturient with sickle cell crisis are controversial. Some favor the approach of systemic analgesia with local infiltration for delivery, but others recommend conduction analgesia/anesthesia. We feel that epidural analgesia/anesthesia is acceptable if the vaso-occlusive crisis is mild or can be aborted with blood infusion. If not, intermittent intravenous analgesia with pudendal block for vaginal delivery is more appropriate. Continuous epidural morphine has also been utilized with success in these patients. For abdominal delivery, general anesthesia appears to be preferable. A Hb A concentration of 50% or more prior to general anesthesia reduces the risk of sickling which can be initiated by hypoxia occurring at the time of induction or as a consequence of other anesthetic complications. Careful monitoring of the patient's vital signs is important during anesthesia so that hypoxemia and acidosis are obviated. Avoidance of hypothermia and hypoxia during labor, as well as in the delivery room, is critical. Persons skilled at neonatal resuscitation should be present at delivery. Consultation with anesthesia and neonatology during labor is important. The use of oxytocic agents for induction/augmentation or an ecbolic agent during the third stage of labor is not contraindicated.

Postpartum

Crises after delivery usually do not develop unless hypovolemia, acidosis or infection occur. On the other hand, patients with Hb S-C are more likely to experience crises postpartum than during pregnancy. The same pitfalls of management applied during the antepartum period are also prudent after birth. Both urinary tract infection and endometritis are common and are frequently associated with crises. There is also a substantial increased risk of pulmonary edema and thromboembolic disease in these patients. Maintenance of isovolemia and high Hb A levels ($> 20\%$) appear to be important points in management.

SUMMARY

Patients with sickle cell disease are more likely to have a vaso-occlusive crisis during gestation than when they are not pregnant. The diagnosis of crisis in these subjects is difficult, because of other medical, surgical and obstetric disorders simulating this problem. A high index of suspicion and good diagnostic acumen is necessary to obtain optimal results in the pregnant patient with sickle cell disease.

REFERENCES

1. Laros RK Jr. The hemoglobinopathies. In Laros RK Jr, ed. *Blood Disorders in Pregnancy*. Philadelphia: Lea & Febiger, 1986:37–61
2. Palmer SM, Sherrill J, Morrison JC. Diseases of the blood. In Danforth DN, Scott JR, eds. *Obstetrics and Gynecology*, 5th edn. Philadelphia: Lippincott, 1986
3. Bunn HF. Pathogenesis and treatment of sickle cell disease. *N Engl J Med* 1997;337:762–69
4. Martin JN, Files J, Morrison JC. Sickle cell crisis. In Clark SL, Phelan JP, Cotton DB, eds. *Critical Care Obstetrics*, 2nd edn. Oradell, NJ: Medical Economics, 1990
5. ACOG. *Hemoglobinopathies in Pregnancy*. ACOG Technical Bulletin No. 185, Washington, DC: ACOG, October 1993
6. Ogedenbe OK, Akinyanju OO. The hemoglobinopathies and pregnancy in Lagos. *Int J Gynecol Obstet* 1988;26: 229–33
7. Schneider RG, Hightower B, Hosty TS, *et al.* Abnormal hemoglobins in a quarter million people. *Blood* 1976;48:629–37

8. Perry KG Jr, Martin JN Jr, Morrison JC. Hematologic and hemorrhagic diseases. In Sweet AY, Brown EG, eds. *Fetal and Neonatal Effects of Maternal Disease.* St Louis: Mosby Year Book, 1991:224–40

9. Martin JN Jr, Martin RW, Morrison JC. Acute management of sickle cell crisis in pregnancy. *Clin Perinatol* 1986;13:853–68

10. Steinberg MH. Management of sickle cell disease. *New Engl J Med* 1999;340:1021–30

11. Serjeant GR. Sickle-cell disease. *Lancet* 1997;350: 725–30

12. Nagel RL, Fabry ME, Pagnier J, *et al.* Hematologically and genetically distinct forms of sickle cell anemia in Africa: the Senegal type and Benin type. *N Engl J Med* 1985;312:880–4

13. Dean J, Schechter AN. Sickle-cell anemia. Molecular and cellular basis of therapeutic approaches. *N Engl J Med* 1978;752:863–70

14. Solovey A, Lin Y, Browne P, *et al.* Circulating activated endothelial cells in sickle cell anemia. *New Engl J Med* 1997;337(22):1584–90

15. Rodgers GP, Noguchi CT, Schecter AN. Irreversibly sickled erythrocytes in sickle cell anemia: a quantitative reappraisal. *Am J Hematol* 1985;20:17–23

16. Wautier J, Galacteros F, Wautier MP, *et al.* Clinical manifestations and erythrocyte adhesion to endothelium in sickle cell syndrome. *Am J Hematol* 1985;19:121–30

17. Rodgers GP, Schechter AN, Noguchi CT, *et al.* Periodic microcirculatory flow in patients with sickle-cell disease. *N Engl J Med* 1984;311:1534–8

18. Pearson HA. Sickle cell anemia and severe infection due to encapsulated bacteria. *J Infect Dis* 1977;136: S25–S30

19. Venkataraman M, Westerman MP. B-cell changes occur in patients with sickle cell anemia. *Am J Clin Pathol* 1985;84:153–8

20. De Ceulaer K, Pagliuca A, Forbes M, *et al.* Recurrent infections in sickle cell disease: hematological and immune studies. *Clin Chim Acta* 1985;148:161–5

21. Adams R, McKie V, Nichols F, *et al.* The use of transcranial ultrasonography to predict stroke in sickle cell disease. *New Engl J Med* 1992;326(9):605–10

22. Shah Y, Kumar A. Differentiating vaso-occlusive crisis and infection in sickle cell anemia. *J Fam Pract* 1981;13: 752–64

23. Rutledge R, Croom RD III, Davis JW Jr, *et al.* Cholelithiasis in sickle cell anemia: surgical considerations. *South Med J* 1986;79:28–30

24. Morrison JC, Pryor JA. Hematologic disorders. In Eden R, Boehm F, eds. *Assessment and Care of the Fetus: Physiologic, Clinical and Medicolegal Principles.* Norwalk, CT: Appleton & Lange, 1990

25. Morrison JC, Ruvinsky ED, Nicolls ET. Sickling and pregnancy: a worrisome combination. *Contemp Obstet Gynecol* 1981;18:125–35

26. Morrison JC, Morrison FS, Floyd RC, *et al.* Use of continuous flow erythrocytapheresis in pregnant patients with sickle cell disease. *J Clin Apheresis* 1991;6:224–9

27. Cunningham FG, Pritchard JA, Mason R. Pregnancy and sickle cell hemoglobinopathies: results with and without prophylactic transfusion. *Obstet Gynecol* 1983; 62:419–24

28. Morrison JC, Douvas SG, Martin JN Jr, *et al.* Erythrocytapheresis in pregnant patients with sickle hemoglobinopathies. *Am J Obstet Gynecol* 1984;149:912–14

29. Koshy M, Burd L, Wallace D, *et al.* Prophylactic red-cell transfusions in pregnant patients with sickle cell disease. *N Engl J Med* 1988;319:1447–52

Section IIIa

Perinatal infections: bacterial infections

18

Gonorrhea infection

J.B. Shumway

The past 30 years have brought about tremendous changes in sexual practices and significant advances in our understanding of sexually transmitted diseases. Epidemic rates of multiple venereal diseases have focused attention on their impact on pregnancy. Gonorrhea, one of the traditional venereal diseases, is still ever-present in any practice.

INCIDENCE

Approximately 700 000 new infections with *Neisseria gonorrhoeae* are estimated to occur in the USA yearly. In 1995, 392 848 cases of *N. gonorrhoeae* were reported, with an estimated 50% of cases not reported. A significant reporting bias exists among persons of minority race/ethnicity who attend public sexually transmitted disease (STD) clinics. This bias may partially explain the large reported race differentials among persons with this disease[1] (Figure 1).

Gonorrhea is the second most common STD in the USA, trailing behind infection with *Chlamydia*[2]. The incidence of gonorrhea infections appears now to be declining rapidly in the USA (Figure 2). Between 1994 and 1995 the rate decreased from 165.1 to 149.5 cases per 100 000 population, and this trend appears to be continuing with 120 cases per 100 000 projected for 1999[2].

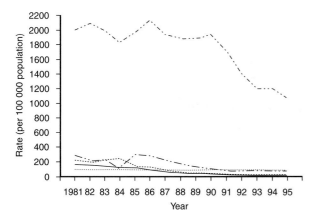

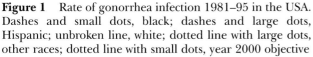

Figure 1 Rate of gonorrhea infection 1981–95 in the USA. Dashes and small dots, black; dashes and large dots, Hispanic; unbroken line, white; dotted line with large dots, other races; dotted line with small dots, year 2000 objective

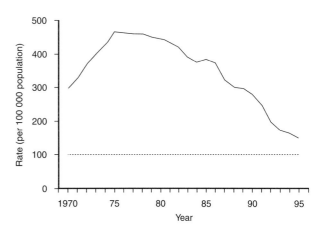

Figure 2 Reported rates of gonorrhea in the USA, 1970–95, unbroken line. Dotted line, year 2000 objective

MICROBIOLOGY AND GENETIC EVOLUTION

Bacteria of the genus *Neisseria* are non-motile, non-spore-forming, Gram-negative diplococci whose stained cells appear characteristically kidney-shaped with their concave sides adjacent to each other. As a result, diplococci sometimes look like small doughnuts. *N. gonorrhoeae* is closely related to *N. meningitidis*, the etiological agent of epidemic meningitis.

The non-pathogenic *Neisseria* (part of the normal flora of the nasopharynx) are slightly larger and easier to grow than the pathogenic species. *N. gonorrhoeae* are fragile and require serum or blood in the growth medium (chocolate blood agar) and a higher concentration of carbon dioxide for optimal growth (hence special collection techniques). The virulence of *N. gonorrhoeae* is correlated with specific colony types, depending on the presence and type of membrane pili. Piliated gonococci are better able to attach to mucosal surfaces. Colonies of types P+ and P++ (formerly T1 and T2, respectively) which contain pili that facilitate attachment to epithelial surfaces are pathogenic[3]. Colonies of type P− (formerly T3,T4) lack pili and are non-pathogenic. *N. gonorrhoeae* also contains specific proteins which enhance its endocytosis by the mucosal cell. After adherence, mediated by the pili, to mucosal columnar or cuboidal cells, porin (formerly protein I) facilitates pinocytosis, and an endotoxin is released, causing local cytotoxic effects[4]. An IgA protease, which destroys secretory immunoglobulins, also enhances gonococcal virulence. Additional proteins Opa and Rmp have specific adherence and immunological effects, which enhance virulence[5]. Rmp can stimulate the production of blocking antibodies[6].

In 1976, strains of *N. gonorrhoeae* with high-level penicillin resistance (penicillinase-producing *N. gonorrhoeae* – PPNG) due to plasmid-mediated production of beta-lactamase were noted[7]. In 1983, other gonococcal subtypes were discovered with a high-level chromosomal resistance to penicillin (CMRNG). In 1985, additional gonococcal strains were discovered with a plasmid-mediated, high-level resistance to tetracycline (TRNG)[8].

Recent evolutionary trends in the gonococcus in the eastern USA involve the development of three virulent isolates of *N. gonorrhoeae*: plasmid-mediated PPNG; high level chromosomal resistant strains (CMRNG) which are resistant to tetracycline, cephalosporins, spectinomysin, aminoglycosides and penicillin; and plasmid-mediated, high-level resistance to tetracycline (TRNG) strains[1] (Figures 3 and 4). In 1995 the percentage of isolates from the Gonococcal Isolate Surveillance Project showing significant antibiotic resistance rose to 31.6%. New strains showing resistance to ciprofloxacin were first identified in 1991, but are rare at present.

EPIDEMIOLOGY AND PATHOGENESIS

N. gonorrhoeae is a fastidious organism requiring particular care to grow in a laboratory setting. Its only natural host is the human. It is a venereal disease that, with few exceptions, is acquired through sexual contact or

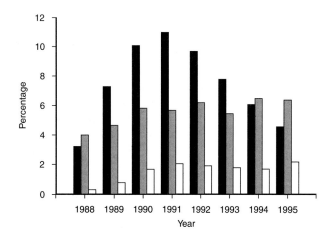

Figure 3 Gonococcal Isolate Surveillance Project: trends in plasmid-mediated resistance to penicillin (black bars, penicillinase-producing *Neisseria gonorrhoeae*) and tetracycline (hatched bars, tetracycline-resistant *N. gonorrhoeae*). Cross-hatched bars, resistance to both

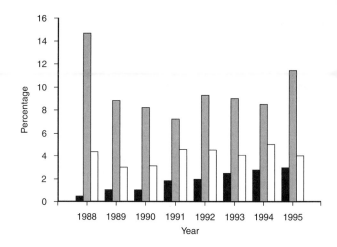

Figure 4 Gonococcal Isolate Surveillance Project: trends in chromosomally mediated resistance to penicillin and tetracycline, 1988–95. Resistance to penicillin denotes a minimum inhibitory concentration (MIC) of ≥ 2 µg/ml and beta-lactamase negativity (black bars); chromosomally mediated resistance to tetracycline corresponds to a MIC of ≥ 2 µg/ml without plasmid-mediated tetracycline resistance (hatched bars). Cross-hatched bars, resistance to both

vaginal birth. The organisms penetrate the mucous membranes of the genital tract, initially causing a localized infection. Other sites of infection include the rectum, pharynx and eye. Localized infection may give rise to hematogenous spread to distant organs resulting in disseminated disease.

National surveys have demonstrated varying prevalence rates for gonorrhea among females, with 1–2% prevalence rates in private physician offices, 5% in public clinics and 25% in STD clinics[9]. Prevalence rates in pregnancy mirror these rates and increase in the young, with the highest prevalence among patients aged 18–24 years. Infection at a young age is associated with failure to use barrier methods effectively and increased risk-taking behavior[10]. Other risk factors include poverty, unmarried status, prostitution, urban residence, early sexual activity and illicit drug use[9,11].

CLINICAL PRESENTATION

Most infected men have symptoms of an acute urethritis, resulting in a purulent discharge and painful urination. The prostate gland and epididymis may also be infected. Asymptomatic infection is rare and the presence of symptomatic infection motivates men to seek timely treatment, leading to the prevention of serious sequelae. Unfortunately, this treatment often occurs after transmission to other sexual partners. The risk of horizontal transmission from an infected male to a female partner has been estimated at 70–80%[12]. Female-to-male transmission is much less common, at 20–25% per sexual encounter[13].

Women infected with gonorrhea often report mild or non-specific symptoms while significant destructive urethral, vaginal, cervical and Fallopian tubal inflammatory processes are active. Genitourinary infection may result in dysuria and purulent discharge after an incubation period of 7–21 days. Infection is much more likely to be asymptomatic in females with the endocervical canal and transition zone of the cervix being favored sites of colonization. Vaginal discharge and dysuria are the most common complaints of symptomatic women, resulting from local infection to the endocervical urethra and cervix. Adnexal and uterine tenderness is seen with ascending infection[14].

Disseminated gonococcal infection may also occur, leading to papular lesions in the skin, heart, eye, meninges, liver and joints. Acute febrile illness with a severe arthritis/tenosynovitis may cause significant pain in disseminated disease and is the most common presentation of disseminated disease[15].

PERINATAL AND NEONATAL INFECTION

Pregnancy appears to make women more susceptible to gonococcal arthritis and other disseminated forms of gonorrhea in all trimesters[16]. The rate of pharyngeal gonococcal infection appears to increase during pregnancy, possibly as a result of altered sexual practices[17]. Associated pregnancy complications include spontaneous abortion, premature rupture of membranes, preterm labor, chorioamnionitis, disseminated gonococcal disease and arthritis[18–21]. First and early second-trimester post-abortion endometritis, salpingitis, pelvic inflammatory disease and sterility are recognized sequelae of untreated infection[22]. Pelvic inflammatory disease is uncommon after the first trimester and its decline is postulated as being due to the products of conception effectively filling the uterine cavity. Performance of elective abortion of chorionic villous sampling should be preceded by appropriate testing for gonorrhea infection.

Endocervical maternal infection may lead to amniotic and fetel infection via transplacental infection. Untreated endocervical gonococcal infection is associated with an increased risk of premature rupture of membranes, preterm delivery and subsequently high infant morbidity and mortality[19–21]. These intrapartum and postpartum complications persist despite antenatal treatment[23]. Acute chorioamnionitis, fetal infection, neonatal sepsis and maternal postpartum endomyometritis are associated with third-trimester gonococcal infection[24].

Although the definitive gonococcal studies may have been confounded by failure to correct for the contributions of group B streptococcal and chlamydial infection in prematurity, recent studies support the association of the gonococcus with preterm labor, premature rupture of membranes, low birth weight and preterm delivery[25,26]. Recent Canadian studies also demonstrate the frequent concomitant coinfection of *Chlamydia* and *N. gonorrhoeae* particularly in young age groups with increased prematurity risks[27,28].

Ophthalmia neonatorum, a neonatal infection of the eye acquired during vaginal birth, was first recognized in the 1700s. By 1881 ophthalmia neonatorum was a complication in up to 10% of births. Ophthalmia neonatorum may be caused by a variety of bacteria; however, *Chlamydia trachomatis* and *N. gonorrhoeae* are more likely to cause serious corneal infection. This is manifested clinically within the first 3–4 weeks of life with bilateral purulent conjunctivitis which, if untreated, leads to corneal ulceration, scarring and blindness. Vertical transmission rates of 30–35% were present in exposed neonates[29]. Legally mandated universal bactericidal treatment for the gonococcus and chlamydia at birth (1% silver nitrate or tetracycline ointment) has largely eliminated neonatal disease, even with the emergence of new virulent penicillinase-producing *N. gonorrhoeae*. Most cases of neonatal gonorrhea occur non-sexually, usually owing to poor hygiene, before the age of 1 year, while later infection is probably sexual[30].

DIAGNOSIS

Isolation of the bacteria is achieved by culturing purulent material from an infected site on selective chocolate or Thayer–Martin media. Colonies usually appear by 48 h. The enzyme immunoassay Gonozyme (Abbott Laboratories, North Chicago, IL) can be used to detect the gonococcal antigen. The high specificity (97%) but moderate sensitivity (60%) make it a suboptimal test for widespread screening in a low-prevalence population. A test that detects gonococcal DNA (Gen-Probe, PACE, San Diego, CA) is being used clinically as a screening test. Culture remains the most reliable method for diagnosis.

Gram staining of a urethral exudate in men with dysuria and purulent discharge is a rapid and reliable diagnostic modality. The Gram stain demonstrates Gram-negative diplococci within leukocytes. In women, a Gram stain is less useful, with only 60% of infected women demonstrating sufficient bacteria to be picked up on a Gram stain. Chronic gonorrhea, particularly in the female, can be difficult to diagnose by Gram staining, since there is little or no discharge and few organisms. Diagnosis in women requires isolation of *N. gonorrhoeae* by culture.

Disseminated gonococcal infection is manifested by arthritis and synovitis. Culture of the aspirated purulent effusion permits identification while blood cultures are usually negative. Cultures should also be obtained from anal and pharyngeal lesions. All sexually active women, particularly in high-risk groups, should be screened during pregnancy. Risk factors include partners with gonorrhea or urethritis, multiple partners, lower genital discharge or pelvic pain and age of less than 24 years. All pregnant women should have a culture for *N. gonorrhoeae* at their initial prenatal visit, and again at 28 weeks for those with high-risk factors. The proper technique for collection of the sample for gonorrhea culture is to keep the swab in the site sampled (e.g. endocervical canal) for 15–30 s to increase the absorption of the gonococcus by the dry cotton swab. Use of specific media and meticulous transport of specimens are critical for reliability and accuracy of results.

In women, a single properly obtained endocervical culture detects 80–90% of uncomplicated anogenital gonorrhea[15]. Optimal yield of *N. gonorrhoeae* detection is accomplished by simultaneously culturing the cervix and the anus. The pharynx is unlikely to be the only site of infection (5%) but should not be overlooked in women reporting oral–genital contact or sore throat.

TREATMENT

Several antibiotic regimens are safe and effective in eliminating *N. gonorrhoeae*, preventing transmission, relieving symptoms and reducing clinical sequelae. As resistance of gonococcal strains to penicillin, ampicillin, amoxicillin and the tetracyclines is common throughout the USA, none of these drugs should be used. Current guidelines of the Centers for Disease Control offer 98% microbiological and clinical efficacy for genital/rectal gonorrhea (Table 1).

Ciprofloxacin 500 mg is safe and effective for uncomplicated gonorrhea and is the least expensive of the recommended options. Ofloxacin is also effective. As for all quinolones, neither ciprofloxacin nor ofloxacin should be used in patients younger than 18 years of age, and both are contraindicated for use during pregnancy and lactation, owing to their erosion of cartilage in weightbearing joints and known teratogenic and embryocidal effects.

Hospitalization is recommended for the initial therapy of patients with disseminated gonorrhea. Patients with gonococcal meningitis, nephritis and endocarditis require extended multiweek therapy with ceftriaxone intravenously (1–2 g every 12 h). They should also be evaluated for complement deficiencies and be managed in consultation with an expert[27,31].

Since up to 40% of women with gonorrhea also demonstrate co-infection with *Chlamydia trachomatis*, a regimen active against *C. trachomatis* should be prescribed[12,13,32,33]. As the use of tetracyclines is not advisable during pregnancy and lactation, the recommended regimen is ceftriaxone and one of the erythromycin derivatives for 7 days. In clinical practice, however, many pregnant women will not tolerate these large erythromycin doses. Alternatively, an extended treatment for 2 weeks with one-half the recommended dose can be offered. It appears that azithromycin is

Table 1　Centers for Disease Control recommended treatment of uncomplicated gonococcal infections in adults (1998) (From reference 15)

Recommended regimens

Ceftriaxone 125 mg IM in a single dose
  or
Cefixime 400 mg orally in a single dose
  or
Ciprofloxacin 500 mg orally in a single dose
  or
Ofloxacin 400 mg orally in a single dose
  plus
A regimen effective against possible coinfection with *Chlamydia trachomatis*, such as doxycycline 100 mg orally twice a day for 7 days or azithromycin 1 g orally in a single dose

Alternative regimens

(1)　Spectinomycin 2 g IM in a single dose
(2)　Injectable cephalosporins such as ceftizoxime 500 mg IM, cefotaxime 500 mg IM, cefotetan 1 g IM and cefoxitin 2 g IM, all as a single dose with probenecid 1 g orally
(3)　Quinolone regimens including enoxacin 400 mg orally, lomefloxacin 400 mg orally, or norfloxacin 800 mg orally as a single dose

IM, intramuscularly

highly effective and well tolerated with minimal side-effects. Sexual partners of infected patients should be examined, cultured and treated for gonorrhea and chlamydia.

Pregnant women who are allergic to ceftriaxone should be treated with spectinomycin, 2 g intramuscularly once, and with 1 g azithromycin orally.

A culture for test of cure should be performed after effective treatment at 4–7 days after therapy. This recommendation is controversial, owing to the rare occurrence of treatment failure[18]. We recommend that all treated women be re-screened at 2–8 weeks after therapy. Careful counselling should be offered regarding contraception and effective sexual barrier methods as appropriate to the clinical setting. Patients should be instructed to refer their sexual partners for evaluation and treatment (Table 2).

PREVENTION AND THE FUTURE

Condoms, properly used, provide effective protection from the acquisition of gonorrhea. It is likely that the female condom is also effective, although the use effectiveness of the device is uncertain. Other barrier methods such as the cervical cap and diaphragm, especially when used with nonoxynol-9 spermicide, afford some protection. Immediate washing, douching, or urinating after exposure have not been shown to have any beneficial effect.

Table 2 Centers for Disease Control special treatment guidelines for gonorrhea

Recommended regimens

(1) Cephalosporin or quinolone allergic
   Treatment with spectinomycin with follow-up throat culture and treatment of pharyngeal gonorrhea if present at 3–5 days post-treatment

(2) Pregnancy
   Cephalosporin or spectinomycin IM with additional erythromycin or amoxicillin or azithromycin for treatment of presumptive *Chlamydia trachomatis*

(3) HIV infection – standard treatment

(4) Gonococcal conjunctivitis
   Ceftriaxone 1 g IM in a single dose and leavage the infected eye with saline solution once

(5) Disseminated gonococcal infection (DGI)
   (Skin lesions, arthralgia, tenosynovitis, arthritis)
   Ceftriaxone 1 g IM or IV every 24 h for 7 days
   Cyrofloxacin 500 mg IV every 12 h for 7 days
   Spectinomycin 2 g IM every 12 h for 7 days
   Treatment for gonococcal meningitis and endocarditis should be undertaken with an expert

(6) Prophylactic treatment for infants born to mothers with untreated gonorrheal infection
   Ceftriaxone 25–50 mg/kg IV or IM not to exceed 125 mg in a single dose

IM, intramuscularly; IV, intravenously

An experimental vaccine against gonorrhea has been developed and its effectiveness has been limited by the extraordinary variability in the antigenitive sites present on the pili, and associated membrane proteins. Work to develop a vaccine against more stable antigens is ongoing[33].

REFERENCES

1. Division of STD/HIV Prevention, US Department of Health and Human Services, Public Health Service. Sexually Transmitted Disease Surveillance, 1995. Atlanta: Centers for Disease Control and Prevention, 1996

2. Centers for Disease Control. Summaries of notifiable diseases in the United States, 1994. *Morbid Mortal Weekly Rep* 1994;43(53):1–80

3. Schoolnik GK, Fernandez R, Tai JY, *et al.* Gonococcal pili: primary structure and receptor binding domain. *J Exp Med* 1984;159:1351–70

4. McGee ZA, Johnson AP, Taylor-Robinson D. Pathogenic mechanisms of *Neisseria gonorrhoea*. Observations on damage to human fallopian tubes in organ culture by gonococci of colony type I or type IV. *J Infect Dis* 1981;143:413–22

5. Blake MS, Gotschlich EC. Gonococcal membrane proteins: speculation on their role in pathogenesis. *Prog Allergy* 1983;33:298–313

6. Rice PA, Vayo HE, Tam MR, Blake MS. Immunoglobulin G antibodies directed against protein III block killing of serum-resistant *Neisseria gonorrhoea* by immune system. *J Exp Med* 1986;164:1735–48

7. Perine PL, Morton RS, Piot P, *et al.* Epidemiology and treatment of penicillinase-producing *Neisseria gonorrhoeae*. *Sex Trans Dis* 1979;6(suppl):152–8

8. Centers for Disease Control and Prevention. Tetracycline-resistant *Neisseria gonorrhoeae* – Georgia,

Pennsylvania, New Hampshire. *Morbid Mortal Weekly Rep* 1985;34(37):563–4,569–70

9. Klass PE, Brown ER, Pelton SI. The incidence of prenatal syphilis at the Boston City Hospital: a comparison across four decades. *Pediatrics* 1994;94:24–8

10. Dallabetta G, Hook EW III. Gonococcal infections. *Infect Dis Clin North Am* 1987;1:25–54

11. Hook EW III, Handsfield HH. Gonococcal infections in the adult. In Holms KK, Mardh PA, Sparling PF, *et al.* eds. *Sexually Transmitted Diseases*. New York: McGraw-Hill, 1990:149–65

12. Hooper RR, Reynolds GH, Jones OG, *et al.* Cohort study of venereal disease: I. The risk of gonorrhea transmission from infected women to men. *Am J Epidemiol* 1978;108:136–44

13. Thin RNY, William IA, Nicol CS. Direct and delayed methods of immunofluorescent diagnosis of gonorrhea in women. *Br J Vener Dis* 1970;47:27–30

14. McCormack WM, Stumacher RJ, Johnson K, Donner A. Clinical spectrum of gonococcal infection in women. *Lancet* 1977;1:1182–5

15. Centers for Disease Control. Sexually transmitted disease treatment guidelines. *Morbid Mortal Weekly Rep* 1998;47:59–69

16. Holmes KK, Counts GW, Beaty HN. Disseminated gonococcal infection. *Ann Intern Med* 1990;74:979–93

17. Corman LC, Levison ME, Knight R, *et al.* The high frequency of pharyngeal gonococcal infection in a prenatal clinic population. *J Am Med Assoc* 1974; 230:568–70

18. ACOG. *Gonorrhea and Chlamydial Infections*, ACOG Technical Bulletin No.190. Washington DC: American College of Obstetricians and Gynecologists, 1994: 169–74

19. Donders GGG, Desmyter J, DeWet GH, Van Assche FA. The association of gonorrhoea and syphilis with premature birth and low birthweight. *Genitourinary Med* 1993;69:98–101

20. Sarrel PM, Pruett KA. Symptomatic gonorrhea during pregnancy. *Obstet Gynecol* 1968;32:670–3

21. Edwards LE, Barrada MI, Hamann AA, Hakansen EY. Gonorrhea in pregnancy. *Am J Obstet Gynecol* 1978;132: 637–41

22. Burkman RT, Tonascia JA, Atienza MF, King TM. Untreated endocervical gonorrhea and endometritis following elective abortion. *Am J Obstet Gynecol* 1976; 126:648–51

23. Amstey MS, Steadman KT. Symptomatic gonorrhea and pregnancy. *J Am Vener Dis Assoc* 1976;3:14

24. Handsfield HH, Hodson A, Holmes KK. Neonatal gonococcal infection. *J Am Med Assoc* 1973; 225:697–701

25. Alger LS, Lovchik JC, Hebel JR, et al. The association of *Chlamydia trachomatis, Neisseria gonorrhoeae,* and group B streptococci with preterm rupture of the membranes and pregnancy outcome. *Am J Obstet Gynecol* 1988;159:397–404

26. Elliott B, Brunham RC, Laga M, et al. Maternal gonococcal infection as a preventable risk factor for low birth weight. *J Infect Dis* 1990;161:531–6

27. Gonorrhea and chlamydial infections. *Int J Gynecol Obstet* 1994;45:69–74

28. Holmes KK. Gonococcal infection. In Remington JS, Klien JO, eds. *Infectious Diseases of the Fetus and Newborn Infant.* Philadelphia: WB Saunders, 1983:616–36

29. Rawstron SA, Bromberg K, Hammerschlag MR. STD in children: syphilis and gonorrhoea. *Genitourinary Med* 1993;69:66–75

30. Judson FN, Werness BA. Combining cervical and anal-canal specimens for gonorrhea on a single culture plate. *J Clin Microbiol* 1980;12:216–19

31. *Infection Protocols for Obstetrics and Gynecology.* Montvale NJ: Medical Economics press, 1992:46

32. Cavenee MR, Farris JR, Spalding TR, et al. Treatment of gonorrhea in pregnancy. *Obstet Gynecol* 1993;81:33–8

33. Tramont RC. Gonococcal vaccines. *Clin Microbiol Rev* 1989;2(suppl):574–7

19

Group B streptococcus infection

H.N. Winn and H. Hamill

Group B streptococcus (GBS) (*Streptococcus agalactiae*), a Gram-positive coccus, is one of the major causes of maternal or neonatal severe infection and sepsis. Maternal infection associated with GBS includes acute chorioamnionitis, endometriosis and urinary tract infection. Neonatal GBS infection is characterized as early-onset if occurring within 7 days of age or late-onset otherwise, and involves bacteremia, pneumonia or meningitis[1,2].

EPIDEMIOLOGY

Of all pregnant women in the USA, 5–40% have recto-vaginal colonization with GBS[3–5]. In patients with preterm labor or preterm premature rupture of membranes (PROM), the incidence of genital colonization of GBS is 15%[6]. Of urinary tract infections, 1–5% result from GBS colonization[7]. The incidence of neonatal GBS infection is 1.8 per 1000 live births[8]. Neonatal colonization of GBS may occur as a result of *in utero* ascending infection from the maternal genital tract or direct contact during delivery. Vertical transmission from the mother to the neonate by either method accounts for up to 75% of cases of neonatal GBS colonization, and 1–2% of these infants will develop early-onset GBS infection[9–13]. The case fatality of early-onset GBS neonatal infection varies from 11% to almost 50%[8,14–16]. Maternal risk factors that predispose a neonate to early-onset GBS infection include preterm delivery, prolonged rupture of membranes (> 18 h), intrapartum fever temperature of at least 38°C or 100.4°F, or prior infant with GBS infection[17]. The risk of neonatal GBS colonization from a GBS-colonized mother is 45.5 per 1000 live births if maternal fever, prolonged rupture of membranes and preterm birth coexist[18]. Late-onset GBS neonatal infection may occur from maternal–neonatal transmission, or nosocomial or community contacts[19,20].

DIAGNOSIS

Group B streptococcal colonization can be detected by either culture or rapid diagnostic tests. Currently, culture remains the gold standard for diagnosing GBS colonization[17]. The yield of positive GBS culture is increased by sampling the anorectum in addition to the vagina, since the gastrointestinal tract is a major reservoir of GBS[5,21]. This can be done in a single swab. Inhibition of competing organisms by using a selective medium such as Todd–Hewitt broth, which contains gentamicin, polymyxin B and validixic acid, also increases the yield of the GBS culture[1]. The main limitation of culture is time. Since culture results are not available for 24–48 h, management may be problematic if delivery is imminent.

Rapid diagnostic tests of GBS directly detect the extracted specific polysaccharide antigen. The available tests use either latex particle agglutinization (LPA), or enzyme immunoassay (EIA). These tests are relatively easy to perform, are generally less expensive than a culture and produce results within a short period of time (usually within 1 h). Although rapid detection tests are highly sensitive in patients who are heavily colonized with GBS, their overall rates of sensitivity and high false-negative results compared to those of cultures prevent their widespread clinical application[22–26]. These drawbacks for the rapid diagnostic tests also exist in the setting of preterm labor or preterm PROM, demonstrating that the rapid latex agglutination test fails to identify GBS neonatal infection in (1) heavily; (2) moderately; and (3) lightly colonized mothers. More importantly, the overall sensitivity of the latex agglutination test in identifying maternal–neonatal pairs at risk for GBS neonatal infection is only 25%[6].

TREATMENT

Intrapartum chemoprophylaxis is effective in reducing the attack rate of early-onset neonatal GBS[18]. The American College of Obstetricians and Pediatricians recommends screening pregnant women at 26–28 weeks and provides intrapartum chemoprophylaxis for those with positive cultures for rectovaginal GBS colonization[27]. In a decision analysis of 19 screening and treatment strategies for the prevention of neonatal GBS sepsis, the three most cost-effective strategies were: (1) universal intrapartum maternal chemoprophylaxis of all pregnant patients without screening for rectovaginal GBS colonization; (2) intrapartum chemoprophylaxis of pregnant patients with risk factors; and (3) universal culture for rectovaginal

GBS colonization at 36 weeks and provision of chemoprophylaxis for those with positive cultures or preterm deliveries[28]. The cost effective analysis was based on the three main outcomes: (1) the incidence of early-onset GBS sepsis; (2) the number of gravidas receiving chemoprophylaxis; and (3) the total cost of cultures, rapid diagnostic tests, maternal antibiotic therapy and treatment of early GBS neonatal sepsis and sequelae.

Another decision analysis, population-based, revealed the following approaches as cost-effective for prevention of early-onset neonatal GBS infection: (1) universal screening of pregnant women at 26–28 weeks and intrapartum administration of antibiotics to parturients who are GBS carriers and have risk factors; (2) no antenatal GBS screening but an intrapartum administration of antibiotics to parturients who are blacks or teenagers (less than 20 years old) and have risk factors; and (3) maternal vaccination with a multivalent vaccination. The most cost-effective approach is maternal vaccination followed by selective intrapartum administration of antibiotics without antenatal screening for GBS genital colonization[29].

Currently, prenatal treatment of symptomatically colonized pregnant patients with oral antibiotics is not recommended, since this approach is unlikely to eradicate maternal genital GBS colonization at the time of labor and delivery. Of pregnant patients who received antenatal ampicillin or aqueous penicillin for genital colonization of GBS, 30–70% remained colonized at delivery[30,31].

The use of antibiotics in preventing early-onset neonatal GBS infection in the setting of PROM with prolonged latent phase remains to be determined. One approach is to initiate antibiotic treatment pending the genital culture result. If the culture is negative, the antibiotic is discontinued; otherwise the antibiotic is continued orally for a total of 1 week. The genital GBS cultures are repeated weekly to determine the additional course of chemoprophylaxis. The patient should receive intrapartum chemoprophylaxis if she ever had genital GBS colonization during her pregnancy, regardless of the results of intervening GBS cultures and/or treatments.

INTRAPARTUM CHEMOPROPHYLAXIS

Aqueous penicillin G is the drug of choice with the initial dose of 5 million units and maintenance dose of 2.5 million units every 4 h. Ampicillin is the alternative with the initial dosage of 2 g and the maintenance dose of 1 g every 4 h. Penicillin G is preferable to ampicillin because of its narrower spectrum of bacterial sensitivity, thus being less likely to cause the selective emergence of other pathogenic bacteria[32]. Clindamycin 600 mg every 8 h or erythromycin

500 mg every 8 h may be substituted in case of penicillin allergy. Intrapartum chemoprophylaxis should be given intravenously until delivery.

SUMMARY

Although controversy exists regarding screening and treatments, there is a consensus that chemoprophylaxis in the intrapartum period dramatically reduces the rate of infection in both the mother and the neonate. At present, the most cost-effective strategy of reducing early-onset GBS infection is the selective intrapartum treatment of patients without antenatal screening who have one of the following risk factors: preterm delivery, prolonged rupture of membranes (>18 h), intrapartum fever or prior infant with GBS infection. Penicillin G is the drug of choice for this purpose and ampicillin is the alternative. Clindamycin and erythromycin may be used if allergy to penicillin exists. Maternal vaccination, being developed, appears to be the most cost-effective measure in preventing early-onset GBS neonatal infection.

REFERENCES

1. Baker CJ. Summary of the workshop on perinatal infections due to group B streptococcus. *J Infect Dis* 1977;136:137–52
2. Faro S. Group B beta-hemolytic streptococci and puerperal infections. *Am J Obstet Gynecol* 1981;139:686–9
3. Anthony BF, Okada DM, Hobel CJ. Epidemiology of group B streptococcus: longitudinal observations during pregnancy. *J Infect Dis* 1978;137:524–30
4. Regan JA, Klebanoff MA, Nugent RP. Vaginal Infections and Prematurity Study Group. The epidemiology of group B streptococcal colonization in pregnancy. *Obstet Gynecol* 1991;77:604–10
5. Dillon HC, Gray E, Pass MA, Gray BM. Anorectal and vaginal carriage of group B streptococci during pregnancy. *J Infect Dis* 1982;145:794–9
6. Winn HN, McLennan M, Amon E. Clinical assessment of the rapid latex agglutination screening test for group B streptococcus. *Int J Gynecol Obstet* 1994;47:289–90
7. Schwartz B, Schuchat A, Oxtoby MJ. Invasive group B streptococcal disease in adults. *J Am Med Assoc* 1991;266:1112–14
8. Zangwill KM, Schuchat A, Wenger JD. Group B streptococcal disease in the United States, 1990: report from a multistate active surveillance system. In *CDC Surveillance Summaries* v. 41. MMWR, 1992, No. SS-6:25–32 (November 20)
9. Jones DE, Kanarek KS, Lim DV. Group B streptococcal colonization patterns in mothers and their infants. *J Clin Microbiol* 1984;20:438–440
10. Francois RA, Knostman JD, Zimmerman RA. Group B streptococcal neonate and infant infections. *J Pediatr* 1973;82:707
11. Hood M, Janney A, Dameron G. Betahemolytic streptococcus group B associated with problems of the perinatal period. *Am J Obstet Gynecol* 1961;82:809

12. Baker CJ, Barrett FF. Transmission of group B streptococci among parturient women and their neonates. *J Pediatr* 1973;83:919

13. Baker CJ, Edwards MS. Group B streptococcus infections: perinatal impact and prevention methods. *Ann NY Acad Sci* 1988;549:193–202

14. Schuchat A, Oxtoby M, Cochi S, *et al*. Population-based risk factors for neonatal group B streptococcal disease: results of a cohort study in metropolitan Atlanta. *J Infect Dis* 1990;102:672–7

15. Dars MA, Gray BM, Khare S, *et al*. Prospective studies of group B streptococcal infections in infants. *J Pediatr* 1979;95:437–43

16. Opal SM, Cors A, Palmer M, *et al*. Group B streptococcal sepsis in adults and infants. *Arch Intern Med* 1988;148:641–5

17. American College of Obstetricians and Gynecologists. *Group B Streptococcal Infections in Pregnancy*. ACOG Committee Opinion Number 173, June 1996

18. Boyer KM, Gotoff SP. Prevention of early onset neonatal group B streptococcal disease with selective intrapartum chemoprophylaxis. *N Engl J Med* 1986;314:1665–9

19. Yow MD, Leeds LJ, Mason EO, *et al*. The natural history of group B streptococcal colonization in the pregnant woman and her offspring. I. Colonization studies. *Am J Obstet Gynecol* 1980;137:34–8

20. Anthony BF, Okada DM, Hobel CJ. Epidemiology of the group B streptococcus: maternal and nosocomial sources for the infant acquisitions. *J Pediatr* 1979;95:431–6

21. Badri MS, Zawaneh S, Cruz AC, *et al*. Rectal colonization with group B streptococcus: relation to vaginal colonization of pregnant women. *J Infect Dis* 1977;135:308–12

22. Kontrick C, Edberg S. Direct detection of group B streptococci from vaginal specimens compared with quantitative culture. *J Clin Microbiol* 1987;25:573–4

23. Wald E, Dashefsky B. Rapid detection of group B streptococci directly from vaginal swabs. *J Clin Microbiol* 1987;25:573–4

24. Skoll MA, Mercer BM. Evaluation of two rapid group B streptococcal antigen tests in labor and delivery patients. *Obstet Gynecol* 1991;77:322–6

25. Gentry YM, Hillier SL. Evaluation of two rapid enzyme immunoassays for detection of group B streptococcus. *Obstet Gynecol* 1991;78:397–401

26. Granab PA, Petosa MT. Evaluation of a rapid screening test for detecting group B streptococci in pregnant women. *J Clin Microbiol* 1991;29:1536–8

27. Committee on Infectious Diseases and Committee on Fetus and Newborn. Guidelines for prevention of group B streptococcal (GBS) infection by chemoprophylaxis. *Pediatrics* 1992;90:775–8

28. Rouse DJ, Goldenberg RL, Cliver SP, *et al*. Strategies for the prevention of early-onset neonatal group B streptococcal sepsis: a decision analysis. *Obstet Gynecol* 1994;83:493–4

29. Mohle-Boetani JC, Schuchat A, Plikaytis J, *et al*. Comparison of prevention strategies for neonatal group B streptococcal infection. *J Am Med Assoc* 1993;270:1442–8

30. Hall RT, Barnes W, Krishnan L, *et al*. Antibiotic treatment of parturient women colonized with group B streptococci. *Am J Obstet Gynecol* 1976;124:630–4

31. Gardner SE, Yow MD, Leeds LJ, *et al*. Failure of penicillin to eradicate group B streptococcal colonization in the pregnant woman: a couple study. *Am J Obstet Gynecol* 1979;135:1062–5

32. Centers for Disease Control and Prevention. Prevention of perinatal group B streptococcal disease: a public health perspective. *Morbid Mortal Weekly Rep* 1996;45:1–24

20

Other bacterial infections: listeria, Lyme disease, granuloma inguinale and chancroid

J.L. Swingler

LISTERIOSIS

Listeriosis during pregnancy can result in unfavorable fetal outcomes and occasional maternal adversities. Pregnancy may lead to a greater risk of infection because of a possibly impaired immune system.

Epidemiology

Major outbreaks of listeriosis in the past decade have contributed much to our knowledge of the disease. Fertilizer manure from listeria-infected sheep contaminated cabbage, and therefore coleslaw, in 1981 in Nova Scotia, resulting in 34 perinatal infection cases and four stillbirths; 27% of the neonates died[1]. A 1983 Massachusetts outbreak associated with pasteurized milk led to seven perinatal infection cases, of which 19% resulted in stillbirth[2]. An outbreak of 142 cases in the Los Angeles area associated with Mexican-style soft cheese was seen in 1985. Although there was no maternal mortality, the perinatal mortality rate was 63%[3].

Most cases of listeriosis are sporadic or confined to smaller outbreaks. The causative organism is ubiquitous in the environment, having been found in dust, soil, sewage, water sources, silage, vegetation and animals, which can exhibit carriage or infection in many species[4]. Epizootics occur in sheep, cattle, poultry, shellfish, crustaceans and some fish, all of which can lead to food contamination. Overall, an estimated 1700 cases of listeriosis occurred in the USA in 1986, according to a study by the Centers for Disease Control (CDC)[4]. The annual incidence estimate was 7.1 cases per 10^6 population. The perinatal case rate was 12.4 cases per 100 000 live births. At least 100 stillbirths per year in the USA may be attributed to listeriosis. Infants may rarely acquire infection by direct exposure to contaminated equipment or facilities in the nursery or delivery room[5-7].

Fecal carriage rates in the population range from 0.6% to 16%[8]. Transperineal spread to the vagina and occasionally to the male partner can be seen; however, this is not a venereal disease[8].

Etiology

Listeriosis is caused by *Listeria monocytogenes,* a Gram-positive motile coccobacillus which resembles normal commensal skin diphtheroids. This resemblance leads to underdiagnosis on Gram stains and cultures. Listeria is a facultative anaerobe, and colonies are β-hemolytic. Sixteen serotypes exist; most human disease is related to types 1 and 4b. Phage typing is useful. The organism can be difficult to isolate in a mixed culture.

Listeria resists environmental extremes but grows quite well at food refrigeration temperatures[9]. It can also survive pasteurization, in some cases salt, preservatives such as nitrite, anaerobic conditions, drying and alkaline pH[9]. Refrigerated, ready-to-eat foods previously cooked are ideal media[9-11]. Reheating via a microwave oven may also allow survival of the organism[12]. This organism is widespread in nature and can easily contaminate food sources and can survive and even multiply under conditions used for processing and storing food.

Pathogenesis

The portal of entry is the gastrointestinal tract. Gastric acidity helps to destroy the organism, but natural buffering by food and antacid permits survival of the organism[11,13]. Entry then occurs through the intestinal mucosa.

The best defense against listeriosis is a competent immune system, particularly the T-cell system which activates macrophages[4]. Without this activation the organism can survive and proliferate within macrophages. Immunosuppressive therapy, steroids, autoimmune disorders, malignancies, acquired immune deficiency syndrome (AIDS), advanced age, pregnancy and neonatal immunoincompetence carry a greater risk of infection due to T-cell suppression.

Maternal infection may give symptoms such as fever, backache, diarrhea, malaise, myalgia and headache and may lead to septicemia and adult respiratory distress syndrome[14]. Transplacental infection may occasionally occur. The role of listeriosis in recurrent pregnancy loss is controversial[15–17].

Infection later in pregnancy can yield the classic early neonatal infection known as granulomatosis infantisepticum, with listerial microabscesses seen in the liver, brain, placenta, spleen, lungs, kidney, gastrointestinal tract, adrenals, pharynx and skin. The infant is often premature and septic. The perinatal mortality rate depends on gestational age, timely initiation of treatment and severity of infection ranging from 3% to 50%[4,18]. Meconium presence and aspiration are noted in many cases. Neonatal respiratory distress and sepsis are apparent within 3 days of birth.

Transplacental infection can lead to colonization of the amniotic fluid and may cause preterm labor and delivery[19–23]. Antibiotic treatment is of cardinal importance if listeriosis is suspected. Many of these fetuses showed abnormalities on electric monitoring such as baseline tachycardia, poor reactivity and late decelerations[20,22,23]. Listeriosis has also been associated with non-immune hydrops fetalis[24].

Late-onset disease is analogous to the group B streptococcal model, in that the infection is acquired by passage through the contaminated birth canal. The onset is from 5 days to several weeks after birth, averaging about 2 weeks[4]. The presentation is generally that of meningitis, and prompt treatment with antibiotics is essential.

Maternal death from listeriosis is rare, but has been reported in one patient with severe lupus nephrosis and subsequent renal failure[25] and in another with AIDS[26].

Diagnosis

The clinical signs are fairly non-specific and resemble urinary tract infection, influenza or gastroenteritis. Listeriosis should be considered in pregnant patients with any flu-like illness and preterm labor. Uterine tenderness and preterm labor indicate an acute chorioamnionitis. Gram stain and culture of the amniotic fluid obtained by transabdominal amniocentesis may show Gram-positive coccobacilli. Selective culture media containing acriflavine and nalidixic acid increase the yield of the organism[8]. Cold enrichment can be carried out, but this slows the result. Listeria may be mistaken for diphtheroids. Listeria has a very characteristic tumbling motility at room temperature, and hence a wet mount examination can be useful.

Serology testing of the patient with listeriosis has not been useful because there is much cross reactivity with other bacteria. A monoclonal antibody probe specific and sensitive for *Listeria monocytogenes* in clinical specimens would be useful. Maternal blood, cervical and fecal cultures may aid in the diagnosis.

Management

Once the diagnosis of listeriosis is made, prompt maternal treatment with antibiotics will usually result in excellent maternal and neonatal outcomes[27–29]. Ampicillin and penicillin are the drugs of choice. Ampicillin can be given in a dose of 2 g intravenously every 6 h until the patient has been afebrile for 24 h, then amoxicillin 500 mg orally every 8 h for a total duration of 7 days. In the case of penicillin allergy, erythromycin 500 mg every 6 h can be used as a substitute. Ampicillin and gentamicin act synergistically and both should be used to treat listeria meningitis or sepsis[30]. Erythromycin may not reach a therapeutic level in the cerebrospinal fluid. Listerias are less susceptible to other agents such as cephalosporins. Delivery is indicated in the presence of acute amnionitis[23,31,32].

Prevention during pregnancy includes proper cooking and storage of food at 3°C[9]. Aged items should be discarded. Milk products should be pasteurized, and no raw milk should be taken. Ready-to-eat salads and other foods incorporating meat or cheese should be inspected for freshness. All refrigerated food should be heated to the point of steaming to kill listerias. The above recommendations are particularly important in pregnant women, to avoid infection.

Finally, listerial culture may be part of the workup of fetal death, as some of these cases may be due to occult perinatal infection[33].

LYME DISEASE

Lyme disease was described as a definite clinical entity in 1977[34]. Patients exhibited a complex of symptoms and stages resembling the syphilitic model. In 1985 it became apparent that pregnancy outcome might be affected[35].

Epidemiology

Although the first cases were described in residents of heavily wooded areas in Connecticut, it is known that Lyme disease has a worldwide distribution. Different vectors and animal reservoirs are involved in different geographic areas. Overpopulation of optimal animal hosts, such as white-tailed deer and white-footed mice, combined with suburban development and utilization of wooded areas, gives larger numbers of cases in certain endemic areas. Sporadic cases can occur elsewhere. The northeastern USA, Wisconsin/Minnesota and California/Oregon regions account for most of the caseload. A CDC study showed 13 795 cases from 1980 to 1988 in 43 different states[36,37].

The majority of infections are noted between May and July, when nymphal ticks are active, but disease can be acquired at other times[38]. Women living in endemic areas and involved in outdoor activities run the risk of contracting the disease during pregnancy.

Etiology

Lyme disease is caused by the spirochete *Borrelia burgdorferi,* which is usually contracted via the bite of an infected *Ixodes dammini* tick[39]. This tick, also known as the deer tick, lays eggs in the spring. Larval ticks develop and feed on mice in the late summer and fall. They molt to become nymphs, which feed on white-footed mice and other hosts including humans from May to July. The larval and nymphal ticks can therefore infect a widespread mouse population and other hosts. The adult ticks must rely on larger animals, such as the white-tailed deer, which are vital in maintaining the overall tick population, but unimportant as a reservoir of infection. Humans and domesticated animals are infected when bitten by the spirochete-laden nymphs, or more rarely adult ticks[38–40]. At least 31 species of mammals and 49 species of birds can serve as hosts; however, the infection of mice and deer is of greater concern. The organism has also been isolated from other insect and tick vectors, such as deerflies, horseflies, mosquitoes, certain fleas and the lone star tick *Amblyoma americanum,* the last being suspected of being a secondary vector[41].

Pathogenesis

The first stage occurs in 60% to 80% of infected individuals with the characteristic erythema migrans rash, which can last for 3 or 4 weeks, and mild flu-like symptoms. The second stage occurs 4–6 weeks after the onset of the first stage and involves dissemination of the spirochetes from the skin site via lymphatic and hematogenous spread, affecting multiple organs. Multisystem disease begins, and includes arthritis, bursitis, myositis, meningitis, Bell's palsy, other neurological symptoms, cardiac blocks, myopericarditis, hepatitis, ocular problems and constitutional symptoms. The third stage develops when infection persists, resulting in a more severe chronic arthritis and neurological disorders[38]. Spirochete damage and the autoimmune response both play a role in the pathogenesis.

Borrelia can cross the placenta and cause fetal infection with adverse outcomes. Maternal infection in early pregnancy has been associated with spontaneous abortion[42–44], preterm delivery[44], cardiac defects such as coarctation of the aorta, patent ductus arteriosus, valvular stenosis and atrial or ventricular septal defects[35,42,44–46], syndactyly, absence of hemidiaphragm and craniofacial abnormalities such as hydrocephalus and meningomyelocele[42,46,47]. Maternal infection in later gestation has been associated with fetal growth retardation, fetal demise and neonatal hyperbilirubinemia[48]. It should be cautioned that a mere association of fetal infection and fetal anomalies does not necessarily mean a cause and effect relationship. A more recent population-based study of approximately 2000 patients reveals that maternal infection with

Lyme disease before pregnancy, evidenced by a positive serology at the first prenatal visit, is not associated with an increased risk of fetal death, intra-uterine growth retardation or major congenital fetal malformations[30].

Diagnosis

The diagnosis can be made from clinical presentation and serology. As these are tiny ticks, there is often no recollection of a bite. Culture of *Borrelia burgdorferi* in a complex liquid medium, Barbour—Stoenner—Kelly medium, is possible but difficult and generally not useful[38].

Both indirect fluorescent antibody (IFA) and enzyme-linked immunosorbent assay (ELISA) serology tests for detection of antibodies to *B.burgdorferi* are available, with ELISA being more sensitive. Testing has not been standardized, and the rates of false positive and negative tests are high, especially in the first stages of the disease. Serology tests for syphilis such as rapid plasma reagin (RPR) or Venereal Disease Research Laboratories (VDRL) should also be simultaneously obtained, because of cross reactivity with *Treponema pallidum* antibodies[38].

The Warthin Starry silver stain can be used to demonstrate spirochetes on biopsy or, more commonly, autopsy tissue.

Management

If a pregnant woman presents with erythema migrans or other Lyme symptomatology, she should be treated pending serology results. Early and prompt treatment may prevent seroconversion in some cases. Tetracycline is used in non-pregnant individuals. During pregnancy the best treatments are with phenosymethyl penicillin (Pen-V) 500 mg orally four times a day[49] or amoxicillin 500 mg three times a day[50]. Erythromycin 250–500 mg orally four times a day can be used for penicillin-allergic patients, although it is less effective. The duration of treatment is 3 weeks[51] because of the long half-life of borrelia, which grows slowly. For individuals exhibiting more serious arthritic, neurological or cardiac complications, ceftriaxone 2 g intravenously once a day for 14 days may be the best therapy[38,50,51].

During pregnancy, avoidance of ticks and efforts at personal protection are important in preventing exposure and subsequent development of Lyme disease[41].

GRANULOMA INGUINALE

Granuloma inguinale, also known as Donovanosis, is often considered a venereal disease. It was first described by McLeod in 1982. Donovan was the first to identify and demonstrate the characteristic Donovan body staining reaction that bears his name.

Epidemiology

This tropical disease is endemic to such areas as New Guinea, Africa, India, the Caribbean and aboriginal Australia. Outbreaks, however, can be found in developed countries such as those seen in the Southeastern United States with documented cases in Atlanta and Houston[52,53]. There are fewer than 100 cases per year in the USA. Poor hygiene and low income are associated with acquisition of the disease. Transmission occurs with close physical contact. Sexual transmission occurs in 20–66% of cases, with a higher rate noted among prostitutes[52-58].

Etiology

The causal organism is *Calymmatobacterium granulomatis*. It is an encapsulated Gram-negative bacterium that exhibits bipolar staining reminiscent of a safety pin. It is found intracellularly inside histiocytes; often 20–30 organisms are sequestered together within a vacuole, best demonstrated by the Giesma stain. The organism cannot be cultured on laboratory media, but has been cultured in chick embryonic yolk sacs[59]. The organism with its capsule and antigenic characteristics shares much in common with the *Klebsiella* species that can induce granulomas[54].

Pathogenesis

After exposure there is an incubation period of 3 days to 6 months. Experimentally produced lesions in volunteers appear in 40 to 50 days[60]. Single or multiple papules soon ulcerate and erode the skin. A beefy-red granulomatous area forms and slowly spreads to adjacent areas. There is no pain, unless there is rare secondary infection. The lesions gradually heal with areas of fibrosis, lymphedema and elephantiasis and may result in severe stricture and disfigurement. There are epithelial changes at the periphery of the lesion which can stimulate carcinoma. Actual cases of carcinoma can be present concurrently within the lesion or at its borders. Extension to the inguinal area or occasionally to the nodes themselves gives pseudobuboes in some cases. Extragenital site involvement can occur by extension or autoinoculation and includes lesions to the scalp, orbits, face, oral cavity, throat, larynx, lungs, neck, axillae, extremities, bone lesions, joints, liver, bladder, spleen and trunk[54,61]. Lymph nodes can also be involved with granulomas[61].

In the female, the upper genital tract can be involved. Spread of granulomatous disease to the cervix, uterus, tubes, ovaries, parametrium and ureters, causing hydronephrosis, has been reported[62]. Rectovaginal and other genital fistulas can form from breakdown of granulomatous tissue. Urethral strictures also may occur.

Vaginal bleeding may result from granulomatous disease involving the uterus, cervix or vagina, and may present as an antepartum hemorrhage from a friable lesion[53,63].

Diagnosis

Diagnosis is aided by the clinical features. Appropriate tests to rule out chancroid, syphilis, lymphogranuloma venereum, genital cancer and, if indicated, genital tuberculosis and amebiasis, are indicated.

Since the organism cannot be readily cultured, the diagnosis is based on biopsy specimens and, in particular, the preparation of a proper tissue smear[54,64], which is then stained with Giesma stain and examined for Donovan bodies at high power. Multiple or repeat tissue smears can be taken to confirm the diagnosis.

Management

Since this condition often involves little pain, patients may present with fairly large lesions that have gone untreated for months or years. For non-pregnant patients, treatments include tetracycline 500 mg by mouth four times a day, streptomycin 1.0–2.0 grams intramuscularly daily, minocycline 100 mg by mouth twice a day, or chloramphenicol 500 mg by mouth four times a day, all for 3 or 4 weeks[65].

For pregnant patients the best choices are trimethoprim/sulfamethoxazole 160 mg/800 mg by mouth twice a day, erythromycin 500 mg four times a day, or ampicillin 500 mg four times a day[53,65]. During pregnancy a combination of erythromycin and lincomycin (2 g of each per day) has been used with good neonatal outcomes[55]. Pregnant patients with granuloma inguinale may respond to trimethoprim/sulfamethoxazole more slowly than non-pregnant patients[65]. Regardless of the antibiotics used, it is important to treat patients for at least 2 weeks after the lesions disappear, to avoid recurrence. Donovan bodies begin to disappear within 5 days of adequate therapy[54].

Other problems encountered in pregnancy include an increased frequency of spontaneous abortion, soft tissue dystocia from scarring, stenosis/obstruction of the birth canal and postpartum infection leading to death, if no treatment has been given[54]. Severe upper genital tract disease may require surgical management including hysterectomy if medical therapy fails[62]. Plastic surgery may be necessary to correct severe scarring or stenosis[66].

Sexual partners of patients with granuloma inguinale should be examined and treated if lesions are present.

CHANCROID

Chancroid is an acute genital disease caused by the organism *Haemophilus ducreyi*. Typically there is a single ulcerated lesion, but multiple lesions can be seen. Concomitantly, painful inguinal lymphadenitis occurs in the majority of cases. These buboes can be quite large and suppurate.

Epidemiology

Chancroid is endemic in many parts of the world. In some developing countries it is one of the most common sexually transmitted diseases[67-69], but in developed countries chancroid is much less common. Several epidemic outbreaks have occurred in North America, including Dallas, Winnepeg, Orange County in California and New York[70-73]. Prostitution is often involved with transmission. There has been a gradual increase in the number of cases seen in the USA over the past decade[74].

Etiology

H. ducreyi is a short, Gram-negative facultative anaerobic bacillus. It requires hemin (X factor) but not NAD (V factor) for growth. On Gram staining, Indian-file chaining or a 'school of fish' pattern is seen. Culture yields are higher if swabs are plated soon after collection and media containing chocolate or blood agar plates supplemented with crystal violet agar (CVA; DIFCO Labs, Detroit, Michigan). Vancomycin can be added to make the medium more selective.

Pathogenesis

After exposure there is an incubation period of 2–11 days. Initially a tender papule forms, becoming pustular and finally ulcerated. Single or multiple lesions of 2–20 mm in size can be found on the labia, fourchette, clitoris, vagina, perineum, thigh or perianal area. About 80% of women with chancroid have multiple lesions[75]. Occasionally, a widespread destructive lesion called phagedemic chancroid may occur as a result of mixed infection of *H. ducreyi* and anaerobes[70]. Extra-genital lesions can be found on the breasts, fingers and mouth.

About 50% of patients develop buboes, which are often unilateral, erythematous and tender. Spontaneous drainage and ulceration of these can result. Infants born to mothers with active disease present at delivery are usually not affected[76].

Diagnosis

The diagnosis of chancroid depends on clinical findings of ulcer and bubo, Gram stain culture and biopsy of the lesions[70,76-78]. The main problem is that the organism may not be isolated in many cases.

Biopsy of the ulcer may be helpful as these ulcers have three characteristic zones[70,76]. Biopsy or culture of the bubo is less diagnostic. A promising diagnostic tool utilizing a DNA probe has been described. This is helpful when clinical suspicion is high while the culture is negative[79].

It is very important to rule out other diseases that cause genital ulcers, by performing herpes simplex culture; dark-field examination and acute and late serology tests for syphilis; and a Giesma stain for Donovan bodies.

Management

Antibiotic resistance mediated via plasmids has been noted particularly in endemic areas. Penicillins, sulfonamides, tetracyclines, chloramphenicol and, more recently, trimethoprim-resistant strains have been isolated[70,77]. During pregnancy, and at other times, the best treatment consists of erythromycin 500 mg, four times a day for 7 days or a single 250-mg dose of ceftriaxone intramuscularly[80]. Quinoline antibiotics such as ciproflexin and corfloxacin are also efficacious, but information about fetal effects is quite limited[81-83].

Aggressive therapy with the addition of anaerobic antibiotic therapy is indicated in phagedemic cases. Buboes are best not excised, but rather aspirated or treated medically[70].

Ulcerative lesions, such as chancroid, significantly increase the risk of transmitting HIV[84], probably owing to disruption of the skin and exposure of immune cells in the ulcer to infectious virus. Compared to North America, developing countries have a much higher incidence of chancroid which may partially explain the greater spread of HIV via heterosexual intercourse in these countries. The pregnant patient with chancroid or other genital ulcers should be screened for HIV. Sexual partners should be examined and treated with the same regimen as mentioned above.

REFERENCES

1. Schlech W, Lavigne P, Bortolusse R, *et al*. Epidemic listeriosis: evidence for transmission by food. *N Engl J Med* 1983;308:203–6
2. Fleming D, Cochi S, MacDonald K, *et al*. Pasteurized milk as a vehicle of infection in an outbreak of listeriosis. *N Engl J Med* 1985;312:404–7
3. Linnan M, Mascola L, Lou X, *et al*. Epidemic listeriosis associated with Mexican-style cheese. *N Engl J Med* 1988;319:823–8
4. Gellin B, Broome C. Listeriosis. *J Am Med Assoc* 1989; 262:1313–20
5. Simmons M, Cockcroft P, Okubadejo O. Neonatal listeriosis due to cross-infection in an obstetric theatre. *J Infect* 1986;13:235–9
6. Florman A, Sundararajan V. Listeriosis among nursery mates. *Pediatrics* 1968;41:784–8
7. Larsson S, Cederberg A, Ivarsson S, *et al*. Listeria monocytogenes causing hospital acquired enterocolitis and meningitis in newborn infants. *Br Med J* 1978;2:473–4
8. Lamont R, Postethwaite R, MacGowan A. *Listeria monocytogenes* and its role in human infection. *J Infect* 1988; 17:7–28
9. Brightman C, Dumbreck A. Listeriosis. *Br J Hosp Med* 1989;42:366–70

10. Schwartz B, Broome C, Brown G, *et al*. Association of sporadic listeriosis with uncooked hotdogs and undercooked chicken. *Lancet* 1988;2:779–82

11. Kerr K, Lacey R. Listeriosis: new problems with an old pathogen. *J Hosp Infect* 1988;12:247–50

12. Lund B, Knox M, Cole M. Destruction of *Listeria monocytogenes* during microwave cooking. *Lancet* 1989;1: 218–19

13. Ho J, Shands K, Friedland G, *et al*. An outbreak of type 4b *Listeria monocytogenes* infection involving patients from eight Boston hospitals. *Arch Intern Med* 1986; 146:520–4

14. Boucher M, Yonekura M, Wallace R, *et al*. Adult respiratory distress syndrome: a rare manifestation of *Listeria monocytogenes* infection in pregnancy. *Am J Obstet Gynecol* 1984;149:686–7

15. Rappaport R, Rabinowitz M, Toaff R, *et al*. Genital listeriosis as a cause of repeated abortion. *Lancet* 1962; 2:484–7

16. Rabau E, David A. *Listeria monocytogenes* in abortion (letter). *Lancet* 1963;1:228

17. Lawler F, Wood W, King S, *et al*. *Listeria monocytogenes* as a cause of fetal loss. *Am J Obstet Gynecol* 1964;89:915

18. Teberg A, Yonekura M, Salminen C, *et al*. Clinical manifestations of epidemic neonatal listeriosis. *Pediatr Infect Dis J* 1987;6:817–20

19. Valkenburg M, Essed G, Potters H. Perinatal listeriosis underdiagnosed as a cause of pre-term labor? *Eur J Obstet Gynecol Reprod Biol* 1988;27:283–8

20. Makar A, Vanderheyden J, DeSchrijver D, *et al*. Perinatal listeriosis; more common than reported. *Eur J Obstet Gynecol Reprod Med* 1989;31:83–91

21. Khong T, Frappel J, Steel H, *et al*. Perinatal listeriosis; a report of six cases. *Br J Obstet Gynaecol* 1986;93: 1083–7

22. Boucher M, Yonekura L. Perinatal listeriosis (early onset); correlation of antenatal manifestations and neonatal outcome. *Obstet Gynecol* 1986;68:593–7

23. Romero R, Winn H, Wan M, *et al*. *Listeria monocytogenes* chorioamnionitis and preterm labor. *Am J Perinatol* 1988;5:286–8

24. Gembruch U, Neisen M, Hansmann M, *et al*. Listeriosis: a cause of non-immune hydrops fetalis. *Prenat Diagn* 1987;7:277–82

25. Fan Y, Pastorek J, Janney F, *et al*. Listeriosis as an obstetric complication in an immunocompromised patient. *South Med J* 1989;82:1044–5

26. Wetli C, Roldan E, Fogace R. Listeriosis as a cause of maternal death: an obstetric complication of the acquired immunodeficiency syndrome. *Am J Obstet Gynecol* 1983;147:7

27. Cruikshank D, Warenski J. First trimester maternal *Listeria monocytogenes* sepsis and chorioamnionitis with normal neonatal outcome. *Obstet Gynecol* 1989;73: 469–71

28. Dick J, Palframan A, Hamilton D. Listeriosis and recurrent abortion in a renal transplant recipient. *J Infect* 1988;16:273–7

29. Hume O. Maternal *Listeria monocytogenes* septicemia with sparing of the fetus. *Obstet Gynecol* 1976;48:33S–34S

30. Strobino B, Willams C, Abid S, *et al*. Lyme disease and pregnancy outcome: a prospective study of two thousand prenatal patients. *Am J Obstet Gynecol* 1993; 169:367–74

31. Espaze E, Reynaud A. Antibiotic susceptibilities of listeria: *in vitro* studies. *Infection* 1988;16:S160–4

32. Marget W, Seeliger H. *Listeria monocytogenes* infections – therapeutic possibilities and problems. *Infection* 1988; 16:S175–7

33. Pitkin R. Fetal death: diagnosis and management. *Am J Obstet Gynecol* 1987;157:583–9

34. Steere A, Malawista S, Snydman D, *et al*. Lyme arthritis: an epidemic of oligoarticular arthritis in children and adults in three Connecticut communities. *Arthritis Rheum* 1977;20:7–17

35. Schesinger P, Duray P, Burke B, *et al*. Maternal–fetal transmission of the Lyme disease spirochete, *Borrelia burgdorferi*. *Ann Intern Med* 1985;103:67–8

36. Centers for Disease Control. Lyme disease Connecticut. *Morbid Mortal Weekly Rep* 1988;37:1–2

37. Tsai T, Bailey R, Moore P. National surveillance of Lyme disease 1987–1988. *Conn Med* 1989;53:324–6

38. Steere A. Lyme disease. *N Engl J Med* 1989;321:586–96

39. Burgdorfer W, Barbour A, Hayes S, *et al*. Lyme disease – a tick borne spirochetosis? *Science* 1982;216:1317–19

40. Anderson J. Ecology of Lyme disease. *Conn Med* 1989; 53:343–6

41. Stafford K. Lyme disease prevention: personal protection and prospects for tick control. *Conn Med* 1989; 53:347–51

42. MacDonald A. Gestational Lyme borreliosis – implications for the fetus. *Rheum Dis Clin North Am* 1989; 15:657–77

43. Carlomagno G, Luksa V, Canduss G, *et al*. Lyme borrelia positive serology associated with spontaneous abortion in an endemic Italian area. *Acta Eur Fertil* 1988; 19:279–81

44. Maraspin V, Cimperman J, Lotric-Furlan S, *et al*. Treatment of erythema migrans in pregnancy. *Clin Infect Dis* 1996;22:788–93

45. MacDonald A, Benach J, Burgdorfer W. Stillbirth following materal Lyme disease. *NY State J Med* 1987; 87:615–16

46. Nadal D, Hunziker U, Bucher H, *et al*. Infants born to mothers with antibodies against *Borrelia burgdorferi* at delivery. *Eur J Pediatr* 1989;148:426–7

47. Markowitx L, Steere A, Benach J, *et al*. Lyme disease during pregnancy. *J Am Med Assoc* 1986;255:3394–6

48. Williams C, Benach J, Curran A, *et al*. Lyme disease during pregnancy: a cord blood serosurvey. *Ann NY Acad Sci* 1988;539:504–6

49. Zaki M. Selective tickborne infections: a review of Lyme disease, Rocky Mountain spotted fever and babesiosis. *NY State J Med* 1989;89:320–35

50. Treatment of Lyme disease. *Med Lett* 1989;31:57–9

51. Luft B, Gorevic P, Halperin J, *et al*. A perspective on the treatment of Lyme borreliosis. *Rev Infect Dis* 1989; 11:S1518–25

52. Rosen T. Donovanosis (letter). *Int J Derm* 1986; 25:668–9

53. Wysoki R, Majmudar B, Willis D. Granuloma inguinale (Donovanosis) in women. *J Reprod Med* 1988;33:709–13

54. Richens J. Donovanosis: a review. *Papua New Guinea Med J* 1985;28:67–74

55. Ashdown L, Kilvert G. Granuloma inguinale in northern Queensland. *Med J Aust* 1979;1:146–8

56. Sehgal V, Jain M. Pattern of epidemics of Donovanosis in the nonendemic region. *Int J Derm* 1986;27:396–9

57. Sehgal V, Prasad A. A clinical profile of Donovanosis in the nonendemic area. *Dermatologica* 1984;168:273–8

58. Lal S, Nicholas C. Epidemiological and clinical features in 165 cases of granuloma inguinale. *Br J Vener Dis* 1970;46:461–3

59. Anderson K. Etiologic considerations of Donovania granulomatis cultured in 3 cases in embryonic yolks. *J Exp Med* 1945;8:451–5

60. Greenblatt R, Dienst R, Pund E, *et al.* Experimental and clinical granuloma inguinale. *J Am Med Assoc* 1939; 113:1109–16

61. Freinkel A. Granuloma inguinale of cervical lymph nodes stimulating tuberculosis lymphadenitis: two case reports and review of published reports. *Genitourin Med* 1988;64:339–43

62. Scrimgeour E, Sengupta S, McGoldrick I. Primary endometrial and endocervical granuloma inguinale (Donovanosis). *Br J Vener Dis* 1983;59:198–201

63. Murigan S, Venkatram K, Renganathan P. Vaginal bleeding in granuloma inguinale. *Br J Vener Dis* 1982; 58:200–1

64. Gallow M, Blums M, Haverkort F. Rapid diagnosis of granuloma inguinale (letter). *Med J Aust* 1986;144:502

65. Lasif A, Mason P, Paraiwa E. The treatment of Dono-vanosis (granuloma inguinale). *Sex Transm Dis* 1988; 15:27–9

66. Parkash S, Radhakrishna K. Problematic ulcerative lesions in sexually transmitted diseases: surgical man-agement. *Sex Transm Dis* 1986;13:127–33

67. Nsanze H, Fast MV, D'Costa LJ, *et al.* Genital ulcers in Kenya: clinical and laboratory study. *Br J Vener Dis* 1981;57:378–81

68. Taylor DN, Duagmani C, Svongse C, *et al.* The role of *Hemophilus ducreyi* in penile ulcers in Bangkok, Thailand. *Sex Transm Dis* 1984;11:148–51

69. Plumner FA, Nsanze H, Karasira P, *et al.* Epidemiology of chancroid and *Hemophilus ducreyi* in Nairobi, Kenya. *Lancet* 1983;2:1293–5

70. McCarley M, Cruz P, Sontheimer R. Chancroid: clinical variants and other findings from an epidemic in Dallas County 1986–1987. *J Am Acad Dermatol* 1988;19:330–7

71. Blackmore C, Limpakarninarat K, Rigau-Perez J, *et al.* An outbreak of chancroid in Orange County California: descriptive epidemiology and disease control measures. *J Infect Dis* 1985;151:840–4

72. Schmid G, Sanders L, Blount J, *et al.* Chancroid in the United States: re-establishment of an old disease. *J Am Med Assoc* 1987;258:3265–8

73. Hammond G, Slutchuk M, Scatliff J, *et al.* Epidemio-logic clinical, laboratory and therapeutic features of an urban outbreak of chancroid in North America. *Rev Infect Dis* 1980;2:867–79

74. Felman Y. Recent developments in sexually transmitted diseases: chancroid epidemiology, diagnosis, and treat-ment. *Cutis* 1989;44:113–14

75. D'Costa L, Bowner I, Nsanze H, *et al.* Advances in the diagnosis of management of chancroid. *Sex Transm Dis* 1986;13:189–91

76. Ronald A, Albritton W. Chancroid and *Hemophilus ducreyi*. In Holmes K, ed. *Sexually Transmitted Diseases*. New York, NY: McGraw-Hill, 1984

77. Morse S. Chancroid and *Hemophilus ducreyi*. *Clin Microbiol Rev* 1989;2:137–57

78. Albritton W. Biology of *Hemophilus ducreyi*. *Microbiol Rev* 1989;53:377–89

79. Parsons L, Shayegani M, Waring A, *et al.* DNA probes for the identification of *Hemophilus ducreyi*. *J Clin Microbiol* 1989;27:1441–5

80. LeSaux N, Ronald A. Role of ceftriazone in sexually transmitted diseases. *Rev Infect Dis* 1989;11:299–309

81. Megran D. Quinolones in the treatment of sexually transmitted diseases. *Clin Invest Med* 1989;12:50–60

82. Bodhidatta L, Taylor D, Chitwarakorn A, *et al.* Evalua-tion of 500 and 1000 mg doses of ciprofloxacin for the treatment of chancroid. *Antimicrob Agents Chemother* 1988;32:723–5

83. Ariyarit C, Mokamukkul B, Chitwarakorn A, *et al.* Clinical and microbiological efficacy of a single dose of norfloxacin in the treatment of chancroid. *Scand J Infect Dis Suppl* 1988;56:55–8

84. Pepin J, Plummer F, Brunham R, *et al.* The interaction of HIV infection and other sexually transmitted diseases: an opportunity for intervention. *AIDS* 1989; 3:3–9

21
Postpartum infections

D. J. Mostello

Problems of the antepartum and intrapartum periods are the primary focus of maternal–fetal medicine, yet significant complications may occur after delivery. The most common postpartum complication is infection. Some factors which place the puerpera at risk for infection include rapid colonization of the postpartum endometrial surface by vaginal flora[1], contamination of the perineal area by vaginal and fecal flora, introduction of bacteria through manipulations or instrumentation employed to effect delivery, as well as the physiological adaptation of the breasts for lactation. Despite these predisposing conditions, the overall incidence of clinical infection in the postpartum period is probably less than 10%. An actual rate of postpartum infection is difficult to assess, as published reports reflect selected populations and use varying criteria to define infection.

The definition of 'standard puerperal morbidity' as a temperature of 38.0°C in any 2 of the first 10 days postpartum, exclusive of the first 24 h, may not be a valid indicator of infection and seems impractical with the current practice of early patient discharge. While transient elevations in temperature occur commonly and resolve spontaneously, a temperature greater than 38.4°C or persistent low-grade fever during the first 24 h postpartum is highly predictive of ensuing infection[2]. Disregarding temperature elevations which do not fit into the standard definition or ignoring signs and symptoms of infection not accompanied by fever may delay proper evaluation and therapy.

Time of onset of symptoms may provide a clue to etiology. Infections occurring within 48 h of delivery commonly involve the uterus and peritoneum following Cesarean section, the urinary tract following catheterization, or the respiratory tract. The micro-organisms responsible for early infection were frequently present or introduced at the time of delivery, and the rate of bacteremia is high. Abdominal and episiotomy wound infections, breast infections, complications of uterine infection, and uterine infection that follows vaginal delivery usually present later in the postpartum period. The rate of bacteremia is low and the organisms associated with late infection may be anaerobic, chlamydial, endogenous or introduced after delivery[3].

Postpartum women are generally young and healthy; however, serious postpartum infections remain a significant cause of maternal morbidity and mortality. The general resilience of the postpartum woman probably accounts for the relatively low rate of infection, but may also impede prompt diagnosis because of underestimation of the risks by patient or physician. Identification and close surveillance of patients at risk allow for timely diagnosis and prompt treatment which may minimize serious sequelae of infection.

ENDOMETRITIS

Endometritis, or infection arising from the uterine cavity, is the most common postpartum infection. The diagnosis, classically heralded by a tender uterus and foul lochia, is usually one of exclusion in the febrile postpartum woman without signs of infection from another source.

Etiology

The pathophysiology of endometritis is thought to be similar to that of other pelvic infections – polymicrobial and ascending from the colonized lower genital tract. Specific risk factors continue to be identified, although none are absolutely predictive. When more than one factor is present, risk may be cumulative[4], but unknowns still exist in the equation that determines who becomes infected.

Endometritis following vaginal delivery occurs in 1–3% of patients. Delivery by Cesarean section increases the incidence 3–30 times when compared to the vaginal route[5,6], thus the vast majority of cases of endometritis follow Cesarean section. The myometrium and peritoneal cavity may be directly inoculated with micro-organisms from amniotic fluid or vagina at the time of surgery. The presence of suture material and surgically devitalized tissue, along with postoperative exudation and fluid collections, create a favorable environment for subsequent bacterial growth[7]. Placement of the uterine incision has no effect on the incidence of postpartum infection[8].

Duration of labor, particularly labor preceding Cesarean section, is the most consistent obstetric risk factor for infection. The length of labor probably accounts for the morbidity attributed to the number of vaginal examinations and duration of internal monitoring[9]. Frank chorioamnionitis is an obvious antecedent of postpartum intrauterine infection, often despite intrapartum antibiotic therapy[10,11]. Increased risk is compounded by the frequency of dysfunctional labor and failure to progress in women with chorioamnionitis, necessitating delivery by Cesarean section[12]. A positive amniotic fluid culture, in the absence of overt signs of infection, is also highly predictive of subsequent endometritis, especially after Cesarean section[13]. Bacterial contamination of amniotic fluid, rare when fetal membranes are intact, is almost always present after 6 h of ruptured membranes[14]. The quantity and virulence of the organisms which colonize the amniotic fluid following membrane rupture are primary determinants of subsequent infection[6,15]. In patients with few or low-virulence organisms, infection is unlikely. Duration of ruptured membranes, accordingly, is a risk factor for endometritis only if significant colonization has occurred. When colonization is not taken into account, the risk from ruptured membranes may be obscured by more potent factors such as duration of labor[16].

The presence of Bacterial vaginosis is a strong indicator of subsequent endometritis[17,18]. After Cesarean section, one-third of women with bacterial vaginosis develop endometritis despite prophylactic antibiotic therapy. The increased vaginal concentration of bacteria, along with the presence of particularly virulent micro-organisms in bacterial vaginosis, are likely sources of the increased risk. Bacterial species associated with bacterial vaginosis have been isolated more frequently from patients with postpartum endometritis than would be expected from the prevalence of bacterial vaginosis among pregnant women[18]. Similarly, untreated carriers of group B streptococci are also more likely to contract endometritis[19].

Obesity, anemia, nulliparity, socioeconomic class, preterm delivery, duration of surgery, skill of the operator, estimated blood loss and intrapartum fever have been associated with an increased risk of endometritis. Their significance is debated as they may represent mere markers for more significant predisposing factors. Administration of glucocorticoids for acceleration of fetal lung maturation does not increase the risk of endometritis or other postpartum infections[20].

Diagnosis and evaluation

The diagnosis of endometritis is usually based upon clinical findings. Fever is the most useful sign and should prompt a physical examination even within the first 24 h postpartum. In the absence of other signs of infection, continued observation may be appropriate, but further evaluation is indicated if fever persists. Endometritis after Cesarean section typically presents within 48 h of surgery. When endometritis follows vaginal delivery, the diagnosis is made within 7 days in 84%, and within 14 days postpartum in 98%[6].

The patient may complain of malaise, chills, abdominal pain or foul-smelling discharge. On physical examination, tachycardia, decreased bowel sounds, lower abdominal tenderness, uterine and adnexal tenderness to bimanual palpation and purulent or foul lochia may be found, although physical findings may be minimal. A pelvic mass on initial examination is unusual. Because the differential diagnosis for fever in the immediate postpartum period includes atelectasis, pneumonia, pyelonephritis, viral syndrome, mastitis and appendicitis, the physical examination should be conducted to exclude these conditions.

If infection is suspected, laboratory evaluation should include blood cultures, complete blood count, urinalysis and urine culture. Routine endometrial cultures are rarely useful, as well chosen antibiotic therapy results in a rapid recovery in most patients despite culture isolates. An endometrial culture may be helpful when hemolytic streptococci or clostridia are suspected or when endometritis develops in patients who have received antibiotic prophylaxis, as unusual or resistant organisms may be present[21]. Prior to obtaining specimens transcervically, preparation by cervical cleansing is recommended to minimize contamination with lower genital tract flora[7]. Multiple lumen sampling devices, although expensive, may reduce contamination. Use of a suction cannula for tissue sampling has also proved effective[22].

Treatment

Choice of antibiotic therapy for acute endometritis is directed by the current understanding of the bacteriology of the infection. Aerobic organisms are found in about 70% of cultures and anaerobic organisms in about 80%[23]. Typically, more than one isolate per culture are identified[22,24]. Gram-negative bacilli, particularly *Escherichia coli*, are the most common aerobes, followed by Gram-positive aerobes such as groups B and D streptococci. Group A streptococci and *Staphylococcus aureus* are recovered in less than 5% of cases. The most common anaerobic isolates are *Bacteroides bivius* and *B. fragilis* as well as the anaerobic streptococci peptococcus and peptostreptococcus. Genital mycoplasmas and chlamydia may be recovered from patients with acute endometritis, but clinical response to antibiotics ineffective against these organisms belies their importance[3].

Empirical therapy with parenteral antibiotics should be initiated as soon as the diagnosis of endometritis has been made and cultures have been taken (Table 1). Most patients will show a clear response to treatment within 48–72 h. Following vaginal delivery, 95% respond to initial administration of a penicillin plus an aminoglycoside, despite incomplete anaerobic coverage. With additional antibiotics in those who fail initial therapy, less than 2% develop

Table 1 First-line therapy for endometritis

After Cesarean delivery

Clindamycin 900 mg intravenously every 8 h plus
  gentamicin 2 mg/kg intravenous loading dose,
  then 1.5 mg/kg intravenously every 8 h*
Clindamycin (as above) plus aztreonam 2 g
  intravenously every 6–8 h*
Metronidazole 500 mg intravenously every 6 h,
  plus gentamicin (as above), plus ampicillin 2 g
  intravenously every 6 h

After vaginal delivery

Ampicillin (as above), plus gentamicin (as above)

*Single agent for mild to moderate cases (after vaginal
or Cesarean delivery)*

Ampicillin–sulbactam 3 g intravenously every 6 h
Cefotaxime 2 g intravenously every 8 h
Cefotetan 2 g intravenously every 12 h
Cefoxitin 2 g intravenously every 6 h
Imipenem 500 mg intravenously every 6 h*
Mezlocillin 4 g intravenously every 6 h
Piperacillin 4 g intravenously every 6 h
Ticarcillin–clavulanic acid 3.1 g intravenously every 6 h

*For penicillin-allergic patients

major infectious complications such as abscess or septic pelvic thrombophlebitis[6]. Only 64–78% of patients with post-Cesarean endometritis respond to initial therapy with a penicillin plus an aminoglycoside, with 4% developing major sequelae despite additional therapy[25–27]. This inferior regimen has been abandoned for initial therapy which is active against anaerobes. Clindamycin plus an aminoglycoside has been proved effective with clinical response in 86–100% of cases and reduction in both the need for a third antibiotic and serious sequelae[7,26]. Metronidazole–penicillin–aminoglycoside and clindamycin–aztreonam may be appropriate choices for post-Cesarean infection as well[7].

Single agents, such as second or third generation cephalosporins, ureidopenicillins, or penicillins combined with a β-lactamase inhibitor are acceptable alternatives for initial therapy of mildly to moderately severe endometritis following vaginal or Cesarean delivery[3,7,16]. A single agent, if used for prophylaxis, should not be continued as therapy after prophylaxis failure. Initial response and failure rates with single-agent therapy are comparable to those with clindamycin plus an aminoglycoside; however, the published experience with single agents must be interpreted with caution. Patient numbers are small, thus a true difference in rare complications may go undetected; the uncommon severely ill patients are likely to have been excluded; and some trials excluded antibiotic prophylaxis failures. Patients with severe endometritis, prophylaxis failure, serious medical conditions or immunosuppression may be best served by combination therapy[3,27].

The appropriate duration of therapy has not been well established. Typically, antibiotics have been continued until the patient has been afebrile for 48 h. Discontinuation of treatment in a non-bacteremic patient when the patient's temperature has been ≤ 37.5°C for at least 24 h has recently been shown to be safe and cost-effective in both private and indigent populations[28,29]. Follow-up oral antibiotics, except in patients with known chlamydial infection, are generally unnecessary[3,16,27].

Failure to respond within 48–72 h warrants re-evaluation of the patient. Common causes of failure include wound infection and resistant micro-organisms. Culture results should be reviewed, if available, and cultures of blood, endometrium and wound collected. Antibiotic therapy should be assessed. Increases in dose or frequency of administration may be required, as pregnancy-related changes in renal function, blood volume and total body water affect elimination and volume of distribution of drugs, usually toward lower serum levels[30]. In patients receiving clindamycin plus an aminoglycoside, aminoglycoside levels should be drawn and ampicillin added to provide coverage against enterococci[21]. Anaerobic coverage should be added if lacking. Single-agent therapy may be changed to clindamycin plus an amnioglycoside plus a penicillin. For proven staphylococcal infection, specific therapy should be added (e.g. nafcillin 1–2 g intravenously every 4–6 h, cefazolin 2 g intravenously every 8 h, or vancomycin 1 g intravenously every 12 h). Wound infection, of course, warrants drainage.

If antibiotic therapy requires no modification, or if changes fail to produce response (80% respond) within another 48–72 h, the case should be scrutinized for sources of continued fever. The differential diagnosis must be broadened to include wound infection, pelvic cellulitis, pelvic abscess, venous thromboembolism, drug fever, septic pelvic thrombophlebitis, enterocolitis, retained placental fragments as well as viral or connective tissue disorders. Pelvic ultrasound may be helpful in visualizing retained placenta or a fluid collection. A computed tomographic (CT) scan may identify ovarian vein thrombosis, abscess, hematoma, or other masses.

Bacteremia

The incidence of documented bacteremia following Cesarean section is 3–4%, compared to 0.1–0.4% in patients who have delivered vaginally. Endometritis accounts for the majority of cases, but wound, respiratory and urinary infections as well as endocarditis may be responsible[31,32]. Bacteremia is more commonly found in post-Cesarean endometritis (8–30%) compared to endometritis following vaginal delivery (5%)[5,6]. Organisms isolated from the blood reflect organisms infecting the endometrium and are found in similar proportions[27]. While blood culture results may guide antibiotic therapy for endometritis, failure to respond to initial therapy does not correlate with a resistant organism in blood culture[31]. Identification of a pathogenic organism resistant to the antibiotics administered warrants broadening the antibiotic coverage despite apparent clinical response. Prolonged therapy may be indicated when *S. aureus* is isolated from the blood to avoid metastatic infection[7,23]. Mortality among obstetric bacteremic patients is extremely low (< 1%) compared to other medical or surgical populations[32].

Prevention

Despite the overwhelming effectiveness of antibiotic therapy, prevention of endometritis is a more desirable alternative. Antibiotic prophylaxis in Cesarean section reduced the rates of subsequent endometrial and wound infections by half in high-risk groups studied[23]; infections in private patients undergoing Cesarean section without prior labor were not significantly decreased[33]. Many antibiotics are effective, and some have been shown to be more efficacious (Table 2)[34]. Newer broad-spectrum agents perhaps should be reserved for treatment of serious infections, as clear benefits over older and cheaper antibiotics have not yet been demonstrated. Delaying the first dose until cord clamping, to avoid clouding evaluation of the newborn, does not significantly change the maternal course. One to three doses of an agent provide adequate prophylaxis[33,34].

Use of prophylactic antibiotics is not without risks. Severe allergic or toxic reactions fortunately are rare, but can occur. Changes in genital and fecal flora, especially increases in enterococci[21], have been demonstrated and may affect treatment of subsequent infection or development of antibiotic-associated diarrhea. Despite the reduction in clinical infections due to prophylaxis, a reduction in serious infectious complications has not been clearly demonstrated[23]. Antibiotic prophylaxis should therefore be reserved for those with a significant risk of infection. A reported reduction in endometritis following operative vaginal delivery from 3.5 to 0%[35], although statistically significant, probably does not justify the use of prophylactic antibiotics for that indication.

Other methods of prevention are available. Mere enforcement of standard infection control measures,

such as handwashing and proper disposal of infected materials, can decrease postoperative morbidity[23]. Intraoperative irrigation with antibiotic solution[23] or administration of methylergometrine for a week following Cesarean section[36] can decrease the rate of endometritis. Saline amnioinfusion in patients at risk for cord compression reduced the rate of endometritis from 19 to 2.4%, although the incidence of Cesarean section was also less in the treated group[37]. The recent identification of bacterial vaginosis as a risk factor has prompted suggestions to prevent endometritis by eliminating bacterial vaginosis prior to labor[18,24]. Clearly, methods aimed at reduction in the rate of postpartum endometritis need continued attention.

Late infection

Late postpartum endometritis, with onset from 7 to 42 days after delivery, is a clinically mild disease which typically occurs in women who have delivered vaginally. Lower abdominal pain and an increasing vaginal discharge with odor are the presenting symptoms; systemic signs are rare. *Chlamydia trachomatis*, uncommon in acute endometritis[24], is isolated from the cervix or endometrium in 30–67% of cases[38]. In women with chlamydial infection detected in the antepartum period, late postpartum endometritis develops in 30–60% if untreated[38]. When late-onset infection is suspected, a cervical or endometrial culture for chlamydia should be obtained. Oral tetracycline (doxycycline 100 mg orally twice a day for 10–14 days) or erythromycin (500 mg orally four times a day for 10–14 days) therapy is clinically effective. Treatment in the antepartum period may prevent late postpartum infection.

PELVIC THROMBOPHLEBITIS

Pelvic thrombophlebitis is a potentially life-threatening complication of the postpartum period. It occurs most commonly after obstetric procedures, but may be associated with pelvic surgery, inflammation, or malignancy. The incidence is reported as one per 600 to 3000 deliveries. In patients with postpartum endometritis, the risk climbs to 0.5–2%[39].

The pathogenesis of pelvic thrombophlebitis rests on Virchow's triad of venous stasis, intimal damage and alterations in coagulation factors. Damage to the intima of pelvic veins may result from direct surgical trauma or from the inflammatory response to an infected uterus. The velocity of blood flow through the dilated ovarian veins declines sharply postpartum. The long veins have multiple valves which are major sites of venous pooling and their thin walls make them subject to external compression. Pregnancy-related increases in levels of clotting factors and platelet adhesiveness, along with possible thromboplastin release from placental fragments and necrotic tissue, may generate a thrombotic process[39].

Table 2   Some alternatives for antibiotic prophylaxis – single dose

Ampicillin 2 g intravenously
Cefazolin 2 g intravenously
Piperacillin 4 g intravenously
Cefotetan 1 g intravenously

Pelvic thrombophlebitis presents in two forms – acute ovarian vein thrombosis and enigmatic fever. In the acute ovarian vein syndrome, the cardinal symptom is lower abdominal or flank pain. Nausea and vomiting may be present. Onset is acute, usually within 2–4 days postoperatively, but may be weeks after delivery. The patient usually appears ill with a low-grade fever, tachycardia, abdominal tenderness with guarding and ileus with abdominal distention. A tender rope-like abdominal mass originating near the uterine cornu and extending cephalad and laterally is palpable in one-half to two-thirds of patients and represents the thrombosed ovarian vein. Ovarian vein thrombosis commonly occurs in association with pelvic infection, but the patient's symptoms worsen, rather than improve, with continued antibiotic therapy. The syndrome may present in the absence of clinical infection, sometimes prompting laparotomy to exclude other disorders. The differential diagnosis includes acute appendicitis, broad ligament hematoma, degenerating fibroid, adnexal torsion, pyelonephritis, ureterolithiasis and abscess.

Postpartum ovarian vein thrombosis is predominantly a right-sided lesion (80%), with bilateral and left-sided lesions unusual (14 and 6%, respectively)[40,41]. The preponderance of right-sided involvement is explained by venous drainage which, in the upright position, flows from the left ovarian vein and uterine venous plexus into the right ovarian vein, increasing venous stasis and the inoculum of pathogens on the right[3].

Septic pelvic thrombophlebitis, with diffuse thrombosis of multiple small pelvic vessels, usually presents with enigmatic fever, and typically follows the diagnosis of endometritis or other pelvic infection. After several days of antibiotic therapy, recurrent high spiking fevers occur despite resolution of other signs and symptoms of infection. The diagnosis is usually presumptive, based on defervescence within 48–72 h after addition of heparin to the antibiotic regimen.

Some diagnostic studies may be of help in evaluating patients with septic pelvic thrombophlebitis. Thrombus in ovarian and larger veins may be visualized by CT scan, ultrasound, duplex Doppler or magnetic resonance imaging (MRI), but imaging techniques do not demonstrate the small uterine and vaginal veins which have commonly been shown at laparotomy to be involved[42]. Findings on intravenous pyelography are supportive but non-specific. Sonography with duplex Doppler has been suggested as an appropriate screening examination in patients at risk for pelvic vein thrombophlebitis, but sonographic findings are frequently non-diagnostic secondary to intervening bowel gas. CT remains the imaging procedure of choice. MRI offers no clinical advantages to balance its increased cost and limited availability. All imaging techniques are helpful only if positive and are inadequate in excluding the diagnosis. Laboratory studies are generally not helpful.

Serious complications of pelvic thrombophlebitis are mainly due to extension of thrombus or embolization. Extension of clot from the ovarian to the renal vein may result in renal vein thrombosis with subsequent nephrotic syndrome and renal insufficiency. Clots in pelvic vessels may fragment, possibly owing to the presence of bacteria, and embolize. Showers of small infected emboli are characteristic with resulting septicemia and metastatic abscesses[43]. Massive involvement of ovarian veins or the vena cava may precipitate large pulmonary emboli with symptoms of venous occlusion; in fact, respiratory distress from pulmonary embolism may be the presenting symptom[41]. Ventilation–perfusion scanning of the lung may be indicated to determine whether pulmonary embolization has occurred, and has been found to be abnormal in one-third of patients tested[39].

The diagnosis of pelvic thrombophlebitis, in either form, may not be confirmed by radiographic study, yet the risk of laparotomy for diagnostic purposes may not be warranted. Clinical response to heparin may secure the diagnosis in both the acute and the enigmatic syndromes. Full anticoagulation with an intravenous infusion of heparin should be continued for 7–10 days along with broad-spectrum antibiotics (Table 3). Micro-organisms have been isolated from resected venous specimens and require treatment to promote resolution of the thrombus[39]. Primary surgical ligation of ovarian veins and vena cava, employed 50 years ago, decreased mortality from 50 to 10%[44], but is fraught with risks of significant hemorrhage, embolization and death[40]. Today, a surgical approach should be reserved for patients who do not respond to anticoagulation plus antibiotics, who experience pulmonary embolization while on therapeutic anticoagulation, or for those in whom the diagnosis is uncertain. If pelvic vein thrombosis is found unexpectedly at postpartum laparotomy, closure of the abdomen without vein ligation and institution of medical therapy is probably the procedure of choice.

The subject of long-term anticoagulation is controversial. No reliable data are available. Some clinicians will extend anticoagulation by adding oral agents for 6 weeks to 6 months, especially if a large clot or septic pulmonary emboli have been documented. Need for

Table 3 Treatment of septic pelvic thrombophlebitis

Full anticoagulation with heparin
  5000–10 000 units loading dose, followed by 800–2000 units/h to maintain the PTT at 1.5–2.5 × baseline value

Continuation of antibiotic therapy
  to complete at least a 7-day course or until the patient is afebrile for 48–72 h

anticoagulation during or after subsequent pregnancy is probably not required.

EPISIOTOMY INFECTIONS

Postpartum infection arising from an episiotomy site is a rare but potentially fatal condition. An episiotomy is a contaminated wound; yet clinical infection manifests in only 0.035–3% of patients[45,46]. Life-threatening infection associated with episiotomy has occurred in 0.5–2 per 100 000 live births, accounting for 20% of maternal mortality. Perineal infection has been classified according to the depth of soft-tissue involvement[47]. Successful management depends on accurate assessment of the infected tissues.

Infection limited to the skin and superficial fascia along the episiotomy incision may be managed conservatively. Episiotomy dehiscence or perineal pain may be the presenting complaint, with edema and erythema confined to the area immediately adjacent to the episiotomy[47]. The previous repair should be taken down to allow careful inspection of the wound to exclude hematoma, abscess or unsuspected rectovaginal communication. Following cleansing and débridement, the wound may be allowed to heal secondarily. With surrounding cellulitis, a course of broad-spectrum parenteral antibiotics (such as suggested in Table 1), in addition to local wound care, may be required. Early repair of episiotomy dehiscence, while contrary to conventional practice, has produced excellent anatomical and functional results[48].

Superficial fascial infection presents with erythema and edema which extend beyond the area of episiotomy to the thigh, buttock or abdominal wall. Appropriate therapy is dependent upon determination of associated necrotizing fasciitis. Diagnosis by inspection is unreliable, thus surgical exploration may be necessary to rule out fascial necrosis. In the absence of obvious signs of necrotic fascia, frozen-section biopsy has been employed to expedite diagnosis and avoid a possible lethal delay in treatment[49]. In the absence of fascial necrosis, severe systemic involvement is uncommon and response to broad-spectrum antibiotics should occur within 24–48 h. Lack of response or progression of the infection during antibiotic therapy may indicate a more severe infection.

When necrotizing fasciitis is present, aggressive management is necessary to avert mortality. Both Camper's and Colles' fascial layers become necrotic with this infection, which spreads along these fascial planes, undermining the skin, and eventually involves all tissues external to the deep fascia[50]. The onset is acute with a rapidly progressive clinical course, systemic toxicity and a fatality rate of 21–76%[47]. Although the condition is classically described in patients with diabetes or atherosclerosis, affected obstetric patients are usually otherwise healthy[51]. The patients appear severely ill, usually with fever and leukocytosis. Erythema with indistinct margins that gradually fade into normal areas may be present. As the disease progresses, skin color becomes blue or brown, with subsequent formation of bullae and gangrene. Progressive brawny edema and induration are evident; vulvar edema, especially unilateral, is characteristic[51]. Marked local tenderness is common initially, but the lesions become hypesthetic or anesthetic as cutaneous nerves become ischemic[50]. Crepitation may be detected. Exudate is serosanguinous 'dirty dishwater' rather than purulent. Anemia due to hemolysis is common[50], but may be masked by massive fluid shifts into the extravascular compartment with resultant hemoconcentration[47]. Hypocalcemia may develop due to saponification of liquified subcutaneous fat[50]. At surgical exploration, the superficial fascia does not bleed and lacks resistance to blunt probing; the skin is easily separated from the underlying deep fascia.

Prompt surgical resection of the involved tissues is essential for effective management of necrotizing fasciitis. Mortality is 100% in patients treated with antibiotics alone or with incision and drainage only[52]. Débridement should extend to where the subcutaneous tissues cannot be separated from the underlying deep fascia or from normal skin. Any tissue that is indurated, edematous or crepitant, or that does not bleed readily when incised, should be removed[50]. More than one surgical débridement may be necessary if subcutaneous necrosis is not arrested. Hyperbaric oxygen is at best an adjunctive measure and should not be substituted for surgical débridement.

Similar to most pelvic infections, necrotizing fasciitis is a polymicrobial disorder. The pathophysiology involves bacterial synergism among various combinations of aerobic and anaerobic organisms[50,52]. Comprehensive antibiotic coverage with a penicillin, clindamycin and an aminoglycoside is recommended as an adjunct to operative intervention until a healthy bed of granulation tissue is apparent. After extensive débridement, these patients resemble those with severe burns. Management in an intensive care setting with invasive monitoring, aggressive fluid management and hemodynamic support may be required[50]. Porcine xenografts may be used to limit fluid and protein loss as well as promote the growth of granulation tissue in preparation for permanent skin grafting[51]. The wound may be allowed to heal secondarily.

Infection beneath the deep fascia produces myonecrosis. A clostridial infection is the most common cause, although myonecrosis can occur from a neglected necrotizing fasciitis which invades deep fascia. Clostridial infection may present early in the postpartum period with severe pain disproportionate to the physical findings. A wound or blood culture positive for clostridia should raise the index of suspicion for myonecrosis. Crepitation or clinical deterioration in the presence of an episiotomy infection warrants surgical exploration and radical excision of involved tissues, supplemented with antibiotic therapy. For clostridial infection, high-dose penicillin (4 million units intravenously every 4 h) is indicated. Polyvalent gas gangrene antitoxin is thought to be ineffective[47]. *Clostridium perfringens* is the most notorious organism associated with myonecrosis. *Clostridium sordellii* has also been identified in serious episiotomy infections, but presents with massive malignant vulvar edema thought to be caused by toxin production and results in death from cardiovascular collapse[53].

WOUND INFECTIONS

Abdominal wound infections occur in 1.6–10% of women delivered by Cesarean section[4,33,46,54]. Patients with a wound infection endure a longer febrile course and a longer hospital stay than patients with endometritis[55].

Determinants of wound infection after other abdominal surgery, such as operation time, estimated blood loss, obesity and pre-existing infection, apply to post-Cesarean wound infections[55]. Other predisposing factors such as patient age, gross spillage from the gastrointestinal tract, duration of preoperative hospitalization and debilitating illnesses are rarely operative in the obstetric population[54]. Specific obstetric variables do play a role in post-Cesarean wound infection and are remarkably similar to risk factors for endometritis[54]. Presence of endometritis is itself a risk factor[3,55]. High wound infection rates occur among women with bacteria present in amniotic fluid at the time of uterine incision[14]. Duration of labor, duration of ruptured membranes, number of vaginal examinations, presence of internal monitors, operation due to dystocia, as well as performance of an emergency procedure[3] are highly correlated with post-Cesarean wound infection[54]. Antibiotic prophylaxis has been shown to reduce the rate of wound infection from 8–10% to 3%[33,55].

The diagnosis of wound infection is based on the findings of local erythema and induration with purulent discharge from the wound. Fever is not always present. Clinical signs typically manifest 4–8 days following delivery. Many patients have had earlier evidence of endometritis and present with recurrent fever after the initial response to antibiotics given for the uterine infection. The majority of wound infections result from extension of polymicrobial contamination of the endometrium and amniotic fluid by vaginal flora to the incision site[55]. Organisms cultured from the wound are frequently similar to endometrial isolates. Staphylococcal wound infections, in contrast, typically develop in women without obstetric risk factors. If wound infection presents with fever and spreading cellulitis within the first 48 h after operation, a single bacterial pathogen, such as group A β-hemolytic streptococci or *Clostridium perfringens*, may be responsible. A Gram stain of material aspirated from the active margin of infection may identify the causative organism.

Treatment for early-onset infection consists of antibiotic therapy such as penicillin 4 million units intravenously every 4 h or cefazolin 2 g intravenously every 6 h, and prompt débridement of necrotic tissue[56]. Late infections usually respond to simple incision and drainage. Hot wet packs may help localize extensive induration into a drainable area[3]. Antibiotics are required only if there is extensive cellulitis, bacteremia, or failure to defervesce within 12–24 h of opening the wound[56]. Débridement under anesthesia is sometimes required[55].

Serious complications of abdominal wound infection include fascial dehiscence and toxic shock syndrome. Wound dehiscence occurs in 0.5% of post-Cesarean patients but has been reported in 7–12.5% Cesarean section patients with wound infections[54,55]. Fascial repair under anesthesia may be necessary. Toxic shock syndrome has been reported to occur in association with post-Cesarean *S. aureus* wound infections from several days to weeks after surgery[3] and requires aggressive supportive care and antibiotic therapy.

Complications of wound infection such as necrotizing fasciitis, synergistic bacterial gangrene and clostridial gas gangrene are extremely rare after Cesarean section but should be suspected if the patient fails to respond following incision and drainage of the wound. Early recognition is essential to prevent mortality from these life-threatening conditions. Necrotizing fasciitis should be suspected if the patient appears critically ill or if the edema and induration surrounding the wound worsen rapidly despite treatment or are accompanied by local anesthesia or crepitus. At surgical exploration, there is undermining of the involved skin surrounding the wound and the superficial fascia lacks resistance to a blunt instrument. Synergistic bacterial gangrene is recognized by a central ulcer, a surrounding deep red zone and peripheral erythema. The process is slowly progressive and often marked by severe pain. Clostridial gangrene presents with sudden onset of severe pain, mild local edema, thin watery drainage from the wound and systemic toxicity. In advanced stages, the skin appears bronzed with bullae, gangrene and crepitation. Gas may be evident on X-ray[56]. These destructive processes require extensive surgical débridement. Aerobic and anaerobic cultures and broad-spectrum parenteral antibiotics are appropriate in the management of these polymicrobial infections. Delays in treatment may lead to maternal mortality.

MASTITIS

Mastitis occurs in 2–3% of breastfeeding women[57], but may rarely occur in women who are not nursing. Most cases are sporadic, presenting commonly in the second or third week following delivery[58,59]. The onset of symptoms is usually abrupt with chills, malaise, generalized achiness and fever as high as 39–40°C. The affected breast is tender, hot, swollen and erythematous in a wedge-shaped segment with its apex at the nipple and its base towards the periphery, demarcated by the divisions between the lobes of the breast. Decreased milk secretion may be noted[60], but expression of pus from the ducts is uncommon[59]. Nipple fissuring and milk stasis are considered to be the primary etiological factors, but the cause of most cases is unclear[57]. Mastitis is no more common among women who are nursing for the first time than among women who have previously nursed. Recurrence in successive pregnancies is not typical. Toxic shock syndrome has been reported in women with puerperal mastitis[61].

Breast infections should be distinguished from segmental breast inflammation due to milk stasis or focal engorgement. Fever and erythema are less marked in the absence of infection. When the diagnosis is uncertain, leukocyte counts from the milk and quantitative bacterial cultures may be helpful in differentiating the non-infected cases from mastitis[60,62]. Cases of milk stasis (sterile culture and counts of less than 10^6 leukocytes/ml of milk) need no specific treatment and resolve in 2–3 days. Inflammation of the breast, with counts of $> 10^6$ leukocytes but $< 10^3$ bacteria/ml of milk, may be treated by regular emptying of the breast. The counts may be repeated if the degree of suspicion for infection permits a delay in treatment[62]. The diagnosis of mastitis may be based on leukocyte counts of $> 10^6$/ml and bacterial counts of $> 10^3$/ml, but patients with obvious signs and symptoms of mastitis should be treated regardless of leukocyte and bacterial counts.

Staphylococcus aureus is the organism isolated in 40–50% of breast infections, and 50–70% show penicillin resistance *in vitro*[57,60,63]. Other common pathogens include coagulase-negative staphylococci, *Escherichia coli*, *Klebsiella pneumoniae* and *Bacteroides fragilis*[60].

Appropriate therapy for mastitis includes routine emptying of the breast and administration of antibiotics. Breastfeeding from both breasts should continue during mastitis. If the infected breast is too sore for nursing, gentle pumping may be employed to reduce congestion. Local hot wet compresses or prone soaks in a hot tub may soften the indurated breast and allow drainage[59]. Weaning may increase the risk of abscess formation[57,59,62]. Choice of antibiotic may be empirical or based on culture of expressed breast milk. Cultures of breast milk may be useful, since mastitis may be protracted or recur in 10–20% of women treated with antibiotics (albeit penicillin) prescribed without susceptibility testing[62–64]. In most cases, antibiotics may be given orally, and hospitalization is not required. Therapy with a penicillinase-resistant penicillin, such as dicloxacillin (250–500 mg orally four times a day), or a first-generation cephalosporin (cefalexin 500 mg orally four times a day) should be started immediately after cultures are obtained. (Erythromycin 500 mg orally four times a day is an alternative in penicillin-allergic patients.) Delay in institution of antibiotic therapy may promote abscess formation[58]. Most patients become afebrile and asymptomatic within 36–48 h of beginning treatment[57]. If the patient is not improved within 48 h, examination for abscess formation is warranted. Therapy should be continued for at least 10 days. Episodes of recurrent mastitis should be treated with continued breastfeeding and a repeat course of antibiotics.

Breast abscesses develop in 4–6% of patients despite appropriate treatment[57,63]. An indurated, fluctuant area may be palpable, usually peripherally, and should be aspirated for culture if suspected. Axillary lymphadenitis is not typical, but the patient may be febrile and tachycardic, with leukocytosis. Bacteremia may occur[65]. *Staphylococcus aureus* is recovered from the majority of abscesses[3]. Incision and drainage is the standard treatment. Radial or circumferential incision is made over the site of maximum tenderness and loculi are broken down, followed by insertion of a dependent drain or pack. Rapid resolution is invariable. Alternative approaches such as curettage and primary obliteration of the cavity[65] or repeated aspiration[66] have produced good results as well.

Antibiotic coverage is recommended preoperatively and susceptibility-directed antibiotic therapy is continued postoperatively[65]. Milk stasis should be prevented by breast pumping to avoid secondary abscess formation. Breastfeeding is contraindicated, as the presence of a staphylococcal breast abscess has been associated with infant deaths from lung abscesses, presumably due to aspiration of a large inoculum. Infants of mothers with breast abscesses should be evaluated by a pediatrician for possible infection and should not breastfeed until the abscess has cleared[3].

Epidemic mastitis is a hospital-acquired infection caused by *Staphylococcus aureus*. During the 1940s and 1950s, when lengthy postpartum hospitalization was practiced, up to 20% of women became infected[3]. The infection involves the lactiferous glands and ducts of the breast, in contrast to the interlobular connective tissue in the sporadic form, and may affect multiple lobes. Abscess formation is common. Epidemic mastitis usually originated in hospital nurseries and was traceable to attendant carriers of the specific phage type that caused the infection[3,58]. Infants suffered significant mortality from staphylococcal pneumonia, meningitis, osteomyelitis and pyoderma during these outbreaks[58,64]. Fortunately, infection control measures and superior antibiotics have made epidemic mastitis an unlikely occurrence today.

URINARY TRACT INFECTION

Immediately postpartum, bacteriuria is found in 15–20% of women, but resolves spontaneously in most[67]. By the third postpartum day, bacteriuria is found in 1.7–4% by suprapubic aspiration. Only one-fourth of women with bacteriuria complain of dysuria, but the symptom is more common following catheterization. Cesarean section, vaginal operative delivery, epidural anesthesia and bladder catheterization significantly increase the risk of bacteriuria[68]. Antibiotic prophylaxis may decrease the incidence of post-Cesarean bacteriuria, but results are variable in the studies reviewed[33].

Treatment for urinary tract infection is similar to that for the non-pregnant woman. High rates of cure are achieved even with a short (3 days) course of therapy[68]. The causative organism is *Escherichia coli* in 80–90% of infections, but may be another coliform or staphylococcal or enterococcal species[3,68]. Culture and susceptibility testing may guide therapy, especially in patients who have recently received antibiotics. Suprapubic aspiration from a full bladder or urethral catheterization may be necessary to obtain samples of urine, as clean-catch midstream collections are frequently (46–69%) contaminated[68].

Treatment of persistent asymptomatic bacteriuria, perhaps unwarranted in the non-pregnant patient, is recommended in the postpartum period. Decreased bladder tone, increased capacity and incomplete emptying, along with a dilated collecting system and an enlarged uterus, capable of mechanical obstruction, may be present for weeks to months postpartum. These pregnancy-related changes predispose to vesicoureteric reflux and development of pyelonephritis. Infection of the urinary tract can be minimized by avoiding routine urethral catheterization of laboring or postpartum women. High-risk patients, who have received antibiotic suppression during the antepartum period to prevent pyelonephritis, should probably continue the regimen for at least 2 weeks postpartum.

UNUSUAL INFECTIONS

Infections resulting from spinal or epidural anesthesia occur following less than one in 10 000 blocks[69]. The diagnosis should be considered in the febrile patient with backache and pain radiating from the spinal area. Evaluation may include neurological examination, cerebrospinal fluid analysis and myelography. Weakness, numbness and finally paralysis will develop if the infection goes untreated[70].

Subgluteal or retropsoal infections have been reported following paracervical or pudendal block[69,71]. Patients presented with poorly localized severe hip pain and limited range of motion. Associated organisms were normal vaginal or bowel flora. Gas in the soft tissues was seen in half the cases, and abscess formation was common. Treatment may be delayed, owing to failure to suspect the diagnosis. In addition to antibiotic therapy, surgical drainage, débridement and diverting colostomy may be necessary for appropriate treatment. Sequelae from these serious infections include persistent discomfort, impaired ambulation and death.

SEPTIC SHOCK

Rarely, septic shock may complicate a postpartum infection. Septic shock is characterized by hypotension and inadequate tissue perfusion, owing to overwhelming infection. The hypotension may be preceded by chills and fever and associated tachycardia, tachypnea, oliguria or mental obtundation. Current theories of pathogenesis and treatment of septic shock are reviewed elsewhere[72] (see Chapter 15).

Micro-organisms causing sepsis incite the formation or release of vasoactive and inflammatory mediators which lead to peripheral vasodilatation, regional microembolization and endothelial cell injury. Severe multiorgan dysfunction involving the lungs, kidneys, liver, heart and central nervous system may result from inadequate perfusion. Aggressive management strategies incorporate broad-spectrum antibiotic coverage, volume replacement, invasive hemodynamic monitoring, inotropic agents and peripheral vasoconstrictors to maintain afterload. Rapid reversal of organ hypoperfusion, improvement in oxygen delivery and correction of acidosis must be achieved for successful stabilization of the patient. A careful search for infected or necrotic foci that may be responsible for persistent bacteremia is warranted. Surgical intervention is sometimes required to remove the underlying cause of sepsis.

Associated complications include adult respiratory distress syndrome, pulmonary edema, disseminated intravascular coagulation, thromboemboli and cardiac arrest. The risk of maternal mortality increases as associated complications become superimposed on the septic hypotension. Fortunately, mortality due to septic shock is thought to be considerably lower than in the non-obstetric population. Early identification of sepsis, prompt institution of antibiotic therapy, volume administration and cardiopulmonary support when needed are essential to prevent complications and minimize mortality.

REFERENCES

1. Gibbs RS, O'Dell TN, MacGregor RR, *et al.* Puerperal endometritis: a prospective microbiologic study. *Am J Obstet Gynecol* 1975;121:919–25
2. Filker R, Monif GRG. The significance of temperature during the first 24 hours postpartum. *Obstet Gynecol* 1979;53:358–61

3. Eschenbach DA. Acute postpartum infections. *Emerg Med Clin North Am* 1985;3:87–115

4. Nielsen TF, Hokegard K-H. Postoperative cesarean section morbidity: a prospective study. *Am J Obstet Gynecol* 1983;146:911–6

5. Gibbs RS. Clinical risk factors for puerperal infection. *Obstet Gynecol* 1980;55:178S–183S

6. Gibbs RS, Rodgers PJ, Castaneda YS, Ramzy I. Endometritis following vaginal delivery. *Obstet Gynecol* 1980; 56:555–8

7. Duff P. Pathophysiology and management of post-cesarean endomyometritis. *Obstet Gynecol* 1986;67:269

8. Blanco JD, Gibbs RS. Infections following classical cesarean section. *Obstet Gynecol* 1980;55:167–9

9. D'Angelo LJ, Sokol RJ. Time-related peripartum determinants of postpartum morbidity. *Obstet Gynecol* 1980;55:319–22

10. Gilstrap LC, Leveno KJ, Cox SM, *et al*. Intrapartum treatment of acute chorioamnionitis: impact on neonatal sepsis. *Am J Obstet Gynecol* 1988;159:579–83

11. Koh KS, Chan FH, Monfared AH, *et al*. The changing perinatal and maternal outcome in chorioamnionitis. *Obstet Gynecol* 1979;53:730–4

12. Gilstrap LC, Cox SM. Acute chorioamnionitis. *Obstet Gynecol Clin North Am* 1989;16:373–9

13. Blanco JD, Gibbs RS, Castaneda YS, St Clair PJ. Correlation of quantitative amniotic fluid cultures with endometritis after cesarean section. *Am J Obstet Gynecol* 1982;143:897–901

14. Gilstrap LC, Cunningham FG. The bacterial pathogensis of infection following cesarean section. *Obstet Gynecol* 1979;53:545–9

15. D'Angelo LJ, Sokol RJ. Determinants of postpartum morbidity in laboring monitored patients: a reassessment of the bacteriology of the amniotic fluid during labor. *Am J Obstet Gynecol* 1980;136:575–8

16. Cox SM, Gilstrap LC. Postpartum endometritis. *Obstet Gynecol Clin North Am* 1989;16:363–71

17. Newton ER, Prihoda TJ, Gibbs RS. A clinical and microbiologic analysis of risk factors for puerperal endometritis. *Obstet Gynecol* 1990;75:402–6

18. Watts DH, Krohn MA, Hillier SL, Eschenbach DA. Bacterial vaginosis as a risk factor for post-cesarean endometritis. *Obstet Gynecol* 1990;75:52–8

19. Christensen KK, Svenningsen N, Dahlander K, *et al*. Relation between neonatal pneumonia and maternal carriage of group B streptococci. *Scand J Infect Dis* 1982;14:261–6

20. Curet LB, Morrison JC, Rao AV. Antenatal therapy with cortiocosteroids and postpartum complications. *Am J Obstet Gynecol* 1985;152:83–4

21. Walmer D, Walmer KR, Gibbs RS. Enterococci in post-cesarean endometritis. *Obstet Gynecol* 1988;71:159–62

22. Martens MG, Faro S, Hammill HA, *et al*. Transcervical uterine cultures with a new endometrial suction curette: a comparison of three sampling methods in postpartum endometritis. *Obstet Gynecol* 1989;74:273–6

23. Gibbs RS. Infection after cesarean section. *Clin Obstet Gynecol* 1985;28:697–10

24. Watts DH, Eschenbach DA, Kenny GE. Early postpartum endometritis: the role of bacteria, genital mycoplasmas, and *Chlamydia trachomatis*. *Obstet Gynecol* 1989;73:52–60

25. Gibbs RS, Jones PM, Wilder CJ. Antibiotic therapy of endometritis following cesarean section. *Obstet Gynecol* 1978;52:31–7

26. DiZerega G, Yonekura L, Roy S, *et al*. A comparison of clindamycin–gentamicin and penicillin–gentamicin in the treatment of post-cesarean section endomyometritis. *Am J Obstet Gynecol* 1979;134:238–42

27. Yonekura ML. Treatment of postcesarean endomyometritis. *Clin Obstet Gynecol* 1988;31:488–500

28. Soper DE, Kemmer CT, Conover WB. Abbreviated antibiotic therapy for the treatment of postpartum endometritis. *Obstet Gynecol* 1987;69:127–30

29. Morales WJ, Collins EM, Angel JL, Knuppel RA. Short course of antibiotic therapy in treatment of postpartum endomyometritis. *Am J Obstet Gynecol* 1989;161:568–72

30. Fortunato SJ, Dodson MG. Therapeutic considerations in postpartum endometritis. *J Reprod Med* 1988;33:101–6

31. Blanco JD, Gibbs RS, Castaneda YS. Bacteremia in obstetrics: clinical course. *Obstet Gynecol* 1981;58:621–5

32. Ledger WJ, Norman M, Gee C, Lewis W. Bacteremia on an obstetric–gynecologic service. *Am J Obstet Gynecol* 1975;121:205–12

33. Swartz WH, Grolle K. The use of prophylactic antibiotics in cesarean section. *J Reprod Med* 1981;26:595–608

34. Faro S, Martens MG, Hammill HA, *et al*. Antibiotic prophylaxis: is there a difference? *Am J Obstet Gynecol* 1990;162:900–9

35. Heitmann JA, Benrubi GI. Efficacy of prophylactic antibiotics for the prevention of endomyometritis after forceps delivery. *South Med J* 1989;82:960–2

36. Iatrakis GM, Sakellaropoulos GG, Kourounis G, Argyroudis E. Methylergometrine and puerperal infections after normal delivery and after cesarean section. *Isr J Med Sci* 1989;25:714–15

37. Owen J, Henson BV, Hauth JC. A prospective randomized study of saline solution amnioinfusion. *Am J Obstet Gynecol* 1990;162:1146–9

38. Hoyme UB, Kiviat N, Eschenbach DA. Microbiology and treatment of late postpartum endometritis. *Obstet Gynecol* 1986;68:226–32

39. Duff P, Gibbs RS. Pelvic vein thrombophlebitis: diagnostic dilemma and therapeutic challenge. *Obstet Gynecol Surv* 1983;38:365–73

40. Khurana BK, Rao J, Friedman SA, Cho KC. Computed tomographic features of puerperal ovarian vein thrombosis. *Am J Obstet Gynecol* 1988;159:905–8

41. Munsick RA, Gillanders LA. A review of the syndrome of puerperal ovarian vein thrombophlebitis. *Obstet Gynecol Surv* 1981;36:57–66

42. Brown CEL, Lowe TW, Cunningham FG, Weinreb JC. Purepreal pelvic thrombophlebitis: impact on diagnosis and treatment using x-ray computed tomography and magnetic resonance imaging. *Obstet Gynecol* 1986; 68:789–94

43. Josey WE, Staggers SR. Heparin therapy in septic pelvic thrombophlebitis: a study of 46 cases. *Am J Obstet Gynecol* 1974;120:228–32

44. Cohen MB, Pernoll ML, Gevirtz CM, Kerstein MD. Septic pelvic thrombophlebitis: an update. *Obstet Gynecol* 1983;62:83–9

45. Thacker SB, Banta HD. Benefits and risks of episiotomy: an interpretative review of the English language literature, 1860–1980. *Obstet Gynecol Surv* 1983;38:322–38

46. Sweet RL, Ledger WJ. Puerperal infectious morbidity. *Am J Obstet Gynecol* 1973;117:1093–110

47. Shy KK, Eschenbach DA. Fatal perineal cellulitis from an episiotomy site. *Obstet Gynecol* 1979;54:292–8

48. Hankins GDV, Hauth JC, Gilstrap LC, *et al*. Early repair of episiotomy dehiscence. *Obstet Gynecol* 1990;75:48–51

49. Stamenkovic I, Lew PD. Early recognition of potentially fatal necrotizing fasciitis. *N Engl J Med* 1984;310:1689–93

50. Addison WA, Livengood CH, Hill GB, *et al*. Necrotizing fasciitis of vulvar origin in diabetic patients. *Obstet Gynecol* 1984;63:473–9

51. Sutton GP, Smirz LR, Clark DH, Bennett JE. Group B streptococcal necrotizing fasciitis arising from an episiotomy. *Obstet Gynecol* 1985;66:733–6

52. Stone HH, Martin JD. Synergistic necrotizing cellulitis. *Ann Surg* 1972;175:702–10

53. McGregor JA, Soper DE, Lovell G, Todd JK. Maternal deaths associated with *Clostridium sordellii* infection. *Am J Obstet Gynecol* 1989;161:987–95

54. Gibbs RS, Blanco JD, St Clair PJ. A case–control study of wound abscess after cesarean delivery. *Obstet Gynecol* 1983;62:498–501

55. Emmons SL, Krohn M, Jackson M, Eschenbach DA. Development of wound infections among women undergoing cesarean section. *Obstet Gynecol* 1988;72:559–64

56. Gibbs RS. Severe infections in pregnancy. *Med Clin North Am* 1989;73:713–21

57. Marshall BR, Hepper JK, Zirbel CC. Sporadic puerperal mastitis. *J Am Med Assoc* 1975;233:1377–9

58. Devereux WP. Acute puerperal mastitis. *Am J Obstet Gynecol* 1970;108:78–81

59. Niebyl JR, Spence MR, Parmley TH. Sporadic (nonepidemic) puerperal mastitis. *J Reprod Med* 1978;20:97–100

60. Thomsen AC, Hansen KB, Moller BR. Leukocyte counts and microbiologic cultivation in the diagnosis of puerperal mastitis. *Am J Obstet Gynecol* 1983;146:938–41

61. Demey HE, Hautekeete ML, Buytaert P, Bossaert LL. Mastitis and toxic shock syndrome. *Acta Obstet Gynecol Scand* 1989;68:87–8

62. Thomsen AC, Espersen T, Maigaard S. Course and treatment of milk stasis, noninfectious inflammation of the breast, and infectious mastitis in nursing women. *Am J Obstet Gynecol* 1984;149:492–5

63. Matheson I, Aursnes I, Horgen M, *et al*. Bacteriological findings and clinical symptoms in relation to clinical outcome in puerperal mastitis. *Acta Obstet Gynecol Scand* 1988;67:723–6

64. Olsen CG, Gordon RE Jr. Breast disorders in nursing mothers. *Am Fam Physician* 1990;41:1509–16

65. Benson EA. Management of breast abscesses. *World J Surg* 1989;13:753–6

66. Dixon JM. Repeated aspiration of breast abscesses in lactating women. *Br Med J* 1988;297:1517–18

67. Marraro RV, Harris RE. Incidence and spontaneous resolution of postpartum bacteriuria. *Am J Obstet Gynecol* 1977;128:722–3

68. Stray-Pedersen B, Solberg VM, Torkildsen E, *et al*. Postpartum bacteriuria. A multicenter evaluation of different screening procedures and a controlled short-course treatment trial with amoxycillin. *Eur J Obstet Gynecol Reprod Biol* 1988;31:163–70

69. Gibbs RS, Wienstein AJ. Puerperal infection in the antibiotic era. *Am J Obstet Gynecol* 1976;124:769–87

70. Baker AS, Ojemann RG, Swartz MN, Richardson EP. Spinal epidural abscess. *N Engl J Med* 1975;293:463–8

71. Hibbard LT, Synder EN, McVann RM. Subgluteal and retropsoal infection in obstetric practice. *Obstet Gynecol* 1972;39:137–50

72. Lee W, Cotton DB, Hankins GDV, Faro S. Management of septic shock complicating pregnancy. *Obstet Gynecol Clin North Am* 1989;16:431–47

22

Syphilis infection

J.B. Shumway

Tremendous variation in sexual practices and significant advances in our understanding of sexually transmitted diseases continue to add to the broad spectrum of syphilitic disease. Epidemic rates of multiple venereal diseases have focused attention on their impact on pregnancy. Syphilis, one of the traditional venereal diseases, is still ever-present in any practice.

EPIDEMIOLOGY

Syphilis is an ancient disease with protean clinical presentations. It has been called the 'great imposter' with its varied natural course. During the period of the 'great pox' that ravaged Eurasia at the close of the 15th century, syphilis was often accompanied by death. Based on historical accounts of the 16th century, it is believed that syphilis was much more severe in the 16th century than it is at present[1]. The mild course of syphilis seen in modern times possibly reflects a more resistant human host, a less virulent syphilis organism, or an alteration in the cofactors (nutrition, sanitation, etc.).

Syphilis is the third most common sexually transmitted disease in the USA. The incidence of syphilis peaked during World War II with nearly 600 000 reported cases yearly. In the late 1980s, after several decades of relative stability, the incidence of syphilis began to rise again among homosexual men. As safe sex practices were instituted among homosexual populations with the advent of acquired immune deficiency syndrome (AIDS), the incidence fell. As a sex-for-drugs culture emerged, a rapid increase in new cases of syphilis was seen in heterosexual populations with a concomitant rise in cases seen in women and neonates[2,3].

In 1995 there were 68 000 adult cases of syphilis and 1500 cases of congenital syphilis[4,5]. These figures do not take into account the non-reporting of syphilis, with only one in four cases of syphilis reported. In the USA, 100 000 new cases of primary and secondary syphilis occur yearly. As noted, a marked increase of syphilis in women and neonates (congenital syphilis) was also noted in patients who exchanged sex for crack cocaine[3]. Prenatal care is often deficient in populations using illicit drugs, and this accounts for an increasing incidence of congenital syphilis. A ten-fold rise over 6 years in congenital syphilis was seen during 1986–92,

with 4500 cases in 1991 and 3850 cases in 1992[4,5,6]. This rapid rise has slowed, with 1500 cases in 1995.

MICROBIOLOGY AND GENETIC EVOLUTION

The treponemal spirochete is tightly coiled, and measures 5–15 μm in length and about 0.09–0.18 μm in diameter. The ends of the spirochetes are tapered, with three fibrils inserted into each end. It moves with a drifting rotary motion with a characteristic flexing or undulating movement.

There are four major human treponemal pathogens: (1) *Treponema pallidum* spp. *pallidum*, the etiological agent of syphilis; (2) *Treponema pallidum* spp. *pertunue*, the cause of yaws; (3) *Treponema carateum*, the cause of pinta; and (4) *Treponema pallidum* spp. *endemicum*, an agent of bejel, non-venereal or endemic syphilis. No metabolic, structural, immunological or virulent marker has been found to distinguish between the four pathogenic treponemes and they are speciated by their associated clinical illness[7]. The spirochete *Treponema pallidum* is also structurally similar to the other pathogenic spirochetes, *Borrelia* and *Leptospira*.

No pathogenic species of *Treponema* has been successfully cultivated on artificial media, although they can be maintained for short periods on highly enriched media.

PATHOGENESIS

With the exception of congenitally acquired syphilis, syphilis is venereally spread. It can be spread by close contact with mucous-membrane lesions, as with kissing, or transmitted through blood transfusions. Localized digital syphilis infection due to direct inoculation by an accidental finger prick with an infected needle or by direct contact with mucous membranes by examining health professionals has been described[8]. In the human, the minimum inoculum dose is unknown but an inoculum of four spirochetes can establish an infection in rabbits[9].

A patient is most infectious when a chancre, condyloma lata, or other skin lesion is present. Four years after acquisition of syphilis, the patient cannot spread syphilis by sexual contact, because so few spirochetes are present peripherally. Congenital syphilis occurs most frequently with transplacental passage *in utero* although the neonate may acquire syphilis by passage through an infected lower genital tract.

The majority of syphilis cases occur within the young, ages 15–30 years, who are the most sexually active cohort. The aggressive treatment of all recently exposed persons is important in syphilis control.

After entering the body through non-apparent breaks in abraded areas of the skin, the spirochete enters the lymphatics within hours. Regional lymph nodes become enlarged and a subsequent hematogenous invasion results in disseminated infection. Virtually any organ in the body, including 'protected sites' such as the fetus and maternal central nervous system, can be infected. With a division rate of once every 30–33 h, clinical lesions appear when 10^7 organisms per gram of tissue are present[10]. This incubation period usually lasts 3 weeks, but may vary from 3 to 90 days, depending on the size of the initial inoculum. A primary chancre will appear at the end of the incubation period usually at the site of initial entrance of the organisms. Multiple chancres can occur, especially in immunosuppressed patients with coexisting HIV infection[11].

CLINICAL PRESENTATION

Following initial infection, the usual course of syphilis is divided into several stages based on the clinical manifestations of the disease.

The primary stage of syphilis consists of the initial incubation and development of the painless chancre, which usually heals spontaneously over 2–8 weeks, although healing may be delayed in the immunocompromised host. Persons with a history of a previous syphilitic infection may fail to develop any lesions or develop a small darkfield-negative papule, depending on how long their natural infection went untreated[10].

Most genital chancres have a clean appearance with no exudate. Oral and anal chancres are most likely to be secondarily infected. They heal at a slower rate and make the diagnosis of syphilis easier to miss. Regional lymphadenopathy with moderately enlarged, firm, non-suppurative, painless lymph nodes or satellite buboes are common in the primary stage.

Secondary syphilis is characterized by widespread lesions. Because of their appearance, syphilis was originally given the name 'the great pox' to differentiate it from smallpox. The lesions are most commonly recognized on the skin and mucous membranes; when hair follicles are involved, a loss of hair, eyebrows, or beard results. The cutaneous lesions may manifest as macular, papular, papulosquamous, pustular, follicular, or nodular lesions. The lesions often appear on the trunk, extremities, palms and soles. The primary chancre may still be visible on examination[12]. Malaise,

anorexia, headache, sore throat, arthralgia and low-grade fever are also common presentations. These lesions are filled with spirochetes easily visualized by dark-field microscopy[1]. Because they are highly infectious, the organisms can be spread by contact in a non-venereal manner. Essentially any organ of the body may be involved, including the central nervous system, eyes, bones and other internal organs, leading to a wide variety of clinical manifestations[1]. Immune-complex glomerulonephritis[13] and arthritis[14] are commonly seen.

After a period of 4–8 weeks, the lesions disappear and the disease becomes latent. During the subsequent 3–4 years, however, relapses may occur, resulting in mucocutaneous lesions, which eventually disappear. This remission represents the host's finally overcoming a treponemal suppression of the cellular immune response. Among the secondary syphilis remissions, approximately one-fourth of these cases appear to be true cures, based on the observation that such persons will lose their antibodies to the treponema. Another one-fourth retain a latent infection for life, with lifelong antibody production without clinical evidence of active disease. The remaining 50% of untreated secondary syphilis remissions reactivate as tertiary syphilis.

Tertiary syphilis may occur 5–50 years after initial infection and is characterized by gummata, which are attributed to an intense cellular immune response to the syphilis organism and its cellular products. The gumma is an agranulomatous lesion consisting of a necrotic, coagulated center and small-vessel obliterative endarteritis. The skin, liver, bones and spleen are the most common sites for gummata. Lesions may occur in the central nervous system, causing paresis. An obliterative endarteritis of the vaso vasorum of the aorta and small blood vessels in the brain accounts for the findings of cardiovascular and meningovascular neurosyphilis.

PERINATAL/NEONATAL INFECTION WITH SYPHILIS

Congenital syphilis has emerged as a significant problem in the late 1980s in the USA owing to a rise in the incidence of syphilis in the heterosexual population. *In utero* infection is more likely in the early primary and secondary syphilitic stages. Infection of the fetus before the 4th month of gestation is uncommon, and abortion prior to 12 weeks is unlikely to be due to congenital syphilis. This is not an absolute rule, as documented passage of *T. pallidum* has been shown as early as 8 weeks of gestational age[15]. Syphilitic endometritis in the first trimester has been sporadically reported[16]. The fetus is at risk throughout gestation for acquiring congenital syphilis. Late infections after 16 weeks may present as late abortion, stillbirth, neonatal death, fetal hepatomegaly, placentomegaly and fetal hydrops[17]. In the absence of fetal hydrops, the diagnosis of fetal infection is difficult to make. Inoculation of amniotic fluid obtained by amniocentesis into rabbit testes or determination of fetal serum IgM antibody specific to *T. pallidum* wall antigen (anti-47-kDa), in the blood obtained by funicentesis, may be used to confirm fetal infection[18–20].

High rates of antenatal complications including preterm labor, premature rupture of membranes and intrauterine growth retardation have also been described in syphilitic mothers, but confounding factors of poverty, poor access to prenatal care and maternal drug use limit interpretation[21]. In one large prospective study a 28% incidence of preterm birth was found in the presence of maternal syphilis of unknown duration[22].

The inoculum of *T. pallidum* in the maternal bloodstream depends on the stage of disease and affects the fetal risk of infection and death. Transmission to the fetus can occur at any gestational age. Transmission of congenital syphilis approaches 100% with 50% perinatal mortality in mothers with primary or secondary syphilis; 40% transmission with 20% mortality with early latent syphilis; and 10% transmission and 11% perinatal mortality in late latent syphilis[23]. If mothers receive regimens recommended by the Centers for Disease Control (CDC) for syphilis during pregnancy, the transmission rate is diminished to 38% with a perinatal mortality rate of 8%, demonstrating not only the modest effectiveness of treatment but also the virulence of *T. pallidum* congenitally[22]. Fetal hydrops may resolve with penicillin therapy, making it one of the treatable causes of non-immune hydrops[17].

Classical neonatal lesions of congenital syphilis include rhinitis (snuffles), which is soon followed by a diffuse maculopapular desquamative rash with extensive sloughing on the palmar, plantar, oral and anal skin. A vesicular rash (unique to congenital syphilis) and bullae may appear. The nose (saddle nose) and metaphysis of the lower extremities (saber shin – anterior bowing) represent a generalized systemic osteochondritis or perichondritis that is often present in congenital infection.

Splenomegaly, anemia, thrombocytopenia, jaundice and subsequent liver failure may occur when the liver is heavily infected. Severe pulmonary hemorrhage, pneumonia, immune-complex glomerulonephritis and liver failure are recognized common, severe and mortal sequelae of congenital infection[24].

CDC case definitions are given in Table 1[25], and criteria for the evaluation of congenital syphilis are given in Table 2[26].

LABORATORY DIAGNOSIS

T. pallidum is a strict anaerobic spirochete. Rabbits are commonly used as laboratory hosts because *T. pallidum*

Table 1 Congenital syphilis case definition (Centers for Disease Control 1998). From reference 25

Confirmed case

Infant in whom *Treponema pallidum* is identified by dark-field microscopy, fluorescent antibody, or other specific stains in specimens from lesions, placenta, umbilical cord, or autopsy material

Presumptive case

(1) Any infant whose mother had untreated or inadequately treated syphilis at delivery, regardless of signs or symptoms

  or

(2) Any infant or child who has a reactive treponemal test for syphilis and any one of the following:
a. Evidence of congenital syphilis on physical examination†
b. Evidence of congenital syphilis on long-bone X-ray
c. Reactive CSF VDRL
d. Elevated CSF cell count or protein‡
e. Reactive test for FTA-ABS-19S-IgM antibody

*Any non-penicillin therapy or penicillin given < 30 days before delivery; †Clinical signs in an infant include hepatosplenomagaly, characteristic rash, condyloma lata, snuffles, jaundice, pseudoparalysis, anemia, thrombocytopenia, or edema. Stigmata in children of > 2 years include interstitial keratitis, nerve deafness, anterior bowing of shins, frontal boring, mulberry molars, Hutchinson's teeth, saddle nose, rhagades, or Clutton's joints. ‡WBC > 5/mm^3 and protein > 50 mg/dl

Table 2 Criteria for evaluation of congenital syphilis. From reference 26

Born to seropositive women who meet the following criteria:
(1) Had untreated syphilis on delivery
(2) Had serological evidence of relapse or re-infection after treatment (i.e. a four-fold or greater increase in Venereal Disease Research Laboratory or rapid plasma reagin tests)
(3) Was treated with erythromycin or other non-penicillin regimen for syphilis during pregnancy
(4) Was treated for syphilis ≤ 1 month before delivery
(5) Did not have a well-documented history of treatment for syphilis
(6) Was treated for early syphilis during pregnancy with the appropriate penicillin regimen, but non-treponemal antibody titers did not decrease four-fold.
(7) Received prior treatment but had insufficient serological follow-up to ensure adequate treatment response and a lack of current infection. This includes a four-fold reduction of titers and a stable non-treponemal titer of ≤ 1 : 4

cannot be cultured *in vitro*. Diagnostic testing for syphilis centers on direct smears and serology testing. A dark-field examination of the serous fluid from the primary chancre which is teeming with treponemes provides the most fundamental laboratory method for an immediate diagnosis.

The corkscrew appearance and spiraling motion are characteristic. A lesion should be considered non-syphilitic only after three negative examinations have been made. Specimens from mouth lesions are worthless, since *T. pallidum* cannot be distinguished from non-pathogenic treponemes by appearance alone. Cleaning of the lesion prior to sampling with antiseptic or bactericidal saline obscures the diagnosis, since dead or non-motile spirochetes are poorly seen. Responses to commonly used serological tests for syphilis are shown in Table 3.

Of children born with congenital syphilis, a third of mothers have no prenatal care, and 50% have had a negative Venereal Disease Research Laboratory test (VDRL) earlier in their pregnancy[27]. Serological testing should be repeated at delivery in high-risk patients[28]. In New York State, mandatory testing of umbilical cord blood or maternal blood at delivery has demonstrated greatly improved diagnosis of congenital infection with the rate of unrecognized congenital syphilis falling from 10% to 1%[29]. Causes for false-positive tests are shown in Table 4. The cost of universal testing and prompt treatment of newborn infants to limit ongoing damage to the central nervous system and bones is clearly less than the cost of treating older children with now irreversible developmental problems resulting from delayed treatment. We strongly advocate mandatory testing of the umbilical cord at delivery. Maternal sera at delivery, neonatal sera at 2–3 days of life and cord sera[30] are the most optimal testing media, in decreasing order.

CLINICAL DIAGNOSIS

Primary syphilis must be differentiated prinicipally from several similar infections such as chancroid, herpes virus and severe genital irritation resulting from poor hygiene or trauma. Other agents such as granuloma inguinale, lymphogranuloma venereum, tularemia, anthrax and mycobacterial infections may also mimic early syphilis.

Chancroid differs from syphilis in that its ulcers are usually painful, contain exudates and are more prone to bleed upon scraping for dark-field viewing. Painful lymphadenopathy is usually present in chancroid. Primary genital herpes is characterized by an erythematous rash with clusters of vesicles and regional lymphadenopathy. A syphilitic rash is almost never vesicular (except possibly in congenital syphilis).

Secondary syphilis usually shows a rash on the palms and soles. Lesions of condyloma lata in warm, moist intertiginous areas represent coalesced papules, which form painless, broad gray–white plaques, and should be searched for with dark-field examination.

Symptoms of low-grade fever, malaise, pharyngitis, laryngitis, anorexia, weight loss, arthralgia and lymphadenopathy are often found in secondary syphilis.

Table 3 Percentage of patients with positive responses to commonly used serological tests (from reference 1)

	Stage		
Test	Primary	Secondary	Late
Non-treponemal (reaginic tests) Venereal Disease Research Laboratory (reaginic) test (VDRL)	70*	99*	56†
Rapid plasma reagin card test (RPR) Automated reagin test (ART)	80	99	56
Specific treponemal tests Fluorescent antibody adsorbed test (FTA-abs)	85	100	98
T. pallidum hemagglutination assay (TPHA, MHA-TP)	65	100	95
Treponemal immobilization test (TPI)	50	97	95

*Percentage of patients with positive serological tests in treated or untreated primary or secondary syphilis; †treated late syphilis

Table 4 Causes for false-positive serological tests (rapid plasma reagin or Venereal Disease Research Laboratory)

Lyme disease
Menses
Chicken pox
Lymphogranuloma venereum
Tuberculosis, leprosy
Chancroid
Malaria, rickettsial disease
Hepatitis
Early HIV infection
Rheumatoid heart disease
Drug addiction
Connective tissue disease
Pregnancy
History of blood transfusions

Renal involvement may be demonstrated by proteinuria or hematuria. Syphilitic hepatitis is characterized by a markedly elevated serum alkaline phosphatase level[31]. The central nervous system is involved in up to 40% of patients, with headache and meningismus being common findings. Analysis of cerebrospinal fluid may inconsistently demonstrate increased protein and lymphocyte counts.

Latent syphilis is characterized by no clinical evidence of disease, normal studies of cerebrospinal fluid, normal chest X-ray but positive fluorescent treponemal antibody adsorption (FTA-abs) and high-titer VDRL or rapid plasma reagin tests. The FTA-abs is usually positive for life, even with treatment[32].

Table 5   Centers for Disease Control 1998 recommended treatment of syphilis. From reference 26

(1) *Primary and secondary syphilis*

  Recommended regimen
    benzathine penicillin G, 2.4 million units IM in a single dose
  Penicillin allergy (non-pregnant)
    doxycycline 100 mg orally 2 times a day for 2 weeks
     or
    tetracycline 500 mg orally 4 times a day for 2 weeks

(2) *Latent syphilis*

  Recommended regimens
    early latent syphilis (< 1 year)
     benzathine penicillin G, 2.4 million units IM in a single dose
    late latent syphilis (> 1 year)
     benzathine penicillin G, 7.2 million units total, administered as 3 doses of 2.4 million units IM each,
    at 1-week intervals
    penicillin allergy (non-pregnant)
     doxycycline 100 mg orally 2 times a day
      or
     tetracycline 500 mg orally 4 times a day
    both drugs administered for 2 weeks in duration < 1 year, otherwise 4 weeks

(3) *Tertiary syphilis*

  Recommended regimen (without neurosyphilis)
    benzathine penicillin G, 7.2 million units total, administered as 3 doses of 2.4 million units IM, at 1-week intervals
  Penicillin allergy
    same as for late latent syphilis

(4) *Neurosyphilis (all should be tested for HIV)*

  Recommended regimen
    18–24 million units aqueous crystalline penicillin G daily, administered as 3–4 million units IV
    every 4 h, for 10–14 days
  Alternative regimen (if compliance assured)
    2.4 million units procaine penicillin IM daily, plus probenecid 500 mg orally 4 times a day, both for 10–14 days

(5) *Syphilis during pregnancy*

  Recommended regimens
    penicillin regimen appropriate for the pregnant woman's stage of syphilis. Some experts recommend additional
    therapy, (e.g. second dose of benzathine penicillin 2.4 million units IM) 1 week after the initial dose, particularly for
    women in the third trimester and for those who have secondary syphilis during pregnancy
  Penicillin allergy
    a pregnant woman with a history of penicillin allergy should be treated with penicillin after desensitization

(6) *Syphilis among HIV-infected patients*

  Primary and secondary syphilis
    recommended benzathine penicillin 2.4 million units IM. Some experts recommend additional treatments such
    as multiple doses of benzathine penicillin G as in late syphilis for three weekly doses. Penicillin-allergic patients
    should be desensitized and treated with penicillin
  Latent syphilis (normal CSF examination)
    benzathine penicillin G 7.2 million units as 3 weekly doses of 2.4 million units each

IM, intramuscular; IV, intravenous; CSF, cerebrospinal fluid

Conversion to a non-reactive FTA-abs status may be seen in HIV-infected patients who received early, effective treatment[33,34]. For most HIV-infected patients, serological tests are accurate and reliable but unusually high, low, delayed, fluctuating, and absent titers have been reported[5]. HIV patients with neurological symptoms should always be evaluated for neurosyphilis. Although latent infections cannot be passed sexually, a pregnant women with late latent syphilis can infect her fetus. Latent syphilitic infection can also be transmitted by transfusion of contaminated blood.

Neonatal congenital syphilis must be differentiated from other generalized congenital infections including toxoplasmosis, cytomegalovirus and rubella. Necrotizing funisitis, an inflammatory process involving the matrix of the umbilical cord characterized by

Table 6 Oral desensitization protocol for penicillin-allergic patients with a positive skin test. From reference 40

Dose no.	Penecillin V suspension (units/ml)	Milliliters	Units	Cumulative dose (units)
1	1 000	0.1	100	100
2	1 000	0.2	200	300
3	1 000	0.4	400	700
4	1 000	0.8	800	1 500
5	1 000	1.6	1 600	3 100
6	1 000	3.2	3 200	6 300
7	1 000	6.4	6 400	12 700
8	10 000	1.2	12 000	24 700
9	10 000	2.4	24 000	48 700
10	10 000	4.8	48 000	96 700
11	80 000	1.0	80 000	176 700
12	80 000	2.0	160 000	336 700
13	80 000	4.0	320 000	656 700
14	80 000	8.0	640 000	1 296 700

Note: Interval between doses 15 min. Each dose given in 30 ml of water and then given orally

perivascular inflammation and obliterative endarteritis, is a finding unique to congenital syphilis. It is seen in approximately one-third of cases[30]. The umbilical cord may appear like a red and white barber-pole[32]. In cases of stillbirth with significant fetal maceration, in which classic findings of syphilis may be masked, spirochetes can be detected using Warthin–Starry silver stains[35,36].

TREATMENT

Patients with a positive dark-field examination, serological evidence with a specific treponemal test, or history of sexual contact with a person with documented syphilis should receive appropriate treatment. The latest CDC guidelines (Table 5) include subtreatment categories for non-pregnant, pregnant and HIV-infected patients. Treatment using CDC guidelines has been shown to be 100% effective in treating primary, secondary, and early latent syphilis infection. Congenital syphilis is eradicated in 98.2% with treatment failures more likely with maternal drug use or HIV infection[37].

In the non-pregnant patient with penicillin allergy, primary or secondary syphilis may be treated with doxycycline or tetracycline for 2 weeks. In the pregnant patient with penicillin allergy, syphilis should be treated with penicillin after desensitization[38]. Treatment of syphilis in the setting of HIV infection is the same as for non-HIV patients, unless involvement of the central nervous system is present. Doxycycline and tetracycline are contraindicated during gestation, owing to fetal effects[39], and erythromycin may not eradicate fetal infection. Desensitization can be performed orally (Table 6) or intravenously and must be performed on an inpatient basis with availability of appropriate equipment for the management of anaphylaxis.

Women who are treated after 20 weeks of gestation are at risk for premature labor and fetal distress if antitreponemal therapy with antibiotics precipitates a Jarisch–Herxheimer reaction. This is a profound systemic reaction that usually occurs 1–2 h after initiation of therapy with an abrupt onset of fever, chills, myalgia, headache, tachycardia, hyperventilation, vasodilatation and mild hypotension. This state often occurs when secondary syphilis is treated (40–50% of cases) and lasts 12–24 h. It is caused by the release of a heat-stable pyrogen from the spirochetes[41]. Patients should be warned of the reaction and in pregnancy, pretreatment with aspirin and prednisone should be considered to abort the reaction and ensure fetal well-being. Fetal monitoring should be utilized as appropriate to the clinical setting[26,42].

Post-treatment clinical and serological studies should be performed at 3 and 6 months in patients with primary or secondary syphilis. Patients with latent or tertiary syphilis require follow-up at 6 and 12 months with a potential of yearly testing. A four-fold fall in quantitative non-treponemal titers demonstrates adequate treatment. Treatment failures require retreatment after evaluation for HIV, including all sexual partners.

REFERENCES

1. Tramont E. *Treponema pallidum*. In Mandell, Douglas, Bennett, eds. *Principles and Practice of Infectious Diseases*. New York: Churchill Livingstone, 1995:2118
2. Ansell DA, Hu T-C, Straus M, *et al*. HIV and syphilis seroprevalence among clients with sexually transmitted diseases attending a walk in clinic at Cook County Hospital. *Sex Transm Dis* 1993;21:93–7
3. Siegal HA, Carlson RG, Falck R, *et al*. High-risk behaviors for transmission of syphilis and human immunodeficiency virus among crack cocaine-using women: a case study from the Midwest. *Sex Transm Dis* 1992;19:266–71
4. Centers for Disease Control. Summary of notifiable diseases, United States, 1992. *Morbid Mortal Weekly Rep* 1993;41:1–73
5. Centers for Disease Control. Summary of notifiable diseases, United States, 1998. *Morbid Mortal Weekly Rep* 1998;47(RR-1):1–141
6. Zenker P. New case definition for congenital syphilis reporting. *Sex Transm Dis* 1991;18:44–5
7. Becker PS, Akins DR, Radolf JD, Norgard MV. Similarity between the 38-kilodalton lipoprotein of *Treponema pallidum* and the glucose/galactose-binding (Mg1B) protein of *Escherichia coli*. *Infect Immun* 1994;62:1381–91
8. Younai FS. Postexposure protocol. *Dent Clin North Am* 1996;40:457–86
9. Cumberland MC, Turner TB. Rate of multiplication of *Treponema pallidum* in normal and immune rabbits. *Am J Syph* 1949;33:201–12

10. Magnuson HJ, Thomas EW, Olansky S, *et al*. Inoculation syphilis in human volunteers. *Medicine* 1956; 35:33–82

11. Chapel TA. The variability of syphilitic cancers. *Sex Transm Dis* 1978;5:68–70

12. Kumpmeier RH. *Essentials of Syphilology*, 3rd edn. Philadelphia: JB Lippincott, 1943

13. O'Regan S, Fong JS, de Chadarevian JP, *et al*. Treponemal antigens in congenital and acquired syphilitic nephritis: demonstration by immunofluorescence studies. *Ann Intern Med* 1976;85:325–7

14. Reginato AJ, Schumacher HR, Jiminez S, Maurer K. Synovitis in secondary syphilis: clinical, light and electron microscopic studies. *Arthritis Rheum* 1979;22:170–6

15. Harter C, Benirschke K. Fetal syphilis in the first trimester. *Am J Obstet Gynecol* 1976;124:705–11

16. Lee WK, Schwartz DA, Rice RJ, Larsen SA. Syphilitic endometritis causing first trimester abortion: a potential infectious cause of fetal morbidity in early gestation. *South Med J* 1994;87:1259–61

17. Barton JR, Thorpe EM Jr, Shaver DC, *et al*. Nonimmune hydrops fetalis associated with maternal infection with syphilis. *Am J Obstet Gynecol* 1992;167:56–8

18. Nathan L, Twickler DM, Peters MT, *et al*. Fetal syphilis: correlation of sonographic findings and rabbit infectivity testing of amniotic fluid. *J Ultrasound Med* 1993;12:97–101

19. Crane MJ. The diagnosis and management of maternal and congenital syphilis. *J Nurse-Midwifery* 1992;37:4–16

20. Hallak M, Peipert JF, Ludomirsky A, Byers J. Nonimmune hydrops fetalis and fetal congenital syphilis: a case report. *J Reprod Med* 1992;37:173–6

21. Ricci JM, Fojaco RM, O'Sullivan MJ. Congenital syphilis: the University of Miami/Jackson Memorial Medical Center experience 1986–1988. *Obstet Gynecol* 1989;74:687–93

22. McFarlin BL, Bottoms SF, Dock BS, Isada NB. Epidemic syphilis: maternal factors associated with congenital infection. *Am J Obstet Gynecol* 1994;170:535–40

23. Fiumara NF, Fleming WJ, Downing JG, Good FL. The incidence of prenatal syphilis at the Boston City Hospital. *N Engl J Med* 1952;247:48–52

24. O'Regan S, Fong JS, de Chadarevian JP, *et al*. Treponemal antigens in congenital and acquired syphilic nephritis: demonstration by immunofluorescence studies. *Ann Intern Med* 1976;85:325–7

25. Zenker P. New case definition for congenital syphilis reporting. *Sex Transm Dis* 1991;18:44–5

26. Centers for Disease Control and Prevention. 1998 Sexually transmitted diseases treatment guidelines. *Morbid Mortal Weekly Rep* 1998;47:28–49

27. Zoler ML. N.Y.'s universal testing has cut congenital syphilis. *Obstetrics* 1996;87:19

28. Chhabra RS, Brion LP, Castro M, *et al*. Comparison of maternal sera, cord blood, and neonatal sera for detecting presumptive congenital syphillis: relationship with maternal treatment. *Pediatrics* 1993;91:88–91

29. Nandwani R, Evans DT. Are you sure it's syphilis? A review of false positive serology. *Int J STD AIDS* 1995;6:241–8

30. Schwartz DA, Larsen SA, Beck-Sague C, *et al*. Pathology of the umbilical cord in congenital syphilis: analysis of 25 specimens using histochemistry and immunofluorescent antibody to *Treponema pallidum*. *Hum Pathol* 1995;26:784–91

31. Drusin LM, Topf-Olstein B, Levy-Zombeck E. Epidemiology of infectious syphilis at a tertiary hospital. *Arch Intern Med* 1979;139:901–4

32. Fojaco RM, Hensley GT, Moskowitz L. Congenital syphilis and necrotizing funisitis. *J Am Med Assoc* 1989;261:1788–90

33. Gourevitch MN, Selwyn, PA, Davenny K, *et al*. Effects of HIV infection on the serologic manifestations and response to treatment of syphilis in intravenous drug users. *Ann Intern Med* 1993;118:350–5

34. Johnson PD, Graves SR, Stewart L, *et al*. Specific syphilis serological tests may become negative in HIV infection. *AIDS* 1991;5:419–23

35. Young SA, Crocker DW. Occult congenital syphilis in macerated stillborn fetuses. *Arch Pathol Lab Med* 1994;118:44–7

36. Qureshi F, Jacques SM, Reyes MP. Placental histopathology in syphilis. *Hum Pathol* 1993;24:779–84

37. Alexander JM, Sheffield JS, *et al*. Efficacy of treatment for syphilis in pregnancy. *Obstet Gynecol* 1999;93:5–8

38. Ray JG. Lues-lues: maternal and fetal considerations of syphilis. *Obstet Gynecol Surv* 1995;50:845–50

39. Egerman RS. The tetracyclines. *Obstet Gynecol Clin North Am* 1992;19:551–61

40. Wendel GD Jr, Stark BJ, Jamison RB, *et al*. Penicillin allergy and desensitization in serious infections during pregnancy. *N Engl J Med* 1985;312:1229–32

41. Young EJ, Weingarten NM, Baughn RE, Duncan WC. Studies on the pathogenesis of the Jarisch–Herxheimer reaction: development of an animal model and evidence against a role for classical endotoxin. *J Infect Dis* 1982;146:606–15

42. Myles TD, Elam G, *et al*. The Jarisch-Herxeimer reaction and fetal monitoring changes in pregnant women treated for syphilis. *Obstet Gynecol* 1998;92:859–64

23
Urinary tract infection

S.R. Allen

Urinary tract infections commonly complicate pregnancy, and are present in as many as 11% of gestations. Asymptomatic bacteriuria is encountered most frequently; less common symptomatic infections are cystitis and pyelonephritis. Of these three infections, the primary impact on pregnancy outcome is from acute pyelonephritis, which is commonly preceded by asymptomatic bacteriuria rather than acute cystitis[1]. Clinical presentation, risk factors, common complications and treatment for these three forms of urinary tract infection are summarized in Table 1.

The bacteria responsible for all three types of urinary tract infections in pregnancy are similar. *Escherichia coli* is the most common isolate, present in 65–85% of positive urine cultures. Bacteria from other genuses of Enterobacteriaceae are next most common: *Klebsiella, Enterobacter, Citrobacter* and *Proteus*. Gram-positive organisms are present in <10% of positive urine cultures, with group B streptococcus the most common member of this group[1–5].

Many risk factors for urinary tract infections in women have been identified, including non-white race, younger maternal age and antepartum genital tract infection[6]. Because of its short length (approximately 4 cm) and its termination beneath the labia and relatively near the anus, the female urethra is at increased risk of colonization by Gram-negative colonic bacteria. Urethral and periurethral bacteria may intermittently enter the bladder, typically after intercourse[7]. Once within the urinary tract, attachment of bacteria to carbohydrate components of urothelial cell surface glycolipids and glycoproteins, perhaps regulated by the expression of blood group antigens, is an important virulence factor[8].

Half of women with urinary tract infections during pregnancy have an enlarged bladder capacity, and 15% have a significant post-void residual volume (50–150 ml)[9]. Normal physiological changes of pregnancy include a mild hydronephrosis and hydroureter, potentially created by both the mechanical compression of the ureter by the enlarging uterus and pelvic blood vessels at the pelvic brim (right greater than left), and the relaxant effect of progesterone on ureteral smooth muscles. In combination, these factors account for the increased rate of both bladder and ascending infections during pregnancy.

CYSTITIS

Acute cystitis in pregnancy has a clinical presentation not unlike that of symptomatic bladder infection outside of pregnancy. The diagnosis is suspected in a patient with urgency, frequency, dysuria, or hematuria, and without evidence of upper urinary tract infection

Table 1 Summary of urinary tract infections during pregnancy

	Acute cystitis	*Asymptomatic bacteriuria*	*Pyelonephritis*
Symptoms	urgency, frequency, dysuria	no symptoms	back or flank pain, fever, chills
Individual risk factors	history of recurrent cystitis, typically after intercourse	parity, non-white race, lower socio-economic status	asymptomatic bacteriuria
Risks	recurrent acute cystitis	pyelonephritis	bacteremia, septic shock, pulmonary edema
Treatment	oral broad-spectrum antibiotic, 3–7 days	oral broad-spectrum antibiotic, 3–7 days	broad-spectrum antibiotic: parenteral until clinically improved, then oral to complete 10–14 day course, followed by oral broad-spectrum antibiotic suppression until 6 weeks postpartum

or systemic illness. The diagnosis is confirmed by a culture of catheterized or mid-stream urine positive for a single organism. Although the traditional diagnosis of urinary tract infection is based upon a quantitative culture containing $\geq 10^5$ bacteria/ml, a lower threshold may be appropriate in the presence of bladder symptoms. Comparing cultures of urine obtained directly from the bladder via suprapubic aspiration or urethral catheterization with those of mid-stream specimens in acutely dysuric (non-pregnant) women, mid-stream samples with $\geq 10^2$ bacteria/ml have a sensitivity of 95% and a specificity of 85% for the detection of coliform bacteria[10].

Acute cystitis occurs much less frequently in pregnancy than asymptomatic urinary tract infections. Harris and Gilstrap[2] found the incidence of cystitis to be 1.3% among a population of military dependents. Two-thirds developed their symptomatic infection after the initial clinic visit, and of these, 95% had negative urine cultures at their first prenatal visit. Although 50% of the patients with cystitis had a history of urinary tract infections, after a 10-day course of antibiotic only 17% had recurrence, and no patients developed pyelonephritis.

The usual treatment for acute cystitis in pregnancy is with a short (usually 3–7 day) course of broad-spectrum antibiotic. In non-pregnant women, without the cited physiological genitourinary tract changes, multiple dose regimens provide better treatment than a single dose of a broad-spectrum antibiotic[11]. A 10-day course of one of the following – ampicillin 250 mg four times a day, nitrofurantoin macrocrystals 100 mg three times a day, sulfisoxazole 500 mg four times a day or cefazolin 250 mg four times a day – is equally effective in pregnancy[2]. Compared to penicillins and cephalosporins, trimethoprim–sulfisoxazole has been proven to be more effective in eliminating cystitis in non-pregnant women, but is generally avoided during pregnancy; trimethoprim, a folate antagonist, may hinder cell replication. Obviously, the selection of antibiotics during pregnancy must include not only a consideration of effectiveness but also of potential fetal effects. Of the antibiotics commonly used for the treatment of urinary tract infections, both nitrofurantoin and sulfisoxazole have theoretical reasons for avoidance in the antepartum period: nitrofurantoin is capable of inducing hemolytic anemia in glucose-6-phosphate dehydrogenase-deficient fetuses, and sulfisoxazole competes with bilirubin for albumin binding and could lead to kernicterus. In practice, however, each of these drugs has been used successfully and safely in the management of acute cystitis and other urinary tract infections in pregnancy. Any one of these drugs may be started empirically for the clinical diagnosis of cystitis, with appropriate changes in selection based on urine culture sensitivity results. A follow-up urine culture may be obtained after initial treatment to confirm

appropriate therapy, but because of the low rate of recurrence, monthly screening urine cultures are not recommended.

Sexual intercourse is a risk factor for recurrent cystitis in some women. Pfau and Sacks[12] showed a 99% reduction from the baseline (pre-pregnant) rate of recurrent cystitis among 33 pregnant women using post-coital cephalexin 250 mg or nitrofurantoin 50 mg. As compared to daily prophylaxis, this form of therapy provides most at-risk women with the convenience and cost benefit of less frequent antibiotic administration.

ASYMPTOMATIC BACTERIURIA

Asymptomatic bacteriuria, silent bacterial colonization of the urinary tract, is the most common urinary tract infection in pregnancy, with an incidence of 2–10%[3,13,14]. Lower socioeconomic status, non-white race and increased parity infer increased risk[13].

Bacteriuria is diagnosed by quantitative bacterial urine culture: two mid-stream urine cultures or a single catheterized urine specimen containing $\geq 10^5$ bacteria/ml. Asymptomatic bacteriuria thus occurs with a positive culture in the absence of symptoms of urinary tract infection. The bacteria identified in asymptomatic bacteriuria are similar to those of other urinary tract infections; however, Wood and Dillon[4] found 29% of bacteriuric gravidas to be infected with group B streptococcus.

The significance of asymptomatic bacteriuria lies not in the primary infection but rather in the potential secondary complications. Subsequent pyelonephritis occurs in approximately 40% of untreated women with asymptomatic bacteriuria[15]. Its effect on pregnancy outcome was assessed by Romero and colleagues[16] with meta-analysis of 19 studies. They identified a positive relationship between untreated asymptomatic bacteriuria and low birth weight/preterm delivery (typical relative risk 0.65 for low birth weight and 0.50 for preterm delivery, abacteriuria vs. untreated bacteriuria), which may be negated by treatment for asymptomatic bacteriuria (typical relative risk 0.56 for low birth weight in treated as compared to non-treated asymptomatic bacteriuria).

Based on 1988 dollar values and a population with an asymptomatic bacteriuria incidence of at least 2%, a cost savings for bacteriuria screening has been predicted if the cost is no greater than $26[17]. However, screening with urine cultures would usually exceed those cost restraints. Therefore, to try to improve the cost effectiveness of screening for bacteriuria, several other less expensive techniques have been evaluated; the performance characteristics of several screening tests are shown in Table 2.

An ideal screening technique should have both a high sensitivity (so few abnormal results are missed)

Table 2 Effectiveness of screening for asymptomatic bacteriuria

Technique	Reference	Sensitivity(%)	Specificity(%)	Positive predictive value(%)	Negative predictive value(%)
Uri-Cult*	14	98–100	33–97	2–81	99–100
Bac-T-Screen[†]	18	96	56	16	99
Limulus amoebocyte lysate	19	89	99	90	99
Nitrite	20–22	37–46	99–99.7	75	96
Leukocyte esterase	20–22	17–52	90–97	25	97
Gram's stain	20	83	95	28	
Uriscreen[‡]	21	100	81	30	100

*Orion Diagnostica, Helsinki, Finland; [†]Marion Laboratories, Kansas City, MO; [‡]Diatech Diagnostics Ltd., Kiryat Weizmann, Ness Ziona, Israel

and a high specificity (so few normal patients are considered abnormal and receive follow-up testing or empirical treatment). None of the indirect screening techniques are as efficacious as urine culture. Yet even screening by urine culture will not identify all patients at risk for pyelonephritis, as a small proportion of women negative on initial screening will later develop bacteriuria and an ascending infection. Recognizing the imperfection and significant cost of screening for bacteriuria, Rouse and co-workers[23] developed a decision analytic model to compare the cost effectiveness of screening with leukocyte esterase–nitrite dipstick or urine culture vs. no screening. Both screening techniques were predicted to be cost effective as compared to no screening. However, the culture strategy was not cost effective compared to the dipstick strategy, as the additional expense of culture screening outweighed the cost of treating the cases of pyelonephritis predicted to be missed by dipstick screening (0.5% incidence).

To accurately interpret the results of a quantitative urine culture, it must have been obtained under conditions known to optimize the yield. Vulval cleansing with chlorhexidine may reduce the bacterial colony counts of a mid-stream urine sample, and cleansing with water provides more representative results. Additionally, the quantity of bacteriuria correlates with the time interval between episodes of voiding; although a first morning void is not necessary, the practice of having patients drink fluid to speed diuresis should be avoided[24].

With the diagnosis of bacteriuria made by urine culture, antimicrobial selection may be guided by susceptibility results. Their low-risk profiles and high rates of effectiveness make ampicillin or nitrofurantoin excellent initial choices. If avoided near term, a sulfonamide such as sulfamethizole may also be used safely and effectively[25]. With the increasing rate of ampicillin resistance recognized in urinary tract infections, other drugs have been examined for their efficacy. Amoxicillin–clavulanic acid and cephalexin were found to be equally effective (80% and 69% cure rates, respectively) in a population with a 42% rate of

resistance to ampicillin[26]. Importantly, there is not a good correlation between *in vitro* antimicrobial sensitivity testing and therapeutic response to antibiotic treatment. Using a conservative definition of effectiveness for antibiotics (expected urinary concentration at least five-fold its minimal inhibitory concentration against the infecting organism) in a non-pregnant population, Fair and Fair[27] found ampicillin to be effective against 76% of *E.coli* samples; cephalexin and nitrofurantoin were effective against 95% of the samples.

Although early protocols used continuous treatment until delivery, by 1977 Whalley and Cunningham[25] had shown that short-term treatment (14 days) combined with surveillance for recurrent bacteriuria provided similar results. At the other extreme from continuous treatment, randomized controlled trials have shown single-dose therapy with amoxicillin (3 g) or sulfamethizole (2 g) to be as effective as longer therapy (4–6 days), with success rates for single-dose treatments of 77% and 59%, respectively[28,29]. Other studies have shown single oral doses of ampicillin (2 g, plus 1 g probenimide), nitrofurantoin macrocrystals (200 mg), sulfisoxazole (2 g), amoxicillin (3 g) and cephalexin (2 g) to be similarly effective[30,31].

Urine cultures and antimicrobial sensitivity studies should be obtained 1–2 weeks after initiation of therapy, and additional screening should be done thereafter, such as once per trimester. Primary treatment failure may be retreated with a 7–14 day course of the same antibiotic if the initial treatment was a single dose, or with another antibiotic of proven efficacy if the first treatment was of multiple doses. Following a recurrent urinary tract infection, broad-spectrum antibiotic suppression for the remainder of the pregnancy is recommended, such as with nitrofurantoin 100 mg every day. For women with recurrent infections, urological examination should be scheduled for 3–6 months postpartum, as up to half of these women will have a urinary tract structural abnormality[9]. Although pyelographic abnormalities are more common in women with a history of asymptomatic bacteriuria, these may be primarily rather than secondarily associated.

Follow-up studies 10–17 years after the index pregnancy have shown a slight decrease in urine-concentrating ability, but no increased risk for urinary tract infection requiring hospitalization, hypertension, persistent bacteriuria or reduction in creatinine clearance[32,33].

PYELONEPHRITIS

Affecting 1–2% of all pregnancies, pyelonephritis is the most common serious medical problem encountered during pregnancy. It will develop in 36–42% of untreated women with asymptomatic bacteriuria; this risk falls to 0–3% with treatment for bacteriuria[15,34]. Pyelonephritis during pregnancy is rare in women abacteriuric at the initial prenatal visit[34]. It occurs most commonly during the second or third trimesters, although up to 8% of infections are diagnosed intrapartum and 8–19% postpartum[1,35]. It is usually an ascending infection, more likely to occur during pregnancy because of the physiological changes predisposing to urinary stasis. Conditions unique to the renal medulla make it particularly vulnerable to infection in the presence of stasis: high urine osmolarity, high urea and sodium concentrations and low pH impair chemotaxis and inhibit polymorphonuclear leukocyte phagocytosis.

Unlike its usual precursor asymptomatic bacteriuria, pyelonephritis is nearly always diagnosed clinically. Patients typically present with the symptoms of back pain and chills (82%); approximately one in four have nausea and vomiting. An elevated temperature is uniformly present, with a temperature of $\geq 40°C$ in 10% of patients. The majority of patients have costovertebral angle tenderness (predominantly right-sided or bilateral)[1]. Because none of these signs or symptoms are pathognomonic for pyelonephritis, the final diagnosis depends on a urine culture positive for a known uropathogen.

To speed treatment while awaiting the urine culture results, microscopic examination of uncentrifuged urine can be performed. One bacterium per high power field indicates a bacterial concentration of at least 10^5/ml. One or more white blood cells per high power field will also usually be seen in pyelonephritis. Although indicative of a urinary tract infection, none of these findings are specific for pyelonephritis. Antibody coating of bacteria, detected by fluorescein-labelled antibody, has been reported to correlate with renal rather than bladder infection[36], but this is a time-consuming and subjective assay not generally available. If the diagnosis of pyelonephritis is suspected, blood cultures may also be obtained before antibiotic treatment is begun. However, the additional cost of blood cultures may not be substantiated by clinical benefit, as the blood culture results of the one of six bacteremic patients with pyelonephritis usually parallel the urine culture results; MacMillan and Grimes[37] changed antibiotic treatment based on blood cultures in only 2% of pregnant patients with pyelonephritis.

Acute treatment for pyelonephritis includes hydration and antibiotics; some patients will also require correction of hyperthermia and the use of tocolytics. Although ampicillin has been used for primary therapy, the increasing resistance of *E. coli* to ampicillin has compromised its status as the drug of choice. Fair and Fair[27] found ampicillin to be effective against 76% of the strains of *E. coli* typical for pyelonephritis, and cephalexin and nitrofurantoin to provide effective treatment against 95% of these samples. Gentamicin is nearly uniformly effective but because of theoretical fetal ototoxicity, associated costs for monitoring serum levels, and the lack of an oral equivalent, it is not usually used for primary therapy. Van Dorsten and associates[38] showed the importance of appropriate initial antibiotic selection, demonstrating a 67% rate of successful treatment with an antibiotic proven effective by routine sensitivity methods, as compared to a 42% rate of successful treatment with an antibiotic to which the isolated bacteria were resistant. Therefore, therapy with a limited-spectrum cephalosporin, such as cefazolin 1–2 g every 8 h, may be the best initial antimicrobial choice, although Sanchez-Ramos and co-workers[39] reported the single daily intravenous administration of ceftriaxone 1 g to be equally effective and less costly.

Traditional management recommendations for acute pyelonephritis in pregnancy include hospitalization and intravenous antibiotic administration until significant clinical improvement allows conversion to oral antibiotics, completing a 10–14-day course of therapy[40]. Recognizing that outpatient oral treatment of acute pyelonephritis in non-pregnant patients has been proven safe and effective[41], Angel and colleagues[42] compared oral vs. intravenous cephalosporin treatment of pyelonephritis in pregnancy. They reported excellent results for both forms of administration (91% and 93% success rate for oral and intravenous, respectively), with no increased risk for complications using oral therapy. Because the sample size was small, all patients were managed as inpatients and the bacteremic patients (14% of total, whose bacteremia could not be predicted) were not included in data analysis, this study cannot conclusively be used to recommend outpatient management of acute pyelonephritis in pregnancy. Millar and colleagues[43] demonstrated the efficacy of outpatient treatment for pyelonephritis in women with pregnancies of less than 24 weeks' estimated gestational age. Compared to women receiving standard hospitalization and intravenous cefazolin, women randomized to receive outpatient treatment received two doses of ceftriaxone 1 g intramuscularly (the first in the hospital and the second as an outpatient); after a 4–24-h period of hospital observation, outpatients received three home visits by a nurse and completed a 10-day course of oral cephalexin 500 mg four times a day. Both groups had approximately a 20% failure for initial treatment, and no unusual complications occurred in the outpatient group.

The importance of chronic antibiotic suppression after primary treatment for pyelonephritis has been demonstrated by Harris and Gilstrap[5], who reduced the 60% risk of recurrent pyelonephritis in their population to 3% by continuing broad-spectrum antibiotic suppression after primary therapy until 2 weeks postpartum. Nitrofurantoin macrocrystals 50 mg every day is an excellent choice for suppression. Note, however, that such suppression is only effective if the primary antibiotic therapy is appropriate for the etiological organism[38].

Following appropriate parenteral antimicrobial therapy, clinical improvement occurs quickly, with resolution of fever anticipated within 48 h in 85% of patients[44]. In the uncommon event of no improvement after 48–72 h of appropriate antibiotic therapy, consideration should be given to complicating factors such as obstruction, cortical abscess, papillary necrosis, or perinephric abscess. A renal ultrasound scan will detect most of the treatable complications which could delay response to therapy.

Transient renal dysfunction has been demonstrated during acute pyelonephritis, with a reduction of endogenous creatinine clearance to ≤ 80 ml/min in 27% of patients, and an incidence of approximately 20% for elevated blood urea nitrogen (> 11 mg/dl) and serum creatinine (>1 mg/dl)[1,45]. The urinary tract is the most common site of origin for Gram-negative sepsis, and bacteremia occurs in up to 14% of patients with pyelonephritis. Bacteremia in the presence of pyelonephritis is usually an incidental finding, but it may also present as septic shock. Cunningham and co-workers[44] reported a 3% incidence of septic shock among gravidas with acute pyelonephritis. Septic shock occurs secondary to endotoxemia or exotoxemia, and may lead to multiple organ failure. Acute renal failure secondary to acute tubular necrosis may further compromise the transient renal dysfunction commonly seen with pyelonephritis. Septic shock complicating pyelonephritis may also cause hemolysis, thrombocytopenia, hepatic dysfunction and adult respiratory distress syndrome. A syndrome of non-cardiogenic pulmonary edema, with or without renal, hepatic, or hematopoietic dysfunction, has been reported in 2% of pregnant patients with pyelonephritis[46]. This syndrome typically appears within 30 h of admission and manifests as dyspnea, tachypnea, hypoxemia and pulmonary effusions and consolidation; 20% of patients require mechanical ventilation, and most recover within 2–3 days.

An association between pyelonephritis and both preterm delivery and increased perinatal mortality was recognized in the pre-antibiotic era; however, appropriate antibiotic therapy appears nearly to eliminate these risks. Gilstrap and co-workers[47] reported a higher rate of low birth weight for women with pyelonephritis (< 2500 g, 15% incidence vs. 10% in controls), but no increase in perinatal mortality rate, and Fan and associates[35] found no increase in low birth weight, size small for gestational age, or preterm delivery.

The long-term prognosis following acute pyelonephritis is not clear. Early studies based on autopsy findings suggested that any renal infection predisposed to chronic pyelonephritis and eventual renal failure, but those studies probably included patients who ingested large quantities of phenacetin, a drug known to cause interstitial nephritis and papillary necrosis. More recently, no pyelographic renal scarring had been documented after pyelonephritis in women[48], and pyelonephritis was considered to create no long-term risks for hypertension or renal dysfunction. This complacency has recently been re-examined; prospectively following 27 patients with acute pyelonephritis, acute and follow-up computed tomography scans have shown a 7% incidence of renal atrophy and a 30% incidence of cortical scarring[49]. The significance of renal scarring detected with this very sensitive technique remains undetermined.

REFERENCES

1. Gilstrap LC III, Cunningham FG, Whalley PJ. Acute pyelonephritis in pregnancy: an anterospective study. *Obstet Gynecol* 1981;57:409–13
2. Harris RE, Gilstrap LC III. Cystitis during pregnancy: a distinct clinical entity. *Obstet Gynecol* 1981;57:578–80
3. Campbell-Brown M, McFadyen IR, Seal DV, Stephenson ML. Is screening for bacteriuria in pregnancy worthwhile? *Br Med J* 1987;294:1579–82
4. Wood EG, Dillon HC Jr. A prospective study of group B streptococcal bacteriuria in pregnancy. *Am J Obstet Gynecol* 1981;140:515–20
5. Harris RE, Gilstrap LC III. Prevention of recurrent pyelonephritis during pregnancy. *Obstet Gynecol* 1974; 44:637–41
6. Schieve LA, Handler A, Hershow R, *et al.* Urinary tract infection during pregnancy: its association with maternal morbidity and perinatal outcome. *Am J Public Health* 1994;84:405–10
7. Buckley RM Jr, McGuckin M, MacGregor RR. Urine bacterial counts after sexual intercourse. *N Engl J Med* 1978;298:321–4
8. Lomberg H, Cedergren B, Leffler H, *et al.* Influence of blood group on the availability of receptors for attachment of uropathogenic *Escherichia coli*. *Infect Immun* 1986;51:919–26
9. Diokno AC, Compton A, Seski J, Vinson R. Urologic evaluation of urinary tract infection in pregnancy. *J Reprod Med* 1986;31:23–6
10. Stamm WE, Counts GW, Running KR, *et al.* Diagnosis of coliform infection in acutely dysuric women. *N Engl J Med* 1982;307:463–8
11. Greenberg RN, Reilly PM, Luppen KL, *et al.* Randomized study of single-dose, three-day, and seven-day treatment of cystitis in women. *J Infect Dis* 1986; 153:277–82

12. Pfau A, Sacks TG. Effective prophylaxis for recurrent urinary tract infections during pregnancy. *Clin Infect Dis* 1992;14:810

13. Turck M, Goffe BS, Petersdorf RG. Bacteriuria of pregnancy. Relation to socioeconomic factors. *N Engl J Med* 1962;266:857–60

14. Van Dorsten JP, Bannister ER. Office diagnosis of asymptomatic bacteriuria in pregnant women. *Am J Obstet Gynecol* 1986;1555:777–80

15. Kincaid-Smith P, Bullen M. Bacteriuria in pregnancy. *Lancet* 1965;1:395–9

16. Romero R, Oyarzun E, Mazor M, *et al*. Meta-analysis of the relationship between asymptomatic bacteriuria and preterm delivery/low birth weight. *Obstet Gynecol* 1989; 73:576–82

17. Wadland WC, Plante DA. Screening for asymptomatic bacteriuria in pregnancy. *J Fam Pract* 1989;29:372–6

18. McNeeley SG, Baselski VS, Ryan GM. An evaluation of two rapid bacteriuria screening procedures. *Obstet Gynecol* 1987;69:550–3

19. Nachum R, Arce JJ, Berzofsky RN. Gram-negative bacteriuria of pregnancy: rapid detection by a chromogenic Limulus ameobocyte lysate assay. *Obstet Gynecol* 1986; 68:215–19

20. Baschman JW, Heise RH, Naessens JM, Timmerman MG. A study of various tests to detect asymptomatic urinary tract infections in an obstetric population. *J Am Med Assoc* 1993;270:1971–4

21. Hagay Z, Levy R, Miskin A, *et al*. Uriscreen a rapid enzymatic urine screening test: useful predictor of significant bacteriuria in pregnancy. *Obstet Gynecol* 1996;87:410–13

22. Pels RJ, Bor DH, Woolhandler S, *et al*. Dipstick urinalysis screening of asymptomatic adults for urinary tract disorders. *J Am Med Assoc* 1989;262:1221–4

23. Rouse DJ, Andrews WW, Goldenberg RL, Owen J. Screening and treatment of asymptomatic bacteriuria of pregnancy to prevent pyelonephritis: a cost-effectiveness and cost–benefit analysis. *Obstet Gynecol* 1995; 86:119–23

24. Roberts AP, Robinson RE, Beard RW. Some factors affecting bacterial colony counts in urinary infection. *Br Med J* 1967;1:400–3

25. Whalley PJ, Cunningham FG. Short-term versus continuous antimicrobial therapy for asymptomatic bacteriuria in pregnancy. *Obstet Gynecol* 1977;49:262–5

26. Pedler SJ, Bint AJ. Comparative study of amoxicillin–clavulanic acid and cephalexin in the treatment of bacteriuria during pregnancy. *Antimicrob Agents Chemother* 1985;27:508–10

27. Fair WR, Fair WR III. Clinical value of sensitivity determinations in treating urinary tract infections. *Urology* 1982;19:565–9

28. Gerstner GJ, Muller G, Nahler G. Amoxicillin in the treatment of asymptomatic bacteriuria in pregnancy: a single dose of 3 g amoxicillin versus a 4-day course of 3 doses 750 mg amoxicillin. *Gynecol Obstet Invest* 1989; 27:84–7

29. Olsen L, Nielsen IK, Zachariassen A, *et al*. Single-dose versus six-day therapy with sulflamethizole for asymptomatic bacteriuria during pregnancy. *Dan Med Bull* 1989;36:486–7

30. Harris RE, Gilstrap LC III, Pretty A. Single-dose antimicrobial therapy for asymptomatic bacteriuria during pregnancy. *Obstet Gynecol* 1982;59:546–8

31. Jakobi P, Neiger R, Merzbach D, *et al*. Single-dose antimicrobial therapy in the treatment of asymptomatic bacteriuria in pregnancy. *Am J Obstet Gynecol* 1987;156:1148–52

32. Zinner SH, Kass EH. Long-term (10 to 14 years) follow-up of bacteriuria of pregnancy. *N Engl J Med* 1971; 285:820–4

33. Birch CD, Fischer-Rasmussen W, Vejlsgaard R. The long-term prognosis of bacteriuria in pregnancy. *Acta Obstet Gynecol Scand* 1987;66:291–5

34. Kass EH. Bacteriuria and pyelonephritis of pregnancy. *AMA Arch Int Med* 1960;105:194–8

35. Fan Y, Pastorek JG II, Miller JM Jr, *et al*. Acute pyelonephritis in pregnancy. *Am J Perinatol* 1987;4: 324–6

36. Jones SR, Smith JW, Sanford JP. Localization of urinary tract infections by detection of antibody-coated bacteria in urine sediment. *N Engl J Med* 1974;290:591–3

37. MacMillan MC, Grimes DA. The limited usefulness of urine and blood cultures in treating pyelonephritis in pregnancy. *Obstet Gynecol* 1991;78:745–8

38. Van Dorsten JP, Lenke RR, Schifrin BS. Pyelonephritis in pregnancy. The role of in-hospital management and nitrofurantoin suppression. *J Reprod Med* 1987;32: 895–900

39. Sanchez-Ramos L, McAlpine JK, Adair CD, *et al*. Pyelonephritis in pregnancy: once-a-day ceftriaxone versus multiple doses of cefazolin. A randomized, double-blind trial. *Am J Obstet Gynecol* 1995;172:129–33

40. Duff P. Pyelonephritis in pregnancy. *Clin Obstet Gynecol* 1984;27:17–31

41. Safrin S, Siegel D, Black D. Pyelonephritis in adult women: in-patient versus outpatient therapy. *Am J Med* 1988;85:793–8

42. Angel JL, O'Brien WF, Finan MA, *et al*. Acute pyelonephritis in pregnancy: a prospective study of oral versus intravenous antibiotic therapy. *Obstet Gynecol* 1990;76:28–32

43. Millar LK, Wing DA, Paul RH, Grimes DA. Outpatient treatment of pyelonephritis in pregnancy: a randomized controlled trial. *Obstet Gynecol* 1995;86:560–4

44. Cunningham FG, Morris GB, Mickal A. Acute pyelonephritis of pregnancy: a clinical review. *Obstet Gynecol* 1973;42:112–7

45. Whalley PJ, Cunningham FG, Martin FG. Transient renal dysfunction associated with acute pyelonephritis of pregnancy. *Obstet Gynecol* 1975;46:174–7

46. Cunningham FG, Lucas MJ, Hankins GDV. Pulmonary injury complicating antepartum pyelonephritis. *Am J Obstet Gynecol* 1987;156:797–804

47. Gilstrap LC, Leveno KH, Cunningham FG, *et al*. Renal infection and pregnancy outcome. *Am J Obstet Gynecol* 1981;141:709–16

48. Huland H, Busch R, Riebel TH. Renal scarring after symptomatic and asymptomatic upper urinary tract infection: a prospective study. *J Urol* 1982;128:682–5

49. Meyrier A, Condamin MC, Fernet M, *et al*. Frequency of development of early cortical scarring in acute primary pyelonephritis. *Kidney Int* 1989;35:696–703

Section IIIb

Perinatal infections: viral infections

24
Cytomegaloviruses

G.R.G. Monif

Taxonomically, the cytomegaloviruses (CMVs) belong to the herpes virus group, which includes herpes simplex viruses types 1 and 2 (HSV-1 and HSV-2), varicella zoster virus and the Epstein–Barr (EB) virus. A CMV viral particle measures approximately 1800–1000 Å in diameter. The viral particle consists of a core single molecule of double-stranded DNA and the sequential layers composed of an icosahedral protein coat and a lipid envelope. The site of viral DNA synthesis is within the host cell nucleus. Consequently, histological evidence of virus replication can be observed in the form of an intranuclear inclusion body which is characterized by both cytoplasmic and nuclear gigantism.

Spread is by intimate contact with biological fluids containing the virus such as tears, saliva, urine, colostrum and blood. The demonstration of CMV in semen and endocervical mucus makes venereal transmission of the infection a distinct possibility.

Infection with CMV results in the establishment of latent infection. Unlike HSV-1, HSV-2 or the varicella zoster virus, clinically overt manifestations of CMV replication are seldom seen. Except in the immunologically compromised individual and in the developing fetus, CMV rarely exhibits virulence for humans.

MATERNAL INFECTION

The incidence of maternal CMV infection is a partial function of socioeconomic status and, indirectly, race. A prospective study of 69 congenitally infected infants demonstrated that age, race and marital status all were strongly associated with congenital CMV infection[1]. The overall incidence rate of congenital CMV infection was 3 per 1000 live births, ranging from 25 per 1000 live births for single black women under age 20 years, to 1.6 per 1000 live births for married or cohabiting white women over the age of 25 years. In another study of 16 218 pregnant women from two socioeconomic groups, 64.5% of the women in the high income group were seronegative for CMV, as opposed to 25% of the women in the lower socioeconomic group. The rates of transmission *in utero* were 3.9% in the high-income group and 3.1% in the low-income group. Only 25% of the congenital infections in the low-income group were associated with primary maternal infection in contrast with 63%

in the high-income group. Infections contracted early and late in gestation had similar rates of transmission *in utero*, but infants who were exposed in the first half of pregnancy were more likely to be symptomatic at birth or develop permanent sequelae at a future date[2].

In immunologically competent adults, infection with CMV is subclinical or asymptomatic. The most common disease pattern observed in pregnant women is that of an infectious mononucleosis-like syndrome characterized by intermittent fever lasting as long as 3 weeks, lethargy, malaise and hematological alterations such as atypical lymphocytosis. Notably absent are tonsillitis or pharyngitis and cervical lymphadenopathy. Patients may have biochemical evidence of hepatitis such as elevation of serum glumatic–oxaloacetic transaminase (SGOT) or serum glutamic–pyruvic transaminase (SGPT).

Clinically overt CMV infection is rare. Anicteric hepatitis occurs primarily in young children. Post-transfusion syndrome (cryptogenic fever, splenomegaly and the hematological and biochemical abnormalities described above) result from a chronic cell-associated viremia occurring 3–8 weeks following transfusion.

Disseminated systemic diseases may occur in chronically debilitated patients with thymomas and patients with secondary impairment of immunological processes (especially human immunodeficiency virus (HIV) infection).

DIAGNOSIS

Traditionally, the diagnosis of primary congenital CMV infection requires greater than a four-fold rise in anticytomegalovirus antibody titer (serological conversion) or the presence of the maternal IgM specific antibody. Antibodies detected by immunofluorescence, indirect hemagglutination and enzyme linked immunosorbent assay appear within 2 weeks after primary infection. Serum CMV-specific IgM antibodies can be demonstrated during the acute phase of primary CMV infection. Recent maternal infection can be inferred from a single serum specimen by the demonstration of IgM specific antibody. IgM antibodies appear early in the course of the disease and persist for 4–8 months, depending upon which test is used. A rise in titer during pregnancy or a single high antibody titer greater than 1:128 does not usually correlate with an ensuing neonatal morbidity, unless IgM maternal antibodies are present[3]. CMV endocervical colonization or viruria is not a reliable marker for probable vertical transmission to the fetus. Non-immune hydrops may be a marker of CMV infection[4]. With amniocentesis, virus isolation or viral antigen demonstration using polymerase chain reaction technology is possible.

CONGENITAL CMV INFECTION

The magnitude of CMV sequelae is a partial function of gestational age; the younger the fetus, the greater the probability of permanent sequelae.

A 7-year prospective study showed that fetal loss occurred in the approximately 15% (four of 26) of gravid women who contracted CMV infection early in gestation as opposed to non-infected individuals, who had an incidence of 2.2% (16 of 744)[5]. Primary, maternal infection led to a congenital infection in instances nine of 46[6]. Two infants developed definitive intellectual impairment after birth[5]. One study prospectively identified 50 infants who had contracted CMV infection *in utero*. Three (6%) had symptoms at birth. Four had no specific abnormalities at birth but developed permanent neurological sequelae including spastic quadriplegia and psychomotor retardation. Five of the seven mentioned above, including one of the infants with neurological manifestations, had sensorineural deafness (which was bilateral in three of the five children). Neurological or sensorineural defects followed exposure to primary maternal infection, as well as recurrent maternal infection, in all trimesters[7].

As a rule of thumb, it is estimated that 15–50% of primary maternal infection results in fetal infection. When maternal CMV antedates pregnancy, the probability of infection is less than 3–5%[5,6]. The overall incidence of congenital CMV infection among progeny of seropositive women is approximately 1.8%. An overall prevalence of 3.4% congenital CMV infection was observed among offspring of women with high levels of preconceptual antibodies[7].

The major organ affected in overt CMV infection is the brain. In a Swedish study involving more than 10 328 newborns, congenital infection was found in 50 cases (0.5%). Nine of the 47 (19%) infected infants with known clinical status at birth had hepatomegaly, splenomegaly, jaundice and/or petechiae. Two of eight (25%) neonatally symptomatic infants and three of the 35 (9%) asymptomatic infants developed neurological sequelae. Of the five infants with neurological sequelae, one had very severe psychomotor retardation and deafness. This child was born with primary infection of the first trimester. One child with moderate retardation and three children with deafness all bore the result of secondary infection[8]. Paraventricular cysts, intraventricular strands and mild ventriculomegaly

as a consequence of congenital infection have been described[9].

About 10% of congenitally infected infants will develop some degree of sensorineural hearing loss or a tendency to subnormal intelligence. Important psychomotor impairment may occur in one out of every 1000 live births as a result of congenital CMV infection[10,11].

Prenatal diagnosis of fetal infection can be accomplished from either amniotic fluid by amniocentesis or fetal blood by funicentesis. Amniotic fluid can be cultured for CMV or analyzed for a specific segment of CMV DNA by the polymerase chain reaction. This combination of tests of amniotic fluid has a sensitivity of 92% in detecting fetal CMV infection. Fetal infection can also be demonstrated by testing for CMV-specific IgM in the fetal blood by means of an enzyme-linked immunosorbent assay (ELISA). This latter approach has a sensitivity of about 70% in detecting fetal CMV infection[3]. Caution should be used when amniocentesis or funicentesis is performed before 21 weeks of gestation, because of a higher rate of false-negative results compared to those performed later[12–14]. This could result from either an immature fetal immune system or a short interval (less than 7.0 weeks) from the time of maternal CMV infection to the initiation of prenatal diagnosis[13]. Therefore, a negative CMV test before 21.0 weeks of gestation may require a repeat test 4–6 weeks later. Culture and polymerase chain reaction are preferable in the amniotic fluid to the fetal blood, because of a higher sensitivity of detecting CMV fetal infection[12,15]. In addition, amniocentesis is associated with fewer fetal complications than is funicentesis.

SIGNIFICANCE OF MATERNAL INFECTION ANTEDATING PREGNANCY

Unlike with other viruses, the birth of one congenitally infected infant does not totally preclude the possibility of congenital infection in subsequent gestations. Neutralization kinetics and restriction enzyme analysis have demonstrated antigenic and genetic homology between viral strains isolated from two siblings consecutively infected *in utero*[16]. The ability to involve more than one progeny renders the current approaches to vaccine development impractical.

THE DANGER OF NOSOCOMIAL SPREAD

The ability to disseminate infection to susceptible individuals in the immediate environment is characteristic of maternal, neonatal and congenital infection. Infants with congenital CMV infection excrete infectious virus from the oropharynx and urinary tract and are often responsible for the lateral spread of disease among individuals who come in intimate contact with them. Consequently, precautionary measures should be instituted to exclude gravidas from intimate contact with a congenitally infected infant.

REFERENCES

1. Preece PM. Congenital cytomegalovirus infection: Predisposing maternal factors. *J Epid Comm Health* 1986;40:205–9
2. Stagno S, Pass RF, Cloud G. Primary cytomegalovirus infection in pregnancy. *J Am Med Assoc* 1986;256:1904–8
3. Haukenes G, Finne PH, Bertnes E. Cytomegalovirus (CMV) and rubella virus infection during pregnancy. *Acta Obstet Gynecol Scand* 1984;63:431–5
4. Katz VL, Cefat RE, McClure BK, *et al*. Elevated second trimester maternal serum alpha-fetoprotein and cytomegalovirus infection. *Obstet Gynecol* 1986;68:580–1
5. Griffiths PD, Baboonian C. A prospective study of primary cytomegalovirus infection during pregnancy. *Br J Obstet Gynaecol* 1984;91:307–15
6. Adler SP. Cytomegalovirus and pregnancy. *Curr Opin Obstet Gynecol* 1992;4:670–5
7. Stagno S, Reynolds DW, Huang ES, *et al*. Congenital cytomegalovirus infection: occurrence in an immune population. *N Engl J Med* 1977;296:1254
8. Preece PM, Pearl KN, Peckham CS. Congenital cytomegalovirus infection. *Arch Dis Child* 1984;59:1120–6
9. Ahlfors K, Ivarsson SA, Johnson T. Congenital cytomegalovirus infection and disease in Sweden and the relative importance of primary and secondary maternal infection. *Scand J Infect Dis* 1984;16:129–37
10. Kumar ML, Gold E, Jacobs IB. Primary cytomegalovirus infection in adolescent pregnancy. *Pediatrics* 1984; 74:493–500
11. Hanshaw JB, Shelmor AP, Mosley AW, *et al*. School failure and deafness after silent congenital cytomegalovirus infection. *N Engl J Med* 1976;295:408
12. Hanshaw JB. Congenital cytomegalovirus infection: a fifteen year perspective. *J Infect Dis* 1971;123:555
13. Donner C, Liesnard C, Content J, *et al*. Prenatal diagnosis of 52 pregnancies at risk for congenital cytomegalovirus infection. *Obstet Gynecol* 1993;82:481–6
14. Nicolini U, Kusterman A, Tassis B, *et al*. Prenatal diagnosis of congenital human cytomegalovirus infection. *Prenat Diagn* 1994;14:903–6
15. Catanzarite V, Dankner W. Prenatal diagnosis of congenital cytomegalovirus infection: false-negative amniocentesis at 20 weeks gestation. *Prenat Diagn* 1993;13:1021–5
16. Hagay Z, Biran G, Ornoy A, *et al*. Congenital cytomegalovirus infection: a long-standing problem still seeking a solution. *Am J Obstet Gynecol* 1996;174:241–5

25

Herpes infection: herpes simplex virus and varicella zoster virus

R.R. Viscarello

HERPES SIMPLEX VIRUS

Over the past two decades, herpes simplex virus type-2 (HSV-2) infections have drawn increasing attention owing to their growing prevalence and the mounting concern generated by the unpredictable clinical course of this chronic sexually transmitted disease. There is no cure available for infection with HSV-2; once infected, a carrier may transmit HSV-2 to sexual partners at any time. The fact that the virus may be transmitted vertically from mother to child with the potential for a highly morbid neonatal outcome only increases the level of anxiety.

While much information has been acquired regarding the natural history of maternal and neonatal HSV-2 infection, the pace of this acquisition has not matched the epidemic spread of the virus, particularly in women of reproductive age. There has been a concomitant rise in neonatal HSV-2 infection among healthy as well as immunocompromised gravidae, the latter group being at exceptionally high risk for severe sequelae. Recommendations for management of pregnancy and parturition for patients with a history of HSV-2 infection have been dramatically revised. Diagnosis has become easier with the utilization of new laboratory methods. Anti-viral therapies may ameliorate some of the morbid sequelae of both maternal and neonatal infection with HSV-2.

Maternal HSV-2 infections are not life-threatening, except in the rare cases of disseminated herpes infection in the setting of concurrent immunocompromise. The changes in cell-mediated immunity associated with advancing pregnancy may be linked to a slight increase in the risk of disseminated HSV-2 disease. Disseminated HSV-2 infection has been associated with a mortality rate of > 50% in both mother and fetus[1]. The frequency of disseminated HSV-2 infections in pregnancy may rise as the population of women with human immunodeficiency virus type-1 (HIV-1) increases.

Herpes infections assume greater significance during pregnancy because of their potential to cause morbidity and mortality in the fetus and neonate. Neonatal HSV-2 infection may vary from subclinical to symptomatic and has the potential to cause severe developmental damage, if unrecognized and untreated. Among HSV-2-infected neonates who develop disease, about half of the survivors will incur permanent ocular impairment or central nervous system (CNS) damage[2].

Epidemiology

HSV-2 infections are common in a variety of populations worldwide. Genital herpes is not subject to mandatory reporting to the Centers for Disease Control (CDC); therefore, no accurate data regarding incidence and prevalence of the disease in the USA are available. However, estimates from the CDC show a dramatic increase in the number of annual private physician visits attributable to genital HSV-2 infection, with 260 000 visits in 1983, a nine-fold rise from 1966 estimates[3]. The number of new cases had increased to 450 000 by 1984, although since that time, annual figures have declined slightly[4]. The incidence of HSV-2 is thought to be 1–2% of the total population[4]. An actual increase in the prevalence, coupled with the increasing recognition of HSV-2 infection, may account for the phenomenal rise in estimates of infected individuals. A concurrent increase in the number of neonatal HSV-2 infections has also been noted, with a four-fold increase seen from 1966 to 1981[5]. Neonatal HSV-2 infection is estimated to occur in one in 5000 deliveries annually[6] (Figure 1).

An increased prevalence of HSV-2 has been noted in older, white, married, well-educated women[7], although HSV-2 infection is noted in most racial, geographic and socioeconomic subsets. HSV-2 infection is correlated with the presence of other sexually transmitted diseases. Projections from serological studies indicate that 50–80% of adults in the USA have antibodies to HSV-1 or HSV-2[4]. Maternal genital herpes virus infection, the most common cause of neonatal herpes infection, is most often caused by the serological subtype HSV-2, although 15% of genital herpes cases are thought to result from herpes simplex virus type-1 (HSV-1)[8]. Antibody to HSV-2 is found in 30–90% of women[4].

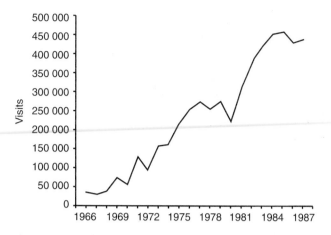

Figure 1 Incidence of private office visits related to herpes simplex virus type-2 infection in the USA during calendar years 1966 to 1987. Reprinted with permission from reference 102

Clinical manifestations

Maternal

Initial exposure to the virus through sex with an infected partner results in acute primary infection with distinct clinical manifestations. Asymptomatic primary infection is rare; however, infection may be acquired from an asymptomatic sexual partner[9]. Acute primary disease is characterized by eruption of numerous, bilaterally distributed, small vesicles on an erythematous base. Characteristically, the lesions are painful, soft, vesicular and ulcerative in appearance. These vesicles may coalesce into bullae with eventual progression to ulcerous lesions that crust and heal, usually without scarring. Fever, pharyngitis, malaise, headaches, myalgia, inguinal lymphadenopathy and severe local pain may accompany the primary herpes lesion. There is an excellent correlation between clinical symptoms and the laboratory diagnosis of HSV-2[10]. The mean duration of an acute episode is about 15 days. Primary HSV-2 infection is often localized in the cervix, although often lesions are oropharyngeal, or anal if infection was contracted through receptive oral or anal sex, respectively. Lesions may be located anywhere on the body, but the oral and genital locations are the most common. Spread of lesions to distal sites such as fingers, back and buttocks may occur via contact transmission. Once infection has occurred, the virus enters a latent stage leaving the patient vulnerable to recurrences that vary in both frequency and severity (Figure 2).

About half of patients diagnosed with primary HSV-2 will experience clinical recurrence within 6 months, although the frequency and risk of recurrence are probably determined by the serotype of HSV-2 (Table 1). Infection due to HSV-2 results in recurrent episodes with 3–4 times the frequency of HSV-1 infections[7]. Patients presenting with recurrences will

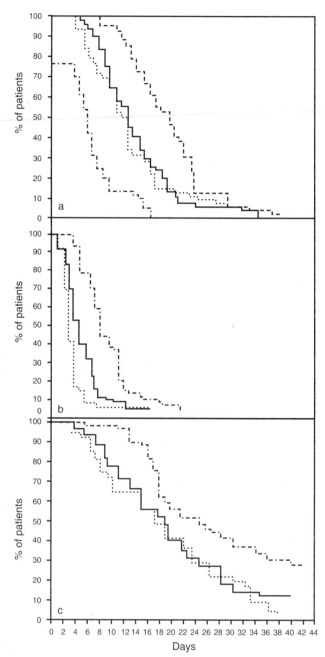

Figure 2 Clinical course of mucocutaneous herpes simplex virus (HSV) infection. Duration of signs and symptoms (a) of primary oral or genital HSV infection; (b) of recurrent HSV infection; (c) in immunosuppressed patients. Reprinted with permission from reference 17. Dashed lines, lesions; unbroken lines, pain; dotted lines, viral shedding; dashed and dotted lines, constitutional symptoms

have fewer, milder lesions without systemic effects lasting about 7–10 days[11]. The duration of both viral shedding and the time to healing are shorter than with primary infection. A 1- or 2-day prodrome may precede recurrences with pruritus, tingling, or pain at the typical lesion site noted (Table 2).

Table 1 Comparison of local and systemic factors that may precipitate recurrent genital herpes outbreak. Modified with permission from reference 102

Systemic factors
Menstruation
Fatigue
Emotional stress
Intercurrent bacterial or viral disease
Immunosuppressive drugs
Malignancy

Local factors
Skin trauma
Chemical burn or irritation
Sunburn
Epilation
Dermabrasion therapy
Ganglion manipulation
Application of retinoic acid
Application of prostaglandin E$_2$

Table 2 Comparison of characteristics of primary genital HSV-2 infection with those of recurrent disease. Modified with permission from reference 14

Characteristics	Primary genital infection	Recurrent genital infection
Incubation period	2–10 days	chronic
Duration of viral shedding	12–14 days	5–7 days
Duration of local symptoms	15–20 days	7–10 days
Number of lesions	greater	fewer
Cervical lesions	common	uncommon
Prodrome	acute	1–2 days
Systemic symptoms	frequent	rare
Fever	often present	usually absent
Malaise	common	rare
Pain	frequent	frequent
Regional lymphadenopathy	often present	usually absent

The estimated rate of HSV-1 or HSV-2 seroconversion in pregnant patients who were seronegative for both HSV-1 and HSV-2 is 3.7%. The estimated rate of HSV-2 seroconversion in patients who were positive for HSV-1 is 1.7%, while that of HSV-1 conversion in patients who were positive for HSV-2 is 0%. This suggests that prior HSV-2 infection may prevent subsequent HSV-1 infection[12]. Prior antibody to HSV-1 may alter the course of infection with HSV-2, resulting in a non-primary, first-episode genital herpes manifestation[13]. Non-primary, first-episode HSV-2 infection has a shorter duration and milder clinical course than true primary, first-episode HSV-2 infection. Brown and co-workers[10] in 1987 noted that women who acquired primary genital herpes during pregnancy tended to be younger, unmarried, and have a younger age at first sexual intercourse and first pregnancy than those who acquired non-primary, first-episode herpes during the gestation noted.

Typically, recurrent episodes of HSV-2 are preceded by prodromal symptoms of pruritus, numbness and/or mild pain at the usual lesion site. Infection with HSV-2 results in recurrence with a frequency of 3–4 times that of HSV-1. Pregnancy does not seem significantly to alter the rate of recurrence[14]. Clinical presentation is characterized by fewer lesions which have a shorter duration (approximately 7 days) than primary episodes. Nearly one-quarter of recurrences may be clinically asymptomatic, although the virus still may be shed concomitantly from the cervix[7]. Maternal asymptomatic shedding of HSV-2 into the genital tract during vaginal delivery is the source of 70% of all neonatal HSV-2 infections[15]. Cervical shedding of HSV-2 is found in 80–86% of women with primary genital HSV-2 infection, in 65% of women with non-primary, first-episode HSV-2 infection, and in 12% of women with recurrent genital HSV-2 lesions[7].

Clinical presentation of HSV-2 may vary in immunocompromised or iatrogenically immunosuppressed patients. There may be deep cutaneous and mucosal involvement. Friability, tissue necrosis, pain, hemorrhage and an inability to ingest food or drink may occur[16,17]. A few case reports of herpes encephalitis in both immunocompromised as well as healthy gravidae exist. Symptoms may include hemiparesis, seizures, amnesia and/or unusual behavior[18]. Disseminated HSV-2 infection may present predominantly as hepatitis with or without CNS infection. Symptoms may include fever, malaise, chills and genital pain[18] (Figure 3).

Maternal HSV-2 infection may be associated with an adverse pregnancy outcome depending on whether the infection is primary or recurrent, the location of the lesions, subclinical viral excretion, the status of the membranes (intact or ruptured) and/or the gestational age at the onset of maternal infection. Neonatal HSV-2 infection, spontaneous abortion, intrauterine growth retardation (IUGR) and prematurity are more strongly associated with primary maternal infections than with recurrent episodes[2,10]. The exact relationship of maternal HSV-2 and prematurity is unclear, but approximately 40% of HSV-2-infected neonates are born before the 36th week of gestation[19]. Premature infants may represent a more susceptible host to HSV-2 infection[2]. Transplacental infection resulting in a congenital herpes syndrome is quite rare and is more likely to be the result of maternal primary infection early in pregnancy. The neonatal mortality rate with congenital herpes infection has been reported to be 31% and results in severe, permanent neurological damage in most survivors[20].

Neonatal HSV-2 infection may be acquired from an infected maternal lower genital tract during vaginal

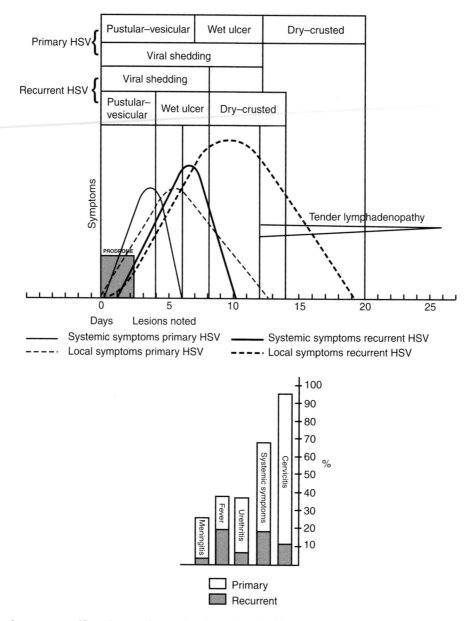

Figure 3   Clinical course, manifestations and complications of genital herpes simplex virus (HSV) type-2 infection. Reprinted with permission from reference 103

delivery. HSV-2 may ascend from an infected cervix, causing neonatal infection during an operative delivery following prolonged labor or following rupture of membranes. The risk of neonatal HSV-2 infection after vaginal delivery with maternal primary genital infection at the time of birth is about 40–60%[10,12,21]. The highest risk of neonatal HSV infection occurs in maternal primary infection without seroconversion prior to delivery[12]. The highest risk of perinatal morbidity is associated with women contracting primary genital HSV-2 during the third trimester of pregnancy[10,21]. Suppressive therapy in patients having primary genital herpes during pregnancy with oral acyclovir 400 mg

three times per day from 36 weeks until delivery significantly reduces the incidence of clinically apparent recurrent genital herpes at delivery, thus the need for Cesarean section[22]. Furthermore acyclovir prophylaxis in preventing neonatal herpes infection appears to be more cost-effective than the approach of Cesarean section for recurrent genital herpes at the time of delivery without antenatal acyclovir prophylaxis[23]. The neonatal attack rate in women with recurrent disease at the time of delivery is much lower, with estimates of a 1–4% risk of neonatal infection. Yeager and Arvin[15] found only one-third of neonates with herpes to have mothers with a history of typical recurrent HSV-2 episodes. Postnatal HSV-2 infection of the newborn may occur as a result of exposure to infected sources. Newborns have acquired HSV-2 infection postnatally from mothers, fathers and health care workers with HSV-1, HSV-2, or herpetic whitlow[6]. HSV-2 has been isolated in breast milk; whether this can serve as a source of neonatal HSV-2 transmission is not clear. Until recently cervical infection with HSV-2 was suspected as a possible etiological agent of cervical carcinoma. Recent research has discounted the role of HSV-2, while indicting human papilloma virus (HPV) as the more likely co-factor in cervical neoplasia[24,25].

Neonatal

Neonatal herpes infections will typically present by 7–10 days postnatally. Neonatal HSV-2 infection may develop on the skin, mucosal membranes and in the CNS or it may be disseminated[6]. Clinical symptoms may include skin lesions appearing initially on the presenting parts, respiratory irregularity, eye involvement, cyanosis, jaundice, convulsions, or disseminated intravascular coagulopathy. At present, viral culture and direct immunofluorescence are the only reliable means of diagnosis of neonatal herpes. Skin lesions characteristic of adult HSV-2 infection may be absent in 30–50% of newborns with culture-proven HSV-2 infection and when present may be confused with pyoderma or diaper rash[26]. Initial skin or mucosal infection will progress to disseminated disease if untreated. Lesions culture-positive for *Staphylococcus aureus* may be concomitantly herpetic. Biopsy by needle aspiration may be necessary to confirm brain involvement[2].

Maternal primary infection during pregnancy may result in transplacental herpes infection with a recognized congenital syndrome, although few cases have been described[20]. Intrauterine HSV-2 infection will present clinically in the neonate's first week of life[27–29]. Hutto and collaborators[20] performed a study of 13 neonates suspected of intrauterine HSV-2 infection. There were scars and lesions present at birth or shortly thereafter, chorioretinitis, microencephaly, hydranencephaly and microphthalmia. Multiple system involvement was found in 92% with CNS infection. Transplacental infection due to cytomegalovirus (CMV), rubella, toxoplasmosis, or syphilis must be excluded from the diagnosis by viral culture or serological means (Table 3).

Etiology

Infection with herpes simplex virus is caused by two separate antigenically related serotypes, HSV-1, known as oral–labial herpes, and HSV-2, or genital herpes. Herpes infections of the genital area are primarily caused by HSV-2, although HSV-1 may infect the

Table 3 Clinicopathological abnormalities in neonatal herpes simplex virus infections. Reprinted with permission from reference 76

Timing of transmission	Abnormality
In utero	skin vesicles, cutaneous scars, cutaneous calcifications, absence of scalp skin, microcephaly, cerebral atrophy, hydranencephaly, cerebral and cerebellar necrosis, intracranial calcifications, hepatosplenomegaly, chorioretinitis, micro-ophthalmia, keratoconjunctivitis, short digits, cataracts, retinal dysplasia, bone abnormalities
Intrapartum or postpartum – acute infection	vesicular rash, hepatitis, seizures, keratoconjunctivitis, chorioretinitis, pneumonia, shock, disseminated intravascular coagulation, poor feeding, temperature instability, bulging fontanelle
Post-infectious complications	microcephaly, hydranencephaly, porencephalic cysts, blindness, seizures, psychomotor retardation, learning disabilities, spasticity, recurrent mucocutaneous herpes, hearing defects

genitals as well[8]. The subtypes and strains can be differentiated by restriction endonuclease analysis, thus yielding valuable information for prognosis of clinical course and frequency of genital recurrences[7,30]. Subtyping is also of value in determining patterns of transmission, which is of greater consequence to epidemiological studies than to management of individual patients[31]. A single patient may be infected with multiple types and strains of herpes, each resulting in separate recurrent episodes[32,33].

Herpes simplex virus is a member of the Herpes Viridae family which includes HSV-1, HSV-2, varicella zoster virus (VZV), CMV, the Epstein–Barr virus (EBV) and the human herpes virus type-6 (HHV-6). These are large viruses with a double-stranded, linear DNA core. Structurally, the genomes of HSV-1 and HSV-2 are about 50% homologous[16]. Covering the virus is a lipid membrane envelope acquired as progeny viral cells bud through the host cell membrane during replication[34]. Viral glycoproteins contained in the lipid envelope facilitate binding to the host cell surface and entrance into the cell membrane[16] (Figure 4).

Pathophysiology

Herpes simplex virus may infect a broad spectrum of tissue-culture cell lines *in vitro*. Infectivity does not always result in massive viral replication, although 50 000 to 200 000 virions per cell may be produced in

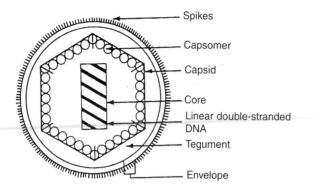

Spikes

Capsomer

Capsid

Core

Linear double-stranded
DNA

Tegument

Envelope

Figure 4 Schematic illustration of herpes simplex virus type-2. Reprinted with permission from reference 102

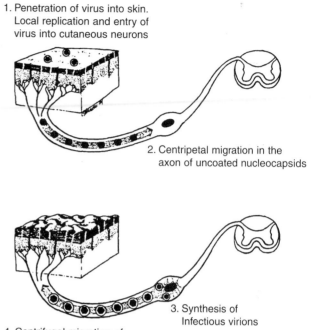

1. Penetration of virus into skin. Local replication and entry of virus into cutaneous neurons

2. Centripetal migration in the axon of uncoated nucleocapsids

3. Synthesis of Infectious virions

4. Centrifugal migration of infectious virions to epidermis

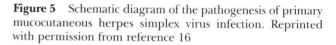

Figure 5 Schematic diagram of the pathogenesis of primary mucocutaneous herpes simplex virus infection. Reprinted with permission from reference 16

permissive cell lines[34]. Host cell death is thought to occur in part because of restraint of cell macromolecular synthesis[16,17]. It is unclear why particular HSV strains are tropic for certain cell types, since the receptor sites are not known at present.

Herpes virus replicates within the nucleus, resulting in Cowdry type-A intranuclear inclusions. The DNA molecules of the herpes simplex virus are linear and double-stranded, each coding for at least 50 different proteins including thymidine kinase and DNA polymerase, the enzymes thought to participate in viral replication[17,35]. Fusion of cell membrane and viral envelope enables the release of nucleocapsid (composed of viral DNA and proteins) into the host cell cytoplasm. Part of the nuclear membrane is acquired in this process. The nucleocapsid then travels to the cell surface where it is released either extracellularly or into proximal cells, where further replication ensues[35]. Virus-coded glycoproteins, some type-specific, can be found on both the infected cell surface and the viral envelope. Particular glycoproteins serve as targets of the host immune response, which may inhibit release of virions by antibody-dependent, cell-mediated cytotoxicity (ADCC)[36] or neutralizing antibody[35].

Specific regions of both herpes virus genomes are known to enable morphological changes of cells *in vitro*. Detection of herpes simplex virus-specific DNA sequences or viral proteins in cervical neoplasias would seem to support the association with cervical carcinoma. However, investigations have implicated human papilloma virus in the etiology of cervical tumors[24].

Primary infection follows exposure to virulent virus at mucosal surfaces or abraded skin. Concomitant infections, burns, trauma, or eczema are thought to increase host susceptibility. Active replication ensues, with spreading of progeny first to adjacent cells, followed by sensory nerve endings. Clinically apparent lesions may or may not develop. Latency is thought to be established once the viral nucleocapsid travels along the axonal pathways to neuronal nuclei in ganglion cells. During latency, active viral replication and cell death do

not result from neural infection, although some viral genomes are maintained by the cells in a repressed state[16,17]. The detection of herpes simplex virus RNA in sensory ganglia supports the theory of limited transcription during latent infection[37] (Figure 5).

Once infection has occurred, latency is lifelong with varying intervals of reactivation of viral replication and resulting recurrence of clinical or silent infection. The frequency and duration of recurrences are probably dependent upon host immune responses. There is no evidence supporting anecdotal reports of total spontaneous termination of recurrences; once latent infection is established the presence of virus in neurons is permanent. It is unclear what mechanism induces recurrent episodes of HSV-2 infection and why they are more frequent than with HSV-1. In the 'ganglion trigger' hypothesis, Corey[13] has theorized that stimuli affecting latently infected ganglia induce productive viral replication resulting in flow of virus down peripheral nerves, spreading into dermal layers and resulting in characteristic herpes lesions. Alternatively, Corey's 'skin trigger' hypothesis surmises that virus regularly produced by ganglia reaches the skin surface, but results in vesicular lesions only if local suppression of immune surveillance mechanisms has occurred. Herpes simplex virus maintaining latency in the neural cells of ganglia may be subject to a wide variety of peripheral stimuli such as ultraviolet light or emotional stressors that may directly influence the neuronal expression of latent HSV-2 genes. There are anecdotal reports linking recurrences with co-factors such as exposure to sunlight or bad music, stress, menstruation, prostaglandins, sexual excitement, concomitant illness, etc[38] (Table 1).

Host humoral response to HSV-2 infection begins with development of IgM, IgG and IgA antibodies directed against viral proteins. While antibody may ameliorate the severity of HSV-2 disease, its role in regulating infection is not understood. Direct cell-to-cell spread of HSV-2 may enable the virus to evade potential neutralization by antibody. Persons with agammaglobulinemia and HSV-2 infection do not display more frequent or severe recurrences. Additionally, specific antibody in a host offers no protection against recurrence or neonatal HSV-2 infection[2]. It is interesting to note a potential ameliorative effect of maternal antibody upon neonatal infection as demonstrated by a lower attack rate of HSV-2 following maternal recurrent vs. primary infection. Interferon (IFN) also plays a part in regulation of HSV-2 infection. Production of γ-IFN may serve as a marker or direct determinant of recurrence of HSV-1[39]. Also, IFN has been shown to be effective in preventing reactivation of HSV-1 infection following surgery on the trigeminal nerve root[40].

The cell-mediated immune response appears to control the course of HSV-2 infection. Studies have established ADCC, natural killer cell (NK), and blastogenic responses to primary and recurrent HSV-2 infection. Deficiencies in cell-mediated immunity, whether congenital, acquired, or iatrogenically induced, result in more frequent, more lengthy and more severe HSV-2 recurrences. However, no consistent defect in immune response has been noted in immunocompromised patients with highly frequent HSV-2 recurrences[35].

Laboratory diagnosis

The presence of HSV-2 should be confirmed by viral culture, which is considered the most sensitive, currently available, diagnostic method. Vesicular fluid is more likely to yield virus in culture than ulcerative or crusted lesions[41]. Positive results can usually be identified by a cytopathic effect typical of HSV-2 within 48–72 h. HSV-2 will survive without loss of titer in transport media at 4°C for up to 2 days[42]. Chancroid, lymphogranuloma venereum and *Chlamydia trachomatis* may be eliminated from the differential diagnosis owing to the absence of suppuration accompanying the lymphadenopathy. Infection with *Treponema pallidum* may be ruled out by the use of dark-field microscopy on samples obtained from genital ulcers and by serological testing[11]. Dual infection can occur. HSV-2 lesions may also be confused with those associated with Behçets and Crohn's diseases (Table 4).

Primary episodes are more likely to be culture-positive than recurrences. The false-negative rate of viral culture for a single HSV-2 culture is approximately 5–30%. Virus can be isolated from cervical HSV-2 lesions less often than from external genital lesions. The cervix is frequently the site of culture-proven, subclinical viral excretion following primary genital herpes infection. The labia are more likely to shed asymptomatically after non-primary, first-episode HSV-2 infection[10]. HSV-2 particles may be detected rapidly (within 1–2 h) by electron microscopy. Sensitivity varies, however, as this method cannot distinguish HSV-2 from VZV. Electron microscopy is not always available and requires technical expertise for consistent evaluation of HSV-2[11].

The widely available Papanicolaou (Pap) smear may show cytopathic changes typical of HSV-2 such as multinucleated giant cells and intranuclear inclusions; however, 50% of results may be false-negative. Other staining methods such as indirect immunoperoxidase and direct immunofluorescence using rabbit-derived anti-HSV-2 antibody are about 20% more sensitive than the Pap smear[43].

The evolution of high-affinity monoclonal antibodies may enable more rapid and accurate methods of laboratory testing to be performed. At present, testing

Table 4 Diseases that cause genital ulcers and inguinal lymphadenopathy. Reprinted with permission from reference 11

Disease	Cause	Type of ulcer	Type of adenopathy
Genital herpes	HSV-2, HSV-1	small, painful when scraped, 'soft'	firm, tender when palpated
Syphilis	*Treponema pallidum*	painless, 'hard', indurated	firm, 'rubbery', non-tender or tender
Chancroid	*Haemophilus ducreyi*	painful, 'soft', indurated, purulent	fluctuant, tender, overlying erythema
Lymphogranuloma venereum	*Chlamydia trachomatis* (L1, L2, L3 subtypes)	usually absent	fluctuant, tender
Granuloma inguinale	*Calymmatobacterium granulomatis*	painless, chronic, spreading	none

by monoclonal antibodies is a less sensitive (78% in a high-prevalence population) method as compared to viral culture[31]. An inadequate number of cells on the direct smear leads to an unacceptable amount of inadequate specimens. Lafferty and co-workers[44] recommended against replacement of viral culture by monoclonal antibody testing for HSV-2, because of the lower predictive value in low-prevalence populations and the better correlation of infectivity with results from viral culture. In addition, monoclonal antibody stains may be only half as sensitive as culture in detecting asymptomatic cervical shedding of HSV-2. Fluorescein-conjugated, monoclonal antibodies may be of specific efficacy during pregnancy. As long as the slides are adequately prepared (> 50 cells per smear), immunofluorescence with monoclonal antibodies is rapid and nearly 100% specific and sensitive, thus possibly having a positive impact upon decisions regarding management of labor during pregnancy complicated by HSV-2 infection.

Enzyme-linked immounosorbent assay (ELISA) tests have been assessed for detection of genital herpes infections. Although it is rapid, the low sensitivity (34%) and a positive predictive value of only 65% limit its utility in areas of low prevalence[45]. A higher specificity (100%) and sensitivity (84%), as well as a greater positive predictive value (89%) were obtained with ELISA in a higher-prevalence population (44%), making a more favorable comparison with viral culture[46]. ELISA was recently found to have a sensitivity of 97.5% and specificity of 98.6% in a study of 563 samples, and compared favorably with viral culture in a population with an HSV-2 prevalence of 12.8%[47].

The Tzanck smear method for detection of multinucleated giant cells characteristic of HSV-2 is widely available but less sensitive than culture. The sensitivity of the Tzanck smear is enhanced by obtaining exudate from multiple vesicles before progression to ulceration has begun. Significant improvement in specificity and sensitivity results from the use of monoclonal antibodies tagged with immunofluorescent markers[48]. The Tzanck smear cannot differentiate HSV-2 from VZV.

Recent infection can be documented by measurement of serum antibodies to HSV-2 shown by a fourfold or greater rise in neutralizing antibody or complement-fixing antibody titers between acute and convalescent sera. This is useful only in seroprevalence studies, however, since only 5% of patients with recurrent HSV-2 infection will show a four-fold rise in titer, rendering serological diagnosis of little clinical use[11].

Management

In view of the high morbidity and mortality of neonatal infection, management of pregnant women should include identification of those with either a personal history or a partner with a history of recurrent HSV-2 infection to minimize the risk of vertical transmission of the disease. Infection of the fetus and newborn occurs presumably because of direct contact with infected material. Most herpetic infections in pregnancy are reactivations of latent disease with incidence of subclinical, maternal lower genital tract infection on the day of delivery estimated at 1.4%[49]. Although asymptomatic shedding of HSV-2 occurs in 0.09–4% of pregnant women[50,51], weekly antenatal cultures have been shown to have poor predictive value of neonatal exposure to asymptomatic infection on the day of delivery[49,52]. Even careful weekly culture cannot prevent neonatal HSV-2 infection[53].

In a study of 6904 deliveries, Prober and co-workers[54] found neonatal exposure to subclinical maternal HSV-2 to be unpredictable. Given the high cost[55], poor predictive value, low correlation of antepartum shedding with viral excretion on the day of delivery, and low attack rate in infants delivered vaginally to women with asymptomatic perinatal HSV-2 infection (none of 34 exposed neonates infected; 95% confidence limit for maximum neonatal infection rate of 8%)[56], weekly viral cultures are not recommended for pregnant women with a history of genital herpes in the absence of genital lesions or a prodrome[57]. Spontaneous vaginal delivery is appropriate for women with a history of herpetic infection without genital lesions or viral prodrome at the time of delivery, unless there are other obstetric indications for operative delivery. Maternal or neonatal viral culture obtained on the day of delivery may aid in the recognition of infants with potential exposure to HSV-2. Maternal isolation is not mandated. The calculated risk of neonatal infection in the absence of maternal genital lesions without weekly cultures and mandatory Cesarean delivery is thought to be about one in 1000[57].

Operative delivery may reduce the risk of neonatal infection for women with genital HSV-2 lesions or who are prodromal at the onset of labor[58]. It used to be thought that the lowest risk of neonatal HSV-2 was associated with Cesarean section performed within 4–6 h of rupture of the fetal membranes, before infected cells could ascend the birth canal during labor[59]. This was based on studies which noted that the risk of neonatal HSV-2 infection associated with maternal clinical HSV-2 infection at the time of delivery was > 40% unless Cesarean section was performed within 4 h of rupture of the membranes[59]. However, since Cesarean section may help prevent neonatal herpes infection in cases of longer intervals after rupture of the membranes[57], operative delivery is now recommended in all cases in which there are active lesions or prodromal symptoms, regardless of the duration of rupture of the membranes.

For women with clinical HSV-2 infection remote from the vulva, vaginal delivery is recommended unless there are other indications for operative delivery, provided that surgical drapes can be placed over the lesions to prevent contamination of the vaginal delivery area. The incidence of concomitant subclinical cervical shedding when there is non-vulvar maternal HSV-2 infection is thought to be low. Wittek and colleagues[52] found only one of 47 women with remote HSV-2 lesions to have a positive cervical culture. Non-invasive modes of intrapartum monitoring should be utilized when possible, owing to the risk of neonatal inoculation with HSV-2. There have been cases suggesting that HSV-2 infections of the newborn may have been introduced or aggravated by the use of fetal scalp electrodes during delivery[60,61].

Premature rupture of membranes in women with recurrent HSV-2 infection poses a dilemma for the clinician when deciding to deliver operatively to avoid possible neonatal HSV-2 infection, or to manage expectantly to maximize fetal development. For pregnancies with a low rate of neonatal morbidity and mortality, Cesarean section would be appropriate if fetal pulmonic maturity could be demonstrated by lecithin/sphingomyelin (L/S) ratio and phosphatidylglycerol level. When the premature rupture of membranes occurs prior to 31–32 weeks of gestation and is complicated by maternal HSV-2, a case-by-case management strategy must be employed. There have been several cases of prolonged premature rupture of membranes with concomitant symptomatic maternal HSV-2 infection where expectant management was successful and neonatal HSV-2 infection was avoided[62,63]. Suspicion of chorioamnionitis, placentitis, labor, fetal distress or documented fetal lung maturity would make delivery advisable[62,63]. The greater risk of neonatal infection associated with maternal primary HSV-1 or HSV-2 infection may indicate operative delivery after premature rupture of membranes during primary maternal infection.

Recommendations for supportive treatment for episodes of HSV-2 during gestation may include sitzbaths, topical anesthetics or acetaminophen and use of a blow-dryer on the cool setting to provide relief from symptoms. In recent years, acyclovir (Zovirax, Burroughs and Wellcome, Research Triangle Park, NC) has been shown to be the first useful anti-viral treatment for HSV-2. A guanosine analog, acyclovir inhibits viral DNA synthesis by selectively interfering with viral thymidine kinase in HSV-2-infected cells. Acyclovir is the recommended treatment for first-episode, symptomatic genital HSV-2 infection, and as a suppressive regimen for immunocompromised patients or for frequent and severe recurrences in the general population, but it is not approved for use in pregnancy (Figures 6 and 7).

In view of its high specificity for HSV-2-infected cells, acyclovir seems unlikely to have adverse fetal effects, although it does cross the placenta. No negative fetal effects related to the use of intravenous acyclovir are known from the limited number of women treated with acyclovir during gestation[18,63–65]. Maternal

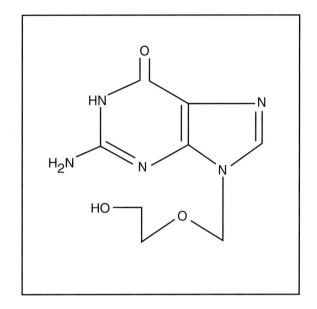

Figure 6   Chemical structure of 9-(2-hydroxyethoxymethyl) guanine (acyclovir)

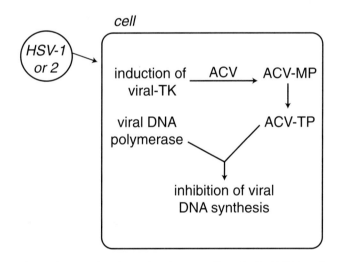

Figure 7   Mechanism of activation of acyclovir (ACV) and inhibition of herpes simplex virus (HSV) DNA polymerase. TK, thymidine kinase; MP, monophosphate; TP, triphosphate. Reprinted with permission from reference 68

acyclovir therapy may not prevent fetal infection[66]. The use of acyclovir during pregnancy should be considered with a risk/benefit analysis employed on an individual basis. Use of oral acyclovir during gestation may be affected by a suboptimal gastrointestinal absorption rate of 20% of that achieved by intravenous dosing combined with the decreased gastrointestinal absorption associated with pregnancy. Oral acyclovir should rarely be used to ameliorate recurrences during pregnancy or as a suppressive regime to avoid HSV-2 reactivation near term, as studies have failed to show that suppressive therapy with acyclovir prevents asymptomatic shedding of HSV-2[67]. Pregnant women with disseminated HSV-2 infections should be treated

Table 5 Recommendations for acyclovir treatment of herpes simplex virus infection. Reprinted with permission from reference 35

Infection	Site	Dose	Route	Schedule	Duration (days)	Comments
Immunocompetent host						
Primary epsiode	oral	—	—	—	—	inadequately tested
	genital	5%	topical	6 × /day	7	decreases virus shedding, very modest decrease in symptoms and time to heal
	genital	200 mg	oral	5 × /day	5–10	shortens duration of virus shedding; modest reduction in symptoms and time to healing
	genital	250 mg/m^2	intravenous	every 8 h	5–7	shortens duration of virus shedding, symptoms and time to healing
Recurrent	oral	5%	topical	6 × /day	7	no significant benefit; not recommended
	genital	5%	topical	6 × /day	7	possible reduction in virus shedding; not recommended
	genital	200 mg	oral	5 × /day	5	modest reduction in virus shedding, symptoms and time to healing
Immunocompromised host						
Primary episode	oral or genital	—	—	—	—	inadequately tested
Recurrent	oral	5%	topical	6 × /day	7	significant reduction in virus shedding, symptoms and time to healing
	oral	200 mg	oral	5 × /day	5–10	more effective than topical therapy
	oral		intravenous	every 8 h	5–10	impressive reduction in virus shedding, symptoms and time to healing
	genital	—	—	—	—	no data available

with parenteral acyclovir, given the > 50% mortality for both mother and fetus associated with this condition. Successful regimens have ranged from 5.0 mg/kg intravenously every 8 h for 5 days to 7.5 mg/kg intravenously every 8 h for 20 doses. Careful monitoring of kidney function should follow, since acyclovir is cleared renally. Acyclovir has demonstrated clinical value in treating maternal primary HSV-2 infection complicated by premature rupture of membranes when expectant management is mandated by fetal prematurity and attendant mortality and morbidity in survivors[63] (Table 5).

There have been a small number of cases of resistance to acyclovir found in immunocompromised patients who developed strains of HSV-2 with altered thymidine kinase activity, some after prolonged suppressive treatment. Of note, there has been no linkage of drug-resistant HSV-2 strains with multiorgan disease or dissemination in immunocompromised patients[68].

Any suspicion of neonatal infection should be aggressively investigated, since anti-viral treatment may prevent progression to disseminated HSV-2 in the newborn[17,69]. Both vidarabine and acyclovir are effective in reducing morbidity and mortality of HSV-2 infections of the newborn. Infants with diagnosed HSV-2 skin infections treated with 30 mg/kg vidarabine or acyclovir do not progress to CNS or disseminated herpes[70]. Neonates with CNS HSV-2 infections are less responsive to either anti-viral drug since symptoms are not likely to present until after extensive and irreversible brain damage has occurred. The prognosis of anti-viral therapy in the neonate with disseminated herpes is also less favorable, since more than 50% will develop fatal infection in spite of acyclovir or vidarabine[26]. Isolation for an infected neonate is recommended to reduce the opportunity for nosocomial spread of HSV-2.

VARICELLA ZOSTER VIRUS

Several of the herpes viruses, particularly CMV and HSV-2, are well-known for their ability to cause fetal, neonatal and maternal illness with teratogenic, morbid, or fatal consequences. The VZV, also a herpes virus, is the etiological agent causing varicella after primary infection in a previously seronegative individual. The course of childhood varicella is generally benign with mild constitutional symptoms followed by the viral exanthem commonly known as 'chickenpox'. If contracted early in gestation, varicella may cause a recognized congenital syndrome. Maternal-to-fetal transmission of the virus later in pregnancy, especially exposure during the last 3 weeks, may result in severe neonatal clinical infection, but will not include the congenital defects found with early first-trimester exposure.

Epidemiology

Varicella is a highly contagious viral exanthem ubiquitous in temperate climates with a secondary household attack rate of more than 90% among susceptible contacts[71]. There are approximately 3 million cases of varicella annually in the USA, with 90% of these cases developing in children between the ages of 1 and 14 years of age[72]. Infection with varicella occurs year-round, although incidence is found to peak in March, April and May in temperate climates[71,72]. Seroepidemiological studies utilizing ELISA have shown immunity in the form of VZV-specific IgG antibodies in 85–90% of young adults living in the USA and the (then) Federal Republic of Germany[73,74]. The percentage of seronegative women raised in tropical or semitropical climates may be much higher[75]. Estimates of incidence of varicella in pregnancy range from one to five per 10 000 gestations; inclusion of mild or asymptomatic cases would probably render the figure higher[1].

Among non-immune adults, the immunosuppressed or compromised, and in the fetus and neonate, infection with varicella can be severely morbid or fatal. Normal adults develop complications from infection with varicella at 25 times greater frequency than children. Gestation does not seem to alter this risk[76]. Adults constitute only 2% of the total number of cases of varicella, yet they account for 25% of the case fatalities, mostly due to varicella pneumonia[71], although disseminated infection can be fatal as well[77]. In one recent study[77] of 43 pregnant women with primary varicella infection, four progressed to symptomatic pneumonia, two of the patients needed ventilatory assistance and one died. Adults with varicella encephalitis have a mortality rate of up to 35%[72]. Varicella is communicable from about 2 days before[78] to about 7 days after the onset of rash[73]. Transmission of VZV occurs presumably via respiratory droplets from an infected source. Transmission may also occur as a result of direct contact with vesicles of either varicella or herpes zoster; crusts are less likely to contain infectious virus[79]. Contagion of varicella from contact with zoster is conceivable, since zoster vesicles are also full of infectious virions. Nearly 99% of all cases of varicella present between the 11th and 20th days after exposure (mean 14–15 days)[73], although the incubation period may be shorter in the immunocompromised patient[71]. Most infections occur from household or institutional contact. VZV infection can be contracted nosocomially; airborne spread of infection in hospitals has also been documented[80].

Table 6 Risk of abnormalities consistent with congenital varicella infection. Numbers in parentheses are those with congenital abnormalities per number of live births. Modified with permission from reference 81

Study	First trimester		Total gestation	
	Observed risk (%)	*95% confidence interval (%)*	*Observed risk (%)*	*95% confidence interval (%)*
Paryani and Arvin (1986)[74]	9.1 (1/11)	0.2–41.3	2.6 (1/38)	0.1–13.8
Siegel (1973)[104]	7.4 (2/27)	0.9–24.3	1.5 (2/135)	0.2–5.6
Enders (1984)[70]	0.0 (0/23)	0.0–14.8	0.0 (0/31)	—
Manson *et al.* (1960)[105]	0.0 (0/70)	0.0–5.1	0.0 (0/288)	0.0–1.5
Balducci *et al.* (1992)[79]	0.0 (0/35)	0.0–8	—	—
Total	1.8 (3/166)	0.5–6.5	0.6 (3/461)	0.1–2.1

Maternal infection with varicella during weeks 8–20 following the last menstrual period may result in the birth of a neonate with a recognizable array of congenital abnormalities. The incidence of varicella in pregnancy in temperate climates is rare, but the occurrence of congenital varicella syndrome is rarer still, with individual observed risk rates of 2.3% with a range of 0.5–6.5% at 95% confidence interval with first-trimester maternal varicella[81]. A recent prospective study involving 40 patients with first-trimester varicella infection yielded a 0% incidence of congenital varicella syndrome and a 3% rate of other congenital anomalies with a range of 0–8.0 at 95% confidence level[82] (Table 6).

About 10% of babies exposed to varicella antenatally will acquire intrauterine infection[71]. Estimates of the risk of symptomatic fetal infection following maternal first-trimester varicella range from 2.3% (3 of 131)[81] to 5%[77]. About 24% of neonates will develop congenital chickenpox following maternal varicella during the last 3 weeks before delivery[83]. Overall case fatality is thought to be 5%[84]. The severity of neonatal disease is directly related to the time of onset of maternal perinatal infection. About one-third of newborns become infected

Transfer of maternal antibody	Period of risk	Antibody response of newborn

-8 -7 -6 -5 -4 -3 -2 -1 0 1 2 3 4 5 6 7 8

↑ Delivery

Day of maternal onset

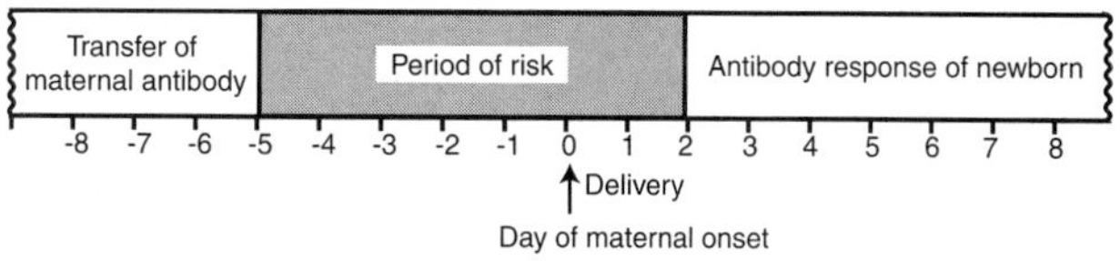

Figure 8 Varicella in newborns. For neonates, the risk of varicella infection and its associated complications is greatest when maternal onset of disease occurs in a 7-day period from 5 days before delivery to 2 days after delivery. Reprinted with permission from reference 71

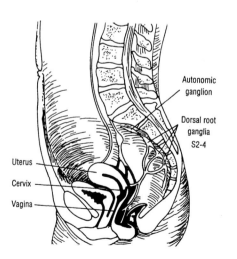

Figure 9 Schematic illustration of the most common reservoirs of latent HSV-2 infection, the sacral ganglia and autonomic ganglion. Reprinted with permission from reference 102

following the onset of maternal rash within 5 days of delivery. If maternal rash appears earlier than 5 days before delivery the rate of transmission to the neonate drops to 18%. Congenital chickenpox presenting between the 5th and 10th days antenatally may result in mortality as high as 20%, presumably owing to the absence of transplacentally acquired antibodies which modify the severity of the disease[1,83]. Maternal rash appearing within the first 2 days postpartum also indicates transplacental exposure to infectious virus without the ameliorating effects of passively acquired maternal antibody, resulting in a 17% risk of congenital varicella in the newborn[71]. Despite some minor controversy[73], VZV seems to have no association with either spontaneous abortion or premature rupture of membranes and no effect upon labor or fetal outcome[79] (Figure 8).

Clinical manifestations

Once infection has occurred, VZV persists in a latent form within satellite cells of sensory nerve ganglia, wherein an infinitesimally small number of viral genes are actively transcribed[38] (Figure 9). Reactivation of latent VZV occurs in 10–20% of people infected with chickenpox as a child and is strongly associated with the decline in cell-mediated immunity resulting from the normal aging process, with immunodeficiency, or immunosuppression. The resulting reactivation of VZV infection is termed herpes zoster, or 'shingles' and is most commonly experienced as a single outbreak in the sixth decade of life[85].

The appearance of a zoster outbreak is often preceded by a 1–4-day prodrome of fever, malaise, dysthesia and head pain. The zoster exanthem develops on one to three adjacent dermatomes, characterized by clusters of vesicles on an erythematous base. The vesicles progress to a pustular state by day 4 and crust over by days 7–10. Healing with scarring due to dermal involvement usually occurs in 2–3 weeks[71]. Zoster is often associated with pain, especially in the form of post-herpetic neuralgia which may persist for months or years. Visceral, ocular, cutaneous and neurological complications of zoster are much less frequent than the pain and may include encephalitis, motor neuropathies including ophthalmoplegia and the Ramsay–Hunt syndrome. While the decline in cell-mediated immunity associated with pregnancy may precipitate an attack of zoster, there is little clinical and no immunological evidence linking maternal zoster with congenital anomalies[73,84] (Table 7).

Etiology

VZV is a large DNA virus, 150–200 nm in diameter. The virus is composed of a nucleocapsid consisting of 162 capsomeres, enclosed by a multilayered, membranous viral envelope punctuated by glycoprotein spikes[71,73]. The double-stranded linear DNA encodes about 75 proteins, including DNA polymerase, ribonucleotide

Table 7 Neurological sequelae of fetal infection with varicella zoster virus. Reprinted with permission from reference 86

Damage to sensory nerves
Cutaneous manifestations
Cicatricial (zigzag) skin lesions
Hypopigmentation

Damage to optic stalk, optic cup and lens vesicle
Microphthalmia
Cataracts
Chorioretinitis
Optic atrophy

Damage to the cervical and lumbosacral cord
Hypoplasia of the upper/lower extremities
Motor /sensory deficits
Absent deep tendon reflexes
Anisocoria/Horner's syndrome
Anal/vesicle sphincter dysfunction

Damage to the brain
Encephalitis
Microcephaly
Hydrocephaly
Calcifications
Aplasia of the brain

reductase, thymidine kinase, and the major DNA-binding protein[71]. The genome is divided into unique long (UL) and unique short (US) regions surrounded by inverted repeat elements. The US region and its repeat element invert during DNA replication, resulting in two isomers of VZV DNA[71] (Figure 10). Although the exact mechanism of VZV viral DNA replication is not clear, the viral origin of replication can be traced to the US region. Amino acid homology with this and other corresponding regions of HSV-2 suggests analogous properties in the enzymes needed for DNA replication. More than 70 RNA transcripts have been recognized and are thought to code for all viral proteins; little is known about the regulation of the viral transcription process[71,73].

The virus occurs as a single serotype without antigenic variation demonstrated among strains of VZV[73].

The structure of the genome itself is relatively unchanging. Molecular studies have shown that variations between unrelated isolates arise from additions or subtractions in the number of small repeated elements in the DNA. It has been hypothesized that discrepancies in the number of amino acid repeats within glycoprotein V (gpV) may correspond to variations in immunogenicity and virulence among differing strains[71]. Minor antigens may be shared with HSV-2[73]. Further study of the five VZV glycoproteins may determine their individual antigenic capacities to elicit host humoral and cell-mediated immune responses[71].

Only humans are susceptible to VZV *in vivo*, an impedance to research and vaccine development; *in vitro*, tissue culture is limited to primate cells. In cultures of human diploid cells and human or simian permanent cell lines, infection with VZV produces giant cells with acidophilic nuclear or cytoplasmic inclusions. Only a small amount of virus is released into the supernatant, resulting in focal arrangement of the characteristic cytopathic effect in culture.

Pathophysiology

In the imunocompetent host, primary infection with VZV is thought to occur in the conjunctivae or nasal mucosa with subsequent local viral replication in cervical lymph nodes followed by primary viremia. Subclinical viremia occurs 1–11 days before onset of exanthem in normal and immunosuppressed patients. This initial viremia is succeeded by viral replication in peripheral blood monocytes and at epithelial sites throughout the body, followed by a secondary viremia with attendant visceral and cutaneous dissemination by way of the capillaries. VZV is both neurotropic and cell-associated; the virus is spread by direct contact to proximal cells. The characteristic pox formed by exudation of clear fluid then occurs at local sites of epithelial degeneration[75,86].

Humoral response to infection with VZV appears 2–5 days after viral exanthem in the form of IgG, IgM

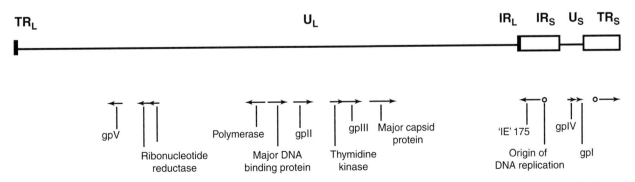

Figure 10 Structure of the varicella zoster virus genome. The unique long sequence (UL) and its flanking terminal (TR_L) and internal repeats (IR_L), and the unique short sequence (US) and its terminal (TR_S) and internal repeats (IR_S) are shown. Origins of DNA replication within IR_S are shown (small open circles), as are the open reading frames and the directions of transcription for several viral gene products including known glycoproteins (gpI–V). Reprinted with permission from reference 71

and IgA antibodies. Maximum antibody titers are reached 14–21 days following onset of rash. Antibody levels diminish thereafter: IgA and IgM are undetectable within 1 year of primary infection; IgG declines, but remains at low numbers[75]. The role of humoral antibody in ameliorating primary infection with varicella is not fully understood. Concomitant agammaglobulinemia in children with varicella does not result in increased morbidity. However, VZV-specific antibody, either maternal in origin or dispensed as zoster immune globulin (ZIG) or varicella zoster immune globulin (VZIG) prophylaxis will lessen the severity of varicella infection, possibly by induction of antibody-dependent cellular cytotoxicity[87], but fails to prevent infection. Those who have experienced primary varicella infection modified by the administration of ZIG, VZIG or maternal antibody may be susceptible to exogenous re-infection resulting in a second primary attack of varicella of more typical clinical course[75].

What implications does this information have for isolation algorithms and management of subsequent pregnancies after maternal primary attack of VZV modified by VZIG or ZIG? Primary infection with VZV results in diminished cell-mediated immunity with reversal of the helper/suppressor T cell ratio[88]. Host ability to launch a cellular immune response to specific antigenic challenge appears to contain VZV in a low-replicative state of quiescence or latency. A depressed cellular immune response, as indicated by diminished or absent response to the lymphocyte proliferation transformation test correlates inversely with the incidence of recrudescent VZV infection or zoster. Diminished cell-mediated immunity decreases with age, is found temporarily in gestation and is a hallmark of infection with HIV-1. Maternal to fetal transmission of VZV is thought to occur transplacentally during the viremia associated with primary VZV infection[77,84]. Garcia's discovery of multiple necrotic foci in the placenta from a spontaneously aborted fetus following varicella in the 4th month of gestation would seem to support this notion[89]. Although infrequent, malformations associated with maternal primary VZV infection in weeks 8–20 of gestation also support the theory of transplacental infection[76]. It has been theorized that the segmental defects arising from the same spinal levels as the cutaneous dermatomal involvement indicate that the fetus develops both varicella and zoster with the segmental deformities secondary to the spinal cord and peripheral nerve involvement associated with zoster[90]. Both primary infection and recrudescence appear to be necessary for the fetus to develop congenital varicella syndrome; thus, maternal varicella infection in the first trimester leaves the exposed fetus most at risk for reactivation (Figure 11).

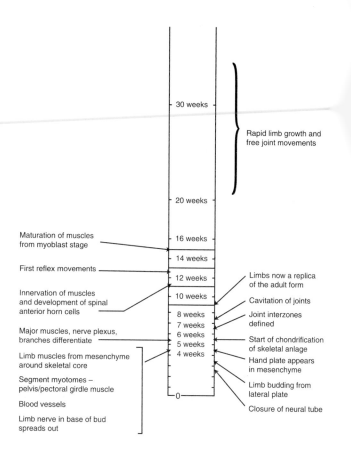

Figure 11 Embryologic events demonstrating the relationship of the timing of maternal varicella infection and subsequent fetal outcome. Reprinted with permission from reference 71

Clinical and laboratory diagnosis

Primary infection with VZV usually manifests as a pruritic, vesicular rash on an erythematous base found on the trunk, face or scalp. Asymptomatic primary infection is rare; subclinical exogenous re-infection as shown by rising antibody titers has been documented. A prodrome of 2–3 days of malaise, joint pain and fever may precede the onset of rash. In typical, uncomplicated varicella, multiple crops of new maculopapules appear for 3–5 days with progression to vesicles, crusting and healing occurring by the 6th day[71]. Complications may include encephalitis, pneumonia, arthritis, localized bacterial super-infections and hemorrhagic varicella[71,76]. Clinical diagnosis is straightforward when history, age, exposure, season and clinical characteristics are evaluated. Differential diagnoses would include visceral or disseminated zoster, disseminated HSV-1, hand-foot-and-mouth disease and rickettsialpox.

Normal and immunosuppressed adults and newborns infected with varicella are far more likely to develop morbid complications than normal children. These may include neurological symptoms such as varicella encephalitis, aseptic meningitis, Guillain–Barré syndrome, transient focal changes and transverse myelitis[71]. Reye's syndrome is more common in children aged 5–14 years. Varicella encephalitis in adults is characterized by sensory alterations, focal neurological signs and seizures. Varicella pneumonia is the most serious complication of primary VZV in an adult. The patient will present 1–6 days after the appearance of the rash with cough, dyspnea, fever and possible pleuritic chest pain. There may be correlation of severe cutaneous disease with higher probability of developing varicella pneumonia[91]. Concomitant high-dose corticosteroid therapy increases the risk of severe infection with VZV[92]. Hepatitis may develop after varicella in immunosuppressed patients. Other less frequent complications may be arthritis, ocular inflammation, carditis and inappropriate antidiuretic hormone syndrome[71].

There does not appear to be any greater risk of morbidity or mortality facing the gravida than the non-pregnant adult woman, although there have been several recent case reports of fatal varicella pneumonia in previously healthy pregnant women[79]. These cases may justify considering pregnant women with varicella pneumonia at grave risk of mortality[71,77]. Even in the absence of a clear history of varicella as many as 75% of adults raised in temperate climates show serological evidence of immunity[93]. The immune status of a patient to varicella when the history is unclear is best determined by indirect ELISA-IgG[71,73]. Complement-fixation titers to VZV tend to decrease over time, making complement fixation insensitive for determining past infection with varicella. Use of the fluorescent antibody against membrane antibody assay (FAMA) may provide the most sensitive detection of past infection with VZV; however, FAMA is not widely available and technically difficult to perform.

Acute infection with VZV is easily detected using vesicular fluid in human diploid cell cultures. Results may be hastened by utilizing the anticomplement immunofluorescence (AC-IF) test for rapid detection of early induced VZV-specific nuclear antigen. Use of counter-current immunoelectrophoresis on vesicular fluid will provide rapid detection of specific antigen, as may direct immunofluorescence staining of cellular material obtained from the base of fresh vesicles[73]. Specific serodiagnosis from two samples 7–10 days apart demonstrating a four-fold or greater rise in IgG antibody titer may be 20% less specific than ELISA, due to cross-reactivity with heterotypic antibody to HSV-2 found following recent primary infection with HSV-2. There is no analogous heterotypic IgM antibody response using the indirect ELISA assay for VZV-specific IgM[73].

Management

The congenital varicella syndrome is characterized by scarred or dermatomal skin lesions, limb hypoplasia, rudimentary digits which are usually unilateral and ipsilateral to the cutaneous involvement, cortical atrophy, chorioretinitis or other ocular or CNS abnormalities, including seizures, brain calcification, Horner's syndrome and mental retardation. The greatest risk of congenital varicella syndrome arises from maternal varicella early in pregnancy with most cases occurring from weeks 8–20 of gestation[77]. Direct proof of maternal varicella as the causative agent of these congenital defects has not yet been established; since virus has not been isolated from these neonates postpartum the link with maternal varicella is based on clinical evidence alone. Other infectious agents such as CMV and *Toxoplasma gondii* should be eliminated from the differential diagnosis by culture and serology[90].

Prenatal diagnosis of the congenital varicella syndrome has been made using ultrasound[94] and with percutaneous umbilical blood sampling (cordocentesis) to detect virus-specific, fetal immune globulin[95]. There is a high correlation of limb defects with brain damage in the congenital varicella syndrome; therefore, therapeutic abortion may be recommended if limb hypoplasia can be visualized by 20 weeks' gestation[96]. Since fetal production of immune globulins may not occur until 20–24 weeks' gestation, assays of fetal blood for antibody response to infection may not be reliable until after 24 weeks, notably too late for those seeking pre-termination confirmation[97]. Chorionic villus sampling and polymerase chain reaction have been used to demonstrate VZV-specific DNA sequences indicating placental infection following maternal varicella; however, this information provides no basis for diagnosis of fetal manifestation of infection[97] (Table 8).

Isolation of virus from vesicular fluid will provide the best means of diagnosis of neonatal VZV infection. Neonatal VZV infection following intrauterine

Table 8 Clinicopathological abnormalities in newborns following maternal gestational varicella infection. Reprinted with permission from reference 76

8–20 weeks of pregnancy
Cicatricial skin lesions, denuded skin, limb hypoplasia, muscular atrophy, dysphagia, rudimentary digits, clubfoot, intrauterine growth retardation, cataracts, nystagmus, optic atrophy, microcephaly, cerebellar and cortical atrophy, seizures, brain calcifications, Horner's syndrome, psychomotor retardation, sensory deficits, micro-ophthalmia, chorioretinitis, herpes zoster, anal sphincter dysfunction, recurrent aspiration pneumonia

Last 3 weeks of pregnancy
Fever, vesicular rash, hemorrhagic rash, cyanosis, respiratory distress, pneumonia, widespread necrotic lesions of the viscera (in fatal cases)

---

transmission of varicella may be clinically asymptomatic, detectable only by immunological means[77]. The clinical course of varicella in the newborn may range from mild illness with a small number of macules and papules appearing for 3–5 days without fever or other symptoms, to a biphasic presentation of several lesions followed by an interval of wellness with a period of generalized eruption of pox later progressing to much more acute illness. There may also be a pattern of prolonged illness with crops of new macules appearing for the first 14 days after birth. Central nervous system involvement is uncommon in neonates. Extensive skin involvement may progress to visceral dissemination and pneumonia; lung involvement in neonates is strongly associated with mortality[98]. Postmortem findings of fatal neonatal varicella have shown areas of focal necrosis, giant cells and intranuclear inclusions throughout the viscera with pulmonic consolidation with edematous fluid and focal necrotic sites[98]. Presentation with herpes zoster in the newborn and infant is also considered evidence of intrauterine VZV infection[98]. Physicians should have a high index of suspicion of intrauterine varicella for any neonate or infant with zoster. Such a patient should be carefully examined for signs of chorioretinitis or dysfunction of the CNS[75].

Therapy

Ideally, pre-conceptual counseling should involve adequate history and screening to determine the patient's immune status. There is a paucity of data regarding the practice and efficacy of offering pre-exposure prophylaxis to non-pregnant women considering conception, especially in the setting of the immunocompromised or immunosuppressed patient. Non-immune pregnant women should be advised to avoid contact with anyone with chickenpox or zoster; although contagion is possible for 2 days prior to the onset of rash, transmission from casual contact does not occur. Given that pregnant women are very likely to have intimate contact with small children, the major reservoir for contagious disease, and the subclinical infectious period characteristic of primary infection with VZV, this advice may be ineffective.

Passive immunization with ZIG or VZIG, which are available from the Red Cross, may ameliorate symptomatic varicella in non-immune persons if administered within 96 h of exposure, although efficacy is thought to be greater with more rapid response. Should the patient's immune status be questionable, results from an ELISA-IgG assay may be available as rapidly as 6 h. Some investigators[71,73,77] advise administration of ZIG (0.2 ml/kg) or VZIG (four 2.0-ml vials intramuscularly) to non-immune pregnant women who have had intimate exposure to varicella or zoster on the basis of maternal risk from varicella pneumonia. No

transmission of hepatitis B or HIV-1 has occurred as a result of use of immune globulins, although there may be transient, passive transfer of antibody to both viruses. No data exist to indicate that post-exposure administration of VZIG or ZIG to pregnant women will eliminate the risk of congenital varicella syndrome. It should be noted that both VZIG and ZIG are extremely expensive, costing over $100. The extremely low risk of congenital varicella syndrome does not make first-trimester maternal varicella an indication for elective abortion. Most women who develop varicella in early pregnancy do not elect termination, owing to the unlikelihood of congenital varicella syndrome[90].

Treatment of uncomplicated maternal varicella should be supportive, with use of an anti-pruritic and cleanliness stressed to prevent bacterial superinfection of lesions. If maternal varicella progresses to pneumonia, many investigators believe that intravenous treatment with the anti-viral acyclovir (7.5 mg/kg every 8 h) is necessary[71,72,81] owing to high maternal morbidity. Although vidarabine (Vira-A) is the only agent approved by the US Food and Drug Administration for the treatment of VZV infections, acyclovir is now believed to be less toxic, more easily administered, owing to the poor solubility of vidarabine, and possibly of greater efficacy. Patient renal function should be monitored. Acyclovir is highly specific for VZV, though a much greater concentration is necessary to inhibit VZV replication *in vitro* than with HSV-2[71], and has been used in a small number of cases of maternal varicella pneumonia with no apparent association with negative fetal outcome[67]. Varicella was the indication for acyclovir for 27 of the 165 women in the USA who were reported to the Acyclovir in Pregnancy Registry[99]. As a category C drug, acyclovir should not be used in gestation unless the potential benefits outweigh the potential fetal risks. Studies of treatment of varicella in immunosuppressed children indicate decreased morbidity from visceral dissemination. More information from collaborative trials is needed to establish the safety and efficacy of acyclovir for maternal varicella pneumonia and for the fetus[67].

VZIG (one 2.0-ml vial intramuscularly)[71,90] or ZIG (2.0 ml/kg)[73] are indicated treatments for neonates of mothers who had onset of varicella less than 6 days before or less than 2 days after delivery to provide some passive antibody to VZV and possibly ameliorate neonatal infection. VZIG and ZIG have no efficacy if administered after the onset of clinical disease[76]. It is important to note that disseminated and fatal cases of congenital chickenpox have occurred despite use of recommended administration of VZIG.

There is speculation that comparable serum acyclovir levels in mother and fetus and high concentration in amniotic fluid would result in greater protection if a maternal acyclovir/neonatal VZIG regimen were adopted[64]. If maternal or neonatal varicella or neonatal zoster develops, contact isolation procedures should be employed in the hospital setting. Any neonate exposed to maternal varicella within 20 days before parturition should also be isolated[79]. Only immune staff should be allowed to interact with a mother or infant with varicella and respiratory isolation is imperative in the case of varicella pneumonia or disseminated varicella[73,96]. Additionally, infants should be isolated from mothers for 5 days following the onset of maternal exanthem[100]. There is no indication for isolating infected newborns from their mothers. There are insufficient data on VZV in breast milk of mothers in either active or convalescent stages of infection[100].

Infants with varicella need careful monitoring; either vidarabine or acyclovir should be started in any case of extensive cutaneous lesions, hepatic enzyme elevation or lung involvement, although neither antiviral therapy is licensed for that use[76]. Non-immune mothers and neonates should avoid home discharge to a setting where there is unavoidable intimate contact with an older sibling who has just developed chickenpox. If no alternative accommodations are available to segregate the susceptible family members, VZIG may be administered at previously mentioned dose levels, especially if the infant was very premature (less than 32 weeks' gestation) or compromised in any way[96].

Prevention of maternal varicella is the only way of eradicating congenital VZV syndrome and varicella in the neonate. There is a live, attenuated varicella vaccine available (Oka strain) but it is as yet unlicensed for use in the USA, although authorized for use in Europe and Japan. Questions remain with the Oka vaccine regarding long-term protective immunity and whether zoster will reactivate at a greater rate in vaccinees, although a prospective study by Lawrence and colleagues[101] indicates the risk of zoster to be lower than that following natural infection with varicella.

ACKNOWLEDGEMENT

I am sincerely grateful to Sandy Kalison-Peccerillo, BS, for her extensive and expert work in all phases of the researching, writing and editing of this manuscript.

REFERENCES

1. Stagno S, Whitley R. Herpesvirus infections of pregnancy. Part II: Herpes simplex virus and varicella-zoster virus infections. *N Engl J Med* 1985;313: 1327–30
2. Whitley R, Nahmias A, Visintine A, *et al*. The natural history of herpes simplex virus infection of mother and newborn. *Pediatrics* 1980;66:489–94
3. Centers for Disease Control and Prevention. Prevention of varicella: recommendations of the Advisory Committee on Immunization Practices (ACIP). *Morbid Mortal Weekly Rep* 1996;45(RR-11): 1–36
4. Baker DA. Herpes virus. *Clin Obstet Gynecol* 1983; 26: 165–72
5. Sullivan-Bolyai J, Hull H, Wilson C, Corey L. Neonatal herpes simplex virus infection in King County, Washinton: increasing incidence and epidemiologic correlates. *J Am Med Assoc* 1983;250:3059–62
6. Nahmias AJ, Keyserling HH, Kerrick G. Herpes simplex. In Remington JS, Klein JO, eds. *Infectious Diseases of the Fetus and Newborn Infant*. Philadelphia: WB Saunders, l983:156–90
7. Corey L, Adams HG, Brown ZA, Holmes KK. Genital herpes simplex virus infections: clinical manifestations, course, and complications. *Ann Intern Med* 1983;98: 958–72
8. Corey L. The diagnosis and treatment of genital herpes. *J Am Med Assoc* 1982;248:1041–4
9. Rooney JF, Felser JM, Ostrove JM, *et al*. Medical intelligence: acquisition of genital herpes from an asymptomatic sexual partner. *N Engl J Med* 1986;314:1561–4
10. Brown Z, Vontver L, Benedetti J, *et al*. Effects on infants of a first episode of genital herpes during pregnancy. *N Engl J Med* 1987;317:1246–51
11. Corey L, Holmes K. Genital herpes simplex virus infections: current concepts in diagnosis, therapy and prevention. *Ann Intern Med* 1983;98:973–83
12. Brown ZA, Selke S, Zeh J. The acquisition of herpes simplex virus during pregnancy. *N Engl J Med* 1997;337:509–15
13. Corey L. Herpes simplex virus. In Holmes KK, ed. *International Perspectives on Neglected Sexually Transmitted Diseases*. Washington, DC: Hemisphere Publishing Corporation, 1983
14. Sweet RL, Gibbs RS. *Infectious Diseases of the Female Genital Tract*, 2nd edn. Baltimore: Williams and Wilkins, 1990:494
15. Yeager A, Arvin A. Reasons for the absence of a history of recurrent genital infections in mothers of neonates infected with herpes simplex virus. *Pediatrics* 1984; 73:188–93
16. Corey L, Spear P. Infections with herpes simplex viruses (Part I). *N Engl J Med* 1986;314:686–91
17. Corey L, Spear P. Infections with herpes simplex viruses (Part II). *N Engl J Med* 1986;314:749–57
18. Lagrew D, Furlow T, Hager W, Yarrish R. Disseminated herpes simplex infection in pregnancy. Successful treatment with acyclovir. *J Am Med Assoc* 1984;252:2058–9
19. Whitley RJ, Hutto C. Neonatal herpes simplex virus infections. *Pediatr Rev* 1985;7:119
20. Hutto C, Arvin A, Jacobs R, *et al*. Intrauterine herpes simplex virus infections. *J Pediatr* 1987;11:97–101
21. Amstey MS, Monif GR. Genital herpes virus infection in pregnancy. *Obstet Gynecol* 1979;44:394
22. Scott LL, Sanchez PJ, Jackson GL, *et al*. Acyclovir suppression to prevent Cesarean delivery after first-episode genital herpes. *Obstet Gynecol* 1996;87:69–73
23. Randolph AG, Hartshorn RM, Washington AE. Acyclovir prophylaxis in late pregnancy to prevent neonatal herpes: A cost-effectiveness analysis. *Obstet Gynecol* 1996;88:603–10
24. Cassai E, Rotola A, Meneguzzi G, *et al*. Herpes simplex virus and human cancer I. Relationship between human

cervical tumors and herpes simplex virus type-2. *Eur J Cancer* 1981;17:685–93

25. Fish EN, Robin SM, Cooter NBE, Papsin ER. Update on the relationship of herpes virus hominis type II to carcinoma of the cervix. *Obstet Gynecol* 1982;59: 220–4

26. Arvin AM, Koropchak CM, Wittek AE. Immunologic evidence for re-infection with varicella-zoster virus. *J Infect Dis* 1983;148:200–5

27. South MA, Tompkins WAF, Morris CR, *et al.* Congenital malformation of the central nervous system associated with genital type (type-2) herpes virus. *J Pediatr* 1969;75:13

28. Florman AL, Gershon AA, Blackett PR, *et al.* Intra-uterine infection with herpes simplex virus: resultant congenital malformations. *J Am Med Assoc* 1973; 225:129

29. Schaffer AJ, Avery ME. *Diseases of the Newborn*, 3rd edn. Philadelphia: WB Saunders, 1971:656

30. Nahmias AJ, Dannenbarger SM. Herpes simplex virus. In Nahmias AJ, Dowdle WR, eds. *The Human Herpes*. New York: Raven Press, 1981

31. Volpi A, Lakeman A, Pereira L, Stagno S. Monoclonal antibodies for rapid diagnosis and typing of genital herpes infections during pregnancy. *Am J Obstet Gynecol* 1983;146:813–5

32. Buchman TG, Roizman B, Nahmias AJ. Demonstration of exogenous genital reinfection with herpes simplex virus type-2 by restriction endonuclease fingerprinting of DNA. *J Infect Dis* 1979; 140:295–304

33. Fife KH, Schmidt O, Remington JS. Primary and recurrent concomitant genital infection with herpes simplex virus type 1 and 2. *J Infect Dis* 1983;147:163

34. Roizman B. An inquiry into the mechanism of recurrent herpes infections of man. *Perspect Virol* 1965; 4:283–301

35. Straus S, Rooney J, Sever J, *et al.* Herpes simplex virus infection: biology, treatment, and prevention. *Ann Intern Med* 1985;103:404–19

36. Shore SL, Nahmias AJ. Immunology of herpes simplex viruses. In Nahmias AJ, O'Rielly RJ, eds. *Immunology of Human Infection*: Part II. *Viruses and Parasites; Immunodiagnosis and Prevention of Infectious Diseases*. New York: Plenum Press, 1981:21–72

37. Galloway DA, Fenoglio C, Shevchufk M, McDougall JK. Detection of herpes simplex RNA in human sensory ganglia. *Virology* 1979;95:265–8

38. Straus S. Clinical and biological differences between recurrent herpes simplex virus and varicella-zoster virus infections. *J Am Med Assoc* 1989;262:3455–8

39. Cunningham AL, Merigan TC. γ-Interferon production appears to predict time of recurrence of herpes labialis. *J Immunol* 1983;130:2397–400

40. Pazin GJ, Armstrong JA, Lam MT, *et al.* Prevention of reactivated herpes simplex infection by human leukocyte interferon after operation on the trigeminal root. *N Engl J Med* 1979;301:225–30

41. Lafferty WE, Coombs RW, Benedetti J, *et al.* Recurrences after oral and genital herpes simplex virus infection: influence of site of infection and viral type. *N Engl J Med* 1987;316:1444

42. Yeager AS, Moris JE, Prober CG. Storage and transport of cultures for herpes simplex virus, type-2. *Am J Clin Pathol* 1979;72:977–9

43. Mosely RC, Corey L, Benjamin D, *et al* . Comparison of viral isolation, direct immunofluorescence, and indirect immunoperoxidase techniques for detection of genital herpes simplex virus infection. *J Clin Microbiol* 1981;13:913–18

44. Lafferty WE, Krofft S, Remington M, *et al.* Diagnosis of herpes simplex virus by direct immunofluorescence and viral isolation from samples of external genital lesions in a high-prevalence population. *J Clin Microbiol* 1987;25:323–6

45. Warford A, Levy R, Rekrut K, Steinberg E. Herpes simplex virus testing of an obstetric population with an antigen enzyme-linked immunosorbent assay. *Am J Obstet Gynecol* 1986;154:21–8

46. Alexander I, Ashley CR, Smith KJ, *et al.* Comparison of ELISA with virus isolation for the diagnosis of genital herpes. *J Clin Pathol* 1985;38:554–7

47. Baker DA, Gonik B, Mitch PO, *et al.* Clinical evaluation of a new herpes simplex virus ELISA: a rapid diagnostic test for herpes simplex virus. *Obstet Gynecol* 1989;73:322–5

48. Lopez C, Roizman B. *Human Herpes Virus Infections*. New York: Raven Press, 1986

49. Arvin A, Hensleigh P, Prober C, *et al.* Failure of antepartum maternal cultures to predict the infant's risk of exposure to herpes simplex virus at delivery. *N Engl J Med* 1986;315:796–800

50. Tejani J, Klein W, Kaplan M. Subclinical herpes simplex genitalis infections in the perinatal period. *Am J Obstet Gynecol* 1979;135:547

51. Scher J, Bottone E, Desmond E, Simons W. The incidence and outcome of asymptomatic herpes simplex genitalis in an obstetric population. *Am J Obstet Gynecol* 1982;144:906–9

52. Wittek A, Yeager A, Au D, Hensleigh P. Asymptomatic shedding of herpes simplex virus from the cervix and lesion during pregnancy. *Am J Dis Child* 1984; 138:439–42

53. Growdon WA, Apodaca L, Cragun J, *et al.* Neonatal herpes simplex virus infection occurring in second twin of an asymptomatic mother. *J Am Med Assoc* 1987;257:508–11

54. Prober C, Hensleigh P, Boucher F, *et al.* Use of routine viral cultures at delivery to identify neonates exposed to herpes simplex virus. *N Engl J Med* 1988;318:887–91

55. Binkin N, Koplan J, Cates W. Preventing neonatal herpes. The value of weekly viral cultures in pregnant women with recurrent genital herpes. *J Am Med Assoc* 1984;251:2816–21

56. Prober C, Sullender W, Yasukawa L, *et al.* Low risk of herpes simplex virus infections in neonates exposed to the virus at the time of vaginal delivery to mothers with recurrent genital herpes simplex virus infections. *N Engl J Med* 1988;316:240–4

57. Gibbs R, Amstey A, Sweet R, *et al.* Management of genital herpes infection in pregnancy. *Obstet Gynecol* 1988;71:779

58. Catalano P, Merritt A, Mead P. Incidence of genital herpes simplex virus at the time of delivery in women

with known risk factors. *Am J Obstet Gynecol* 1991; 164:1303–6

59. Nahmias AJ, Josey WE, Naib ZM, *et al.* Perinatal risk associated with maternal genital herpes simplex virus infection. *Am J Obstet Gynecol* 1971;110:285

60. Goldkrand J. Intrapartum inoculation of herpes simplex virus by fetal scalp electrode. *Obstet Gynecol* 1982;59:263–5

61. Parvey L, Ch'ien L. Neonatal herpes simplex virus infection introduced by fetal-monitor scalp electrodes. *Pediatrics* 1980;65:1150–3

62. Ray D, Evans A, Elliott J, Freeman R. Maternal herpes infection complicated by prolonged premature rupture of membranes. *Am J Perinatol* 1985;2:96–100

63. Utley K, Bromberger P, Wagner L, Schneider H. Management of primary herpes in pregnancy complicated by ruptured membranes and extreme prematurity: case report. *Obstet Gynecol* 1987;69:471–3

64. Cox S, Phillips L, DePaolo H, Faro S. Treatment of disseminated herpes simplex virus in pregnancy with parenteral acyclovir. *J Reprod Med* 1986;31:1005–7

65. Chazotte C, Anderson H, Cohen W. Disseminated herpes simplex infection in an immunocompromised pregnancy: treatment with intravenous acyclovir. *Am J Perinatol* 1987;4:363–4

66. Berger SA, Weinberg M, Treves T, *et al.* Herpes encephalitis during pregnancy: failure of acyclovir and adenine arabinoside to prevent neonatal herpes. *Isr J Med Sci* 1986;22:41

67. Brown Z, Baker D. Acyclovir therapy during pregnancy. *Obstet Gynecol* 1989;73:526–31

68. Dorsky D, Crumpacker C. Drugs five years later: acyclovir. *Ann Intern Med* 1987;107:859–74

69. Whitley RJ, Alford CA, Hirsch MS, *et al.* Vidarabine versus acyclovir therapy in herpes simplex encephalitis. *N Engl J Med* 1986;314:144–9

70. Whitley RJ, Arvin A, Corey L, *et al.* Vidarabine versus acyclovir therapy of neonatal herpes simplex virus, HSV, infection. *Pediatr Res* 1986;20:323A

71. Straus S, Ostrove J, Inchauspe' G, *et al.* Varicella-zoster virus infections. *Ann Intern Med* 1988;108:221–37

72. Preblud S. Varicella: complications and costs. *Pediatrics* 1986;78:728–35

73. Enders G. Varicella-zoster virus infection in pregnancy. *Progress* 1984;29:166–96

74. Prober CG, Arvin AM. Varicella zoster and herpes simplex virus infection. *Eur J Clin Microbiol* 1987;6:245

75. Weller T. Varicella and herpes zoster: changing concepts of the natural history, control and importance of a not-so-benign virus (Part I of II). *N Engl J Med* 1983; 309:1362–8

76. Freij B, Sever J. Herpesvirus infections in pregnancy. *Clin Perinatol* 1988;15:203–31

77. Paryani S, Arvin A. Intrauterine infection with varicella-zoster virus after maternal varicella. *N Engl J Med* 1986;314:1542–6

78. Brunell PA. Transmission of chickenpox in a school setting prior to the observed exanthem. *Am J Dis Child* 1989;143:1451–2

79. Young N, Gershon A. Chickenpox, measles and mumps. In Remington J, Klein J, eds. *Infectious Diseases*

of the Fetus and Newborn Infant, 2nd edn. Philadelphia: WB Saunders, 1983:375–427

80. Leclair J, Zaia J, Levin M, *et al.* Airborne transmission of chickenpox in a hospital. *N Engl J Med* 1980;302: 450–3

81. Preblud S, Cochi S, Orenstein W. Varicella-zoster infection in pregnancy (letter). *N Engl J Med* 1986; 315:1416–17

82. Balducci J, Rodis J, Rosengren S, *et al.* Pregnancy outcome following first-trimester varicella infection. *Obstet Gynecol* 1992;79:5–6

83. Meyers J. Congenital varicella in term infants: risk reconsidered. *J Infect Dis* 1974;129:215–17

84. Paryani SG, Arvin AM. Consequences of varicella or herpes zoster during pregnancy for mother and infant. *Twenty-fourth Interscience Conference on Antimicrobial Agents and Chemotherapy* Washington, DC, 1984

85. Straus S, Reinhold W, Smith H. Endonuclease analysis of viral DNA from varicella and subsequent zoster infection in the same patient. *N Engl J Med* 1984; 311:1362–4

86. Grose C, Itani O. Pathogenesis of congenital infection with three diverse viruses: varicella-zoster virus, human parvovirus, and human immunodeficiency virus. *Semin Perinatol* 1989;13:278–93

87. Gershon AA, Steinberg SP. Inactivation of VZV *in vitro*: effect of leukocytes and specific antibody. *Infect Immunol* 1981;33:507–11

88. Bertotto A, Gentili F, Vaccaro K. Immunoregulatory T cells in varicella. *N Engl J Med* 1982;307:1271–2

89. Garcia A. Fetal infection in chickenpox and alastrim, with histopathologic study of the placenta. *Pediatrics* 1963;32:895–901

90. Gershon AA. Viral infections of infancy. *Comp Ther* 1983;9:9–14

91. Grose C, Itani O, Weiner C. Prenatal diagnosis of fetal infection: advances from amniocentesis to cordocentesis–congenital toxoplasmosis, rubella, cytomegalovirus, varicella virus, parvovirus and human immuno-deficiency virus. *Pediatr Infect Dis J* 1989;8:59–68

92. Zaia JA. Clinical spectrum of varicella-zoster virus infection. In Nahmias AJ, Dowdle WR, Schinazi RE, eds. *The Human Herpesviruses: an Interdisciplinary Perspective*. New York: Elsevier, 1981:10–19

93. Gershon A. Live attenuated varicella vaccine. *Annu Rev Med* 1987;38:41–50

94. Byrne J, Ward K, Kochenour N, Dolcourt J. Prenatal sonographic diagnosis of fetal varicella syndrome. *Am J Hum Genet* 1990;47:A270

95. Cuthbertson G, Weiner C, Giller R, Grose C. Prenatal diagnosis of second-trimester congenital syndrome by virus-specific immunoglobulin M. *J Pediatr* 1987;111: 592–5

96. Prober C, Gershon A, Grose C, *et al.* Consensus: varicella-zoster infections in pregnancy and the perinatal period. *Pediatr Infect Dis J* 1990;9:865–9

97. Isada N, Paar D, Johnson M, *et al. In utero* diagnosis of congenital varicella zoster virus infection by chorionic villus sampling and polymerase chain reaction. *Am J Obstet Gynecol* 1991;165:1727–30

98. Brunell P. Varicella in the womb and beyond. *Pediatr Infect Dis J* 1990;9:770–2

99.   Andrews E, Yankaskas B, Cordero J, *et al*. Committee. TAiPRA. Acyclovir in pregnancy registry: six years' experience. *Obstet Gynecol* 1992;79:7–13

100. Brunell P. Fetal and neonatal varicella-zoster infections. *Semin Perinatol* 1983;7:47–56

101. Lawrence R, Gershon A, Holzman R, Steinberg S, Group NVVCS. The risk of zoster after varicella vaccination in children with leukemia. *N Engl J Med* 1988;318:543–8

102. Millikan LE. *Topics in Clinical Dermatology – Sexually Transmitted Diseases*. New York: Igaku-Shoin Medical Publishers, 1990:115

103. Driscoll CE. Genital herpes: etiology, diagnosis, and management. *Female Patient* 1984;9:42

104. Siegel M. Congenital malformations following chickenpox, measles, mumps, and hepatitis: results of a cohort study. *J Am Med Assoc* 1973;226:1521–4

105. Manson MM, Logan WPD, Loy RM. Rubella and other virus infections during pregnancy. In *Reports on Public Health and Medical Subjects* (no. 101). London: Her Majesty's Stationery Office, 1960

26

Human immunodeficiency virus

S.A. Gall

ETIOLOGY

The human immunodeficiency virus (HIV-1) was first isolated and implicated as the etiological agent in the acquired immunodeficiency syndrome (AIDS) in 1984[1]. This virus was also previously labeled as the human T lymphotropic virus-3 (HTLV-3) or as leukemia-associated virus-1 (LAV-1)[2]. HIV-1 is a single-stranded RNA retrovirus, with a cylindrical core surrounded by a glycoprotein-studded lipid coat[1,2]. The virus is approximately 100 nm in size[2]. The core consists of genomic RNA, reverse transcriptase and core proteins[1]. The principal core proteins are p18 and p24; the principal surface glycoproteins are gp120 and gp41[2].

EPIDEMIOLOGY

The first cases of AIDS were reported in 1981[2]. Initially this infection was appreciated in male homosexuals, but was quickly recognized in other 'high-risk' groups including intravenous drug abusers, hemophiliacs with multiple blood transfusions and Haitians. The disease is now recognized in all categories of patients including heterosexual partners of homosexuals and intravenous drug abusers, children of HIV-positive women and in patients without any known risk factors.

By the end of 1994, more than 500 000 cases of AIDS had been reported to the Center for Disease Control[3]. Conservative estimates are that 14% of AIDS cases are in women, and it is estimated that 79% of affected women are between the ages of 13 and 39 years and are of reproductive age[1]. Women with AIDS are predominantly from minority groups with over 70% from the black or Hispanic communities[1,4]. It is estimated that over 90% of pediatric AIDS patients are children born to HIV-positive women and virtually all new cases in children are from perinatal transmission[5].

As there is an asymptomatic period of time following initial infection with HIV and seroconversion prior to disease progression to AIDS, those patients who manifest symptoms of AIDS represent the 'tip of the iceberg'.

Primary infection with HIV follows direct viral contact with susceptible cells, i.e. CD4 receptor-positive cells[1]. Activities that result in the breaching of normal skin, mucous membranes, and blood barriers lead to infection[1]. HIV has been isolated from a variety of body fluids including blood, semen, vaginal fluids, saliva, tears and breast milk. Activities that would place an individual at risk for exposure to HIV include intravenous drug use with shared contaminated needles, transfusion of blood products contaminated with HIV, or intercourse that would expose rectal or vaginal mucosa to contaminated body fluids[1].

PATHOPHYSIOLOGY

As noted above, a cell is considered susceptible to HIV infection if it has surface expression of a specific glycoprotein antigen, CD4 (also OKT4A, Leu 3A), recognized by the 'comparable' glycoprotein gp120 noted on the surface of the HIV virus[1]. Cells which demonstrate the CD4 antigen and which may therefore be susceptible include helper–inducer T lymphocytes (T4 cells), B lymphocytes, monocytes, macrophages, Langerhans cells, endothelial cells, astrocytes, oligodendrogliocytes and neuroretinal cells[1]. The virus attaches to the CD4 receptor of the cell and enters the cell for replication. Reverse transcriptase is employed in the formation of double-stranded DNA. The newly formed DNA becomes circular and enters the host cell nucleus where it becomes integrated into the cell's DNA[1,2]. The fusion of the virus to the cell membrane is pH independent[1]. Once DNA transcription is initiated, viral proteins are synthesized and ultimately viral RNA and proteins are assembled at the cell surface. New virons are formed by budding. These virons demonstrate the glycoproteins gp120 as well as additional transmembrane protein gp41[1] (Figure 1). It is thought that the glycoprotein gp41 may be responsible for cell-to-cell fusion resulting in multinucleated giant cell formation, cellular swelling and eventual host cell death[1]. Each infected cell ultimately dies or is unable to continue to function in a normal capacity. The length of time to cell death is variable, with some cells, e.g. monocytes and macrophages[1], demonstrating less frequent syncytium formation and cell death.

It is through the destruction of the helper T4 lymphocytes and subsequent loss of cellular immune functions that HIV demonstrates its true pathogenesis. The impaired T4 lymphocyte is unable to recognize antigens and replicate in response, or incite other cells of the immune system to respond appropriately[1]. The infected monocyte can pass through the blood–brain barrier and can be found in other organs, including the lung and bone marrow. In the brain, the release of monokines and proteolytic enzymes is toxic to neural and glial tissues[1,2]. Infected macrophages do not show proper chemotaxis, and the infected B cell will have a poor response to a new antigen but will release high levels of immunoglobulin[1]. Decreased cellular immune function leaves the infected host susceptible to opportunistic infections and malignancies that lead to host death.

DIAGNOSIS

Detection of HIV antibody for diagnosis is through either enzyme-linked immunosorbent assay (ELISA) or through Western blot. The ELISA method is used as an initial screening test with the Western blot used as a confirmatory test[2]. To be considered positive, the Western blot test must detect antibody to multiple virus-specific bands, i.e. p24, p31 and either gp41 or gp160[2]. If these criteria are not met, the test is considered indeterminate. To be interpreted as negative by Western blot, no bands should be detected[2]. Sever[2] reported that up to 15–20% of tests on a low-risk population may be indeterminate, with a very low false-positive or false-negative rate. Diagnosis in the newborn child is problematic in that maternal IgG HIV antibody is known to cross the placenta and will result in a positive test in the uninfected infant for up to 15 months[6].

Maternal IgG may persist in the neonatal circulation for up to 15 months. A reliable test for HIV-specific IgM has not yet been developed, and culture for HIV may take up to 4 weeks to complete. The measurement of p24 antigen in plasma is an insensitive marker of infection, with sensitivity of 50%[7].

The polymerase chain reaction (PCR) takes 2–3 days to complete. If the PCR is negative, the neonate is very unlikely to have HIV[7–9]. The concordance rate ranges from 96 to 100% for culture and PCR[6–8]. Five of seven neonates and six of six infants who tested positive in the postnatal period (> 28 days) later developed AIDS[7]. An active replication of HIV may ensue during the first weeks of life, reflecting the occurrence of late contamination[10].

Prior to the availability of antibody identification, the diagnosis of AIDS, the end-stage manifestation of HIV infection, was on a clinical basis. Current classification by the Center for Disease Control (CDC)[11] permits a diagnosis by the following criteria without laboratory confirmation and exclusion of other causes of immunodeficiency.

(1) Candidiasis of the esophagus, trachea, bronchi, or lungs;

(2) Extra-pulmonary cryptococcoses;

(3) Cryptosporidiosis with diarrhea persisting longer than 1 month;

(4) Cytomegalovirus infection of an organ other than liver, spleen, or lymph nodes in a patient over 1 month of age;

(5) Herpes simplex virus infection causing a mucocutaneous ulcer that persists longer than 1 month, or bronchitis, pneumonitis, or esophagitis for any duration affecting a patient over 1 month of age;

(6) Kaposi's sarcoma affecting a patient under 60 years of age;

(7) Lymphoma of the brain affecting a patient under 60 years of age;

(8) Lymphoid interstitial pneumonia or pulmonary lymphoid hyperplasia affecting a child under 13 years of age;

(9) Disseminated *Mycobacterium avium* or *M. Kansasii* disease;

(10) *Pneumocystis carinii* pneumonia;

(11) Progressive multifocal leukoencephalopathy; or

(12) Toxoplasmosis of the brain affecting a patient over 1 month of age.

With laboratory confirmation of HIV infection regardless of other causes of immunodeficiency:

(1) Multiple or recurrent bacterial infections caused by *Haemophilus*, *Streptococcus* or other pyogenic bacteria affecting a child under 13 years of age;

(2) Disseminated coccidiomycosis;

(3) HIV encephalopathy;

(4) Disseminated histoplasmosis;

(5) Isoporiasis with diarrhea persisting longer than 1 month;

(6) Kaposi's sarcoma at any age;

(7) Lymphoma of the brain at any age;

(8) Other non-Hodgkin's lymphoma of B cell or unknown immunological phenotype, and small non-cleaved lymphoma or immunoblastic sarcoma of histological type;

(9) Any disseminated mycobacterial disease caused by species other than *M. tuberculosis*;

(10) Extra-pulmonary *M. tuberculosis* infection;

(11) Recurrent *Salmonella* septicemia; or

(12) HIV wasting syndrome.

It is generally recognized that there are three stages to HIV infection. The initial infection may be asymptomatic and the only evidence of infection may be positive immunological testing. Other infected individuals may demonstrate a self limited and brief febrile illness similar to mononucleosis and complain of fatigue and malaise. Rarely, neurological symptoms will be seen;

these include seizures, encephalitis and peripheral neuropathy[1]. These symptoms are self limited.

Following initial infection there is an asymptomatic incubation state. This state is variable in length but may last up to 10 years, and may depend upon the age, nutritional status and general health of the individual. Although the infection is asymptomatic, viral replication occurs and the virus can be found in body fluids and secretions, rendering these individuals infectious[6].

The second stage of HIV infection is a more severe and symptomatic form previously described as AIDS-related complex (ARC). The most common clinical manifestation of ARC is a persistent and generalized lymphadenopathy with lymph node enlargement noted in two or more sites other than the groin for a duration of over 3 months. Other signs and symptoms include night sweats, fever, diarrhea, weight loss and fatigue. Unusual infections may develop, such as oral candidiasis or herpes zoster[1]. It has been estimated that after 2 years in this condition 20% of individuals will progress to AIDS and that, following 4.5 years, approximately 30% of patients will show progression to AIDS[1].

The third and most severe stage of HIV infection is the complete syndrome, AIDS. As noted above in the CDC classification, this stage is characterized by opportunistic infections, uncommon or unusual malignancies and cachexia.

Early reports of pregnancy in the AIDS patient suggested that pregnancy had a detrimental effect and resulted in a more rapid progression of this disease. These reports were possibly biased by delayed diagnosis, however, and involved HIV-positive patients identified on a retrospective basis following the birth of infected infants. These patients may have represented a population of patients in a state of advanced disease prior to diagnosis[1]. The true effect of pregnancy on AIDS or HIV infection is still not known[1,12].

PERINATAL TRANSMISSIONS

The effect of HIV on pregnancy is not well established. Positive HIV serostatus in itself has not been shown to have a major negative effect on the outcome of pregnancy, but may help identify a group of patients with a variety of risk factors associated with complications[11]. It has been well established that vertical transmission from the gravid patient to her fetus does occur, but the rate of vertical transmission is not completely clear[12]. In their review, Landesman and colleagues[12] estimated the risk of perinatal transmission by transplacental infection to be between 30% and 73%. Transplacental transmission of HIV is the major route of infection in infants and has been reported as the route of infection for approximately 75–80% of pediatric AIDS cases[12]. Two factors have been cited as being important as predictors of vertical transmission. The first factor is previous vertical transmission to a fetus, and the second factor is severely depressed immune function[1]. It should be noted that twin pregnancies may be discordantly infected and that women who have previously delivered an HIV-positive infant have subsequently delivered persistently HIV-negative children[1,6,11–13]. HIV has been isolated from amniotic fluid at a variety of gestational ages and from fetal tissue at 14 weeks[1]. Concurrent maternal syphilis infection is significantly associated with vertical perinatal HIV-1 transmission[14].

Typically, most infants delivered to HIV-positive patients will be asymptomatic at birth[6]. Maternal IgG will be present at birth but will gradually decline[6]. Some infants who have lost maternal IgG and fail to form IgM may be infected and viral culture and/or PCR testing is necessary to confirm infection[6]. In most circumstances the infected infant will demonstrate neonatal derived anti-HIV IgG antibody in 4–8 weeks[6].

It should be noted that the pattern of clinical infection in infants differs from that seen in adults. Infants will demonstrate opportunistic infections, fever and weight loss as seen in adults, but will also show an increased incidence of bacterial sepsis, lymphoid interstitial pneumonitis and a low risk of Kaposi's sarcoma[6]. The infected infant will show an inability to respond to neoantigens such as standard bacterial toxoids and a defective ability to develop a primary immune response to common antigens[6]. Neurological manifestations of infection in the pediatric patient include a static or progressive encephalopathy with loss of developmental milestones and intellectual ability, progressive weakness with pyramidal tract signs and impaired brain growth[6].

A dysmorphic syndrome has been described by Marion and co-workers[15] in infants and children with HIV infection, presumably following viremia early in fetal development[6]. Features of this syndrome include growth failure, microcephaly and craniofacial abnormalities (ocular hypertelorism, box-like forehead, flat nasal bridge, upward or downward obliquity of the eyes, long palpebral fissures, blue sclera, short nose with flattened columella, triangular philtrum and patulous lips)[6,15].

MANAGEMENT

Management of the HIV-seropositive patient should be directed at decreasing risk to the fetus and therapy to decrease opportunistic infections. In order to identify those pregnant women who are HIV seropositive, a policy of universal testing of all pregnant women is highly desirable. In addition to routine antenatal testing, a baseline CD4 T-cell count should be obtained as well as HIV RNA titer, and serology for toxoplasmosis, herpes simplex virus, and syphilis. The CD4 count and HIV RNA titer should be repeated in each trimester. The purpose of the CD4 count is to use it as a guide to the initiation of other prophylactic therapy. Patients with CD4 counts under 200 cells/μl or less than 20% of their total lymphocyte count carry a significant risk of opportunistic infection, particularly *P. carinii* pneumonia.

The mainstay of management is the initiation of zidovudine therapy during pregnancy and labor and in the infant. Data from the pediatric AIDS clinical trial group protocol 076 and 185 indicate that zidovudine should be administered during pregnancy and labor and to the neonate[16,17].

The pediatric AIDS clinical trial group protocol (PACTG) 076 was a randomized double-blinded placebo-controlled study of the efficacy and safety of zidovudine (ZDV) in reducing the risk of perinatal transmission of HIV. The protocol is summarized in Table 1. This protocol was limited to pregnant patients with CD4+ T-lymphocyte counts above 200 cells/μl and no prior ZDV therapy. Analysis of the results of 419 infants showed that 7.6% of the infants in the ZDV group were infected compared to 22.6% of the infants in the placebo group, a 66% reduction in the risk of perinatal transmission[16]. Another protocol, PACTG 185, studied pregnant patients with advanced HIV-1 disease, low CD4+ T-lymphocyte counts, and prior antiretroviral therapy. The protocol was similar to the one described in Table 1, with the addition of intravenous infusion of either hyperimmune HIV-1 immunoglobulin (HIVIgG) or standard immunoglobulin (IgG) without HIV-1 antibodies, monthly during pregnancy and at 6 weeks, 3 months, 6 months, 12 months, and 18 months postpartum. The perinatal transmission rates were 10% and 3.6% for patients with CD4+ T-lymphocyte counts < 200 cells/μl and > 200 cells/μl respectively. There was no significant difference in the perinatal transmission rates regarding the timing of ZDV therapy (before vs. during pregnancy) or the type of immunoglobulin transfusion (HIVIgG vs. IgG groups)[17]. This study also demonstrated the effectiveness of ZDV prophylaxis in reducing perinatal HIV transmission in patients with advanced HIV-1 disease[17]. Maternal administration of ZDV does not appear to increase the fetal risks

of congenital anomalies or postnatal problems such as malignancies, growth, neurodevelopment and immunologic status. Similarly, the maternal CD4+ T-lymphocyte counts and clinical status at 18 months postpartum are not affected by maternal administration of ZDV for reduction of perinatal transmission[18].

The mechanism by which zidovudine reduces the risk of perinatal HIV transmission has not been well established. Possible factors include diminished fetal exposure to HIV virus from a reduction of viral load in the maternal circulation, conversion of ZDV into an active metabolite by the placenta, and pre-exposure chemoprophylaxis of the infants[18]. A recent study demonstrated that in patients who received ZDV during pregnancy, the maternal plasma HIV-1 RNA level was the best predictor of the risk of perinatal transmission of HIV-1 infection, with minimal risk associated with maternal HIV-1 RNA level less than 500 copies/ml[19].

Despite therapy some infants treated with zidovudine became infected. These infections could have occurred as the result of (1) HIV transmission before treatment; (2) inefficient suppression of viral replication with zidovudine; (3) non-compliance with the protocol; or (4) a unique strain of HIV with increased resistance to zidovudine.

The severity of immune dysfunction in the AIDS patients can also be followed by assessment of the T4/T8 ratio. However, normal pregnancies show a decreased ratio from the normal non-pregnant range of 1.7–2.3 to a normal pregnancy range of 0.9–1.92[1]. The T4 depression in pregnant, HIV-seropositive patients can result in ratios as low as 0.1–0.8[1].

In addition to the above laboratory determinations, the HIV-seropositive patient is at higher risk for other sexually transmitted diseases and tuberculosis, and should be tested for these during her antepartum course.

As noted above, those patients with severe immune depression should receive *Pneumocystis carinii* pneumonia prophylaxis as there is a 5–20% mortality rate associated with the patient's first episode, and without prophylaxis there is a high recurrence rate[20]. The two most common agents used for prophylaxis are oral

Table 1 Pediatric AIDs Clinical Trials Group (PACTG) 076 zidovudine (ZDV) regimen

Time of ZDV administration	Regimen
Antepartum	Oral administration of 100 mg ZDV five times daily, initiated at 14–34 weeks' gestation and continued throughout the pregnancy
Intrapartum	During labor, intravenous administration of ZDV in a 1-hour initial dose of 2 mg/kg body weight, followed by a continuous infusion of 1 mg/kg body weight/hour until delivery
Postpartum	Oral administration of ZDV to the newborn (ZDV syrup at 2 mg/kg body weight/dose every 6 hours) for the first 6 weeks of life, beginning at 8–12 hours after birth. (Note: intravenous dosage for infants who can not tolerate oral intake is 1.5 mg/kg body weight intravenously every 6 hours)

trimethoprim–sulfamethoxazole or aerosolized pentamidine[20]. Oral trimethoprim–sulfamethoxazole, one double-strength tablet twice daily with folinic acid, 5 mg once daily, is effective but often poorly tolerated. Reactions such as fever, rash, neutropenia or elevated transaminase levels will dictate a change to a low-dose regimen[20]. A low-dose regimen of one tablet three times a week without folinic acid is better tolerated and reported to be effective[20].

Monthly treatment with aerosolized pentamidine is also effective if given in a dose of 300 mg. This regimen has been associated with both local and systemic failure, is expensive, and requires a system that allows delivery of the drug to the alveoli and yet protects others from aerosolized contamination. Toxicity most commonly associated with pentamidine causes cough and bronchospasm. Other reactions include neutropenia, anemia, liver function abnormalities, renal insufficiency and hyper- and hypoglycemia[20].

Management of the HIV-seropositive patient beyond appropriate laboratory monitoring and prophylactic therapy should include frequent examination for neurological and constitutional symptoms as well as for evidence of premature labor and intrauterine growth retardation[6]. Invasive tests such as funicentesis or amniocentesis should be avoided for fear of increasing the risk of transmission of HIV to the fetus[1,6,12]. Although intrapartum management should not be compromised, the use of fetal scalp electrodes and scalp pH determinations should be limited for the same reason[6,12]. It is unclear whether Cesarean section reduces perinatal transmission[12,21]. However, 'bloodless Cesarean section' with utmost attention to hemostasis and minimal contact of infant to maternal blood during the operation reduces the relative risk of perinatal transmission to 73.4% in patients who do not receive ZDV therapy during pregnancy[21].

As HIV can be transmitted through breast milk, the patient should be discouraged from breast-feeding her infant. There is no need for isolation of the patient or her infant.

Finally, efforts must be focused on the prevention of spread through a variety of activities, including patient education and the use of universal precautions with all patients. The seropositive patient should be counseled regarding the availability of abortion in early pregnancy and the use of proper contraceptives as well as measures that will help prevent the spread of her disease. Occupational exposure of the health care worker is minimized by the use of universal precaution. As of June 1997, 52 US health care workers (HCWs) with documented seroconversion temporally associated with an occupational HIV exposure were reported. The majority of these infections were through percutaneous exposure (87%). The average risk for HIV transmission from a percutaneous exposure or a mucous membrane exposure to HIV-infected blood is about 0.3% or 0.1% respectively. The risk of HIV transmission after a skin exposure to HIV-infected blood is unknown but likely to be less than 0.1%[22,23].

Just as the health care worker is concerned over the possible acquisition of disease from an occupational exposure, recent publicity of transmission from the health care provider to the patient has caused some concern in the uninfected patient. As of May 1993, there was no evidence of transmission of HIV from HIV-infected health care workers to patients except the six patients who received dental care from a single Florida dental practice[24].

REFERENCES

1. Wenstrom KD, Gall SA. HIV infection in women. *Obstet Gynecol Clin North Am* 1989;16:627
2. Sever JL. HIV: biology and immunology. *Clin Obstet Gynecol* 1989;32:423
3. Center for Disease Control. The first 500,000 AIDS cases – United States. *Morbid Mortal Weekly Rep* 1995;44:849–53
4. Willoughby A. AIDS in women: epidemiology. *Clin Obstet Gynecol* 1989;32:429
5. Davis SF, Byers RH, Lindegren ML, *et al.* Prevalence and incidence of vertically acquired HIV infection in the United States. *J Am Med Assoc* 1995;294:952–5
6. Gall SA. Human immunodeficiency virus infection in pregnancy. *Immunol Allergy Clin North Am* 1990;10:133
7. Krivine A, Yakudima A, Le May M, *et al.* A comparative study of virus isolation, PCR, and antigen detection in children of mothers infected with HIV. *J Pediatr* 1990;116:372–6
8. Rogers MF, Ou CY, Rayfield M, *et al.* Use of PCR for early detection of the proviral sequences of HIV in infants born to seropositive mothers. New York City Collaborative Study of Maternal HIV Transmission and Montefiore Medical Center HIV Perinatal Transmission Study Group. *N Engl J Med* 1989;320:1649–54
9. Fang G, Burger H, Grimson R, *et al.* Maternal plasma human immunodeficiency virus type I RNA level: a determinant and projected threshold for mother to child transmission. *Proc Natl Acad Sci USA* 1995;92:12100–4
10. Krivine A, Firstion G, Cao L, *et al.* HIV replication during the first weeks of life. *Lancet* 1992;339:1187
11. Center for Disease Control. Revision of the CDC surveillance case definition for acquired immunodeficiency syndrome. *Morbid Mortal Weekly Rep* 1987;36:4S–5S
12. Landesman SH, Kalish LA, Burns ON, *et al.* Obstetrical factors and the transmission of human immunodeficiency virus tupe I from mother to child. *N Engl J Med* 1996;334:1617–23
13. Goedert JJ, Duliege AM, Amos CI, *et al.* High risk of HIV-1 infection for first-born twins. The International Registry of HIV-exposed twins. *Lancet* 1991;338:1471
14. Lee M-J, Hallmark RJ, Frenkel LM, *et al.* Maternal syphilis and vertical perinatal transmission of human immunodeficiency virus type-1 infection. *Int J Gynaecol Obstet* 1998;63:247–52

15. Marion RW, Wiznia AA, Hutcheon RG, *et al*. Human T-cell lymphotrophic virus type III (HTLV-III) embryopathy. *Am J Dis Child* 1986;140:638

16. Sperling RS, Shapiro DE, Coombs RW, *et al*. Maternal viral load, zidovudine treatment, and the risk of transmission of human immunodeficiency virus type 1 from mother to infant. *N Engl J Med* 1996;335:1621–9

17. Stiehm ER, Lambert JS, Mofenson LM, *et al*. Efficacy of zidovudine and human immunodeficiency virus (HIV) hyperimmune immunoglobulin for reducing perinatal HIV transmission from HIV-infected women with advanced disease: results of Pediatric AIDS Clinical Trials Group protocol 185. *J Infect Dis* 1999;179:567–75

18. Public Health Service Task Force. Recommendations for the use of antiretroviral drugs in pregnant women infected with HIV-1 for maternal health and for reducing perinatal HIV-1 transmission in the United States. *Morbid Mortal Weekly Rep* 1998;47 (RR-2):1–30

19. Mofenson LM, Lambert JS, Stiehm ER, *et al*. Risk factors for perinatal transmission of human immunodeficiency virus type 1 in women treated with zidovudine. Pediatric AIDS Clinical Trials Group Study 185 Team. *N Engl J Med* 1999;341:385–93

20. Sperling RS, Stratton P. Treatment options for human immunodeficiency virus-infected pregnant women. *Obstet Gynecol* 1992;79;443–8

21. Towers CV, Deveikis A, Asrat T, *et al*. A "bloodless cesarean section" and perinatal transmission of the human immunodeficiency virus. *Am J Obstet Gynecol* 1998;179:708–14

22. Center for Disease Control. Surveillance for occupationally acquired HIV infection – United States, 1981–1992. *Morbid Mortal Weekly Rep* 1992;41:823

23. Public Health Service Guidelines for the management of health-care worker exposures to HIV and recommendations for postexposure prophylaxis. *Morbid Mortal Weekly Rep* 1998;47(RR-7):1–33

24. Update: investigations of persons treated by HIV-infected health-care workers – United States. *Morbid Mortal Weekly Rep* 1993;42(RR-17):329–31, 337

27
Other viral infections

S.A. Gall

CONDYLOMA ACUMINATA

Etiology

It has been well established in recent years that condyloma acuminata, fibroepithelial tumors of the anogenital region, are secondary to infection with the papilloma virus. These viruses are members of the papovavirus family, all characterized by a circular, double-stranded DNA genome, and an icosahedral capsid[1]. The papilloma virus particle has a diameter of 55 nm, and lacks a lipid membrane envelope[1]. The viral genome is approximately 7900 base pairs in length[1].

Not only are the members of the papovavirus family host specific but each identified subtype is also highly tissue specific. At present there are at least 68 distinct human papilloma virus (HPV) subtypes, each with a significant difference in the DNA sequence of its genome[1]. The HPV subtypes most commonly associated with anogenital lesions are HPV 6, 11, 16, 18, 31, 33, 35, 39, 42, 43 and 44[1].

Epidemiology

The prevalence of genital HPV infection in sexually active adults is approximately 1% for visible genital warts and at least 15% for subclinical infection as detected by HPV DNA[2]. In general, transmission of HPV responsible for condyloma acuminata is by sexual contact. These viral particles are, however, partially stable to heat and desiccation, which may allow for infection in some cases without direct contact between individuals[1]. Autoinoculation to either distant sites or tissue adjacent to a primary infection does occur.

Most investigators agree that there must be direct contact between fully formed and viable virions and squamous epithelial membranes for infection to occur. As will be noted below, the primary infection is seen in the basal cells of the epidermis, indicating that inoculation must occur through abrasions, fissures or minute tears in the epithelial membranes[1,3].

Early estimates of prevalence rates of clinically evident HPV infection in pregnancy are approximately 1.5%[1,3]. However, there are recent estimates that 20% of the population is affected. The investigator reported that by the filter *in situ* hybridization technique, 28% of cytologically negative pregnant women were positive for HPV DNA[4]. Of special interest is the concurrent finding that only 12.5% of non-pregnant women were positive for HPV DNA by the same technique[4].

Pathophysiology

The papilloma virus primarily infects the keratinocyte of the squamous epidermis and will induce acanthosis or hyperplasia of the intermediate layers of the epidermis[1]. Histological examination of infected tissue will demonstrate koilocytes, cells demonstrating perinuclear vacuolization and nuclear hyperchromasia and convolution[1]. Koilocytes are seen in the more superficial layers of the epidermis, presumably where new viral particles are assembled[1].

Human papilloma virus DNA is present in a majority of cervical cancers, with the viral DNA integrated into the DNA of the host cell[1]. The association between HPV 16 and 18 and invasive carcinoma to the cervix is well established. Fortunately the incidence of cancer of the cervix in pregnancy is low and estimated at one per 1500 or less[3]. More commonly, HPV infection is associated with cervical intraepithelial neoplasia (CIN), especially subtypes 6 and 11.

Of particular concern in pregnancy is the possible transmission of any maternal infection to the fetus. Intrauterine infection with HPV has not been documented[3]. Evidence from both electron microscopic examination and clinical observations has suggested a link between maternal anogenital papilloma and subsequent juvenile laryngeal papilloma (JLP)[5]. Transmission via intrapartum events is thought to be by viral DNA in vaginal secretions[3]. The papilloma virus subtype most consistently linked to JLP is HPV 6[3].

The higher rate of both prevalence and incidence of HPV in pregnancy, as well as an increased rate of viral replication in pregnancy, may be secondary to the altered immunocompetence of normal pregnancy, or secondary to increased levels and influence of sex steroid hormones noted in pregnancy[3].

Diagnosis and management

Diagnosis of condyloma acuminata is often made by clinical examination. Lesions are commonly found on the cervix, vagina, clitoris, vulva, perineal body and urethra or in the perineal region. Infection is also often subclinical and demonstrated only in abnormal cytology, e.g. CIN, vaginal intraepithelial neoplasia, vulvar intraepithelial neoplasia, or in the presence of invasive squamous cell carcinoma of the genital tract. Diagnosis of flat condyloma is often made only after colposcopic examination or colposcopic directed biopsy. Although the typical lesions of condyloma acuminata are multiple and polymorphic, biopsy may be necessary to make the diagnosis in a persistent or atypical lesion. If a lesion demonstrates rapid growth, friability or bleeding, or if it is particularly painful, biopsy should be performed to rule out invasive carcinoma. Lesions identified by abnormal cytology or by colposcopic examination warrant biopsy to establish the grade of CIN or to rule out invasive disease.

Included in the differential diagnosis of condyloma acuminata are condyloma lata of secondary syphilis, granuloma inguinale, carcinoma of the vulva, fibroepitheliomas, seborrheic keratosis and molluscum contagiosum.

Condyloma acuminata may be sufficiently large to result in significant discomfort and pruritus, may become secondarily infected or be the source of significant bleeding[3]. Infectious complications may subsequently be a source of premature spontaneous rupture of the membranes, chorioamnionitis or intrapartum fetal infection[3]. Extremely large condyloma may obstruct vaginal delivery or result in increased obstetric hemorrhage.

The subset of patients who have abnormal cytology or CIN, as noted above, warrant colposcopic evaluation and follow-up at 2–3-month intervals[3]. Treatment for CIN can be delayed until the patient is 2–3 months postpartum in most cases[3]. If the diagnosis of invasive carcinoma is made, management is based on the gestational age at diagnosis and the desires of the patient, and is beyond the scope of this chapter.

Genital condyloma acuminata have been noted to show spontaneous resolution near term and postpartum in many individuals[3]. Safe treatment modalities during pregnancy include trichloracetic acid, electrocoagulation, electrodesiccation, cryotherapy and ablation with the carbon dioxide laser[3,6]. Agents commonly used in the non-pregnant patient such as podophyllin, 5% 5-fluorouracil cream or bleomycin are contraindicated during pregnancy because of possible systemic absorption and possible significant side-effects and morbidity in both the mother and the fetus[3,6]. The use of interferon or autologous vaccine injection for treatment in pregnancy has not been fully evaluated and is currently contraindicated.

The exposed neonate may develop condyloma of the conjunctiva or the anogenital regions[3]. Of more concern is the previously noted risk of JLP. Laryngeal papilloma manifests clinically as an abnormal cry or hoarseness. This process may eventually lead to respiratory distress and stridor[5]. Laryngeal papillomas are multiple and occur most frequently on the true vocal cords. Extensive laryngeal papillomas may involve the supraglottic endolarynx, subglottic area, trachea and bronchi[5]. Juvenile laryngeal papillomas are often resistant to therapy with frequent recurrences necessitating repeated treatments or procedures[3]. Treatment modalities for JLP include repeated forceps removal, cryotherapy, electrocautery, electrodiathermy, ultrasound therapy, radiotherapy and carbon dioxide laser vaporization combined with interferon injections[3].

In the pregnancy complicated by the presence of genital condyloma acuminata, the estimated risk of transmission of HPV to the newborn is between 1 in 80 and 1 in 1500[3]. No cases of JLP were found in 55 000 mother–baby pairs of the national Perinatal Collaborative Study after 5 years of follow-up. Juvenile laryngeal papillomatosis has been reported after Cesarean section in at least one case[3]. A more recent study of 151 pregnant women having HPV infection, using polymerase chain reaction (PCR) to detect HPV deoxyribonucleic acid (DNA) in the infants up to 3 years of age, revealed that the upper 95% confidence interval of the risk of perinatal HPV transmission to the newborn was 2.8%[7]. In addition, no infant had any clinical manifestation of HPV infection[7]. The association between maternal condyloma acuminata and subsequent JLP is not strong enough to dictate Cesarean section when maternal HPV clinical infection is present.

MOLLUSCUM CONTAGIOSUM

Epidemiology

Molluscum contagiosum is a disease of humans with a worldwide distribution, and is found in patients of all ages. This disease is spread by sexual intercourse or by fomites[8].

Etiology

The poxvirus responsible for molluscum contagiosum is a large virus, 250–320 nm in diameter, containing double-stranded DNA. This virus has a long incubation period of 2 weeks to 2 months[8].

Pathophysiology

The disease molluscum contagiosum is secondary to viral infection and replication of the poxvirus in the cytoplasm of both basal and parabasal keratinocytes[9,10]. The infection results in a usually benign and self-limited disorder of the skin. The lesions typical of molluscum contagiosum are characterized by a complete lack of any immunocompetent cells in the epithelial component of these lesions[9]. The surrounding epidermis demonstrates an increase of normal Langerhans cells[9].

Atypical cases of severe and refractory eruptions secondary to molluscum contagiosum have been seen in the immunocompromised host, e.g. in the patient with acquired immunodeficiency syndrome (AIDS), chronic lymphocytic leukemia, sarcoidosis, atopic eczema, malignant thymoma and congenital immunodeficiency[10]. Atypical infection can follow iatrogenic immunosuppressive therapy[10]. In the immunosuppressed host, spontaneous resolution of molluscum contagiosum may not occur[10].

Diagnosis and management

The primary sites of infection with molluscum contagiosum include the eyelids, face, trunk and anogenital regions[8]. The disease is easily recognized by the characteristic clinical features, that is, small discrete waxy, flesh-colored umbilicated papules[11]. If biopsied, intracytoplasmic molluscum bodies are seen on microscopic examination, but may be obscured on occasion by dense inflammatory infiltrates[8].

The differential diagnosis of molluscum contagiosum includes lichen planus, verrucous papules, basal cell epithelioma and pyogenic granuloma[8].

Lesion may persist for months to several years, but following regression, recurrences are rare. Sharp curettage or expression of the porous material will aid in healing without scar formation[8].

There are no reports that would indicate that infection with molluscum contagiosum has an adverse effect on pregnancy, or results in any significant disease in the neonate. Similarly, pregnancy does not significantly alter the natural course or treatment of molluscum contagiosum.

INFLUENZA

Etiology

The influenza viruses are members of the orthomyxovirus family and are an RNA-containing capsid surrounded by a glycoprotein envelope[12,13]. Three major serotypes have been identified. The most clinically important and virulent serotype is type A which is responsible for most epidemics and pandemics. Type B is of less importance, usually resulting in disease of lesser severity than serotype A, and is rarely seen as the etiology of epidemics[12]. Type C is rarely responsible for severe disease and is of little clinical importance.

The surface antigens of the glycoprotein are important in identification of the influenza virus and are used in subclassification. Four classes of hemagglutinins have been identified (H0, H1, H2 and H3), and two classes of neuraminidase subtypes are known (N1 and N2)[12–14]. Each strain of influenza is classified according to the major antigen, the geographic location where it was first isolated, laboratory sample number, year of isolation and by hemagglutination and neuraminidase

subtype[12,14]. As an example, the pandemic of 1957 was secondary to influenza A/Japan/305/57 (H2N2).

Epidemiology

Transmission of the influenza virus, like other respiratory viruses, is by nebulized respiratory droplets from one individual to another. Outbreaks of influenza by the identical subtype may occur simultaneously worldwide, as seen in pandemics in 1918, 1957 and 1958[14]. These viruses are highly contagious. Epidemics follow major 'shifts' in the antigenic determinants, whereas minor changes in the antigens are referred to as 'drifts'[12,13].

Pathophysiology

With distribution by aerosolized droplets, the virus is deposited on the nasopharyngeal mucosa or the lower bronchial tree. The usual incubation period is from 1 to 5 days. If symptomatic, the acute illness will last from 3 to 7 days, though complete convalescence may take weeks[12–14]. Viral shedding following incubation will last for 3 to 5 days[13].

Viral replication takes place in the ciliated columnar epithelial cells and results in local inflammation, cell death and contiguous spread. The subsequent denudation of the tracheobronchial tree may result in impaired ciliary clearance, decreased mucus production and mucosal edema. These changes may lead to small airway obstruction with debris and subsequently decreased ventilation and diffusion capacity[13]. Viremia has been documented but is thought to be both rare and transient[13].

While influenza may be asymptomatic, complications may also occur that will lead to host death. The most common, potentially fatal complication is secondary bacterial pneumonia, particularly with *Streptococcus pneumoniae*, *Staphylococcus aureus*, *Haemophilus influenzae* and *Klebsiella pneumoniae*[12,13]. Viremia with dissemination may lead to primary influenza pneumonia, myositis, myocarditis, encephalitis and transplacental infection[13].

Transplacental infection was confirmed by McGregor and co-workers[15]. Although the virus was cultured from the amniotic fluid, the infant was disease-free at birth. A higher rate of congenital malformations secondary to maternal influenza infection has been suggested by multiple reports. However, these reports have not shown a consistent pattern of malformations and have not been supported by later studies, especially studies documenting infection by serology[12]. Each epidemic of influenza is associated with increased stillbirths and prematurity[13]. These complications are seen primarily with severe maternal infection, and are without doubt multifactorial[13].

Each epidemic has been associated with higher morbidity and mortality in the pregnant patient than in the non-pregnant population. In the 1918 pandemic, the maternal mortality rate in the USA was approximately 30%, and was noted to be as high as 60% if infection occurred in the third trimester[12,13]. Although a similar pattern was seen in 1957 and 1958, mortality rates were not as high. With improved antibiotic therapy and intensive care, fatal infection is now rare[14]. Women who are at greatest risk of complications include those with heart disease, pulmonary disease, immunocompromised states or who are in the last trimester of pregnancy[12,13]. More specifically patients who have congenital heart disease, rheumatic heart disease, severe asthma, bronchiectasis, tuberculosis, cystic fibrosis, chronic renal disease with azotemia or nephrotic syndrome, insulin dependent diabetes, neuromuscular or orthopedic disorders that impair ventilation, hemoglobinopathies, or immunodeficiency states are at particular risk[12,13].

Cell-mediated immunity is important in recovery from influenza, particularly T lymphocyte-mediated cytotoxicity. Alterations in maternally mediated immunity may contribute to the increased risk of complications for the gravid patient[13]. In addition, the increased blood volume and decreased serum albumin, normal to pregnancy, may predispose the pregnant patient to pulmonary complications of influenza[13].

Diagnosis and management

During an epidemic or pandemic, the diagnosis of influenza is not difficult to make. While patients may be asymptomatic, the usual symptoms of influenza are those of any viral respiratory infection, with cough, sore throat, fever, malaise, headache and acute debilitation[12–14]. The discrepancy between symptomatology and serological confirmation is demonstrated by reports that 39–60% of asymptomatic women will show seroconversion during pregnancy[14]. Definitive diagnosis of influenza can be made by serology or demonstration of viral antigens in nasopharyngeal epithelial cells or by isolation of virus in culture[14]. Confirmation of influenza infection by serology requires positive virus-specific IgM antibodies, or a four-fold rise in virus-specific IgG antibody titers. The most commonly utilized serological tests for influenza are complement fixation, hemagglutination inhibition, or enzyme-linked immunosorbent assay (ELISA)[12,14]. Viruses can be isolated from throat washings during the first 3 days of illness[12]. Neither serological antibody testing nor viral isolation is recommended in the uncomplicated patient.

Management of the uncomplicated patient involves reassurance and symptomatic relief. The patient should have liberal fluids, and should be prescribed acetaminophen for analgesia and antipyretic. If the diagnosis is pneumonia, the patient should be hospitalized and intravenous antibiotic therapy provided to cover a broad spectrum of possible secondary bacterial pneumonias as noted above[12]. If delivery is indicated for either obstetric or fetal considerations, local anesthetics are preferred for vaginal deliveries, and epidural anesthesia for Cesarean sections[12]. Potential pulmonary complications must be considered prior to the use of β-mimetics[12]. Route of delivery should be determined on obstetric criteria.

Amantadine and rimantadine are chemical agents, which have been shown to be effective against influenza A. They provide some improvement in pulmonary function and a shortened course of disease in the non-pregnant patient[12]. Amantadine in high doses has been shown to be embryotoxic and teratogenic in animal studies. These agents in general are contraindicated in the pregnant patient[12]. Several authors have suggested that, during an epidemic, amantadine may be appropriate in the selected high-risk patient. Examples of such high-risk patients include the non-immune patient with marginally compensated cardiac disease and chronic lung disease[12,13]. As amantadine does appear in breast milk, its use during lactation should be restricted[12].

Influenza vaccine contains three inactivated virus strains (two type A and one type B) which are likely to circulate in the United States. There is no evidence that influenza vaccination is of any significant risk to either the expectant mother or her fetus, and immunization should be encouraged in all patients who are pregnant during the influenza season[13]. Influenza vaccine produces hemagglutination-inhibition antibodies which are protective against illness caused by strains similar to those in the vaccine or the related variants. The vaccine also produces protective antibodies against influenza in HIV-infected patients who have minimal AIDS-related symptoms and high CD4+ T-lymphocyte counts[16]. The influenza vaccine does not cause influenza because it contains only inactivated viruses. Side-effects of immunization include fever, malaise and myalgia and minor local reactions. Contraindications to influenza vaccination include a history of allergy to egg proteins and other vaccine components[16].

PARVOVIRUS

Etiology

Most references to human parvovirus primarily refer to the B19 strain, as this is the single strain most consistently studied. A second strain, RA-1, has been identified and associated with rheumatoid arthritis, but will not be discussed further in this text[13,14].

The human parvovirus B19 is a member of the DNA virus family Parvoviridae, originally known as Pincodnaviruses[14]. This virus is one of the smallest know DNA viruses, approximately 18–25 nm in size, about 5.5 kb in length, with single-stranded DNA[13,14]. This virus lacks an envelope, but does code for at least two major structural or capsid proteins, and at least one non-structural protein[14].

Epidemiology

The human parvovirus B19 was first discovered by British investigators in 1975 while they were screening blood for hepatitis B antigen. Subsequently, B19 was associated with aplastic anemia crisis and erythema infectiosum or 'fifth disease'[17,18]. This virus has also been associated with chronic bone marrow suppression, arthritis or arthropathy, fetal hydrops and, most recently, purpura[17].

Infection with parvovirus B19 has been noted worldwide, and is commonly seen in children aged 5–14 years[17]. Outbreaks are most common in winter and spring, and there is a year to year variation in incidence as well[17,18]. Estimates of positive seroprevalence rates in adults range from 28 to 72%, with most authors indicating a seroprevalence of approximately 50%[18-20].

A population-based cohort study of 30 946 pregnant patients in Denmark revealed that 65% of patients had past infection prior to pregnancy and that the risks of seroconversion during the endemic and epidemic periods were 1.5% and 13.0%, respectively[21]. The risk of past infection increased with the number of siblings and a difference of less than 2 years between the patient's age and that of the nearest sibling. The risks of past infection and seroconversion increased with number of children in the household and varied with the ages of the children. The 6.8% risk of seroconversion during pregnancy occurred in the highest group of households having children in the age group of 5–7 years. The risk of seroconversion from occupational exposure, mainly nursery school teachers and persons in contact with children aged 5–7 years, was 6%[21].

Transmission of the virus is by respiratory droplets. The incubation period is 4–14 days. Viremia develops 7–8 days after initial inoculation, lasting approximately 4 days[18]. The rash associated with parvovirus B19 appears following viremia. The primary host is no longer infectious once the rash appears. Initial infection and seroconversion provide the host with lifelong immunity, and reinfection is rare.

Pathophysiology

Parvovirus B19 viral replication and encapsidation take place in the host cell nucleus[17,18]. Replication is accomplished via self-priming palindromic loops found at either end of the DNA strand[17]. Host cell enzymes are used in viral replication. Rapidly dividing cells are preferentially infected, perhaps a product of the S phase of cell replication, a requirement for viral growth. The parvovirus B19 is particularly trophic and cytotoxic for erythroid progenitor cells[17,18].

Following initial incubation and viremia, there is a transient inhibition of erythropoiesis and reticulocytopenia in an infected host[17]. Similar changes are seen in other blood cell lines but to a lesser degree. This bone marrow depression is first seen approximately 7 days after initial infection and lasts for approximately another 7 days[17]. In the host with normal red blood cell survival or in a non-immunocompromised state, this bone marrow depression is usually asymptomatic and self limited. Aplastic crisis is seen particularly in the patient with abnormally shortened red blood cell survival, in conditions such as sickle cell anemia, hereditary spherocytosis, pyruvate kinase deficiency, thalassemia, dyserythropoietic anemia and autoimmune hemolytic anemia[17,18]. The immunocompromised host may develop chronic bone marrow suppression of all cell lines secondary to an inability to clear the virus[17].

Transplacental fetal infection, and subsequent fetal anemia, may result in fetal hydrops and demise[17]. The fetus is an ideal host for human parvovirus B19 because of an immature immune system and accelerated erythropoiesis with a markedly shortened red blood cell life span[17,18]. The pathogenesis of non-immune fetal hydrops may be multifactorial. In addition to anemia from extensive hemolysis, it has been suggested that hemosiderin deposits may lead to hepatic fibrosis and extramedullary hematopoiesis that may result in portal hypertension. It has also been proposed that the marked fetal anemia observed may lead to tissue anoxia and subsequent high output or hypoxic cardiac failure[19]. While transplacental infection may lead to fetal anemia and hydrops, parvovirus B19 is not a common cause of birth defects or neonatal disease[18,19]. The period of peak fetal morbidity following maternal infection is approximately 4–6 weeks after maternal symptoms[19]. The fetal loss rate following maternal infection has been estimated to be as low as 2.5%[20].

The rash associated with human parvovirus B19 infection occurring at 17–21 days after infection is probably secondary to antigen–antibody reaction[17]. Arthritis or arthropathy, probable postinfection phenomena, may last for months or years[17]. Parvovirus B19 infection may manifest with a purpuric rash-like illness, often associated with other signs of vasculitis. This rash may begin as a vesiculopustular eruption and often is distributed on the buttocks and lower extremities, similar to Henoch–Schönlein purpura[17].

Diagnosis and management

As with many viral infections, infection with human parvovirus B19 may be asymptomatic or carry symptoms of only a mild flu-like illness[18]. The rash may be absent or impossible to distinguish from other childhood rashes[14]. While the rash is more common in children than in adults, adults are more likely to develop arthritic complaints[17,18]. The rash is characterized as a lacy rash especially on the face, providing the 'slapped cheek' appearance. Following this initial rash, a variable rash may appear on the extremities and has morbilliform, confluent, circinate, or annular appearance. With central clearing of the annular lesions, the rash takes a reticular pattern. The rash usually does not involve the trunk, palms or soles, and may be pruritic. The rash usually disappears within 1–2 weeks but may recur especially with stress, exercise, sunlight, or bathing[17,18].

Cultured human parvovirus B19 requires bone marrow cells, and is therefore clinically impractical. Enzyme-linked immunoassay for B19 antigen and antibodies is available to aid in diagnosis. Diagnosis can be made through DNA hybridization techniques including DNA amplification via the polymerase chain reaction (PCR)[17–19]. Maternal IgM antibodies can be detected 3–4 days after the onset of clinical illness, whereas IgG antibodies are seen within 7 days. IgM antibodies persist for 3–4 months, and IgG antibodies are present for years[18,20]. Patients who demonstrate positive IgG with a negative IgM are considered immune and carry little risk from exposure to parvovirus B19. Those patients who have had an acute infection will have a positive IgM and are at significant risk for an adverse fetal outcome[20].

Fetal infection can be monitored by ultrasound for evidence of fetal hydrops and percutaneous umbilical blood sampling to diagnose fetal anemia and the preserve of parvovirus B19[20]. Demonstration of parvovirus B19 antigens or parvovirus-specific IgM antibody DNA will confirm the diagnosis. Infection is strongly suggested if eosinophilic inclusion and marginated chromatin are seen in the infected fetal erythroid precursors[20].

If the initial ultrasound examination of the fetus is normal, the fetus should be followed by serial ultrasound examinations up to approximately 12 weeks after maternal symptoms[17,20]. Ultrasound-documented fetal hydrops resolves spontaneously in some cases of transplacental infection[19]. Transplacental infection and hydrops fetalis treated through intrauterine exchange transfusion have subsided[17,20].

If the serological status of a pregnant patient with known or suspected exposure to parvovirus B19 is unknown, antibody testing should be performed as soon as possible. Those patients who are seronegative, immunocompromised, or have chronic hemolytic anemia are advised to avoid exposure[17]. In practice, however, this recommendation is impractical, as infected individuals will usually demonstrate clinically recognizable signs only in the postinfectious state. Vaccines or antiviral therapies specific against parvovirus B19 have not yet been developed[17].

Maternal serum α-fetoprotein levels are elevated in association with intrauterine infection prior to the development of fetal hydrops as detected by ultrasound[17,18,20]. The value of this test is limited because of its non-specific nature. Similarly, the value of intravenous gamma globulin for postexposure prevention of infection has not been fully evaluated.

ENTEROVIRUSES

Etiology

Human enteroviruses are members of the family of RNA Picornaviridae and are some of the most common of human viruses[22–25]. There are at least 72 serotypes of enterovirus. Original classification of the enteroviruses divided these serotypes into four classes based on their growth characteristics in laboratory animals and cell cultures[22,23]. The four recognized classes of enterovirus are poliovirus, coxsackie A virus, coxsackie B virus and echovirus. To date, there are three poliovirus serotypes, 23 coxsackie A serotypes, six coxsackie B serotypes and more than 30 echovirus serotypes[22,23]. Echovirus serotype 72 has been identified as hepatitis A. Because of the relative elimination of poliovirus infection, this review will focus on non-polio enteroviruses.

Viruses of the genus enterovirus are small (27 nm), single-stranded RNA viruses with approximately 7500 bases. These viruses are icosahedral, and lack an envelope. Enteroviruses do have a nucleocapsid that is composed of 60 structural subunits[22,23].

Epidemiology

As infections with enterovirus are not reported on a national basis, the true incidence of disease secondary to these agents is not known. As noted above, these viruses are thought to be one of the most common pathogens of humans[22,23]. Between 50 and 80% of infections are thought to be asymptomatic. Infection may occur throughout the year, and is most prevalent from June to October in temperate climates[22,23]. Serotypes vary by region or year. The usual route of transmission is by either respiratory droplets or by the gastrointestinal route[22,23].

Of all enterovirus infections, 80–90% are in children and adolescents 16 years old or younger[24]. Adults account for approximately 8% of non-polio enteroviral infections[24]. Neonatal infections within the first month of life are common. In one study 12.8% of newborns acquired enterovirus infection within 1 month of life[22], and all infants recovered without difficulty.

Women contracting enteroviral infections in late pregnancy are usually asymptomatic; displayed symptoms are mild and non-specific[22,23]. Perinatal infections commonly follow infection with the following serotypes: echovirus serotypes 5, 7, 9, 11, 17, 18, 19 and 22; coxsackie B serotypes 1–5[22].

Pathophysiology

Diseases attributed to infection with non-polio enterovirus include aseptic meningitis, encephalitis, myocarditis, hepatitis and pneumonia pleurodynia orchitis[22–24]. Though often asymptomatic, infection may manifest with rashes, pharyngitis and conjunctivitis, parotitis, pericarditis and pancreatitis. Rarely the infection may be fulminant and fatal.

Following initial infection, viral replication occurs in the submucosal lymphoid tissue, and within 1–3 days can be identified in regional lymph nodes[22]. With subsequent viremia, the virus can be found in distant lymphoreticular organs, i.e. the liver, spleen and bone marrow[22]. After replication in the lymphoreticular tissue, a more generalized infection with inflammation occurs, affecting multiple organs or tissues such as the central nervous system (CNS), striated muscle and the heart[22]. This disease process may be exacerbated by concurrent pregnancy, steroid administration, irradiation, exercise or cold stress. Animal studies have demonstrated a shorter incubation period and higher virus titers in pregnancy. Susceptibility to infection appears to increase with gestational age, but reverts rapidly to that of the non-pregnant state following delivery[22,23]. Sites of primary infection in the gastrointestinal tract do not show evidence of this destructive process, therefore diarrhea will not ensue in most patients.

The host immune response to enterovirus infection includes the production of both humoral and mucosal antibodies, and a cytotoxic T-lymphocyte cellular response[22].

Most perinatal infections occur secondary to transmittal of the virus to the neonate during parturition or immediately in the postnatal period[23]. Vertical transmission of non-polio enterovirus by transplacental infection is rare but has been documented[22,23]. As in infection of children and adults, the severity of disease in the neonate may range from mild to fatal, causing diseases of the CNS, liver or heart[23]. The neonate who has acquired an enteroviral infection by vertical transmission in the immediate peripartum period is thought to be at greater risk of serious illness when compared to the infant who has gained infection following postnatal transmission[22,23].

Little is known about neonatal infection with coxsackie A virus. Though there are case reports of *in utero* fetal death with disseminated coxsackie A virus, it is rare for coxsackie A to be passed to the fetus[24]. There appears to be no association between echovirus or coxsackie B virus infection and an increased spontaneous abortion rate[22,23]. Stillbirth late in pregnancy increases with both maternal echovirus and coxsackie B virus[22,23]. The association between maternal coxsackie B virus infection and a slightly higher risk of fetal urogenital defects and congenital heart defects is tenuous at least[22,23]. Coxsackie B virus, particularly serotypes B3 and B4, have been implicated in neonatal myocarditis[26].

Diagnosis and management

Typical presenting symptoms of maternal enteroviral infection are those of an upper respiratory tract infection such as fever of a few days' duration with or without rash. Infection may also produce abdominal pain of such intensity that it may be mistaken for abruptio or chorioamnionitis in the pregnant patient[22,23]. Rarely the patient presents with aseptic meningitis or myopericarditis[22,23]. A presumptive diagnosis can be made by demonstrating virus-specific IgM antibodies, or by documenting rising IgG titers in maternal serum. Definitive diagnosis requires culturing of the virus from either respiratory secretions or stool.

If maternal infection is established more than 5–7 days prior to delivery, the maternal immune response provides IgG antibody that crosses the placenta and protects against serious neonatal illness[22,23]. In the absence of maternally derived antibody when enterovirus infection occurs close to delivery, a more severe and complicated infection may follow[22,23]. Multiple studies have indicated that when the neonate has severe echovirus or coxsackie B virus infection, approximately 60% of the gravid patients will have been symptomatic during the perinatal period, usually within 1 week of delivery[22,23].

There is no specific treatment, effective vaccine, or reliable immune globulin immunization for enterovirus infection. Vertical transmission at birth causes the most neonatal harm. Owing to the absence of passive immunization via maternal antibodies, some suggest delaying delivery for over 1 week after maternal onset of the disease.

MUMPS

Etiology

The mumps virus is an RNA virus in the Paramyxovirus family. The virus has a lipid membrane envelope with both neuraminidase and hemagglutinin. The envelope carries an 'S' antigen; however, the antigen does cross react with other paramyxoviruses. The core antigen 'V' is more specific to the mumps virus[14].

Epidemiology

Mumps may be found worldwide, and the virus is spread by respiratory droplets or fomites[14]. Epidemics may occur, especially in urban settings or where susceptible individuals are in close quarters. The incubation period may range from 7 to 23 days but more typically is about 14–18 days[14,27]. The infected individual is contagious from 6 days prior to and up to 9 days after the onset of disease[27]. The virus may be isolated from the throat, saliva and urine during the first 3 days of illness and may be found in the urine up to 2 weeks after it has disappeared from other sites[14]. The virus may also be isolated from blood, breast milk and the testes[14].

The incidence of mumps has fallen dramatically from the pre-vaccination era. A live virus vaccine was introduced in 1967 and has found widespread use since 1977[28]. The incidence dropped from 185 691 in 1967 to 2982 in 1985; a resurgence occurred from 1985 to 1987[28].

As in the pre-vaccine era, mumps is predominantly a disease of school-age children (ages 5–14 years)[28]. Immunization of children from 1967 to 1977 was scant, with less than 50% of children immunized up to 1976[28]. This practice has left a population of susceptible adolescents and young adults, and outbreaks can be seen in high school, college campuses and some occupational settings[27].

The incidence of mumps in pregnancy is estimated to be between 0.8 and 10 cases per 10 000 pregnancies[14].

Pathophysiology

Mumps is usually a benign and self-limited disease. Following infection and incubation, viremia occurs. The disease is asymptomatic in 30–60% of patients. Most patients experience moderate debilitation[14,28]. Typical symptoms include fever, malaise and swelling of one or both parotid glands. If the parotids are swollen, other salivary glands may also be involved[14]. With dissemination of the virus, viral replication occurs in multiple organs. Pancreatitis, nephritis, arthritis and myocarditis are rare complications[14,27]. Approximately 20% of postpubertal males will have orchitis. Infection of the thyroid and breast may occur in the postpubertal female[14].

The virus may be cultured from cerebrospinal fluid in the asymptomatic patient and meningeal signs can be seen in 5–25% of infections[14,28]. The incidence of mumps encephalitis may be as high as 5 per 1000 reported cases[27]. The cranial nerves may be involved, and the most common residual CNS symptom is deafness[14].

Symptomatic reinfection has been known to occur[27]. Although mumps infection may be fatal, the mortality rate is extremely low. Fatal cases of mumps are more common in adults, with approximately one-half of mumps-associated deaths in patients 20 years of age or older[28].

The mumps virus can infect the placenta and infection can cause transplacental infection. Mumps has increased the spontaneous abortion rate, reported at 27% with first-trimester maternal infection in one study, double the rate seen in control[14,28]. Mumps has not been associated with prematurity.

Diagnosis and management

The diagnosis of mumps may be made on clinical symptoms if present. The diagnosis can be confirmed in both symptomatic or exposed, susceptible asymptomatic patients by serological studies demonstrating virus-specific IgM or a rising titer of virus-specific IgG. The virus can be easily cultured in African green monkey kidney cells, embryonated hens' eggs and human cells[14].

In contrast to other viral infections, such as influenza or varicella zoster, mumps does not demonstrate increased virulence or severity in the pregnant patient[14]. Treatment is supportive. The patient should be observed for potential complications.

Special precautions and delivery in isolation if possible has been suggested when the obstetric patient has overt mumps or if the patient has had proven or suspected onset of mumps within the 10 days preceding delivery[27]. These same recommendations are suggested for the non-immune patient exposed in the 3 weeks prior to labor[27]. Postpartum care should be provided in isolation, though there is no need to separate the patient and her infant, and breast-feeding should be permitted[27]. It has been estimated that approximately one-half of newborns delivered to patients with overt mumps will acquire asymptomatic disease and may be contagious up to the age of 4 weeks if hospitalized[27]. Non-immune hospital personnel should not care for the patient with mumps and if exposed should not take care of other non-immune patients.

An effective attenuated live virus vaccine is available but contraindicated in pregnancy. The risk to the fetus following immunization in pregnancy is theoretical. Women should avoid pregnancy for 3 months following vaccination[28]. Inadvertent immunization during pregnancy is not an indication for termination of pregnancy[28]. Immune globulin has not been shown to be effective in the prevention of disease, and is not recommended[27,28].

MEASLES

Etiology

Measles is an exanthematous disease caused by a member of the Paramyxovirus family. This virus differs from other members of this family in that it does not demonstrate a neuramidase[14].

Epidemiology

Prior to the development and introduction of measles vaccination in 1963, epidemics of measles were seen approximately every 2–3 years, with an average of 500 000 cases reported annually[14]. In this era there were approximately 400–500 deaths attributed to complications of measles[14]. In the 1980s, however, reported incidence of measles fell to 1500–3000 cases per year[14]. Prior to the era of widespread vaccination, measles was primarily a disease of children under the age of 10 years, with its highest incidence between the ages of 2 and 6 years[14]. Despite vaccination, measles remains predominantly a pediatric disease. However, from 1976 to 1980, 46% of cases were in children over the age of 10 years, and approximately 25% of cases were seen in children 4 years old or less[14]. The incidence of measles in pregnancy is rare with estimates ranging from 6 to 40 cases per 100 000 pregnancies[14,29]. Congenital measles is rare[30].

In the susceptible population, prior to vaccination, measles is very contagious, with an attack rate of approximately 90% in the non-immune patient[29]. Transmission from one individual to another is by respiratory droplets, with the mucosa of the nose, oropharynx or conjunctivae as the portal of entry[14,31]. The usual incubation period is 10–14 days, but may be as short as 7 days[14,29,31]. The patient is infectious for 2–3 days prior to symptoms and 3–4 days after the appearance of the rash[31].

Pathophysiology

After initial infection and incubation, viremia occurs and the patient demonstrates symptoms of an upper respiratory infection. There is usually a 3-day prodromal period with fever, inflammation of mucosal membranes, cough and coryza. Examination of the pharyngeal mucous membranes may reveal pathognomonic Koplik's spots. Subsequently the patient develops a generalized maculopapular exanthema and malaise[14,29,31].

Complications of measles do occur. In children the most common complication is otitis media. Secondary bacterial pneumonia may follow measles viremia and is the most common lethal complication. Encephalitis may be seen in patients of all ages and occurs in approximately 1 in 1000 cases[14]. If encephalitis complicates measles, it usually appears within 3–7 days after the appearance of the rash and carries a mortality rate of approximately 10%[14]. Subacute sclerosing panencephalitis is an extremely rare late neurological complication which usually occurs in preschool children[31]. The overall mortality rate of measles is estimated at less than 0.1% but is higher in children less than one year[14].

Diagnosis and management

In a community epidemic of measles, the clinical signs and symptoms noted above may allow the clinician to make a diagnosis. The differential diagnosis of measles includes a number of viral exanthematous diseases, however, and the diagnosis may be difficult to make.

Immunity is demonstrated by IgG antibody by ELISA or the hemagglutination-inhibition test. Measles antigen can be detected in nasopharyngeal secretions in the first 3–4 days of illness by immunofluorescence or ELISA. Rising measles-specific IgG titers in paired serum ELISA, hemagglutinin inhibition or complement fixation will document acute infection. However, IgM will also allow diagnosis of an acute infection. IgM antibody will usually appear 2–5 days after the appearance of the exanthem[31].

There appears to be a higher rate of complications and a higher mortality in the gravid patient when compared to the non-pregnant patient[14]. Pneumonia has been noted to be the most frequent fatal complication[14].

The virus infrequently crosses the placenta. Gestational measles has been linked to a higher incidence of premature labor and abortion but is not an indication for termination of pregnancy. Maternal measles may lead to premature labor and delivery, and therefore increased neonatal mortality. Pregnancies complicated by measles have not been firmly associated with consistent congenital malformations or a higher rate of malformations[14,31]. Newborns are provided passive immunity to measles by maternally derived IgG measles-specific antibody secondary to either maternal infection or immunization[31]. Rarely, measles within a week of delivery may result in measles in the infant within a few days of birth[31]. If maternal antibodies exist prior to delivery, most transplacental cases of neonatal measles are mild.

Non-immune patients can be protected against measles following exposure if they are provided with passively acquired immunoglobulin preferably within 3 days of exposure. The recommended dose of immune serum globulin is 0.2 ml/kg body weight intramuscularly[31]. Passive immunization with 0.04 ml/kg body weight will mitigate serious illness[31].

Measles vaccine is a live attenuated vaccine available either alone or in combination with mumps and rubella live virus vaccines (MMR). As it is a live virus vaccine, pregnancy is a contraindication to vaccination. Inadvertent vaccination during pregnancy has not been associated with fetal damage, therefore this is not an indication for termination of pregnancy[31].

In 1985, Gazala and colleagues[30] reported the outcome of five pregnancies at 28–34 weeks' gestation, complicated by a measles epidemic in Israel from December 1981 to May 1982. All five pregnancies were complicated by premature delivery with a mean duration between onset of illness and delivery of 3.5 days. The infants demonstrated low birth weight, and three of four live births had severe respiratory distress. The fifth infant was stillborn and had multiple congenital malformations. Each of the live-born infants received immune serum globulin intramuscularly at a dose of 0.2 ml/kg on day 1 of life. None of the infants demonstrated any clinical signs or symptoms of measles. However, an addendum to this report noted a 1985 delivery at 36 weeks to a patient with measles. The infant developed mild clinical measles at 7 days, despite prophylactic immune serum globulin at birth[30].

In summary, although there is no specific therapy for measles, management of the non-immune gravid patient exposed to measles should include prophylactic passive immunization with IgG, and close observation for premature labor or other complications such as secondary bacterial pneumonia. If the pregnant patient delivers with active disease, immunization of the neonate seems to protect the infant against severe measles.

RUBELLA

Etiology

The rubella virus is a member of the togavirus group and is a spherical, enveloped, RNA virus 50–70 nm in diameter[32].

Epidemiology

Rubella has a worldwide distribution. Prior to the era of vaccination, pandemics occurred approximately every 20 years, with epidemics occurring on a 6–9 year cycle[32,33]. Rubella is endemic throughout the year but in temperate climates demonstrates a peak incidence from March to May[32]. Following the licensed availability of rubella vaccine in the USA in 1969, there has been a dramatic decrease in incidence of the disease. Prior to widespread vaccination rubella was primarily a disease of children from the ages of 5–9 years[32,33]. In the post-vaccination era, however, there has been a major shift in the age of infected individuals. Data from the Center for Disease Control in 1986 indicated that of 551 cases of rubella, 58% were in individuals aged 15 years or older[33]. It is estimated that 12–24% of post-pubertal individuals are not immune to rubella[33].

Transmission of rubella from one individual to another is by aerosolized respiratory droplets. The usual incubation period is commonly 16–18 days but may range from 14 to 21 days[32,33]. The infected individual may shed the virus for 1 week prior to and for approximately 1 week after the appearance of the typical rash[32,33]. The virus may be isolated from respiratory secretions throughout this period of time but may also be present in urine and blood prior to the rash[33]. A mild prodrome of malaise, low-grade fever, headache and conjunctivitis may precede the rash by 1–5 days[33]. Over one-half of infectious cases are subclinical, with a ratio of 2 : 1 for asymptomatic to symptomatic illness[32].

Pathophysiology

With initial infection, the rubella virus implants on the respiratory mucosa where primary viral replication

occurs. The virus is also present and undergoes early replication in local lymph nodes[32]. During incubation, approximately 1 week prior to the onset of the rash the virus can be isolated from leukocytes, the conjunctiva, urine and stool[32].

The immune response of the host to infection is both a humoral and cell-mediated response. Viral-specific antibodies may be detected within 24–48 h of the onset of the rash[32].

Infection with rubella is usually self-limited and mild. Postauricular, suboccipital and posterior cervical lymphadenopathy are distinguishing features of this exanthematous disease[32,33]. This adenopathy will often herald the onset of the typical rash and is usually seen with a subsequent rash.

The most significant and devastating complication of rubella occurs secondary to transplacental vertical transmission of the virus to the fetus during maternal viremia. *In utero* infection may occur at any state of pregnancy[33]. The virus may infect the placenta and results in granulomatous changes and necrosis of chorionic villi[32]. Fetal rubella infection may result in spontaneous abortion or stillbirth. Once established, fetal infection is chronic and persists well beyond birth[32,33]. The rubella virus may be persistent in the most severely affected infants for up to 1 year[33]. The exact pathological mechanism of fetal infection and subsequent tissue and organ damage is not well understood. Rubella is not cytolytic like measles, and inflammation is not a prominent feature of infected tissues[32,33]. Infected cells do show reduced mitotic activity[33].

The rate of congenital infection and the effect of transplacental infection appear to vary with the gestational age at the time of infection. In a prospective study of 1016 women with confirmed rubella infection conducted by Miller and co-workers, the rate of congenital infection was 81% in the first 12 weeks, 54% at 13–16 weeks, 36% at 17–22 weeks, 30% at 23–30 weeks, 60% at 31–36 weeks and 100% from 37 weeks to delivery[33]. No congenital rubella defects were seen if infection occurred after 16 weeks. In a similar prospective evaluation, there were no anomalies seen if maternal infection occurred after 17 weeks' gestation[34,35].

The congenital rubella syndrome (CRS) involves a wide spectrum of clinical features. Clinical manifestations of CRS in order of decreasing frequency are hearing loss, mental retardation, cardiac malformations and ocular defects[32–35]. The risk to the fetus is greatest if maternal infection occurs in the first trimester. Multiple defects are not commonly seen if maternal infection occurs later. Congenital anomalies of the heart, eye and CNS have been seen only if maternal infection occurred between 3 and 12 weeks[34,35]. As noted above, deafness was the most common anomaly occurring in 58% of affected offspring overall and in 40% as a single defect[34]. Patent ductus arteriosus was the most common cardiac defect and accounted for

79% of the cardiac anomalies seen[34,35]. Although a complete discussion of CRS is beyond the scope of this chapter, other features seen include intrauterine growth retardation, hepatosplenomegaly, jaundice, thrombocytopenic purpura and radiolucencies of the long bones[27]. Infants born with multiple defects at birth secondary to CRS have a poor prognosis with a high mortality rate in the first year of life[32].

More than half of newborns with features of CRS are normal at birth but display delayed manifestations of disease later in life, particularly auditory, ocular and CNS abnormalities[32,33]. Delayed manifestations call for continued follow-up. Ten per cent of CRS patients develop additional forms of eye damage, such as glaucoma, keratoconus and spontaneous lens resorption[33]. By age 35 years, 20% of these patients will have diabetes mellitus, and 5% will experience thyroid dysfunction[33]. Progressive rubella panencephalitis, though rare, is uniformly fatal, and may occur in the second decade of life[32,33].

Diagnosis and management

The diagnosis of rubella, as in other exanthematous diseases, may be difficult to make. As noted above, the patient who is symptomatic may experience a prodrome of malaise, low-grade fever and tender and swollen lymphadenopathy of the suboccipital, postauricular and posterior cervical lymph nodes prior to the onset of a rash[32]. Rarely the patient will have a cough, coryza, or conjunctivitis[32]. The rash of rubella initially appears over the face and posterior to the ears as a small, faint, pink circular macular rash that eventually spreads to the neck, trunk and extremities[32,33]. The rash may also appear as a general blush in the face or may be described as petechial or purpuric[32]. The patient's symptoms will show improvement within 1–2 days, and the rash generally will disappear in 3 days[32].

Clinical history and examination are not reliable for making a diagnosis and should not be trusted to establish a history of prior disease or probable immunity. The rubella virus may be cultured, but this process is expensive and slow, and is not clinically recommended. The diagnosis of rubella infection is typically confirmed by serological antibody detection by a variety of methods. Currently rubella-specific IgM and IgG may be detected by hemagglutination inhibition, ELISA, complement fixation, hemolysin in gel, passive hemagglutination, immunofluorescence and radioimmunoassay[32,33]. Cross reactions have been noted between rubella and human parvovirus-specific IgM, and therefore one must use caution in interpretation of these results if these levels are reported as low or equivocal[33]. As in other diseases, the presence of IgM indicates acute illness, as does a four-fold rise in IgG. IgM will disappear after 4–6 weeks[32].

All obstetric patients should be screened for rubella immunity on their first visit. A history of prior disease is unreliable, in that the differential diagnosis of rubella is large, and more than half of naturally occurring disease that will provide immunity is asymptomatic. Prior vaccination does not guarantee immunity[32]. This screen will determine susceptibility. If a patient suspects possible exposure, and her immunity has not been established, serology should be obtained as soon as possible. If the exposed patient is non-immune her serum should be tested approximately 3 weeks later concurrently with the first specimen[32]. The patient who has a confirmed infection with rubella may have an evaluation for fetal infection by reverse transcription and nested polymerase chain reaction of the chorionic villi, amniotic fluid or fetal blood[36]. The patient should be informed about the sequelae of fetal infection and the option of pregnancy termination if fetal infection occurs prior to 20 weeks of gestation. It should be noted that reinfection with rubella may occur, but in the presence of antibodies the risk of viremia and hence the risk to the fetus is minimal[32,33].

Vaccination for rubella was licensed in the USA in 1969, with two attenuated live virus vaccines, HPV77/DE5 vaccine and the Cendehill vaccine[32]. In 1980 a third vaccine was introduced: RA 27/3 marketed as Meruvax II[32]. The RA 27/3 vaccine demonstrated a higher rate of seroconversion and persistent immunity and is now the only vaccine available in the USA[32]. Current recommendation for vaccination includes vaccination of all infants between 12 and 15 months, and vaccination of susceptible adolescents and young adults[32]. All patients identified as non-immune as a result of an obstetric antenatal screen should be immunized postpartum. There is little risk to the postpartum patient from vaccination and minimal risk to the breast-fed infant, even though the virus can be isolated in breast milk after maternal inoculation[33]. Contraindications to immunization include pregnancy, febrile illness, immunodeficiency states or receipt of immune serum globulin within the preceding 3 months[32].

The risk to the fetus from inadvertent administration of the vaccine in pregnancy is not exactly known and appears to be theoretical. In a review by Freij and colleagues[33], it was noted that there were no defects compatible with the congenital rubella syndrome in 522 infants born to 635 women who inadvertently received the RA 27/3 vaccine during pregnancy. The virus in this vaccine is capable of crossing the placenta and has been shown to produce a subclinical infection in 1–2% of infants born to these patients. Women who have received vaccination within 3 months prior to or during pregnancy should not be considered candidates for therapeutic abortion as the risks to the fetus are minimal[34].

REFERENCES

1. Smotkin D. Virology of human papilloma virus. *Clin Obstet Gynecol* 1989;32:117–26
2. Koutsky L. Epidemiology of genital human papillomavirus infection. *Am J Med* 1997;102:3–8
3. Ferenczy A. HPV-associated lesions in pregnancy and their clinical implications. *Clin Obstet Gynecol* 1989;32:191–9
4. Schneider A, Hotz M, Gissmann L. Increased prevalence of human papillomaviruses in the lower genital tract of pregnant women. *Int J Cancer* 1987;40:198–201
5. Cook TA, Brunschwig JP, Butel JS, *et al.* Laryngeal papilloma: etiologic and therapeutic considerations. *Ann Otol Rhinol Laryngol* 1973;82:649–55
6. Ferenczy A. Treating genital condyloma during pregnancy with the carbon dioxide laser. *Am J Obstet Gynecol* 1984;148:9
7. Watts DH, Koutsky LA, Holmes KK, *et al.* Low risk of perinatal transmission of human papillomavirus: results from a prospective cohort study. *Am J Obstet Gynecol* 1998;178:365–73
8. Davis BD, Dulbecco R, Elsen HN. Other pox viruses that infect man. In *Microbiology*, 2nd edn. Hagerstown, MD: Harper and Row, 1973:1275
9. Viac J, Churdonnet Y. Immunocompetent cells and epithelial cell modifications in molluscum contagiosum. *J Cutan Pathol* 1990;17:202–5
10. Cotton DWK, Cooper C, Barrett DF, *et al.* Severe atypical molluscum contagiosum infection in an immunocompromised host. *Br J Dermatol* 1987;116:871–6
11. Pennys NS, Matsuo S, Mogollon R. The identification of molluscum infection by immunohistochemical means. *J Cutan Pathol* 1986;13:97–101
12. Larson JW. Influenza and pregnancy. *Clin Obstet Gynecol* 1982;25:599–603
13. Lee RV. Influenza. In *Principles and Practice of Medical Therapy in Pregnancy*, 2nd edn. Norwalk, CT: Appleton and Lange, 1992:656–59
14. Korones SB. Uncommon virus infections of the mother, fetus, and newborn: influenza, mumps and measles. *Clin Perinatol* 1988;15:259
15. McGregor JA, Burns JC, Levin MJ, *et al.* Transplacental passage of influenza A/Bangkok (H3N2) mimicking amniotic fluid infection syndrome. *Am J Obstet Gynecol* 1984;149:856–9
16. Prevention and control of influenza: recommendations of the Advisory Committee on Immunization Practices (ACIP). *Morbid Mortal Weekly Rep* 1996;45(RR-5):1–24
17. Rotbart HA. Human parvovirus infections. *Annu Rev Med* 1990;41:25–34
18. Thurn J. Human parvovirus B19: historical and clinical review. *Rev Infect Dis* 1988;10:1005–11
19. Torok TJ. Human parvovirus B19 infections in pregnancy. *Pediatr Infect Dis J* 1990;9:772–6
20. Rodis JF, Quinn DL, Gary WG, *et al.* Management and outcomes of pregnancies complicated by human B19 parvovirus infection: a prospective study. *Am J Obstet Gynecol* 1990;163:1168–71
21. Valeur-Jensen AK, Pedersen CB, Westergaard T, *et al.* Risk factors for parvovirus B19 infection in pregnancy. *J Am Med Assoc* 1999;281:1099–105
22. Modlin JF, Kinney JS. Perinatal enterovirus infections. *Adv Pediatr Infect Dis* 1987;2:57–78
23. Modlin JF. Perinatal echovirus and group B coxsackie virus infections. *Clin Perinatol* 1988;15:233–46
24. Torfasion EG, Reimer CB, Keyserling HL. Subclass restriction of human enterovirus antibodies. *J Clin Microbiol* 1987;8:1376–9
25. Amstey MS, Miller RK, Menegus MA, *et al.* Enterovirus in pregnant women and the perfused placenta. *Am J Obstet Gynecol* 1988;158:775–82
26. Rosenberg HS. Cardiovascular effects for congenital infections. *Am J Cardiovasc Pathol* 1987;1:147–50
27. Sterner G, Grandien M. Mumps in pregnancy at term. *Scand J Infect Dis* 1990;71(suppl):36–8
28. Watson JC, Hadler SC, Dykewicz CA, *et al.* Measles, mumps, and rubella – vaccine use and strategies for elimination of measles, rubella, and congenital rubella syndrome and control of mumps: recommendations of the Advisory Committee on Immunization Practices (ACIP). *Morbid Mortal Weekly Rep* 1998;47(RR-8):1–57
29. Amstey MS. Measles. In *Principles and Practice of Medical Therapy in Pregnancy*, 2nd edn. Norwalk, CT: Appleton and Lange, 1992:659–61
30. Gazala E, Karplus M, Liberman JR, *et al.* The effect of maternal measles on the fetus. *Pediatr Infect Dis* 1985;4:203–41
31. Grandeim M, Sterner G. Measles in pregnancy. *Scand J Infect Dis* 1990;71(suppl):45–8
32. Horstmann DM. Rubella. *Clin Obstet Gynecol* 1982;25:585–97
33. Miller E, Cradock-Watson JE, Pollock TM. Consequences of confirmed maternal rubella at successive stages of pregnancy. *Lancet* 1982;2:781–4
34. Munro ND, Sheppard S, Smithers RW, *et al.* Temporal relations between maternal rubella and congenital defects. *Lancet* 1987;2:201–4
35. Gall SA. Rubella in pregnancy. *Obstet Gynecol Rep* 1990;2:161–9
36. Tanemura M, Suzumori K, Yagami Y, *et al.* Diagnosis of fetal rubella infection with reverse transcription and nested polymerase chain reaction: a study of 34 cases diagnosed in fetuses. *Am J Obstet Gynecol* 1996;174:578–82

Section IIIc

Perinatal infections: chlamydia infection

28
Chlamydia infection

J.B. Shumway

Chlamydia trachomatis is a sexually-transmitted disease of epidemic proportions, infecting an estimated 4 million people a year[1]. The economic costs related to its treatment are estimated to exceed 3 billion dollars annually[1,2]. *C. trachomatis* is an ancient insidious disease with significant morbidity. It is the most common sexually-transmitted pathogen in the United States. Of the 155 000 infants in the USA exposed to chlamydia during delivery each year, approximately 100 000 become infected[3]. Vertical transmission during vaginal delivery occurs in 50–70% of infants causing neonatal conjunctivitis, bronchiolitis or chlamydia pneumonia. In addition, maternal infection *per se* may have severe consequences for the mother. The causes of maternal morbidity include infertility, ectopic pregnancy, adverse pregnancy outcome with increased risk of urethritis, pelvic inflammatory disease and, potentially increased risk for stillbirth, and preterm deliveries[4–8]. Ectopic pregnancy is responsible for 11% of maternal deaths with *C. trachomatis* being a significant etiologic pathogen for salpingitis and subsequent tubal scarring.

On a global perspective, *C. trachomatis* is a significant cause of trachoma, a chronic conjunctivitis affecting at least 500 million people in developing countries and resulting in the blindness of 10 to 12 million people annually. In some communities, all are infected by 2 years of age. In industrial nations, however, the mode of transmitting *C. trachomatis* is sexual, unlike the direct transmission by touch or contaminated clothing that occurs in endemic areas of trachoma. Like all sexually-transmitted diseases, Chlamydia trachomatis has reached epidemic levels in Western societies causing significant impaired fertility and perinatal complications, and in developing societies,

significant ocular disease. Lymphogranuloma venereum, a chronic vulvar disease found worldwide and caused by *C. trachomatis* serotypes LI, L2, L3, also causes significant maternal morbidity.

EPIDEMIOLOGY

Studies of the prevalence and risk factors for *C. trachomatis* are flawed by imprecision in diagnosis due to difficulty of culturing in McCoy's media, failure to study large and well-characterized populations, selection bias and failure to correct for selection bias. Many studies lack a clear description of the population screened. Most of these groups (i.e. college students, gynecologic clinic patients, obstetrical patients, etc.) are neither homogenous nor representative of the population at large. Thus, the generalizability of these studies and conclusions are limited.

The prevalence of infection with *C. trachomatis* varies widely from 3% in asymptomatic women to as high as 20% in patients attending sexually-transmitted disease clinics. As seen in Table 1, in pregnancy, widely divergent prevalence rates have been published[9]. In a large study of obstetrical clinic patients in Memphis, Ryan *et al.*[10] reported a 21% prevalence of *C. trachomatis* cervical infection in pregnant women studying a population of 11 544 women. Most published studies have a clear selection bias toward high-risk populations and the national (USA) average for chlamydia infection of the cervix is 5% in sexually-active women[11].

Risk factors of chlamydia infection in pregnancy

High-risk groups for cervical chlamydia studies have been characterized. Chlamydial infection in pregnancy

Table 1 Prevalence of cervical infection with *Chlamydia trachomatis* during pregnancy

Investigators	Site	Positive test	%
Alexander *et al.* 1983	New Mexico	139	27
Harrison *et al.* 1983	Gallup, NM	48/200	24
Ismail *et al.*[23] 1985	Chicago, IL	44/201	21
Gravett *et al.*[6] 1986	Seattle, WA	47/534	9
Ryan *et al.*[10] 1990	Memphis, TN	2424/11 544	21
Alary *et al.*[50] 1993	Quebec City, CAN	136/772	18
Hardy *et al.* 1993	Baltimore, MD		37

has been associated with presence of other sexually-transmitted diseases in the patient or in their partner, marital status, age < 20 years, sterile pyuria (acute urethral syndrome) and late/absent prenatal care[12]. These studies, however, do suffer from the same inadequacies as the aforementioned prevalence studies, i.e. imprecise and technically-difficult diagnostic testing, non-randomly assembled and inadequately defined patient populations (selection bias), and failure to correct for interrelated variables (confounding bias).

In a large case control study of 672 pregnant patients in Quebec City, Canada, young age, nulliparity and a new sexual partner in the last year were all factors independently associated with infection (values were all at least < 0.001). For two groups of women aged less than 20, and ages 20–25 years, the odds ratio of *C. trachomatis* is 8.1 and 6.0. Routine screening of all women below 25 years of age may be necessary to optimize use of specific diagnostic tests[3]. In a large Japanese study of 10 980 married pregnant women and 1792 unmarried pregnant women seeking voluntary termination of pregnancy, the detection rate among the married women was 5.6%. In the unmarried group, the rate was 15.2% (272 of 1792 cases). They also noted an increase in detection in both married and unmarried as the age of the subjects decreased. Young, unmarried women were at highest risk[13,14]. Young age < 20 also is predictive of recurrent chlamydial colonization during pregnancy[14]. Up to 45% of women with gonorrheal infection have coexisting chlamydial infection[15–17].

MICROBIOLOGY

The order Chlamydiales, which includes *Chlamydia psittaci*, *Chlamydia pneumoniae* and *Chlamydia trachomatis* species are obligate intracellular bacteria. It has a unique reproductive cycle which involves ingestion by a specific host cell and inhibition of phagolysosomal fusion. Once inside the cell, the chlamydia elementary body (which is the infectious agent) reorganizes and transforms into an active replicating form, using ATP furnished by the host cell, called a reticulate body. These reticulate bodies then produce 300–500 progeny. At the end of 48 h, the growth cycle is complete, the cell wall is broken and the new spore-like elementary bodies are released to initiate new infectious cycles. Chlamydia bacteria divide by binary fusion and are similar to Gram-negative bacteria in the content of their cell wall. Like viruses, they are obligate intracellular parasites requiring viable cells for survival.

C. trachomatis may be differentiated into 18 serotypes. Serotypes A, B, Ba and C cause trachoma, an endemic chronic ocular infection in the developing world. Serotypes LI, L2 and L3 cause lymphogranuloma venereum (LGV) leading to a chronic granulomatous change of the vulvar region. LGV occurs sporadically in Western societies, but is endemic to Africa, India, Asia and South America. In its final stages, LGV leads to inguinal lymphadenitis, buboes and progressive tissue destruction. Its course is not affected by pregnancy. Its perinatal significance involves possible transmission to the neonates during birth through an infected vagina. *C. trachomatis* serotypes D–K are responsible for the genital and ocular infections seen in Western industrialized societies (Table 2).

The incubation period for genital infection is 6–14 days with the primary site of infection being the female endocervix. The majority of infected patients are asymptomatic, which along with a persistent carrier state facilitates the high prevalence of chlamydial

Table 2 *Chlamydia trachomatis* serotypes

Organism	Inclusions stain with iodine	Origin(s)	Serotype(s)	Disease(s)
Chlamydia trachomatis	Yes	Mostly of human origin	A, B, Ba, C	Hyperendemic blinding trachoma
			D, E, F, G, H, I, J, K	Inclusion, conjunctivitis, cervicitis, nongonoccocal urethritis, salpingitis, proclitis, epididymitis, pneumonia of newborn
			L1, L2, L3	Lymphogranuloma vencreum
Chlamydia pneumoniae	No	Respiratory tract infections in humans	TWAR	Upper and lower respiratory tract infections
Chlamydia psittaci	No	Common pathogen in birds and lower mammals	Many	Psittacosis

infections. Most cases are discovered only through epidemiologic contact tracing of treated patients or through incidental health screening procedures. A wide spectrum of diseases have been attributed to *C. trachomatis* including pelvic inflammatory disease (PID), mucopurulent cervicitis, endometritis, acute salpingitis, proctitis, urethritis and acute urethral syndrome. Asymptomatic infection, which occurs primarily in women, exacts a heavy health toll in chronic sequelae of infertility and ectopic pregnancy resulting from ascending infection to the upper genital tract. Exposure to conserved chlamydial antigens through reinfection or persistent infection results in chronic inflammation and tubal scarring. The key antigenic proteins in this process are chlamydial heat shock protein Hsp 60 and Hsp 10, which are capable of eliciting intense mononuclear inflammation.

Unusual presentations of chlamydial infection include Reiter syndrome which is an immune-mediated systemic illness that occurs most often in men who posses the HLA-B27 haplotype. It is characterized by a classic triad of urethritis, conjunctivitis and arthritis appearing approximately 4 weeks after genital infection sequelae. Endocarditis, pleuritis, hepatic infection and dilated cardiomyopathy have also been described with chlamydial infection. Among men, the primary site of chlamydial infection includes urethritis, epididymitis, proctitis and possibly acute prostatitis.

PERINATAL RISKS OF CHLAMYDIAL INFECTION

It is uncertain if adverse pregnancy outcomes such as preterm delivery, premature rupture of the membranes, low birthweight, perinatal death and late onset postpartum endometritis are associated with chlamydial genital infection[4,6,19]. In other surveys, no significant association was seen. Sweet *et al.*[11], however, demonstrated that antepartum cervical infection with *C. trachomatis*, as shown by rising IgM serology, was a risk factor for premature rupture of the membranes, preterm delivery or low birth weight. In a study by Cohen *et al.*[20] the risk of premature rupture of the membranes, preterm labor, IUGR, and preterm delivery were reduced significantly by the aggressive treatment of maternal cervical chlamydial infections. More recent data confirm these findings[21].

The multicenter VIP study (Vaginal Infection and Prematurity Study) with interim results published in 1993 showed a modest trend toward low birthweight and preterm delivery in those women infected with *C. trachomatis*. This study reported on 7566 women who enrolled in the first 32 months of the study who had delivered and for whom culture information was available. *C. trachomatis* was isolated in specimens from 8.2% of the women. Univariate analysis indicated that both preterm delivery (OR 1.6; 95% CI 1.3–2.0) and

low birthweight (OR 1.6; 95% CI > 1.3–2.1) were more likely to occur in the presence of *C. trachomatis*. After controlling for age, marital status, ethnicity and other organisms (*M. hominis, U. ureulyticum and T. vaginalis*) with backward-stepping logistic regression analysis, there was an adjusted odds ratio of 1.53 (95% CI 1.21–1.93) for preterm delivery in the presence of *C. trachomatis*[22].

It appears that an adverse pregnancy outcome, such as preterm delivery, is more likely in the presence of chlamydial infection. The magnitude of this association may in part be related to the timing of initial infection and pregnancy. It had been suggested that genital chlamydial infection may shorten the latency period and predispose to a higher incidence of chorioamnionitis and early endometritis in patients with preterm premature rupture of membranes (PROM). However, in a prospective study of conservative management of 178 patients with premature rupture of membranes (PROM) between weeks 22 and 35 weeks of gestation, the presence of chlamydia had no effect on latency, chorioamnionitis or endometritis[23].

The vertical transmission role of chlamydia has been estimated at 60–70% with vaginal delivery[24–26]. Based on serologic assessment of infants born to mothers with untreated cervical chlamydial infection, some 50–80% of exposed infants develop serologic evidence of chlamydial infection. Infants born by Cesarean section with PROM have a decreased risk of vertical transmission (20%) compared to vaginal delivery (53%)[27]. It has been thought that in-utero transmission does not occur, however, recent case reports demonstrate that fetal infection occurs despite Cesarean section while the membranes were intact[28–30]. This suggests the capability of transmembranous or transplacental passage of chlamydia to the fetus. Fetal infection with chlamydia has been associated with fetal demise[5,29].

The most common manifestations of neonatal infection are conjunctivitis and pneumonia; *C. trachomatis* is the most common form of conjunctivitis in the newborn. Approximately 18–50% of exposed infants develop conjunctivitis within the first 2 weeks of life, 11–18% develop pneumonia in the first 3–11 weeks of life. It is important that infants receive prophylaxis with topical treatments such as erythromycin ointment. Silver nitrate drops, although effective in treating gonorrhea are ineffective in treating chlamydial conjunctivitis. Spontaneous resolution usually occurs although conjunctival scarring may ensue. Serologic evidence of infection is found in 50–80% of exposed infants born to mothers with untreated infection.

Infants who develop a chlamydial pneumonia may recover if untreated, although the course will be protracted with resolution over a period of weeks. Pneumonia in the first 6 months of life may be associated with reactive airway disease later in childhood.

DIAGNOSIS

The diagnosis and isolation of *C. trachomatis* has been difficult. It is technically challenging because the organism requires a susceptible tissue culture cell line. The cycloheximide-treated McCoy cell is the one most employed with sensitivity of 80–90% and specificity of 99% in optimal conditions. Because of the technically arduous procedure of inoculation and then reexamination at 24 hours and then 72 hours later for inclusions, other methods of testing have been developed. These include detection by fluorescent monoclonal antibody testing to chlamydial or 'elementary bodies', enzyme-linked immunosorbent assay (ELISA), DNA probes to specific ribosomal RNAs31 and PCR testing using primers directed against the major outer membrane protein gene and the trachomatis-specific cryptic plasmid[32].

These new technologies are rapidly altering the use of the 'gold standard' labor-intensive and expensive McCoy cell cultures. Antigen detection kits are widely available and represent a less costly alternative to culture. Recent improvements have increased sensitivity and specificity in these new tests to 93% or better[31]. The recent PCR tests appear to be even more sensitive than McCoy cell culture in some situations[32]. Recent studies to detect chlamydia specimens from the vaginal introitus (as opposed to the posterior vaginal vault and endocervix) using PCR technology during pregnancy were highly sensitive and specific. This technique is clinically useful because a speculum examination is not necessary[33]. Diagnosis of fetal infection with chlamydia trachomatis has recently been described using polymerase chain reaction-reaction methods on chorionic villi[34]. As with all screening tests, their best use is in populations with a high prevalence of chlamydia infection. The positive predictive value of these tests is diminished in low prevalence populations.

The identification of proper screening populations during pregnancy for chlamydia is controversial. All sexually active women should be screened, especially during pregnancy. Young, nulliparous women and those having a new sexual partner within the past year are particularly at risk and should be tested[3]. Adolescent pregnancies are also high risks for reinfection and may require serial screening[14,35,36]. Any woman undergoing tests for unexplained infertility needs chlamydial testing because atypical or subclinical pelvic inflammatory disease due to chlamydia is now more prevalent[37]. Even one single episode of treated chlamydia will cause infertility in 7.8% of women[38].

Serologic testing is a useful epidemiologic tool to assess the incidence of prior infection with chlamydia, particularly when used as a periodic survey. Recent studies show no serologic evidence to link past chlamydial infection to miscarriage[39,40] although its link

to late pregnancy complications and infertility is well established[11,20,41–43]. Virtually all infected individuals will develop a measurable antibody response. An individual with paired acute and convalescent serum titers demonstrating a four-fold rise in IgG or the presence of IgM antibodies could be considered acutely infected. In practice, however, the high background rate of anti-chlamydial antibodies and the chronic nature of many chlamydial infections renders serodiagnosis not clinically useful except as an epidemiologic tool (Table 3).

It is clear that a single infection will not result in immunity. Homo and heterotypic multiple infections are common with some level of immunity developing after serial infections. Both antibody and cell-mediated immunity are important in host resistance and clearance of primary infection[44,45].

TREATMENT AND MANAGEMENT

Chlamydia trachomatis is susceptible to a wide range of antibiotics. Tetracyclines and erythromycin are generally the drugs of choice for chlamydial genital tract infections. Resistance to these agents has never been shown naturally. All documented treatment failures have demonstrated the recovered agents being susceptible. A relative resistance to erythromycin has developed, but is not yet clinically significant[46].

The newly approved azalide drug, azithromycin, given as a single 1 g oral dose is as effective as doxycycline and improves patient compliance. Azithromycin is a treatment option in women who cannot tolerate erythromycin[47]. Penicillin is effective against chlamydial infection in large doses, clindamycin and rifampin are also very active. However, resistance to penicillin, clindamycin and rifampin in laboratory settings develops rapidly.

Because chlamydia occurs concomitantly in 30–50% of women with gonorrhea, treatment for chlamydia is recommended for any patient with gonorrhea[15–17]. Erythromycin or amoxicillin are the treatments of choice in pregnancy and in childhood. Recent studies showed that amoxicillin is more effective and more tolerated in pregnancy[48,49]. Treatment of the mother is effective in preventing vertical transmission to the infant with the eradication rates of 95–98% for erythromycin or amoxicillin[25,51]. Clindamycin is a potential third line agent, but is not as effective as erythromycin. Tetracyclines and quinolones are contraindicated in pregnancy due to their potential adverse effect on fetal bones and teeth[52]. The large dose of erythromycin required to treat genital chlamydial infection represents a major problem with compliance with 30–70% of patients describing gastrointestinal distress. If the 7-day erythromycin regimen is not tolerated, a lower dose of 250 mg for 14 days appears effective. Erythromycin estolate is

Table 3 Diagnosis of common *C. trachomatis* infection in women

Associated findings	Clinical criteria	Laboratory criteria presumptive	Diagnostic
Mucoprurulent cervicitis	Mucoprurulent cervical discharge, ectopy and edema, friable cervix	Cervical GS with > 30 PMN/HPF	Positive culture, antigen test, or PCR
Acute urethral syndrome	Dysuria-frequency in young sexually active women; recent new sexual partner; more than 7 days of symptoms	Pyuria, no bacteriuria	Positive culture, antigen detection, or PCR (cervix or urethra)
PID	Lower abdominal pain; adnexal and cervical motion tenderness; evidence muco-purulent cervicitis often present	Cervical GS > 30 PMN/HPF; endometritis on endometrial biopsy	Positive culture, antigen detection, or PCR from cervix, endometrium, or tube
Perihepatitis	Right upper quadrant pain, nausea, vomiting, fever; young sexually active women; evidence of PID	As for MPC and PID	High-titer IgM or IgG antibody to *C. trachomatis*

Reprinted with permission from Stamm WE. Diagnosis of *Chlamydia trachomatis* genitourinary infections. *Ann Intern Med* 1988;108: 710–17. GS, Gram stain; MPC, mucoprurulent cervicitis; PMN, polymorphonuclear neutrophils; HPF, high power field, PCR, polymerase chain reaction

contraindicated during pregnancy because of a drug-related hepatotoxicity[53]. All sexual contacts within the previous 30 days should be examined, treated and counseled regarding safer sex practices[37] (Table 4).

If chlamydial urethritis or cervicitis persists after treatment with good patient compliance, a repeated course of erythromycin is usually effective. The persistent symptoms may be due to another as yet undefined pathogen.

PREVENTION AND FUTURE RESEARCH

Vaccination against *Chlamydia trachomatis* is the source of ongoing research study. This development is hampered by the need to generate a superior immune response than that which occurs after natural infection (as multiple episodes of infection are needed to confer immunity in a natural setting). Furthermore, the pathogenesis of chlamydia is not well understood, particularly the mechanism for chronic inflammation leading to tissue damage[37]. It is thought that the antigen-antibody reactions to chlamydial heat-shock proteins may be an important link to the morphological scarring seen with chlamydia[18,43]. The cause and mechanism of tissue damage from persistent infection leading to infertility or ectopic pregnancy in addition to the risks of preterm labor[53], PROM or fetal growth retardation are fertile grounds for further study. However, it is clear that effective

Table 4 Treatment recommendations for chlamydial infection in pregnant women

Recommended regimens
  Amoxicillin 500 mg orally 3 times daily
    for 7 days; or
  Erythromycin base 500 mg
    orally 4 times daily for 7 days
Alternative regimens
  Azithromycin 1 g orally; or
  Erythromycin base 250 mg orally 4 times daily
    for 14 days; or
  Erythromycin ethylsuccinate 800 mg orally
    4 times daily for 7 days; or
  Erythromycin ethylsuccinate 400 mg orally
    4 times daily for 14 days

From Centers for Disease Control and Prevention (CDC). 1998 guidelines for sexually transmitted diseases. *MMWR Morb Mortal Wkly Rep* 47(RR–1):1, 1998

treatment is available and can improve perinatal outcomes[54].

REFERENCES

1. Much DH, Yeh SY. Prevalence of chlamydia trachomatis infection in pregnant patients. *Public Health Reports* 1991;106:490–3

2. Centers for disease control and prevention (CDC): Recommendations for the prevention and management of Chlamydia trachomatis infection 1998. *MMWR Morb Mort Weekly* 47:52–60

3. Alary M, Joly JR, Moutqiun JM, LaBrecque M. Strategy for screening pregnant women for chlamydial infection in a low-prevalence area. *Obstet Gynecol* 1993;82: 339–404

4. Martin DH, Koutsky L, Eschenbach DA, *et al*. Prematurity and perinatal mortality in pregnancies complicated by maternal Chlamydia trachomatis infections. *J Am Med Assoc* 1982;247:1585–8

5. Koskiniemi M, Ammala P, Narvanen A, *et al*. Stillbirths and maternal antibodies to Chlamydia trachomatis – A new EIA test for serology. *Acta Obstet Gyn Scand* 1996;75:657–61

6. Gravett MG, Nelson HP, DeRoues T, *et al*. Independent associations of bacterial vaginosis and Chlamydia trachomatis infection with adverse pregnancy outcome. *J Am Med Assoc* 1986;256:1899–1903

7. Gencay M, Koskiniemi M, Saikku P, *et al*. Chlamydia trachomatis seropositivity during pregnancy is associated with perinatal complications. *Clin Infect Dis* 1995;21:424–6

8. Claman P, Toye B, Peeling RW, *et al*. Perinatal complications with perinatal infection with *Chlamydia trachomatis*. *Can Med Association J* 1995;153:259–62

9. Stamm WE, Holmes, KK. Chlamydia trachomatis infection of the adult. In Holmes KK, March P-A, Sparling PF, Wiesner PJ, eds. *Sexually Transmitted Diseases*, 2nd edition. New York: McGraw Hill, 1990:181–93

10. Ryan GM, Abdella TN, McNeeley SG, *et al*. Chlamydia trachomatis infection in pregnancy and effect of treatment on outcome. *Am J Obstet Gynecol* 1990;162:34–39

11. Sweet RL, Landers DV, Walker C, *et al*. Chlamydia trachomatis infection and pregnancy outcome. *Am J Obstet Gynecol* 1987;156:824–33

12. Centers for Disease Control. Chlamydia trachomatis infections: Policy guidelines for prevention and control. *MMWR* 1985;34(S3):53S–74S

13. Koroku M, Kumamoto Y, Hirose T, *et al*. Epidemiologic study of Chlamydia trachomatis infection in pregnant women. *Sex Trans Diseases* 1994;21:329–31

14. Miller JM. Recurrent chlamydial colonization during pregnancy. *Am J Perinatology* 1998;15:307–9

15. Centers for Disease Control and Prevention. Sexually transmitted disease treatment guidelines. *MMWR* 1993;42(RR–14):1–102

16. Centers for Disease Control and Prevention. Sexually transmitted disease treatment guidelines. *MMWR* 1989;38(S8):1–43

17. Christmas JT, Wendell GD, Bawdon RE, *et al*. Concomitant infection with Neisseria gonorrhoeae and Chlamydia trachomatis in pregnancy. *Obstet Gynecol* 1989;74(3 pt 1):295–8

18. LaVerda D, Kalayoglu MV, Byrne GI. Chlamydial heat shock proteins and disease pathology: new paradigms for old problems? *Infect Dis Obstet Gynecol* 1999;7:64–71

19. McGregor JA, French JI, Richter R, *et al*. Antenatal microbiologic and maternal risk factors associated with prematurity. *Am J Obstet Gynecol* 1990;163:1465–73

20. Cohen I, Veille JC, Calkins BM. Improved pregnancy outcome following successful treatment of chlamydial infection. *J Am Med Assoc* 1990;263:3160–3

21. Ryan GM, Abdella TN, McNeeley SG, *et al*. Chlamydia trachomatis infection in pregnancy and effect on outcome. *Am J Obstet Gynecol* 1990;162:34

22. Carey JC, Yaffe SJ, Catz C. The vaginal infections and prematurity study: an overview. *Clin Obstet Gynecol* 1993;36:809–20

23. Ismail MA, Pridjian G, Hibbard JU, *et al*. Significance of positive cervical cultures for Chlamydia trachomatis in patients with preterm premature rupture of membranes. *Am J Perinatol* 1992;9:368–70

24. Arya OP, Mallinson H, Goddard AD. Epidemiological and clinical correlates of chlamydial infection of the cervix. *Br J Vener Dis* 1981;57:118–24

25. Tait IA, Rees E, Hobson D, *et al*. Chlamydial infection of the cervix in contacts of men with nongonococcal urethritis. *Br J Vener Dis* 1980;56:37–45

26. Schachter J, Grossman M, Sweet RL, *et al*. Prospective study of perinatal transmission of Chlamydia trachomatis. *J Am Med Assoc* 1986;255:3374–77

27. Smith JR, Taylor-Robinson D. Infection due to Chlamydia trachomatis in pregnancy and the newborn. *Baillier Clin Obstet Gynaecol* 1993;7:237–55

28. Shariat H, Young M, Abedin M. An interesting case presentation: a possible new route for perinatal acquisition of Chlamydia. *J Perinatol* 1992;12:300–2

29. Thorp JM Jr, Katz VL, Fowler LJ, *et al*. Fetal death from chlamydial infection across intact amniotic membranes. *Am J Obstet Gynecol* 1989;161:1245–6

30. Shariat H, Young M, Abedin M. An interesting case presentation: a possible new route for perinatal acquisition of Chlamydia. *J Perinatol* 1992;12:300–2

31. Hosein IK, Kaunitz AM, Craft JJ. Detection of cervical Chlamydia trachomatis and Neisseria gonorrhoeae with deoxyribonucleic acid probe assays in obstetric patients. *Am J Obstet Gynecol* 1992;167:588–91

32. Talley AR, Garcia-Ferrer F, Laycock KA, *et al*. Comparative diagnosis of neonatal chlamydial conjunctivitis by polymerase chain reduction and McCoy cell culture. *Am J Ophthalmol* 1994;117:50–7

33. Witkin SS, Inglis SR, Polaneczky M. Detection of Chlamydia trachomatis and Trichomonas vaginalis by polymerase chain reaction in introital specimens from pregnant women. *Am J Obstet Gynecol* 1996;175:165–7

34. Dong ZW, Li Y, Zhang LY, Liu RM. Detection of chlamydia trachomatis intrauterine infection using polymerase chain reaction on chorionic villi. *Int J Gynaecol Obstet* 1998;61:29–32

35. Oh MK, Cloud GA, Baker Sl, *et al*. Chlamydial infection and sexual behavior in young pregnant teenagers. *Sex Trans Dis* 1993;20:45–50

36. Allaire AD, Huddleston JF, Graves WL, Nathan L. Initial and repeat screening for Chlamydia trachomatis during pregnancy. *Infect Dis Obstet Gynecol* 1998;6:116–22

37. Paavonen J. Immunopathogenesis of pelvic inflammatory disease and infertility – What do we know and what shall we do? *Hum Reprod* 1996;11(2 Suppl S):42–45

38. Westrom LV. Chlamydia and its effect on reproduction. *Hum Reprod* 1996;11(2S):23–30

39. Osser S, Persson K. Chlamydial antibodies in women who suffer miscarriage. *Br J Obstet Gynecol* 1996;103:137–41

40. Rae R, Smith IW, Liston WA, Kilpatrick DC. Chlamydial serologic studies and recurrent spontaneous abortion. *Am J Obstet Gynecol* 1994;170:782–5

41. Lan J, van den Brule AJ, Hemrika DJ, *et al.* Chlamydia trachomatis and ectopic pregnancy: retrospective analysis of salpingectomy specimens, endometrial biopsies, and cervical smears. *J Clin Path* 1995;48:815–9

42. Claman P, Toye B, Peeling RW, *et al.* Serologic evidence of Chlamydia trachomatis infection and risk of preterm birth. *Can Med Assn J* 1995;153:259–62

43. Witkin SS. Immunity to heat shock proteins and pregnancy outcome. *Infect Dis Obstet Gynecol* 1999;7:35–8

44. Williams DM, Schachter J, Grubbs B, Sumaya CV. The role of antibody in host defense against the agent of mouse pneumonitis. *J Infect Dis* 1982;145:200–5

45. Williams DM, Grubbs B, Schachter J. Primary murine Chlamydia trachomatis pneumonia in B-cell deficient mice. *Infect Immun* 1987;55:2387–90

46. Mourad A, Sweet RL, Sugg N, Schachter J. Relative resistance to erythromycin in Chlamydia trachomatis. *Antim Agen Chemother* 1980;18:696–8

47. Bush MR, Rosa C. Azithromycin and erythromycin in the treatment of cervical chlamydial infection during pregnancy. *Obstet Gynecol* 1994;84:61–3

48. Wehbeh HA, Ruggeirio RM, Shahem S, *et al.* Single-dose azithromycin for Chlamydia in pregnant women. *J Reprod Med* 1998;43:509–14

49. Turrentine MA, Newton ER. Amoxicillin or erythromycin for the treatment of antenatal chlamydial infection: a meta-analysis. *Obstet Gynecol* 1995;86:1021–5

50. Alary M, Joly JR, Moutquin JM, *et al.* Randomised comparison of Amoxicillin and erythromycin in treatment of genital chlamydial infection in pregnancy. *Lancet* 1994;344(8935):1461–5

51. Crombleholme WR, Schachter J, Grossman M, *et al.* Amoxicillin therapy for Chlamydia trachomatis in pregnancy. *Obstet Gynecol* 1990;75:752–6

52. Egerman RS. The tetracyclines. *Obstet Gynecol Clin N Am* 1992;19:551–61

53. Ngassa PC, Egbe JA. Maternal genital Chlamydia trachomatis infection and the risk of preterm labor. *Int J Gynecol Obstet* 1994;47:241–6

54. Gonorrhea and Chlamydial infections. *ACOG Technical Bulletin* #90 March 1994

Section IIId

Perinatal infections: protozoan infection

29

Protozoan infection: toxoplasmosis, trichomoniasis, lice and scabies

E.R. Newton

TOXOPLASMOSIS

Although toxoplasma encephalitis[1] has gained worldwide recognition as a major cause of death and morbidity in immunodeficient individuals, especially those with acquired immunodeficiency syndrome (AIDS), the fetus and child remain the major victims of toxoplasmic infection. Approximately 3500–4000 pregnant women per year are infected with *Toxoplasma gondii* and 10–60% of their fetuses will be infected. Although the majority (80–90%) appear asymptomatic at birth, recent studies suggest that a significant proportion (40–60%) will demonstrate subsequent defects consistent with chronic toxoplasmosis. These defects include chorioretinitis, hydrocephalus, deafness and mental retardation. Unfortunately, problems in primary prevention, diagnosis, treatment and follow-up limit the effectiveness of intervention programs.

Biology

Toxoplasma gondii is a ubiquitous coccidian whose effects are felt in many animals in addition to humans. The organism has three distinct forms: sporozoites within an oocyst, tachyzoites (also called endozoites or trophozoites) and brachyzoites (or cystozoites) within a tissue cyst.

The life cycle of *T. gondii* is outlined in Figure 1. Members of the cat family, Felidae, are the only known

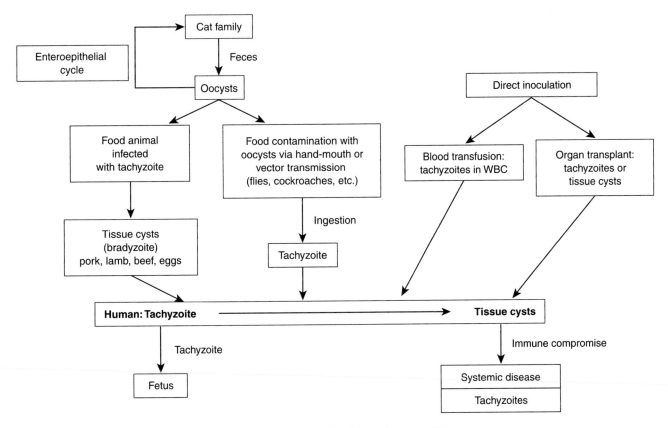

Figure 1 Life cycle of *Toxoplasma gondii*

303

definitive hosts. The sexual reproductive cycle occurs in the villi of the cat ileum. The time from primary inoculation to oocyst appearance in the feces varies by the mode of primary infection: ingestion of tissue cysts (chronic infection in prey animals), 3–5 days; ingestion of fecal oocysts, 20–24 days; or ingestion of tachyzoites, 7–10 days. Oocysts are shed for 1–3 weeks with peak production at 5–8 days[2,3]. Millions of oocysts are shed in a single day. Most cats are infected primarily at 6–12 weeks of age[4], corresponding to weaning and the development of hunting skills. Once a cat has been infected, its immune system severely curtails or eliminates future oocyst production. The previously infected cat may therefore be a safer pet than a seronegative cat whose behavior is curtailed.

After excretion with feces, the zygote within the oocysts (13×11 μm) undergo sporulation. The zygote divides into two sporoblasts that form two sporocysts within the larger oocyst. Each sporoblast undergoes two divisions to produce four sporozoites (8×3 μm). Sporulation takes 1–21 days (average, 3–4 days), depending upon temperature, moisture and oxygenation. The oocysts can remain infectious for months[2,3].

After elimination and within the 3–4 days prior to sporulation, the fecal oocysts are not infectious[2,3,5]. As a result, human infection from direct contact with a shedding cat is unusual. The major role of cats in human toxoplasmosis is transiently to pollute the environment with massive numbers of oocysts that may remain infectious for months or years. The likelihood of human toxoplasmosis is related to environmental conditions that enhance or reduce oocyst survival, the prevalence of feline toxoplasmosis within that region and culinary habits of the population at risk.

Higher rates of seropositivity to toxoplasmosis are associated with warm, moist climates: Brazil, 72%[6]; Alabama, 69%[7]; Denver, Colorado, 3%[8]; Oslo, Norway, 1%[9]. These observations are supported by experimental data concerning oocyst survival related to humidity and temperature. Oocysts remain infectious for at least 17 months in water, at least 32 days in 100% relative humidity (at 22–26 °C) and 11 days at 37% relative humidity, and they lose their ability to infect at less than 19% relative humidity and when the moisture content of feces drops to 0–1%[2,3,10].

Ambient temperatures affect both sporulation (infectivity) and survival of the oocysts. Unless combined with low relative humidity (< 20%), extremes in environmental temperature will not completely eliminate *T. gondii* from contaminated soil.

Survival and infectivity of sporulated oocysts after application of various cleaning agents has been examined experimentally by Frenkel and Dubey[3]. High concentrations of ammonia (33%) and iodine (7%) killed all oocysts within 30 min, whereas ammonia (1.7%) and iodine (2%) were no more effective than drying alone. Household ammonia (4–6%) requires more than 60 min of exposure to sterilize cat feces. Smaller particles of fecal matter (empty, uncleaned litter pan) exposed to water heated to boiling and poured into the pan (75–80 °C) are sterilized rapidly.

Despite strong experimental evidence, a direct relationship between oocyst shedding and human toxoplasmosis is not clear from epidemiological studies. Although 14–50% of cats in the USA are seropositive, oocysts are found in the feces of less than 1% of cats examined, perhaps due to the limited age range and short duration (1–3 weeks) of oocyst shedding[11,12]. Likewise, the presence of oocysts in the soil correlates poorly with seropositivity in humans[11,12]. Additionally, serological studies of veterinarians and cat owners do not support a strong relationship between a long, intensive exposure to cats and a greater risk of acute toxoplasmosis[13–15]. Indeed, persons who report no contact with cats have seropositivity rates of 5–40%[13–15].

The latter discrepant information raises questions concerning the role of direct contact with cats and acute toxoplasmosis and our present methods of ascertaining the association. The correlation between seropositivity and house cats may be too crude to reveal a relationship. Studies limited to exposure to sick, young or feral cats may identify a relationship.

On the other hand, oocysts may be so widely distributed in the environment and direct contact with a cat that is shedding oocysts so rare, that the risk of acute toxoplasmosis through oocysts is a function of age and non-specific contact, such as outdoor gardening, culinary habits, food preparation, presence of insect vectors and personal hygiene.

The tachyzoite form of the parasite is seen in the acute stage of the infection. Tachyzoites result from ingestion of oocysts (food contamination) or tissue cysts (infected food source). The liberated parasites can survive for 1–3 h in pepsin–hydrochloric acid (stomach fluid) and 4–6 h in trypsin (intestinal fluid) – enough time for transmural migration into the host. The tachyzoites are spread hematogenously and can be identified by Wright's or Giemsa stains. Every cell type is susceptible to penetration.

The tachyzoite requires an intracellular habitat to survive. The intracellular, intravascular tachyzoite undergoes multiplication, endodyogeny, every 4–6 h to form rosettes. These intracellular collections (tissue cysts) vary in size, but may contain as many as 3000 organisms and are 200 μm in size. Rupture of the host cell results in continuing infection and tissue destruction. As the host develops an immune response to the parasite, parasitemia and systemic infection with tachyzoites decreases. In their 'protected' intracellular cysts, the tachyzoites evolve into brachyzoites (cystozoites).

The latent or chronic stage is manifested by tissue cysts in most organs. The brain, skeletal muscle, cardiac muscle and placenta are the most common sites for tissue cysts, which may be identified by periodic acid-Schiff stain. Recurrent parasitemia is rare in immune-competent individuals. However, under immunodepressed states, especially acquired immunodeficiency syndrome (AIDS), the cysts may reactivate and cause parasitemia and tissue destruction.

The ingestion of tissue cysts in undercooked or uncooked meat is an important source of infection in the USA. Serological evidence of past infection and potential for tissue cyst inoculation[16,17] is present in 15% of cattle, 15% of sheep, 30% of pigs and 43% of goats. The reported frequency of tissue cysts in common cuts of meat is less frequent: fresh beef, less than 1%; lamb, 5%; mutton, 10%; and pork, 30%[16,17]. However, these studies may underestimate the risk. The selected samples used were too few and too small to estimate the prevalence accurately. It is also probable that modern farming techniques, intensive pen raising and processed commercial feed reduce the risk.

There is clear evidence to support the relationship between infected meat ingestion and acute toxoplasmosis. Butchers and meat handlers have a higher seropositivity rate than does the general population, through oral ingestion or inoculation of open wounds. In 1965, Desmonts and colleagues[18] reported a definitive study supporting the meat-to-human hypothesis. Seroconversion rates rose in response to adding undercooked mutton (as a part of therapy) to the diets of children in a French sanitarium. More recently, acute toxoplasmosis was associated with ingestion of undercooked hamburger[19].

Experimental data suggest that attention to food preparation will reduce transmission of tissue cysts. Cleansing food preparation surfaces and utensils with warm soapy water after meat preparation will limit contamination of other foodstuffs. Salting (2% NaCl for 24 h), drying (24 h at 18–20 °C), freezing (–15 °C for 12–24 h) or heating (to 60 °C for 15–20 min) sterilizes the meat[20].

Clinical presentations

Acute infection

Toxoplasmosis is asymptomatic or very mild (lymphadenopathy and/or fatigue) in 80% of immune-competent individuals. Cervical, suboccipital, supraclavicular, axillary or inguinal lymph nodes are commonly enlarged. An enlarged single posterior cervical node is highly suspicious. In cases associated with a virulent strain of *T. gondii* or in cases associated with immunosuppressive therapy, acquired or congenital immunodeficiency syndromes (e.g. AIDS) or an immature fetus, clinical signs or symptoms are present in 30–100% of infections.

The clinical syndrome in presumably immune-competent individuals is best illustrated by an epidemic that was related to oocyst exposure in a riding stable[21]. Of 37 patients with serologically proven toxoplasmosis, 80% had fever, headache and lymphadenopathy (flu-like syndrome). Myalgia, stiff neck and anorexia were associated with 50–70% of patients. Additionally, arthralgia, rash, mental confusion and hepatitis were more common than in controls. Interestingly, only 3/25 (12%) of patients were correctly diagnosed by their physicians. The combination of lymphadenopathy, fatigue, malaise, atypical lymphocytosis and/or occasional liver/spleen involvement is similar to mononucleosis or Epstein–Barr infections.

In immunocompromised patients, (AIDS, cancer therapy, transplant patients), reactivation of tissue cysts from prior infection leads to local tissue destruction and, ultimately, systemic parasitemia. As the central nervous system is a common site for tissue cysts, the clinical manifestations include central nervous system abscesses, encephalitis, cognitive impairment, headache and chorioretinitis. Toxoplasma encephalitis occurs in 30–40% of AIDS patients[1].

Most pregnant women are immune-competent, and clinical expression of the infection ('flu' or lymphadenopathy) is mild and occurs in a minority (5–15%). Serological evidence of maternal infection varies by maternal age and locale[6,22]. The age-related incidence is 20% at less than 25 years, 23% at 26–35 years and 35% at more than 36 years old. Warm, moist climates have high seropositivity rates (40–60%) and cold, dry climates have much lower rates (10–20%). These observations support the theory that toxoplasmosis is related to the ubiquitous distribution of infectious oocysts and/or food contamination with tissue cysts.

Table 1 describes the variation by locale and the risks of fetal infection. Between 45 and 87% of women

Table 1 Prevalence of pregnant women at high risk for toxoplasmosis

Place	Year	Test	n	Seronegative	High risk*	Fetal infection
Melbourne, Australia[83]	1983	ELISA	3463	54.6%	0.5%	—
Oslo, Norway[6]	1980	DT	8043	87.1%	0.7%	4/11
New York, NY[6]	1971	DT/CFT	4048	68.3%	0.6%	3/23
USA (NCPP)[22]	1959–65	IHA	22 848	61.3%	2.3%	2/15
Brussels, Belgium[48]	1976–86	IHA/CFT	6549	45.4%	1.2%	—

ELISA, enzyme-linked immunosorbent assay; DT, Sabin–Feldman dye test; IHA, indirect hemagglutinin test; CFT, complement fixation test; NCPP, National Collaborative Perinatal Project
*Seroconversion, four-fold increase in titer (≥ 1 : 256), high initial titer (≥ 1 : 1024)

will be seronegative and at risk for primary infection during pregnancy. Between 0.5 and 2.3% of pregnant women will be described as being at high risk for fetal infection (probable maternal infection) as indicated by maternal seroconversion, four-fold increase in paired titers or high initial titers (greater than 1:1025 by an indirect hemagglutination test). Of these, 5–18% demonstrate fetal infection documented by neonatal signs or symptoms and/or positive neonatal *T. gondii*-specific IgM titers.

Although standard *in vitro* tests have shown little if any difference in humoral or cellular immunity between pregnant and non-pregnant women, latent infection by certain organisms (e.g. varicella, human papilloma virus) may be reactivated during pregnancy. The combination of latent HIV (or organ transplantation with immunosuppression), latent toxoplasmosis and pregnancy often leads to maternal and fetal concerns of reactivation of toxoplasmosis. In AIDS patients, reactivation usually occurs with CD4 counts of < 100 cells/mm³. It appears that pregnant women have no greater risk than that defined by low CD4 counts. Among 48 pregnant women receiving immuno-suppressive therapy after organ transplantation, no cerebral toxoplasmosis was recorded. Among 105 HIV-positive women, only one case of cerebral toxoplasmosis occurred[23], with a CD4 count of 20 cells/mm³. Prophylactic treatment to prevent maternal reactivation and vertical transmission is not indicated for CD4 counts of > 100 cells/mm³. At CD4 counts under l00 cells/mm³ the risk is still small, but prophylaxis may be justified, although benefit is not proven. These observations raise a serious question of whether reactivation of latent toxoplasmosis occurs in immunocompetent pregnancies. Seroconversion, rather than high or rising titers, may be the major serological marker for fetal infection.

In a recent study by Zadik and associates[24], the rate of primary infection with toxoplasma was assessed by seroconversion; 1621 women had paired serum more than 500 days apart. Primary infection was determined by seroconversion alone. In 160 patients (9.9%), initial titers were positive. Only one seroconversion was detected in 2966 woman-years. The projected rate for primary infections was 0.23 (95% CI 0.0059–1.3) per 1000 pregnancies. This rate of maternal infection is much lower than predicted by combined serological methods (e.g. high titer, rising titer, etc.). On the other hand, the neonatal infection rate may be higher, as it is a primary infection and true infection is better defined.

Experimental infection of rhesus monkeys showed that transmission of *T. gondii* occurred in four of nine (44%) in second-trimester maternal infections, and three of nine (33%) in the third trimester[25]. Another four fetuses of mothers infected in the third trimester were probably infected, but the organism could not be

isolated. The overall infection rate was 61%. Likewise, pregnant cats were orally inoculated with *T. gondii*[26]. Among eight animals euthanized at 10 or 31 days after inoculation, seven of 33 (21%) fetuses from all litters had *T. gondii* isolated. Eight additional pregnant cats were allowed to reach parturition and nurse their kittens. Twenty-six of 40 (65%) kittens from all eight litters had *T. gondii* isolated from tissues; 25 of 26 kittens were severely ill by 24 days of life. It is apparent that in susceptible specimens (cats, rhesus monkeys and humans) the rate of intrauterine fetal infection is 40–70%.

Fetal infection is a combination of acute and persistent infection due to relative immune incompetence and reduced passive IgG transfer from the mother. Prior to 30 weeks' gestation, the fetal immune system is of little help; IgM, IgG and cellular responses are limited and functionally immature[27]. For example, in proven cases of *in utero* infection with toxoplasmosis in the first trimester, funicentesis at 20–24 weeks demonstrated four out of nine with toxoplasma-specific IgM[28]. Placental transfer of maternal IgG is limited by gestational age and target antigen. Immunoglobulin G transport has been noted by 8 weeks, but remains less than 100 mg/dl until 20 weeks. Subsequently, the fetal levels of maternal IgG rise until they are greater than maternal levels.

Acute fetal toxoplasmosis results from initial placental involvement and subsequent systemic fetal parasitemia and infection. The most consistent histological placental finding is chronic inflammation in the decidua capsularis and focal reaction in the villi. Tissue cysts as well as tachyzoites may be seen. Systemic involvement results in splenomegaly, hepatomegaly, jaundice, anemia, thrombocytopenia, chorioretinitis and encephalitis. Persistent infection due to limited immune response leads to extramedullary hematopoiesis in the liver and decreased plasma protein production. When it is coupled with cardiac involvement, non-immune hydrops may result. Widespread tissue destruction manifests as clinically apparent growth restriction. The most characteristic damage in the central nervous system is extensive necrosis of brain parenchyma secondary to vasculitis; microcephaly is a common sequela. Periventricular and periaqueductal vasculitis is common in toxoplasmosis. Subsequent calcification of these areas is apparent on roentgenographic or ultrasonographic examinations. Obstruction of the aqueduct and/or meningeal involvement leads to hydrocephalus. Chorioretinitis may be present at birth or may develop in the first two decades after birth through recrudescence or persistence of the disease.

Table 2 shows the incidence of organ system involvement in 210 congenitally infected neonates who were followed prospectively for 1 year[29]. Twenty-one (10%) of the infants (including one death) had severe congenital toxoplasmosis with central nervous system involvement. Seventy-one (34%) had a normal clinical examination except for peripheral retinal scarring or isolated asymptomatic intracranial calcifications. One hundred and sixteen (55%) were normal. Caution should be exercised when evaluating the incidence of injury. Most series are populations of referred neonates and represent a population with more clinically apparent diseases. Unless all pregnant women and neonates are screened and all infected neonates are systematically examined, the risk is lower than is published.

The timing of acute fetal toxoplasmosis greatly affects the sequelae[30] (Table 3). When it occurs early in gestation, the infection is more widespread and destructive. The immaturity of the fetal immune system and limited passive transfer of toxoplasma-specific maternal IgG prior to 30 weeks cannot limit the infection. Additionally, immune tolerance to toxoplasma antigen due to early exposure may play a role in persistent or recurrent infection, i.e. chorioretinitis.

Table 2 Sequelae (%) of fetal toxoplasmosis (*n* = 210). Adapted from reference 29

Prematurity (≤ 2500 g)	4
Intrauterine growth restriction	6
Jaundice	10
Hepatosplenomegaly	4
Thrombocytopenia	2
Anemia	4
Eosinophilia	2
Microcephaly	5
Hydrocephalus	4
Hypotonia	6
Seizures	4
Psychomotor retardation	5
Intracranial calcifications	11
Abnormal cerebrospinal fluid	35
Microphthalmia	3
Bilateral chorioretinitis	6
Unilateral chorioretinitis	16
Normal	55

Table 3 Time of maternal infection and the frequency (%) of fetal infection. Adapted from reference 30

	Time of maternal infection		
	First trimester (*n* = 126)	Second trimester (*n* = 246)	Third trimester (*n* = 128)
No infection	86	71	41
Perinatal death	5	2	0
Fetal infection	9	27	59
severe	6	2	0
mild	1	5	6
subclinical	2	20	53

Chronic infection

Early reports of follow-up indicated that children with clinically apparent disease at birth had a poor prognosis: mental retardation, 93%; seizures, 81%; spasticity or palsies, 70%; impaired vision, 61%; hydrocephalus or microcephaly, 32%; deafness, 15%; and normal, 11%[31]. Fortunately, many infants with congenital toxoplasmosis are completely normal at birth (40–55%). The prognosis in mildly affected or asymptomatic infection appears to be much better (Table 2).

A continued risk of damage is apparent in 20-year follow-up of congenitally infected children and in epidemiological studies. Koppe and co-workers[32] followed 11 children for 20 years. One of five asymptomatic and treated infants and four of six (two with severe disabilities) symptomatic infants developed new chorioretinitis by the age of 20 years. Wilson and associates[33] followed 23 children with subclinical infections at birth for 1.25–17.25 years. Nineteen of 23 (83%) had one or more episodes of chorioretinitis, 11 (48%) had unilateral or bilateral blindness and 12 (53%) had a new diagnosis of central nervous system disorders. Sever and colleagues[22] performed a multivariate analysis of 22 845 patients in whom toxoplasmosis titers were correlated with poor outcomes during a standardized examination at 7 years of age. The results were controlled for race, maternal age and socioeconomic index. Visual impairment, microcephaly, co-ordination problems, right and left identification and soft neurological signs correlated with toxoplasmosis titer. Bilateral deafness, extra-ocular movement and IQ of < 70 correlated with the interaction variable, toxoplasmosis titer × maternal age.

Diagnosis
Isolation of the parasite

Isolation of the parasite from the mother or infant provides unequivocal proof of infection. The parasite (bradyzoite or tachyzoite) can be isolated from blood, muscle, brain, amniotic fluid or placental tissue through inoculation of mice or tissue culture. The frequency of isolation from the placenta varies by the trimester in which toxoplasmosis was acquired and untreated[34]: first trimester, 25%; second trimester, 54%; third trimester, 65%; and overall, 50%. However, the placenta may be negative in the presence of a congenitally infected fetus. Parasitemia in infected newborns varies by clinical stage: acute/generalized, 71%; neurological or ocular, 17%; and subclinical, 52%[35]. When the diagnosis is attempted by funicentesis in the second trimester, the fetal blood is positive in 70% of cases[28]. Overall (term and preterm), the amniotic fluid sediment will contain toxoplasma in 60% of samples from fetuses with congenital infection. Although isolation of the organism is a powerful investigational tool, it requires time (6 weeks) and specialized laboratories not readily available to the practicing physician.

Molecular genetics

Molecular genetics has provided a powerful new tool in antigen identification: the polymerase chain reaction (PCR)[36,37]. In 43 cases, PCR was compared to mouse inoculation (tissue/amniotic fluid cultures) and IgM immunosorbent agglutination (IgM-ISAGA) on fetal blood. PCR correctly diagnosed toxoplasmosis as positive in eight out of ten samples with no false-positive diagnosis[37]. Hohlfeld and colleagues[36] compared a competitive PCR test of amniotic fluid to conventional diagnostic methods (ultrasonography, fetal blood sampling and serological diagnosis) in 339 women who had acquired toxoplasmosis during pregnancy (combined serological diagnosis). Conventional methods identified 34 of 37 (sensitivity 91.9%) neonates with serologically or pathologically confirmed toxoplasmosis at birth. The PCR test identified 36 of 37 infants (sensitivity 97.3%). The PCR test on amniotic fluid is now the standard method for diagnosis of fetal toxoplasmosis.

Serological testing

The majority of infected pregnant women are asymptomatic, and a combination of testing for IgG, IgM and IgA antibodies is used to diagnose toxoplasmosis. These tests include the Sabin–Feldman dye test, complement fixation, indirect hemagglutination test, indirect fluorescence antibody test, agglutination test, double-sandwich IgM enzyme-linked immunosorbent assay (IgM-ELISA) and the IgM immunosorbent agglutination assay (IgM-ISAGA).

Although the Sabin–Feldman dye test is the time-honored 'gold standard', its technical complexity (mouse inoculation and observation of a biological response) limits application outside research settings. In the indirect hemagglutination test, red blood cells tagged with toxoplasma antigen agglutinate when exposed to serum containing IgG and IgM antibodies to toxoplasma. This response occurs several months after an infection. As a result, as many as 50% of infants with fetal infection will have negative indirect hemagglutination tests in the first 6 months of life. Complement fixing antibodies appear later than dye test antibodies and, depending on the antigen employed, the results vary. The agglutination test uses parasites fixed in formalin and is very sensitive to IgM antibodies. Non-specific agglutination may occur due to 'naturally' occurring IgM (in mothers negative for toxoplasma-specific IgG and IgM antibodies). Unless the laboratory corrects for these antibodies, false-positives can occur. The indirect fluorescence antibody test uses slide preparations of fixed toxoplasma that are washed with the patient's serum at different dilutions and cross-reacted with fluorescein-tagged antiserum prepared against IgG (anti-IgG). Although this test is equal to the dye test in specificity, patients with connective tissue disorders, e.g. positive rheumatoid factor, may test false-positive. Positive tests should be confirmed with a dye test or indirect hemagglutination test.

The IgM titer is measured in three ways: IgM–indirect fluorescent antibody (IgM-IFA), IgM-ELISA and IgM-ISAGA. IgM-IFA relies on antiserum specific to IgM. A titer of > 1:160 is diagnostic of an acute infection. If the antiserum cross-reacts with IgG, which occurs with some testing kits, the results may be false-positive. Additional problems include an inhibitory effect of high maternal IgG titers on fetal IgM titers and false-positives created by autoimmune antibodies, e.g. rheumatoid factor.

The conventional IgM-ELISA may also be false-positive in patients with chronic infection or autoimmune disease. As a result, Naot and co-workers[38] developed a double-sandwiched IgM-ELISA. In a direct comparison with IgM-IFA in 55 serum samples from neonates with proven toxoplasmosis, the double-sandwich IgM-ELISA was more likely to be positive (81% vs. 25%) than was IgM-IFA.

The IgM-ISAGA combines the advantages of direct agglutination and double-sandwich ELISA. The IgM-ISAGA does not use an enzyme conjugate and avoids cross-reactivity with rheumatoid factor. It is more sensitive than the IgM-IFA or the IgM-ELISA and will be positive 1–2 weeks earlier than the latter tests. However, this is a new test that needs to be evaluated in the clinical setting.

The maternal antibody response is normal; IgM appears first and the level rises sharply for 1–2 weeks and is sustained for 4–6 months (IgM-IFA) or 6–12 months (when measured by more sensitive methods: double-sandwiched IgM-ELISA). The IgG level rises slowly for 1–3 weeks (2–50 IU/ml, 1:10–1:200). After 3–6 weeks, the IgG antibody level rises sharply to > 400 IU/ml or titers of > 1:1000. In 2–4%, the titers are > 1:4000 (indirect hemagglutinin test) and persist at high levels for years. Again, IgG tests vary in their sensitivity.

Seroconversion, four-fold rise in titer (IgG or IgM) and/or a persistent high titer (> 1:1024, by indirect hemagglutinin test) are used to classify women at high risk for fetal infection. Seroconversion provides unequivocal evidence of infection occurring between the two tests. However, most women become pregnant without knowledge of their antibody status and diagnosis must rely on rising antibody titers or, occasionally, persistent high titers. Unfortunately, the numerous tests used to measure antibody responses have considerable inter- and intra-test variability.

The documentation of IgM or IgA antibody is associated with recent infection. The presence of any IgG titer in the absence of IgM antibody indicates a toxoplasma infection antedating pregnancy in most cases; the risk of fetal infection is very low. Although it is extremely rare, the presence of a high level of IgM in the absence or low levels of IgG defines an early infection. Simultaneous high IgG and IgM titers, the usual scenario, signify an infection within 4–12 months, depending on the test used to measure IgM. A four-fold rise in titer can help date the onset of infection within 6–10 weeks. Rising titers are defined by repeating the same screening test, in the same laboratory, on a portion of the original sample and another sample that is taken 3 weeks later. A four-fold rise in titer on paired samples documents a recent infection.

An antibody capture agglutination assay was used for *T. gondii*-specific IgA and IgM[39] in 260 patients with acquired toxoplasmosis, 94 fetuses with suspected congenital toxoplasmosis and 30 infected children. *T. gondii*-specific IgA antibody appears to be a slightly more sensitive test on cord blood than *T. gondii*-specific IgM (75% vs. 61%) and may persist for longer than 24 months after birth. The *T. gondii*-specific IgA assay (if available) should be one of several tests to confirm congenital toxoplasmosis.

Antenatal diagnosis

The advent of sophisticated ultrasound diagnosis and invasive fetal testing (funicentesis) has heralded new options in the diagnosis and management of toxoplasmosis. Although serological testing may identify 0.5–2.5% of pregnant women at high risk of fetal toxoplasmosis, only 4–20% of maternal infections in the first 20 weeks of pregnancy result in fetal infection, usually with severe consequences (Table 3). Access to fetal tissues (amniocytes, chorionic villi, or fetal blood) allows unequivocal fetal diagnosis and treatment. *In utero* fetal infection may be diagnosed through demonstration of toxoplasma antigens (parasites or DNA), fetal immune response (IgM), or physical or laboratory evidence of fetal infection. Inoculation of mice or tissue

cultures with fetal specimens is 50–70% sensitive in documenting fetal infection. PCR identification of toxoplasma DNA significantly reduces the time and laboratory requirements for antigen detection. However, adequate laboratory support is essential. Currently, there is limited access and availability.

The demonstration of a fetal IgM response is limited by gestational age. Prior to 24 weeks, the upper age limit for abortion in the USA, less than half of fetuses will mount an IgM response[28]. Ultrasound findings include fetal hydrops, ascites, hydrocephalus, microcephaly, growth restriction or intracranial calcifications. Abnormal laboratory findings on fetal blood include elevated white cell count, eosinophil count, monocytes, γ-glutamyl transpeptidase and lactic dehydrogenase activity (Table 4).

Universal screening

The frequency of maternal (0.8%) and fetal (0.32%) infection, the frequency of long-term disability after fetal infection (50–90%) and the cost of caring for those disabilities ($60 000–100 000 per case) describe the potential benefits of a universal screening program. This potential benefit compares favorably with other universal screening programs: for syphilis, gonorrhea, phenylketonuria or maternal serum α-fetoprotein. Commercial laboratories would easily and happily accommodate the demand for serological testing in a universal screening program. Finally, respected researchers endorse the concept of universal screening[40].

On the other hand, the cost, unreliability in testing and the inadequacy and cost of resources to interpret, diagnose and treat fetal infection are major obstacles to implementation. The immunofluorescent antibody test, which is used in 80% of commercial laboratories[41], costs $40–60. Each patient would require two or three tests: two tests to document seroconversion and three tests (in 40% of patients) to document a rising titer

Table 4 Antenatal diagnosis of fetal toxoplasmosis

	Daffos et al.[28]	*Foulon et al.*[87]	*Total*
Number of high-risk mothers	746	50	796
Fetal infection	42	6	48/796 (6%)
Diagnosed *in utero*	39/42	5/6	44/48 (92%)
Positive specific IgM	9/42	1/3	10/45 (22%)
Elevated total IgM	22/37	—	59%
Elevated white blood cell count	16/39	—	41%
Eosinophilia	8/33	2/3	10/36 (28%)
Elevated lactic dehydrogenase	7/35	3/3	10/38 (26%)
Elevated γ-glutamyl transpeptidase	24/34	3/3	27/37 (73%)
Abnormal ultrasound scan			
ascites	2/42	0/3	2/45 (4%)
ventricular dilatation	17/42	1/3	18/45 (40%)
intracranial calcification	—	1/3	33%

(paired samples or IgM). Universal serological screening would cost an estimated $320 million to $720 million.

A cost–benefit analysis based on data from a Finnish prospective study[42] and on Finnish cost data was performed to compare the no-screening and screening alternatives for primary toxoplasma infection during pregnancy[43]. Given 20.3% seropositivity and an incidence of fetal infection of 2.4/1000 seronegative pregnancies, the total annual costs of congenital toxoplasmosis without screening were $128 per pregnancy per year (US dollars). With screening the cost would be $95. The authors concluded that universal screening, plus health education, would be cost-effective if the incidence of maternal primary infection exceeded 1.1/1000 pregnancies and the effectiveness of treatment was greater than 22%.

The diagnosis of fetal infection in high-risk mothers would be necessary unless the practitioner and patient were willing to abort or treat 9–15 uninfected fetuses for each infected fetus. Amniocentesis and/or funicentesis would be needed in 29 600 (0.8% × 3.7 million) women per year, with each ultrasound-guided procedure costing a minimum of $500. The necessary expertise, laboratory support and financial resources are not available for this demand.

In summary, universal screening for toxoplasmosis is not warranted at this time in USA. However, serological screening should be considered when the patient has a 'flu'-like syndrome and/or has lymphadenopathy, or when the fetus, on ultrasonographic examination, has growth restriction, non-immune hydrops, ascites, hydrocephalus, microcephaly, or intracranial calcification.

Antibiotic therapy

Couvreur, in close cooperation with Desmonts, Daffos and colleagues, has the largest clinical experience with the treatment of pregnant women with infected fetuses. One of their recommended regimens is alternating 3-week courses of either pyrimethamine 50 mg/day plus sulfadiazine 3 g/day or spiramycin 1.5 g twice a day until delivery. Folic acid in the form of leucovorin calcium (10 mg/day) should be used during pyrimethamine therapy[28,34].

Pyrimethamine, a substituted phenylpyrimidine antimalarial drug, cures toxoplasmosis in laboratory animals through folic acid antagonism. Pyrimethamine produces a reversible, dose-related bone marrow depression. Thrombocytopenia, with its associated bleeding sequelae, is the most common toxic affect, but anemia and leukopenia may occur as well. A semi-weekly complete blood cell and platelet count should be obtained while the patient is being treated.

Sulfadiazine (or sulfapyrazine, sulfamethazine, or sulfamerazine) acts synergistically with pyrimethamine with a combined activity against toxoplasmosis much greater than a merely additive affect. Like pyrimethamine, sulfa drugs disrupt folic acid metabolism in bacterial species. Renal toxicity (crystalluria and hematuria), toxic dermal reaction (Stevens–Johnson syndrome) and blood dyscrasias are reported with sulfa drug therapies. However, these agents are well tolerated in most individuals. In the neonate, sulfa drugs displace bilirubin from albumin, and kernicterus may occur. The risk of neonatal kernicterus from maternal intake of sulfa drugs is quite small.

The evaluation of antibiotic efficacy depends on the time between the onset of infection and initiation of therapy. In human studies, the timing of fetal toxoplasmosis is very difficult to determine because the infection is usually asymptomatic. Experimental inoculation of non-human primates and rhesus monkeys, and treatment with anti-toxoplasmosis antibiotics provides powerful insight into the pharmacokinetics of pregnancy and the efficacy of the antibiotics.

Schoondermark-Van de Ven and colleagues[44] established the dosage regimen for pyrimethamine and sulfadiazine in pregnant rhesus monkeys. The distributions of both drugs followed a one-compartment model. The maximum concentration in serum was 88.7 μg/nl and 0.22 μg/nl for sulfodiazine and pyrimethazine, respectively. The serum elimination half-life was much greater for pyrimethamine (44.4 h) than sulfadiazine (5.2 h).

Subsequent to the latter experiment, the authors used the dosage regimen to treat six rhesus monkeys who were infected with *T. gondii* at 90 days' gestation (second trimester)[44]. Four similarly infected pregnant monkeys were used as controls. Infection was documented by isolation of *T. gondii* from amniotic fluid samples. The treated animals received pyrimethazine l mg/kg body weight and sulfadiazine 50 mg/kg per day for the remainder of the pregnancy. *T. gondii* was present at birth in three of four untreated neonates. In all animals treated with pyrimethazine and sulfadiazine, no parasite was identified in the amniotic fluid 10–13 days after initiation of therapy. No neonate demonstrated *T. gondii* at birth.

Spiramycin, a macrolide antibiotic, has an antibacterial spectrum similar to that of erythromycin and is active against toxoplasmosis in laboratory animals. With spiramycin 2 g/day, the concentrations were as follows: maternal serum, l.19 μg/nl; umbilical cord, 0.63 μg/nl; and placenta, 2.75 μg/nl. With spiramycin 3 g/day the concentrations were: maternal serum, l.69 μg/nl; umbilical cord serum, 0.78 μg/nl; and placenta, 6.2 μg/nl[45]. Persistent, high tissue levels account for its greater activity against toxoplasmosis than is shown by erythromycin. During pregnancy, spiramycin is concentrated in placental tissue at 2–4 times serum levels, an important advantage, as placental infection is sentinel to fetal infection. Spiramycin seems to be well tolerated. When it is used as an antineoplastic agent in doses greater than 35 mg/kg, some patients experienced vertigo, nausea, vomiting and anorexia. No impairment of the heart, blood, liver or kidneys was noted[46].

Schoondermark-Van de Ven and co-workers[47] inoculated eight rhesus monkeys at 90 days' gestation (second trimester). The parasite was found in five of eight amniotic fluid samples at subsequent sampling. These monkeys with documented fetal infection were treated with intravenous spiramycin 20 mg/kg per day in two divided doses. At 14 days after initiation of spiramycin treatment, *T. gondii* was still detectable by PCR analysis, but not by mouse inoculation in four of five amniotic fluid samples. In four monkeys who had received spiramycin for 7 weeks, no *T. gondii* was detected by PCR or mouse inoculation in the placenta, amniotic fluid or neonatal organs. One fetus who delivered prematurely after 2 weeks of spiramycin treatment had *T. gondii* associated with its placenta found on PCR results alone. Spiramycin accumulated in extra-central nervous system tissues at concentrations 5–28 times umbilical cord concentrations; but no spiramycin was found in fetal/neonatal brains. These data suggest that in primates early treatment with spiramycin may eliminate fetal infection with moderate success, but if there is fetal central nervous system involvement, spiramycin is likely to be ineffective.

Treatment

Prevention

Primary prevention has the potential for greatly reducing the medical and economic costs of congenital toxoplasmosis. A combination of public education – in the high school curriculum, preconceptual counselling and early prenatal counselling – would be most effective in reducing congenital toxoplasmosis. In addition to material concerning the risks of toxoplasmosis, the role of cats and the general guidelines are listed in Table 5.

Foulon and co-workers[48] evaluated the reduction in the incidence of congenital toxoplasmosis using a primary prevention scheme (education) and a secondary prevention scheme (screening and treatment). Among 11 286 consecutive pregnant women, primary prevention reduced the seroconversion rate by 63% ($p = 0.013$). Among 76 women who were thought to be at risk for delivering a child with congenital toxoplasmosis, eight (11%) infected fetuses were detected by prenatal fetal diagnosis. Of these, secondary prevention (antibiotics) reduced the incidence of congenital toxoplasmosis by an additional 40%.

Medical therapy

Although pyrimethamine plus sulfadiazine and spiramycin cure toxoplasmosis in laboratory animals

Table 5 Primary prevention of toxoplasmosis during pregnancy

Oocyst exposure

Avoid the purchase of a new cat just prior to or during pregnancy
Avoid sick or feral cats
Use gloves for gardening
Have other family members clean the litter box
Clean the litter pan daily
Sterilize the empty litter pan with boiling water for 20 min
Prevent flies and other vectors from contaminating food
Thoroughly wash fruits and vegetables

Tissue cyst exposure

Cook meat to 150 °F (66 °C)
Cleanse the preparation surface immediately after meat preparation
Wash hands immediately after meat preparation
Avoid contact with mucous membranes of the mouth and eyes while handling raw meat

in controlled trials, the efficacy of treatment regimens in humans has been studied only in retrospective, descriptive studies that have used historical controls. The results of these studies must be interpreted with the following limitations: treatment regimens may be mixed; doses may change within a series; and fetuses are of different gestational ages at onset, diagnosis and therapy. Diagnosis during pregnancy has become more accurate and easier than was diagnosis in the 1960s and 1970s, and work-up and follow-up vary within and between series. In addition, the study populations have changed through the institution of national screening programs (France, Belgium). Early diagnosis and subsequent abortion eliminate the population at greatest risk for clinical disease. Antibiotic therapy may appear to reduce fetal infection because milder cases are being treated.

The outcome of antibiotic therapy for fetal toxoplasmosis is reviewed in Table 6. Additionally, Desmonts and colleagues[49] reported a series of 278 women at risk for giving birth to a child with congenital toxoplasmosis. Five women terminated their pregnancies prior to fetal diagnosis, and 273 women underwent fetal diagnosis. All patients were treated with spiramycin 3 g/day until delivery. Nine (3.3%) of the fetuses were diagnosed with fetal toxoplasmosis; all mothers had therapeutic abortions. The remaining 264 women continued antibiotics until delivery. A total of 199 infants were examined in follow-up; one (0.5%) had congenital toxoplasmosis and 3/157 of the placental cultures were positive.

The same group[50] compared 52 patients treated with a combination of pyrimethamine and a sulfa drug to 51 patients treated with spiramycin alone (see Table 6). The results exemplify *in utero* therapy of fetal

Table 6 Treatment of fetal toxoplasmosis

Study	Antibiotic	Treated		Untreated		Abortion	Comment
		n	%	n	%		
Desmonts and Couvreur[88]	spiramycin 2 or 3 g/day	24/98	24	36/82	44	11	spontaneous abortion only
Daffos *et al.*[28]	spiramycin 3 g/day + P/S	6/15	40	—	—	24	
Hohlfeld *et al.*[89]	spiramycin 3 g/day + P/S, folic acid	10/54	19	—	—	34	
Foulon *et al.*[87]	spiramycin 3 g/day + P/S	39/65	60	—	—	1	
Couvreur *et al.*[34]	spiramycin 2–3 g/day	51/269	19	26/52	50	—	placental isolation
	spiramycin 2 g/day	48/53	91	—	—	—	placental isolation
	spiramycin 3 g/day + P/S > 14 days	89/118	75	12/14	86	—	placental isolation
	spiramycin 3 g/day < 15 days	16/18	89	—	—	—	placental isolation
Berrebi *et al.*[90]	spiramycin 9 million units per day + P/S in 23	27/162	17	—	—	0	ten infants with CNS lesion
Couvreur *et al.*[50]	spiramycin 3 g/day + P/S	22/52	42	—	—	0	placental isolation specific IgM at birth
	spiramycin 3 g/day	31/51	61	—	—	0	spiramycin + P/S 17.6% spiramycin alone 69%

P/S, pyrimethamine plus sulfadiazine

toxoplasmosis. Combination chemotherapy appears to be superior, but, despite early therapy, at least one in five will be infected at birth. A critical missing piece of information is the efficacy of antibiotics, especially spiramycin, in eliminating fetal/neonatal central nervous system disease.

Summary

The medical costs of maternal toxoplasmosis warrant the development of effective programs in primary prevention, diagnosis and therapy. Maternal toxoplasmosis occurs in 0.5–1% of pregnancies, and 10–60% of their fetuses will be infected. While the majority (80–90%) of infected neonates will be asymptomatic at birth, a large proportion (20–90%) will develop one or more disabilities. These include hydrocephalus, microcephaly, chorioretinitis, mental retardation and deafness.

Primary prevention through education and monitoring of food sources has an unfulfilled potential. The effectiveness of primary prevention is measured by changes in behavior and seroconversion rates. A universal screening program, especially preconceptual screening, will improve diagnosis and allow abortion as an option. However, the lack of standardized tests and poor correlation between maternal infection and fetal infection may result in many unnecessary abortions.

Fetal diagnosis allows more focused therapy. It will significantly reduce unnecessary abortion and antibiotic therapy. Unfortunately, fetal diagnosis requires sophisticated clinical skills, equipment and laboratory support, currently available only at major medical centers.

The inability to pinpoint the onset or severity of fetal toxoplasmosis limits the effectiveness of antibiotic regimens used to treat fetal toxoplasmosis. Despite therapy, 10–50% of fetuses infected in the first half of pregnancy will manifest injury. This failure rate may be related to an ineffective antibiotic regimen or inadvertently delayed treatment. Comparative trials of antibiotics are critically important to the management of fetal toxoplasmosis in the future.

TRICHOMONIASIS

Most clinicians recognize the sexually transmitted protozoan, *Trichomonas vaginalis*, as a common cause of vulvovaginitis and cervicitis. Although trichomoniasis is considered to be a nuisance disease by most practitioners, a growing body of evidence describes *T. vaginalis* as a major obstetric pathogen. The treatment of trichomoniasis during pregnancy has been limited by perceived unimportance of the infection and concerns about metronidazole and fetal injury. This section describes the biology, clinical presentation and treatment of *T. vaginalis*.

Biology

The pathogen *T. vaginalis* is one of three highly site-specific trichomonad parasites that infect humans: *T. tenax* in the mouth, *T. hominis* in the gastrointestinal tract and *T. vaginalis* in the urogenital tract. *T. vaginalis* is an actively mobile tetraflagellated protozoan with an anterior nucleus, anterolateral undulating membrane and prominent axostyle. The organism is oval or fusiform and, under ideal conditions, slightly longer than a leukocyte, 12–16 μm. Under more adverse conditions, it may be larger, 20–30 μm, or smaller, 7–13 μm. The organism is most robust when its milieu is at 35–37 °C and pH is 5.5–5.8. The organism is killed by drying, freezing, or raising the temperature to 50°C for 4 min. The induction of clinical trichomoniasis in human volunteers[51] was facilitated by pre-existing abnormal vaginal flora, anaerobic conditions and few lactobacilli (bacterial vaginosis).

The organism is a facultative anaerobe and can utilize a variety of sugars. It phagocytizes bacteria, erythrocytes and epithelial cells[52,53]. The organism reproduces by binary fission, and no spore or cyst form has been recognized. *T. vaginalis* appears to damage epithelial cells by direct contact and to cause microulcerations[54,55]. The organism can effectively resist the host response. Most women will not eradicate *T. vaginalis* and are often asymptomatic (60–90%). The ability of *T. vaginalis* to resist eradication may allow other pathogenic organisms to survive. In addition, *T. vaginalis* may act as a vector for bacteria to reach the upper genital tract[56].

Trichomoniasis is a sexually transmitted disease. Three million American women contract trichomoniasis every year. The incidence is highest among women with multiple partners and those with other venereal diseases. The incubation period is 1–4 weeks, and 30–80% of male consorts of infected women will harbor the organism. *T. vaginalis* is recovered in 60–100% of female consorts of infected males[57]. About 15% of female neonates will harbor the protozoan in the vaginal vestibule for 3–4 weeks after passage through an infected birth canal[58]. Occasionally, neonatal respiratory distress can occur[59].

Clinical presentation

Wølner-Hanssen and co-workers[60] provide the most complete description of the signs and symptoms in non-pregnant women who harbor *T. vaginalis* in their genital tract. The authors randomly selected 779 women who were attending a sexually transmitted disease clinic in Seattle, Washington. They compared 118 women with *T. vaginalis* colonization to 667 without

the organism. *T. vaginalis* colonization was associated with multiparity, unemployment, smoking, black race and not using barrier or oral contraceptives. *T. vaginalis* infection was associated with *Neisseria gonorrhoeae* (31% vs. 11%), *Mycobacterium hominis* (75% vs. 45%), bacterial vaginosis (75% vs. 45%) and a mucopurulent cervicitis (44% vs. 31%). The positive predictive value of *T. vaginalis* colonization and the following symptoms and signs are: yellow discharge, 28%; vulvar itching, 18%; colpitis macularis, 90%; purulent discharge, 30%; frothy discharge, 62%; vulvar erythema, 19%; and vaginal erythema, 33%.

A purulent vaginal discharge is an important clinical clue to *T. vaginalis* and other sexually transmitted diseases. The likelihood of sexually transmitted organisms being present in patients with purulent discharge compared to patients without purulent discharge (odds ratio) was *T. vaginalis*, 8.0; *Chlamydia trachomatis*, 3.1; *N. gonorrhoeae*, 1.8; and herpes simplex, 5.1. The positive predictive value of purulent discharge for infection with any of these organisms was 70%.

The incidence of *T. vaginalis* in unscreened antenatal patients varies between 3 and 60% with most between 3 and 10%[61–68]. Many patients (50%) have few or no complaints which discriminate *T. vaginalis* infection from the increase in vaginal discharge normally seen during pregnancy. However, the association between *T. vaginalis* and other sexually transmitted diseases is valid during pregnancy. The independent risks of the other sexually transmitted diseases and the risk of behavior often associated with sexually transmitted diseases, i.e. drug abuse, add to the risk associated with *T. vaginalis* in pregnancy.

Clinical signs and symptoms are non-specific for *T. vaginalis* and serve to render a population, where all subjects are screened for *T. vaginalis*, in which the prevalence of the disease is higher: 9% in asymptomatic women and 50% in symptomatic women. Further laboratory tests are needed to confirm the diagnosis. A wet mount is simple, inexpensive and reasonably accurate. A drop of secretion is mixed with saline and examined for the typical, motile morphological types. Culture for trichomonads is easy. A swab-full of secretions is incubated for 5 days in Diamond's or Kupferberg medium. A sample is examined daily for motile trichomonads. Table 7[69–71] describes the comparison of several diagnostic techniques using culture results as a 'gold standard'. Newer antibody techniques may replace wet mount/culture as the diagnostic tests of choice.

Until recently, the data were inconclusive and scarce regarding the association between *T. vaginalis* and adverse pregnancy outcome. Mason and Brown[72] reported no association between *T. vaginalis* and adverse outcome. Hardy and associates[67] reported more infants of low birth weight (< 2500 g) among inner-city black adolescents who harbored *T. vaginalis*, compared to similar adolescents who did not (18% vs. 6.7%).

Table 7   Diagnosis of trichomonas

Authors	How selected	n	Positive culture	Papanicolaou smear		Wet smear		Monoclonal antibody	
				n	%	n	%	n	%
Krieger *et al.*[69]	random	600	88	49	56	53	60	76	86
McLennan *et al.*[70]	symptomatic	1000	192	159	83	168	88	—	—
Spence *et al.*[71]	consecutive	100	48	35	73	25	52	—	—

Minkoff and colleagues[66] associated *T. vaginalis* with premature rupture of membranes (odds ratio 1.4).

Between 1984 and 1988, 13 816 subjects were enrolled in six centers at 23–26 weeks' gestation (Vaginal Infections in Prematurity Study). Each patient had an extensive history taken, a physical examination and vaginal cultures. After control for sociodemographic, medical and microbiological confounders, *T. vaginalis* was associated with preterm delivery, RR 1.3 (1.1–1.4); and low birth weight, RR 1.3 (1.1–1.5)[73]. In light of this information, treatment of *T. vaginalis* after the first trimester is warranted.

Treatment

Lossick[74,75] has reviewed the treatment of *T. vaginalis* infection. The most effective treatment for *T. vaginalis* is metronidazole or related 5-nitroimidazole derivatives. The two treatment regimens are a single dose of 2 g or a regimen of 500 mg twice a day for 7 days.

T. vaginalis has been identified in about 13–58% of steady sex partners of infected women and in 80% of men after their first contact with a partner with vaginal trichomonas[57,74]. This suggests a necessity to treat consorts. Lyng and Christensen[76] demonstrated, through a double-blind study, that treatment (tinidazole) of sex partners reduced the relapse rate from 24% to 5%. Relapse rates of 6–15% have been reported in descriptive studies of pregnant women whose sex partners were not treated[57,74]. A single 2-g dose of metronidazole is recommended for treatment of sex partners[57,74].

Metronidazole interrupts nucleic acid and DNA synthesis in *T. vaginalis*. *In vivo* susceptible trichomonads exposed to 1–4 µg of metronidazole/ml die within 8 h[75]. Metronidazole is absorbed 95–100%, and peak levels (17.4 ± 3.2 µg/ml) occur 1–3 h after a 1-g oral dose[76]. Pregnant women have slightly lower peak levels. The half-life after a 1-g dose was 7.7 h after ingestion. Metronidazole rapidly crosses the placenta[77–79].

Breast milk of mothers who have received a 2-g dose of metronidazole will contain a moderate amount of the drug. The milk/maternal serum ratio is about 1 : 1, and the infant will receive about 25 mg of the drug. Its plasma levels will be about 25% of maternal levels. Metronidazole is reluctantly given to newborns. In most cases the mother may elect to pump and discard her milk for 12 h after a 2-g dose of metronidazole.

Side-effects of metronidazole are dose-related and self-limited[74,75]. The common complaints include nausea and/or vomiting (10–25%), cephalgia/dizziness (10%), reversible leukopenia (5–10%) and reversible peripheral neuropathy (rare). The combination of ethyl alcohol and metronidazole may produce disulfiram-like effects.

The interaction between metronidazole and DNA synthesis raises potential concerns about carcinogenesis or mutagenesis. Indeed, in the 1970s chronic high-dose metronidazole was associated with tumor growth in laboratory animals[74,75,80]. Since the latter observations, numerous tumor studies have failed to identify an increased risk of cancer[74,75,80]. As the latent period for carcinogenesis after *in utero* exposure may be 10–30 years, a certain amount of caution must be maintained.

Mutagenesis has been reported in a distinct minority of studies using various animal models. Studies of pregnant women with *T. vaginalis* infection treated with metronidazole do not indicate a higher incidence of congenital abnormalities when treatment is administered during the first trimester[81–85]. In laboratory animals the ingestion of alcohol with metronidazole seems to potentiate the risk of developmental defects. Most studies do not account for this powerful covariate.

The antifungal agent clotrimazole is effective against *T. vaginalis in vitro*. Between 50 and 80% of patients will have short-term cures with 100 mg intravaginal doses daily for 6 days[75]. There is minimal maternal or fetal risk associated with this drug.

Summary

Trichomoniasis is usually asymptomatic, but may manifest as vulvovaginitis with a purulent discharge. The diagnosis is based on clinical signs and symptoms, wet smear and culture. The adverse pregnancy outcomes associated with *T. vaginalis* result from the independent effects of the organism, the behaviors associated with sexually transmitted diseases (multiple partners, drug abuse) and the presence of other obstetric pathogens (*N. gonorrhoeae*, chlamydia, etc.). If *T. vaginalis* occurs during pregnancy, the patient and her sex partner(s) should be treated with one 2-g dose of metronidazole after the first trimester.

SCABIES AND LICE

Ectoparasites, scabies and lice, commonly creep into the clinical experience of most practitioners. Any condition that promotes multiple, close personal contacts within a family or community may increase the incidence. Although non-sexual contact often results in spread of the disease, the epidemic of ectoparasites is largely due to the changing sexual mores of the last 40 years.

Sarcoptes scabiei var. *hominis* is a host-specific human mite that is nearly microscopic. The female is 0.35–0.40 mm long, and the male is half that size. The life cycle of the sarcoptic mite is 45–50 days. After copulation on the skin surface, the female burrows into the stratum corneum, and the male dies. As she burrows 0.5–5 mm/day for the duration of her life (30 days), she lays 2–3 large eggs per day. These hatch in 3–5 days, to emerge as adults in 17 days[86].

Scabies presents with a combination of pruritus (nocturnal), burrows and a symmetrical, polymorphous eruption of red papules, vesicles and pustules. The itching starts about 4 weeks after exposure. The burrows are best seen on the wrists, finger webs and finger sides. The upper back, neck, face, scalp, palms and soles are usually spared. Excoriation and secondary infection often obscure the burrows.

The history, physical examination and documentation of burrows are the best ways to diagnose scabies. A history of symptomatic family members, severe pruritus and the demonstration of a polymorphous eruption are usually sufficient to make the diagnosis. The burrow ink test may be helpful in questionable cases. The underside of an ink pen is rubbed over a suspicious papule, and the ink is quickly wiped off with alcohol. The ink tracks down the burrow and describes a dark, zigzagged line.

The treatment of choice is 1% lindane (Kwell®). A single application is usually curative. The medication is applied sparingly to most of the body; 28 g will cover the trunk and extremities of an adult. There has been recent concern about neurotoxicity associated with its use. However, animal studies have demonstrated minimal effects[86]. The package insert recommends against use in pregnancy. Crotamiton 10% (Eurax®), sulfur (6%) in petrolatum and benzyl benzoate are reasonably effective alternatives. These require more than one application, and little information is available concerning their use in pregnancy.

Scabies cannot be transmitted 24 h after the application. Pruritus may persist for 2–4 weeks after treatment. Antihistamines or local application of steroid creams provide symptomatic relief.

Humans are the only natural host for the head louse (*Pediculosis capitis*), the body louse (*Pediculosis corporis*)[86] and the pubic or crab louse (*Pediculosis pubis*)[86]. All are highly site-specific. Although the head and body louse can live 10–14 days on the human host, the crab louse can exist for only 12 h without the warmth and food of the host. The average body population of these organisms is less than 50.

Severe pruritus is the most common presenting symptom, usually beginning about 30 days after infestation. Examination reveals excoriations and secondary pyoderma. Rarely, hemorrhagic papules or macules exist at sites where they have fed. The finding of mites in clothing (body lice) or hair (head or pubic lice) confuses the diagnosis.

Treatment of lice can be limited to the affected area, thus reducing toxicity. Lindane, malathion, carbaryl (Sevin®) or crotamiton (Eurax®) and pyrethrins (RID®) are used to treat lice. Although ineffective in scabies infestation, the pyrethrins with piperonyl butoxide provide potentially safer alternatives in the treatment of pregnant women with lice. Their topical absorption is poor, so potential toxicity should be less than that of lindane.

REFERENCES

1. Luft BJ, Remington JS. Toxoplasmic encephalitis. *J Infect Dis* 1988;157:1–6
2. Dubey JP, Miller NL, Frenkel JK. The *Toxoplasma gondii* oocyst from cat feces. *J Exp Med* 1970;132:636–62
3. Frenkel JK, Dubey JP. Toxoplasmosis and its prevention in cats and man. *J Infect Dis* 1972;126:664–73
4. Dubey JP, Hoover EA, Walls KW. Effect of age and sex on the acquisition of immunity to toxoplasmosis in cats. *J Protozool* 1977;24:184–6
5. Dubey JP, Frenkel JK. Experimental toxoplasma infection in mice with strains producing oocysts. *J Parasitol* 1973;59:505–12
6. Feldman HA. Epidemiology of toxoplasma infections. *Epidemiol Rev* 1982;4:204–13
7. Hunter K, Stragno S, Capps E, Smith RJ. Prenatal screening of pregnant women for infections caused by cytomegalovirus, Epstein–Barr virus, herpes virus, rubella, and *Toxoplasma gondii*. *Am J Obstet Gynecol* 1983;145:269–73
8. Hershey DW, McGregor JA. Low prevalence of toxoplasma infection in a Rocky Mountain prenatal population. *Obstet Gynecol* 1987;70:900–2
9. Stray-Pedersen BA. A prospective study of acquired toxoplasmosis among 8043 pregnant women in the Oslo area. *Am J Obstet Gynecol* 1980;136:399–406
10. Yilmaz SM, Hopkins SH. Effects of different conditions on duration of infectivity of *Toxoplasma gondii* oocysts. *J Parasitol* 1972;58:938–9
11. Dubey JP. Toxoplasmosis in cats. *Feline Pract* 1986;16:12–45
12. Dubey JP. Toxoplasmosis. *J Am Vet Med Assoc* 1986;189:166–70
13. Behymer RD, Harlow DR, Behymer DE, Franti CE. Serologic diagnosis of toxoplasmosis and prevalence of *Toxoplasma gondii* antibodies in selected feline, canine, and human populations. *J Am Vet Med Assoc* 1973;162:959–63
14. Sengbusch HG, Sengbusch LA. Toxoplasma antibody prevalence in veterinary personnel and a selected

population not exposed to cats. *Am J Epidemiol* 1976; 103:595

15. Ganley JP, Comstock GW. Association of cats and toxoplasmosis. *Am J Epidemiol* 1980;111:238–46

16. Jacobs L, Remington JS, Melton ML. A survey of meat samples from swine, cattle, and sheep for the presence of encysted toxoplasma. *J Parasitol* 1960;46:23–8

17. Krogstad DJ, Juranek DD, Walls KW. Toxoplasmosis: with comments on risk of infection from cats. *Ann Intern Med* 1972;77:773–8

18. Desmonts G, Couvreur J, Alison F, *et al.* Étude épidémilogique sur la toxoplasmose: de l'influence de la cuisson des viandes de boucherie sur la fréquence de l'infection humaine. *Rev Fr Étud Clin Biol* 1965;l0: 952–8

19. Kean BH, Kimball AC, Christianson WN. An epidemic of acute toxoplasmosis. *J Am Med Assoc* 1969;208:1002

20. Jacobs L, Remington JS, Melton ML. The resistance of the encysted form of *Toxoplasma gondii*. *J Parasitol* 1957; 46:11–21

21. Teutsch SM, Juranek DD, Sulzer A, *et al.* Epidemic toxoplasmosis associated with infected cats. *N Engl J Med* 1979;300:695–9

22. Sever JL, Ellenbery JH, Ley AC, *et al.* Toxoplasmosis: maternal and pediatric findings in 23,000 pregnancies. *Pediatrics* 1988;82:181–92

23. Biedermann K, Flepp M, Fierz W, *et al.* Pregnancy, immunosuppression and reactivation of latent toxoplasmosis. *J Perinat Med* 1995;23:191–203

24. Zadik PM, Kudesia G, Siddons AD. Low incidence of primary infection with toxoplasma among women in Sheffield: a seroconversion study. *Br J Obstet Gynaecol* 1995;102:608–10

25. Schoondermark-Van de Ven E, Melchers W, Galama J, *et al.* Congenital toxoplasmosis: an experimental study in rhesus monkeys for transmission and prenatal diagnosis. *Exp Parasitol* 1993;77:200–11

26. Dubey JP, Lappin MR, Thulliez P. Diagnosis of induced toxoplasmosis in neonatal cats. *J Am Vet Med Assoc* 1995; 207:179–85

27. Wilson CB. Developmental immunology and the role of last defense in neonatal susceptibility. In Remington JS, Klein JO, eds. *Infectious Disease of the Fetus and Newborn Infant*, 3rd edn. Philadelphia: WB Saunders, 1990:17–67

28. Daffos F, Forestier F, Capella-Pavlovsky M, *et al.* Prenatal management of 746 pregnancies at risk for congenital toxoplasmosis. *N Engl J Med* 1988;318:271

29. Couvreur J, Desmonts G, Tournier G, *et al.* Étude d'une série homogène de 210 cases de toxoplasmose congénitale chéz des nourrissons âgés de 0 a 11 mois et dépistes de façon prospective. *Ann Pediatr* 1984;31:855

30. Remington JS, Desmonts G. Toxoplasmosis. In Remington JS, Klein JO, eds. *Infectious Disease in the Fetus and Newborn Infant*, 4th edn. Philadelphia: WB Saunders, 1995:140–267

31. Eichenwald H. A study of congenital toxoplasmosis. In Siim JC, ed. *Human Toxoplasmosis*. Copenhagen: Munksgaard, 1960:41–9

32. Koppe JG, Loewer-Sieger DH, deRoever-Bonnet H. Results of 20-year follow-up of congenital toxoplasmosis. *Lancet* 1986;1:254–6

33. Wilson CB, Remington JS, Stagno S, *et al.* Development of adverse sequelae in children born with

34. Couvreur J, Desmonts G, Thulliez PH. Prophylaxis of congenital toxoplasmosis: effects of spiramycin on placental infection. *J Antimicrob Chemother* 1988;22: 193–200

35. Desmonts G, Couvreur J. Toxoplasmosis: epidemiologic and serologic aspects of perinatal infection. In Krugman S, Gershon AA, eds. *Infections of the Fetus and the Newborn Infant. Progress in Clinical and Biological Research*, vol. 3. Alan R. Liss: New York, 1975:115–32

36. Hohlfeld P, Daffos F, Costa JM, *et al.* Prenatal diagnosis of congenital toxoplasmosis with a polymerase-chain-reaction test on amniotic fluid. *N Engl J Med* 1994; 331:695–9

37. Grover CM, Thulliez P, Remington JS, Boothroyd JC. Rapid prenatal diagnosis of congenital toxoplasma infection by using polymerase chain reaction and amniotic fluid. *J Clin Microbiol* 1990;28:2297–301

38. Naot Y, Desmonts G, Remington JS. IgM enzyme-linked immunosorbent assay test for the diagnosis of congenital toxoplasma infection. *J Pediatr* 1981;98:32–6

39. Bessieres MH, Roques C, Berrebi A, *et al.* IgA antibody response during acquired and congenital toxoplasmosis. *J Clin Pathol* 1992;45:605–8

40. Wilson CB, Remington JS. What can be done to prevent congenital toxoplasmosis? *Am J Obstet Gynecol* 1980;138:357–63

41. Sever JL. TORCH tests and what they mean. *Am J Obstet Gynecol* 1985;152:495–9

42. Lappalainen M, Koskela P, Hedman K, *et al.* Incidence of primary toxoplasma infections during pregnancy in southern Finland: a prospective cohort study. *Scand J Infect Dis* 1992;24:97–104

43. Lappalainen M, Sintonen H, Koskiniemi M, *et al.* Cost–benefit analysis of screening for toxoplasmosis during pregnancy. *Scand J Infect Dis* 1995;27:265–72

44. Schoondermark-Van de Ven E, Melchers W, Camps W, *et al.* Effectiveness of spiramycin for treatment of congenital *Toxoplasma gondii* infection in rhesus monkeys. *Antimicrob Agents Chemother* 1994;38:1930–6

45. Remington JS, Desmonts G. Toxoplasmosis. In Remington JS, Klein JO, eds. *Infectious Diseases of the Fetus and Newborn Infant*, 2nd edn. Philadelphia: WB Saunders, 1983:143–263

46. Back N, Ambrus JL, Velasco H, *et al.* Clinical and experimental pharmacology of parenteral spiramycin. *Clin Pharmacol Ther* 1962;3:305–13

47. Schoondermark-Van de Ven E, Galama J, Camps W, *et al.* Pharmacokinetics of spiramycin in the rhesus monkey: transplacental passage and distribution in tissue in the fetus. *Antimicrob Agents Chemother* 1994;38:1922–9

48. Foulon W, Naessens A, Derde MP. Evaluation of the possibilities for preventing congenital toxoplasmosis. *Am J Perinatol* 1994;11:57–62

49. Desmonts G, Forestier F, Thulliez PH, *et al.* Prenatal diagnosis of congenital toxoplasmosis. *Lancet* 1985; 8427:500–4

50. Couvreur J, Thulliez P, Daffos F, *et al. In utero* treatment of toxoplasmic fetopathy with the combination pyrimethamine–sulfadiazine. *Fetal Diagn Ther* 1993;8:45–50

51. Hesseltine HC, Wolters SL, Campbell AJ. Experimental human vaginal trichomoniasis. *J Infect Dis* 1942;71:127

52. Lehker MW, Chang TH, Dailey DC, Alderete JF. Specific erythrocyte binding is an additional nutrient acquistion system for *Trichomonas vaginalis*. *J Exp Med* 1990;171:2165–70

53. Alderete JF, Demes P, Gombosova A, *et al*. Specific parasitism of purified vaginal epithelial cells by *Trichomonas vaginalis*. *Infect Immun* 1988;56:2558–62

54. Alderete JF, Garza GE. Identification and properties of *Trichomonas vaginalis* proteins involved in cytadherence. *Infect Immun* 1988;56:28–33

55. Krieger JN, Ravdin JI, Rein MF. Contact-dependent cytopathogenic mechanisms of *Trichomonas vaginalis*. *Infect Immun* 1985;50:778–86

56. Keith LG, Berger GS, Edelman DA, *et al*. On the causation of pelvic inflammatory disease. *Am J Obstet Gynecol* 1984;149:215–19

57. Rein MF. *Trichomonas vaginalis*. In Mandel GL, Douglas GR, Bennett IE, eds. *Principles and Practice of Infectious Disease*, 4th edn. New York: Churchill Livingstone, 1995

58. Al-Salihi FL, Curran JP, Wang JS. Neonatal *Trichomonas vaginalis*: report of three cases and review of the literature. *Pediatrics* 1974;53:196–200

59. McLaren LC, Davis LE, Healy GR, James CG. Isolation of *Trichomonas vaginalis* from the respiratory tract of infants with respiratory disease. *Pediatrics* 1983;71:888–90

60. Wølner-Hanssen P, Krieger JN, Stevens CE, *et al*. Clinical manifestations of vaginal trichomoniasis. *J Am Med Assoc* 1989;261:571–6

61. Cassie R, Stevenson A. Screening for gonorrhoea, trichomoniasis, moniliasis and syphilis in pregnancy. *J Obstet Gynaecol Br Commonw* 1973;80:48–51

62. Sparks RA, Williams GL, Boyce MH, *et al*. Antenatal screening for candidiasis, trichomoniasis, and gonorrhoea. *Br J Vener Dis* 1975;51:110–5

63. Hurley R, Leask BGS, Faktor JA, Fonseka CI. Incidence and distribution of yeast species and of *Trichomonas vaginalis* in the vagina of pregnant women. *J Obstet Gynaecol Br Commonw* 1973;80:252–7

64. Ross SM, Hoosen AA, Sheik AI. Diagnosis and treatment of vaginal discharge in pregnancy. *S Afr Med J* 1980;58:757–9

65. de Louvois J, Hurley R, Stanley VC. Microbial flora of the lower genital tract during pregnancy: relationship to morbidity. *J Clin Pathol* 1975;28:731–5

66. Minkoff H, Grunebaum AN, Schwarz RH, *et al*. Risk factors for prematurity and premature rupture of membranes: a prospective study of the vaginal flora in pregnancy. *Am J Obstet Gynecol* 1984;150:965–8

67. Hardy PH, Nell EE, Spence MR, *et al*. Prevalence of six sexually transmitted disease agents among pregnant inner-city adolescents and pregnancy outcome. *Lancet* 1984;8398:333–7

68. Ross SM, Middelkoop AV. Trichomonas infection in pregnancy – does it affect perinatal outcome? *S Afr Med J* 1983;63:566–7

69. Krieger JN, Tam MR, Stevens CE, *et al*. Diagnosis of trichomoniasis: comparison of conventional wet-mount examination with cytologic studies, cultures, and monoclonal antibody staining of direct specimens. *J Am Med Assoc* 1988;259:1223

70. McLennan MT, Smith JM, McLennan CE. Diagnosis of vaginal mycosis and trichomoniasis: reliability of cytologic smear, wet smear and culture. *Obstet Gynecol* 1972;40:231–4

71. Spence MR, Hollander DH, Smith J, *et al*. The clinical and laboratory diagnosis of *Trichomonas vaginalis* infection. *Sex Transm Dis* 1980;7:168–71

72. Mason PR, Brown Z Trichomonas in pregnancy (letter). *Lancet* 1980;2:1025

73. Cotch MF, Pastorek JC II, Nugent RP, *et al*. *Trichomonas vaginalis* associated with low birth weight and preterm delivery. The vaginal infections and prematurity study group. *Sex Transm Dis* 1997;24:353–60

74. Lossick JG. Treatment of sexually transmitted vaginosis/vaginitis. *Rev Infect Dis* 1990;12:S665–S681

75. Lossick JG. Treatment of *Trichomonas vaginalis* infections. *Rev Infect Dis* 1982;4:S801–S818

76. Lyng J, Christensen J. A double-blind study of the value of treatment with a single dose tinidazole of partners to females with trichomoniasis. *Acta Obstet Gynecol Scand* 1981;60:199–201

77. Amon I, Amon K, Franke G, Mohr C. Pharmacokinetics of metronidazole in pregnant women. *Chemotherapy* 1981;27:73–9

78. Heisterberg L. Placental transfer of metronidazole in the first trimester of pregnancy. *J Perinat Med* 1984;12:43–5

79. Karhunen M. Placental transfer of metronidazole and tinidazole in early human pregnancy after a single infusion. *Br J Clin Pharmacol* 1984;18:254–7

80. Roe FJ. Toxicologic evaluation of metronidazole with particular reference to carcinogenic, mutagenic, and teratogenic potential. *Surgery* 1983;93:158–64

81. Morgan I. Metronidazole treatment in pregnancy. *Int J Gynaecol Obstet* 1978;15:501–2

82. Piper JM, Mitchel EF, Ray WA. Prenatal use of metronidazole and birth defects: no association. *Obstet Gynecol* 1993;82:348–52

83. Burtin P, Taddio A, Ariburnu O, *et al*. Safety of metronidazole in pregnancy: a meta-analysis. *Am J Obstet Gynecol* 1995;172(2 Pt 1):525–9

84. Caro-Paton T, Carvajal A, Martin de Diego I, *et al*. Is metronidazole teratogenic? A meta-analysis. *Br J Clin Pharmacol* 1997;44:179–82

85. Czeizel AE, Rockenbauer M. A population based case-control teratologic study of oral metronidazole treatment during pregnancy. *Br J Clin Pharmacol* 1998;105:322–7

86. Gurevitch AW. Scabies and lice. *Pediatr Clin North Am* 1985;32:987–92

87. Foulon W, Naessens A, Mahler T, *et al*. Prenatal diagnosis of congenital toxoplasmosis. *Obstet Gynecol* 1990;76:769–72

88. Desmonts G, Couvreur J. Congenital toxoplasmosis: a prospective study of 378 pregnancies. *N Engl J Med* 1974;290:1110–16

89. Hohlfeld P, Daffos F, Thulliez P, *et al*. Fetal toxoplasmosis: outcome of pregnancy and infant follow-up after *in utero* treatment. *J Pediatr* 1989;115:765–9

90. Berrebi A, Kobuch WE, Bessieres MH, *et al*. Termination of pregnancy for maternal toxoplasmosis. *Lancet* 1994;344:36–9 Comments: *Lancet* 1994;344:540–1

Section IIIe

Perinatal infections:
other infections and issues

30

Bacterial vaginosis in pregnancy: evidence-based approaches

J.A. McGregor and J.I. French

'Infection in the female reproductive tract (especially in the cervix) can cause premature rupture of membranes and induce premature labor ... this process is responsible for many preventable infant deaths.'

Knox and Hoerner, 1950[1]

INTRODUCTION

Bacterial vaginosis is the commonest cause of vaginal discharge among women of reproductive age[2]. Symptoms and findings of bacterial vaginosis have been recognized for centuries. This condition has also been termed *Gardnerella* vaginitis, non-specific vaginitis and anaerobic colpitis. Studies performed worldwide show that bacterial vaginosis is associated with preterm birth, preterm labor, premature rupture of membranes, chorioamnionitis, amniotic fluid infection, postpartum endometritis and Cesarean section infectious morbidity[3-15]. Many of these adverse effects can be prevented by screening and treating bacterial vaginosis early in pregnancy[15-18]. Of these complications, the evidence is most compelling for prevention of significant numbers of preterm birth by screening and treating bacterial vaginosis early in pregnancy. Review of evidence from many centers regarding preterm birth and bacterial vaginosis now satisfies Bradford Hill's modified criteria for causality[19]:

(1) Consistent associations;
(2) Plausible pathophysiological mechanisms;
(3) Effective etiology-specific intervention strategies;
(4) Demonstration of cost savings based on these strategies.

We will review each of these causality criteria and justify the following clinical recommendations:

(1) All pregnant women should be screened and treated for bacterial vaginosis (as well as other prevalent genitourinary microbial conditions) during their initial antenatal visit;

(2) Treatment should be with oral medication (metronidazole or clindamycin) so as to ensure suppression or eradication of susceptible upper-tract micro-organisms;

(3) A test of cure should be completed approximately 1 month after treatment;

(4) Women with a prior history of preterm birth, who have a low body mass index (BMI < 50 kg), or who have early gestational bleeding, will receive the greatest benefits from treatment;

(5) Asymptomatic as well as symptomatic women should be treated and receive tests of care.

Indeed, each of the randomized, double-blind placebo-controlled intervention trials reviewed here excluded symptomatic patients, as symptomatic patients were all promptly treated and excluded from study[16,18]. These recommendations, as well as screening and treatment of other prevalent urogenital infections, are already considered a matter of due medical diligence in many centers.

MICROBIOLOGY AND PATHOGENESIS OF BACTERIAL VAGINOSIS

Bacterial vaginosis consists of a dynamic microecological alteration in which a characteristic set of bacterial species greatly expand their populations within the vagina. This 'blooming' causes dramatic alterations in the biochemical make-up of vaginal fluid (Table 1)[20,21]. An analogous occurrence is a so called 'red tide', in which there is a similar, often odiferous, blooming of microbes in large bodies of water.

In the healthy vagina, between five and 15 microbial species are usually recoverable. High concentrations (10^5–10^6/g of fluid) of lactic acid-producing acidophilic facultative lactobacilli are normally the predominant microflora found throughout the menstrual cycle[20-22]. Until recently, *Lactobacillus acidophilus* was thought to predominate in the vagina. However, advances in microbiological identification techniques indicate that *Lactobacillus crispatus, Lactobacillus jensenii, Lactobacillus fermentum* and *Lactobacillus gasseri* represent the predominant vaginal species[21]. Many of these produce H_2O_2 as well as lactic acid. Other bacteria account for

Table 1 Biochemical factors in bacterial vaginosis and their potential pathophysiological effects

Vaginal fluid constituent	Known or potential actions	Potential effects in pregnancy
↑ pH	↑ attachment of anaerobic bacteria and ↓ *Lactobacillus* species attachment	↑ numbers of pathogenic anaerobic bacteria
↑ Succinic acid	impairs neutrophil phagocytic killing and response to chemotactic stimuli	↓ vaginal fluid host defenses
↑ Butyrate	toxic to fibroblasts in cell culture	? effects on cervical connective tissue and amniochorion
↑ Mucinase ↑ Sialidase	degrades protective surface mucin, ↑ bacterial attachment to epithelial cells	↓ cervical mucus barrier
↑ IgA protease	degrades IgA proteins	↓ cervical IgA
↑ Collagenase ↑ Non-specific proteases	degrades collagen types	↑ cervical ripening, amniochorion weakening
↑ Phospholipase A_2	induces matrix metalloproteinases, induces prostaglandins	↑ cervical ripening, amniochorion weakening and uterine contractions

approximately 10% of the bacteria recovered from the healthy vagina[20–22].

Bacterial vaginosis is characterized by, first, decreased numbers or the absence of normal lactobacilli and, second, high concentrations (10^8–10^{11} colony-forming units/g of fluid or greater) of potentially pathogenic bacteria, most notably *Prevotella* species (formerly *Bacteroides* species), *Peptostreptococcus* species, *Porphomonas* species and *Mobiluncus* species, along with *Gardnerella vaginalis*, *Mycoplasma hominis* and *Ureaplasma urealyticum*[20,21].

Vaginal biophysical changes associated with bacterial vaginosis include elevated pH (> 4.5), reduced redox potential, increased fluid concentrations of diamines, polyamines and organic acids, as well as increased concentrations of enzymes, including mucinases, sialidases, IgA proteases, collagenases, non-specific proteases and phospholipases A_2 and C[21,23–29]. Endotoxin (lipopolysaccharide), cytokine interleukin-1α, and prostaglandins E_2 and F_2α are also increased in the vaginal fluid of women with bacterial vaginosis[30,31]. These virulence factors promote tissue attachment, overcome host defense mechanisms and facilitate entrance of micro-organisms and associated factors into the upper reproductive tract. Vaginal fluid protease and phospholipases probably play roles in bacterial vaginosis pathogenesis and ascent of microbes and their associated substances into the uterus during pregnancy. Mucinases and sialidases are well-established gastrointestinal tract bacterial virulence factors. These enzymes lyse protective mucin and promote bacterial attachment, allowing invasion and subsequent spread to underlying epithelial cells. These enzymes probably play roles in disruption of cervical mucus and other host defenses, leading to upper-genital-tract spread of bacterial vaginosis-associated microflora[25].

During pregnancy, bacterial phospholipases A_2 and C, as well as non-specific proteases, can act on cervical and amniochorion tissues and probably promote cervical ripening and amniochorion weakening[27]. In addition, phospholipases A_2 and C may promote the release of arachidonic acid and prostaglandins, thus furthering the processes leading to preterm birth[27]. Thus, these bacterial substances directly contribute to the initiation of a number of bacterial vaginosis-associated obstetric complications[25–29].

Amines, primarily trimethylamine, putrescine and cadaverine, are produced during amino-acid metabolism by bacterial vaginosis-associated anaerobic bacteria[24,32]. These volatile amines are released as pH increases and are responsible for the 'sharp' or 'fishy' odor sometimes noticed in the presence of bacterial vaginosis[24,32]. Several short-chain fatty acids, including succinate, acetate, propionate, isobutyrate, butyrate and isovalerate, are also increased in bacterial vaginosis[21]. *In vitro* studies demonstrate that increased succinic acid dramatically impairs neutrophil phagocytic killing, response to chemotactic stimuli and generation of respiratory bursts required for bacterial killing[33]. Butyrate inhibits lymphocyte activation by release of an exotoxin and is toxic to human fibroblast and mouse neuroblastoma cells in culture[33,34]. Each of these 'signature' chemicals characteristic of bacterial vaginosis fluid is also found in abscess fluid.

In addition to their role in maintaining an acidic vaginal environment, lactobacilli, particularly H_2O_2-producing strains, play roles in the maintenance of a healthy, self-sustaining vaginal ecosystem[35,36]. The acidic environment in the healthy vagina is maintained by microbial metabolism of glucose, produced by vaginal epithelial cells from glycogen, to lactic acid[35]. *In vitro* experiments demonstrate that *Lactobacillus* species inhibit growth of other bacterial species in part by producing antimicrobial factors, including acidolin and lactacin B, in addition to H_2O_2[37–40]. Hydrogen peroxide-producing *Lactobacillus* species are predominant in the vaginal fluid of healthy women[40]. The microbicidal action of H_2O_2 is further enhanced in the presence of a halide ion, such as chloride, from cervical mucus, and peroxidase enzymes, such as myeloperoxidase, produced by neutrophils and monocytes[36]. Each of these factors is present in the vaginal fluid of healthy women in sufficient concentrations to produce *in vitro* bactericidal effects[36].

How bacterial vaginosis becomes established is a matter of interest. Do bacterial vaginosis-associated bacteria become established in the vagina because of the absence of H_2O_2-producing lactobacilli? Or does invasion of abnormal bacteria or other factors cause a subsequent decline in the numbers of lactobacilli? In a longitudinal study, Hillier and colleagues[41] found that women without H_2O_2-producing lactobacilli more often developed bacterial vaginosis and more frequently relapsed after successful treatment. These findings support the hypothesis that an absence of H_2O_2-producing lactobacilli precedes the development of bacterial vaginosis[41]. Other recent findings suggest that, first, lytic bacterial phages (viruses) can account for reduced lactobacilli populations in some women and, second, young females may have never acquired protective lactobacilli from their mothers or the environment as children[42]. Women lacking protective lactobacilli may be susceptible to inoculation of bacterial vaginosis-associated microflora from an infected partner or possibly from environmental sources[40].

Other etiological possibilities for acquisition of bacterial vaginosis include primary pH and/or biochemical alterations. Increased pH tends to displace lactobacilli from receptor sites on vaginal epithelial cells and maximizes adherence of *G. vaginalis* and other bacterial vaginosis-associated micro-organisms[43,44]. Elevations in vaginal pH following intercourse, douching with basic solutions or antenatal bleeding have been suggested as processes contributing to the initiation of bacterial vaginosis. Elevated vaginal fluid pH is directly implicated in preterm premature rupture of the membranes and preterm birth[45].

Acquisition of bacterial vaginosis frequently is related to sexual behavior[46]. Bacterial vaginosis may be related to acquisition of a new male sexual partner[47,48]. In general, bacterial vaginosis occurs more frequently among women who have initiated sexual activity at an early age, among women reporting more sexual partners and among women with concurrent or prior sexually transmitted infections[23,47]. Bacterial vaginosis is also noted among sexually abused children and among lesbian couples[49,50]. Microbiological examination of male partners of women with bacterial vaginosis demonstrates that bacterial vaginosis-associated micro-organisms, including *M. hominis*, *G. vaginalis*, *Peptostreptococcus* species, *Mobiluncus* species and *Bacteroides* species, are recovered from 17–52% of urethral cultures[50]. Foreskin cultures yield even higher rates of recovery of associated micro-organisms. Furthermore, the same *G. vaginalis* biotypes are isolated within couples[51]. Holst[48] suggests that urethral carriage of these micro-organisms in males originates and is sustained by exposure to female partners. Bacterial vaginosis microflora were no longer recovered from male partners following 2 weeks of condom use[48]. Holst further suggests that the anaerobic component of bacterial vaginosis microflora originates in the gastrointestinal tract[48]. Detection of bacterial vaginosis among virginal women and children, even though the occurrence is low, weighs against sexual transmission as the exclusive means for acquisition of bacterial vaginosis[49]. Results of trials demonstrating the recurrence of bacterial vaginosis among women, despite treatment of male contacts, further supports the concept of non-sexual acquisition[52].

EPIDEMIOLOGY AND NATURAL HISTORY OF BACTERIAL VAGINOSIS

Numerous studies have prospectively examined bacterial vaginosis among populations of pregnant women and demonstrated prevalences ranging from 6–32% (Table 2)[4,6,8–12,17,53,54]. Studies from Sweden and Denmark both report bacterial vaginosis among 14% of pregnant women[55,56], which is similar to the 16% prevalence reported in the largest US study[12]. In the USA, the prevalence of bacterial vaginosis is highest among African American women and lowest among Asian American women; furthermore, it is highest among women with multiple sexual partners and lowest among women with no history of heterosexual contact[4,17,46]. Smoking and bacterial vaginosis are commonly associated. Among non-pregnant women of reproductive age, bacterial vaginosis is detected more often among those not using any method of contraception and among women using an intrauterine contraceptive device[23,47].

The natural history of bacterial vaginosis is increasingly well characterized. Studies in pregnancy show that most women with bacterial vaginosis remain positive unless treated[11,46,55,57]. Among pregnant women initially negative for bacterial vaginosis in the first trimester, only 2.9% of British women and no Swedish women developed bacterial vaginosis by the follow-up examination at 28 weeks' gestation[55,57]; 47–55% of initially positive women continued to have findings of bacterial vaginosis at the third-trimester follow-up visit[55,57]. A further 2.4% of women without bacterial vaginosis in the first trimester had developed bacterial vaginosis by term[55,57]. Similarly, only 7.3% of Indonesian women developed bacterial vaginosis between their initial examination at 16–20 weeks' gestation and the follow-up examination at approximately 28 weeks' gestation[11]. Bacterial vaginosis developed

Table 2   Prevalence of bacterial vaginosis in pregnant women followed prospectively

Study population	Diagnostic method	Prevalence
USA		
Seattle, Washington[9,84]	gas–liquid chromatography	14–28%
	clinical	6–21%
	Gram stain	12–21%
Denver, Colorado[12,25]	Gram stain	18.7–23%
	clinical	32%
Vaginal Infections and Prematurity Study[18]	Gram stain and pH > 4.5	16%
Halifax, Nova Scotia, Canada[83]	clinical	23%
Finland[15]	quantitative cultures	21.4%
Harrow, UK[16]	Gram stain	12–14%
Adelaide, Australia[14]	*G. vaginalis* culture (heavy growth)	28%
Jakarta, Indonesia[17]	Gram stain	17%

among 12% and 13% of American women between 23–26 weeks' gestation and follow-up after 28 weeks' gestation in two US studies which provided longitudinal follow-up[18,46]. In addition, in 31% of untreated women with bacterial vaginosis, the condition resolved during this interval[46]. Importantly, Joesoef and co-workers[11] determined that women with bacterial vaginosis at 16–20 weeks' gestation suffered increased risk for preterm birth, even if they no longer had findings of bacterial vaginosis at the later follow-up visit (28–32 weeks' gestation).

Prospective treatment studies show that bacterial vaginosis frequently recurs in pregnancy, regardless of initial successful treatment[25]. Well-controlled treatment trials document bacterial vaginosis recurrences among 30–40% of non-pregnant women within 3 months of oral metronidazole therapy[58,59]. McGregor and colleagues[25] examined the effectiveness of 2% vaginal clindamycin cream for bacterial vaginosis during pregnancy, between 16 and 26 weeks' gestation. One week post-treatment, 4% of women continued to have findings of bacterial vaginosis; however, bacterial vaginosis gradually recurred during the pregnancy, with approximately 10% of women having findings of bacterial vaginosis 8 weeks post-treatment and approximately 20% having recent bacterial vaginosis by 36 weeks' gestation[25]. Other authorities report recurrence of bacterial vaginosis in up to 80% of women within 9 months of initially effective treatment[60]. The individual factors which predispose to acquisition, persistence, resolution and/or recurrence of bacterial vaginosis require further elucidation, but probably involve failure of H_2O_2-producing lactobacilli to recolonize and re-establish a normal, protective vaginal ecosystem following treatment[40,41].

DIAGNOSIS OF BACTERIAL VAGINOSIS

The polymicrobial nature of bacterial vaginosis means that simple cultures are not helpful[23]. The current clinical 'gold standard' was established in 1983 by Amsel and colleagues[23] and is based upon a combination of simple-to-determine clinical criteria. A variety of other diagnostic techniques have been developed in the attempt to reduce reliance on possibly subjective clinical criteria. These include:

(1) Identification of clue cells on a Papanicolaou's smear sampled from the posterior fornix, often in combination with elevated vaginal fluid pH[61];

(2) Gram stains of vaginal fluid interpreted using one of several systems[62–64];

(3) Identification of several different vaginal fluid biochemicals (amines and proline aminopeptidase)[24,65];

(4) Ratio of normal biochemicals to abnormal biochemicals[4,5,21];

(5) Culture or DNA probes for a predominant microorganism (i.e. *G. vaginalis*)[66];

(6) Quantitative microbiological cultures[8,9].

None of these has supplanted Amsel's criteria.

Clinical diagnosis

Accurate clinical diagnosis is based on the presence of three of four clinical criteria:

(1) Homogeneous, thin vaginal fluid that adheres to the vaginal walls;

(2) Vaginal fluid pH> 4.5;

(3) Release of amine odor with alkalinization of vaginal fluid, the 'whiff test';

(4) Presence of vaginal epithelial cells with borders obscured by adherent, small bacteria, called 'clue cells'.

Of the four Amsel's criteria, the presence of clue cells on saline wet-mount examination is the most specific and sensitive indicator of bacterial vaginosis. Identification of clue cells accurately predicts 85–90% of women with clinical bacterial vaginosis (positive predictive value)[67]. Identification of clue cells may be hindered by adherence of normal bacteria, cellular debris, and availability and quality of the microscopy[66]. Clue cells can be microscopically distinguished from normal vaginal epithelial cells by their characteristic stippled and ragged appearance (Figure 1). The cell borders are obscured by adherent small coccobacilli-type bacteria, in contrast to normal vaginal epithelial cells where the cell borders are distinct and clearly seen (Figure 2). In addition to the presence of clue cells, the bacterial flora appear grossly altered on microscopic examination when bacterial vaginosis is present. The characteristic long rods, or normal *Lactobacillus* morphotypes, are absent or rare. Background bacterial flora appear greatly increased in number and short rods and coccobacillary forms predominate. *Mobiluncus* species may be identified by their characteristic spiral or serpent-like motility[68].

The 'whiff test' is similarly specific for the diagnosis of bacterial vaginosis, but may also be positive in trichomoniasis. Alkalinization of vaginal fluid releases volatile amines, putrescine, cadaverine and trimethylamine, which give off a characteristically 'fishy' or sharp odor[24,32]. This odor may be released spontaneously by other agents which raise the vaginal pH, such as sexual intercourse, douching or menses. Presence of an amine odor is highly predictive of bacterial vaginosis. However, putrescine is also present in semen, and other anaerobic infections, including trichomoniasis, can result in a positive amine test[24]. Therefore, the 'whiff test' is the least sensitive of the criteria; conversely, absence of odor by history does not negate the presence of bacterial vaginosis[2].

Normal vaginal pH from menarche to menopause ranges between 3.8 and 4.2[23]. Amsel and colleagues[23] determined that vaginal fluid pH over 4.5 discriminated easily between bacterial vaginosis and normal vaginal fluid. Identification of pH over 4.5 is highly sensitive for the diagnosis of bacterial vaginosis, but it is not specific[2,23,67]. Other factors may raise vaginal pH, including semen, cervical mucus, menses, trichomoniasis and possibly recent douching. Samples for examination of vaginal fluid pH must be obtained from the lateral vaginal side-wall or posterior fornices in order to reflect accurately vaginal, and not cervical, pH. Similarly, the pH indicator paper must allow distinction between the normal vaginal pH (3.8 to 4.2) from

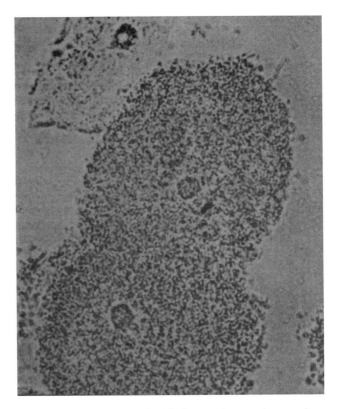

Figure 1 'Clue cells' identified on microscopic examination of saline preparation

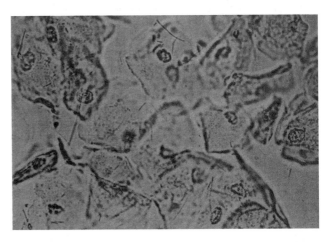

Figure 2 Normal vaginal epithelial cells identified on microscopic examination of saline preparation

pH over 4.5. The characteristic thin, homogeneous and adherent vaginal fluid is the most subjective indicator of bacterial vaginosis.

Gram-stain diagnosis

Gram stains of vaginal fluid are used in research settings to identify the shift from predominance of *Lactobacillus* morphotypes to predominance of coccobacillary morphotypes and Gram-negative rods characteristic of bacterial vaginosis. The Gram-stain diagnosis

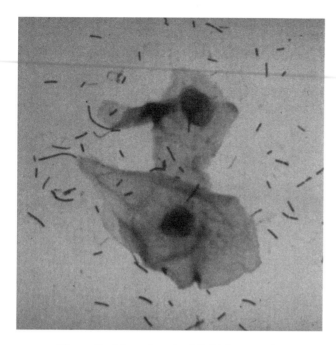

Figure 3   Normal vaginal fluid Gram stain

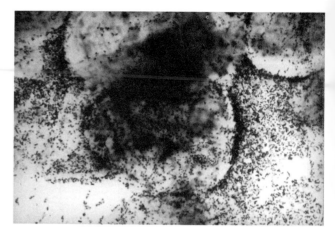

Figure 4   Gram stain of bacterial vaginosis

of bacterial vaginosis is not based upon examination for clue cells; rather, quantitative estimations of the types of bacteria in the vaginal fluid are evaluated[62–64].

Normal vaginal fluid is described by a predominance of large Gram-positive rods, considered *Lactobacillus* morphotypes, with or without smaller Gram-variable bacilli, considered *Gardnerella* morphotypes (Figures 2, 3)[62]. A pattern of mixed vaginal flora, which includes *Gardnerella* morphotypes, Gram-negative rods, fusiforms, curved rods, Gram-positive cocci and absent or reduced numbers of *Lactobacillus* morphotypes (less than five per high-power field), is consistent with bacterial vaginosis (Figure 4)[62]. The technique of Nugent and co-workers[64] examines four bacterial morphotypes and assigns a summary score to the vaginal specimen based on the semi-quantitative assessment for *Lactobacillus* morphotypes, *G. vaginalis*, *Prevotella* morphotypes and *Mobiluncus* morphotypes. A score of 7–10 is considered to indicate bacterial vaginosis[64]. Compared with other diagnostic methods, this standardized scheme has superior reproducibility[69].

Microbial culture

Culture for *G. vaginalis* is both an inaccurate and expensive way to diagnose bacterial vaginosis. Clinical cultures should not be used to diagnose bacterial vaginosis. *G. vaginalis* can be recovered from up to 60% of women[2,53]. Therefore, non-quantitative cultures for *G. vaginalis* would misdiagnose up to 60% of healthy women as having bacterial vaginosis[2,23,53]. Even semi-quantitative examination for heavy colony growth (3+, 4+), suggesting the presence of high concentrations of

G. vaginalis, accurately predicts as few as 41–49% of women with the composite clinical criteria for bacterial vaginosis among populations with low prevalence[2,53]. More than one-half of women with clinical bacterial vaginosis would remain undetected using this method. Quantitative aerobic and anaerobic vaginal cultures have been used in clinical research studies to evaluate bacterial vaginosis, but this technique is costly and impractical for clinical use[8,9].

New diagnostic techniques

New techniques, including nucleic-acid probes to detect high concentrations of *G. vaginalis*, have recently become available[66,69]. The Affirm VP III Microbial Identification Test (Becton Dickinson and Company, Sparks, MD) may provide a less subjective test for bacterial vaginosis than other current methods. Briselden and Hillier[66] reported accurate detection of 95–97% of women with clinical criteria for bacterial vaginosis (sensitivity) using the Affirm VP III test. Specificity for this test ranged from 71–98%[66,69]. Briselden and Hillier[66] noted that the false-positive tests (compared with clinical criteria) occurred most often among women with Gram-stain findings consistent with bacterial vaginosis, suggesting that the Affirm test most closely replicates Gram-stain findings.

OBSTETRIC COMPLICATIONS ASSOCIATED WITH BACTERIAL VAGINOSIS

Preterm birth

Associations between bacterial vaginosis and increased risk for adverse pregnancy outcomes have been investigated through case–control, cross-sectional, prospective cohort studies and randomized, controlled treatment trials (Table 3)[3–12,16–18,25,54,70–74]. Despite differences in study design, definitions of preterm birth

Table 3   Review of prospective cohort studies evaluating bacterial vaginosis and adverse pregnancy outcomes

Outcome and reference	Gestational age when tested (weeks)	Number of positive outcomes	Number of negative outcomes	Relative risk (95% CI)
Preterm Birth (< 37 weeks)				
Minkoff et al. 1984[54]	13	ND	ND	2.3 (0.96–5.5)[*]
McGregor et al. 1990[6]	24	1/24 (4.2%)	3/110 (2.7%)	1.5 (0.2–14.2)
McDonald et al. 1992[8]	22–28	31/135 (23%)	97/651 (14.9%)	1.8 (1.01–3.2)
Kurki et al. 1992[9]	8–17	11/162 (6.8%)	6/571 (1.0%)	6.9 (2.5–18.8)
Joesoef et al. 1993[11]	16–20	17/84 (20.2%)	48/406 (11.8%)	2.0 (1.0–3.9)
	28–32	11/67 (16.4%)	50/395 (12.7%)	1.5 (0.7–3.0)
McGregor et al. 1994[25]	16–26	14/129 (10.9%)	4/122 (3.3%)	3.3 (1.2–9.1)
Hay et al. 1994[10]	< 16	7/57 (12.3%)	9/384 (2.3%)	5.2 (2.0–13.5)
	< 24	8/83 (9.6%)	18/616 (2.9%)	3.3 (1.5–7.4)
McGregor et al. 1995[17]	18	31/165 (18.8%)	37/380 (9.7%)	1.9 (1.2–3.0)
Meis et al. 1995[73]	24	ND	ND	1.4 (0.9–2.0)[†]
	28	ND	ND	1.8 (1.2–3.0)[†]
Hillier et al. 1995[12]	23–26	77/1218 (6.3%)	291/6978 (4.2%)	1.4 (1.1–1.8)[‡]
Preterm premature rupture of the membranes				
Gravett et al. 1986[4]	32	22/102 (21.6%)	44/432 (10.2%)	2.0 (1.1–3.7)
McDonald et al. 1992[8]	22–28	ND	ND	2.7 (1.1–6.5)
Kurki et al. 1992[9]	8–17	6/162 (3.7%)	3/571 (0.5%)	7.3 (1.8–29.4)
McGregor et al. 1994[25]	16–26	6/128 (4.7%)	1/121 (0.8%)	5.7 (0.9–36.1)
McGregor et al. 1995[17]	18	10/144 (6.9%)	7/350 (2.0%)	3.5 (1.4–8.9)
Hillier et al. 1995[12]	23–26	35/1132 (3.1%)	182/6617 (2.8%)	1.1 (0.8–1.6)
Preterm labor				
Minkoff et al. 1984[54]	13	14/66 (21.2%)	21/152 (13.8%)	1.5 (0.8–2.8)[*]
Gravett et al. 1986[4]	32	24/102 (23.5%)	53/432 (12.3%)	2.0 (1.1–3.5)
McGregor et al. 1990[6]	24	6/23 (26.1%)	11/111 (9.9%)	2.6 (1.1–6.5)
Kurki et al. 1992[9]	8–17	17/162 (10.5%)	25/571 (4.4%)	2.6 (1.3–4.9)
McGregor et al. 1994[25]	16–26	23/129 (17.8%)	15/122 (12.3%)	1.5 (0.8–2.6)
Low birthweight				
Gravett et al. 1986[4]	32	24/102 (23.5%)	65/432 (15.0%)	1.7 (1.0–2.9)
McGregor et al. 1994[25]	16–26	11/128 (8.6%)	10/119 (8.4%)	1.0 (0.4–2.3)
Spontaneous abortion				
Hay et al. 1994[10]	< 16	4/57 (7.0%)	5/384 (1.3%)	5.4 (1.5–19.5)[*]
McGregor et al. 1995[17]	< 22	16/305 (5.2%)	11/767 (1.4%)	3.1 (1.4–6.9)
Postpartum endometritis				
Watts et al. 1990[13]	ND[§]	ND	ND	5.8 (3.0–10.9)
Amniotic fluid infection				
Silver et al. 1989[14]	39	22/32 (68.8%)	43/93 (46.2%)	1.5 (1.1–2.0)[*]
Krohn et al. 1995[74]	23–26	43/1296 (3.3%)	183/8741 (2.1%)	1.5 (1.2–2.2)

ND, not described; [*]risk ratio and 95% confidence intervals calculated from data provided; preterm birth defined as [†]< 35 weeks' gestation; [‡]< 37 weeks' gestation and low birth weight; [§]examined at admission for labor

and the techniques used to identify bacterial vaginosis, research from around the world repeatedly supports the association between bacterial vaginosis and increased risk of preterm labor, preterm birth and preterm premature rupture of the membranes (Table 3)[4–12,17,25,70]. Crucially, bacterial vaginosis and associated micro-organisms appear to increase the risk of preterm birth at the lowest viable gestational ages[7]. Two published studies report an association between pre-viable second-trimester pregnancy loss and bacterial vaginosis, suggesting that pathophysiological processes associated with bacterial vaginosis cause a

continuum of both pre-viable loss and birth of severely premature newborns[10,17].

Multiple prospective studies indicate that bacterial vaginosis may be detected months prior to the onset of preterm labor or preterm birth[4,6,8–12]. Eschenbach and colleagues[3] and Gravett and co-workers[4,5] were the first to implicate bacterial vaginosis as a risk factor for preterm labor and low birth weight. Bacterial vaginosis was identified using gas–liquid chromatography among 19% of 534 pregnant women studied[4]. The presence of bacterial vaginosis in the mid-third trimester (mean 32.6 weeks) was associated with increased risk for preterm labor [odds ratio (OR) 2.0, 95% confidence interval (CI) 1.1–3.5] and preterm premature rupture of the membranes (OR 2.0, 95% CI 1.1–3.7)[4]. McDonald and colleagues[8] examined bacterial vaginosis (culture for heavy colonization with *G. vaginalis*) earlier in gestation (22–28 weeks) and demonstrated similar risks for preterm birth following labor (OR 1.8) and preterm premature rupture of the membranes (OR 2.7).

Studies which examine for bacterial vaginosis at the earliest gestational ages and carefully control for intervening antimicrobial treatment demonstrate the strongest association between bacterial vaginosis and preterm birth (Table 3)[9,10]. The highest relative risks (seven-fold increase) between bacterial vaginosis and preterm birth and premature rupture of the membranes were noted in Finnish women who were initially examined in the first trimester[9]. In an insightful analysis, Joesoef and colleagues[11] examined risk of preterm birth for women found to have bacterial vaginosis between 16 and 20 weeks' gestation and/or between 28 and 32 weeks' gestation[11]. Women with bacterial vaginosis in the early second trimester experienced a two-fold increase in premature birth compared with women without bacterial vaginosis[11]. Women with bacterial vaginosis at 28–32 weeks' gestation experienced somewhat less increased risk for premature birth (OR 1.5, 95% CI 0.7–3.0). Women who developed bacterial vaginosis between the screening intervals (i.e. those negative at 16–20 weeks' gestation and positive at 28–32 weeks' gestation) were not at increased risk for preterm birth (10.7% preterm birth among women developing bacterial vaginosis versus 11.8% among women never positive for bacterial vaginosis; calculated OR 0.9)[11]. As discussed, women with findings of bacterial vaginosis at 16–20 weeks' gestation were at increased risk for preterm birth, even if they no longer had findings of bacterial vaginosis at the later follow-up visit (20.5% preterm birth among women with bacterial vaginosis at both visits and 20.5% preterm birth among women with bacterial vaginosis only at the first visit, versus 11.8% preterm birth among women without bacterial vaginosis)[11]. These findings suggest that physiological processes present or initiated at, or prior to, 16 to 20 weeks' gestation are important for the subsequent development of preterm birth. These authors concluded that 'only bacterial vaginosis in early pregnancy plays a major role as a risk factor for preterm delivery'[11].

How many preterm births might be prevented by prompt identification and effective treatment of bacterial vaginosis in pregnancy? McGregor and colleagues[17] identified 22% of preterm births in their inner-city population in Denver, Colorado, as attributable to bacterial vaginosis. In a prospective study, we reduced occurrences of preterm birth and rupture of membranes by 50% by treating bacterial vaginosis and

other prevalent genitourinary infections during initial antenatal care[17]. Most recently, results of a large prospective cohort study from the National Institute of Child Health and Human Development-sponsored Vaginal Infections and Prematurity Study Group[12] demonstrated a 40% increase in risk of delivering a preterm low-birth-weight infant (born at less than 37 weeks' gestation and weighing less than 2500 g) and a 10% increase in risk of preterm premature rupture of the membranes among women with bacterial vaginosis detected between 23 and 26 weeks' gestation. These authors calculated a 9% attributable risk for prematurity in this study of over 10 000 subjects[12]. Other populations could receive more or less benefits, depending on the prevalence of bacterial vaginosis.

Antimicrobial treatment trials for the prevention of preterm birth

Well-controlled, prospective treatment trials to prevent preterm birth demonstrate reductions in the rate of preterm birth among women with both symptomatic and asymptomatic bacterial vaginosis during pregnancy[16,17]. McGregor and colleagues[17] identified bacterial vaginosis using standard clinical criteria among 32% of pregnant women in an unselected population in Denver. Risk of preterm birth was reduced by 50% among women with bacterial vaginosis who received oral clindamycin treatment compared with untreated observational controls[17]. Morales and co-workers[16] randomized pregnant women with both bacterial vaginosis and a prior preterm birth to receive either oral metronidazole or placebo. This placebo-controlled trial demonstrated a similar 50% reduction in the rate of preterm birth among metronidazole-treated women compared with those who received placebo[16]. Subsequently, Hauth and colleagues[18] presented results from an antenatal trial of prophylactic metronidazole and erythromycin versus dual placebos among women considered to be at increased risk for preterm birth because of a prior preterm birth or because of low maternal weight. Subset analyses showed that only women with bacterial vaginosis achieved important reductions in the rates of preterm birth compared with women given placebos[18]. In contrast, two randomized, placebo-controlled trials to prevent preterm birth by treatment of bacterial vaginosis with 2% intravaginal clindamycin cream failed to demonstrate reduced incidence of preterm birth, despite apparently adequate treatment for bacterial vaginosis[25,72].

Why second-trimester intravaginal treatment is not effective in preventing preterm birth is becoming clarified. McGregor and colleagues[25] suggest that bacterial vaginosis-associated micro-organisms gain access to the lower uterine segment and are present within the decidual tissues early in pregnancy or before pregnancy. They suggest that systemic treatment is required for effective eradication and reduction in the risk of preterm birth[17,25]. An alternative explanation would be that women receiving placebo are more likely to continue to have bacterial vaginosis and have this condition subsequently detected and treated by their care providers[25]. Use of non-study, effective, oral antimicrobial therapy among the placebo recipients would probably reduce the incidence of preterm birth, similar to the decreases noted in the treatment arms of clinical trials using oral medications. Finally, Hillier and colleagues[75] demonstrated a transient increase in the recovery of *Escherichia coli* and *Enterococcus* species for up to 1 month following intravaginal clindamycin cream treatment. *E. coli* has also been associated with increased risk for preterm birth, especially when acquired mid-pregnancy[71]. Joesoef and colleagues[72] speculate that this change in the vaginal flora (to *E. coli*, *Enterococcus* species and other gastrointestinal flora) may have further increased the risk for preterm birth among studied women who received clindamycin vaginal cream.

Overall, the information from these treatment trials supports the concept that early pregnancy screening and standard oral treatment for bacterial vaginosis prevents important numbers of preterm births safely and inexpensively.

Intrapartum and postpartum infections

Bacterial vaginosis has been linked with clinical chorioamnionitis, amniotic fluid infection, as well as postpartum endometritis and Cesarean section infection. These associations were first suggested by observations that the micro-organisms frequently recovered from women with these complications often include the common constituents of bacterial vaginosis, i.e. *Prevotella bivius*, *G. vaginalis*, *M. hominis*, *U. urealyticum* and *Peptostreptococcus* species[5,13–15]. Clinical studies have examined bacterial vaginosis, identified by either Gram stain or gas–liquid chromatography, and shown that women with clinical amniotic fluid infection more commonly have findings of bacterial vaginosis compared with women without clinical infection[5,14,15]. Among the 286 (2.4%) women from the Vaginal Infections and Prematurity Study who developed amniotic fluid infection, antenatal carriage (23–26 weeks' gestation) of bacterial vaginosis (relative risk 1.5, 95% CI 1.2–2.2) and bacterial vaginosis-associated micro-organisms were significantly associated with amniotic fluid infection[74]. This increase in risk for amniotic fluid infection associated with bacterial vaginosis was independent of duration of labor, duration of rupture of membranes, concurrent infection with *Neisseria gonorrhoeae*, *Chlamydia trachomatis*, *Trichomonas vaginalis*, group B streptococcus and effective antimicrobial treatment[74]. Future large studies will need to determine if successful antenatal treatment for bacterial

vaginosis or intrapartum screening and treatment for bacterial vaginosis are of benefit in reducing rates of chorioamnionitis and amniotic fluid infection.

Postpartum endometritis occurs following 2–5% of vaginal births and 10–20% of Cesarean deliveries[76]. These infections are polymicrobial in nature for over 80% of affected women[77]. In a series of 161 women with postpartum endometritis described by Watts and colleagues[77], the common constituents of bacterial vaginosis (i.e. *G. vaginalis*, *P. bivius*, *Peptostreptococcus* species and *Bacteroides* species) were recovered from endometrial cultures in up to 60% of women. Wound infections developed among 18% (16/79) of women with endometrial bacterial vaginosis-associated flora and among 8% (4/53) of women with other bacteria recovered from the endometrium[77]. Subsequent work by Watts[13] demonstrated a 5.8-fold increased risk for post-Cesarean section endometritis among women with bacterial vaginosis. Strategies under evaluation to reduce the risk of intrapartum and postpartum infections include:

(1) Identification and treatment of bacterial vaginosis at the initial antepartum examination, followed by periodic tests of cure;

(2) Treatment of bacterial vaginosis prior to birth;

(3) Use of chemoprophylaxis which treats bacterial vaginosis-associated micro-organisms in women requiring Cesarean section.

BACTERIAL VAGINOSIS TREATMENT IN PREGNANCY

Oral (systemic) treatment with either metronidazole or clindamycin is preferred for the treatment of bacterial vaginosis during pregnancy. Only oral treatments provide adequate antimicrobial levels in both uterine and vaginal tissue and are associated with improved pregnancy outcome in published studies. Cure rates are similar to those obtained among non-pregnant women[17,78]. Initial cure rates within 1–2 weeks following completion of treatment are generally 25–35% higher than those among women examined 4–5 weeks post-treatment[58,78].

Oral metronidazole, 500 mg twice daily for 7 days, continues to be the standard therapy recommended by the Centers for Disease Control in the USA for treatment of bacterial vaginosis[79]. Resolution of bacterial vaginosis occurs among 85–100% of studied women examined approximately 1 week following completion of oral metronidazole treatment[58]. The percentage of women without bacterial vaginosis 4–5 weeks following completion of treatment ranges from 60–95% and averages approximately 80%[58,78]. Similarly, bacterial vaginosis was cured among 76% of Australian women 4 weeks following treatment with oral metronidazole and among 70% of women in

Birmingham, Alabama, following treatment with metronidazole and erythromycin[18,78]. Different regimens of oral metronidazole have been examined in trials and observational reports; in general, cure rates at 4 weeks post-dosing with a single 2-g dose of metronidazole range from 45–69%[58].

Traditionally, metronidazole has been avoided during early pregnancy, owing to mutagenicity in bacterial (Ames) testing and tumor production in specific animal models given high doses of drug. However, after 30 years of clinical use, teratogenic and carcinogenic effects in humans have not been established. Several retrospective studies and a meta-analysis have examined the pregnancy outcomes for women who received metronidazole during pregnancy without evidence of teratogenicity[80,81].

Clindamycin is also effective treatment for bacterial vaginitis, as well as its associated microflora, including some genital mycoplasmas. Greaves and co-workers[82] examined 49 women 7–10 days following completion of a 7-day course of oral clindamycin, 300 mg twice daily, and demonstrated a cure rate of 94% for bacterial vaginosis. McGregor and associates[17] examined 194 pregnant women and found a cure rate of 92% 2–4 weeks post-treatment[17]. Importantly, among a subgroup of women who received treatment early in pregnancy and were followed for the remainder of the pregnancy, 90% remained cured for up to 11 weeks (McGregor, unpublished data). Oral treatment with clindamycin may be used throughout pregnancy, including the first trimester; it provides resolution of bacterial vaginosis equivalent to that of oral metronidazole. Intravaginal treatments for bacterial vaginosis are similarly effective, but did not improve pregnancy outcomes in the available studies; these studies initiated treatment well into the second trimester (16–26 weeks' gestation), after which intrauterine transfer of micro-organisms may have already occurred[25,72,83,84].

Other treatments for bacterial vaginosis have been evaluated: ampicillin, augmentin, ofloxacin, erythromycin, triple sulfa cream and vaginal acidification[58,59]. These treatments are less effective than both oral and vaginal preparations of metronidazole or clindamycin and are not recommended. Similarly, probiotic therapy with microbial products commercially available in the USA, such as lactobacillus powders and capsules, should be avoided at this time; many of the non-dairy products are contaminated with potentially harmful bacteria such as *Clostridium sporogenes* and *Enterococcus* species[86]. Therapy with yogurt or acidophilus milk is also likely to be of little benefit, since the *L. acidophilus* strains are not easily established in the vagina[87].

Treatment of sexual partners of women with bacterial vaginosis is unnecessary: randomized controlled trials which examined co-treatment of male partners failed to demonstrate reduced recurrence rates of bacterial vaginosis for women[52,88].

Adverse effects from treatment

An unpleasant taste is the most common complaint after generic oral metronidazole, occurring in between 35 and 50% of patients[89,90]. Nausea, vomiting, abdominal pain, headache and dizziness are also noted and are reported on frequently with use of proprietary products. Incidence of yeast vaginitis following oral metronidazole treatment varies from 5 to 22%[89,90]. Among women receiving oral treatment with clindamycin, nausea (12%) and yeast vaginitis (8.5–24%) are the most common complaints[17,82]. Complaints of loose stools or diarrhea occur in similarly small numbers of women receiving oral clindamycin (6.3%) and among women given a single 2-g dose of oral metronidazole (8.8%)[17]. Adverse side-effects from intravaginal treatments occur less often than among orally treated women, with the exception of yeast vaginitis[83,84].

Cost savings analysis

Recent economic models of preterm birth have focused on direct economic savings of screening and treating bacterial vaginosis. Other genitourinary tract infections, such as trichomoniasis, chlamydial endocervitis and gonorrhea, as well as asymptomatic bacteriuria are routinely identified and treated in most centers. Using conservative assumptions (585 000 cases of bacterial vaginosis in US pregnant women in 1995; diagnosis and treatment $28), Oleen-Burkey and Hillier[91] concluded that, in 1993, direct savings for preventing bacterial vaginosis-caused preterm birth to be $150 million yearly. Bloom and Lee[92] calculated a direct cost-saving ratio of 25 : 1 for identifying and treating bacterial vaginosis among 'high-risk' women. In this study, costs for diagnosis were assumed to be $20 for evaluating Amsel's clinical criteria[23,92]. Neither analysis took into account costs incurred after infant discharge or increased liability costs due to avoidable adverse pregnancy outcomes. It is likely that change in medical-care financing and incentives currently taking place will lead to more comprehensive calculation of the benefits of preventing preterm birth.

CONCLUSION

Bacterial vaginosis is the commonest cause of vaginal discharge in pregnant and non-pregnant women. This common condition represents massive microbial (*G. vaginalis*, anaerobes, mycoplasmas, etc.) and biochemical (pH, phospholipases, proteases, sialidase, etc.) perturbations of lower-reproductive-tract microecology. Diagnostic tests (Amsel's criteria) are easily and inexpensively performed in symptomatic and asymptomatic women. Treatments include oral treatment with relatively inexpensive generic agents, i.e. metronidazole or clindamycin. Descriptive and intervention studies carried out world-wide demonstrate, first increased risks of preterm birth associated with bacterial vaginosis and, second, that preterm birth, and possibly other adverse consequences, can be reduced by screening and systematically treating bacterial vaginosis in women at risk in both selected and unselected populations. These studies evaluated only asymptomatic women – women with symptoms were treated and excluded from study. Economic analysis of direct costs demonstrates cost savings from screening and treating bacterial vaginosis. Most clinicians consider the cost savings of preventing preterm birth 'obvious' when long-term sequelae, costs and liability are considered. Providers, patients and payers now have evidence-based, etiology-directed and cost-saving opportunities to prevent important numbers of preterm births, as well as individual children's suffering from being born 'too soon'.

REFERENCES

1. Knox IC, Hoerner JK. The role of infection in premature rupture of membranes. *Am J Obstet Gynecol* 1950; 59:190–4
2. Eschenbach DA, Hillier SL, Critchlow C, *et al*. Diagnosis and clinical manifestations of bacterial vaginosis. *Am J Obstet Gynecol* 1988;158:819
3. Eschenbach DA, Gravett MG, Chen KCS, *et al*. Bacterial vaginosis during pregnancy. An association with prematurity and post partum complications. In Mårdh PA, Taylor-Robinson D, eds. *Bacterial Vaginosis*. Stockholm: Almqvist and Wiksill, 1984:213–22
4. Gravett MG, Nelson HP, DeRouen T, *et al*. Independent associations of bacterial vaginosis and *Chlamydia trachomatis* infection with adverse pregnancy outcome. *J Am Med Assoc* 1986;256:1899–903
5. Gravett MG, Hummel D, Eschenbach DA, Holmes KK. Preterm labor associated with subclinical amniotic fluid infection and with bacterial vaginosis. *Obstet Gynecol* 1986;67:229–37
6. McGregor JA, French JI, Richter R, *et al*. Antenatal microbiologic and maternal risk factors associated with prematurity. *Am J Obstet Gynecol* 1990;163:1465–77
7. Hillier SL, Martius J, Krohn MA, *et al*. A case–control study of chorioamnionic infection and histologic chorioamnionitis in prematurity. *N Engl J Med* 1988; 319:972–8
8. McDonald HM, O'Loughlin JA, Jolley P, *et al*. Prenatal microbiological risk factors associated with preterm birth. *Br J Obstet Gynaecol* 1992;99:190–6
9. Kurki T, Sivonen A, Renkonen O-V, *et al*. Bacterial vaginosis in early pregnancy and pregnancy outcome. *Obstet Gynecol* 1992;80:173–7
10. Hay PE, Lamont RF, Taylor-Robinson D, *et al*. Abnormal bacterial colonization of the genital tract and subsequent preterm delivery and late miscarriage. *Br Med J* 1994;308:295–8
11. Joesoef MR, Hillier SL, Utomon B, *et al*. Bacterial vaginosis and prematurity in Indonesia: association in early and late pregnancy. *Am J Obstet Gynecol* 1993;169: 175–8
12. Hillier SL, Nugent RP, Eschenbach DA, *et al*. for the Vaginal Infections and Prematurity Study Group. Association between bacterial vaginosis and preterm delivery of a low-birth-weight infant. *N Engl J Med* 1995;333:1737–42
13. Watts DH, Krohn MA, Hillier SL, Eschenbach DA. Bacterial vaginosis as a risk factor for post Cesarean endometritis. *Obstet Gynecol* 1990;75:52–8
14. Silver HM, Sperling RS, St Clair P, Gibbs RS. Evidence relating bacterial vaginosis to intramniotic infection. *Am J Obstet Gynecol* 1989;161:808–12
15. Hillier SL, Krohn MA, Cassen E, *et al*. The role of bacterial vaginosis and vaginal bacteria in amniotic fluid infection in women in preterm labor with intact fetal membranes. *Clin Infect Dis* 1995;20(Suppl 2): S276–8
16. Morales WJ, Schorr S, Albritton J. Effects of metronidazole in patients with preterm birth in preceding pregnancy and bacterial vaginosis: a placebo-controlled, double-blind study. *Am J Obstet Gynecol* 1994;171:345–9
17. McGregor JA, French JI, Parker R, *et al*. Prevention of premature birth by screening and treatment for common genital tract infections: results of a prospective controlled evaluation. *Am J Obstet Gynecol* 1995; 173:157–67
18. Hauth JC, Goldenberg RL, Andrews WW, *et al*. Reduced incidence of preterm delivery with metronidazole and erythromycin in women with bacterial vaginosis. *N Engl J Med* 1995;333:1732–6
19. Hill AG. *Principles of Medical Statistics*, 9th edn. New York: Oxford University Press, 1953:309–23
20. Spiegel CA. Bacterial vaginosis. *Clin Microbiol Rev* 1991;4:485–502
21. Spiegel CA, Amsel R, Eschenbach D, *et al*. Anaerobic bacteria in nonspecific vaginitis. *N Engl J Med* 1980; 303:601–7
22. Giorgi A, Torriani S, Dellaglio F, *et al*. Identification of vaginal lactobacilli from asymptomatic women. *Microbiologica* 1987;10:377–84
23. Amsel R, Totten PA, Spiegel CA, *et al*. Nonspecific vaginitis. Diagnostic criteria and microbial and epidemiologic associations. *Am J Med* 1983;74:14
24. Chen KCS, Amsel R, Eschenbach DA, Holmes KK. Biochemical diagnosis of vaginitis: determination of diamines in vaginal fluid. *J Infect Dis* 1982;145:337–47
25. McGregor JA, French JI, Jones W, *et al*. Bacterial vaginosis is associated with prematurity and vaginal fluid sialidase: results of a controlled trial of topical clindamycin cream. *Am J Obstet Gynecol* 1994;170:1048–60
26. Glasson JH, Woods WH. Immunoglobulin proteases in bacteria associated with bacterial vaginosis. *Aust J Med Lab Sci* 1988;9:63–5
27. McGregor JA, French JI, Jones W, *et al*. Association of cervico/vaginal infections with increased vaginal fluid phospholipase A_2 activity. *Am J Obstet Gynecol* 1992; 167:1588–94
28. McGregor JA, Lawellin D, Franco-Buff A, Todd JK. Phospholipase C activity in microorganisms associated with reproductive tract infection. *Am J Obstet Gynecol* 1991;164:682–6
29. McGregor JA, Lawellin D, Franco-Buff A, *et al*. Protease production by microorganisms associated with reproductive tract infection. *Am J Obstet Gynecol* 1986;154:109

30. Platz-Christensen JJ, Brandberg A, Wiqvist N. Increased prostaglandin concentrations in the cervical mucus of pregnant women with bacterial vaginosis. *Prostaglandins* 1992;43:133–41

31. Platz-Christensen JJ, Mattsby-Baltzer I, Thomsen P, Wiqvist N. Endotoxin and interleukin-1α in the cervical mucus and vaginal fluid of pregnant women with bacterial vaginosis. *Am J Obstet Gynecol* 1993;169:1161–6

32. Brand JM, Galask RP. Trimethylamine: the substance mainly responsible for the fishy odor often associated with bacterial vaginosis. *Obstet Gynecol* 1986;68:682–5

33. Rotstein OD, Pruett TL, Fiegel VD, *et al*. Succinic acid, a metabolic by-product of *Bacteroides* species, inhibits polymorphonuclear leukocyte function. *Infect Immunol* 1985;48:402–8

34. Singer RE, Buckner BA. Butyrate and propionate: important components of toxic dental plaque extracts. *Infect Immunol* 1981;32:458–63

35. Redondo-Lopez V, Cook RL, Sobel JD. Emerging role of lactobacilli in the control and maintenance of vaginal bacterial microflora. *Rev Infect Dis* 1990;12:856–72

36. Klebanoff SJ, Hillier SL, Eschenbach DA, Waltersdorph AM. Control of the microbial flora of the vagina by H_2O_2-generating lactobacilli. *J Infect Dis* 1991;164:94–100

37. Mårdh P-A, Soltesz LV. *In vitro* interactions between lactobacilli and other microorganisms occurring in the vaginal flora. *Scand J Infect Dis* 1983;40(Suppl):47–51

38. Barefoot SF, Klaenhammer TR. Detection and activity of lactacin-b, a bacteriocin produced by *Lactobacillus acidophilus*. *Appl Environ Microbiol* 1983;45:1808–15

39. Chan RCY, Reid G, Irvin RT, *et al*. Competitive exclusion of uropathogens from human uroepithelial cells by lactobacillus whole cells and cell wall fragments. *Infect Immunol* 1985;47:84–9

40. Eschenbach DA, Davick PR, Williams BL, *et al*. Prevalence of hydrogen peroxide-producing *Lactobacillus* species in normal women and women with bacterial vaginosis. *J Clin Microbiol* 1989;27:251–6

41. Hillier SL, Krohn MA, Rabe LK, *et al*. The normal vaginal flora, H_2O_2-producing lactobacilli, and bacterial vaginosis in pregnant women. *Clin Infect Dis* 1993;16(Suppl 4):S273–81

42. Mou SM, Pavlova SI, Kilic AO, Tao L. Phage infection in vaginal lactobacilli: an *in vitro* model. Presented at *Annual Meeting Infectious Diseases, Obstetrics/Gynecology Society*, Bever Creek, CO, 14–17 August 1996

43. Paavonen J. Physiology and ecology of the vagina. *Scand J Infect Dis* 1983;40:31–5

44. Peeters M, Piot P. Adhesion of *Gardnerella vaginalis* to vaginal epithelial cells: variables affecting adhesion and inhibition by metronidazole. *Genitourin Med* 1985;61:391–5

45. Ernest JM, Meis PJ, Moore ML, Swain M. Vaginal pH: a marker of preterm premature rupture of the membranes. *Obstet Gynecol* 1989;74:734–8

46. Hillier SL, Krohn MA, Nugent RP, Gibbs RS, for the Vaginal Infections and Prematurity Study Group. Characteristics of three vaginal flora patterns assessed by Gram stain among pregnant women. *Am J Obstet Gynecol* 1992;166:938–44

47. Barbone F, Austin H, Louv WC, Alexander WJ. A follow-up study of methods of contraception, sexual activity, and rates of trichomoniasis, candidiasis and bacterial vaginosis. *Am J Obstet Gynecol* 1990;163:510–14

48. Holst E. Reservoir of four organisms associated with bacterial vaginosis suggests lack of sexual transmission. *J Clin Microbiol* 1990;28:2035–9

49. Hammerschlag MR, Cummings M, Doraiswamy B, *et al*. Nonspecific vaginitis following sexual abuse in children. *Pediatrics* 1985;75:1028–31

50. Berger BJ, Zenelman JM, Feldman J, McCormack WM. Bacterial vaginosis in lesbians: a sexually transmitted disease. *Clin Infect Dis* 1995;21:1402–5

51. Piot P, Van Dyck E, Peeters M, *et al*. Biotypes of *Gardnerella vaginalis*. *J Clin Microbiol* 1984;22:677–9

52. Vejtorp M, Bollerup AC, Vejtorp L, *et al*. Bacterial vaginosis: a double-blind randomized trial of the effect of treatment of the sexual partner. *Br J Obstet Gynaecol* 1988;95:920–6

53. Krohn MA, Hillier SL, Eschenbach DA. Comparison of methods for diagnosing bacterial vaginosis among pregnant women. *J Clin Microbiol* 1989;27:1266–71

54. Minkoff H, Grunebaum AN, Schwarz RH, *et al*. Risk factors for prematurity and premature rupture of membranes: a prospective study of the vaginal flora in pregnancy. *Am J Obstet Gynecol* 1984;150:965–72

55. Platz-Chritensen JJ, Pernevi P, Hagmar B, *et al*. A longitudinal follow-up of bacterial vaginosis during pregnancy. *Acta Obstet Gynecol Scand* 1993;72:99–102

56. Thorsen P, Jensen IP, Molsted K, *et al*. An epidemiologic study of bacterial vaginosis in a population of 3600 pregnant women: first antenatal visit. Presented at *11th Annual meeting of the International Society for STD Research*, New Orleans, Louisiana, 27–30 August 1995: abstr 204

57. Hay PE, Morgan DJ, Ison CA, *et al*. A longitudinal study of bacterial vaginosis during pregnancy. *Br J Obstet Gynaecol* 1994;101:1048–53

58. Larsson P-G. Treatment of bacterial vaginosis. *Int J STD AIDS* 1992;3:239–47

59. Sobel JD, Schmitt C, Meriwether C. Long-term follow-up of patients with bacterial vaginosis treated with oral metronidazole and topical clindamycin. *J Infect Dis* 1993;167:783–4

60. Hillier SL, Holmes KK. Bacterial vaginosis. In Holmes KK, Mardh PA, Sparling PF, *et al*. eds. *Sexually Transmitted Diseases*, 2nd edn. New York: McGraw-Hill Information Services Company, 1990:547–59

61. Platz-Christensen JJ, Larsson P-G, Sundstrom E, Bondeson L. Detection of bacterial vaginosis in Papanicolaou smears. *Am J Obstet Gynecol* 1989;160:132–3

62. Spiegel CA, Amsel R, Holmes KK. Diagnosis of bacterial vaginosis by direct Gram stain of vaginal fluid. *J Clin Microbiol* 1983;18:170–7

63. Hay PE, Taylor-Robinson D, Lamont RF. Diagnosis of bacterial vaginosis in a gynaecology clinic. *Br J Obstet Gynaecol* 1992;99:63–6

64. Nugent RP, Krohn MA, Hillier SL. Reliability of diagnosing bacterial vaginosis is improved by a standardized method of Gram stain interpretation. *J Clin Microbiol* 1991;29:297–301

65. Thomason JL, Gelbart SM, Wilcoski LM, *et al*. Proline aminopeptidase activity as a rapid diagnostic test to

confirm bacterial vaginosis. *Obstet Gynecol* 1988; 71: 607–11

66. Briselden AM, Hillier SL. Evaluation of Affirm VP microbial identification test for *Gardnerella vaginalis* and *Trichomonas vaginalis*. *J Clin Microbiol* 1994;32: 148–52

67. Thomason JL, Gelbart SM, Anderson RJ, *et al.* Statistical evaluation of diagnostic criteria for bacterial vaginosis. *Am J Obstet Gynecol* 1990;162:155–60

68. Thomason JL, Schreckenberger PA, Spellacy WN, *et al.* Clinical and microbiological characterization of patients with non-specific vaginosis having motile, curved anaerobic rods. *J Infect Dis* 1984;149:801–7

69. Joesoef MR, Hillier SL, Josodiwondo S, Linnan M. Reproducibility of a scoring system for Gram stain diagnosis of bacterial vaginosis. *J Clin Microbiol* 1991; 29:1730–1

70. McDonald HM, O'Loughlin JA, Jolley P, *et al.* Vaginal infection and preterm labour. *Br J Obstet Gynaecol* 1991; 98:427–35

71. McDonald HM, O'Loughlin JA, Jolley PT, *et al.* Changes in vaginal flora during pregnancy and association with preterm birth. *J Infect Dis* 1994;170:724–8

72. Joesoef MR, Hillier SL, Wiknjosastro G, *et al.* Intravaginal clindamycin treatment for bacterial vaginosis: effects on preterm delivery and low birth weight. *Am J Obstet Gynecol* 1995;173:1527–31

73. Meis PJ, Goldenberg RL, Mercer B, *et al.* The preterm prediction study: significance of vaginal infections. *Am J Obstet Gynecol* 1995;173:1231–5

74. Krohn MA, Hillier SL, Nugent RP, *et al.* for the Vaginal Infections and Prematurity Study Group. The genital flora of women with intraamniotic infection. *J Infect Dis* 1995;171:1475–80

75. Hillier S, Krohn MA, Watts DH, *et al.* Microbiologic efficacy of intravaginal clindamycin cream for the treatment of bacterial vaginosis. *Obstet Gynecol* 1990;76:407–13

76. Gibbs RS. Infection after Cesarean section. *Clin Obstet Gynecol* 1985;28:697–710

77. Watts DH, Eschenbach DA, Kenny GE. Early postpartum endometritis: the role of bacteria, genital mycoplasmas, and *Chlamydia trachomatis*. *Obstet Gynecol* 1989;73:52–9

78. McDonald HM, O'Loughlin JA, Vigneswaran R, *et al.* Bacterial vaginosis in pregnancy and efficacy of short-course oral metronidazole treatment: a randomized controlled trial. *Obstet Gynecol* 1994;84:343–8

79. Centers for Disease Control. 1993 Sexually transmitted diseases treatment guidelines. *Morbidity Mortality Weekly Rev* 1993;42 (no. RR-14)

80. Piper JM, Mitchel EF, Ray WA. Prenatal use of metronidazole and birth defects: no association. *Obstet Gynecol* 1993;82:348–52

81. Burtin P, Taddio A, Ariburnu O, *et al.* Safety of metronidazole in pregnancy: a meta analysis. *Am J Obstet Gynecol* 1995;172:525–9

82. Greaves WL, Chungafung J, Morris B, *et al.* Clindamycin versus metronidazole in the treatment of bacterial vaginosis. *Obstet Gynecol* 1988;72:799–802

83. Livengood CH III, McGregor JA, Soper DE, *et al.* Bacterial vaginosis: efficacy and safety on intravaginal metronidazole treatment. *Am J Obstet Gynecol* 1994; 170:759–64

84. Ferris DG, Litaker MS, Woodward L, *et al.* Treatment of bacterial vaginosis: a comparison of oral metronidazole, metronidazole vaginal gel, and clindamycin vaginal cream. *J Fam Pract* 1995;41:443–9

85. Covino JM, Black JR, Cummings M, *et al.* Comparative evaluation of ofloxacin and metronidazole in the treatment of bacterial vaginosis. *Sex Trans Dis* 1993;20: 262–4

86. Hughes VL, Hillier SL. Microbiologic characteristics of *Lactobacillus* products used for colonization of the vagina. *Obstet Gynecol* 1990;75:244–8

87. Wood JR, Sweet RL, Catena A, *et al. In vitro* adherence of *Lactobacillus* species to vaginal eipthelial cells. *Am J Obstet Gynecol* 1985;153:740–3

88. Moi H, Erkkola R, Jerve F, *et al.* Should male consorts of women with bacterial vaginosis be treated? *Genitourin Med* 1989;65:263–8

89. Schmitt C, Sobel JD, Meriwither C. Bacterial vaginosis: treatment with clindamycin cream versus oral metronidazole. *Obstet Gynecol* 1992;79:1020–3

90. Fischbach F, Petersen EE, Weissenbacher ER, *et al.* Efficacy of clindamycin vaginal cream versus oral metronidazole in the treatment of bacterial vaginosis. *Obstet Gynecol* 1993;82:405–10

91. Oleen-Burkey MA, Hillier SL. Pregnancy complications associated with bacterial vaginosis and their estimated costs. *Infect Dis Obstet Gynecol* 1995;3:149–57

92. Bloom BS, Lee DW. Costs of preventing preterm birth [Letter]. *N Engl J Med* 1996;331:1338

31
Candidiasis and helminthic infection

J.M. Piper and E.R. Newton

CANDIDIASIS IN PREGNANCY

Introduction

Yeast infection in pregnancy is an important issue in women's health, even though systemic fungal infection is exceedingly rare in women of child-bearing age. The dysuria, itching and inflammation that accompany genital fungal infection may be severe enough to interrupt daily activities and prompt the patient to seek medical attention[1]. This chapter reviews the prevalence, pathophysiology, diagnosis and therapy of vulvovaginal candidal infection, as well as systemic candidiasis, prenatal/neonatal complications and resistant/recurrent infection.

The first description of human yeast infection was penned by Hippocrates in about 400 BC when 'white patches' were noted on the mucous membranes of those with debilitating disease[2]. In 1849, Wilkinson made the connection between the presence of fungi and vaginal infection. The term 'monilia vulvovaginitis' was coined in 1931 and *Candida albicans* was officially named in 1954[2]. More than 100 species of *Candida* have since been identified, with many further classified to the strain level[3].

The presence of *Candida* organisms is almost universal. Three-fourths of all women have had symptomatic *Candida* vulvovaginitis and almost half of those with an initial attack have additional episodes[1]. *Candida* organisms are also isolated in cultures of 8% of asymptomatic females[4]. Thus, the prevalence of candidal colonization/infection is quite high, occupying an important portion of gynecological and obstetric care.

The role of sexual contact in the spread of *Candida* is not resolved. Davidson[5] found positive penile cultures for *Candida* in 15% of males seen at a walk-in clinic for sexually transmitted diseases. The culture-positive rates were the same in both circumcised (14%) and uncircumcised males (17%); however, there was a much higher rate of symptomatic *Candida* infection in uncircumcised men[5]. The female sexual contacts of these men were also evaluated. Partners of culture-negative males had positive *Candida* cultures 32% of the time, whereas 80% of contacts of culture-positive males had positive cultures[5]. Even though this shows correlation between partners, there is no direct evidence of transmission of *Candida* through sexual contact. Diseases known to be sexually transmitted (herpes, chlamydia, gonorrhea and syphilis) frequently occur concomitantly. The lack of association of *Candida* with these diseases provides evidence against labelling it as a sexually transmitted disease.

Pathophysiology of *Candida* infection

Of the more than 100 species of *Candida* identified, only seven are identified frequently in human clinical cultures. *Candida albicans* and *C. tropicalis* form 80% of all clinical isolates[6,7]. *Candida glabrata* and *C. parapsilosis* comprise an additional 10–15%, leaving 5–10% distributed among other species[7,8]. Species differentiation is based on subculture characteristics. Germ tube and chlamydospore formation are elicited by culture for 24–48 h on chlamydospore agar. *Candida albicans* exhibits both germ tube and chlamydospore growth[3]. *Candida parapsilosis*, *tropicalis* and *glabrata* produce neither. Further, differentiation of these species is based on characteristic ability to assimilate and ferment sugars in subculture[3,8].

The species breakdown in vulvovaginal infection is different from that in overall laboratory isolates. *Candida albicans* is identified in 80–85% of all positive vaginal cultures. *Candida glabrata* is seen in 10–15% of cases, with minimum identification of other species. *Candida glabrata*, previously known as *Torulopsis glabrata*, is one of the more recently characterized species. The rising diagnostic rate of this species in genital candidiasis may be related to improved detection, as its role as a pathogen is more widely understood[1].

All *Candida* are dimorphic organisms with blastospore and mycelial forms. The blastospore form (budding yeast) is associated with transmission and colonization, and is the form found in the bloodstream in systemic infection. Germinated yeast with mycelia and pseudohyphae is the tissue-invasive form that causes symptomatic disease.

The *Candida* life cycle is one of rapid budding, maturation and degeneration. Budding occurs as a new cell outgrowth from the mother blastospore. Following mitosis, a septum partitions the two cells and budding resumes in each cell. Mycelium formation begins as a cylindrical outgrowth from the cell wall. Septae are laid down behind the apical tip as the hyphae shoot lengthens. Blastospores are then produced just behind the newly created septae. Pseudohyphae are a morphological derivative between budding and hyphael growth that is found in all *Candida* species[9].

The attachment of *Candida* to vaginal cells has been reported to be mediated by mannose-containing receptors on the surface of the mucosal epithelial cells[3]. The effect of estrogen in increasing vaginal epithelial avidity for candidal adherence may involve these surface receptors[1]. Intracellular receptors for estradiol and corticosteroids have been identified in *C. albicans* and *C. glabrata*[10,11]. Although the mechanisms of action of these receptors have not yet been elucidated, high levels of estrogens and corticosteroids are associated with increased candidal virulence and tissue invasion.

The human host defense mechanism against candidal vaginitis is primarily based on the natural bacterial flora of the vagina, particularly lactobacilli. Cell-mediated immunity also plays a role in preventing infection. Monocytes and leukocytes prevent deep tissue invasion and systemic infection. IgG and IgM are elicited systemically and IgA is secreted in cervical mucus in response to acute candidal infection. Infection rates, however, are not increased in patients with isolated immunoglobulin deficiencies[1].

Factors that predispose a patient to candidal vulvovaginitis can be categorized as systemic, localized or exogenous. Systemic conditions associated with genital candidiasis include diabetes, non-diabetic glucosuria, endocrinopathies, debilitating disease, older age and pregnancy[1,4,12]. Vaginal colonization with yeast occurs in 30–40% of all pregnancies. The attack rate is higher in the third trimester and symptomatic recurrence is more common than in non-pregnant patients. The cause of increased prevalence in pregnancy is not known, but theories include fungal growth promotion via estrogen receptors on the vaginal mucosa and within the yeast cells, as well as improved fuel for growth due to higher mucosal glycogen content[1].

Local conditions that alter the barrier function of the perineal epithelium allow higher infection rates. Occlusion via tight pants or nylon undergarments creates excess moisture accumulation, causing tissue maceration. Urinary leakage, as seen in stress incontinence or late in pregnancy, inflames the external genitalia, decreasing its resistance. Skin thinning, as occurs in menopause or with chronic topical steroid use, decreases the barrier function as well.

A variety of commonly prescribed medications lower a women's resistance to candidiasis. Antibiotics, especially tetracycline, ampicillin and oral cephalosporins, allow vaginal colonization rates to triple from 10% to 30%. The effect of antibiotics on *Candida* colonization is theorized to be due to elimination of the normal vaginal flora, particularly lactobacilli, allowing overgrowth of the yeast. Lactobacillus is thought to decrease fungal growth via competition for nutrients, mechanical interference with candidal mucosal adherence and chemical inhibition by lactobacillus secretions[1]. There may also be direct stimulation of *Candida* cells by antibiotic compounds.

Immunosuppressive agents and systemic steroids decrease local systemic resistance to fungal infections[4]. Alteration of cell-mediated immunity allows *Candida* to act as an opportunistic pathogen, with increased risk of deep invasion. Oral contraceptives were previously thought to increase fungal colonization and infection rates, but recent studies with the low-dose combination pills have shown no effect[1].

Clinical presentations of candidal infections

Most *Candida* infections of the female genital tract do not progress to systemic disease. Their importance, instead, is related to their annoying symptomatology. Vulvovaginal itching or irritation, the most common symptom, is reported by 60% of women with positive yeast cultures[13]. External dysuria and vaginal discharge are the other typical complaints.

One-third of females with positive vaginal cultures for yeast have no symptoms, while one-fourth of women with negative cultures do have symptoms[13]. The vaginal discharge associated with *Candida* is white to beige, curdled in appearance and has a slight yeasty odor[14]. It is comprised of yeast cells, mycelia and epithelial cells[15]. The patient's presentation may fall in a spectrum from acute and exudative (sudden onset, heavy discharge loaded with yeast) to progressive and inflammatory (minimal discharge, few organisms, severe itching)[1]. The pruritus may be a hypersensitivity reaction, and worsens with occlusive clothing and in the premenstrual phase of the cycle[15].

Classic physical findings for *Candida* vulvovaginitis are bright erythema and skin erosions with satellite pustules[4]. The pustules are non-follicular and are scattered around the eroded areas. The erosions are superficial with a narrow white border of scale. In advanced cases, the entire perineum may appear scalded and oozing, with excoriations and fissures. Edema may be a finding in both early and advanced disease[12]. Inguinal lymphadenopathy may accompany perineal involvement.

Vaginal examination reveals inflamed, erythematous, edematous mucosa with white thrush patches and pooling of the thick, white, curd-like discharge in the posterior fornix[12]. The cervix becomes red, inflamed and quite friable. Papanicolaou smear should be delayed until therapy is completed, as inflammation complicates its interpretation and bleeding may occur.

Males with *Candida* balanitis (inflammation of the glans penis) have swelling, itching and burning of the glans and shaft of the penis. Symptoms are more common in uncircumcised males (75%); circumcised men with positive yeast cultures are usually asymptomatic (90%)[4].

Physical findings in the male with *Candida* balanitis include edema, erythema and peeling of the glans penis and scrotum[4]. Transient non-progressive penile inflammation following intercourse may be due to a hypersensitivity reaction to *Candida* in the female partner's genital tract[4].

Although the diagnosis of *Candida* infection is generally suspected on the basis of physical findings, confirmation should be obtained. The use of saline or potassium hydroxide (KOH) wet mounts of the vaginal secretions is the most rapid and least expensive confirmatory test. If a saline preparation is used, dark-field or phase-contrast microscopy may aid in visualization of the fungal elements[16]. Potassium hydroxide (10–20% solution) lyses the epithelial cells, allowing the *Candida* to be seen more easily. Wet-mount analysis is highly specific, but sensitivity is poor. One study revealed that only 20% of women with a positive culture for *Candida* had visible yeast on either saline or KOH wet mount[13].

Other microscopic methods of *Candida* detection include Gram stain of smears or touch preps and Papanicolaou smears[16]. Tissue biopsy may well reveal candidal infection when other lesions were suspected (biopsy is not recommended if *Candida* is suspected). The appearance on biopsy is that of partial or total destruction of the surface epithelium with filaments of fungus extending into the underlying tissues, covered by a thick film composed of inflammatory cells, necrotic debris, yeast cells and pseudohyphae[16].

In patients with clinical evidence of *Candida* vaginitis but negative wet mounts, a trial of therapy is warranted, owing to its low cost. If the symptoms persist, further investigation is mandatory prior to repetitive therapy.

When microscopic analysis is negative and symptoms persist through a trial of therapy, culture diagnosis is utilized. A swab of the infected secretions is transported moist to the laboratory. *Candida* can be cultured on many different media, but Sabouraud's dextrose slants or Nickerson's medium have the highest sensitivity (90%) and specificity (70%) for *Candida* strains[14]. Tube incubation is preferred, owing to decreased contamination with other fungal elements (especially *Coccidioides immitis*). *Candida* species will grow at any pH, but prefer low to neutral pH and a temperature range of 25–37°C[3].

Candida grows more rapidly than other fungi and molds in culture, often within 24 h. Isolates from sterile sources should be subcultured and identified to the species level. For vaginal specimens, categorization to either 'albicans' or 'not albicans' is sufficient[3].

Culture of yeast from blood specimens is more difficult. Automated systems such as the Bactec radiometric system (Johnston Laboratories, Towson, MD) can detect *Candida* in 2–4 days. Use of biphasic media improves sensitivity, but requires 5–9 days for adequate growth[3]. Debilitated patients may succumb to systemic candidiasis prior to detection of *Candida* in blood cultures.

Therapy of vulvovaginal candidiasis

Therapy of vaginitis in the early 1900s involved douching with lactic acid, carbolic acid, mercury or potassium permanganate, followed by glycerine coverage of the vaginal epithelium; if ulceration occurred, silver nitrate was applied[17]. This regimen was quite caustic, capable of inducing rectovaginal and vesicovaginal fistulas. It did, however, also kill yeast.

Painting the affected areas with Gentian violet was the mainstay of therapy from 1935 to 1955[2]. Application of a 1% solution two or three times a week provided rapid symptomatic relief, but was quite inconvenient, owing to staining of skin and clothing. The side-effects included vaginal drying, inflammation, hypersensitivity reactions and even ulcerations. Gentian violet is fungicidal via interference with fungal enzymes[2].

Nystatin, a polyene antifungal antibiotic, was a breakthough in antifungal therapy in 1955. Nystatin (Mycostatin®) could be formulated as a tablet or cream. One tablet (100 000 units), inserted intravaginally twice a day for 15 days, provided a 65–80% cure rate at 30 days[18]. The polyene antifungals bind to sterols in the fungal membrane, causing membrane incompetence and allowing intracellular components to leak out[2]. Polyenes are not well absorbed orally or via mucous membranes.

The next advance in antifungal therapy was the introduction of the imidazole antifungal agents in the early 1970s. Miconazole (Monistat®) allowed reduced dosing and shortened therapeutic regimens, improving patient compliance. Imidazoles inhibit fungal cell wall synthesis and are absorbed in small amounts through mucous membranes[2]. Miconazole cream (100 mg) daily for 14 days was compared with nystatin (100 000 units) twice a day for 15 days in two 1974 clinical trials. Miconazole showed a 15–20% improvement in 30-day cure rate over nystatin in both pregnant and non-pregnant patients[18,19].

Clotrimazole (Gyne-lotrimin®, Mycelex®), another topical imidazole, allowed further simplification of the treatment requirement. Fleury and colleagues[20], in 1985, reported a comparison of two clotrimazole dosage plans – a single-dose 500-mg vaginal tablet vs. two 100-mg vaginal tablets daily for 3 days – and found 30-day cure rates of 79% and 74%, respectively, in non-pregnant patients. Lebherz and co-workers[21] completed an identical study, in pregnant women, with 30-day cure rates of 65% and 74%. Evaluation of vaginal secretions revealed that therapeutic levels persist for 3 days following insertion of one 500-mg clotrimazole tablet[22].

Butoconazole cream (Femstat®) and tablets followed soon after clotrimazole. The tablets were shown to be equally as effective as clotrimazole tablets in a 3-day regimen[23]. Butoconazole cream (Femstat®) was likewise not significantly different from miconazole cream in a trial of therapy with 6-day regimens[24].

Ketoconazole (Nizoral®), an oral imidazole antifungal, has also been recommended for vulvovaginal candidiasis in recurrent or resistant cases. When taken daily (400 mg for 14 days, then 100 mg for 6 months), ketoconazole reduced the recurrence rate from 71% (placebo) to 5%[25]. Its use is limited to difficult cases, because of gastrointestinal side-effects and ability to cause idiosyncratic hepatitis.

The most recent azole formula introduced for vaginal antifungal use is terconazole, a triazole compound (Terazol®). Hirsch compared terconazole to clotrimazole, with no significant difference in cure rates with either cream or suppositories[26]. Thomason[27] found both terconazole and miconazole to be more effective than placebo, but showed no difference between terconazole and miconazole in either cream or suppository form (30-day cure rates 61–76%).

The most recent advance in therapy was the approval of single dose, oral fluconazole (Diflucan®) for the treatment of acute vaginal candidiasis in 1994. Fluconazole as a single oral dose (150 mg) has been shown to be as effective as intravaginal clotrimazole (200 mg/day for 3 days)[28], intravaginal miconazole (1200 mg single dose)[29] and oral ketoconazole (400 mg/day for 5 days)[30]. Short-term response rates of 94% (symptomatic) and 85% (mycological) have been reported[31].

Boric acid powder placed in capsules has also been used to treat *Candida* vaginitis, with a 30-day cure rate of 72% when given at 600 mg daily for 14 days[32]. There is some absorption of borate through the mucous membranes (less than 1 µg/ml serum levels), therefore the use of boric acid is not recommended in pregnancy. Outside of pregnancy, boric acid therapy provides a very low-cost alternative for therapy of yeast vaginitis.

The safety of the other treatment modalities in pregnancy varies. Gentian violet is not recommended for use in pregnancy because no adequate studies have been performed to judge its safety (Pregnancy Category C)[33]. The topical azole antifungals have been extensively studied in human pregnancy with no adverse effects or increase in congenital malformations noted (Pregnancy Category B)[33]. Ketoconazole given orally has been shown to increase abortion and fetal loss in mice and rats, with no adequate human studies to document its effect on human pregnancy; therefore, its use for vaginitis in pregnancy is not recommended (Pregnancy Category C). Fluconazole, likewise, is associated with fetal loss in animal studies with no adequate human studies to document safety; therefore, it is not recommended for use in pregnancy (Pregnancy Category C). Polyene antifungals have

been studied extensively in pregnancy and found to be safe for use (Pregnancy Category B)[33].

For many years, nystatin was the primary drug used for *Candida* vulvovaginitis in pregnancy because its extremely poor absorption was felt to improve its safety. As studies have proven the safety and increased efficacy of the azole antifungal agents, miconazole, clotrimazole, butoconazole and terconazole have become the mainstays of therapy. Studies have shown no clear leader from this group in terms of efficacy and patient satisfaction, so selection may be based on availability and cost for an azole antifungal agent for use in pregnancy.

The most frustrating aspect of treating vulvovaginal candidiasis for both physician and patient is the high rate of recurrence. Almost one-half of women with an initial infection will have additional episodes. The subsequent attacks may be newly acquired cases or persistent infection due to incomplete eradication.

Studies of culture-proven vaginal candidiasis with appropriate antifungal therapy show persistence of the same *Candida* strain in 20–25% of patients at 4–6-week follow-up[1]. An intracellular phase of candidal growth could evade topical antifungal therapy to re-enter the extracellular environment after therapy ceases[34].

Recurrent candidal vaginitis may also be due to chronic anovaginal transmission, if intestinal colonization is present. Prior studies have shown 100% strain-specific correlation between vaginal and rectal yeast cultures, supporting this source of infection. More recent studies, with fastidious techniques for sample collection, have shown a much lower, but still significant, rectal colonization rate (40%)[1]. According to this theory, eradication of intestinal yeast should lower recurrence rates. Oral nystatin lowered the intestinal carriage rate, but left the recurrence rate unchanged[35]. Six-month therapy with oral ketoconazole eliminated intestinal yeast completely, but did not prevent recurrent vaginitis[25]. Although intestinal *Candida* may play some role in recurrent vaginal infection, it is not a major factor.

The role of male-partner penile colonization in promoting recurrent vaginitis is unresolved. Evidence in favor of a role for this includes a four-fold higher rate of asymptomatic penile colonization and the presence of *Candida* in the ejaculate of partners of women with recurrent vaginitis[1]. Evidence against this includes the lack of documentation of sexual transmission previously outlined and the lack of improved recurrence rates following treatment of the male partner. Attention to hygiene should be recommended in all cases of *Candida* vaginitis. A trial of therapy in the male partner may be attempted if other therapy is unsuccessful in resolving recurrent infections.

All patients with recurrent episodes of vulvovaginal candidiasis without an obvious precipitating factor, such as pregnancy or antibiotic therapy, should be evaluated for underlying systemic disease. Blood glucose evaluation to rule out diabetes and HIV testing to rule out acquired immunodeficiency syndrome should be performed. Physical examination to rule out endocrinopathy or debilitating disease is likewise important, as is careful questioning of the patient with regard to medications, particularly the application of over-the-counter or 'home' remedies for the perineal and vaginal areas. Many of these compounds (steroid creams, Lysol® douches, etc.) alter the vaginal flora and weaken the natural resistance of the mucosa.

Patients with continued pruritis without evidence of organisms may be experiencing an allergic reaction, not only to the *Candida*, but also to the antifungal medications. The inflammation should improve following completion of therapy if it has hypersensitivity as its etiology.

Refractory vaginitis is a multifocal problem with no single solution. Adequate evaluation, with therapy aimed at the individual components, is the most logical approach. Inadequate therapy, resistant organisms, intestinal colonization, male-partner colonization, vaginal flora abnormalities, immunodeficiency, hypersensitivity reaction and hampered barrier function may all be involved to a differing extent in individual patients with recurrent candidal infections.

Systemic candidiasis

Although systemic candidiasis is exceedingly rare in women of child-bearing age, it may occur in debilitated patients with diabetes, acquired immunodeficiency syndrome, intravenous drug use, malignancies, chemotherapy, prolonged antibiotic or steroid therapy and intravenous hyperalimentation[36]. Systemic infection can be subdivided into disseminated infection, fungemia and single-organ infection (meningitis, endocarditis, pneumonia, arthritis, peritonitis, laryngitis, endophthalmitis and urinary tract infections)[36]. Systemic candidal infection is usually associated with an indwelling foreign body (intravenous catheter, Foley catheter, endotracheal tube, etc.). Symptoms are variable; however, persistent fever, in spite of broad-spectrum antibiotic coverage, is the most frequent clue[36]. Hypotension and mental status changes (confusion to obtundation) are also commonly seen. The fever may be masked in patients on adrenal steroids.

The diagnosis of disseminated candidiasis may be difficult. Blood cultures may be negative in 40–60% of cases proven by autopsy. Tissue biopsy, culture of fluids from sterile spaces and urine cultures augment blood cultures in the detection of candidiasis in the patient at risk. Survival rates are still poor, ranging from 0 to 50%, and correlate with immunocompetence and renal function[36]. Amphotericin B given intravenously is the drug of choice in all levels of systemic infection[36]. Amphotericin B is a macrolide antifungal that acts by interrupting cell membranes. Amphotericin B is limited, by its considerable toxicity, to use

in systemic infection. Major complications of therapy include hypotension, hypertension, hypokalemia, renal toxicity, anaphylaxis, cardiac arrhythmias and even cardiac arrest[36]. Side-effects that are minor in comparison, but may be repetitive, include fever, chills, anorexia, diarrhea, malaise and phlebitis at the injection site. Amphotericin B therapy must be preceded by a test dose to avoid anaphylaxis. 5-Fluorocytosine may be added to amphotericin therapy in life-threatening cases, to provide a second mechanism of fungicide. 5-Fluorocytosine is converted to 5-fluorouracil by susceptible fungal cells and inhibits protein synthesis by altering DNA[36]. The treatment of systemic candidiasis is not altered by pregnancy. Amphotericin B has been used in pregnancy without reported evidence of teratogenicity; however, no controlled studies have been performed[37].

Maternal/neonatal complications of candidal infection in pregnancy

Intra-amniotic infection with yeast is exceedingly rare with intact membranes, but can be seen in the presence of a foreign body, such as a cerclage or an intrauterine device (IUD). The infection may cause preterm labor or spontaneous abortion by invading the umbilical cord and major fetal organs[2].

Although intra-amniotic infection is rare, up to 80% of infants that pass through an infected birth canal are colonized with yeast[38]. The vast majority of these infants have either oral colonization (thrush) or diaper dermatitis, both easily treated with local therapy. Congenital cutaneous candidiasis is a disseminated papulovesicular to pustular dermatitis involving mainly the head, neck, palms and soles[38]. It resolves rapidly with topical antifungal therapy and carries little risk of progression to systemic infection in normal neonates.

Summary

Candida vulvovaginitis is an epithelial infection that very rarely progresses to systemic or life-threatening disease in immunocompetent adults. There are generally no adverse effects on maternal or fetal outcome in pregnancy. The symptoms, however, may be quite disturbing. Therapy with topical azole antifungals is effective in the majority of cases and is not contraindicated in pregnancy. Recurrent infection is common, particularly in pregnancy, and is multifactorial in origin.

HELMINTHIC INFECTION IN PREGNANCY

Introduction

Helminths are parasitic worms that spend at least a portion of their life cycle in an animal or human host. Helminths include cestodes (tapeworms), trematodes (flukes) and nematodes (round worms). Helminthic infection has a worldwide distribution, but is more prevalent in underdeveloped countries. Even so, it was estimated that there were 54 million cases of helminthic infection in the USA in 1972 (the last cumulative estimate available)[39]. Although the prevalence rates have since fallen, helminthic infection has by no means disappeared. Life-threatening parasitic infection in pregnancy is uncommon in industrial nations of the world, but may be seen in individuals who have recently immigrated from less developed areas.

The effects of helminthic infection on pregnancy, although generally benign, should be recognized and treated. Anemia is a common feature of intestinal parasitic infection (owing to intestinal blood loss) and may compound anemia of pregnancy. Malnutrition may occur as a result of competition for nutrients. Chronic helminthic infection may lead to a debilitated state, with the possibility of superimposed bacterial infection. Most helminthic infections in pregnancy are only mildly symptomatic, and may be conservatively managed until postpartum, when definitive therapy can be given. Each organism, however, has to be considered individually for therapeutic recommendations.

The diagnosis of helminthic infection must be individualized, but may be suspected on the basis of gastrointestinal symptoms (nausea, vomiting, diarrhea) and a history compatible with exposure. With notable exceptions, helminthic infection is diagnosed by demonstration of eggs or larvae in feces. In heavy infection, eggs and larvae may be seen directly in saline wet mounts. To evaluate lighter infections, concentration must be performed via zinc sulfate flotation or formalin–ether sedimentation prior to saline wet-mount examination. Traditionally, examination of stool specimens from three consecutive days has been recommended to detect ova and parasites. However, a recent retrospective study found single-specimen evaluation as effective as multiple testing[40]. If this result is borne out by prospective trials, single-specimen examination would markedly decrease the cost of parasitic screening.

A description of the classification system for helminths is followed by review of the more commonly identified helminths. The chapter is completed by a discussion of the antiparasitic agents and their availability for use in pregnancy. Much of the discussion of the individual parasites will pertain to non-pregnant as well as pregnant patients.

Classification

All helminths are classified as Platyhelminthes (flatworms) or Nematoda (roundworms). Flatworms are further divided into cestodes and trematodes (Table 1). Cestodes, or tapeworms, have segmented bodies consisting of proglottids attached via the neck zone to a head or scolex. The scolex provides attachment and locomotion via grooves, suckers and hooks extending from its surface (Figure 1). Tapeworms are hermaphroditic, with both male and female reproductive organs contained in each segment. There is no organized digestive tract; nutrients are absorbed via the integument. Excretory and nervous systems are present, but only in primitive form[41].

Trematodes, or flukes, have a flattened, leaf-like body with one or more ventral muscular suckers to provide attachment. Flukes are monoecious (hermaphroditic), with separate male and female reproductive organs that connect at the common genital atrium. Trematodes have a more advanced alimentary canal, nervous system and excretory system (Figure 2). All trematodes require a period of external development in a snail host[41].

Nematodes are unsegmented worms with an external cuticle, developed internal organ structures and somatic musculature (Figure 3). Most nematodes are dioecious (heterosexual), with male and female sexual differentiation and mating required for reproduction. The alimentary, excretory and nervous systems of nematodes are more differentiated that those of other helminths. Most nematodes undergo four moults, with shedding or resorption of the old external cuticle, and formation of a new cuticle[41].

Taenia saginata and Taenia solium

Taenia saginata and *T. solium* have a worldwide distribution and cause taeniasis or tapeworm infection. Adult taenia are 3–8 m in length and comprise a small scolex (1–2 mm) and multiple proglottids, each about 0.5 cm × 1–2 mm in size[42]. Taenia eggs are yellow to brown and spherical, with thick shells (Figure 4).

The life cycle of the taenias involves a definitive host (humans) and an intermediate host (*T. saginata*, cattle; *T. solium*, pigs). Eggs are passed in feces and reach pastures where they are ingested by the intermediate host. The larvae hatch and migrate to the muscle tissue, where they remain until the raw beef or pork is ingested by the definitive host. The infective form (cysticerci) require 3–5 months to mature to adulthood. Taenia adult worms may live in the human small intestine for 25 years[42].

T. solium eggs can be directly infective if ingested by humans, causing cysticercosis. Extreme care must be taken in handling all specimens with taenia eggs, as *T. solium* are not easily distinguished from *T. saginata*[42]. Cysticercosis is the disease caused by larval migration throughout the body. Cysticercosis may be severe, even fatal, due to inflammation of vital organs, particularly cardiac muscle.

The clinical effects of taeniasis are usually minimal, but a minority of cases report abdominal discomfort, vomiting and diarrhea[41]. Rare cases of appendicitis and intestinal obstruction do occur.

The diagnosis of taenia infection is based on identification of eggs or proglottid segments in the patient's

Table 1 Classification of helminths

Platyhelminthes		Nematodes
Cestodes (tape worms)	Trematodes (flukes)	(round worms)
Taenia saginata	*Schistosoma mansoni*	*Enterobius vermicularis*
Taenia solium	*Schistosoma japonicum*	*Trichuris trichiura*
Diphyllobothrium latum	*Schistosoma haematobium*	*Trichinella spiralis*
Hymenolepis nana	*Schistosoma intercalatum*	*Ascaris lumbricoides*
Hymenolepis diminuta	*Fasciola hepatica*	*Capillaria hepatica*
Echinococcus granulosus	*Fasciola gigantica*	*Capillaria philippinensis*
Echinococcus multicularis	*Fasciolopsis buski*	*Strongyloides*
Multiceps multiceps	*Clonorchis sinensis*	*Ancyclostoma*
Dipylidium caninum	*Opisthorchis felineus*	*Necator*
	Opisthorchis viverrini	*Tricostrongylus*
	Gastrodiscoides hominis	*Toxocara*
	Watsonius watsoni	*Ternidens*
	Heterophyes heterophyes	*Angiostrongylus*
	Metagonimus yokogawai	*Metastrongylus*
	Paragonimus westermani	*Anisakis*
		Lagochilascaris
		Gongylonema
		Thelazia
		Gnathostoma
		Wucheria
		Brugia
		Onchocerca
		Loa Loa
		Dipetalonema
		Mansonella
		Dracunculus
		Dirofilaria

stool specimen[42]. Taenia infection generally has minimal effects on pregnancy and can thus be left untreated until the postpartum period, unless a symptomatic infection with *T. solium* is diagnosed (owing to the risk of cysticercosis). The treatment of choice is niclosamide (single 2-g dose), regardless of pregnancy status; paromomycin is the best alternative[43]. Paromomycin may be used in lactation without interruption[44]. Niclosamide is poorly absorbed; however, there are inadequate data to recommend uninterrupted breastfeeding during its use.

Diphyllobothrium latum

Diphyllobothrium latum, or fish tapeworm, is found in northern Europe, North America and Japan, specifically in temperate areas with cold, clear lakes. *D. latum* adult worms are 4–10 m long, with a small scolex (3 × 1 mm) and wide, short proglottids[42]. The eggs are yellow to brown and ovoid, with an operculum (a lid-like structure).

The life cycle begins as eggs are passed in feces into water, where they hatch two weeks later, with coracidium released. The coracidium are ingested by copepods, where they develop to the procercoid stage. Following ingestion of the copepod host by fish, the infective form (plerocercoid or sparganum) matures to await ingestion of raw fish by humans or other carnivores. *D. latum* migrates to the small intestine, where it attaches and matures to an adult. The adult worm may survive for up to 25 years, releasing its eggs in the feces[42].

Fish tapeworm infection may be asymptomatic, or may have mild to severe gastrointestinal symptoms. Diagnosis is based on finding eggs in feces[43].

Diphyllobothriasis may cause vitamin B_{12} deficiency in pregnancy, owing to malabsorption; therefore vitamin B_{12} supplementation is recommended. Unless infection is severe, antihelminthic therapy is delayed until the postpartum period. Niclosamide (2-g dose) and paromomycin are the first and second choices for therapy[43]. Paromomycin may be used in lactation without interruption[44]. Niclosamide is poorly absorbed; however, there are inadequate data to recommend uninterrupted breastfeeding during its use.

Hymenolepis nana

Hymenolepiasis or dwarf tapeworm infection is cosmopolitan in distribution. *Hymenolepis nana* adult

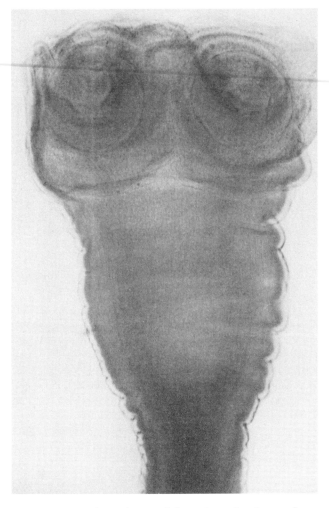

Figure 1 *Taenia saginata* adult scolex, showing suckers. From reference 42 with permission, (p. 223, figure 1)

worms are small tapeworms measuring 2 × 4 cm, with short wide proglottids[42]. The eggs are spherical with a thin hyaline shell (Figure 5).

The definitive hosts of *H. nana* are mice and humans; beetles are intermediate hosts. The life cycle involves passage of eggs in feces with subsequent ingestion by beetles. The beetles are eaten by mice in the natural life cycle. Humans can be infected directly, by ingestion of the eggs. In humans, the eggs hatch, cysticercoids develop in the wall of the small intestine and tapeworms emerge into the lumen of the intestine to mature to adulthood. Eggs are then passed in feces to restart the cycle[42].

The clinical effect of dwarf tapeworm infection in humans is variable. There may be no symptoms or gastrointestinal complaints (diarrhea, nausea, anorexia or vomiting)[41]. The course is generally not severe. Hymenolepiasis is diagnosed by the finding of characteristic eggs in feces[42].

Pregnancy is not threatened by hymenolepiasis, and treatment is deferred to the postpartum period.

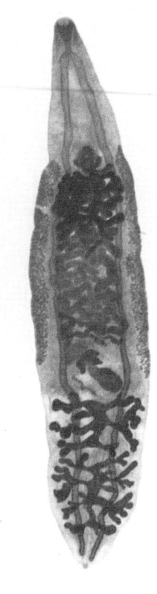

Figure 2 *Clonorchis sinensis* adult fluke (Carmine stain). From reference 42 with permission, (page 213, figure 4)

Niclosamide (2-g dose), praziquantel and paromomycin are the drugs of choice for postpartum therapy[43]. Paromomycin can be used in breastfeeding mothers[44].

Echinoccoccus granulosus, Echinococcus multilocularis and Multiceps multiceps

The definitive hosts of echinococcus and multiceps species are dogs and wild carnivores. On occasion, humans are an incidental host, infected by the ingestion of infective eggs. The embryos hatch in the intestine, and migrate through the body to various organs, where cysts develop. Symptoms occur as the cysts enlarge and create a space-occupying lesion[41]. *Multiceps multiceps* cysts are commonly located in the

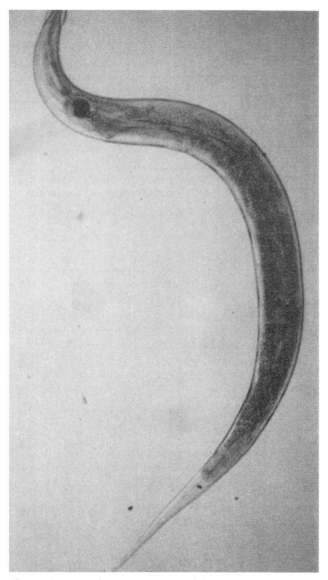

Figure 3 *Enterobius vermicularis* adult female. From reference 42 with permission, (page 133, figure 1)

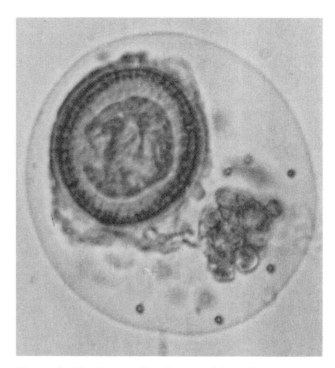

Figure 4 Taenia egg (*T. solium* and *T. saginata* eggs are indistinguishable). From reference 42 with permission, (page 225, figure 2)

subarachnoid space, and may cause meningitis[41]. Clinical diagnosis is based on biopsy of the cyst/granuloma area, or on immunological testing.

Pregnancy can be threatened if the echinococcal cysts are located in the uterine muscle. Intrauterine growth retardation and even impairment of labor may result from uterine cysts. Migration and encystment in vital organs can be life-threatening. Treatment is immediate, regardless of pregnancy status. Surgery to resect the cyst is the best therapy, but mebendazole treatment (100 mg twice a day) can be attempted prior to surgery, once the patient is postpartum[43]. If surgery is not feasible and antepartum therapy is needed, praziquantel can be used in pregnancy[45]. It is not as effective in reducing cyst size. In lactating women, use of mebendazole or praziquantel requires temporary cessation of breastfeeding with pumping and discarding of milk until maternal drug levels have cleared (1–2 days).

Schistosoma mansoni, Schistosoma japonicum and Schistosoma haematobium

Schistosomiasis or bilharziasis is mainly seen in the Middle East, Africa and South America, but can be found in immigrant populations worldwide. Adult flukes are 0.5–2 cm in length, with females longer than males. Male flukes are wider with a posterior fold, the gynecophoric canal, in which the female rests. All schistosoma eggs are non-operculate with a transparent shell and either a lateral spine (*Schistosoma mansoni*) or terminal spine (*S. japonicum*)[42].

Schistosoma adult worms live in the small blood vessels of the pelvic venous plexi. The female lies within the canal of the male for copulation and oviposition. The eggs migrate through the vessel wall and intervening tissues to reach the bladder or bowel, from which the eggs are excreted. If passed into water, the eggs hatch into a miracidial form that can penetrate and infect snails, the intermediate host. While in the snail, the miracidia mature to cercariae. The cercariae burst out of the snail host into water, where they directly infect humans through skin penetration. The schistosomule is transported via the venous system, through the heart and pulmonary vessels, to be propelled into the arterial system by the left ventricle. The schistosomules mature in the large vessels prior to migration to the terminal vascular beds, where the life cycle is completed[46].

Initial infection (schistosome penetration) results in itching and papular rash. The migration of immature flukes causes fever, cough, allergic symptoms and gastrointestinal complaints 2–4 weeks after initial exposure. Chronic schistosomiasis may cause anemia, cirrhosis and urogenital disease. In females, this may include obstructive uropathy, abdominal pain, menorrhagia, salpingitis, oophoritis, sterility and ectopic pregnancy[46].

Schistosome infiltration of the placenta has been reported, but is quite rare[46]. Infection of a fetus with schistosomiasis was last reported in 1920[46]. Although direct involvement is rare, chronic schistosomiasis may be detrimental to pregnancy with systemic disease causing abortions and preterm labor due to maternal debilitation.

Diagnosis of schistosomal infection is based on the finding of eggs in urine, feces or vaginal secretions, or the identification of adult worms or eggs in biopsy of the granulomas. Most infections do not threaten pregnancy, so treatment is postponed to the postpartum period. All therapies destroy only the flukes and have no effect on the migrating eggs[46]. The first and second drugs of choice are metrifonate (10 mg/kg, three doses

2 weeks apart) and oxamniquine (12–15 mg/kg), but neither is recommended in pregnancy. Praziquantel (40 mg/kg) can be used during pregnancy, if therapy is indicated. Praziquantel is excreted in breastmilk, therefore breasts should be pumped and milk discarded for 1–2 days following each dose in lactating women.

Enterobius vermicularis

Enterobiasis or pinworm infection is universally distributed, and is mainly seen in children. Adult male worms are small (2–3 mm) and females are larger (8–13 mm), both with long pointed tails[42]. Pinworm eggs are elongated with one flat side, and have thick, colorless shells (Figure 6).

The definitive hosts for *Enterobius vermicularis* are humans. The female pinworms exit the rectum to lay eggs on the perianal skin overnight. The eggs embryonate in 4–6 h to become infective. Eggs are ingested, hatch and develop in the lower intestinal tract (the cecum, appendix and colon). Ingestion is facilitated by hand-to-mouth transmission or fomites. The adult worms may live for several months in the colon and rectum[42].

The symptoms of pinworm infection are all related to the perianal egg deposition. Insomnia, restlessness, perianal itching/inflammation and perianal bacterial infection (secondary to excoriation) are the common clinical effects[41]. Diagnosis is based on clinical suspicion and cellulose tape prep from perianal skin. Eggs are not found in feces. Cellulose tape prep is performed by taking clear cellulose tape, touching it to

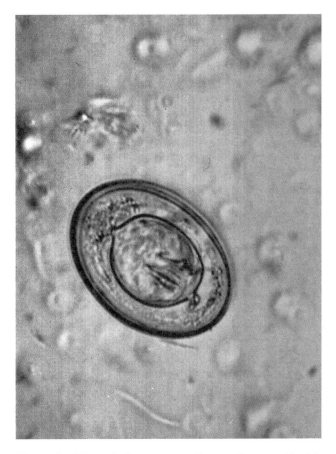

Figure 5 *Hymenolepis nana* egg. From reference 42 with permission, (page 227, figure 1)

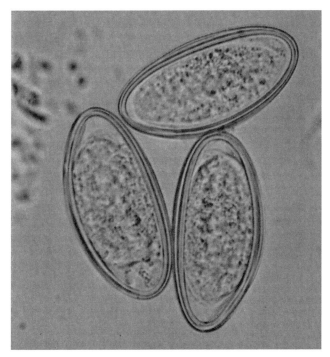

Figure 6 *Enterobius vermicularis* eggs. From reference 42 with permission, (page 131, figure 4)

the perianal skin and then adhering it to a microscope slide for examination[42]. The tape prep is most accurate if done immediately upon arising, prior to bathing.

Pinworms can migrate through the vagina, uterus and Fallopian tubes, but no detrimental effect on the fetus or the pregnancy has been reported[47]. Therapy is delayed until after delivery, unless the psychological pressure or symptoms are too great. Pyrantel pamoate (30 mg/kg, two doses 14 days apart) can be used after the first trimester[47]. The entire family should be treated simultaneously, and clothing and bedding should be washed with hot water or chlorine bleach. Pyrantel pamoate is considered safe for use while breast-feeding[47].

Trichuris trichiura

Trichuriasis, or whipworm infection, is cosmopolitan in warm, moist areas. Adult whipworms are 3–5 mm long, with a slender, whip-like anterior end used to thread its way into the colonic mucosa[42]. Whipworm eggs are barrel-shaped, with a thick shell and plugs at each end (Figure 7).

Humans are the definitive host for *Trichuris trichiura*. Whipworm eggs pass in feces into the soil for further development. Infective eggs are ingested and hatch. The larvae migrate to the large intestine, where they mature to adulthood. The adult worms may remain in the colon for more than 10 years[42].

Symptoms vary from none, in light infection, to colitis with bloody, mucous diarrhea in heavier infestation[41]. Chronic infection can result in rectal prolapse, due to inflammation. Whipworm infection is diagnosed by finding eggs in feces[42].

The impact of whipworm infection on pregnancy is mainly anemia due to increased gastrointestinal blood loss. Fetal infection has not been reported. Therapy is performed postpartum with mebendazole (100 mg twice a day for 3 days) or thiabendazole (20 mg/kg twice a day for 2 days), both of which are relatively contraindicated in pregnancy and breastfeeding, owing to

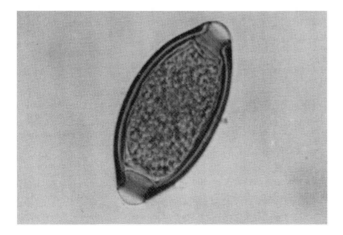

Figure 7 *Trichuris trichiura* egg. From reference 42 with permission, (page 139, figure 2)

teratogenesis and mutagenesis[47]. If therapy is needed prior to cessation of lactation, breasts should be pumped and the milk discarded until the maternal drug levels have cleared (1–2 days).

Trichinella spiralis

Trichinosis has a worldwide distribution, but is most prevalent in Europe and North America. The adult *Trichinella spiralis* are 1–4 mm in length[42]. The female is viviparous, delivering larvae; thus, there is no external egg stage. All carnivorous species, including humans, are the definitive hosts. Most human infections result from ingestion of inadequately cooked meat. Bear, wild pig, boar, horse and dog meat are the usual sources, but pork is the most common cause in the USA[48].

Adult worms, living in the small intestine, release larvae into the mucosal epithelium. The larvae enter the bloodstream and migrate to muscle tissue, where they embed and mature to the infective stage. A cyst envelops the larva, and it remains infective until the cyst calcifies, killing the larva. When meat containing encysted larvae is ingested, the cysts are dissolved by gastric secretions, and the infective larvae are released. Within 36 h, maturation occurs, and within a wee larvae are produced, to become encysted in this new host[42].

The clinical effects of trichinosis in humans range from no symptoms to fatality. The initial ingestion of infected meat may cause diarrhea and gastroenteritis. The majority of symptomatology results from the larval migration and the resultant inflammatory response. Fever, edema, dyspnea, urticaria, weakness and myositis are common manifestations[41]. The ocular muscles are generally the most severely affected, but myocardial involvement is the most common cause of death[48].

Trichinosis in pregnancy typically follows a moderate course, but hospitalization is recommended, regardless of symptomatology, due to the risk of abortion, preterm labor or intrauterine fetal death[48]. Intrauterine infection has been reported twice, resulting in fetal/neonatal death[48].

Diagnosis of trichinosis is based on history of ingestion of undercooked meat, and a compatible clinical picture[42]. Definitive diagnosis requires muscle biopsy finding encysted larvae[41]. Therapy is a combination of pyrantel pamoate (30 mg/kg per day for 4 days), corticosteroids, anti-inflammatory agents and supportive care[49]. Mebendazole (100 mg twice a day for 3 days) and thiabendazole (20 mg/kg twice a day for 2–4 days) can be used in non-pregnant, non-breastfeeding patients. Antihelminthics destroy adult worms, not the larvae; however, once larval production ceases the disease is self-limited; symptoms resolve as soon as all larvae are encysted.

Ascaris lumbricoides

Ascariasis or roundworm infection is most prevalent in warm, moist climates, but can be seen anywhere. Adult worms are quite large (15–30 cm long), with males longer and thinner than females[42]. Ascaris eggs have thick, bile-stained shells (Figure 8). Humans are the definitive host.

The life cycle begins as eggs are passed in feces into soil or water. The infective eggs are then ingested, with larvae released in the small intestine. The larvae migrate through the venous system to the lungs, where they cross into alveoli and climb the bronchial tree. The larvae are then swallowed, and return to the small intestine, to mature into adults[42]. The life span of adult ascaris is less than 1 year[47].

There are two types of clinical disease related to ascariasis. Loefflers' syndrome is heralded by inflammation and pulmonary symptoms due to the migration of the larvae. Migration of the adult worms may cause obstruction of the bile duct or the appendix[47]. Migration of adult females into the hepatic duct allows eggs to be released into the liver, resulting in multifocal abscess formation[41]. Most patients, however, have minimal or no symptoms. Ascariasis is diagnosed by finding eggs in feces or on barium enema, when elongated filling defects occur[41].

Ascariasis in pregnancy is generally asymptomatic. Transplacental infection has been reported, but is quite rare[47]. Pregnant women should, however, be treated prior to labor or Cesarean section, because of the risk of adult worm migration, stimulated by the stress of labor or general anesthetics. Pyrantel pamoate (15–60 mg/kg) should be given about 1 month prior to anticipated delivery[47]. Treatment earlier in pregnancy is not recommended, unless the patient is symptomatic, owing to the benign course and possibility of reinfection. Piperazine citrate (95 mg/kg) can be used in pregnancy if pyrantel pamoate is not available[47]. Mebendazole (100 mg twice a day for 3 days) can be used in non-pregnant patients. Pyrantel pamoate can be used in breastfeeding women.

Capillaria hepatica, *Capillaria philippinensis*

Hepatic capillariasis has a worldwide distribution, whereas intestinal capillariasis is seen mainly in the Philippines and Thailand. The adult worms are 2–4 mm long[42]. *Capillaria hepatica* adults live in the liver parenchyma, whereas *C. philippinensis* adults remain in the small intestine. *Capillaria* eggs have striated shells and are unembryonated. Humans are incidental hosts; birds and rodents are the definitive hosts. The *C. hepatica* life cycle involves passage of eggs in feces, which then embryonate and are ingested by rodents (or humans). The larvae hatch and migrate to the liver to mature. The adult worms deposit eggs in the liver, where they remain until the rodent is consumed by a carnivore. In digestion, the eggs are released from the liver and pass in the carnivore's feces to restart the cycle[42]. *C. philippinensis* eggs pass into water, where they are ingested by fish, and develop to the infective stage. Birds (or humans) are infected by eating raw fish. The adult worms live in the bird's (or human's) intestine and pass eggs in its feces[42].

Hepatic capillariasis is quite uncommon in humans and requires liver biopsy for diagnosis. Intestinal capillariasis is more common and can be diagnosed by finding eggs in feces[42]. The clinical course resembles sprue, with diarrhea and severe gastrointestinal symptoms[41]. Human autoinfection can occur, worsening the prognosis significantly.

Capillariasis in pregnancy may be left untreated until postpartum if symptoms are mild. Severe cases must be treated antepartum. Mebendazole (100 mg twice a day for 3 days) is the drug of choice, regardless of pregnancy status[49]. Mild cases should not be treated until breastfeeding is completed. If therapy is needed prior to cessation of lactation, breasts should be pumped and the milk discarded until the maternal drug levels have cleared (1–2 days).

Strongyloides stercoralis

Strongyloidiasis has a worldwide distribution, but is most common in warm climates with a high water table. Adult worms are all females. They measure 2–3 mm in length, and live in the small intestine. *Strongyloides* eggs are thin-shelled[42].

Female worms deposit eggs in the intestinal mucosa, where they hatch, releasing larvae. The larvae migrate into the lumen and pass in the feces into soil. Following maturation in the soil, infective larvae infect humans through direct skin penetration. The larvae then migrate, via the venous system and lungs, to the

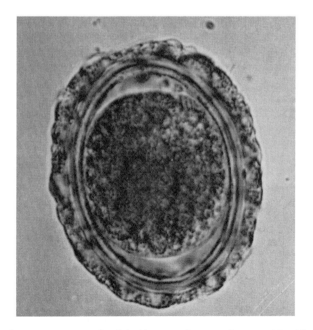

Figure 8   *Ascaris lumbricoides* egg. From reference 42 with permission, (page 135, figure 1)

intestine, where they mature to adulthood and lay eggs. The entire life cycle may occur outside the body (in soil) or inside the body (internal autoinfection)[42].

The clinical effects of *Strongyloides stercoralis* infection include rash or pruritus (penetration phase); pneumonitis and cough (migration phase); and abdominal pain, diarrhea, nausea and vomiting (intestinal phase)[41]. Immunosuppressed patients are at high risk from fulminant autoinfection.

Strongyloidiasis is difficult to diagnose. Fecal concentration techniques are required to find larvae in feces, owing to the low number present. Piperazine is the drug of choice for use in pregnancy[50]. Thiabendazole (20 mg/kg twice a day for 2 days) can be used in severe cases after the first trimester[51]. If therapy is needed prior to cessation of lactation, breasts should be pumped and the milk discarded until the maternal drug levels have cleared (1–2 days).

Necator americanus, Ancylostoma duodenale

Hookworm infection is common throughout Africa, Asia and the South Pacific. Adult worms are small (7–11 mm in length), with females being larger than males. Hookworm eggs are thin-shelled and colorless[42].

Adult hookworms may live in the human intestine for 5–15 years, with the eggs being passed in feces[42]. The eggs enter soil, hatch and mature to third-stage (infective) larvae (Figure 9). Infective larvae directly penetrate human skin and migrate, via the lungs, to the small intestine, where they mature to adulthood[47].

Light hookworm infection is asymptomatic. Heavy infection produces hypochromic macrocytic anemia, due to intestinal blood loss[41]. Hookworm infection is diagnosed by finding eggs in feces[42].

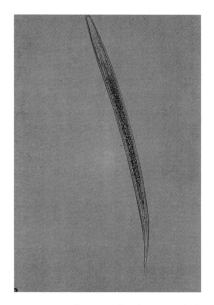

Figure 9   *Necator/Ancylostoma* (hookworm) infective third-stage larva. From reference 42 with permission, (page 151, figure 2)

Prior to modern therapy, severe hookworm infection in pregnancy was associated with significant maternal (27%) and perinatal (23%) mortality[47]. Maternal anemia, if untreated, may result in debilitation and heart failure[52]. This maternal morbidity may cause fetal loss through abortion, preterm delivery or stillbirth. Congenital infection has been reported[47].

If severe hookworm infection is diagnosed in pregnancy, it should be treated immediately with pyrantel pamoate (30 mg/kg one or two doses, or 60 mg/kg single dose). Otherwise the resultant anemia should be treated and antihelminthic therapy delayed until postpartum. Pyrantel pamoate can be used while breastfeeding[47].

Trichostrongylus

Trichostrongylosis has a worldwide distribution, but is most common in Iran and Iraq. The adult worms are small and slender, measuring 2–9 mm in length. *Trichostrongylus* eggs are thin-shelled and colorless, tapering at one end. Humans are incidental hosts; herbivorous animals are definitive hosts[42].

Trichostrongylus eggs pass into soil, where the larvae hatch and mature. Animals (or humans) ingest the larvae, which migrate to the small intestine, mature into adults and lay eggs[42].

Human trichostrongylosis is typically asymptomatic, but may involve anemia, diarrhea and abdominal pain. The diagnosis is based on finding characteristic eggs in feces[41]. Pyrantel pamoate can be used to treat severe trichostrongylosis in pregnancy or while breastfeeding. Mebendazole (100 mg twice a day for 3 days) can be used postpartum, if the patient is not breastfeeding.

Toxocara canis

Toxocara canis (visceral larva migrans) is cosmopolitan, with dogs as the definitive host. The adult worms are 4–10 cm long and inhabit dog intestines. Toxocara eggs are thick-shelled and spherical. Humans are incidental hosts[42].

Toxocara eggs pass into soil, mature and are ingested by rodents. Upon ingestion, the larvae are released and migrate throughout the body. Dogs ingest infected meat, with release of larvae in the stomach and maturation in the intestine. Human infection, called visceral larva migrans, occurs via ingestion of infective eggs with subsequent larval release and migration[42].

Human infection generally occurs in children who have contact with outdoor pets. The clinical syndrome includes hepatomegaly, inflammation and hypereosinophilia. Diagnosis is based on history of contact with a pet and clinical examination. Tissue biopsy demonstrating larvae is required for definitive diagnosis; however, clinical diagnosis is suffficient for treatment[42].

Steroids and anti-inflammatory medications are used to reduce the inflammation associated with migration of the larvae. Thiabendazole (20 mg/kg twice a day for 7 days) can be used as an adjunct to anti-inflammatory agents, once the patient is beyond the first trimester of pregnancy. Prolonged thiabendazole use is not recommended during lactation as there is inadequate time for drug clearance between doses, so breastfeeding must be interrupted throughout the course of therapy.

Antihelminthic agents

Antihelminthic agents are quite effective, with cure rates of 70–100% following a single course of therapy[43]. Niclosamide, paromomycin, praziquantel, pyrantel pamoate and piperazine are the antihelminthic agents commonly used in pregnancy (Table 2). Mebendazole and thiabendazole are avoided, if possible, owing to teratogenicity in rat and rabbit models. Bithionol use is not recommended in pregnancy or while breastfeeding, because no data exist on its safety[42]. (Bithionol is available only by special request to the Centers for Disease Control). Table 3 summarizes the classification of antihelminthic agents for use in pregnancy or lactation.

Pyrantel pamoate, a pyrimidine derivative, acts by paralyzing nematodes, allowing them to be expelled. Its action is similar to depolarizing neuromuscular blocking agents[47]. Pyrantel pamoate is very poorly absorbed, with half remaining in the intestinal tract unabsorbed. This poor absorption is the basis for its recommendation as first-line therapy in pregnancy. Blood levels of pyrantel pamoate are quite low, but it is not known whether it crosses the placenta. Animal teratology studies were negative, and no human malformations have been reported. Pyrantel pamoate is considered safe for use while breastfeeding, due to its low absorption. Side-effects (gastrointestinal complaints) are generally minimal and are not increased in pregnancy. Pyrantel doses can be calculated from the pamoate form or the free base (1 mg base = 2.9 mg pamoate form). Antihelminthic doses are 5–10 mg/kg pyrantel base or 15–30 mg/kg pyrantel pamoate (maximum dose, 1 g pyrantel base)[47].

Piperazine also acts by inducing neuromuscular blockade; however, its mechanism is quite different – that of an anticholinergic effect[47]. Piperazine citrate is readily absorbed and rapidly excreted. Animal teratology studies have not yet been reported. Piperazine use without complications has been reported in early pregnancy. There are no reports of human malformations. Piperazine should be used only if pyrantel is not available, owing to rare, but severe, neurotoxicity. The transport of piperazine across the placenta and into breastmilk is unknown. Interruption of breastfeeding with pumping and discarding of milk following piperazine therapy is necessary until maternal serum clearance of the drug occurs.

Niclosamide, a salicylanilide, inhibits oxidative phosphorylation in the cestode mitochondria, killing

Table 2   Summary of antihelminthic therapy in pregnancy

	First choice	*Alternative*
Cestodes		
*Taenia**	niclosamide	paromomycin
*Diphyllobothrium**	vitamin B_{12}+ niclosamide	paromomycin
Hymenolepis[†]	niclosamide	praziquantel/paromomycin
*Echinococcus**	surgery	mebendazole[††]
Trematodes		
*Schistosoma**	praziquantel	metrifonate[††]
Fasciola[†]	praziquantel	bithionol[††]
Fasciolopsis[†]	niclosamide	praziquantel
*Clonorchis**	praziquantel	
*Opisthorchis**	praziquantel	
*Paragonimus**	praziquantel	bithionol[††]
Nematodes		
Enterobius (pinworm)[†]	pyrantel pamoate	mebendazole[††]
Trichuris (whipworm)[†]	mebendazole[††]	piperazine
Trichinella[‡]	steroids + pyrantel pamoate	thiabendazole[‡‡]
*Ascaris***	pyrantel pamoate	piperazine
Capillaria	mebendazole	
*Strongyloides**	piperazine	thiabendazole[‡‡]
Ancylostoma (hookworm)*	pyrantel pamoate + iron	piperazine/mebendazole[‡‡]
Necator		
Trichostrongylus[†]	pyrantel pamoate	mebendazole[††]
Toxocara (visceral larva migrans)*	steroids	thiabendazole[‡‡]

*Treat postpartum unless severe; [†]treat postpartum; [‡]treat immediately; **treat prior to delivery; [††]use only postpartum; [‡‡]use only after first trimester the worm on contact. Niclosamide has been shown to have no teratogenic effect in rat and rabbit studies[44]. No human malformations have been reported. The drug is poorly absorbed, but no information is available on niclosamide levels in breastmilk, or on its ability to cross the placenta. There are inadequate data to assure the safety of uninterrupted breastfeeding following niclosamide therapy. Since single-dose therapy is used, temporary interruption (24 h) of breastfeeding with disposal of milk can accommodate this therapy.

Paromomycin is an aminoglycoside antibiotic similar to streptomycin and kanamycin[53]. It is poorly absorbed orally. If absorbed, paromomycin carries risks of nephrotoxicity and ototoxicity, similar to those of other aminoglycosides. Animal teratogenicity studies in rat and guinea pig models are negative. There are no reports of human teratogenicity with paromomycin; kanamycin and streptomycin, however, have been associated with deafness. Paromomycin levels in breastmilk are proportional to maternal blood levels (very low if paromomycin is given orally), therefore use while breastfeeding is not contraindicated[53].

Praziquantel is the drug of choice for most trematode infections in pregnancy[43]. An isoquinoline, it is well tolerated with minimal side-effects[46]. Studies of teratogenicity have been negative in mice, rats and rabbits[54,55]. There are no reports of human malformations. Praziquantel is secreted in breastmilk at 29% of the maternal serum level[43]. If therapy is needed prior to cessation of lactation, breasts should be pumped

and the milk discarded until the maternal drug levels have cleared (1–2 days).

Mebendazole and thiabendazole (benzimidazole derivatives) are the drugs of choice for treatment for most nematode infections outside pregnancy. Mebendazole use is contraindicated in pregnancy, due to known teratogenicity in animal studies[47]. Human studies are limited, with inconclusive data. Mebendazole use in lactation requires interruption of breastfeeding with disposal of pumped milk until maternal drug levels are cleared (1–2 days).

Thiabendazole is recommended for use in pregnancy only after the first trimester for severe infection with *Strongyloides*, *Trichinella* or *Toxocara*[43]. Thiabendazole also has proven teratogenicity in animal models[56], with no human studies reported. The use of thiabendazole is recommended only when alternative therapy is inadequate, and maternal disease is felt to outweigh possible fetal risks[43]. In lactating women, use of thiabendazole requires a temporary cessation of breastfeeding until the mother can clear the drug from her system (1–2 days). She may use a breast pump to assure continued milk production.

REFERENCES

1. Sobel JD. Pathophysiology of vulvovaginitis candidiasis. *J Reprod Med* 1989;34:572–9
2. Hill LVH, Embil JA. Vaginitis: current microbiologic and clinical concepts. *Can Med Assoc J* 1986;134:321–31
3. Hopfer RL. Mycology of *Candida* infections. In Bodey GP, Fainstein V, eds. *Candidiasis*. New York: Raven Publishers, 1985
4. McKay M. Cutaneous manifestations of candidiasis. *Am J Obstet Gynecol* 1988;158:991–3
5. Davidson F. Yeasts and circumcision in the male. *Br J Vener Dis* 1977;53:121–2
6. Higashide A, Aman R, Yamamuro O. Clinical characteristics correlated with different fungi causing vulvovaginal mycosis. *Mycoses* 1988;31:213–25
7. Oriel JD, Partridge BM, Denny MJ, Coleman JC. Genital yeast infections. *Br J Med* 1972;4:761–4
8. Redondo-Lopez V, Lynch M, Schmitt C, *et al. Torulopsis glabrata* vaginitis: clinical aspects and susceptibility to antifungal agents. *Obstet Gynecol* 1990;76:651–5
9. Robertson WH. Mycology of vulvovaginitis. *Am J Obstet Gynecol* 1988;158:989–91
10. Powell BL, Frey CL, Drutz DJ. Identification of a 17β-estradiol binding protein in *Candida albicans* and *Candida glabrata*. *Exp Mycol* 1984;8:304–13
11. Loose DS, Schurman DJ, Feldman D. A corticosteroid binding protein and endogenous ligand in *C. albicans* indicating a possible steroid receptor system. *Nature* (London) 1981;293:477–9
12. Fleury FJ. Vulvovaginal candidiasis, clinical history and symptomatology. *J Reprod Med* 1989;34:650–2
13. McCormack WM, Starko KM, Zinner SH. Symptoms associated with vaginal colonization with yeast. *Am J Obstet Gynecol* 1988;158:31–3
14. Kaufman RH. Establishing a correct diagnosis of vulvovaginal infection. *Am J Obstet Gynecol* 1988;158:986–8

Table 3 Summary of pregnancy/lactation recommendations

Antihelminthic agent	Pregnancy use category	Recommendations for breastfeeding women
Pyrantel pamoate	C	I
Piperaine	B	III
Niclosamide	B	II
Paromomycin	∇	I
Praziquantel	B	II
Mebendazole	C	II
Thiabendazole	C	II
Bithionol	∇	III

Pregnancy category definitions: A, studies in humans failed to demonstrate risk; **B**, either negative animal studies with no human studies, or positive animal studies with negative humans studies; **C**, either positive animal studies with no human studies, or neither human nor animal studies available; **D**, positive evidence of human risks limits use to cases where maternal benefit outweighs risk; **X**, positive evidence of human risk outweighs any positive benefit; ∇, not yet classified

Breastfeeding recommendations:

I, no significant amount can be detected in breastmilk; **II**, small amounts may be secreted in breastmilk for 1–3 days following each dose. Therapy may be postponed until lactation ceases or breastmilk may be pumped and discarded until drug has cleared (1–3 days); **III**, inadequate data exist to establish extent of secretion. Use alternative therapy or postpone treatment until breastfeeding has been concluded

15. Gentry LO, Price MF. Urinary and genital *Candida* infections. In Bodey GP, Fainstein V, eds. *Candidiasis*. New York: Raven Publishers, 1985

16. Luna MA, Tortoledo ME. Histologic identification and pathologic patterns of disease due to *Candida*. In Bodey GP, Fainstein V, eds. *Candidiasis*. New York: Raven Publishers, 1985

17. Brown D. Therapeutic alternatives and new treatment modalities in vulvovaginal candidiasis. *J Reprod Med* 1989;34:653–4

18. Culbertson C. Monistat: a new fungicide for treatment of vulvovaginal candidiasis. *Am J Obstet Gynecol* 1974; 120:973–6

19. Davis JE, Frudenfeld JH, Goddard JL. Comparative evaluation of Monistat and mycostatin in the treatment of vulvovaginal candidiasis. *Obstet Gynecol* 1974;44:403–6

20. Fleury F, Hughes D, Floyd R. Therapeutic results obtained in vaginal mycoses after single-dose treatment with 500 mg clotrimazole vaginal tablets. *Am J Obstet Gynecol* 1985;152:968–70

21. Lebherz T, Guess E, Wolfson N. Efficacy of single- versus multiple-dose clotrimazole therapy in the management of vulvovaginal candidiasis. *Am J Obstet Gynecol* 1985;152:965–8

22. Ritter W. Pharmacokinetic fundamentals of vaginal treatment with clotrimazole. *Am J Obstet Gynecol* 1985; 152:945–7

23. Adamson GD. Three-day treatment of vulvovaginal candidiasis. *Am J Obstet Gynecol* 1988;158:1002–5

24. Jacobson JB. Butoconazole versus miconazole: European clinical experience. *J Reprod Med* 1986;31:661–3

25. Sobel JD. Recurrent vulvovaginal candidiasis: a prospective study of the efficacy of maintenance ketoconazole therapy. *N Engl J Med* 1986;315:1455–8

26. Hirsch HA. Clinical evaluation of terconazole: European experience. *J Reprod Med* 1989;34:593–6

27. Thomason JL. Clinical evaluation of terconazole: the United States experience. *J Reprod Med* 1989;34:597–601

28. Brammer KW. A comparison of single-dose oral fluconazole with 3-day intravaginal clotrimazole in the treatment of vaginal candidiasis. *Br J Obstet Gynaecol* 1989;96:226–32

29. Van Heusden AM, Merkus HM, Corbeij RS, *et al.* Single-dose oral fluconazole versus single-dose topical miconazole for the treatment of acute vulvovaginal candidosis. *Acta Obstet Gynecol Scand* 1990;69:417–22

30. Kutzer E, Oittner R, Leodolter S, Brammer KW. A comparison of fluconazole and ketoconazole in oral treatment of vulvovaginal candidiasis; report of a double-blind multicentre trial. *Eur J Obstet Gynecol Reprod Biol* 1988;29:305–13

31. De Los Reyes C, Edelman DE, De Bruin MF. Clinical experience with single-dose fluconazole in vaginal candidiasis: a review of the worldwide database. *Int J Gynecol Obstet* 1992;37(suppl):9–15

32. Van Slyke KK, Michel VP, Rein MF. Treatment of vulvovaginal candidiasis with boric acid powder. *Am J Obstet Gynecol* 1981;141:145–8

33. Briggs GG, Freeman RK, Yaffe SJ, eds. *Drugs in Pregnancy and Lactation*, 2nd edn. Baltimore, MD: Williams and Wilkins, 1986

34. McKay M. Immunological considerations in recurrent candidal vulvovaginitis. *J Reprod Med* 1986;31:651–4

35. Nystatin Multicenter Study Group. Therapy of candidal vaginitis: the effect of eliminating intestinal *Candida*. *Am J Obstet Gynecol* 1986;155:651–5

36. Bodey GP, Fainstein V. Systemic candidiasis. In Bodey GP, Fainstein V, eds. *Candidiasis*. New York: Raven Publishers, 1985

37. Ismail MA, Lerner SA. Disseminated blastomycosis in a pregnant woman. *Am Rev Respir Dis* 1982;126:350–3

38. Rosen T. Cutaneous candidiasis. In Bodey GP, Fainstein V, eds. *Candidiasis*. New York: Raven Publishers, 1985

39. Warren KS. Helminthic diseases endemic in the United States. *Am J Trop Med Hyg* 1974;23:723–30

40. Gyorkos TW, MacLean JD, Lae CG. Absence of significant differences in intestinal parasite prevalence estimates after examination of either one or two stool specimens. *Am J Epidemiol* 1989;130:976–80

41. Zaman V. *Atlas of Medical Parasitology*. Boston, MA: ADIS Health Science Press, 1978

42. Ash LR, Orihel TC. *Atlas of Human Parasitology*, 3rd edn. Chicago: ASCP Press, 1990

43. MacLeod CL. *Parasitic Infections of Pregnancy and the Newborn*. New York: Oxford University Press, 1988

44. Goldsmith R, Markell EK. Other trematode infections. In MacLeod CL, ed. *Parasitic Infections of Pregnancy and the Newborn*. New York: Oxford University Press, 1988

45. Vuitton D. Alveolar echinococcosis of the liver: a parasitic disease in search of treatment. *Hepatology* 1990; 12:617–8

46. McNeely DF, Magu MR. Schistosomiasis. In MacLeod CL, ed. *Parasitic Infections of Pregnancy and the Newborn*. New York: Oxford University Press, 1988

47. MacLeod CL. Intestinal nematode infections. In MacLeod CL, ed. *Parasitic Infections of Pregnancy and the Newborn*. New York: Oxford University Press,1988

48. Kociecka W. Trichinosis. In MacLeod CL, ed. *Parasitic Infections of Pregnancy and the Newborn*. New York: Oxford University Press, 1988

49. Youssef FG, Mikhail EM, Mansour NS. Intestinal capillariasis in Egypt: a case report. *Am J Trop Med Hyg* 1989;40:195–6

50. Young RL, Zund G, Mason BA, Faro S. Pelvic inflammatory disease complicated by massive helminthic infection. *Obstet Gynecol* 1989;74:484–6

51. Ellis CJ. Antiparasitic agents in pregnancy. *Clin Obstet Gynaecol* 1986;13:269–75

52. Langer A, Hung CT. Hookworm disease in pregnancy with severe anemia. *Obstet Gynecol* 1973;42:564–7

53. MacLeod CL, Carden GA. Amoebiasis. In MacLeod CL, ed. *Parasitic Infections of Pregnancy and the Newborn*. New York: Oxford University Press, 1988

54. Frohberg H, Schencking MS. Toxicological profile of praziquantel, a new drug against cestode and schistosome infections, as compared to some other schistosomicides. *Arzneimittelforsch* 1981;31:555–65

55. Frohberg H. Results of toxicological studies on praziquantel. *Arzneimittelforsch* 1984;34:1137–44

56. Tsuchiya T, Tanaka A. *In vivo* inhibition of adenosine triphosphate (ATP) synthesis associated with thiabendazole-induced teratogenesis in mice and rats. *Arch Toxicol* 1985;57:243–5

32

Immunizations in pregnancy

J.E. Deaver

INTRODUCTION

Active immunization, or vaccination, is the introduction of an antigen in order to stimulate an immune response with the effect of preventing, abbreviating or ameliorating natural infection. Currently available vaccines are listed in Table 1.

They are made of live attenuated or inactivated whole organisms, modified exotoxins (toxoids), viral subunits, capsular polysaccharides, or other pure components such as the outer surface protein A of the Lyme disease-causing spirochete.

Passive immunization is the transfer of protective antibodies from immune individuals by parenteral administration of pooled human or equine serum or by placental transfer of immunoglobulin G (IgG) antibodies from mother to fetus. Equine serum is the source of specific antitoxins (e.g. *Clostridia botulinum* antitoxin) and will not be discussed further. Current human globulins and their indications are listed in Table 2.

Table 1 Organisms in current vaccines

Live virus
  Measles
  Mumps
  Rubella
  Varicella
  Poliovirus, oral (OPV)
  Yellow fever
  Adenovirus
  Venezuelan equine encephalitis
Live bacteria
  Bacillus of Calmette and Guerin (BCG)
  Typhoid (Ty21a oral)
Inactivated virus
  Influenza
  Hepatitis A
  Japanese encephalitis
  Poliovirus, inactivated (IPV)
  Rabies
Inactivated bacteria
  Anthrax
  Cholera
  Typhoid (parenteral)
  Pertussis (whole cell)
  Plague
Toxoids
  Diptheria
  Tetanus
Capsular polysaccharides
  Meningococcus
  Pneumococcus
  Haemophilus influenzae type b
  Group B streptococcus (Phase I trials)
Viral subunit
  Hepatitis B (surface antigen)
Other subunits
  Acellular pertussis (bacterial components)
  Borrelia burgdorferi (outer surface protein A)

Table 2 Human immune globulins

Immunobiologic	Indication
Cytomegalovirus immune globulin, IV (CMV-IGIV)	Bone marrow and kidney transplant recipients
Immune globulin (IG)	Hepatitis A pre- and postexposure prophylaxis; measles postexposure prophylaxis; rubella postexposure prophylaxis
Immune globulin, intravenous (IGIV)	Medical problems such as ITP, immune deficiency, Kawasaki disease
Hepatitis B (HBIG)	Hepatitis postexposure prophylaxis, prevention of vertical hepatitis B transmission
Rabies immune globulin (HRIG)	Postexposure prophylaxis
Tetanus immune globulin (TIG)	Postexposure prophylaxis
Vaccinia immune globulin (VIG)	Treatment of vaccinia necrosum, eczema vaccinatum, and ocular vaccinia
Varicella zoster immune globulin (VZIG)	Postexposure prophylaxis of immunocompromised persons, certain pregnant women, and perinatally exposed neonates
Bacterial polysaccharide immune globulin (BPIG)	Groups at high risk for *Haemophilus influenzae* type b infection

Circumstances for which vaccination during pregnancy may be considered are travel to endemic areas, military service, occupational exposure, scheduled booster or primary vaccination, postexposure prophylaxis and cases of extraordinary risk from common infections such as in immunosuppressed patients. Recommendations for vaccination during pregnancy are based on consideration of maternal and fetal risks and benefits, comparing those of natural infection to those of vaccination.

The risk of natural infection depends on the incidence and severity of infection, including the probability and consequence of vertical transmission to the fetus. Theoretically, maternal risk of infection may be increased since pregnancy represents an immunocompromised state[1]. With the possible exceptions of influenza[2] and varicella-zoster[3], however, there is little evidence that natural infections are worse in pregnant compared to non-pregnant women.

Potential risks of vaccination during pregnancy include altered immunogenicity or an increased rate of adverse reactions which have not been convincingly demonstrated for any vaccine. The risk of fetal infection is a concern for attenuated live-virus vaccines, the routine use of which are contraindicated in pregnancy. However, none of the vaccines are proven to be teratogenic. Risk-benefit considerations may dictate the use of certain live virus vaccines in pregnancy under special circumstances, e.g. yellow fever and oral polio vaccine in travellers[4]. Inactivated virus vaccines are indicated in women, regardless of pregnancy, in settings where there are increased risks of exposure or complications of natural infection[4]. Likewise, there is little justification for withholding toxoid vaccines during pregnancy if they are otherwise indicated[4]. There is a theoretical risk that immune unresponsiveness (tolerance) may develop as a result of fetal exposure to vaccines that cross the placenta, although this has not been observed for a number of polysaccharides and proteins[5,6]. Indeed, antigens that cross the placenta may actively immunize the fetus, as has been observed for tetanus toxoid[7].

Benefits of vaccination are determined by the efficacy of the vaccine, including the potential for passive transfer of immunity to the fetus. Vaccination during pregnancy can increase the amount of maternal IgG available for placental transport and passive protection of the neonate[5]. Passive immunity acquired from the mother may be especially important for serious infections, such as group B streptococcal and *Haemophilus influenzae* type b that occur early in life, when active immunization of the neonate is prone to failure because of immune system immaturity[5].

Breastfeeding is never a contraindication to any vaccine. The only vaccine virus that has ever been isolated from breast milk is rubella and there is no good evidence that breast milk from women immunized against rubella is harmful to infants[8].

Following are discussions of individual vaccines by organisms grouped according to vaccine types (live virus, inactivated virus, etc.). The risk-benefit considerations important to deciding whether to recommend vaccine use during pregnancy are presented. There is also discussion relevant to counseling women who are inadvertently vaccinated during pregnancy or around the time of conception. Passive immunization has important uses during pregnancy. The use of immune globulins for specific infections is also presented.

LIVE ATTENUATED VIRUS VACCINES
Rubella

Rubella is a short-lived viral exanthem of little concern except for the potentially tragic consequences of infection during early pregnancy. Gregg reported the first association of maternal rubella with neonatal cataracts in 1941[9], after which the triad of congenital rubella syndrome (CRS) consisting of cardiac lesions, cataracts and hearing loss was recognized. The rubella pandemic of 1962–64 resulted in approximately 20 000 infants affected with CRS in the US alone[10].

Rubella vaccines are prepared from live attenuated viruses. The Cendehill and HPV-77 strains were licensed for use in 1969. The RA 27/3 strain, the only rubella vaccine currently available in the USA, was introduced in 1979. Rubella vaccination has resulted in a decrease in CRS from nearly 4 per 100 000 pregnancies in 1969, the year the original vaccine was licensed, to approximately 0.5 per 100 000 during the early 1990s[11]. Only four confirmed CRS cases were reported to the CDC in 1995 and two were reported in 1996[12].

Despite recommendations for vaccination of all 15-month olds and prepubertal girls[13], 10–33% of reproductive-age women remain susceptible to rubella[14,15]. In addition, 44% of congenital rubella infections occur in first pregnancies[16], cases not preventable by a program of postpartum immunization. An epidemiological study of 21 cases of CRS in four Southern California counties from January 1990 to January 1991 revealed that 57% of these women had missed opportunities for rubella screening or vaccination[17]. The missed opportunities included marriage, previous pregnancies, induced abortions and the postpartum period. Therefore, to reduce the incidence of CRS, screening and vaccination of susceptible women should be offered at the family-planning and abortion clinics in addition to the postpartum period[13,17].

Arthralgia is a frequently reported adverse reaction to rubella vaccine that does not appear to be increased in women vaccinated in the postpartum period compared to those vaccinated at other times[18]. Rubella vaccination has been unsuccessful following blood transfusion, owing to the existence of rubella antibody, and can be delayed for 6 weeks after transfusion[19].

The Advisory Committee on Immunization Practices, however, recommends that rubella vaccination not be delayed because anti-Rho immunoglobulin or other blood or blood products were received during the last trimester or at delivery[20]. If possible, such women should be retested for immunity in 3 months[20].

Rubella vaccination is contraindicated during pregnancy because of the theoretical teratogenic risk. The vaccine virus strain has been isolated from 3–20% of abortion products following periconceptional exposure[21], including a case in which the virus was cultured from the fetal eye[22]. In approximately 2% of normal-appearing infants born after exposure to vaccine virus, there is rubella IgM in cord blood, indicating subclinical fetal infection[23]. There was evidence of fetal infection in a case of vaccination as long as 7 weeks before conception[22]. Therefore, contraception for 3 months following vaccination is essential.

Between 1971 and 1989, the Centers for Disease Control (CDC) followed to delivery 321 known pregnant women who were exposed to rubella vaccine within 3 months before until 3 months after conception[12]. There were no malformations consistent with CRS in any of the 324 infants of these mothers. Five had serologic evidence of subclinical infection. Likewise, periconceptional exposure to rubella vaccine in Germany and Britain has not been associated with CRS[24,25]. The CDC estimates that the theoretical maximum vaccine-related risk of CRS is 1.2%[12].

The vaccine virus is not transmitted person-to-person. Children of pregnant women may be vaccinated[26]. Asymptomatic infection of infants with the rubella vaccine virus during breastfeeding does occur in some cases[27]. However, breastfeeding should not be considered a contraindication to postpartum maternal rubella immunization[12]. There is no evidence that rubella vaccine virus exposure during breastfeeding alters the response to subsequent childhood immunizations[28].

Although serum immune globulin may prevent clinical rubella, there is little evidence that such treatment prevents CRS[29]. Routine postexposure prophylaxis with immune globulin during pregnancy is not recommended[26]. The only potential use is for a patient exposed to the wild-type virus who will not consider termination of pregnancy[4].

Measles

Measles is a highly contagious seasonal viral exanthem affecting nearly everyone during childhood in the absence of vaccination. Occasionally, encephalitis and pneumonia develop. The number of reported cases has declined from nearly a million in 1941, before vaccine availability, to 138 cases in 1997[30]. There may be an increased risk of spontaneous abortion and prematurity in association with measles infection during pregnancy[31]. Neonatal measles infection following

intrauterine exposure may be severe[31]. Measles infection has not been confirmed as a cause of congenital malformations[12], even when it occurs in the first trimester[32].

An inactivated measles vaccine was licensed in 1963 and withdrawn in 1967. Currently, measles immunization is accomplished with a live attenuated Enders-Edmonston measles virus strain in combination with mumps and rubella (MMR)[12]. Vaccination has led to a 94% reduction in risk of contracting measles in the US[31]. Susceptible adults born after 1956 who are more than 17-years-old should be vaccinated with one dose of measles vaccine (using MMR) unless they are pregnant or have another contraindication. Adults born before 1957 who are at increased risk of exposure or transmission should also be vaccinated, including college students, international travellers, and health care workers[12].

Because it is a live attenuated virus with theoretical teratogenic risks, measles vaccine should not be given during pregnancy[33]. Limited experience with woman who became pregnant within 3 months of vaccination with live virus vaccine suggests that no teratogenic effect exists, however[34]. Despite being counseled to avoid vaccination for possible pregnancy, two among 1913 vaccinated adolescents[34] and 11 per 1000 female Air Force recruits[35] were unknowingly pregnant when vaccinated. Such patients should be counseled that, on the basis of limited evidence, the risk of congenital anomalies does not appear to differ from the background risk[20]. The Advisory Committee on Immunization Practices recommends asking women if they are pregnant, excluding those who are, and explaining the risk to the others before vaccination[20]. Measles vaccination may be offered during the postpartum period to susceptible women[4]. Patients should obtain adequate contraception for 3 months following vaccination with MMR and for one month if vaccinated with monovalent measles vaccine[20].

Immune globulin, which affords 80% protection from measles infection[31], is preferred for the prophylaxis of measles in susceptible pregnant women during epidemics[19,31,33]. If immune globulin has been administered, vaccination should be deferred for 3 months[31].

Mumps

Mumps is an acute contagious viral illness producing parotitis and orchitis in addition to infecting the salivary glands, pancreas, joints, myocardium and kidneys. Mumps virus has been isolated from fetal tissues and placentas of induced and spontaneous abortions following mumps infection in pregnancy[36]. Mumps virus has also been isolated from a newborn following maternal mumps in the days before delivery[37]. However, a teratogenic influence of mumps virus infection has not been observed. Mumps in the first trimester may be followed by a greater than expected rate of spontaneous abortion[32].

Mumps vaccine, currently consisting of the Jeryl Lynn attenuated live virus strain, is usually administered as a single dose in combination with measles and rubella. Almost all (98%) of vaccinees produce antibody[38].

Vaccination of susceptible adults and children after the first year of life with a single dose in combination with measles and rubella is recommended[39]. Most patients are immune from natural or subclinical infection by adulthood. The need to vaccinate an adult should arise only rarely.

Because of the theoretical risk of fetal infection from live attenuated virus, mumps vaccine is contraindicated during pregnancy[33]. The Jeryl Lynn strain has been isolated from the placenta in two of three vaccinated patients following therapeutic abortion[40]. However, two cohort studies of term pregnancies following mumps vaccine[32,41] identified a risk of congenital anomalies no greater than the background rate. Vaccination should not be considered an indication for termination of pregnancy[20].

Poliovirus

The majority of poliovirus infections are mild or asymptomatic. Paralytic disease is uncommon. The number of poliomyelitis cases reported in the USA decreased from 20 000 in 1954, before the Salk vaccine was introduced, to 1000 in 1962, when the Sabin vaccine became widely available[42]. Poliovirus infection is presently a concern only for international travellers and their contacts. The last case of indigenously acquired wild-type polio infection in the USA was in 1979[43]. The last recorded case was in Peru in 1991[44]. In 1994, the World Health Organization certified that the western world was free of indigenous wild poliovirus[45]. Whether pregnant women are more susceptible to wild poliovirus infection[46] or whether they simply experience more exposure from their children is debated[33]. Pregnancy does not alter the course of polio and mortality from polio is the same in pregnant and nonpregnant women[47]. Poliovirus does not appear to be teratogenic, but the rate of spontaneous abortion may be increased[48]. There have been cases of neonatal paralysis following maternal poliomyelitis, suggesting that vertical transmission around the time of birth does occur[47].

The original Salk polio vaccine, introduced in 1955, was an inactivated poliovirus vaccine (IPV) that produces immunity after four doses to all three poliovirus types in 95% of recipients[49]. The first enhanced potency inactivated virus preparation was licensed for use in the USA in 1987[50]. Two such IPVs are currently licensed in the USA, IPOL (Pasteur Merieux Serums and Vaccines, Lyon, France) and POLIOVAX

(Connaught Laboratories, Willowdale, Ontario, Canada). Almost all (99–100%) of vaccinees develop protective antibodies to all three types of poliovirus after three doses of enhanced potency IPV[50]. Protection is expected to be long-lasting[50].

The Sabin attenuated live oral polio virus vaccine (OPV) was introduced in 1961. A trivalent formulation (Orimune, Lederle Laboratorie, Pearl River, NY), active against all three human poliovirus strains, became available in 1963 and is the only OPV licensed in the US. The oral vaccine has the advantage of infecting the normal portal of entry, the gastrointestinal tract, from where the attenuated virus is spread from person to person, resulting in nearly 100% of the population being immune. The disadvantage of OPV is the rare instance of vaccine-associated paralytic poliomyelitis (VAPP), with an incidence of one in 2.6 million doses[51]. Between 1980 and 1994, there were 125 cases of VAPP reported to the CDC[50]. The vaccine produces long-lasting protection.

For children, the Advisory Committee on Immunization Practices currently recommends a four-dose primary series consisting of two doses of IPV followed by two doses of OPV[50]. However, a three-dose OPV-only primary series may enhance compliance and is an acceptable alternative[50]. A three-dose IPV-only primary series should be used for immunocompromised persons and their family contacts[50].

Adults in the USA are frequently immune and have a low risk of exposure to poliovirus infection. Therefore, routine vaccination is not recommended[50]. Travelers to areas in which polio is endemic, members of communities in which poliovirus diseases occur, laboratory workers handling poliovirus, health care workers in contact with patients who may be excreting poliovirus, and unvaccinated adults whose children will be receiving OPV should be vaccinated[50]. In adults, use of IPV is recommended because of the slightly increased risk of vaccine-associated paralysis in adults compared to children administered the oral vaccine[52]. Because the recommended schedule requires three doses of IPV administered over 6 months, there may not be enough time before protection is needed. The alternatives are an accelerated schedule of three doses over at least 8 weeks or an abbreviated schedule or two doses four weeks apart. If less than 4 weeks are available before protection is needed, then a single dose of OPV or IPV may be administered[50].

Spread of oral vaccine virus to household contacts of oral polio vaccine recipients is known to occur[53]. However, pregnant women should not alter their unprotected children's immunization schedules.

Oral polio vaccine has been administered to a large number of pregnant women without evidence that it produces congenital anomalies or abortion[54]. However, it is suspected that damage to the fetus can occur as a result of the vaccine and some authors advise against its use[55]. OPV, since it is a live virus, is of theoretical concern and its routine use is not recommended during pregnancy[50]. However, inadvertent exposure does not by itself dictate termination of pregnancy. If a pregnant woman requires immediate protection against poliovirus infection, she may be administered IPV or OPV in accordance with the usual schedule for adults[50].

Varicella

Varicella zoster virus (VZV) is a herpesvirus that causes chickenpox due to primary infection. Herpes zoster (shingles) is due to reactivated latent infection. Nearly everyone in the USA contracts the primary infection, usually during childhood. For that reason, more than 90% of adults are immune[56]. There are 3–4 million new cases each year[57]. Varicella, which is highly contagious, is spread from person-to-person through direct contact or through contact with respiratory secretions of infected patients. Primary infection in children is a mild illness lasting 4–5 days characterized by fever, malaise, and a generalized vesicular rash. Adolescents, adults, and immunocompromised persons generally have more severe disease and are at high risk of serious complications. From 1990 to 1994, adults accounted for only 5% of reported cases of varicella infection, but they accounted for 55% of the varicella-related deaths[58].

Varicella infection occurs in 0.05–0.07% of pregnancies[59]. In addition to the concern for fetal and neonatal infection, maternal morbidity may be severe. 10–20% of pregnant women with varicella develop varicella pneumonitis with maternal mortality as high as 40%[3]. Congenital varicella syndrome, clinical neonatal varicella, or clinical zoster during infancy or early childhood can result from vertical transmission. Congenital varicella syndrome is characterized by low birthweight, cutaneous scarring, limb hypoplasia, microcephaly, cortical atrophy, and ocular abnormalities. The risk of congenital varicella syndrome is 0.5% to 2% of pregnancies complicated by maternal varicella infection[56,57]. The risk of congenital varicella syndrome is higher for maternal infection in the second trimester compared to the first[56]. When maternal illness occur between 5 days before until 2 days after delivery, severe neonatal varicella infection will develop in 17–30%[56].

The OKA strain of varicella virus, used as a vaccine for many years in Japan, was used to manufacture the live attenuated virus vaccine, VARIVAX (Merck and Co., Inc.), that was licensed by the FDA in 1995 for use in the US[57]. The vaccine affords long-lasting protection and is effective, producing a 93% reduction, on average, in the incidence of childhood varicella cases[56]. When natural infection occurs, despite vaccination, it is milder and associated with fewer life-threatening complications than infection in unvaccinated patients[57]. Five per cent of children and 8% of adolescents develop a mild varicella-like rash after vaccination[57]. No concerns about vaccine safety have been identified after more than two million doses of the original OKA strain vaccine in Japan, Korea and certain European countries[56].

Children without chickenpox histories are usually susceptible[57]. The vaccine should be administered routinely to all children at 12 to 18 months of age except those with chickenpox histories[56,57]. Susceptible healthy individuals more than 12 years of age should also be vaccinated with priority given to those who are at high risk of exposure or who are more likely to transmit infection to other susceptible persons at high-risk of severe or complicated infections. Those who might transmit infection to persons at risk of serious complications include health care workers and family members of immunocompromised persons[56]. Those at high-risk for exposure include teachers and daycare center workers, college students, employees and residents of institutions, military personnel, nonpregnant women of childbearing age, and international travellers persons[56]. Persons over 12 years of age with reliable histories of chickenpox are considered immune. Unlike children, adults without reliable chickenpox histories are also usually immune[56,57]. Therefore, it may be cost-effective to identify susceptible adolescents and adults in need of vaccination by performing serologic testing for antibodies to varicella[57]. Susceptible individuals more than 12-years-old, based on negative results of antibody testing, require two doses of vaccine separated by 4–8 weeks[57]. Varicella vaccination should be delayed for 5 months following blood products, immune globulin or VZIG[57]. There is no current role for giving the vaccine for post-exposure prophylaxis[56,57].

The overall risk of vaccine virus transmission from healthy vaccinees to their healthy siblings is at most 2.1% and is rare unless the vaccinee has a varicella-like rash[57]. Transmission from a healthy vaccinee to another individual was never conclusively documented during clinical trials[60]. In contrast, there is an 80–90% chance that naturally infected children will transmit the infection to their household contacts[57]. Since the risk of transmission is low and the severity of vaccine virus infection is mild, vaccination of household contacts of susceptible high-risk individuals is recommended. This includes vaccinating the household contacts of pregnant women[61]. The Committee on Infectious Diseases of the American Academy of Pediatrics stated that a pregnant mother or other household member is not a contraindication for vaccination of the child[60]. However, vaccination of household contacts may be deferred until after the first half of gestation when the susceptible person is at risk because of pregnancy[57,62]. Susceptible pregnant mothers might avoid contact during the rash stage of varicella-like illness following vaccination of children living with them[62] or, if varicella is absent in the community, vaccination of household contacts might be avoided until after pregnancy[62]. Salzman *et al.*[62] reported a well-documented case of varicella vaccine virus transmission from a healthy 1-year-old vaccinee to his pregnant mother. No cases of fetal infection with vaccine virus due to exposure to a vaccinee have yet been reported. Long calculated that the maximal risk of congenital varicella due to vaccination of the healthy child of a susceptible pregnant woman was no higher than 1 in 10 000 and probably was exponentially lower or even zero since 'attenuated VZV is not known to be embryopathic'[63].

Varicella vaccine is contraindicated during pregnancy because of the theoretical concern for fetal infection with live attenuated vaccine virus[56,60]. However, inadvertent administration of the vaccine usually should not be considered a reason to terminate pregnancy[56,60]. In order to disseminate information concerning the risk of vaccination during pregnancy, the manufacturer has established the VARIVAX Pregnancy Registry. Cases of vaccine exposure during pregnancy can be reported by calling + 800 986 8999. Non-pregnant women should avoid becoming pregnant for 1 month following vaccination[56,60] although the manufacturer recommends waiting for at least 3 months[57].

Whether varicella is secreted in breast milk or whether nursing infants can be infected is unknown[56]. Since most live vaccine viruses are not excreted in breast milk and since there have been no symptomatic infections in nursing infants related to any vaccine virus, varicella administration to nursing mothers may be considered[56], especially when there is a high risk for exposure to natural VZV[61].

Varicella zoster immune globulin (VZIG) (US Biologics Laboratories, Massachusetts) given to healthy children within 72 hours of exposure prevents infection[56]. VZIG lowers the rate of infection in immunocompromised children when given within 96 hours of exposure[56]. The infection rate in neonates whose mothers contracted clinical varicella infection within 5 days of delivery and who received VZIG is more than 30%, not different from the rate of infection in those neonates similarly exposed but not treated[56]. However, the rate of fatal illness is significantly lower in neonates administered VZIG[56]. Preterm neonates have immature immune systems. Whether, as a consequence, the course of postnatally acquired varicella is worse in preterm neonates is unknown. However, it is recommended that preterm neonates who have substantial postnatal exposure and whose mothers are varicella-susceptible be given VZIG[56]. VZIG is intended to compensate for an immature immune system and the lack of protection from maternal antibodies.

Those exposed preterm neonates born before 28 gestational weeks or with birthweights less than 1000 grams should receive VZIG regardless of the maternal antibody status since maternal antibody is not likely to have crossed the placenta in any substantial amounts[56]. Postnatally exposed term infants are not at increased risk and should not receive VZIG, regardless of whether maternal antibodies are present[56]. VZIG use should also be considered for susceptible pregnant women who have been exposed to natural varicella infection[56]. VZIG will not interrupt vertical transmission. The risk of congenital varicella syndrome or neonatal varicella infection is unchanged[56,64]. The primary benefit of VZIG during pregnancy is to limit the severity of the maternal infection[56]. VZIG is not recommended for high-risk individuals, including pregnant women, exposed to the varicella-like illness that sometimes follows vaccination[56].

Yellow fever

Yellow fever, occurring in tropical regions of Africa and Central and South America, is an epidemic febrile viral illness characterized by prostration, jaundice, vomiting and diffuse pain. Monkey or human hosts are infected with the virus by the *Aedes aegypti* mosquito vector. Although not rigorously assessed, natural infection does not appear to be the cause of congenital anomalies[65].

The current vaccine is a live attenuated form of the 17D virus strain, isolated from a patient in Senegal in 1927. Since 1975, the World Health Organization (WHO) has stipulated that any vaccine must be derived from the 17D strain. The vaccine is efficacious, providing life-long immunity.

Yellow fever vaccine is required for travel to areas where the disease is prevalent[42]. There is no indication for vaccination within the USA.

During more than 50 years of use, and despite extensive retrospective examination of worldwide experience, the vaccine has not been implicated as the cause of fetal damage[42]. However, a case of transplacental infection with the vaccine virus has been reported[66].

Travel to endemic areas is to be discouraged during pregnancy[47]. As with all live virus vaccines, there is a theoretical risk to the developing fetus. However, when pregnant women are at risk of significant exposure, due to unavoidable travel to regions where yellow fever is endemic, the vaccine can be administered[4,67].

Adenovirus

Adenovirus epidemics that may affect 80% of a population and result in hospitalization of 20% have been common in military recruits[42]. Adenovirus types 3, 4 and 7 account for most epidemics. A live attenuated virus vaccine, active against types 4 and 7, was made available in 1980. Since then it has been used only in the military, where adenovirus type 4 and 7 epidemics are now rare. As with live vaccines in general, adenovirus vaccine is best avoided during pregnancy.

Venezuelan equine encephalitis (VEE)

The VEE virus is distributed in South and Central America and Texas. Equines are the usual hosts for the organism, which is transmitted by mosquitoes. Human illness includes a spectrum from asymptomatic to significant central nervous system symptoms with nuchal rigidity and seizures. Administration of a live attenuated virus vaccine, TC-83, is recommended for some laboratory workers. Concerns regarding possible teratogenicity of wild virus and the vaccine virus have been raised[68]. Pregnancy is a contraindication to TC-83 vaccine[68].

INACTIVATED VIRUS VACCINES

Influenza

Influenza is an acute febrile illness associated with headaches, myalgias, upper airway respiratory complaints and gastrointestinal symptoms. Primary influenza pneumonia, which is usually fatal, may occur in those with cardiopulmonary disease. Most fatalities associated with influenza are due to secondary bacterial pneumonia, however. The epidemiology of influenza is characterized by seasonal epidemics with occasional pandemics. Human influenza is caused by influenza virus types A and B. There are three influenza A subtypes determined by the surface glycoproteins, hemaglutinin (HA) and neuraminidase (NA), referred to as H1N1, H2N2 and H3N2. HA and NA contribute to epidemics by a process of evolution, or antigenic drift, to produce unique virus strains to which immunity in the population is nonexistent. Antigenic shift, in which one influenza subtype replaces another, accounts for other epidemics. Every 10–40 years, new strains are so antigenically novel that pandemics occur. The natural infection has no proven causal relationship to congenital defects[69]. Viremia, a requirement for transplacental infection, is strongly suspected to occur during influenza infection, however[69]. Whether the fetus is more prone to spontaneous abortion, low birth weight and prematurity in association with influenza in pregnancy is controversial[19,70]. The attack rate appeared to be increased in pregnant women during the 1957 pandemic[70]. During pandemics, women in late gestation may be at increased risk of severe illness and mortality[2,69,70]. The effect of influenza on pregnant women is controversial, however[71]. Studies of morbidity and mortality from influenza since 1957 may not support an increased risk for pregnant women[72]. The CDC concluded, however, that the relative risk of hospitalization may be 4.7 times greater in pregnant compared to nonpregnant women[73].

There are three types of inactivated influenza vaccine (killed whole virus, detergent-disrupted split-viruses and purified subunits of HA and NA). Only the split virus and whole virus preparations are manufactured in the US. Influenza vaccine must be administered annually so as to produce immunity to the latest strains. Each year's influenza vaccine contains three virus strains (two type A and one type B) that are likely to circulate during the upcoming flu season[73]. The effectiveness of the vaccine in preventing or alleviating the course of the illness depends on the age and immunocompetence of patients and the similarity between the virus strains in the vaccine and circulating viruses. The vaccine is effective in about 70% of healthy patients less than 65 years of age and in about 30–60% of older patients[2].

The Advisory Committee on Immunization Practices recommends vaccination to: (1) high-risk groups (patients at increased risk for influenza-related complications); (2) health care providers and household members of the high-risk groups; and (3) anyone who desires vaccination. High-risk groups include: (1) persons of 65 years of age or older; (2) residents of nursing homes or other chronic-care facilities: (3) persons with chronic pulmonary (e.g. asthma) or cardiovascular diseases; and (4) persons with chronic metabolic diseases (including diabetes mellitus), renal dysfunction, hemoglobinopathies and immunosuppression; (5) children receiving long-term aspirin therapy who are at risk of developing Reye Syndrome after influenza; and (6) pregnant women who will be in the second or third trimester during the influenza season[73]. It is estimated that an average of 1–2 hospitalizations can be prevented for every 1000 pregnant women immunized[73].

Pregnant women respond to a monovalent influenza vaccine in a manner equivalent to that of non-pregnant women[70,71]. Although experience is limited, inactivated influenza vaccine does not appear to be associated with an increased rate of adverse pregnancy outcomes[69,71,74] or fetal production of vaccine-specific IgM antibodies. No teratogenic influence is suspected. Placental transfer of maternal IgG influenza antibodies does occur and may theoretically confer protection on the fetus and neonate[71,74]. The merit of immunizing mothers for the purpose of eliminating them as sources of viral exposure to infants, as suggested by Sumaya and Gibbs[71], has not been determined. Influenza vaccine does not affect the safety of breast-feeding nor does breastfeeding alter the immune response to the vaccine[73].

Hepatitis A

Hepatitis A, spread person-to-person by the fecal–oral route, is usually a self-limited illness although recovery takes 4–6 weeks. Epidemics occur approximately every

10 years in the USA[75]. There is no chronic carrier state or chronic liver disease associated with hepatitis A. The highest rates occur in native Americans, in the western USA, and settings where living conditions are crowded[75]. Rates are higher in children than in adults[75]. The most common sources of infection are household or sexual contacts, children or employees of day care centers or their contacts, international travellers, food- or water-borne outbreaks, drug users, and men who have sex with other men[75]. Hepatitis A is endemic in Southeast Asia, Africa, Central America, Greenland, Mexico and the Middle East[76]. Food handlers increase the risk of transmitting hepatitis A. Patients with chronic liver disease are at increased risk of fulminant severe infection. Only isolated cases of perinatal infection have been reported[77]. Therefore, unless the mother becomes severely ill, hepatitis does not pose a serious risk to the fetus[77].

Hepatitis A vaccine (HAV) was first licensed for use in the USA in 1995. Two hepatitis A vaccines are currently available in the USA, HAVRIX (SmithKline Beecham) and VAQTA (Merck and Co.). Both are inactivated virus vaccines. The ability to induce seroconversion and prevent infection is the same for both vaccine preparations[78].

Vaccination is recommended for individuals at increased risk and for anyone desiring immunity[75]. Individuals at increased risk who should be vaccinated include[75]:

1.   International traveller's to areas where hepatitis A is endemic at high or intermediate levels
2.   Children living in communities with high rates of hepatitis A virus infection
3.   Men who have sex with other men
4.   Illegal drug users
5.   Persons with occupational risk, specifically those handling non-human primates that are infected with hepatitis A or those working with hepatitis A in a research setting
6.   Individuals with chronic liver disease
7.   Individuals with clotting factor disorders who receive clotting factor concentrates.

Presently, there is no recommendation for vaccination of day care attendees or staff, the institutionalized, food handlers, or for other occupations[78].

According to the CDC's Advisory Committee on Immunization Practices, the safety of hepatitis A vaccine during pregnancy has not been established[75]. The American College of Obstetricians and Gynecologists stated that hepatitis A vaccine may be taken during pregnancy[76] and Duff concluded that the vaccine is safe for use during pregnancy[77]. The vaccine is an inactivated virus so no risk to the fetus would be expected. The risk of the vaccine should be weighed against the risk of illness in women who are at high risk for exposure to hepatitis A[75,78].

The vaccine replaces immune globulin (IG) for pre-exposure prophylaxis[75]. Immune globulin should still be used in susceptible individuals for post-exposure prophylaxis. Hepatitis A vaccine should be given to travellers 4 weeks before departure. Travellers who must depart in less than 4 weeks should receive the vaccine and IG at different sites[75]. IG is not necessary for persons who received the vaccine at least one month before exposure[78]. IG interferes with response to live virus but not to inactivated virus vaccines[78]. IG can be given at same time as HAV if the injections are made at different sites[75]. Current indications for post-exposure prophylaxis with IG include[78]:

1.   Household contacts of patients with hepatitis A
2.   Attendees and staff at same day care center as hepatitis A-infected person
3.   Other food handlers at same restaurant as infected person
4.   Close contacts of institutionalized person with hepatitis A

Immune globulin can be safely used during pregnancy and during lactation[78]. Postpartum mothers who are rubella non-immune are candidates for combined live virus mumps, measles, and rubella (MMR) vaccine. Mothers who receive IG less than 2 weeks after MMR vaccine need to be revaccinated with MMR 5 months following IG[78]. The newborn delivered of a mother with acute hepatitis A infection should receive IG to reduce the risk of horizontal transmission[77].

Rabies

Rabies is a nearly 100% fatal viral encephalitis that is transmitted to humans by the bite or scratch of rabid animals, including domesticated and wild canines and felines in addition to mongooses, skunks, raccoons and bats.

By the end of the 19th century, Pasteur had developed a live bovine rabies virus vaccine attenuated by intracerebral passage through rabbits. His first vaccinee was 9-year-old Josef Meister who survived 14 bites from a rabid dog. Modern vaccines are viruses inactivated by a modification of the Simple method[79]. There are three currently available vaccines in the USA for pre-exposure and post-exposure administration: human diploid cell vaccine (HDCV), rabies vaccine adsorbed (RVA) propagated in fetal rhesus diploid cells, and purified chick embryo cell culture (PCEC) vaccine[80]. The combination of pet control and vaccination in the USA has nearly eliminated human rabies[42].

Like tetanus toxoid, rabies vaccine is indicated for pre-exposure and post-exposure prophylaxis[42]. Candidates for pre-exposure prophylaxis are laboratory workers and veterinarians, spelunkers and travellers to endemic areas where rabies vaccine may not be available[42]. Post-exposure prophylaxis is indicated in individuals bitten by a rabid or potentially rabid animal. Human rabies immune globulin (HRIG) and the first dose of rabies vaccine are provided immediately following the injury[42]. Five doses of rabies vaccine are recommended by the Immunization Practices Advisory Committee to be given initially and at days 3, 7, 14, and 28 following rabies exposure[79]. The World Health Organization recommends a sixth dose on day 90[79].

The inactivated rabies vaccines should not present a fetal risk and limited experience with an older vaccine, duck embryo vaccine (DEV), and HDCV during pregnancy supports this assumption[79].

Given the mortality associated with rabies and the efficacy of the vaccine, rabies vaccine should be administered to exposed pregnant women. Pre-exposure candidates would best avoid the area or activity for the duration of pregnancy, if possible.

Japanese encephalitis

The Japanese encephalitis virus is an endemic cause of viral encephalitis in the Far East. The only indication for the vaccine is to protect travellers and military personnel. It is appropriate to give three doses to travellers to rural areas of endemic regions if they will be staying for more than 2 weeks during summer months[42]. The safety of the vaccine in pregnancy is unknown. As with other inactivated virus vaccines, the theoretic risk to pregnancy is minimal. However, administration during pregnancy should be considered only when travel to an endemic region is unavoidable in which case the risk of natural infection probably outweighs the risk of the vaccine.

TOXOIDS

Tetanus

Clostridium tetani is an anaerobic spore-forming bacillus. Spores germinate under anaerobic conditions to produce bacilli which elaborate toxin with characteristic effects on the central nervous system. In developing countries, neonatal tetanus is the most common form of the disease, accounting for 10–30% of all tetanus cases[81]. The case-fatality rate of neonatal tetanus ranges from 20 to 100%[81]. In Bangladesh, between 1975 and 1977, the infant death rate due to tetanus alone was 25 per 1000 live births[82].

Tetanus vaccine, like diphtheria vaccine, is a toxoid. Tetanus and diphtheria vaccines are usually administered concomitantly. In the USA, current recommendations are for primary vaccination with three doses of toxoid to be followed by booster injections every 10 years[83]. In the setting of a potentially infected but otherwise clean and minor wound, no treatment is necessary if the patient has had a tetanus booster within the past 10 years and has completed the primary series of three doses of adsorbed tetanus toxoid[83]. Otherwise, a single dose of tetanus combined with diphtheria toxoid is recommended[83]. In the case of an extensive injury or wound contamination, the recommendations are the same, except that the interval should be 5 years since the last booster[83]. In these complicated cases, human tetanus immune globulin should also be administered if the patient has not had the primary vaccine series[83].

Fetal vaccine risks are minimal since tetanus toxoid has little teratogenic potential. Experience with mass vaccination during pregnancy in Bangladesh identified no unexpected adverse fetal effects of the vaccine[82]. In many parts of the world, maternal tetanus vaccination contributes to the reduction of neonatal tetanus. Although the high levels of antibody acquired from the mother may interfere with neonatal active immunization, protection at birth is so beneficial that it clearly outweighs this disadvantage[84]. Tetanus toxoid, which crosses the placenta, may actively immunize the fetus if administered in the last trimester[7]. The recommendations for vaccination of adults in the US are not altered by pregnancy. If a tetanus booster is due, then it should be administered[4]. To confer passive immunity on the neonate, it is necessary to administer the first dose of a two-dose primary series of toxoid at least 60 days before and the second dose at least 20 days before delivery[81].

Diphtheria

Diphtheria is a bacterial respiratory infection caused by Gram-positive *Corynebacterium diphtheriae*. Release of an exotoxin during the acute infection results in damage to the kidneys, nervous system and myocardium. More than 200 000 cases, 5–10% of which were fatal, were reported in 1921[83]. During the 4-year period, 1980–1983, only 15 cases of respiratory diphtheria were reported, attesting to the effectiveness of vaccination programs[83]. The rarity of diphtheria makes its effects on pregnancy difficult to ascertain.

Diphtheria toxoid exists in two dosages, 'D' (normal dose) for use in children less than 7-years-old and 'd' (reduced dose) for use in adults. The reduced-dose adult form is necessary because the number and frequency of adverse reactions to diphtheria toxoid increase with age.

Diphtheria toxoid is normally administered in combination with tetanus and acellular pertussis (DTaP) to children as a primary series of four doses. Persons over 7-years-old should routinely receive dT every 10 years and whenever tetanus booster is otherwise indicated[83]. Adults who have not received primary vaccination should receive a primary series of three doses every 4–8 weeks using dT[83]. Close contacts of diphtheria patients should receive diphtheria toxoid if they have not had a booster injection within 5 years[83].

Diphtheria toxoid has no known effect on pregnancy or organogenesis. Pregnancy is not a contraindication to toxoid vaccines. If the patient is due for diphtheria booster, she should be vaccinated regardless of pregnancy[1,4].

VIRAL SUBUNIT

Hepatitis B

Groups at risk of hepatitis B virus (HBV) infection include people with multiple sexual partners, intravenous drug users, blood or blood product recipients, caretakers and residents in institutions for the developmentally disabled, and the sexual and household contacts of those at risk[76]. Other high-risk groups are medical care personnel, hemodialysis patients, homosexual men, and infants of HBV carrier mothers[42]. Some include in the high-risk group persons with histories of sexually transmitted diseases and household members having contact with HBV carriers[4]. Mothers who are positive for hepatitis B surface antigen (HBsAg) have a 10–20% chance of neonatal transmission[76]. Infants born to mothers who are positive for both HBsAg and hepatitis B e antigen (HBeAg) have a 90% chance of acquiring HBV infection at birth[76]. Ninety per cent of neonates infected at birth will develop a chronic carrier state compared to only 10–20% of toddlers and 5–10% of adults[85]. There is a 50% estimated lifetime risk of developing hepatocellular carcinoma among male chronic carriers[86].

There is no evidence that pregnancy influences the course of hepatitis B infection or that infection affects pregnancy. The major risk of natural infection during pregnancy is vertical transmission to the neonate.

The first vaccine for hepatitis B in the USA (Heptavax-B), licensed in 1981 but no longer available, was HBsAg purified from pooled HBV carrier sera. In 1984, a recombinant HBV vaccine was introduced which uses a plasmid carrying the gene for HBsAg inserted into brewer's yeast. There are two such recombinant vaccines available in the USA, Recombivax-HB (Merck and Co.) and Engerix-B (SmithKline Beecham Pharmaceuticals). They are equally efficacious and can be used interchangeably[77]. 95% to 99% of healthy vaccine recipients develop protective levels of antibody after all three doses[77]. Groups at risk of exposure should be immunized, including pregnant women. The American College of Obstetricians and Gynecologists recommends not only that pregnant women receive the vaccine but that they be specifically targeted for vaccination[76]. No unusual untoward reactions to the vaccine have been reported during pregnancy. Data are not available to establish the fetal safety of the vaccine during pregnancy with certainty. However, since the vaccine contains a noninfectious viral component, the theoretical risks are minimal.

In addition, pregnancy is not a contraindication to hepatitis B immune globulin (HBIG)[76]. Pregnant women in high-risk groups who are HBsAg-negative should receive the vaccine. Pregnant women who have household or sexual exposure to persons with HBV infection should receive HBIG in addition to the vaccine[76]. If the exposure is sexual, then one dose of HBIG is sufficient. If the exposure involves mucus membrane or skin penetration, then a second dose, one month after the first, is recommended[76]. Universal vaccination of all neonates in the USA, beginning at birth, is currently recommended[87]. Neonates of HBsAg-negative mothers need only vaccine. Neonates of HBsAg-positive mothers should receive both the vaccine and passive immunization with HBIG[87]. Identification of maternal HBsAg carriers, in order to permit passive as well as active immunization of their neonates, is a requirement of prenatal care. Selective screening based on risk factors will miss approximately half of the neonates at risk in inner city areas[88]. Therefore, universal screening for HBsAg is recommended by the Centers for Disease Control[88] and the American College of Obstetricians and Gynecologists (ACOG)[76]. HBIG and the vaccine should be given simultaneously at different sites within 12 hours of birth to those neonates whose mothers are HBsAg-positive or whose HBsAg status is unknown[76]. The rate of HBV carriers among neonates born to mothers who are both HBeAg-positive and HBsAg-positive is reduced from 70–90% to 5–10% as a result of combined active and passive immunization, an efficacy of 80–90%[89].

CAPSULAR POLYSACCHARIDE VACCINES

Group B streptococcus

Infection with invasive group B streptococcus (GBS) of strain types I, II, III, and V has an incidence of 3 per 1000 live births[90]. Absence of GBS type III capsular polysaccharide antibody is more frequent in women whose neonates develop early onset disease[91], characterized by onset within the first 7 days of life, pneumonia and a case-mortality rate of 5–20%[92]. Preterm infants acquire proportionally lower levels of maternal immunoglobulin G, which may be the mechanism for a higher rate of symptomatic GBS infections in neonates born before 36 weeks gestation[92]. Since GBS affects the neonate, whose immune system is immature, a prevention strategy other than active immunization has been pursued. GBS type III polysaccharide vaccine administered to pregnant women induced sufficient antibody capable of crossing the placenta and conferring passive protection on the neonate in only 63% of cases[90]. Antibody appeared to persist for at least 3 months in the majority of neonates[90], comparable to the degree of passive immunity conferred by other polysaccharide vaccines. Vaccines composed of types I, II, III, and V polysaccharides covalently linked to protein carriers, such as tetanus toxoid, are being developed to improve immunogenicity[92]. Passive neonatal immunization by administering immunoglobulin G after delivery has not proved successful in preventing GBS disease of neonates[92].

Haemophilus influenzae type b

Haemophilus influenzae type b (Hib) is the major cause of meningitis in children, and an important cause of pneumonia and septicemia, especially among native American populations. In high-risk groups, the majority of infections occur before the age of 1 year, 40% in the first 6 months after birth[93]. Although polyribose phosphate (PRP) vaccine, the Hib capsular polysaccharide, was licensed in 1985 for universal administration at 2 years of age, this vulnerable period remained unprotected.

An important strategy has been the development of increasingly immunogenic vaccines sufficient to provoke responses even from immature immune systems[5]. These vaccines are PRP conjugated to diphtheria toxoid (PRP-D), diphtheria CRM197 protein (HbOC) and meningococcal outer membrane protein (PRP-OMP). PRP-D, HbOC and PRP-OMP are efficacious and currently licensed for use as a primary series beginning as early as 2 months of age to be followed by a booster dose at 15 months[94]. In 1993, Tetramune, the first combination vaccine against diphtheria, tetanus, pertussis and Hib diseases, was licensed for clinical use[94]. It consists of HbOC and DTP vaccine.

Another strategy is to enhance neonatal passive immunization by maternal vaccination[5,6]. Maternal active immunization results in much higher levels of antibodies than in control women; this is reflected in high levels of antibody in the neonatal circulation when the maternal vaccine is administered in the late third trimester[6]. A third strategy is to confer passive immunization by administration of bacterial polysaccharide immune globulin (BPIG) prepared from the pooled plasma of adult donors immunized with Hib, pneumococcal and meningococcal vaccines[93]. BPIG is effective in preventing Hib bacteremia and meningitis which suggests that it should be used prophylactically in groups at high risk, including infants[93].

Pneumococcus

Pneumococcal infection accounts for 10–20% of all cases of bacterial meningitis[95] and 25–35% of all cases of community-acquired pneumonia requiring hospitalization in the USA[96]. Especially in the elderly and those with chronic disease, mortality remained high despite antibiotics, lending impetus to the development of an effective preventive agent. The current pneumococcal vaccine is composed of the purified capsular polysaccharide from 23 different serotypes of the bacterium in a formulation designed to protect against 90% of pneumococcal infections[95]. Case-control studies suggest an efficacy of approximately 60–70% in USA populations targeted for the vaccine[97]. Current populations for whom routine vaccination is recommended are persons 65-years-old or older and persons 2 to 64 years old with cardiovascular or pulmonary disease, diabetes mellitus, alcoholism, chronic liver disease, cerebrospinal fluid leak, functional or anatomic asplenia, or living in special setting or social environments (e.g. certain native American populations)[96]. Persons less than 65-years-old at last vaccination should be revaccinated every 5 years[96]. A more immunogenic pneumococcal vaccine preparation is needed, particularly for children less than 2-years-old. The development of a protein-polysaccharide conjugate vaccine for selected capsular types holds promise[96]. The safety of pneumococcal vaccine for pregnant women has not been evaluated[97]. Ideally, women at high risk of pneumococcal disease should be vaccinated before pregnancy[97]. However, as with the other purified polysaccharide vaccines, the risk is theoretical and presumably minimal. The American College of Obstetricians and Gynecologists recommends the use of pneumococcal vaccine in women at high risk for pneumococcal infection, such as in women who have undergone splenectomy[4].

Meningococcus

Neisseria meningitidis has become the leading cause of bacterial meningitis in children and young adults in the USA with a case-fatality rate of 13%[98]. Large epidemics are often the result of infection with *N. meningitidis* serotypes A and C. A quadrivalent capsular polysaccharide vaccine against meningococcal groups A, C, Y and W-135 is available in the USA. Immunization is indicated for persons with complement deficiencies, functionally or anatomically asplenic patients, travellers to endemic areas, and research, industrial or clinical laboratory personnel who are routinely exposed to *N. meningitidis*[98]. Vaccination of entire populations, including pregnant women, has been achieved during epidemics without any demonstrable untoward effect on the fetus[99]. The Advisory Committee on Immunization Practices states that vaccination during pregnancy has not documented adverse effect among pregnant women or neonates; altering meningococcal vaccination recommendations during pregnancy is not necessary[98].

OTHER SUBUNITS
Pertussis

Bordetella pertussis is a cause of severe respiratory illness in children, producing whooping cough, pneumonia and occasional deaths. Pertussis infection in adults is more likely to produce mild non-specific respiratory illness. For the past decade, there have been several thousands cases of pertussis annually[100]. The effects of pertussis on pregnancy are unknown.

Whole cell pertussis vaccine is associated with severe local reactions, mild systemic events, and rarely with convulsions, hypotonic episodes, and acute encephalopathy[101]. Acellular pertussis contains inactivated pertussis toxin and one or more other bacterial components[101]. The acellular preparation has fewer local and systemic reactions than the whole-cell vaccine[101]. The US Food and Drug Administration first approved an acellular pertussis vaccine in 1996[102]. There are presently three diptheria-tetanus-acellular pertussis (DTaP) vaccines (Tripedia, Infanrix, and ACEL-IMUNE) that are licensed by the FDA for at least the first four doses of the five dose series (ACEL-IMUNE is licensed for all five doses)[101]. Whole cell pertussis (in DTP) is still available.

Because the incidence and severity of pertussis declines with age and because the vaccine may cause side-effects and adverse reactions, pertussis vaccination is not recommended after the age of 7 years except for those with chronic pulmonary disease exposed to children with pertussis[83].

There has been no experience with the vaccine in pregnancy, but the acellular preparation should not have an effect on organogenesis. Pertussis vaccination during pregnancy should rarely be absolutely necessary.

Borrelia burgdorferi (Lyme disease)

Lyme disease is the most common vector-borne disease in the USA[103]. Patterns of Lyme disease prevalence reflect the geographic distribution of *Ixodes scapularis* (deer tick)[103]. Ninety per cent of cases occur in ten states located in the upper midwest, mid-Atlantic, and northeast where the deer tick is common[104]. 85% of patients have a characteristic early-stage rash, erythema migrans. The early stage of illness is easily treated with inexpensive antibiotics. Drugs of choice are amoxicillin, ceftriaxone, and doxycycline[103]. Mortality from Lyme disease is negligible. However, the disease can progress to musculoskeletal, neurologic and cardiac complications in the absence of early treatment.

The Food and Drug Administration licensed a vaccine, LYMErix (SmithKline Beecham Biologicals, Reixensart, Belgium), in December 1998[105]. The vaccine is made from recombinant DNA coding for the outer surface protein A (OspA) of the causative spirochete. The vaccine is administered at baseline and again at 1 and 12 months[106,107]. Efficacy is 76% to 92% in the year following the third injection[106,107]. The vaccine is safe in persons more than 15-years-old, causing no serious adverse events and only mild local discomfort[106,107]. There are a number of concerns related to the vaccine. It is unknown how long protection lasts, but antibody levels decrease rapidly[104]. Annual booster shots may become necessary[104]. Because the third dose is given at 12 months, complete protection is not available during a single season. A shorter interval between the second and third doses is expected in the future[104]. No efficacy or safety studies have been done in children who account for a significant percentage of Lyme disease cases. There is concern that vaccination may only mask the early stage of disease and result in more late complications of Lyme disease[104]. Lyme disease is not spread from person-to-person so that the vaccine cannot control spread of the disease through herd immunity[104]. The vaccine may not be cost-effective and may be unnecessary since there is a recognizable and easily and inexpensively treated early stage of illness[104].

Universal use is not recommended[104]. Candidates for the currently available vaccine might be persons 15 to 65 years of age who spend time out-of-doors in regions where Lyme disease is highly endemic[104].

Vaccine use is not recommended for pregnant women as pregnant women were excluded from phase III trials[104].

LIVE BACTERIA
Tuberculosis

In some parts of the world, the risk of acquiring tuberculosis is as high as 2% per annum with 80% of persons becoming tuberculin-positive by young adulthood[108]. From 1953, when national surveillance for TB began, until 1985, TB was on the decline in the USA. There followed a resurgence of TB between 1985 and 1992. In 1992, TB prevalence was 10.5 cases per 100 000 population. Since 1992, TB cases have again been on the decline[109].

Calmette and Guerin developed an attenuated strain of *Mycobacterium bovis*, the bacillus of Calmette and Guerin (BCG). More than a billion doses of BCG vaccine have been administered, mostly in the developing world. Although BCG is more than 80% effective in preventing serious TB infection in children, its effectiveness in adolescents and adults is variable and equivocal. In addition, reactivity to the tuberculin test after previous BCG vaccination interferes with management of patient who may be asymptomatically infected with *M. tuberculosis*. In the USA, BCG vaccination is not routinely recommended as a method of controlling TB. Rather, the fundamental strategy in controlling TB involves early detection and treatment of patients with active or asymptomatic infection with *M. tuberculosis*. Asymptomatic infection can be related with isoniazid or rifampin, the latter for isoniazid-resistant *M. tuberculosis*[109].

BCG may be considered for children continually exposed to patients with pulmonary tuberculosis and selected health care workers in endemic settings[109].

The risks of vaccine in pregnancy are unknown. However, because the vaccine is a live attenuated mycobacterium strain, the potential for fetal infection exists. BCG should not be administered to persons whose immunological responses are either impaired or suppressed[109]. Therefore, BCG vaccination during pregnancy is not recommended[109].

INACTIVATED BACTERIA

Cholera

Cholera caused by the El Tor type of Vibrio cholerae has been epidemic throughout much of Asia, the Middle East and Africa and in some parts of Europe. Infection is usually by consuming contaminated food and water. Cholera vaccines reduce the incidence of clinical disease by 50% and then only for a short time[110]. Vaccination against cholera is not required by the USA Public Health Service for visitors from cholera-endemic areas of the world. Nor does the World Health Organization recommend vaccination of international travellers to cholera-endemic areas[110]. The only reason to vaccinate against cholera is for travel to those countries that require proof of cholera vaccination for entry. There is no information concerning the safety of cholera vaccine during pregnancy[110]. Since the vaccine is an inactivated organism, the theoretical risk is low. There should rarely be a need to consider cholera vaccination during pregnancy. However, if travel to a country requiring cholera vaccination is unavoidable during pregnancy, the vaccine may be given.

CONCLUSION

Pregnant women should routinely be administered diphtheria and tetanus toxoids (as dT) if it has been more than 10 years since their last injection. Those at risk should receive hepatitis B, influenza, and pneumococcus vaccines. Unavoidable international travel during pregnancy may require hepatitis A, measles, poliovirus, yellow fever, Japanese encephalitis, meningococcus, and/or cholera vaccination. None of these are known teratogens, but several are live viruses. Patients should be counseled about the theoretical concerns of fetal infection, especially regarding live virus vaccines. Use of other vaccines should be individualized.

Under certain circumstances, passive immunization with VZIG, HBIG, and immune globulin (for hepatitis

A and rubella exposure) may be warranted for exposed pregnant women.

Pregnant women with young children at home should not alter their children's vaccination schedules. The possible exception might be varicella vaccination, in which case household contacts of pregnant women might wait until the last half of pregnancy or until after pregnancy.

All expectant mothers should have serology for rubella and should have hepatitis B screening. Mothers who are negative for rubella IgG should receive MMR vaccine postpartum if they will avoid pregnancy for 3 months. Blood and blood products may interfere with seroconversion in response to live virus vaccines. Mothers who receive blood or blood products in the third trimester, at delivery, or postpartum, including anti-Rho globulin for Rh-negative patients, should be retested for immunity in 3 months following MMR administration, if possible.

Infants of mothers who are HBsAg-positive or whose HBsAg status is unknown should receive HBIG within 12 hours of birth. All neonates should be vaccinated with hepatitis B. An infant of a mother who has an outbreak of varicella zoster infection between 5 days before until 2 days after delivery should receive VZIG. Certain preterm newborns should receive VZIG for postnatal exposure to varicella.

No vaccine given during the preconceptional period or during the first trimester is considered a reason to recommend termination of pregnancy. Mothers should be counseled concerning the theoretical risk. In cases of rubella vaccine given between 3 months before until 3 months after conception, the CDC calculated that the theoretical maximum risk of congenital rubella syndrome (CRS) was 1.2%. The observed risk was zero after observing 324 exposed neonates.

Breastfeeding is never a contraindication to any vaccine nor should breastfeeding be abandoned because of vaccine administration.

REFERENCES

1. Amstey MS. Immunization in pregnancy. *Clin Obstet Gynecol* 1976;19:47–54
2. Advisory Committee on Immunization Practices. Prevention and control of influenza. *MMWR* 1996; 45(RR-5):1–25
3. Paryani S, Arvin A. Intrauterine infection with varicella-zoster after maternal varicella. *N Engl J Med* 1986;314: 1542–6
4. ACOG Technical Bulletin No. 160: *Immunization During Pregnancy*. Washington, DC: American College of Obstetricians and Gynecologists, 1991
5. Insel RA. Maternal immunization to prevent neonatal infection. *N Engl J Med* 1989;319:1219–20
6. Amstey MS, Insel R, Munoz J, Pichichero M. Fetal-neonatal passive immunization against haemophilus influenzae type b. *Am J Obstet Gynecol* 1985;153:607–11

7. Gill 3rd T, Repetti CF, Metlay LA, *et al*. Transplacental immunization of the human fetus to tetanus by immunization of the mother. *J Clin Invest* 1983; 72:987–96

8. Centers for Disease Control. General Recommendations on Immunization: Recommendations of the Advisory Committee on Immunization Practices (ACIP). *MMWR* 1994;43(RR-1):1–38

9. Gregg NM. Congenital cataract following German measles in the mother. *Trans Opthal Soc Aust* 1941;3: 35–46

10. Orenstein W, Bart K, Hinman A, *et al*. The opportunity and obligation to eliminate rubella from the United States. *J Am Med Assoc* 1984;251:1988–94

11. Cooper L, Preblud S, Alford Jr. C. Rubella. In: Remington J, Klein J, eds. *Infectious Diseases of the Fetus and Newborn Infant*, 4th Edition. Philadelphia: WB Saunders Company, 1995

12. Centers for Disease Control. Measles, mumps, and rubella—vaccine use and strategies for elimination of measles, rubella, and congenital rubella syndrome and control of mumps. *MMWR* 1998;47(RR-8): 1–57

13. Centers for Disease Control. Rubella prevention. *MMWR* 1984;33:301–18

14. Shlian DM. Screening and immunization of rubella–susceptible women: experience in a large prepaid medical group. *J Am Med Assoc* 1978;240:662–3

15. Cohen ZB, Rice LI, Felice ME. Rubella seronegativity in a low socioeconomic adolescent female population. *Clin Pediatr* 1985;24:387–9

16. Marshall WC, Peckham CS, Dudgeon JA, *et al*. Parity of women contracting rubella in pregnancy. Implications with respect to rubella vaccination. *Lancet* 1976; 1(7971):1231–3

17. Lee SH, Ewert DP, Frederick PD, Mascola L. Resurgence of congenital rubella syndrome in the 1990s: report on missed opportunities and failed prevention policies among women of childbearing age. *J Am Med Assoc* 1992;267:2616–20

18. Preblud SR. Some current issues relating to rubella vaccine *J Am Med Assoc* 1985;254:253–6

19. Hart RJC. Immunization. *Clin Obstet Gynaecol* 1981;8:421–30

20. Centers for Disease Control. Update: vaccine side effects, adverse reactions, contraindications, and precautions. Recommendations of the advisory Committee on Immunization Practices. *MMWR* 1996; 45(RR-12):1–35

21. Preblud SR, Stetler HC, Frank Jr. JA, *et al*. Fetal risk associated with rubella vaccine. *J Am Med Assoc* 1981; 246:1413–17

22. Fleet Jr. WF, Benz Jr. EW, Karzon DT, *et al*. Fetal consequences of maternal rubella immunization. *J Am Med Assoc* 1974;227:621–7

23. Centers for Disease Control. Rubella vaccination during pregnancy – United States, 1971–1988. *J Am Med Assoc* 1989;261:3374–83

24. Sheppard S, Smithells RW, Dickson A, Holzel H. Rubella vaccination and pregnancy: preliminary report of a national survey. *Br Med J* (Clin Res) 1986;292:727

25. Enders G. Rubella antibody titer in vaccinated and nonvaccinated women and results of vaccination during pregnancy. *Rev Infect Dis* 1985;7(suppl 1): S103–S107

26. ACOG Technical Bulletin No. 171: *Rubella and Pregnancy*. Washington, DC: American College of Obstetricians and Gynecologists, 1992

27. Landes RD, Bass JW, Millunchick EW, Oetgen WJ. Neonatal rubella following postpartum maternal immunization. *J Pediatr* 1980;97:465–7

28. Krogh V, Duffy LC, Wong D, *et al*. Postpartum immunization with rubella virus vaccine and antibody response in breastfeeding infants. *J Lab Clin Med* 1989; 113:695–9

29. Doege TC, Kim K. Studies of rubella and its prevention with immune globulin. *J Am Med Assoc* 1967;200: 104–10

30. Centers for Disease Control. Measles – United States, 1997. *MMWR* 1998;47:273–6

31. Preblud SR, Katz SL. Measles vaccine. In: Plotkin SA, Mortimer Jr. EA, eds. *Vaccines*. Philadelphia: WB Saunders, 1988

32. Siegel M. Congenital malformations following chicken-pox, masles, mumps, and hepatitis. *J Am Med Assoc* 1973;226:1521–4

33. Levine MM, Edsall G, Bruce-Chwatt LJ. Live-virus vaccines in pregnancy. Risks and recommendations. *Lancet* 1974;2:34–8

34. Mann JM, Montes JM, Hull HF, *et al*. Risk of pregnancy among adolescent schoolgirls participating in a measles mass vaccination program. *Am J Public Health* 1983;73:527–9

35. Blouse LE, Lathrop GD, Dupuy HJ, Ball RJ. Rubella screening and vaccination program for US Air Force trainees: an analysis of findings. *Am J Public Health* 1982;72:280–3

36. Garcia AG, Pereira JM, Vidigal N, *et al*. Intrauterine infection with mumps virus. *Obstet Gynecol* 1980;56: 756–9

37. Jones JF, Ray CG, Fulginiti VA. Perinatal mumps infection. *J Pediatr* 1980;96:912–14

38. Weibel RE, Stokes Jr. J, Buynak EB, *et al*. Live attenuated mumps virus vaccine. 3. Clinical and serologic aspects in a field evaluation. *N Engl J Med* 1967;276: 245–51

39. Advisory Committee on Immunization Practices. Mumps prevention. *MMWR* 1988;38:388–400

40. Yamauchi T, Wilson C, St Geme Jr. JW. Transmission of live, attenuated mumps virus to the human placenta. *N Engl J Med* 1974;290:710–2

41. Manson M, Logan W, Loy RM. Reports on Public Health and Medical Subjects, No. 101: *Rubella and Other Virus Infections in Pregnancy*. London: Ministry of Health, 1960

42. Quinnan J. Immunization against viral diseases. In: Galasso G, Whitley R, Merigan T, eds. *Antiviral Agents and Viral Disease of Man*, 3rd Edition. New York: Raven Press, 1990

43. Strebel P, Sutter R, Cochi S, *et al*. Epidemiology of poliomyelitis in the United States one decade after the last reported case of indigenous wild virus–associated disease. *Clin Infect Dis* 1992;14:568–79

44. Centers for Disease Control. Update: Eradication of paralytic poliomyelitis in the Americas. *MMWR* 1992; 41:681–2

45. Centers for Disease Control. Certification of poliomyelitis elimination — the Americas. *MMWR* 1994;43:720–f2

46. Siegel M, Greenberg M. Incidence of poliomyelitis in pregnancy. *N Engl J Med* 1955;253:841–7

47. Blanco JD, Gibbs RS. Immunizations in pregnancy. *Clin Obstet Gynecol* 1982;25:611–17

48. Siegel M, Greenberg M. Poliomyelitis in pregnancy: effect on fetus and newborn infant. *J Pediatr* 1956;49: 280–8

49. Salk J, Drucker J. Noninfectious poliovirus vaccine. In: Plotkin S, Mortimer Jr. EA, eds. *Vaccines*. Philadelphia: WB Saunders, 1988

50. Centers for Disease Control. Poliomyelitis prevention in the United States: introduction of a sequential vaccination schedule of inactivated poliomyelitis vaccine followed by oral poliomyelitis vaccine. Recommendations of the Immunization Practices Advisory Committee. *MMWR* 1997;46 (RR-3):1–25

51. Nkowane BM, Wassilak S, Orenstein WA, *et al*. Vaccine-associated paralytic poliomyelitis. United States: 1973 through 1984. *J Am Med Assoc* 1987;257: 1335–40

52. Terry L. *The Association of Cases of Poliomyelitis with the Use of Type III Oral Poliomyelitis Vaccines: A Technical Report of the United States Surgeon General*. Washington, DC: US Department of Health, Education and Welfare, 1962

53. Melnick JL. Live attenuated poliovaccines. In: Plotkin SA, Mortimer Jr. EA, eds. *Vaccines*. Philadelphia: WB Saunders, 1988

54. Harjulehto T, Aro T, Hovi T, Saxen L. Congenital malformations and oral poliovirus vaccination during pregnancy. *Lancet* 1989;1:771–2

55. Burton AE, Robinson ET, Harper WF, *et al*. Fetal damage after accidental polio vaccination of an immune mother. *J R Coll Gen Prac* 1984;34:390–4

56. Centers for Disease Control. Prevention of varicella: recommendations of the advisory committee on Immunization Practices. *MMWR* 1996;45(RR-11): 1–36

57. Arvin AM. Live attenuated varicella vaccine. *Pediatr Ann* 1997;26:384–8

58. Centers for Disease Control. Varicella-related deaths among adults – United States, 1997. *MMWR* 1997; 46:409–12

59. Gershon AA, Raker R, Steinberg S, *et al*. Antibody to varicella-zoster in parturient women and their offspring in first year of life. *Pediatrics* 1976;58:692–6

60. American Academy of Pediatrics Committee on Infectious Diseases. Recommendations for the use of live attenuated varicella vaccine. *Pediatrics* 1995;95: 791–6

61. Holmes SJ. Review of Recommendations of the Advisory Committee on Immunization Practices, Centers for Disease Control and Prevention, on Varicella Vaccine. *J Infect Dis* 1996;174(Suppl 3): S342–S344

62. Salzman MB, Sharrar RG, Steinberg S, LaRussa P. Transmission of varicella-vaccine virus from a healthy 12-month-old child to his pregnant mother. *J Pediatr* 1997;131:151–4

63. Long SS. Toddler-to-mother transmission of varicella-vaccine virus: how bad is that? *J Pediatr* 1997;131: 10–12

64. Seidman DS, Stevenson DK, Arvin AM. Varicella vaccine in pregnancy: routine screening and vaccination should be considered. *Br Med J* 1996; 313(7059): 701–2

65. Freestone DS. Yellow fever vaccine. In: Plotkin SA, Mortimer Jr. EA, eds. *Vaccines*. Philadephia: WB Saunders, 1988

66. Tsai TF, Paul R, Lynberg MC, Letson GW. Congenital yellow fever virus infection after immunization in pregnancy. *J Infect Dis* 1993;168:1520–23

67. Centers for Disease Control. Yellow Fever Vaccine. Recommendations of the Immunization Practices Advisory Committee. *MMWR* 1990;39(RR-6):1–6

68. Casamassina AC, Hess LW, Marty A. TC-83 Venezuelan equine encephalitis vaccine exposure during pregnancy. *Teratology* 1987;36:287–9

69. MacKenzie JS, Houghton M. Influenza infections during pregnancy: association with congenital malformations and with subsequent neoplasms in children, and potential hazards of live virus vaccines. *Bact Rev* 1974; 38:356–70

70. Murray DL, Imagawa DT, Okada DM, St Geme Jr. JW. Antibody response to monovalent A/New Jersey/8/76 influenza vaccine in pregnant women. *J Clin Micro* 1979;10:184–187

71. Sumaya CV, Gibbs RS. Immunization of pregnant women with influenza A/New Jersey/76 virus vaccine: reactogenicity and immunogenicity in mother and infant. *J Infect Dis* 1979;140:141–146

72. McKinney W, Volkert P, Kaufman J. Fatal swine influenza pneumonia during late pregnancy. *Arch Intern Med* 1990;150:213–5

73. Centers for Disease Control. Prevention and Control of Influenza: Recommendations of the Advisory Committee on Immunization Practices. *MMWR* 1997;46(RR-9):1–25

74. Englund JA, Mbawuike IN, Hammill H, *et al*. Maternal immunization with influenza or tetanus toxoid vaccine for passive antibody protection in young infants. *J Infect Dis* 1993;168:647–56

75. Centers for Disease Control. Prevention of hepatitis A through active or passive immunization: recommendations of the Advisory Committee on Immunization Practices. *MMWR* 1996;45(RR-15):1–30

76. ACOG Educational Bulletin No. 248: Viral *Hepatitis in Pregnancy*. Washington, DC: American College of Obstetricians and Gynecologists, 1998

77. Duff P. Hepatitis in pregnancy. *Sem Perinatol* 1998; 22:277–83

78. Levy M, Herrera J, DiPalma J. Immune globulin and vaccine therapy to prevent hepatitis A infection. *Am J Med* 1998;105:416–23

79. Nicholson KG. Rabies vaccine. In: Zuckerman AJ, ed. *Recent Developments in Prophylactic Immunization*. London: Kluwer Academic Publishers, 1989

80. Centers for Disease Control. Availability of a new rabies vaccine for human use. *MMWR* 1998;47:12,19

81. Chen ST, Edsall G, Peel MM, Sinnathuray TA. Timing of antenatal tetanus immunization for effective protection of the neonate. *Bull World Health Org* 1983;61:159–65

82. Rahman M, Chen LC, Chakraborty J, *et al*. Use of tetanus toxoid for the prevention of neonatal tetanus. 1. Reduction of neonatal mortality by immunization of non-pregnant and pregnant women in rural Bangladesh. *Bull World Health Org* 1982;60:261–7

83. Advisory Committee on Immunization Practices. Diptheria, tetanus, and pertussis: guidelines for vaccine prophylaxis and other preventive measures. *MMWR* 1985;34:405–26

84. Habig WH, Tankersley DL. Tetanus. In: Cryz Jr. SJ, ed. *Vaccines and Immunotherapy*. New York: Pergamon Press, 1991

85. Magriples U. Hepatitis in pregnancy. *Sem Perinatol* 1998;22:112–17

86. Beasley R, Hwang L, Lin C, Chien C. Hepatocellular carcinoma and HBV: a prospective study of 22,707 men in Taiwan. *Lancet* 1981;2:1129–33

87. Centers for Disease Control. Hepatitis B virus: a comprehensive strategy for eliminating transmission in the United States through universal childhood vaccination: recommendations of the Immunization Practices Advisory Committee. *MMWR* 1991;40 (RR-13):1–25

88. Advisory Committee on Immunization Practices. Prevention of perinatal transmission of hepatitis B virus: prenatal screening of all pregnant women for hepatitis B surface antigen. *MMWR* 1988;37:341–51

89. Stevens C. In utero and perinatal transmission of hepatitis viruses. *Pediatr Ann* 1994;23:152–8

90. Baker CJ, Rench MA, Edwards MS, *et al*. Immunization of pregnant women with a polysaccharide vaccine of group B streptococcus. *N Engl J Med* 1988;319:1180–5

91. Baker CJ, Kasper DL. Correlation of maternal antibody deficiency with susceptibility to neonatal group B streptococcal infection. *N Engl J Med* 1976;294:753–6

92. McKenna D, Iams J. Group B streptococcal infections. *Sem Perinatol* 1998;22:267–76

93. Santosham M, Reid R, Ambrosino D, *et al*. Prevention of Haemophilus influenzae type B infections in high-risk infants treated with bacterial polysaccharide immune globulin. *N Engl J Med* 1987;317:923–9

94. Centers for Disease Control. Recommendations for use of Haemophilus b conjugate vaccines and a combined diphtheria, tetanus, pertussis, and Haemophilus b vaccine: recommendations of the Advisory Committee on Immunization Practices (ACIP). *MMWR* 1993;42:1–15

95. Shapiro ED. Pneumococcal vaccine. In: Cryz Jr. SJ, ed. *Vaccines and Immunotherapy*. New York: Pergamon Press, 1991

96. Centers for Disease Control. Prevention of pneumococcal disease: recommendations of the Advisory Committee on Immunization Practices. *MMWR* 1997;46(RR-8):1–24

97. Advisory Committee on Immunization Practices. Pneumococcal polysaccharide vaccine. *MMWR* 1989;38:64–76

98. Centers for Disease Control. Control and prevention of meningococcal disease: recommendations of the Advisory Committee on Immunization Practices. *MMWR* 1997;46(RR-5):1–11

99. McCormick JB, Gusmao HH, Nakamura S, *et al*. Antibody response to serogroup A and C meningococcal polysaccharide vaccines in infants born of mothers vaccinated during pregnancy. *J Clin Invest* 1980;65:1141–4

100. Centers for Disease Control. Resurgence of pertussis – United States, 1993. *MMWR* 1993;42:952–3

101. Centers for Disease Control. Pertussis vaccination: use of acellular pertussis vaccines among infants and young children. *MMWR* 1997;46(RR-7):1–25

102. Centers for Disease Control. Approval of an acellular pertussis vaccine for the initial four doses of the diptheria, tetanus, and pertussis vaccination series. *MMWR* 1996;45:676–7

103. Centers for Disease Control. Lyme Disease – United States, 1996. *MMWR* 1997;46:531–5

104. Gardner P. Lyme disease vaccines. *Ann Intern Med* 1998;129:583–5

105. Centers for Disease Control. Availability of Lyme disease vaccine. *MMWR* 1999;48:35–6,43

106. Steere AC, Sikand VK, Meurice F, *et al*. Vaccination against Lyme disease with recombinant Borrelia burgdorferi outer-surface lipoprotein A with adjuvant. *N Engl J Med* 1998;339:209–15

107. Sigal LH, Zahradnik JM, Lavin P, *et al*. A vaccine consisting of recombinant Borrelia burgdorferi outer-surface protein A to prevent Lyme disease. *N Engl J Med* 1998;339:216–22

108. Snider DE. The tuberculin test. *Am Rev Resp Dis* 1982;125:S108–S118

109. Centers for Disease Control. The role of BCG vaccine in the prevention and control of tuberculosis in the United States: a joint statement by the Advisory Council for the Elimination of Tuberculosis and the Advisory Committee on Immunization Practices. *MMWR* 1996;45(RR-4):1–18

110. Centers for Disease Control. Cholera vaccine. Recommendations of the Immunization Practices Advisory Committee. *MMWR* 1988;37:617–8,623–4

Section IV

Maternal medical disorders

33
Cardiac diseases

P. Cole

INTRODUCTION

Major hemodynamic alterations in the cardiovascular system occur during normal pregnancy, labor and delivery. In addition, because of advanced surgical techniques and improved diagnostic and therapeutic alternatives, greater numbers of women with congenital and acquired heart disease are surviving to the childbearing years. Therefore, management of the pregnant patient, especially those with underlying cardiovascular disease, requires a thorough understanding of both the normal cardiovascular adjustments to pregnancy, as well as the predicted response of the abnormal cardiovascular system to the hemodynamic stresses of pregnancy.

NORMAL CARDIOPULMONARY ADJUSTMENTS DURING PREGNANCY

Symptoms and signs

Symptoms that occur during pregnancy may mimic those of pathological conditions. Frequently reported symptoms include fatigue, dyspnea and decreased exercise tolerance as well as peripheral edema and hyperventilation. Lightheadedness and occasionally syncope can also occur, and are thought to be due in part to a normal fall of systemic arterial pressure. Paroxysmal nocturnal dyspnea and hemoptysis are not normal findings in pregnancy and should be investigated.

On examination, the point of maximum impulse will be laterally displaced, owing to the displacement of the heart by the gravid uterus. Jugular venous pulsations may be unusually prominent.

The first heart sound (S1) will have an increased amplitude and a wide splitting of the two components (mitral and tricuspid) due to early closure of the mitral valve. The second heart sound (S2) is little affected, but the majority of patients (84%) will develop a third heart sound (S3). A fourth heart sound is an unusual finding in pregnancy, present in only 4% of patients. The majority of pregnant women (96%) will have a soft ejection murmur in mid-systole. Half of these are right-sided in origin, with the majority becoming manifest during the second trimester. The presence of a new diastolic murmur during pregnancy is infrequent, and warrants further evaluation.

Cardiovascular hemodynamics

The heart rate increases throughout pregnancy, with a mean increase of 15 beats/min above non-pregnant levels at term, with most of this increase occurring during the first trimester. Twin pregnancies are associated with an even greater increase and, like most hemodynamic measurements, the heart rate is affected by position, with increases in heart rate seen in the sitting or standing position.

Blood pressure appears to be related to both age and parity; mean blood pressure is inversely correlated with parity for any given maternal age, and a rise in both mean systolic and mean diastolic blood pressures is seen as age increases for pregnant patients within each level of parity[1].

Many of the changes in cardiac output and systemic vascular resistance occur during the first 8 weeks of pregnancy[2]. By completion of the embryonic period, systemic vascular resistance can fall to 70% of its preconceptional value. Cardiac output increases up to 20% and 39% above the prepregnancy values by 8.0 weeks and 12 weeks of gestation, respectively. The change in the cardiac outputs from the first trimester to the second trimester is variable and appears to depend on the method of measurement. The change in cardiac outputs from the second trimester to the third trimester is also variable, irrespective of the methods of measurement[3]. Cardiac output may be position-dependent and falls with the supine position. Increase in stroke volume, representing a 22% change over preconception values at 8 weeks in one study, is related to an increase in end-diastolic volume[2]. The point at which cardiac changes regress to preconception levels is debatable; normal levels have been reported from 5 to over 12 weeks postpartum[4,5]. Blood, plasma and red blood cell volume increase up to 50% in correlation with placental weight, number of fetuses, age and parity. Plasma volume increases proportionately more than red blood cell mass, resulting in 'physiological anemia of pregnancy'. The mechanism for expansion in blood volume is not clearly understood, but may be related to hormonal alterations. Uterine blood flow at term may reach 500 ml/min, 10–20 times higher than in the first semester. Renal, mammary, limb and skin blood flow increase markedly, while liver and brain blood flow remain constant.

Alterations during normal labor and delivery

Numerous cardiovascular changes take place during labor and delivery, and these changes are affected by a wide range of variables including anesthesia, analgesia, pain sensation and mode of delivery.

During labor, transient increases in cardiac output occur with each contraction, as well as increases in blood pressure, both systolic and diastolic. These changes are attenuated by anesthesia, with the minimum alterations occurring with spinal or epidural anesthesia, and with the greatest alterations seen during balanced general anesthesia.

Changes in blood volume during delivery are primarily a function of blood loss, with greater loss occurring after Cesarean section rather than vaginal delivery.

These major perturbations in cardiovascular hemodynamics that occur during pregnancy, labor and delivery rapidly revert to normal, and by 5 weeks postpartum are essentially equivalent to the non-pregnant state.

SPECIFIC CARDIOVASCULAR ABNORMALITIES OF LOWER RISK TO THE PREGNANT PATIENT

Atrial septal defect

Ostium secundum atrial septal defect (ASD) is the most common congenital cardiovascular defect seen in pregnancy. Most women are asymptomatic, with an examination that is characterized by a right ventricular heave and a loud systolic ejection murmur at the left sternal border, in addition to a fixed widely split second heart sound. The electrocardiogram (EKG) may show right ventricular hypertrophy and right bundle branch block with a normal axis; the chest X-ray roentgenogram will demonstrate increased pulmonary vascularity and large right-sided chambers. Despite the obligate volume overload in the second trimester, pregnancy is usually well tolerated in the pregnant patient with an ASD.

Numerous reports suggest that pregnancy is safe[6], although there are reports of the development of congestive heart failure and arrhythmias in these patients[7]. The presence of congestive heart failure despite maximum medical therapy is considered to be an indication for surgical repair[8]. Unless the ASD has been repaired using a prosthetic patch, antibiotic prophylaxis during delivery is not indicated.

A small proportion of patients with an ASD will develop pulmonary hypertension and Eisenmenger's syndrome (shunt reversal to a right-to-left shunt due to the development of suprasystemic pulmonary artery pressures). These patients have a markedly higher morbidity and mortality from pregnancy[9] and should be counselled carefully.

Ventricular septal defect

Women who reach childbearing years with an uncorrected ventricular septal defect (VSD) generally have smaller defects that are well tolerated, since the clinical picture is largely determined by the size of the defect; larger defects often require repair in childhood. These patients have physical examinations consistent with a left-to-right shunt, including a holosystolic thrill and murmur along the left sternal border, a loud first heart sound and often a diastolic rumble consistent with increased flow across the mitral valve in diastole. With a small VSD the EKG may be normal but may show evidence of left ventricular hypertrophy and right ventricular hypertrophy with larger defects. The chest X-ray usually shows evidence of right ventricular and left atrial enlargement and, as with as ASD, a contrast echocardiogram can reveal evidence of shunting with detection of bubble turbulence flowing across the defect in a left-to-right fashion.

Pregnancy is usually very well tolerated in women with a VSD[10], possibly because the pregnancy-induced fall in systemic vascular resistance tends to decrease left-to-right shunting. Morbidity and mortality is related to the presence of pulmonary hypertension, with a higher complication rate in those patients with Eisenmenger's physiology[7]. Patients with a VSD complicated by pulmonary hypertension are at risk of significant cardiac decompensation in the immediate postpartum period, when a transient fall in blood pressure and blood volume may cause shunt reversal. Immediate attention to fluid resuscitation and the judicious use of pressors is indicated in this setting.

Patent ductus arteriosus

With improved pediatric surgical techniques, most patients with a patent ductus arteriosus are surgically corrected during infancy and childhood, so it is a rare finding in pregnancy. Many patients are asymptomatic unless there is associated pulmonary hypertension. The physical examination is characterized by a 'machinery' or continuous murmur in the second intercostal space. Both left and right ventricular hypertrophy may be seen on EKG, and the chest radiograph is remarkable for left ventricular and left atrial enlargement, in addition to increased pulmonary vascularity. As with other shunt lesions, Doppler and contrast echocardiography are useful in defining chamber dimensions and shunt detection.

The patient with a patent ductus arteriosus generally tolerates pregnancy well, whether surgically corrected[10] or uncorrected[6,7], but the presence of pulmonary hypertension increases the morbidity and mortality. As with other left-to-right shunt lesions, care should be taken to avoid shunt reversal owing to hypotension and blood loss during the peripartum period.

Mitral regurgitation

The causes of mitral regurgitation are myriad, but in young women of childbearing age the most common etiologies are rheumatic (almost always seen in association with mitral stenosis) and as a component of Barlow's syndrome (click–murmur or mitral valve prolapse syndrome).

The characteristic finding on examination is a holosystolic murmur at the apex which radiates to the axilla, and the EKG may show evidence of left atrial enlargement. Atrial fibrillation is an uncommon finding unless there is marked left atrial enlargement.

In general, pregnancy is very well tolerated, since the normal pregnancy-induced fall in peripheral resistance serves to 'unload' the ventricle. If severe mitral regurgitation results in pulmonary congestion, medical management should include diuresis and prophylactic digoxin, to prevent a rapid ventricular response should atrial fibrillation develop.

Aortic insufficiency

As with mitral regurgitation, aortic insufficiency is seen infrequently in women of childbearing age, and the usually etiology is rheumatic, almost always seen in association with mitral valve disease. An uncommon cause of aortic insufficiency is Marfan's syndrome and it is imperative to evaluate the pregnant patient with aortic insufficiency in association with Marfan's syndrome.

Aortic insufficiency is characterized by a widened pulse pressure, and a diastolic murmur ('blow') heard at the upper sternal border. The murmur is best heard in the sitting position at end-expiration. With long-standing aortic insufficiency, there may by evidence of left ventricular enlargement on the EKG and chest radiograph.

For reasons similar to those of mitral regurgitation, aortic insufficiency is generally well tolerated during pregnancy, and these patients remain essentially asymptomatic from a cardiovascular point of view.

Tricuspid and pulmonary valve lesions

Tricuspid regurgitation is an extremely common finding in normal pregnancy[11] and is rarely clinically important. The exception is tricuspid regurgitation seen in association with Ebstein's anomaly, which increases the morbidity of pregnancy. Tricuspid stenosis and pulmonary insufficiency are uncommon findings in pregnancy, and there are few published data on the outcome of pregnancy in these patients.

Pulmonary stenosis represents a common congenital cardiac defect and is seen both alone and as part of the syndrome of tetralogy of Fallot. Isolated pulmonary stenosis is usually detected in childhood; both surgical and, more recently, non-surgical (with balloon valvuloplasty) repairs are often curative. Patients with all but the severest forms of pulmonary stenosis often tolerate pregnancy well.

Physical findings of pulmonary stenosis include a prominent 'A' wave in the jugular venous pressure, a right parasternal lift, and often a pulmonary ejection click that varies with respiration. A crescendo–decrescendo murmur can often be heard along the upper left parasternal area. The EKG may remain normal unless severe pulmonary stenosis results in evidence of right ventricular hypertrophy and right axis deviation. The chest X-ray will demonstrate a large right ventricle and evidence of prominent central pulmonary arteries.

Pregnancy is generally well tolerated, even in patients with uncorrected pulmonary stenosis[7,12,13]. The incidence of inherited cardiac defects in the offspring of these patients appears to be high[14]. Although percutaneous balloon valvuloplasty is the treatment of choice for pulmonary stenosis, if refractory heart failure persists during pregnancy, surgical repair is preferred over balloon technology, since the latter results in an unacceptable level of radiation to the fetus[15].

Mitral valve prolapse

Mitral valve prolapse is a common cardiac condition, seen in up to 15% of the general population[16]. Less frequently, it is associated with other cardiac conditions including Marfan's syndrome, atrial septal defect and rheumatic heart disease.

Although the majority of patients with mitral valve prolapse are asymptomatic, some patients may experience palpitations, fatigue and chest pain. On physical examination, there may be multiple mid-systolic ejection clicks, and a murmur of mitral regurgitation. The diagnosis can be made by M-mode or two-dimensional echocardiography. The chest X-ray and EKG are usually normal unless severe mitral regurgitation results in left atrial enlargement. Pregnancy is generally well tolerated in patients with mitral valve prolapse[17] and the cardiovascular changes of pregnancy result in an attenuation of the click and murmur towards term. If a murmur is present in association with the click, most sources recommend antibiotic prophylaxis for the delivery, whether by Cesarean section or the vaginal route.

SPECIFIC CARDIOVASCULAR ABNORMALITIES OF MODERATE RISK TO THE PREGNANT PATIENT

Mitral stenosis

A common etiology for mitral stenosis in a woman of childbearing years is rheumatic heart disease, and mitral stenosis represents the most common rheumatic valvular lesion. Because of the obstruction of outflow from the left atrium to the left ventricle, normal cardiovascular changes of pregnancy, such as increases in blood volume, heart rate and cardiac output, can pose hazards to successful completion of pregnancy. Left ventricular filling occurs during diastole. The increase in heart rate seen in pregnancy shortens the diastolic filling time, which in turn compromises left ventricular filling. Concomitant increases in left atrial size and pressure predispose to the development of atrial fibrillation, often with a rapid ventricular response, which can have catastrophic consequences. In addition, the patient with mitral stenosis may have an elevated pulmonary blood volume; the normal pregnancy-induced increases in blood volume and cardiac output may spur an onset of pulmonary edema.

These patients may have symptoms of fatigue and dyspnea. Physical examination may reveal evidence of pulmonary congestion and a diastolic murmur at the apex associated with an opening snap. The EKG usually shows left atrial enlargement and the chest X-ray may demonstrate enlargement of the left atrium and pulmonary vascular redistribution.

It is not uncommon for women with occult mitral stenosis to become symptomatic during pregnancy, usually by mid-pregnancy, when the pregnancy-induced hemodynamic changes are at the maximum. The risk of pulmonary edema exists from this period until several days after delivery.

Morbidity and mortality during pregnancy are a function of the severity of heart failure, with 'mild' mitral stenosis having a low mortality[8] but 'severe' mitral stenosis (New York Heart Association Class III–IV) having a 4–5% maternal mortality; the mortality is even higher if atrial fibrillation is present[18].

Improved diagnostic techniques, better prenatal management and effective cardiac drugs have improved the outcome of these patients. Prophylactic digoxin is often recommended, especially in patients who are in normal sinus rhythm with an enlarged left atrium by echocardiogram, to prevent a rapid ventricular response should atrial fibrillation develop. β-blockers are effective in slowing the heart rate of patients in normal sinus rhythm, and are generally considered safe for the fetus. Diuretics should be withheld unless symptoms of pulmonary congestion develop despite bed rest. If pulmonary congestion fails to respond to medical management, corrective surgery for mitral valve stenosis should be strongly considered. Both open surgical mitral valve replacement[19] and closed mitral valvotomy[20] have been performed successfully during pregnancy. Percutaneous balloon valvuloplasty for mitral valve stenosis is gaining acceptance as the treatment of choice for young people with a pliable valve and has been successfully attempted during pregnancies with good maternal and perinatal outcomes[21,22]. The maternal and perinatal benefits of the procedure probably outweigh the small risk of fetal exposure to the radiation. Fetal radiation exposure can be minimized by shielding the maternal abdomen and pelvis during the procedure. The average fluoroscopy time using the Inoue single-balloon catheter technique is 9.2 min[21].

Aortic stenosis

Aortic stenosis is not a commonly seen valvular abnormality in pregnancy, because it is usually prevalent in an older population. However, patients with aortic stenosis who have a bicuspid aortic valve may become symptomatic in their twenties and thirties. Aortic stenosis represents an obstruction to outflow from the left ventricle. Patients may be asymptomatic until the valve narrows significantly, then may present with symptoms of angina, syncope and congestive heart failure. The physical examination reveals a crescendo–decrescendo systolic murmur at the upper sternal border, and in severe cases, a single or absent second heart sound. The carotid upstroke may be delayed. Left ventricular hypertrophy may be present on the EKG and the cardiac silhouette on the chest radiograph will be enlarged.

Pregnancy can usually be successfully carried to term in all but the most severe cases of aortic stenosis; reported maternal mortality in severe aortic stenosis is 17%[23]. A more recent review of 12 studies demonstrated an average maternal mortality of 6.6% and an average perinatal mortality of 4%[24]. The fetal risks of congenital heart diseases range from 17% to 26%[25,26]. As a result, a fetal echocardiogram during the second trimester is recommended. Complications arise when the already low forward output is compromised further by reduced preload from either hypovolemia or peripheral vasodilatation. The mainstay of therapy in these patients is strict bed rest and the maintenance of adequate blood volume. Management during labor includes central monitoring with a Swan–Ganz catheter and avoidance of hypotension. Spinal or epidural anesthesia should be used with extreme caution in patients with severe aortic stenosis, because of its propensity to cause hypotension.

When feasible, symptomatic aortic stenosis should be corrected prior to pregnancy, although urgent aortic valve replacement during pregnancy with favorable outcomes has been reported[27]. Balloon valvuloplasty of the aortic valve has been successfully and safely accomplished during pregnancy with excellent maternal and perinatal outcomes[28,29].

Coarctation of the aorta, uncomplicated

Coarctation of the aorta is a stenosis of the aorta, usually located just distal to the left subclavian artery at the ligamentum arteriosum (fetal ductus arteriosus). The narrowing produces an obstruction to outflow and is often seen in association with other congenital abnormalities including patent ductus arteriosus, congenital bicuspid aortic valve and aneurysms of the circle of Willis.

The hallmark of coarctation is an asymmetry of limb blood pressures with a markedly decreased pressure in the lower extremities as left ventricular hypertrophy is apparent on physical examination, EKG and the chest X-ray. Patients who have had coarctation of the aorta corrected prior to pregnancy and no other associated anomalies usually tolerate the pregnancy well. These patients, however, are still at a higher risk for cardio-vascular compromise compared to non-pregnant patients.

Complications associated with uncorrected coarcta-tion of the aorta include hypertension, congestive heart failure and aortic dissection. The mainstay of therapy is adequate rest, control of hypertension and avoidance of hypovolemia during the peripartum period. In cases of aortic dissection or severe conges-tive heart failure unresponsive to medical therapy, sur-gical repair has been successfully attempted during pregnancy[30,31]. Fetal morbidity and mortality are high because of decreased placental blood flow from hyper-tension or reduced cardiac output and increased inci-dence of fetal cardiac anomalies[10].

Marfan's syndrome, normal aortic root

Marfan's syndrome is an autosomal dominant condi-tion with defective collagen synthesis affecting the ocu-lar, skeletal and cardiovascular abnormalities with variable severity. The defective gene is located on chromosome 15[32]. The cardiovascular manifestations include mitral valve prolapse with resulting mitral regurgitation, and aneurysmal dilatation of the proxi-mal aorta; the latter may be occasionally associated with aortic regurgitation and dissection.

Pregnancy seems to increase the risk of aortic rup-ture in patients with Marfan's syndrome. The maternal morbidity and mortality depends on whether there are aortic root dilatation or valvular abnormalities[33,34]. Maternal mortality from aortic rupture or dissection may be up to 50% when the aortic root diameter is greater than 40 mm[34]. On the other hand, pregnancy in patients who have normal aortic root diameter and no valvular involvements can be successfully carried to term with minimal maternal mortality or morbidity. Patients should be advised of the risk and should be closely followed for signs and symptoms of aortic dis-section. Serial echocardiograms during pregnancy are recommended to assess the cardiac status, especially the aortic root, and the presence of valvular regurgita-tion. In selected patients, β-blockers may lower the risk of progressive aortic dilatation by reducing the pul-satile pressure on the aortic wall[35,36].

Prior history of myocardial infarction

Coronary artery disease is rare in women of childbear-ing years and there are only a few reports of pregnan-cies in women who have sustained myocardial infarctions prior to pregnancy. The pregnancy out-comes of these patients is related to left ventricular performance as well as the amount of residual ischemia in the non-infarcted myocardium. Myo-cardial infarction during pregnancy poses a much higher risk.

SPECIFIC CARDIOVASCULAR ABNORMALITIES OF HIGH RISK TO THE PREGNANT PATIENT

Eisenmenger's syndrome

This syndrome involves the presence of high pul-monary artery pressures resulting in right-to-left shunting as a result of a communication between the right and left circulations. In these patients, progres-sive pulmonary hypertension, approaching systemic levels, results in a reversal of shunting from left-to-right circulation to right-to-left circulation and causes hypoxemia and death. These patients may present with peripheral cyanosis, congestive heart failure and hemoptysis. Any congenital defect involving a left-to-right shunt such as ASD, VSD, or patent ductus arte-riosus with progressive pulmonary hypertension can result in Eisenmenger's physiology.

This condition is associated with a very high mater-nal mortality (23-50%) which may occur during the pregnancy or the postpartum period[9,37]. The patient should be informed about the risk and offered the options of termination or continuation of pregnancy.

If the patient continues the pregnancy, the manage-ment may include strict bed rest, continuous oxygen, digoxin, invasive hemodynamic monitoring during the peripartum period and shortening of the second stage of labor with low or outlet forceps delivery. Hospitalization is necessary. Maternal Pao_2 should be maintained above 70% to ensure adequate fetal oxygenation[38]. Since the incidence of intrauterine growth retardation and fetal death is high[37], close fetal monitoring with serial ultrasound examinations and non-stress tests and/or biophysical profiles is recommended.

The peripartum period is a precarious time, owing to a rapid shift in blood volume and chance of hemor-rhage. Measures should be taken to avoid a reduction in preload such as hypotension or hemorrhage, since severe hypoxemia and death may ensue from decreased cardiac output and pulmonary artery hypoperfusion. The patients should be closely monitored in the hos-pital setting for a week after delivery, since the signifi-cantly increased risk of maternal mortality still persists during this period.

Primary pulmonary hypertension

Primary pulmonary hypertension (PPH) is a specific pathological entity involving an abnormal thickening and constriction of the arterial media of the pulmonary arteries resulting in intimal fibrosis and occasionally thrombi. The disease of unknown etiology is primarily seen in young women and results in a progressive increase in pulmonary artery pressures. Presenting symptoms include dyspnea, fatigue, palpitations and occasional syncope.

The physical examination is characterized by a prominent 'A' wave of the jugular venous pulse, a right ventricular heave and often a palpable second heart sound. There may be a systolic ejection click, and, if right ventricular dilatation is present, a murmur of tricuspid insufficiency due to tricuspid annular dilatation. In advanced stages, evidence of right ventricular failure (elevation of jugular venous pressure, hepatomegaly and peripheral edema) may be present.

Associated studies may show polycythemia, abnormal liver function tests, right ventricular hypertrophy and right axis deviation on the EKG, and an enlarged right ventricle on chest X-ray. A prominent finding on the chest X-ray is enlargement of the central pulmonary vasculature with peripheral 'pruning'.

Pregnancy is poorly tolerated in patients with PPH, with maternal mortality in excess of 40%[15]. This excess mortality appears to be present even in patients who were asymptomatic or only mildly symptomatic prior to becoming pregnant. In addition, there appears to be a high incidence of fetal and neonatal deaths associated with maternal PPH. Patients with PPH often come to clinical attention during the second trimester, when the hemodynamic changes of pregnancy are maximum, and the presenting symptoms are often those of right ventricular failure.

Considering the high morbidity and mortality of pregnancy in patients with PPH, counseling should be directed toward the avoidance of pregnancy. If pregnancy occurs, elective termination during the first trimester may be offered. If, despite the risks, the patient with PPH chooses to continue the pregnancy, therapy should be aimed at strict bed rest, preferably in the hospital setting during the third trimester, early treatment of congestive heart failure with digoxin and diuretics and careful electrocardiographic and hemodynamic monitoring (with an indwelling Swan–Ganz catheter) during labor and delivery. Frequent measurement of arterial blood gases with oxygen supplementation should be instituted[39].

Pregnancy represents a hypercoagulable state, and anticoagulation may be an important adjunct in improving the prognosis of patients with PPH[15,40]. Intravenous adenosine and high-dose oral nifedipine may be beneficial in patients with severe pulmonary hypertension by probably reducing the pulmonary vascular resistance[41]. Pulmonary hypertension *per se* is not an indication for Cesarean section.

Complex cyanotic congenital heart disease

Many children with complex cyanotic congenital heart disease die during infancy and childhood, and do not reach childbearing age, but, with greatly improved surgical techniques, a larger number of these patients are surviving into adulthood. Specific congenital lesions of interest include: (1) tetralogy of Fallot (pulmonary stenosis, VSD, over-riding aorta and right ventricular hypertrophy); (2) Ebstein's anomaly (displacement of the tricuspid valve into the right ventricular cavity, resulting in a small right ventricle and poor forward output, often associated with right-to-left shunting through an ASD; (3) truncus arteriosis (single outflow tract and outflow valve distal to both ventricles, often associated with a VSD); (4) transposition of the great vessels (separate pulmonary and systemic circulations operating in parallel with communication via a VSD; and (5) tricuspid atresia (absent tricuspid orifice, small non-functional right ventricle and a connection between the pulmonary and systemic circulations. These lesions represent many of the important cyanotic congenital heart lesions, and individual lesions may be variable in severity.

In general, patients with uncorrected cyanotic congenital heart defects do not survive long enough to become pregnant; those who do survive should be counseled against pregnancy. Despite the high morbidity and mortality of pregnancy in these patients, there are case reports of successful completion of pregnancy in patients with these congenital lesions[15]. If the cardiac abnormality has been surgically corrected, maternal morbidity and mortality during pregnancy appears to be related to residual cardiac defects, with a marked improvement in prognosis for those who have undergone successful complete correction.

In all cases, these patients should be carefully monitored during labor and delivery, given supplemental oxygen and treated aggressively for the presence of symptoms of congestive heart failure. Attempts should be made to shorten the second stage of labor, and to avoid peripartum hypotension induced by anesthesia or hypovolemia. In all cases, antibiotic prophylaxis should be administered during delivery.

Marfan's syndrome associated with an abnormal aortic root

Marfan's syndrome, discussed earlier in this chapter, is an autosomal dominant congenital defect in collagen synthesis. In the absence of cardiac or great vessel involvement, pregnancy carries only a moderate risk.

If there is evidence of a dilated aortic root, valvular regurgitation or dissection, maternal and fetal mortality is markedly increased. Transesophageal echocardiography is superior to transthoracic echocardiography in diagnosing aortic root dilatation and aortic dissection. Preventive replacement of the ascending aorta with a graft has been recommended in patients with the aortic root diameter of at least 60 mm prior to pregnancy[42]. Patients who contemplate pregnancy may consider preventive replacement of the ascending aorta when the aortic root dilatation is progressive and approaching 55 mm in diameter[36]. If pregnancy occurs in patients with significant aortic root dilatation, therapeutic termination during the first trimester may be offered. If the patient chooses to continue the pregnancy, careful assessment of the patient throughout pregnancy should include evaluation for aortic dissection and use of β-blockers during pregnancy to reduce the incidence of dissection. The patient should be encouraged to limit physical activity, including consideration of bed rest during the third trimester. Every attempt should be made to shorten the second stage of delivery and urgent delivery and vascular repair should be undertaken if clinical evidence of dissection occurs, regardless of the viability of the fetus.

Myocardial infarction during pregnancy

The epidemiology of coronary artery disease is such that myocardial infarction is extremely rare in women of childbearing years, estimated to occur in 1 in 10 000 pregnancies[43]. Recent case reports of myocardial infarction during pregnancy reveal good maternal and perinatal outcomes with both conservative management and transluminal coronary angioplasty[43–49]. Risk factors for coronary heart disease in pregnant women are the same as those for the general population and include cigarette smoking, hyperlipidemia, diabetes mellitus and hypertension. The causes of occlusion or stenosis of the coronary arteries include thrombus, atherosclerosis and vasospasm[45,48,49].

The patient who develops an acute myocardial infarction during pregnancy should be managed conservatively if possible, with bed rest, supplemental oxygen, nitrates and β-blockers. A Swan–Ganz balloon-tipped pulmonary artery catheter can be placed percutaneously often without the use of fluoroscopy and may be beneficial in the hemodynamic management of these patients. A more invasive approach including cardiac catheterization, balloon angioplasty or cardiac surgery should be reserved for those who are refractory to conservative medical management. Successful vaginal deliveries without further myocardial injury have been reported[46–49]. Therefore, myocardial infarction is not a contraindication for a vaginal delivery. Vacuum extraction or outlet forceps delivery can be attempted to shorten the second stage of labor. Cesarean section delivery should be performed for obstetric indications. Alleviation of pain with either pain medications or epidural anesthesia is important in the management of patients with myocardial infarction during labor and delivery.

CARDIOMYOPATHIES
Peripartum cardiomyopathy

This entity involves the development of heart failure during the last month of pregnancy or in the first 6 postpartum months, without obvious etiology. In the USA, the incidences vary from 1 in 4000 deliveries to 1 in 1500 deliveries, peak during the second postpartum month, and increase among older, multiparous black females. The overall maternal mortality ranges from 25 to 50%[50,51].

Although the etiology of peripartum cardiomyopathy is not known, various factors have been suggested to play a role in its development, including hypertension[52], viral illness[53], an immunological reaction[54] and vitamin deficiency[55]. A more recent report shows that the incidence of myocarditis in patients with peripartum cardiomyopathy is 8.4%, which is comparable to that found in patients undergoing transplantation for idiopathic dilated cardiomyopathy among non-pregnant patients[56]. There is a higher incidence reported in Nigeria, where postpartum custom involves ingestion of large amounts of salt. Non-invasive evaluation with echocardiograms demonstrates high cardiac output and preserved left ventricular function in this group, suggesting that it probably represents a different syndrome[57].

Presenting clinical symptoms include those of left-sided heart failure (orthopnea, dyspnea, weakness) as well as peripheral edema, palpitations and occasionally hemoptysis. On physical examination these patients may have pulmonary rales, cardiomegaly, a gallop rhythm, distended neck veins and peripheral edema. The EKG may be characterized by abnormal ST segments and T wave changes, in addition to various types of rhythm disturbances. Cardiomegaly and pulmonary venous congestion are typical chest X-ray findings.

Echocardiography is helpful in ruling out a valvular or pericardial etiology for the clinical presentation. In addition, echocardiography can demonstrate cardiac chamber size and overall left ventricular function.

Treatment should include bed rest and avoidance of exercise, as well as vigorous therapy for congestive heart failure such as digoxin and diuretics. These patients are at risk for thromboembolic disease, so prophylactic anticoagulation with heparin should be considered. If congestive heart failure is refractory to medical management, early delivery should be considered.

The prognosis appears to be related to the course following pregnancy. Patients who have persistent cardiomegaly have a poor prognosis[58], whereas a return to normal heart size within 6–12 months postpartum predicts a more favorable outcome[59]. Although most sources caution patients with peripartum cardiomyopathy to avoid further pregnancies, successful subsequent pregnancies have been reported in patients who have a return to normal heart size[60,61]. For patients who have a refractory downhill course following the diagnosis of peripartum cardiomyopathy, cardiac transplantation should be considered. Case reports of successful completion of pregnancy following cardiac transplantation have been published[62–66].

Congestive cardiomyopathy

Congestive heart failure is a clinical syndrome characterized by an inability of the heart to generate the forward output necessary to meet the metabolic requirements of the body. This syndrome is the end result of a wide variety of pathophysiological conditions, including peripartum cardiomyopathy and valvular heart disease. The presenting symptoms are those of biventricular heart failure (fatigue, dyspnea, orthopnea and pedal edema). The physical examination, chest X-ray and echocardiography usually demonstrate dilated and poorly contractile cardiac chambers with evidence of volume overload. Pulmonary edema may result when the heart cannot accommodate the overload state of pregnancy. Prognosis depends on the etiology for congestive cardiomyopathy. Some causes of congestive heart failure are treatable medically or surgically. General measures for the pregnant patient with congestive heart failure should include bed rest, avoidance of exercise, digoxin and diuretics, in addition to invasive hemodynamic monitoring during labor and delivery. Patients with severe congestive cardiomyopathy should be counseled against pregnancy, and those who present early in pregnancy may be offered termination of pregnancy.

Hypertrophic cardiomyopathy

Hypertrophic cardiomyopathy is a general term that refers to a primary muscle abnormality characterized by hypertrophy, either concentric or segmental, of the cardiac muscle. It appears to have an autosomal dominant inheritance pattern with a widely variable penetrance, but sporadic cases occur as well.

The clinical presentation in hypertrophic cardiomyopathy is characterized by dyspnea, atypical chest pain, angina, dizziness and syncope, although many patients may remain asymptomatic. Occasionally, sudden death is the presenting symptom. If the patient does not have aortic outflow obstruction, the physical examination may be normal, although the EKG may show left ventricular hypertrophy, ST abnormalities and inferior or lateral Q waves. In patients with outflow obstruction, a loud systolic murmur and thrill can be detected along the left sternal border. Maneuvers that increase venous return or chamber size (handgrip, squatting) decrease the intensity of the murmur. The remainder of the physical examination is characterized by a bifid carotid pulse, prominent 'A' waves in the jugular venous pulse and occasionally a single or absent second heart sound. An apical holosystolic murmur consistent with mitral regurgitation is also commonly heard.

The echocardiogram shows a thickened left ventricular wall, often with a septal wall that is thick out of proportion to the posterior wall, as well as a small intraventricular cavity. There may be Doppler documentation of an outflow gradient, as well as mitral regurgitation.

The published experience on the outcome of pregnancy in patients with hypertrophic cardiomyopathy has been summarized by Kumar and Elkayam[67]. They review the data published on 82 pregnancies and conclude that the outcome of pregnancy is generally favorable, although worsening of symptoms may occur.

If a pregnant patient is asymptomatic, management involves avoiding situations or medications which decrease cavity size or increase contractility (hypovolemia, vasodilatation, increased sympathetic tone), as this may provoke outflow obstruction. For symptomatic pregnant patients, treatment should be aimed at alleviating symptoms. Drugs that increase inotropy (such as digoxin) or cause hypovolemia (such as diuretics) are relatively contraindicated. Poor diastolic relaxation (one of the hallmarks of hypertrophic cardiomyopathy) may be improved by treatment with β-blockers or calcium channel blockers. Arrhythmias, both atrial and ventricular, occur frequently in patients with hypertrophic cardiomyopathy. Arrhythmias should be evaluated in all pregnant patients with the condition, by means of a Holter monitor. Although patients with hypertrophic cardiomyopathy and arrhythmias may be more prone to sudden death, there is little evidence to suggest that treatment of the arrhythmias alters the prognosis.

General measures during labor and delivery in these patients include laboring in the left lateral decubitus position to maximize venous return to the heart, avoidance of hypovolemia and a shortened second stage of labor. Prostaglandins, such as PGE_2 (because of their vasodilatory effect), and β-adrenergic stimulants should be avoided in these patients. In addition, hemodynamic monitoring with an indwelling pulmonary artery (Swan–Ganz) catheter and rhythm monitoring are of value during labor and delivery in most patients with hypertrophic cardiomyopathy.

ARRHYTHMIAS

Tachyarrhythmias

Cardiac arrhythmias may be classified as supraventricular or ventricular, and may occur during pregnancy either spontaneously or related to pre-existing heart disease. Mendelsohn[68] reviewed 92 000 pregnancies and determined the incidence of sustained arrhythmias to be 0.05%, most of which were atrial in origin. Sinus tachycardia is a frequent occurrence during pregnancy, as are premature atrial and ventricular contractions. The hormonal and hemodynamic changes of pregnancy may predispose women, even those with normal cardiovascular systems, to frequent ectopic beats.

Atrial fibrillation is a rapid irregular supraventricular rhythm usually seen in the setting of rheumatic mitral stenosis. The volume overload of pregnancy and subsequent left atrial chamber enlargement may predispose patients with mitral stenosis to develop atrial fibrillation. Two important considerations in pregnancy are the following. (1) If the ventricular rate is rapid, the diastolic filling time shortens, resulting in a fall in both stroke volume and forward output. This can cause decreased placental perfusion and fetal compromise. For this reason, women who are at risk for developing atrial fibrillation during pregnancy should be maintained on prophylactic digoxin or a β-blocker to prevent the rapid ventricular response, should atrial fibrillation develop. (2) Atrial fibrillation predisposes to systemic embolization. Although anticoagulation reduces the risk of embolic events, anticoagulant therapy is not without side-effects. Therapy for each patient should be individualized.

Other supraventricular rhythms such as atrial flutter and paroxysmal supraventricular tachycardia are relatively uncommon during pregnancy. Rapid ventricular response may compromise placental blood flow by lowering cardiac output.

Often the rhythm can be abruptly terminated by vagal maneuvers such as carotid sinus massage, submerging the face in cold water, or a Valsalva maneuver. If these vagal maneuvers are unsuccessful, intravenous adenosine or verapamil should be tried. Although reserved for resistant tachycardia, electrical cardioversion has been used successfully during pregnancy for reversion to sinus rhythm[69].

Ventricular tachycardia is an abnormal ectopic rhythm originating in the ventricles. It is rare during pregnancy, but may represent a more ominous sign than atrial tachycardia. Ventricular tachycardia often accompanies structural heart disease. If the ventricular tachycardia is slow (< 100–120 beats/min) or nonsustained (self-terminating within 30 s), and there is no apparent structural heart disease, the prognosis is excellent and further therapy with antiarrhythmic drugs is usually not necessary. Patients with ventricular tachycardia who have organic heart disease, or those with symptomatic episodes of ventricular tachycardia warrant treatment. The urgency of treatment depends on the presenting symptoms. Rapid ventricular tachycardia in the pregnant patient who is demonstrating significant hemodynamic compromise should be treated urgently with electrical cardioversion, to maintain the fetal blood supply. Patients who are hemodynamically stable can be treated with intravenous procainamide or lidocaine, both of which have been shown to be safe for the fetus. Once sinus rhythm has been re-established, a thorough evaluation should be undertaken to determine the cause of the ventricular tachycardia before long-term therapy is initiated.

Bradyarrhythmias, conduction blocks

Despite the fact that sinus bradycardia and Wenckebach morphology (Type I second-degree atrioventricular block) have been observed during pregnancy, labor and delivery[70], conduction blocks are not a normal finding in pregnancy. Type II second-degree atrioventricular block and third-degree atrioventricular block are associated with an increased incidence of sudden death and should be treated with a permanent pacemaker. The exception to this is congenital complete heart block which is generally well tolerated, and, because it carries a good prognosis, usually does not need to be treated with a pacemaker, unless it is symptomatic.

CARDIAC SURGERY

Cardiac surgery during pregnancy

Certain patients with acquired or congenital heart disease may develop refractory symptoms during pregnancy that necessitate cardiac surgical procedures. In some cases, surgery may be life saving for the mother, albeit resulting in increased fetal mortality.

As early as the 1950s, surgery for relief of mitral stenosis was being successfully performed. In 1961, cardiopulmonary bypass was first used successfully during pregnancy[71]. Over the ensuing four decades, numerous pregnant patients with mitral stenosis have undergone commissurotomy (both open and closed) successfully, with a minimum of maternal and fetal morbidity and mortality.

Valve replacement has been successfully completed during pregnancy for both aortic and mitral valve disease[72–74]. Although this procedure has been shown to be relatively safe and effective, it carries a high fetal mortality and should be reserved for patients refractory to medical management. Other successful intracardiac procedures during pregnancy include pulmonary valvuloplasty, ASD and VSD repair, excision of left atrial myxomas and, as an emergency, repair of an aortic dissection. In addition, there have been several successful coronary artery bypass graft procedures carried out during pregnancy, for patients with unstable angina[72,74].

A recent review of the world literature between 1975 and 1991 reveals no maternal mortality, but embryo-fetal mortality of 12.5% from the cardiopulmonary bypass performed during pregnancy. Interestingly, embryofetal mortality occurs only when hypothermia is used. Hypothermia may cause fetal hypoxia by decreasing oxygen exchange through the placenta[74]. Fetal bradycardia is common during the procedure and can be corrected by infusing sodium nitroprusside to lower the placental vascular resistance[75]. In addition, preterm labor is a frequent complication[74,75]. Uterine contractions can be suppressed by intravenous magnesium sulfate.

Patients who undergo cardiac surgery during pregnancy should undergo invasive intraoperative monitoring, including placement of a Swan–Ganz pulmonary artery catheter, frequent arterial blood gas determinations and electrocardiographic monitoring. The utmost care should be taken to avoid wide swings in blood volume or blood pressure, and fetal heart rate monitoring should be continued throughout the procedure.

Pregnancy following cardiac surgery

Many congenital cardiac defects are detected and successfully repaired in childhood or young adulthood. As a result, there are increasing numbers of women with corrected lesions reaching childbearing years. The outcome of pregnancy in women with corrected congenital heart disease depends on many factors including the success of the surgical repair, the extent of residual cardiac lesions and the need for cardiovascular medications such as coumadin. In addition, some maternal cardiac defects are associated with an increased incidence of congenital fetal cardiac and non-cardiac defects which may affect fetal prognosis. Pregnancies following a heart transplant are usually not complicated[63–66]. Vaginal delivery can be attempted without damage to the transplanted heart[64]. Peripartum cardiomyopathy may not recur after the heart transplant[63].

Patients with successfully corrected cardiac lesions without sequelae have a good prognosis during pregnancy, and, except for antibiotic prophylaxis against endocarditis, can often be managed the same as a non-cardiac patient. Patients with residual stenosis, or residual pulmonary hypertension, are at a greater risk of having maternal and fetal complications during pregnancy, especially during the second and third trimesters, when major hemodynamic changes take place. Each patient needs to be evaluated individually with regard to prenatal counseling and management during pregnancy, labor and delivery. Careful prepregnancy evaluation is important. These patients need to be closely monitored at every stage of pregnancy, to assure the optimal outcome. Management of the patient during labor and delivery will often include careful electrocardiographic monitoring, placement of a balloon-tipped pulmonary wedge catheter (Swan–Ganz) for hemodynamic monitoring, adequate analgesia and shortening of the second stage of labor.

Women who have had valve replacement with a mechanical prosthesis (usually for rheumatic valve disease) pose a special problem, owing to the need for anticoagulation. Anticoagulation in the setting of mechanical heart valves is recommended, because of potential valve thrombosis. Since oral anticoagulation with coumadin has been associated with a constellation of fetal anomalies, namely 'warfarin embryopathy', full-dose anticoagulation with heparin (usually subcutaneous) during the periconception period and through the first trimester (period of organogenesis) is used. Controversy exists as to the optimal form of anticoagulation (heparin or coumadin) during the second and third trimesters, but many authors feel that heparin should be continued throughout the entire pregnancy. Extremely close attention must be paid to the level of anticoagulation, since the metabolism of the anticoagulant may change during pregnancy, and over- or under-anticoagulation could have catastrophic consequences.

Management of the pregnant patient with a bioprosthetic valve is not markedly different from that of patients with native valves, because the valve does not require anticoagulation. These patients should receive antibiotic prophylaxis during delivery. Pregnancy does not adversely affect the incidence of structural valve degeneration of the bioprostheses. The absence of valve-related mortality in previously pregnant patients at 10 and 15 years after valve replacement stands at 92%, which does not significantly differ from the rate in never-pregnant patients[76].

MEDICATIONS
Cardioactive drugs
Digoxin

Digoxin is a weak inotrope that has important effects on slowing the conduction through the atrioventricular node, and can be extremely useful in the management of certain arrhythmias. Digoxin can be given orally or intravenously, and is excreted via the kidneys. Digoxin has a narrow toxic–therapeutic range, so dosing must be careful. Digoxin toxicity may result in nausea, visual disturbances, a wide variety of arrhythmias and various conduction blocks.

Digoxin readily crosses the placenta and can be measured in fetal tissue, amniotic fluid and the breast milk of lactating women. There are several reports of successful treatment of fetal tachycardia by maternal digoxin administration[77,78]. Although there are anecdotal reports of fetal problems, such as electrocardiographic changes and low birth weight, digoxin is widely considered to be safe during pregnancy.

β-Blockers

Blockers of β-adrenergic receptors are widely used for the treatment of hypertension, arrhythmias and migraine headaches, among other conditions. Although much of the physiology of β-blockade in pregnancy was described in the ewe, there is a large body of data on the use of β-blockers during pregnancy in humans. Extensive clinical testing with propranolol (non-selective), metoprolol and atenolol (cardioselective), pindolol (β-blocker with intrinsic sympathomimetic activity) and labetolol (both α- and β-blocking properties) has shown that these drugs are both safe and effective for use during pregnancy[79,80]. Possible neonatal side-effects such as respiratory depression[81], bradycardia[82] and hypoglycemia[82] may occur.

Antihypertensive agents

There is no clear consensus concerning the level at which blood pressure should be treated during pregnancy. Normally, the blood pressure falls during gestation, so a blood pressure that is 'normal' in the non-pregnant state may represent hypertension during pregnancy. Despite this, there is no clear consensus concerning the risks to the fetus of mild or moderate maternal hypertension.

Numerous antihypertensive therapies are available. Diuretics, especially thiazide diuretics, have for years been the mainstay of therapy for hypertension in the non-pregnant patient. Adverse metabolic effects (hypokalemia, hyperlipidemia) and the transient nature of the effects on blood volume have limited their use as antihypertensive agents. They are no longer considered to be the first drug of choice. In general, diuretic use during pregnancy is not advocated, except for intractable volume overload states.

α-methyldopa (Aldomet®) is an effective antihypertensive agent that works best in conjunction with diuretics, since it expands vascular volume. Aldomet has been shown to be safe and effective in pregnancy[83,84].

Angiotensin-converting enzyme (ACE) inhibitors such as captopril are very useful antihypertensives. Their use during pregnancy in animals has been associated with an increased incidence of fetal demise[85]. There may be a role for them as an antihypertensive of last resort during pregnancy.

Calcium channel blockers (nifedipine, verapamil, diltiazem) are newer agents in the treatment of hypertension, but appear to be effective. Since there is limited clinical information on the safety of these agents to treat hypertension in pregnancy, calcium channel blockers should be reserved for those patients refractory to other forms of medical therapy.

For acute hypertensive emergencies during pregnancy, urgent blood pressure lowering is of the utmost importance. Several agents including hydralazine and nitroprusside have been shown to be safe, effective, rapidly acting antihypertensive agents. For patients resistant to these agents, diazoxide, labetolol or nitroglycerin may be considered. In treating these patients, care should be taken not to lower the blood pressure to the point that would compromise placental perfusion.

Antiarrhythmics

Treatments of arrhythmias during pregnancy involves both attention to the underlying condition predisposing the patient to the arrhythmia, and use of the lowest possible effective dose of the antiarrhythmic agent. Rhythm disturbances (both tachyarrhythmias and bradyarrhythmias) may place the fetus in jeopardy, because of rate-related changes in hemodynamics, resulting in compromised placental blood flow.

There is a wide variety of antiarrhythmic agents available. The reader is referred to Rotmensch and colleagues[86] for an extensive discussion.

Quinidine and procainamide have both been shown to be safe and effective for use in controlling pregnancy-associated tachyarrhythmias, although quinidine has been associated with transient neonatal thrombocytopenia[87]. Both of these agents are useful for atrial as well as ventricular dysrhythmias, and the dosage can be adjusted according to the measurement of therapeutic blood levels. Digoxin toxicity may occur when digoxin is administered with quinidine, as quinidine displaces digoxin from binding sites, resulting in a higher serum level. Since the use of procainamide has been associated with the development of antinuclear antibodies and a lupus-like syndrome, it should be used only if quinidine fails to control the rhythm abnormality.

Disopyramide is an effective antiarrhythmic agent useful for the treatment of both supraventricular and ventricular arrhythmias. It is a negative inotrope, so should be used cautiously in patients with depressed left ventricular function. The main side-effects of this agent are those related to its anticholinergic action (constipation, urinary retention, dry mucous membranes), which may preclude use during pregnancy. There are numerous case reports suggesting the safety of disopyramide in pregnancy but, because of limited pharmacokinetic information, it should be reserved for use in patients who are refractory to other antiarrhythmic agents.

Lidocaine, and its newer oral analog mexilitene, are useful agents in the treatment of ventricular arrhythmias. Numerous reports have documented the safety of lidocaine during pregnancy. Since there is little information concerning the safety of mexilitene during pregnancy, its use should be reserved for those patients with rhythm disturbances refractory to other forms of therapy.

Amiodarone is a newer class III antiarrhythmic agent useful for both supraventricular as well as ventricular rhythm disturbances. A very long half-life of action, complicated pharmacokinetics and side-effects (pulmonary toxicity, thyroid and corneal abnormalities, photosensitivity) have limited its usefulness. It is used as an antiarrhythmic drug of last resort. There have been anecdotal reports associating the use of amiodarone during pregnancy with neonatal QT prolongation. However, rare case reports of successful outcomes of pregnancies during which amiodarone was administered suggest that in selected patients it may serve as useful therapy.

There is virtually no information available on the use during pregnancy of new antiarrhythmic drugs such as flecanide, encainide and propafenone. These drugs should be avoided until such information is available.

Careful monitoring of drug levels when feasible is recommended, since standard dosing regimens of antiarrhythmics may alter during pregnancy as body mass, bioavailability and volume of drug distribution change.

Anticoagulation

Certain medical conditions such as venous thrombosis of the proximal venous system, or certain types of prosthetic valves, necessitate anticoagulation during pregnancy. As with other therapy during pregnancy, the risks arising from the untreated condition must be weighed against the risks and side-effects of the treatment. For conditions such as metal prosthetic valve, anticoagulation is a necessity.

Coumadin

Coumadin (warfarin) is an oral anticoagulant that is a vitamin K antagonist, resulting in a decrease in thrombin formation. Coumadin crosses the placenta and has been associated with increased risk of spontaneous abortion, and 'warfarin embryopathy' characterized by hypoplasia of the nasal bone, and a wide variety of central nervous system abnormalities including optic atrophy, mental retardation, deafness and microcephaly[88–90]. In addition, coumadin predisposes both the mother and her fetus to hemorrhagic complications including fetal intracranial hemorrhage[91–94]. In general, coumadin is contraindicated during the first trimester and during delivery. A woman requiring anticoagulation who is planning a pregnancy should be advised to switch from coumadin to heparin prior to becoming pregnant. Some authors advocate the use of coumadin during the 12th week to the 9th month with heparin used at the beginning and end of pregnancy. Successful management of pregnant patients requiring anticoagulation requires both maximum patient compliance and the physician's vigilance.

Heparin

Heparin appears to be a safer alternative than coumadin for anticoagulation during pregnancy. It is a large molecule that does not cross the placenta and has little effect on the fetus. Heparin can be administered by continuous intravenous infusion or by intermittent subcutaneous doses (every 8–12 h). Adequate anticoagulation can be obtained by either schedule. Patients should be instructed to avoid all aspirin products while on heparin.

Antibiotic prophylaxis

Certain cardiac conditions result in a predisposition to bacterial endocarditis during procedures which result in transient bacteremia. The American Heart Association[95] recommends antibiotic prophylaxis for the following conditions: (1) prosthetic cardiac valves; (2) a history of bacterial endocarditis, even in the absence of heart disease; (3) most congenital heart diseases; (4) rheumatic and other acquired valvular dysfunction, even after valvular surgery; (5) hypertrophic cardiomyopathy; and (6) mitral valve prolapse with valvular regurgitation. Patients with one of the above conditions who undergo obstetric procedures such as Cesarean section, vaginal delivery, especially in the presence of infection, dilatation and curettage, or therapeutic abortion should receive prophylactic antibiotics. In general, the incidence of subacute bacterial endocarditis is relatively low during uncomplicated vaginal delivery. The following regimen has been recommended by the American Heart Association[95]:

(1) Ampicillin, 2.0 g intravenously or intramuscularly plus gentamicin, 1.5 mg/kg (not to exceed 80 mg), given 30 min before the procedure. The same regimen may be repeated once, 8 h after the initial doses;

(2) Vancomycin, 1.0 g given intravenously over hour, can be used in place of ampicillin in patients who are allergic to penicillin.

MANAGEMENT DURING LABOR AND DELIVERY

As discussed elsewhere in this chapter, a number of profound cardiovascular changes take place during labor and delivery, and these changes are affected by numerous variables including type of delivery (vaginal vs. Cesarean), level of pain and anesthesia.

With contractions during labor, there is an increase in cardiac output, the level of which depends on the force of contraction and the level of anxiety and pain[1]. Numerous other hemodynamic changes also take place, including increases in heart rate and blood pressure, both systolic and diastolic. There is an even larger increase in cardiac output that occurs immediately postpartum and persists early in the postpartum period, but reverts to prepregnant levels by the end of 4 weeks[2]. Cardiovascular hemodynamics are also affected by the type and amount of anesthesia. Spinal or epidural anesthesia results in a decline in cardiac output and blood pressure; larger alterations in hemodynamics occur with balanced general anesthesia.

The major alterations in hemodynamics that occur during pregnancy, labor and delivery essentially revert to normal by 5 weeks postpartum.

The pregnant patient with cardiovascular disease may tolerate these hemodynamic alterations only marginally and will need close medical supervision during labor and delivery. The intensity of the clinical management will depend on the severity of the cardiac condition, the types of cardiac pathology and the functional class of the patient.

General guidelines for the management of pregnant cardiac patients include induction of labor at term with favorable cervix and laboring in the lateral position. All patients should have nasal oxygen, and a running intravenous line. In selected situations, placement of a Swan–Ganz pulmonary catheter the day before planned induction of labor may be indicated so that hemodynamics can be optimized prior to the onset of labor.

Patients with mitral stenosis often tolerate tachycardia and a volume load poorly. The heart rates of these patients should be controlled (≤ 90 beats/min) during labor and delivery with intravenous propranolol or esmolol (ultra-short-acting intravenous β-blocker).

Strong consideration should be given to administration of intravenous lasix immediately following delivery, to offset the large increases in cardiac output and volume redistribution that occurs at delivery.

Maintenance of cardiac output is critical in aortic stenosis, so the pulmonary capillary wedge pressure should be maintained at ≥ 16 mmHg, and diuretics should be used cautiously and only if there is frank pulmonary congestion.

Patients with pulmonary hypertension are at greatest risk immediately following delivery and should be maintained at high pulmonary capillary wedge pressures with attention paid to avoidance of hypotension. Oxygen administration in these patients is critical.

CARDIAC DIAGNOSTIC TESTING DURING PREGNANCY

Tests not involving ionizing radiation

Electrocardiogram

The EKG can be enormously helpful in diagnosing a wide variety of abnormalities, including arrhythmias, and poses no risk to either the mother or the fetus. A wide range of EKG changes occur during pregnancy, including change in rate, rhythm, axis, intervals and waveform morphology. Premature atrial and ventricular complexes are benign and seen frequently, and a wide variety of brady- and tachyarrhythmias have been documented during labor[96].

Echocardiography

Echocardiography utilizes sound waves to evaluate cardiac function in a non-invasive fashion. Currently, echocardiographic technology includes M-mode, two-dimensional and Doppler (including color flow Doppler) imaging; each version provides slightly different information about the size and function of the heart. Echocardiography has been widely used and poses no risk to either the mother or the fetus.

Magnetic resonance imaging

Magnetic resonance imaging (MRI) is a technique that produces tomographic imaging of the body by use of a magnetic field. It is useful in cardiovascular imaging because of the ability to differentiate flowing blood from stationary structures without the use of contrast media.

The potential risks of MRI have been studied in detail and no apparent long-term adverse effects have been demonstrated on the fetuses of pregnant mice. Despite the lack of demonstrable adverse effects, the current recommendation is that women avoid being scanned during the first trimester of pregnancy[97].

Cardiac diagnostic tests involving ionizing radiation

Ionizing radiation, depending on the dose and the gestational age, may pose risks to the fetus. During the first few weeks after conception, a maternal dose of 0.1 Gy results in a 0.1% increase in abortions over the naturally occurring spontaneous abortion rate of 25–50%. The period of organogenesis (2–8 weeks) is critically important. A dose of 0.1 Gy is estimated to produce a 1% increase in the frequency of congenital fetal abnormalities[98]. After 8 weeks' gestation, the primary effect of radiation exposure is an increased incidence of childhood leukemia. A dose of 0.01 Gy may increase the frequency of malignant disease by up to 11 cases per 1 000 000 live births[98].

Fetal exposure of 0.1 Gy or greater may increase the rise of childhood leukemia and fetal abnormalities such as microcephaly[99]. Some limit the safe fetal dose to 5 mGy. Occasionally, the need arises during pregnancy for cardiac diagnostic testing that involves ionizing radiation. If the information obtained is crucial for the management of the patient, the test should be performed in such a way as to minimize exposure to the fetus.

Chest radiograph

A chest X-ray delivers approximately 0–0.05 mGy to the fetus, which is considered a negligible amount. In addition, the abdomen of the pregnant patient can often be shielded during the test, to minimize exposure. An inadvertent chest X-ray during early pregnancy poses little, if any, risk to the fetus.

Radionuclide ventriculogram

A radionuclide ventriculogram (RVG) involves administration of a radioactive tracer injected intravenously, and detection of radioactive activity by a γ camera during various phases of the cardiac cycle. This produces a scintillation angiogram depicting regional wall motion and ejection fraction. A variation, called a 'first pass' RVG, can demonstrate a left-to-right shunt by detecting early recirculation of tracer over the lung fields.

A RVG delivers a whole-body radiation dose of 2.9 mGy with an unknown (but lesser) exposure to the fetus[100]. Shunt detection and wall motion can now be carried out accurately, owing to improvement in two-dimensional and Doppler echocardiography, the diagnostic tool of choice.

Cardiac catheterization

There are cardiac events during pregnancy that require cardiac catheterization and obligate exposure to ionizing radiation. Examples include: (1) unsuspected pulmonary hypertension where the diagnosis is critical for patient management; and (2) suspected aortic dissection or myocardial infarction during pregnancy where the diagnosis is critical for continued patient management. Under these circumstances, the risk of fetal exposure to ionizing radiation is justified to obtain necessary information.

Cardiac catheterization delivers up to 5 mGy of radiation[101], depending on the length of the procedure, but exposure to the fetus can be minimized by shielding the abdomen with lead, and by careful attention to the duration of fluoroscopy. As with other tests, catheterization should be avoided unless the critical information cannot be obtained in other ways.

REFERENCES

1. Cole PL, St John Sutton M. Normal cardiopulmonary adjustments to pregnancy. *Cardiovascular Health and Disease in Women. Cardiovascular Clinics* 1988;18:37–56
2. Capless EL, Clapp JF. Cardiovascular changes in early phase of pregnancy. *Am J Obstet Gynecol* 1989;161:1449
3. van Oppen ACC, Stigter RH, Bruinse HW. Cardiac output in normal pregnancy: a critical review. *Obstet Gynecol* 1996;87:310–18
4. Cole PL, Plappert T, Saltzman DH, St John Sutton M. Changes in left ventricular geometry, load and function following pregnancy. *J Am Coll Cardiol* 1987;9:43A
5. Capless EL, Clapp JF. When do cardiovascular parameters return to their preconception values? *Am J Obstet Gynecol* 1991;165:883
6. Metcalfe J, McAnulty JH, Ueland K. *Heart Disease and Pregnancy, Physiology and Management*. Boston: Little, Brown, 1986:223
7. Schaefer G, Arditi LI, Solomon HA, Ringland JE. Congenital heart disease and pregnancy. *Clin Obstet Gynecol* 1968;11:1048
8. Szekely P, Snaith L. Heart disease in pregnancy. In *The Evolution and Clinical Course of Chronic Rheumatic Heart Disease*. London: Churchill Livingstone, 1974:48
9. Gleicher N, Midwall J, Hochberger D, Jaffin H. Eisenmenger's syndrome and pregnancy. *Obstet Gynecol Surv* 1979;34:721
10. Whittenmore R, Hobbins JC, Engle MA. Pregnancy and its outcome in women with and without surgical treatment of congenital heart disease. *Am J Cardiol* 1982;50:641
11. Limacher MC, Ware JA, O'Meara ME, *et al*. Tricuspid regurgitation during pregnancy: two dimensional and pulsed Doppler echocardiogram observations. *Am J Cardiol* 1985;55:1059
12. Mendelson CL. *Cardiac Disease in Pregnancy*. Philadelphia: F.A. Davis, 1960
13. Neilson G, Galea EG, Blunt A. Congenital heart disease and pregnancy. *Med J Aust* 1970;1:1806
14. Nora JJ, Nora AH. The evolution of specific genetic and environmental counselling in congenital heart diseases. *Circulation* 1978;57:205
15. Elkayam U, Gleicher N. *Cardiac Problems in Pregnancy*, 2nd edn. New York: Alan R Liss, 1990
16. Savage D, Garrison R, Devereux R, *et al*. Mitral valve prolapse in the general population. I. Epidemiologic features: the Framingham study. *Am Heart J* 1983;106:571
17. Rayburn WF, Fontana ME. Mitral valve prolapse and pregnancy. *Am J Obstet Gynecol* 1981;141:9
18. Szekely P, Snaith L. Atrial fibrillation and pregnancy. *Br Med J* 1961;5237:1407
19. Vosa C, Renzulli A, Festa M, *et al*. Cardiac valve replacement during pregnancy. Report of two cases. *Ital J Surg Sci* 1988;18:175
20. Vosloo S, Reichart B. The feasibility of closed mitral valvotomy in pregnancy. *J Thorac Cardiovasc Surg* 1987;93:675
21. Patel JJ, Mitha AS, Hassen F, *et al*. Percutaneous balloon mitral valvotomy in pregnant patients with tight pliable mitral stenosis. *Am Heart J* 1993;125:1106
22. Mangione JA, Zuliani MF, Del Castillo JM, *et al*. Percutaneous double balloon mitral valvuloplasty in pregnant women. *Am J Cardiol* 1989;64:99–102
23. Arias F, Pineda J. Aortic stenosis and pregnancy. *J Reprod Med* 1978;20:229
24. Lao TT, Sermer M, MaGee L, *et al*. Congenital aortic stenosis and pregnancy – a reappraisal. *Am J Obstet Gynecol* 1993;169:540–5
25. Rose V, Gold RJM, Lindsay G, Allen M. A possible increase in the incidence of congenital heart defects among the offspring of affected parents. *J Am Coll Cardiol* 1985;6:376–82

26. Whittemore R, Hobbins JC, Engle MA. Pregnancy and its outcome in women with and without surgical treatment of congenital heart disease. *Am J Cardiol* 1982;50:641–51

27. Korsten H, VanZundert A, Mooij P, *et al*. Emergency aortic valve replacement in the 24th week of pregnancy. *Acta Anaesth Belg* 1989;40:201

28. Banning AP, Pearson JF, Hall RJC. Role of balloon dilatation of the aortic valve in pregnant patients with severe aortic stenosis. *Br Heart J* 1993;70:544–5

29. Lao TT, Adelman AG, Sermer M, Colman JM. Balloon valvuloplasty for congenital aortic stenosis in pregnancy. *Br J Obstet Gynaecol* 1993;100:1141–2

30. Goodwin JF. Pregnancy and coarctation of the aorta. *Lancet* 1958;1:16–20

31. Wachtel HL, Czarnecki SW. Coarctation of the aorta and pregnancy. *Am Heart J* 1966;72:251

32. Kainulainen K, Pulkkinen L, Savolainen A, *et al*. Location on chromosome 15 of the gene defect causing Marfan syndrome. *N Engl J Med* 1990;323:935–9

33. Pyeritz RE. Maternal and fetal complications of pregnancy in the Marfan syndrome. *Am J Med* 1981;71:784

34. Pyeritz RE. The Marfan syndrome. *Am Fam Physician* 1986;34:83

35. Pyeritz RE. Propranolol retards aortic root dilatation in the Marfan syndrome. *Circulation* 1983;68:111

36. Elkayam UE, Ostrzega E, Shotan A, Mehra A. Cardiovascular problems in pregnant women with the Marfan syndrome. *Ann Intern Med* 1995;123:117–22

37. Avila WS, Grinberg M, Snitcowsky R, *et al*. Maternal and fetal outcome in pregnant women with Eisenmenger's syndrome. *Eur Heart J* 1995;16:460–4

38. Sobervilla LA, Cassinelli MT, Carcelen A, *et al*. Human fetal and maternal oxygen tension and acid base status during delivery at high altitude. *Am J Obstet Gynecol* 1971;111:1111

39. Salvin AG. Importance of hyperbaric oxygenation for a favorable outcome of labor in primary pulmonary hypertension patients. *Vopr Okhr Materin Det* 1979;24:64

40. Fuster V, Steele PM, Edwards WD, *et al*. Primary pulmonary hypertension: natural history and the importance of thrombosis. *Circulation* 1984;70:580

41. Nootens M, Rich S. Successful management of labor and delivery in primary pulmonary hypertension. *Am J Cardiol* 1993;71:1124–5

42. Gott VL, Pyeritz RE, Magovern GJ Jr, *et al*. Surgical treatment of aneurysms of the ascending aorta in the Marfan syndrome. Results of composite-graft repair in 50 patients. *N Engl J Med* 1986;311:1070–4

43. Ascarelli MH, Grider AR, Hsu HW. Acute myocardial infarction during pregnancy managed with immediate percutaneous transluminal coronary angioplasty. *Obstet Gynecol* 1996;88:655–7

44. Nolan TE, Hankins GD. Myocardial infarction in pregnancy. *Clin Obstet Gynecol* 1989;32:68–75

45. Glazier JJ, Eldin AM, Hirst JA, *et al*. Primary angioplasty using a urokinase-coated hydrogel balloon in acute myocardial infarction during pregnancy. *Cathet Cardiovasc Diagn* 1995;36:216–19

46. Sheikh AU, Harper MA. Myocardial infarction during pregnancy: management and outcome of two pregnancies. *Am J Obstet Gynecol* 1993;169:279–84

47. Shalev Y, Ben-Hur H, Hagay Z, *et al*. Successful delivery following myocardial ischemia during the second trimester of pregnancy. *Clin Cardiol* 1993;16:754–6

48. Fujito T, Inoue T, Mizoguchi K, *et al*. Acute myocardial infarction during pregnancy. *Cardiology* 1996;87:361–4

49. Taylor GW, Moliterno DJ, Hillis LD. Peripartum myocardial infarction. *Am Heart J* 1993;126:1462–3

50. Homans DC. Peripartum cardiomyopathy. *N Engl J Med* 1985;312:1432

51. Veille JC. Peripartum cardiomyopathies: a review. *Am J Obstet Gynecol* 1984;148:805

52. Brockington IF. Postpartum hypertensive heart failure. *Am J Cardiol* 1971;27:650

53. Faruque AA. Acute fulminating puerperal myocarditis. *Br Heart J* 1965;27:139

54. Becker FF, Taube H. Myocarditis of obscure etiology associated with pregnancy. *N Engl J Med* 1962;266:62

55. Blegen SD. Postpartum congestive heart failure: Beriberi heart disease. *Acta Med Scand* 1965;178:515

56. Rizeq MN, Rickenbacker PR, Fowler MB, Billingham ME. Incidence of myocarditis in peripartum cardiomyopathy. *Am J Cardiol* 1994;74:474–7

57. Sanderson JE, Adesayna CO, Anjarin FI, Parry E. Postpartum cardiac failure due to volume overload? *Am Heart J* 1979;97:613

58. Walsh JJ, Burch GE, Black WC, *et al*. Idiopathic myocardiopathy of the puerperium (postpartal heart disease). *Circulation* 1965;32:19

59. Demakis JF, Rahimtoola SH, Sutton GC, *et al*. Natural course of peripartum cardiomyopathy. *Circulation* 1971;44:1053

60. St John Sutton M, Cole P, Plappert M, *et al*. Effects of subsequent pregnancy on left ventricular function in peripartum cardiomyopathy. *Am Heart J* 1991;121:1776

61. Cole P, Cook F, Plappert T, *et al*. Longitudinal changes in left ventricular architecture and function in peripartum cardiomyopathy. *Am J Cardiol* 1987;60:871

62. Hedon B, Montoya F, Cabrol A. Twin pregnancy and vaginal birth after heart transplantation. *Lancet* 1990;335:476

63. Carvalho AC, Almeida D, Cohen M, *et al*. Successful pregnancy, delivery and puerperium in a heart transplant patient with previous peripartum cardiomyopathy. *Eur Heart J* 1992;13:1589–91

64. Lowenstein BR, Vain NW, Perrone SV, *et al*. Successful pregnancy and vaginal delivery after heart transplantation. *Am J Obstet Gynecol* 1988;158:589–90

65. Key TC, Resnik R, Dittrich HC, Reisner LS. Successful pregnancy after cardiac transplantation. *Am J Obstet Gynecol* 1989;160:367–71

66. Camann WR, Goldman GA, Johnson MD, *et al*. Cesarean delivery in a patient with a transplanted heart. *Anesthesiology* 1989;71:618–20

67. Kumar A, Elkayam U. Hypertrophic cardiomyopathy in pregnancy. In Elkayam U, Gleicher N, eds. *Cardiac Problems in Pregnancy*. New York: Alan R Liss, 1990:129

68. Mendelsohn CL. Disorders of the heart beat during pregnancy. *Am J Obstet Gynecol* 1956;72:1268

69. Schroeder JS, Harrison DC. Repeated cardioversion during pregnancy. *Am J Cardiol* 1971;27:445

70. Copeland GD, Stern TN. Wenckebach periods in pregnancy and puerperium. *Am Heart J* 1958;56:291

71. Leyse R, Ofstun M, Diller DH, Merendino KA. Congenital aortic stenosis in pregnancy corrected by extracorporeal circulation. *J Am Med Assoc* 1961; 176:1009

72. Becker RM. Intracardiac surgery in pregnant women. *Ann Thorac Surg* 1983;36:453

73. Vosa C, Renzulli A, Festa M, *et al.* Cardiac valve replacement during pregnancy. *Ital J Surg Sci* 1988;18:175

74. Pomini F, Mercogliano D, Cavatelli C, *et al.* Cardiopulmonary bypass in pregnancy. *Ann Thorac Surg* 1996; 61:259–68

75. Parry AJ, Westaby S. Cardiopulmonary bypass during pregnancy. *Ann Thorac Surg* 1996;61:1865–9

76. Jamieson WRE, Miller C, Akins CW, *et al.* Pregnancy and bioprosthesis: influence on structural valve deterioration. *Ann Thorac Surg* 1995;60:S282–7

77. Harrigan JT, Kangos JJ, Sikka A, *et al.* Successful treatment of fetal congestive heart failure secondary to tachycardia. *N Engl J Med* 1981;304:1527

78. Heaton FC, Vaughan R. Intrauterine supraventricular tachycardia: cardioversion with maternal digoxin. *Obstet Gynecol* 1982;60:749

79. Frishman WH, Chesner M. Use of beta-adrenergic blocking agents in pregnancy. In Elkayam U, Gleicher N, eds. *Cardiac Problems in Pregnancy*. New York: Alan R Liss, 1990

80. Langer A, Hung CT, McNulty JA, *et al.* Adrenergic blockade: a new approach to hyperthyroidism during pregnancy. *Obstet Gynecol* 1974;44:181–6

81. Goodlin RC. Beta blockers in pregnancy-induced hypertension. *Am J Obstet Gynecol* 1982;143:237

82. Rubin PC. Beta-blockers in pregnancy. *N Engl J Med* 1981;305:1323–6

83. Redman CWG, Geilin LJ, Bonnar J, Ounsted MK. Fetal outcome in trial of anti-hypertensive treatment in pregnancy. *Lancet* 1976;2:753

84. Redman CWG, Bielin LJ, Bonner J. The treatment of hypertension in pregnancy with methyldopa. Blood pressure control and side effects. *Br J Obstet Gynaecol* 1977;84:419–26

85. Pipkin FM, Turner SR, Symonds EM. Possible risk with captopril in pregnancy: some animal data. *Lancet* 1980;1:1256

86. Rotmensch HH, Pines A, Donchin Y. Antiarrhythmic drugs in pregnancy. In Elkayam U, Gleicher N, eds. *Cardiac Problems in Pregnancy*. New York: Alan R Liss, 1990

87. Mauer AM, Devaux LO, Lahey ME. Neonatal and maternal thrombocytopenic purpura due to quinidine. *Pediatrics* 1957;19:84

88. Hall JG, Pauli RM, Wilson KM. Maternal and fetal sequelae of anticoagulation during pregnancy. *Am J Med* 1980;68:122–40

89. Baillie M, Allen ED, Elkington AR. The congenital warfarin syndrome: a case report. *Br J Ophthalmol* 1980;64:633–5

90. Harrod MJE, Sherrod PS. Warfarin embryopathy in siblings. *Obstet Gynecol* 1981;57:673–6

91. Chen WWC, Chan CS, Lee PK, *et al.* Pregnancy in patients with prosthetic heart valves: an experience with 45 pregnancies. *Q J Med* 1982;51:358–65

92. Vallenga E, Van Imhoff GW, Aarnoudse JG. Effective prophylaxis with oral anticoagulants and low-dose heparin during pregnancy in an antithrombin III deficient woman. *Lancet* 1983;2:224

93. Michiels JJ, Stibbe J, Vellenga E, Van Vliet HHDM. Prophylaxis of thrombosis in antithrombin III-deficient women during pregnancy and delivery. *Eur J Obstet Gynecol Reprod Biol* 1984;18:149–53

94. Oakley C. Pregnancy in patients with prosthetic heart valves. *Br Med J* 1983;286:1680–3

95. Dajani AS, Bisno AL, Chung KJ, *et al.* Prevention of bacterial endocarditis: recommendations by the American Heart Association. *J Am Med Assoc* 1990;264:2919

96. Upshaw CB. A study of maternal electrocardiograms recorded during labor and delivery. *Am J Obstet Gynecol* 1970;107:17

97. Underwood R, Firmin D. *An Introduction to Magnetic Resonance of the Cardiovascular System*. London: Current Medical Literature, 1988

98. Bushong SC. Management of the pregnant employee and the pregnant patient. *Radiol Manage* 1984;6:8

99. Swartz HM, Reichling BA. Hazards of radiation exposure for pregnant women. *J Am Med Assoc* 1978;239: 1907

100. Metcalfe J, McAnulty JH, Ueland K, eds. *Burwell's & Metcalfe's Heart Disease and Pregnancy: Physiology and Management*. Boston: Little, Brown, 1986

101. Wagner LK, Lester RG, Saldana LR. *Exposure of the Pregnant Patient to Diagnostic Radiation*. Philadelphia: JB Lippincott, 1985

34
Dermatologic diseases

A.G. Martin and S. Leal-Khouri

DERMATOLOGIC DISEASES AND PREGNANCY

The skin during pregnancy undergoes profound changes that are associated with the numerous metabolic, immunologic and hormonal adjustments of this state. Pregnant patients may develop physiologic or endocrine-induced skin changes, dermatoses specifically related to pregnancy and all of the skin diseases seen in the non-pregnant state. The 'physiologic' changes occur with such regularity during pregnancy that they are considered almost normal, but they may become pathologic when severe; they often occur in the general population but are increased in frequency among pregnant women, and most regress postpartum. Some of the skin changes may not be primarily hormonal in origin. The most common 'physiologic' changes are pigmentary alterations, stretch marks, vascular spiders and telogen effluvium (Table 1).

The specific dermatoses of pregnancy include herpes gestationis, pruritic urticarial papules and plaques of pregnancy, impetigo herpetiformis, prurigo gravidarum, papular dermatitis of pregnancy, pruritic folliculitis of pregnancy and autoimmune progesterone dermatitis of pregnancy (Table 2). These diseases are discussed later in the chapter.

PHYSIOLOGIC CHANGES ASSOCIATED WITH PREGNANCY

Pigmentary changes

Ninety per cent of pregnant patients develop hyperpigmentation that is usually mild and generalized. There is accentuation of normally hyperpigmented regions such as the areolae, nipples, axillae, genitalia, perineum, anus and inner thighs[1-3]. The skin surrounding the areolae darkens producing what are known as secondary areolae. The linea alba often darkens and changes its name to linea nigra; this is most marked in dark-complexioned women. Pigmentary demarcation lines, which are borders of abrupt transition between more deeply pigmented skin and that of lighter pigmentation, may occur on the lower limbs during pregnancy[4]. Severe generalized hypermelanosis is rare and its occurrence suggests hyperthyroidism.

Table 1 Physiologic skin changes of pregnancy

Pigmentary changes
  hyperpigmentation
  melasma
Hair changes
  hirsutism
  telogen effluvium
  male pattern baldness
Nail changes
  transverse grooving
  distal onycholysis
Striae distensae
Vascular and hematologic changes
  spider angiomas
  palmar erythema
  varicosities
  non-pitting edema
Mucous membrane changes
Cutaneous tumors
  granuloma gravidarum
  hemangiomas
  molluscum gravidarum
Glandular activity

Table 2 Dermatoses of pregnancy

Herpes gestationis
Pruritic urticarial papules and plaques of pregnancy
Impetigo herpetiformis
Prurigo gravidarum
Papular dermatitis of pregnancy
Pruritic folliculitis of pregnancy
Autoimmune progesterone dermatitis of pregnancy

Freckles, melanocytic nevi and recent scars may also darken. An increase in size or change in color of a nevus is always of concern, but the question whether pregnancy or oral contraceptives affects the incidence or prognosis of melanoma remains unknown. Recent studies have demonstrated that women who are pregnant or on oral contraceptives have an increased number of estrogen and progesterone receptors on their nevi cells similar to those observed in melanoma and severely dysplastic nevi[5]. Histopathologic evaluation of melanocytic nevi in pregnancy have suggested mild atypia or 'activation', but never of sufficient degree to result in diagnostic confusion[6].

Generally, hyperpigmentation appears during the first trimester, progresses until delivery and regresses postpartum. However, the affected sites usually do not return to their previous color. The cause of hyper-pigmentation is controversial. Most investigators agree that an increase in output of pituitary, placental and ovarian hormones is responsible[7-9]. Melanocyte-stimulating hormone (MSH), estrogen and proges-terone are strong melanogenic stimulants and may play an important role. MSH is increased during pregnancy and decreases postpartum[10-12].

Melasma (chloasma), or the 'mask of pregnancy', presents as symmetric, blotchy brown pigmentation of the face; it occurs in up to 75% of pregnant women and in up to 34% of women taking oral contracep-tives[13,14]. Melasma usually begins during the second trimester and is more common in dark-complexioned individuals. The causative agent for melasma is unknown. Contributing factors aside from pregnancy and oral contraceptives include genetics, race, sunlight, nutrition, hepatic diseases and parasitosis. Sanchez and colleagues reported an association between melasma and cosmetic usage, but no specific chemical has been implied. Preventive measures such as avoidance of sun, usage of sunscreens and non-allergenic cosmetics rather than perfumed preparations are recommended. Gestational melasma regresses, usually within a year of delivery, but pigmentation due to oral contraceptives tends to persist. Topical combinations of tretinoin, hydroquinone and dexamethasone have been success-fully used in some cases of persistent melasma[15].

Striae distensae

Striae distensae or stretch marks are linear pink to violaceous atrophic lines that develop opposite to the skin tension lines on the abdomen, breast, upper arms, lower back, buttocks, thighs and groin. Stretch marks develop in 90% of pregnant women during the 6th and 7th months[1-3,16-18]. The cause is unknown but probable contributing factors include increased adrenocortical activity, relaxin and estrogens, as well as stretching and familial factors. Postpartum, the striae greatly improve becoming flesh-colored or hypopigmented, but they never disappear entirely.

Hair and nail changes

Some degree of hirsutism develops in most women early in pregnancy, and is most pronounced in women with pre-existing abundant body hairs or dark hair. Hirsutism is most pronounced on the face, however the arms, legs, back and suprapubic areas can be involved. Within 6 months postpartum, the excess lanugo hairs disappear, but the coarse terminal hairs may remain.

The cause of hirsutism is unknown. It could be due to increased ovarian androgen secretion or increased adrenocorticotropic hormone secretion[19,20]. Patients with marked persistent hirsutism should have virilizing tumors excluded. Therapy consists of reassuring the patient, but when hirsutism persists more than 6 months postpartum, electrolysis or cosmetic treatment should be considered.

Lynfield reported an increase proportion of anagen hair follicles (the growth phase) during pregnancy which is thought to be secondary to a decreased rate of conversion of anagen to telogen hairs (the resting phase), producing a thicker than normal growth[21]. Postpartum, a greater than usual number of hairs enter the telogen phase resulting in telogen effluvium. During telogen effluvium, shedding of hairs begins 1 to 5 months postpartum and usually ceases within 15 months. The causes of postpartum telogen effluvium include the stress of delivery, and changes in the hor-mone balance[21]. Treatment involves reassurance since complete spontaneous recovery almost always occurs.

A mild degree of frontoparietal recession in a male pattern distribution may develop toward the end of pregnancy. This usually reverts postpartum. Diffuse thinning of the hair during the last trimester can also occur. The causes of male pattern baldness and hypotrichosis is unknown, but inhibition of gonado-tropic activity secondary to the high steroid levels that occur late in pregnancy may play an important role.

Nail changes seen during pregnancy include Beau's lines (transverse grooving), brittleness or softening, distal onycholysis, subungual keratosis and accelerated nail growth[1-3,19,22]. The pathogenesis of these changes is unknown. Treatment consists of keeping nails trimmed and avoiding external sensitizers and infections.

Vascular and hematologic changes

Vascular changes occur during pregnancy and are rela-ted to distention, fragility and proliferation of vessels. Spider angiomas are macular or papular, red, telan-giectatic puncta with radiating branches and surround-ing erythema. They appear most commonly in areas drained by the superior vena cava. These changes appear in 67% of white and 11% of black women between the 2nd and 5th months of pregnancy and regress within 3 months postpartum in 75% of cases[23]. Elevated levels of circulating estrogens and/or angio-genesis factors are believed to be important in the pathogenesis of spider angiomas, palmar erythema, hemangiomas and pyogenic granuloma. Persistent spider angiomas can be treated with electrodesiccation.

Palmar erythema can be localized to the thenar or hypothenar area, or can present as a diffuse mottling of the hand with cyanosis and pallor. It can occur in 66% of white and 33% of black women begin-ning in the first trimester[1-3]. The erythema usually resolves 1 week postpartum. Diffuse palmar erythema is indistinguishable from that seen in hyperthyroidism and hepatic cirrhosis.

Varicosities involving the saphenous, vulvar and hemorrhoidal veins appear in 40% of women starting from the 3rd month of pregnancy[2,3,17]. A familial tendency for increased elastic tissue fragility in conjunction with increased venous pressure may account for varicosities. Partial regression tends to occur postpartum. Phlegmasia alba dolens and phlegmasia cerulea dolens due to venous occlusion are rare. Cutis marmorata and livedo reticularis of the legs, facial flushing and pallor are presumably due to vasomotor instability secondary to increased estrogens. Patients with pre-existing Raynaud's phenomena may improve because of the vasomotor relaxation.

Non-pitting edema of the eyelids, face, hands and feet is common during the third trimester. The edema tends to decrease during the day. The edema is due to sodium and water retention in conjunction with increased capillary permeability. Purpuric lesions on the legs secondary to increased capillary permeability are common during the last half of pregnancy.

Mucous membrane changes

Pregnancy gingivitis is present in up to 80% of pregnant women and begins in the 2nd month of pregnancy[1-3,24]. The gingivae enlarge, darken, become red, swollen and may bleed spontaneously. The cause is unknown, but poor hygiene, local irritation, nutritional deficiencies and progesterone-induced vascular proliferation are thought to be important in the pathogenesis.

Cutaneous tumors

Proliferation of capillaries in hypertrophied gingivae can result in granuloma gravidarum (pyogenic granuloma of pregnancy, pregnancy tumor). In 27% of women it appears as a deep-red mass arising from the gingiva during the 2nd to 5th month of pregnancy[24]. Clinically and histologically it is identical to pyogenic granuloma in non-pregnant women, but it tends to regress postpartum. Molluscum gravidarum (skin tags) may appear on the neck, chest, axillae and inframammary areas in the latter stages of pregnancy. Occasionally the tumors regress postpartum; however, if persistent they may need to be excised.

Hemangiomas, hemangioendotheliomas, glomangiomas, glomus tumors, neurofibromas, dermatofibromas and leiomyomas may arise during gestation. Except for neurofibromas, they tend to regress postpartum, and all may recur during subsequent pregnancies. Keloids may grow rapidly and desmoid tumors may also develop. Desmoid tumors should be treated by wide local excision since they may be locally destructive.

Glandular activity

Eccrine sweating progressively increases during the third trimester accounting for occasional hyperhidrosis, increased incidence of miliaria and dyshidrotic eczema. The cause is unknown, but some believe that the changes are due to increased thyroid activity. On the other hand, palmar sweating is decreased, which may be secondary to increased adrenocortical activity. If eccrine sweating is significantly increased it can be treated with a solution of 20% aluminum chloride hexahydrate in ethyl alcohol applied every night for 1 week, and then as necessary. Apocrine gland activity decreases during pregnancy, relieving pre-existing Fox–Fordyce disease and hidradenitis suppurativa, but there may be a rebound postpartum. Sebaceous gland activity increases in some patients during the third trimester. Acne and oily skin may develop but the effects of pregnancy on acne are unpredictable. Sebaceous glands associated with lactiferous ducts on the areolae hypertrophy in 30–50% of women, beginning during the 6th week of gestation, and appear as elevated brown papules called Montgomery's tubercules[1-4,20]. The cause of the glandular changes is unknown but estrogen, progesterone and cortisol are implicated. Breast changes during pregnancy include enlargement, tenderness, erect nipples, hyperpigmentation of nipples and areolae, prominence of veins, striae and Montgomery's tubercules. Most of these changes regress postpartum.

DERMATOSES OF PREGNANCY

Herpes gestationis

Herpes gestationis is an autoimmune skin disease of pregnancy and the puerperium characterized by an intensely pruritic, blistering eruption. The disease is most commonly associated with pregnancy, although rare occurrences have been reported with hydatidiform mole and choriocarcinoma[25,26]. The incidences of herpes gestationis range from 1 per 1700 deliveries to one per 50 000 deliveries[27-29]. The name is a misnomer and reflects its 'herpetic' appearance to J.L. Milton in 1872[30]. It is not related to any known viral infection, and most authors agree the name is anachronistic. Mayou and colleagues have proposed that the term 'pemphigoid gestationis' is more appropriate given its clinical and histologic resemblance to bullous pemphigoid[31]. Both names can be found in the literature.

Mounting evidence is accumulating to support an autoimmune pathogenesis of herpes gestationis. It is associated with C4Q0 allele, Class II antigens HLA-DR3, HLA-DR4 and anti-HLA antibodies[32,33]. Circulating material autoantibodies react with an 'antigenic' constituent of the cutaneous basement membrane as well as the chorionic epithelilum and amnion of the placenta. This antigen is a normal constituent of the basement membrane and may be found in the placenta as early as the second trimester. Subepidermal blisters develop from tissue damage incurred by this antigen–antibody reaction with resultant complement activation. A recent finding of abnormal expression of paternal major histocompatibility complex (MHC) II region molecules in the placenta suggests that the maternal immune system evokes an allogenic reaction[34].

Herpes gestationis presents as an extremely pruritic, blistering eruption that may begin at any time during the pregnancy, but most commonly occurs during the second and third trimesters. It frequently begins during the first pregnancy and has a tendency to recur earlier and with greater vengeance in subsequent pregnancies. Initial onset in the postpartum period has also been well documented and is often explosive, occurring within hours of delivering. A frequent observation is a relative remission in the weeks predelivery followed by a postpartum flare as well as flares with the first few postpartum menstrual periods.

Early lesions of herpes gestationalis begin as erythematous, edematous papules and plaques that develop into vesicles and bullae (Figure 1). The lesions may be grouped and develop into erosions with crusting. The eruption begins in and around the umbilicus in the majority of patients and then spreads to involve the abdomen and thighs (Figure 2). The back, breast, palms and soles are frequently affected. The head and mucosa are involved less frequently. A constant feature of herpes gestationis is pruritis. The itching is often extreme and may begin days or weeks prior to the appearance of clinical lesions.

Histology of an early urticaria-like lesion shows a perivascular infiltrate consisting of mononuclear cells and many eosinophils. There is dermal papillary edema, with spongiosis and intracellular edema of the overlying epidermis. Histology of a bulla reveals basal cell necrosis with a resultant subepidermal bulla. There is a pronounced inflammatory infiltrate containing many eosinophils.

Using a direct immunofluorescence assay, patients with herpes gestationis will have linear deposition of complement 3 (C3) along the basement membrane in clinically normal and involved skin[35]. This finding traditionally has been a hallmark of the disease. Immunoglobulin G (IgG) deposition is seen as well (30–40% of patients), and less frequently IgA and IgM. The sera of patients with herpes gestationis contain an antibody to a basement membrane constituent of normal skin. This antibody, known as herpes gestationis factor, avidly binds complement and is an IgG1 molecule[36]. Using conventional immunofluorescence, only 25% of patients show evidence of herpes gestationis factor, and usually in low titers. Today indirect assays using more sensitive and specific monoclonal antibodies against the IgG subclass reveal that all patients possess circulating anti-IgG antibodies directed against

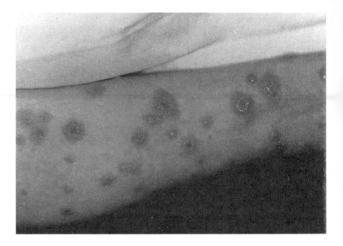

Figure 1   Early lesions of herpes gestationis

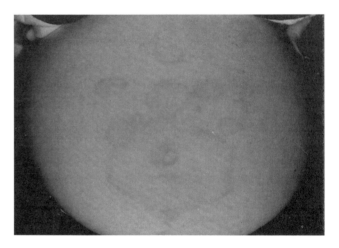

Figure 2   Periumbilical distribution of herpes gestationis

cutaneous basement membrane. Chemically split skin studies reveal the immunoreactants to localize the epidermal side of the lamina lucida[37]. Placental studies reveal a similar deposition of C3 and immunoglobulin along the amniotic basement membrane. As in lesional skin and plasma, IgG1 is the most frequently found immunoglobulin[38].

The herpes gestationis antigen has been characterized as a 180 kDa glycoprotein found in the lamina lucida of the basement membrane of skin and placenta[39,40]. It is most interesting that herpes gestationis antigen may first appear in placenta during the second trimester of pregnancy, coinciding with the time-course of the development of herpes gestationis[41]. Recently, it has been shown that there is abnormal expression of MHC II region molecules within the placenta of patients with herpes gestationis[42]. The authors contend that a particular breakdown of the fetoplacental unit occurs allowing the maternal immune system to participate in an autoimmune response to a placental basement membrane antigen. These IgG1 subclass maternal antibodies cross-react with skin, are capable of fixing complement, and draw forth a cascade of inflammatory cells and mediators to produce the characteristic lesion of herpes gestationis, the subepidermal bullae. The placenta, which is capable of absorbing the IgG1 antibody and depositing it in the placental basement membrane, in essence, protects the fetus.

The main disease entity in the differential diagnosis of herpes gestationis is pruritic urticarial papules and plaques of pregnancy (PUPPP). There is clinical overlap between the two diseases in that they are both pruritic dermatoses of pregnancy that present with urticarial plaques, wheals and vesicles. Herpes gestationis is distinctive, however, in developing bullae (PUPPP occasionally is vesicular), in its initial periumbilical distribution (PUPPP arises in abdominal and thigh striae), and its earlier appearance within the second trimester (PUPPP begins in the third trimester). Histologically, one cannot definitively differentiate them. Direct immunofluorescence of herpes gestationis, however, is always positive for C3 at the basement membrane, while PUPPP is always negative.

Other vesiculobullous diseases, such as dermatitis herpetiformis, bullous pemphigoid and bullous erythema multiforme, are easy to differentiate from herpes gestationalis by clinical presentation and routine immunoflourescence. Bullous pemphigoid has many similarities to herpes gestationis both in its clinical appearance and ultrastructural findings. However, bullous pemphigoid is a disease of the elderly and would rarely be seen in the reproductive years.

Systemic steroids are the mainstay of therapy for moderate to severe herpes gestationis. Mild cases of herpes gestationis often respond to roica fluorinated steroids and antihistamines. As the dosage becomes more aggressive, a prednisone dose of 20–40 mg/day is necessary. One can frequently then taper to a daily 10 mg/day maintenance dose. Fortunately, the use of low-dose systemic steroids in the second- and third-trimester of pregnancy is not associated with increased risk of congenital anomalies, although the mother needs careful monitoring for gestational diabetes and hypertension[43]. Plasmapheresis and cyclophosphamide can be useful alternatives should corticosteroids be ineffective or contraindicated[44,45].

The usual course of herpes gestationalis is complete remission several weeks after delivery with a possible mild flare with resumption of menses. Rarely, severe cases of herpes gestationis will persist far beyond the postpartum period, and require corticosteroid therapy. Monthly perimenstrual flares, ovulatory flares and flares with the use of birth control pills or estrogen therapy have all been reported, and patients should be warned. These reports support the contention that once herpes gestationis is initiated, it is hormonally mediated. Once a patient has herpes gestationis, there is a clear tendency for it to recur in subsequent pregnancies with an earlier onset and more severe disease.

The impact of herpes gestationis on perinatal mortality and morbidity is controversial. While Lawley and colleagues noted an increase in fetal mortality and morbidity[46], Shornick and co-workers found no increase in maternal or fetal complications[28]. More recent data suggested an increase in preterm delivery and fetal growth retardation[47,48]. In any case, good obstetrical and perinatal care gives a favorable outcome in the great majority of cases. Rarely do infants born to mothers with herpes gestationis have vesicles or bullae. When present, the eruption is mild and transient. There appear to be no ill-effects on the child nor evidence of increased incidence of other autoimmune diseases[35].

Pruritic urticarial papules and plaques of pregnancy

Pruritic urticarial papules and plaques of pregnancy (PUPPP) is the most common of the gestational dermatoses with an incidence varying from one in 120 to one in 240 pregnancies[49]. While the etiology is unknown, current speculation favors an inflammatory reaction to connective tissue damage within striae[50]. Recent studies suggest an association of PUPPP with skin distention due to excessive weight gain which leads credence to this viewpoint[51]. Hormonal modulation may be involved as well. The entity is not associated with pre-eclampsia, herpes gestationalis, or autoimmune disease.

In the first report of PUPPP, a woman was described with all the clinical features as we know them: a pruritic, urticarial eruption developing within abdominal striae during the third trimester and generalizing to the thighs and buttocks. While it was termed toxemic rash of pregnancy, there is no association of PUPPP with pre-eclampsia, and this terminology was not accepted[52]. In 1979, Lawley and colleagues[53] reported seven cases in which they carefully defined the clinical features of PUPPP and gave it its widely accepted, yet controversial, name of pruritic urticarial papules and plaques of pregnancy. Later Holmes and Black[54] suggested the name polymorphic eruption of pregnancy based on the varying morphology of the lesions. Both names are now found in the literature.

The onset of PUPPP varies from as early as 17 weeks to 1 week postpartum, with the majority of patients presenting within the third trimester. The mean duration of the disease is 6 weeks but can last as long as 16 weeks. It begins with urticarial-like papules usually in association with striae. Other type lesions seen are papulovesicles, polycyclic wheals and occasionally targetoid lesions. The eruption most frequently begins in the striae of the lower abdomen, sparing the periumbilical region (Figure 3). The thighs and extensor

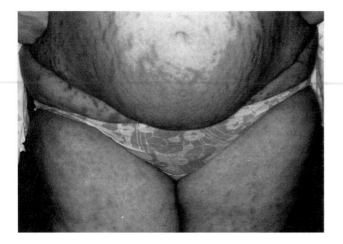

Figure 3 Pruritic urticarial papules and plaques of pregnancy (PUPPP) developing in striae

surfaces of the arms are frequently involved, while the face, palms and soles are rarely involved.

Histopathologic findings of an early urticarial lesion reveal epidermal and upper dermal edema with a superficial lymphodistiocytic perivascular infiltrate. Eosinophils often are present in the infiltrate, however blood eosinophilia is a less usual feature. Vesicles are present in the most florid examples, in which case intense focal spongiosis is seen in the epidermis. Immunofluorescence studies are negative.

Treatment of PUPPP is symptomatic as the disease itself is self-limiting and without serious outcomes. Management of pruritis with medium-potency topical steroid preparations, the use of Aveeno baths and antihistamines such as diphenhydramine have all been successful. Most important is reassurance to the patient that this is a common disease of pregnancy that will terminate in a few weeks, and will have no ill-effect on the outcome of the fetus.

Maternal and fetal prognosis is felt to be entirely normal with PUPPP. The risk of developing PUPPP during a second pregnancy appears to be small, and in cases of recurrence, the disease is attenuated. It has been noted that a second episode occurs earlier in the pregnancy and resolves prepartum.

Impetigo herpetiformis

Impetigo herpetiformis (IH) is rare, with fewer than 100 cases reported. It was first described by Von Hebra in 1872, and it consists of an eruption resembling pustular psoriasis that arises suddenly in a patient without prior history of psoriasis[55]. The disease is associated with pregnancy, but has been reported in male patients[56]. IH begins usually during the last trimester of pregnancy but it may occur as early as the 3rd month. The disease is characterized by prodromal symptoms of malaise, fever, delirium, diarrhea, vomiting and

occasionally tetany secondary to hypocalcemia[56]. Mildly pruritic, circinate, erythematous macules or plaques with pustules advancing peripherally appear preferentially in intertriginous areas. It can spread to mucous membranes as well as to the entire integument, sparing only the face, hands and feet. The lesions heal with non-scarring postinflammatory hyperpigmentation. Severe systemic toxicity may occur resulting in death of the mother or fetus. Usually the illness remits spontaneously postpartum, only to recur in subsequent pregnancies.

Histologically, IH is identical to pustular psoriasis, and is characterized by parakeratosis, elongation of the rete ridges and the spongiform pustule of Kogoj. Leukocytosis, high sedimentation rate, hypocalcemia and hyperphosphatemia may be present. Cultures from the sputum and blood, and immunofluorescence studies are negative.

The etiology of IH is unknown. It may represent an outbreak of pustular psoriasis in a latent psoriatic patient that may be triggered by either hypocalcemia or pregnancy[56,57]. Symptomatic therapy is indicated as well as systemic corticosteroids.

Prurigo gravidarum

Prurigo gravidarum (PG), also known as recurrent cholestasis of pregnancy, is characterized by intense, generalized pruritis in the absence of primary cutaneous lesions, although secondary excoriations may occur (Figure 4). It occurs during the third trimester in 66% of cases, abates quickly after delivery, only to recur with successive pregnancies. The incidence of this disorder ranges from 0.02% to 3%[7,58].

PG may be due to intrahepatic cholestasis, resulting in elevated levels of bile acids in the serum and in the skin, in genetically predisposed women. Minimal abnormalities may be noted on liver function test, including an increase in bilirubin[8]. The intensity of the pruritis varies from mild to severe and may be intermittent initially, occurring only at night. Pruritis may be localized to the abdomen, trunk, or extremities, but it tends to become generalized. Occasionally, the patients may have anorexia, nausea, vomiting and diarrhea. Jaundice is usually mild and becomes detectable 2–4 weeks after the onset of pruritis. There are cases where jaundice is absent. The urine may become dark and the stools light colored. The symptoms resolve rapidly but may recur in subsequent pregnancies or with the use of oral contraceptives. Patients with PG may be at increased risk for having premature and low birth weight infants, as well as postpartum hemorrhage, cholelithiasis and cholecystitis.

Mild pruritis may be treated with emollients and antihistamines. In patients with intense pruritis, cholestyramine, 4 g one to six times daily, given with supplemental fat soluble vitamins may be effective.

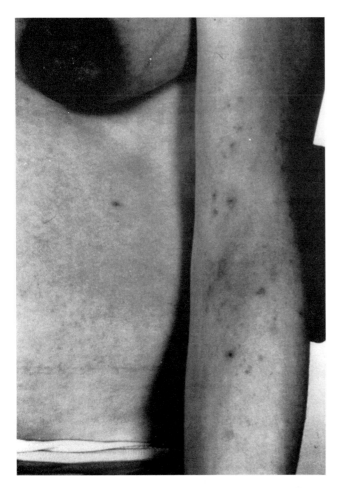

Figure 4   Excoriations in pruritus gravidarum

gonadotropin, reduced plasma cortisol and reduced urinary estriol. Whether the disease is a separate entity of its own is highly doubtful since the biochemical abnormalities observed were not compared to those seen in pregnancies in general or other pregnancy-related dermatoses. The risk of fetal mortality has been reported as high as 30%. This calculation of fetal deaths included possible first-trimester fetal losses occurring prior to development of skin eruption[61]. PDP most likely represents a variant of PUPPP, or pruritis gravidarum in an atopic individual. Systemic administration of corticosteroids such as prednisone has been recommended.

Pruritic folliculitis of pregnancy

The term 'pruritic folliculitis of pregnancy' was first used by Zoberman and Farmer[62] in 1981 to describe a widespread pruritic follicular eruption developing in the latter half of pregnancy. The histology was one of an acute folliculitis and maternal and fetal prognosis were normal. While the incidence of this disorder is unknown it may not be uncommon. Similar to steroid-induced acne, this eruption can take on a monomorphic type of appearance with pustules. This is most likely a form of hormonally induced acne rather than a specific dermatosis of pregnancy. The lesions clear spontaneously at delivery or postpartum. Topical erythromycin gel or solution 2% may be palliative.

Autoimmune progesterone dermatitis of pregnancy

Bierman[63] in 1973 reported the first and only case of autoimmune progesterone dermatitis of pregnancy (APDP). The patient in two successive pregnancies developed an eruption characterized by papules and pustules on the extensor surface of the extremities and buttocks associated with arthritis involving the metacarpophalangeal joints, wrist, knees and ankles. The acneiform rash occurred early in both pregnancies and terminated in spontaneous abortions during the 2nd and 3rd months, followed by resolution of the skin lesions. No premenstrual flares occurred. Usage of oral contraceptives caused recurrence of the rash and the arthritis.

The pathophysiology of APDP is not known, but it seems to represent a hypersensitivity reaction to endogenous progesterone. Biopsy revealed a moderately dense intraepidermal and dermal mixed infiltrate composed predominantly of eosinophils. A lobular panniculitis with abscess formation and a large number of eosinophils were present. Elevated levels of serum IgG and IgM were present. Direct and indirect immunofluorescence were negative. Eosinophilia was present.

Jaundice may develop during the third trimester of pregnancy and may occur alone or in association with pruritis and gastrointestinal symptoms (nausea and vomiting). The increased levels of estrogen, pregnane-diol and progesterone during pregnancy inhibit the enzyme glucuronyl transferase, resulting in impaired bilirubin conjugation and excretion which causes intrahepatic cholestasis. Increased levels of alkaline phosphatase, leucine aminopeptidase, and impaired clearance of bromsulphalein are also observed[59]. Significant elevation of bilirubin or of the transaminases does not occur.

Papular dermatitis of pregnancy

Papular dermatitis of pregnancy (PDP) is a rare generalized pruritic eruption of pregnancy described by Spangler and colleagues in 1962[60]. It can occur anytime during pregnancy and is characterized by discrete, excoriated, urticarial-like papules widely disseminated over the body. Distinguishing features include raised levels of urinary human chorionic

REFERENCES

1. Wong RC, Ellis CN. Physiologic skin changes in pregnancy. *J Am Acad Dermatol* 1984;10:929–40
2. Winton GB, Lewis CW. Dermatoses of pregnancy. *J Am Acad Dermatol* 1982;6:977–98
3. Hellreich PD. The skin changes of pregnancy. *Cutis* 1974;13:82–6
4. James WD, Meltzer MS, Guill MA, *et al.* Pigmentary demarcation lines associated with pregnancy. *J Am Acad Dermatol* 1984;11:438–40
5. Ellis DL, Wheeland RG. Increased nevus estrogen and progesterone ligand binding related to oral contraceptives or pregnancy. *J Am Acad Dermatol* 1986;14:25–31
6. Foucar E, Bentley TJ, Laube DW, *et al.* A histiopathic evaluation of nevocellular nevi in pregnancy. *Arch Dermatol* 1985;121:350–4
7. Wade TR, Wade SL, Jones HE. Skin changes and diseases associated with pregnancy. *Obstet Gynecol* 1978;52:233–42
8. Sasseville D, Wilkinson RD, Schnader JY. Dermatoses of pregnancy. *Int J Dermatol* 1981;20:223–41
9. Callen JP. Pregnancy's effects on the skin: common and uncommon changes. *Postgrad Med* 1984;75:138–45
10. Clark D, Thody AJ, Shuster S, *et al.* Immunoreactive alpha-MSH in human plasma in pregnancy. *Nature* 1978;273:163–4
11. Thody AJ, Plummer NA, Burton JL. Plasma beta-melanocyte-stimulating hormone levels in pregnancy. *J Obstet Gynaecol Br Commonw* 1974;81:875–7
12. McGuinness BW. Melanocyte-stimulating hormone: a clinical and laboratory study. *Ann NY Acad Sci* 1963;100:640–57
13. Sanchez NP, Pathak MA, Sato S, *et al.* Melasma: a clinical, light microscopic, ultrastructural, and immunofluorescence study. *J Am Acad Dermatol* 1981;4:698–710
14. Smith AG, Shuster S, Thody AJ, *et al.* Chloasma, oral contraceptives, and plasma immunoreactive beta-melanocyte stimulating hormone. *J Invest Dermatol* 1976;68:367–76
15. Kligman AM, Willis I. A new formula for depigmenting human skin. *Arch Dermatol* 1975;111:40–8
16. Demis DJ, Dolson RL. Disorders of pregnancy. In Demis DJ, ed. *Clinical Dermatology*, Vol. 4. New York: Harper & Row, 1987:1–15
17. Benson RC. *Current Obstetric and Gynecologic Diagnosis and Treatment.* Los Altos: Lange Medical Publications, 1982
18. Liu DTY. Striae gravidarum. *Lancet* 1974;1:625
19. Cumming K, Derbes VJ. Dermatoses associated with pregnancy. *Cutis* 1967;3:120–6
20. Demis DJ. Skin conditions during pregnancy. In Demis DJ, ed. *Clinical Dermatology*, Vol 2. New York: Harper and Row, 1987:1–9
21. Lynfield YL. Effect of pregnancy on the human pair cycle. *J Invest Dermatol* 1960;35:323–7
22. Benson RC. *Current Obstetric and Gynecologic Diagnosis and Treatment.* Los Altos: Lange Medical Publications, 1982:581
23. Barnhill RS, Wolf JE Jr. Angiogenesis and the skin. *J Am Acad Dermatol* 1987;16:1226–42
24. Goldman HS, Marder MZ. *Physician's Guide to the Diseases of the Oral Cavity.* New Jersey: Medical Economics Co., 1982:118–20
25. Dupont C. Herpes gestationis with hydatiform mole. *Trans St Johns Hosp Dermatol Soc* 1974;60:103
26. Slazinski L, Degefu S. Herpes gestationis associated with choriocarcinoma. *Arch Dermatol* 1982;118:425–8
27. Kolodny RC. Herpes gestationis: a new assessment of incidence, diagnosis, and fetal prognosis. *Am J Obstet Gynecol* 1969;104:39–45
28. Shornick JK, Bangert JL, Freeman RG, *et al.* Herpes gestationalis: clinical and histiologic features of twenty-eight cases. *J Am Acad Dermatol* 1983;8:214–24
29. Roger D, Vaillant L, Fignon A, *et al.* Specific pruritic diseases of pregnancy. A prospective study of 3192 pregnant women. *Arch Dermatol* 1994;130:734–9
30. Milton JL. *The Pathology and Treatment of Diseases of the Skin.* London: Robert Hardwicke, 1872
31. Mayou SC, Black MM, Holmes RC. Pemphigoid (herpes) gestationis. *Semin Dermatol* 1988;7:104–10
32. Shornick JK, Artlett CM, Jenkins RE, *et al.* Complement polymorphism in herpes gestationis: association with C4 null allele. *J Am Acad Dermatol* 1993;29:545–9
33. Shornick JK, Jenkins RE, Briggs DC, *et al.* Anti-HLA antibodies in pemphigoid gestationis (herpes gestationis). *Br J Dermatol* 1993;129:257–9
34. Borthwick GM, Holmes RC, Stirrat GM. Abnormal expression of class II MHC antigens in placenta from patients with pemphigoid gestationis: analysis of class II MHC subregion product expression. *Placenta* 1988;9:81–94
35. Shornick JK: Herpes gestationis. *J Am Acad Dermatol* 1987;17:539–56
36. Kelly SE, Cerio R, Bhogal BS, *et al.* The distribution of IgG subclass in pemphigoid gestationis. PG factor is an IgG autoantibody. *J Invest Dermatol* 1989;92:695–8
37. Yaoita H, Gullino M, Katz SI. Herpes gestationis: ultrastructure and ultrastructural localization of in vivo-bound complement: modified tissue preparation processing for horseradish peroxidase staining of skin. *J Invest Dermatol* 1976;66:383–8
38. Fine JD, Smith LT, Holbrook KA, *et al.* The appearance of four basement membrane zone antigens in developing human fetal skin. *J Invest Dermatol* 1984;83:66–9
39. Kelly SE, Bohogal BS, Black MM, *et al.* Western blot analysis of the antigen pemphoid gestationis. *J Invest Dermatol* 1988;(abstr)91:397
40. Morrison LH, Labib RS, Zone JJ, *et al.* Herpes gestationis autoantibodies recognize a 180 kD human epiderma antigen. *J Clin Invest* 1988;81:2023–6
41. Kelly SE, Black MM. Pemphigoid gestationis: placental interactions. *Semin Dermatol* 1989;8:12–17
42. Kelly SE, Black MM, Flemming S. Pemphigoid gestationis: a unique mechanism of initiation of an auto-immune response by MHC class II molecules? *J Pathol* 1989;158:81–2
43. Schatz M, Patterson R, Zeitz S, *et al.* Corticosteroid therapy for the pregnant asthmatic patient. *J Am Med Assoc* 1975;233:804
44. Van De Weil A, Hart HC, Flinterman J, *et al.* Plasma exchange in herpes gestationis. *Br Med J* 1980;281:1041–2
45. Castle SP, Mather-Mondrey M, Bennion S, *et al.* Chronic herpes gestationis and antiphospholipid antibody syndrome successfully treated with cyclophosphamide. *J Am Acad Dermatol* 1996;34:333–6

46. Lawley TJ, Stingl G, Katz SI. Fetal and maternal risk factors in herpes gestationis. *Arch Dermatol* 1978; 114:552–5

47. Holmes RC, Black MM. The fetal prognosis in pemphigoid gestationis (herpes gestationis). *Br J Dermatol* 1984;110:67–72

48. Shornick JK, Black MM. Fetal risks in herpes gestationis. *J Am Acad Dermatol* 1992;26:63–8

49. Lawley TJ, Hertz KC, Wade TR, *et al.* Pruritic urticarial papules and plaques of pregnancy. *J Am Med Assoc* 1979;241:1696–9

50. Holmes RC. Polymorphic eruption of pregnancy. *Semin Dermatol* 1989;8:18–22

51. Cohen LM, Capeless EL, Krusinski PA, *et al.* Pruritic urticarial papules and plaques of pregnancy and its relationship to maternal-fetal weight gain and twin pregnancy. *Arch Dermatol* 1989;125:1534–6

52. Bourne G. Toxemic rash of pregnancy. *Proc R Soc Med* 1962;55:462–4

53. Lawley TJ, Hertz KC, Wade TR, *et al.* Pruritic urticarial papules and plaques of pregnancy. *J Am Acad Dermatol* 1984;10:473–80

54. Holmes RC, Black MM. The specific dermatoses of pregnancy. *J Am Acad Dermatol* 1983;8:405–12

55. Von Hebra F. On some affections of the skin occurring in pregnant and puerperal women, *Wien Med Wchnschr.* 1872;48:1197; abstracted *Lancet* 1872;1:399 *Am J Syph Dermatol* 1873;4:156

56. Sauer GC, Geha BJ. Impetigo herpetiformis. *Arch Dermatol* 1961;83:119–26

57. Lotem M, Katzenelson V, Rotem A, *et al.* Impetigo herpetiformis: a variant of pustular psoriasis or a separate entity? *J Am Acad Dermatol* 1989;20:338–41

58. Dacus JV, Muram D. Pruritis in pregnancy. *South Med J* 1987;80:614–17

59. Rencoret RH, Aste H. Jaundice during pregnancy. *Med J Aust* 1973;1:167–9

60. Spangler SA, Reddy W, Bardawil WA, *et al.* Papular dermatitis of pregnancy: a new clinical entity? *J Am Med Assoc* 1962;181:577–81

61. Michaud RM, Jaconson D, Dahl MV. Papular dermatitis of pregnancy. *Arch Dermatol* 1982;118:1003–5

62. Zoberman E, Farmer ER. Pruritic folliculitis of pregnancy. *Arch Dermatol* 1981;117:20–2

63. Bierman SM. Autoimmune progesterone dermatitis of pregnancy. *Arch Dermatol* 1973;107:896–901

35

Diabetes mellitus

D.R. Coustan

EPIDEMIOLOGY OF DIABETES IN PREGNANCY

Pre-existing diabetes mellitus complicates approximately 0.3% of all pregnancies in the USA[1], while gestational diabetes complicates 2–5%[2]. Although type 2 diabetes, characterized by the typical clinical presentation of obesity, insulin resistance and no tendency toward diabetic ketoacidosis, is roughly 10 times more prevalent in the American population than is type 1 diabetes, the latter is more likely during pregnancy. This is due to the characteristic younger age of onset with type 1 diabetes, so that a woman in the child-bearing years is apt to have this ketosis-prone form of diabetes, characterized by insulinopenia rather than insulin resistance. It is important to point out that the term 'insulin-dependent diabetes' (type 1) requires that the patient be dependent upon exogenous insulin to prevent ketoacidosis. Thus, individuals with type 2 diabetes may take insulin, but would not go into diabetic ketoacidosis (DKA) in its absence.

ETIOLOGY

Diabetes mellitus is a heterogeneous group of disorders all characterized by hyperglycemia. Type 2 diabetes, as described above, appears commonly to be related to obesity, and to run in families. Some data suggest that the tendency to type 2 diabetes may be inherited as a dominant trait[3]. It is not yet clear whether insulin resistance alone is sufficient to cause type 2 diabetes, or whether there must also be an element of relative insulinopenia. Type 1 diabetes, on the other hand, is generally believed to be an autoimmune disorder in which the immune system is directed against the islet cells in the pancreas. There is clearly a genetic predisposition toward such pancreatic destruction, as evidenced by the preponderance of specific HLA antigens in individuals with type 1 diabetes. However, the genetic predisposition is not sufficient to bring about the disease, as evidenced by the less than 50% concordance of identical twins for this disorder[3].

Gestational diabetes is a condition of 'carbohydrate intolerance of variable severity with onset or recognition during pregnancy'[4]. There is evidence to suggest that women with gestational diabetes are at increased risk, compared to the general population, for the subsequent development of type 2, and in some cases type 1, diabetes[5]. One possible explanation is that the metabolic changes brought about by pregnancy induce transient carbohydrate intolerance in individuals whose metabolism is at some point along a continuum ultimately leading to diabetes[6].

PATHOPHYSIOLOGY

Pregnancy has profound effects on maternal metabolism. It is useful to think of these effects as being designed to assure a plentiful supply of fuel (glucose, gluconeogenic amino acids) and structural material (various amino acids) for the building of a fetus. When the gravida has fasted, circulating glucose and amino acid levels are lower than in non-pregnant fasting women[7]. While it is tempting to speculate that this relative hypoglycemia is secondary to fetal consumption of fuel, the change occurs relatively early in pregnancy, when the fetus cannot yet utilize enough fuel to account for the observed phenomenon. The fall in glucose levels during fasting is associated with a rise in circulating levels of ketone bodies, to an extent greater than is observed in the non-pregnant state. This fall in glucose and rise in ketones has been termed 'accelerated starvation', which is a useful concept. Insulin levels after an overnight fast are significantly higher than in the non-pregnant individual, despite lower glucose values. Such apparent insulin resistance is believed by many to be the underlying cause of gestational diabetes, as will be discussed below.

When the pregnant woman ingests glucose, particularly after an overnight fast, her circulating glucose level increases somewhat more slowly, but to a greater amplitude, than in the non-pregnant state, despite the fact that her insulin level is quite a bit higher than in non-pregnant women[7]. This 'insulin resistance' is present in both the liver and the periphery. Nevertheless, in the context of the usual day-to-day ingestion of mixed meals, it appears that normal pregnant women maintain their circulating glucose levels within a rather narrow range[7,8].

The insulin resistance mentioned above is most probably the cause of the appearance of gestational diabetes in 2–3% of women in the USA. Whether there is also a relative deficiency of insulin production in such individuals remains to be determined.

Individuals with pre-existing diabetes, usually but not always type 1, who become pregnant are impacted dramatically by the increase in insulin resistance brought about by the pregnancy. Those with type 2 diabetes are likely to require markedly increased doses of insulin in order to maintain relative euglycemia. Those with type 1 diabetes generally experience a two- to three-fold increase in insulin requirements as pregnancy progresses[9].

Most importantly, despite a tendency toward hypoglycemia during the first trimester, individuals with type 1 diabetes are significantly more likely to experience DKA during the second half of pregnancy than at other times. This proclivity toward DKA appears to be related to the insulin resistance of pregnancy. The most important causes of DKA are absolute or relative insulinopenia and glucagon excess, resulting in hyperglycemia from hepatic glycogenolysis and gluconeogenesis and hyperketonemia due to uninhibited lipolysis and increased hepatic production of ketone bodies[10]. When DKA is present, hepatic glucose production is increased as much as three-fold, accounting for marked hyperglycemia even in patients who have not eaten for a considerable length of time. The maternal effects of hyperglycemia during DKA include osmotic diuresis, which may result in dehydration. The resultant hypovolemia can cause hypotension, renal dysfunction, mental aberrations and shock. Electrolytes, particularly total body sodium and potassium, become depleted. Because ketone bodies are moderately strong acids the maternal pH falls, the serum bicarbonate level falls and an anion gap ([serum sodium] – [serum bicarbonate + serum chloride] > 10–15 mEq/l) results, indicative of metabolic acidosis. The acidosis is the cause of the characteristic tachypnea and increased tidal volume known as Kussmaul's respirations. Nausea and vomiting frequently accompany the acidosis, further exacerbating the hypovolemia and electrolyte depletion. The fetus is particularly at risk, with fetal mortality rates historically reported to be in the range of 50–90% when maternal DKA occurs[10]. Explanations for this high rate of fetal death include hypoxia due to uterine hypoperfusion resulting from maternal hypovolemia and the possible fetal effects of the rapid transport of hydrogen ions across the placenta. More recent studies[11] report lower perinatal mortality rates of between 10 and 20%, suggesting some improvement in management of this complication over the years. During pregnancy, common causes of DKA appear to be similar to those seen in the non-pregnant state: intercurrent infection and omission of insulin injections. However, in addition, iatrogenic causes may contribute, including the use of betamimetic agents for tocolysis and corticosteroids for the enhancement of fetal pulmonary maturity. DKA is not caused by the administration of exogenous glucose unless there is simultaneous underinsulinization.

Even in the absence of DKA, hyperglycemia is associated with perinatal morbidity and mortality in diabetic pregnancy. In fact, according to the 'Pedersen hypothesis'[12], all of the problems comprising 'diabetic fetopathy' are related to fetal hyperinsulinemia, which results from hyperglycemia transmitted from the maternal to the fetal compartment. This concept was extended by Freinkel[13] as the 'modified Pedersen hypothesis' to acknowledge the probable role of non-glucose secretagogues in stimulating fetal pancreatic insulin production and release.

There is a body of experimental evidence to support the Pedersen hypothesis with regard to both pre-existing and gestational diabetes. Although a randomized, prospective trial of loose vs. strict metabolic control in diabetic pregnancy has not been carried out, existing data on human pregnancy support the concept that near-normalization of maternal circulating glucose levels strongly predicts favorable perinatal outcome. Karlson and Kjellmer[14] demonstrated that diabetic women whose average blood glucose level in the third trimester exceeded 150 mg/dl manifested a 24% perinatal mortality rate, compared to 4% in those whose average third-trimester glucose level was less than 100 mg/dl. Virtually every series published since that time in which near-normalization of glucose levels was attempted has reported a perinatal mortality rate of less than 5%. The pathophysiology of the relationship between maternal hyperglycemia and perinatal death is yet to be determined. However, studies in laboratory animal models have demonstrated that fetal hyperinsulinemia can lead to hypoxia, acidosis and fetal death[15]. Morbidity, such as fetal macrosomia, neonatal hypoglycemia, respiratory distress syndrome, plethora and jaundice have likewise been linked to fetal hyperinsulinemia[15].

It has long been appreciated that infants of diabetic mothers suffer from birth defects at a rate 2–3 times that in the general population. Because virtually all structural anomalies in infants of diabetic mothers have taken place by 8–10 weeks after the last menstrual period[16], the cause(s) of such anomalies in humans have been difficult to study. Laboratory investigations have demonstrated that maternal hyperglycemia during organogenesis can induce fetal anomalies in rodent embryos[17]. In human pregnancies, first-trimester glycosylated hemoglobin levels have been positively correlated with the likelihood of anomalies, raising the possibility of a cause-and-effect relationship between hyperglycemia (or some other aspect of poor metabolic control) and birth defects[18–20]. In the Diabetes in Early Pregnancy (DIEP) Study, an observational study in which women were asked to perform multiple daily self glucose monitoring tests, an approximate halving of the rate of congenital anomalies (4.9%) was noted in diabetic individuals registering for care prior to conception or during very early pregnancy compared to those enrolled after 8 weeks (9%), even though no specific goals for glucose control were imposed[21]. In this study, offspring of diabetic women registering early for care still had an approximate doubling of the malformation rate compared to control children of non-diabetic mothers. Furthermore, no correlation could be found between level of glucose control and malformation rate, a finding possibly attributable to the paucity of pregnancies with either very good or very poor control in the series. In an interventional study Fuhrmann and co-workers[22] demonstrated a malformation rate of 2–3% in offspring of diabetic mothers who were given intensive pre-pregnancy and early pregnancy care, a rate similar to that in the general population and considerably lower than the 8% rate among offspring of mothers registering for care after the 8th week of gestation. Kitzmiller and colleagues[23] reported a major malformation rate of 1.2% among the offspring of 84 diabetic women who entered a preconception care program, compared to 10.9% among the offspring of 110 diabetic women presenting for prenatal care at 6 weeks' gestation or later. Average ambient glucose levels during organogenesis were considerably lower in the preconception care group than in the women participating in the DIEP Study cited above. Poor maternal metabolic control has also been linked to spontaneous abortion in diabetic pregnancy[20,24,25]. It therefore seems likely that there exists a continuum of reproductive damage related to aberrations of metabolism in early diabetic pregnancy. This ranges from spontaneous abortion when poor control is very early and/or severe, to anomalies when it comes somewhat later, is less severe, or happens at a critical time. As described above, aberrations of metabolic control occurring later in pregnancy, after organogenesis has been completed, appear capable of inducing a wide range of problems which may be called, collectively, 'diabetic fetopathy'.

The above pathophysiological mechanisms appear to be operative in gestational diabetic pregnancy, as well as in pregnancy complicated by overt diabetes, albeit to a lesser degree. Because the metabolic alterations seen in gestational diabetes are generally, but not always, less severe than those of pre-existing diabetes, perinatal mortality is distinctly less likely with the milder forms of diabetes, particularly if the condition is identified and treated in some way. However, studies of *undiagnosed* and *untreated* gestational diabetes suggest a marked increase in the perinatal mortality rate[26,27]. Even in gestational diabetic pregnancies maintained in reasonably good metabolic control there is an excess of fetal macrosomia[28]. Furthermore, childhood and young adult obesity has been reported in infants of gestational diabetic mothers[29–31], suggesting the possibility that the intrauterine milieu may have profound and long-lasting effects on adipose

tissue formation. Strengthening this hypothesis is the finding of a significant relationship between maternal response to a glucose challenge during pregnancy and the likelihood of the offspring developing diabetes, and of the female offspring developing gestational diabetes[32].

DIAGNOSIS

By definition, pre-existing or overt diabetes has been diagnosed prior to pregnancy; it is gestational diabetes, therefore, that is the subject of this section. The diagnostic criteria currently accepted in the USA utilize a 100-g, 3-h oral glucose tolerance test and are based on the work of O'Sullivan and Mahan[33], in which normative data were collected for 752 consecutive prenatal patients. Various thresholds derived from these data were then applied to a separate group of subjects who underwent the test during pregnancy and then were followed for 7 years. The criteria recommended were the most efficient predictors of subsequent diabetes. According to these criteria, gestational diabetes is diagnosed if at least two of the four glucose tolerance test values meet or exceed thresholds two standard deviations above the means for their respective specific time intervals. In O'Sullivan's original study[33] venous samples of whole blood were utilized, and the Somogyi–Nelson technology was applied for glucose measurement. The resultant thresholds were: fasting, 90 mg/dl; 1 h, 165 mg/dl; 2 h, 143 mg/dl; and 3 h, 127 mg/dl. These were rounded off to the nearest 5 mg/dl for ease of recall.

In the 1970s most clinical laboratories switched to venous plasma or serum, which yield values approximately 15% higher than whole blood samples. Accordingly, in 1979 the National Diabetes Data Group (NDDG)[34] attempted to convert the O'Sullivan and Mahan criteria to plasma values by adding approximately 15% to each threshold. The resultant criteria have been promulgated by the American Diabetes Association (ADA)[35] and the American College of Obstetricians and Gynecologists (ACOG)[36], and are currently widely utilized in the USA. The recommended thresholds for plasma or serum glucose samples are: fasting, 105 mg/dl; 1 h, 190 mg/dl; 2 h, 165 mg/dl; and 3 h, 145 mg/dl. This is for the 100-g, 3-h oral glucose tolerance test; gestational diabetes is diagnosed if two or more samples meet or exceed the above thresholds.

In addition to the change from whole blood to plasma or serum samples, another alteration in glucose testing occurred in the 1970s. The Somogyi–Nelson method, which measures approximately 5 mg/dl of reducing substances other than glucose, was replaced by more specific enzymatic methods such as glucose oxidase and hexokinase. Consequently in 1982[37] our group published suggested thresholds to take into account both methodological advances: fasting, 95 mg/dl; 1 h, 180 mg/dl; 2 h, 155 mg/dl; and 3 h, 140 mg/dl.

While the NDDG criteria are currently most widely accepted, one study[38], in which the original methodology of O'Sullivan and Mahan was compared directly with current technology, found that the NDDG criteria were above the 95% confidence limits of the O'Sullivan criteria at three of the four glucose tolerance testing intervals, whereas the proposed criteria of Carpenter and Coustan were within such confidence intervals at all times. This suggests that the thresholds most widely used at the present time may be too high to be considered accurate conversions of the O'Sullivan and Mahan criteria.

It is important to point out that the relationship between glucose intolerance and perinatal morbidity and mortality is, in all likelihood, continuous. Magee and colleagues[39] found a similar level of perinatal morbidity in pregnancies in which gestational diabetes diagnosed by the Carpenter and Coustan conversion of O'Sullivan and Mahan's criteria, but not the NDDG conversion criteria, were met; both groups manifested significantly more morbidity than did the general population. Naylor and associates[40] compared patients known to their caregivers to have gestational diabetes (NDDG criteria), patients whose caregivers were blinded to the diagnosis of gestational diabetes (Carpenter and Coustan criteria) and normoglycemic controls. Both groups of patients with gestational diabetes had a greater likelihood of delivering by Cesarean section than did normal controls. However, in the patients with undiagnosed, milder gestational diabetes, Cesarean section was related to an increased likelihood of macrosomia. In the patients with known gestational diabetes, the treatment apparently lowered the macrosomia rate to that of the normal controls, but high Cesarean section rates persisted, possibly because of the caregivers' expectations of macrosomia[41].

The 3-h, 100-g oral glucose tolerance test is too time-consuming and expensive to apply to all patients. Therefore, some screening procedure is necessary in order to choose which patients should be tested. It was at one time traditional to use the taking of a history as the screening test. Patients who reported the presence of certain risk factors (e.g. family history of diabetes, previous macrosomic baby or stillbirth, etc.) would undergo glucose tolerance testing. Unfortunately, this method of screening is too insensitive for clinical use, identifying only approximately 50% of women with gestational diabetes[42]. For this reason both the ADA[35] and the ACOG[36] have recommended the use of a 50-g, 1-h glucose challenge, administered without respect to the time of the last meal, as a screening test for gestational diabetes. The test is administered at 24–28 weeks, and a plasma or serum glucose level of ≥ 140 mg/dl is considered by these two organizations to be an

indication for the full 3-h, 100-g oral glucose tolerance test. In our center we use a threshold of 130 mg/dl, since we have determined that 10% of women with gestational diabetes manifest screening test values of 130–139 mg/dl[42]. Currently the ACOG[43] acknowledges that the benefits to a population of screening for gestational diabetes have not been proven, but suggests that if screening is to be perfomed it be done universally. Exceptions would be populations in which the prevalence is unusually high or low. In high-prevalence populations, such as the Pima Indians, it may make most sense to omit the screening test and go right to the full 3-h oral glucose tolerance test (OGTT), since the likelihood of having gestational diabetes by virtue of being a Pima is higher than that imparted by a positive screening test. In low-prevalence populations, such as attendees to an adolescent pregnancy clinic, screening based on risk-factors may be appropriate. In 1997 the ADA promulgated similar recommendations[44].

MANAGEMENT

The management of diabetes in pregnancy brings together advances in internal medicine, obstetrics, pediatrics, physiology and metabolism. Although there are marked similarities in the management of pregnancies complicated by pre-existing diabetes and those complicated by gestational diabetes, the differences in degree of risk and maternal glycemic stability make it most convenient to consider each separately.

Pre-existing diabetes – medical management

Preconception care

As discussed above, diabetic pregnancy presents a rare opportunity to prevent congenital anomalies[45]. Preconception care should begin at the time diabetes mellitus is diagnosed in a female prior to or during the age of reproduction. Pediatricians, internists, family doctors and others caring for such patients should educate young diabetic women about the need for planning prior to pregnancy, and the increased risk of congenital anomalies when a pregnancy begins prior to the institution of reasonable metabolic control. Various approaches to contraception should be discussed[46] in order to minimize the likelihood of inadvertent pregnancy.

Once the individual with diabetes has decided to attempt pregnancy, a thorough evaluation of her medical status should be undertaken. This could include renal function tests, cardiac assessment, hemogram, immunity testing for hepatitis and rubella, blood type, Rh and antibody testing, and the offer of HIV testing. A thorough physical examination is appropriate, as is an expert ophthalmological examination in patients whose diabetes is not of recent onset. Once risk factors have been assessed, the patient should be counselled as to their significance. This is a good time to suggest that the patient obtain more information about diabetic pregnancy. One good resource, *Diabetes and Pregnancy: What To Expect*, is a book available from the ADA[47]. If pregnancy is to be initiated, intensive management aimed at near-normalization of circulating glucose levels should be instituted. There is not widespread agreement as to the most appropriate goals for glycemic control during the preconception period and during the time of organogenesis in early pregnancy. In our center we attempt to maintain fasting and 2-h postprandial glucose levels, measured at least four times a day, at under 150 mg/dl during this time period. Although we strive for tighter glucose control later in pregnancy, the periconceptional period is of uncertain duration and hypoglycemic reactions appear to be more likely than in the second half of pregnancy. Glycosylated hemoglobin levels are followed at 1–2-month intervals. Once they fall within 2 to 4 standard deviations of the mean for the method being employed, and glucose control appears to be stable, we inform the patient that it is reasonable to discontinue contraception and attempt pregnancy. Preconception care has been shown to be cost effective[48], and an outline of its contents has been published by the ADA[49,50].

Care during early pregnancy

Unfortunately the majority of diabetic women do not present for care until after conception. Furthermore, most of those presenting when already pregnant are not in optimum metabolic control. Because organogenesis has been virtually completed by the 8th to 10th week after the last menstrual period[16], patients who register prior to this time may benefit from attempts to normalize glycemia as rapidly as possible. Often, this means a brief period of hospitalization. Patients who commence care after organogenesis has been completed will also benefit from near-normalization of circulating glucose levels, but the degree of urgency is less and outpatient management can usually accomplish the needed improvement in glycemia without unnecessarily interrupting the patient's life style.

If the patient has not had the benefit of preconceptional care, the baseline evaluation described earlier should be carried out at the time of the first visit in pregnancy. Patients with pre-existing diabetes will benefit from a team approach to management of diabetic pregnancy, including physicians with special expertise in diabetes management and high-risk pregnancy management, as well as dieticians, nurse educators, social workers and subspecialists as needed. Frequent contact with the health care team is essential in order to respond to problems as they arise.

Blood glucose monitoring

Glycemic control can best be assessed by daily self blood glucose monitoring, using glucose oxidase impregnated test strips and reflectance meters[8]. There are a number of different approaches, including measuring fasting and preprandial glucose prior to each meal, 1-h postprandial glucose measurements and 2-h postprandial measurements. No method has been demonstrated to be superior to the others. In our center we currently advise our patients to measure glucose in the morning prior to breakfast and 2 h after each meal, at a minimum. Depending upon the clinical circumstances glucose may be measured at other times, including the middle of the night if the Somogyi effect or the 'dawn phenomenon' is suspected[51].

Goals for metabolic control utilized in our center include the maintenance of fasting values below 100 mg/dl, 1-h values below 130–140 mg/dl and 2-h postprandial values below 120 mg/dl, with glucose levels under 60 mg/dl being viewed as unnecessarily low. All pregnant patients with pre-existing diabetes, and their significant support persons, should be familiar with the appropriate responses to hypoglycemia, including the use of glucagon injections. While hypoglycemia has not yet been demonstrated to be clearly harmful to the fetus, it carries risk enough for the mother that its frequency and severity should be minimized to the extent possible, compatible with the achievement of good metabolic control during pregnancy.

Insulin management

A number of different approaches to insulin administration have been used successfully[52] during pregnancy. Rarely, if ever, does a single daily injection of intermediate-acting insulin suffice to establish and maintain near-normoglycemia. In our center we tend to start with simpler regimens and increase the complexity if the need arises. Based upon the insulin secretion patterns of normal pregnant women in the third trimester[53] we begin with twice daily injections of mixed intermediate- and short-acting insulins. The morning total dose, administered before breakfast, is twice the evening total dose, administered before dinner. The proportion of intermediate- to short-acting insulins is 2 : 1 in the morning and 1 : 1 in the evening[54]. Once a patient has been started on this 'split, mixed' regimen, the various doses can be adjusted to improve the appropriate glucose measurement. Many patients require the evening dose to be 'split up', so that the intermediate insulin is given at bedtime to avoid morning hyperglycemia. Another approach is the use of short-acting insulin before each meal, with long-acting insulin given daily at bedtime, or in the morning, or at both times. In some centers the subcutaneous insulin infusion pump is used by pregnant women with diabetes, although a randomized trial has demonstrated no distinct advantage for this approach compared to intensive conventional therapy[55]. The specific regimen is probably less important than the degree of familiarity, understanding and comfort of both caregiver and patient.

Dietary management

Approaches to dietary management of diabetic pregnancy have varied greatly over the years[56], and there is no single generally accepted dietary prescription. Research is ongoing as to the advisability of caloric restriction in obese women with type 2 diabetes in pregnancy, but there is concern about the possible adverse fetal effects of ketonemia induced by relative starvation[57]. In our center we advise a diet[54] consisting of 30–35 kcal per kg of ideal body weight, with three meals and three snacks. Dinner is the largest meal of the day, and breakfast the smallest. The diet is high in protein (125 g per day if the patient does not have nephropathy), and low in refined sugars. The most important aspect of the diet is the consistency with which it is followed. Dieticians should take into account the ethnic and cultural food preferences of their patients.

Vascular complications

Women with diabetes are at risk for a number of vascular complications, including nephropathy, retinopathy, neuropathy, coronary heart disease and macrovascular disease. A detailed discussion of these specific problems is beyond the scope of the present chapter, but may be found elsewhere[58-60]. It is not clear whether pregnancy has an independent effect on vascular complications of diabetes. Although one prospective study has demonstrated an independent effect of pregnancy on worsening retinopathy[61], it is possible that the adverse effect was due not to pregnancy itself, but to the rapid institution of tight metabolic control coincident with pregnancy. It is important that these complications be diagnosed and managed promptly and effectively even in the non-pregnant individual, and appropriate care becomes even more important when pregnancy co-exists. For example, patients with diabetic nephropathy generally manifest increasing hypertension and almost invariably develop increasing proteinuria as pregnancy progresses[62]. It may be exceedingly difficult to distinguish nephropathy from pre-eclampsia. In our center the worsening of hypertension, or its new appearance, are considered grave complications in diabetic pregnancy and necessitate hospitalization and intensive monitoring of mother and fetus. While proliferative retinopathy does not pose a particular threat to the fetus, it poses a serious risk of maternal blindness. Laser photocoagulation is safe to perform during pregnancy, and should be applied using the usual ophthalmological indications.

Pre-existing diabetes – obstetric management

Obstetric and neonatal complications

In addition to perinatal mortality as described earlier, a number of obstetric complications occur with greater frequency in diabetic than non-diabetic pregnancies[15,63]. Among these are hypertensive disorders, urinary tract infections, hydramnios and possibly preterm delivery. Particular care should be exercised in treating diabetic women with betamimetic agonist tocolysis because of the possibility of severe hyperglycemia and ketoacidosis developing[10]. Cesarean section is more common in diabetic pregnancies, and respiratory distress syndrome occurs with greater frequency at any given gestational age, possibly related to poor metabolic control. Neonatal hypoglycemia, plethora, jaundice and hypocalcemia are also more common than in the offspring of non-diabetic mothers.

Fetal surveillance

Because of the increased perinatal mortality and morbidity risks described above, a number of different modalities of fetal surveillance are brought to bear on diabetic pregnancy. The increased risk for congenital malformations, particularly in cases registering for care after pregnancy has been established and among those whose metabolic control is suboptimal, merits screening for birth defects. Maternal serum α-fetoprotein testing is generally recommended in diabetic pregnancy. The laboratory performing the α-fetoprotein and other screening tests should be informed of the patient's diabetic status, as adjustments in interpretation are sometimes necessary. Furthermore, directed ultrasound examination may be appropriate when metabolic control during organogenesis has been poor or undocumented, even in the presence of normal α-fetoprotein levels.

Serial ultrasound examinations for fetal growth and amniotic fluid volume may be helpful during the third trimester. Antepartum testing is usually performed, but there is not agreement as to which test is ideal, what gestational age is appropriate for commencement of testing, and with what frequency testing should be carried out. In our center we use the non-stress test as our primary approach because of its simplicity of application. In patients with clear high risk for fetal death, such as those with known growth retardation and oligohydramnios, we may commence testing as early as 24–26 weeks, although the danger of a false-positive test is magnified in such early gestations in which delivery has a high inherent perinatal mortality and morbidity risk. Patients with hypertensive disorders likewise may be started on early testing. On the other hand, patients with excellent metabolic control and no other complications may delay the onset of testing until as late as 35 weeks, particularly if daily fetal movement determinations are made. When there is a high level of concern about the fetal condition, we tend to increase the frequency of surveillance to twice weekly or even daily, depending upon the circumstances. Similarly, contraction stress testing or biophysical profiles may be more sensitive under such circumstances.

Timing of delivery

Although diabetic pregnancies formerly were routinely delivered as early as 4–6 weeks prior to term, owing to concern about the possibility of unanticipated fetal death, current surveillance practices have improved the identification of fetuses in jeopardy. In addition, improvements in metabolic control appear to be effective in preventing fetal death[64]. Therefore, automatic early delivery is no longer necessary. However, it may be appropriate to deliver those patients whose metabolic control is poor or undocumented as soon as lung maturity can be documented. In most cases we await the spontaneous onset of labor. If the cervix is 'ripe', consideration may be given to inducing labor at 38 weeks or beyond in order to diminish the inconvenience and expense of continued testing, as well as the anxiety inherent in such high-risk pregnancies. In our center we attempt to document pulmonary maturity by amniocentesis, even when the patient is near term, provided that the amniotic fluid is abundant and accessible[65]. We have allowed diabetic pregnancies to proceed past 40 weeks, but only rarely. In such cases we maintain intensive fetal surveillance and induce labor as soon as the cervix ripens.

Mode of delivery

Maternal diabetes is not an indication for Cesarean section, but its complications may be[66]. Complications such as hypertensive disorders may require early delivery, increasing the likelihood of unsuccessful labor. Fetal macrosomia may also make Cesarean section more likely. Problems such as shoulder dystocia appear to occur more frequently in diabetic pregnancies than in others. Although there is not general agreement on the subject, we tend to deliver by primary Cesarean section without a trial of labor in cases of diabetic pregnancy in which the estimated fetal weight is 4500 g or more[66]. If the estimate is between 4000 and 4999 g we individualize the decision based upon past obstetric history, clinical pelvimetry and events during labor. Unfortunately, our ability to estimate fetal weight by ultrasound is less than ideal, rendering any rigid protocol problematic.

Management of gestational diabetes

The maternal and fetal implications of gestational diabetes differ from those of pre-existing diabetes only by degree. Glucose control is generally accomplished more easily in gestational diabetes, and many patients can be managed with dietary intervention alone. The recommendations of the ADA[35] and ACOG[43] are that fasting glucose values be maintained below 105 mg/dl and 2-h postprandial values be below 120 mg/dl. Unlike patients with pre-existing diabetes, women with gestational diabetes do not universally perform self glucose monitoring. Although self testing has clear benefits in diabetes, the brief interval from diagnosis to delivery in most cases of gestational diabetes, and the mild degree of hyperglycemia manifested by many such patients, make the purchase of equipment, training and supervision needed to pursue this methodology unnecessary for many such patients. However, if self monitoring is not performed, it is important that regular testing of circulating glucose levels be carried out. In our center each woman with gestational diabetes who opts not to perform self glucose monitoring has a weekly 'set' of glucose determinations, fasting and 2 h after breakfast and lunch. If the fasting value exceeds 100 mg/dl or the postprandial value exceeds 120 mg/dl during the third trimester, insulin therapy is begun in a dose of 20 units NPH mixed with 10 units regular insulin each morning prior to breakfast. A number of studies[67,68], including one randomized trial[69], have demonstrated that postprandial glucose measurements are better predictors of macrosomia and perinatal morbidity than are fasting or preprandial values. We feel that it is important to respond immediately to an elevated glucose value. If the patient is not willing to begin insulin, she is urged to start daily self glucose monitoring or to return to our clinic within 1–2 days for repeat glucose testing. The opportunity for therapeutic intervention in gestational diabetic pregnancy is very short; waiting a week to decide whether to act does not seem reasonable.

Although there are data to suggest that women with uncomplicated gestational diabetes do not require fetal surveillance other than fetal movement determinations until term[70], in our center we institute weekly non-stress testing at 36 weeks in order to avoid inadvertently missing gestational diabetic women with risk factors being discovered retrospectively. We prefer to document fetal pulmonary maturity prior to elective delivery, as in pre-existing diabetes.

It should be remembered that fetal macrosomia can complicate gestational diabetic pregnancy despite apparently near-normal blood glucose levels[28]. A number of possible explanations exist, primarily centering around the likelihood that our definitions of 'near-normoglycemia' are not really normal, but rather approximate two standard deviations above the mean. Various approaches to preventing macrosomia have been developed[71]. One randomized trial[72] demonstrated that ultrasonographic demonstration of a large fetal abdominal circumference at 29–33 weeks could select fetuses who would benefit from maternal insulin therapy, decreasing the likelihood of neonatal macrosomia, even though the maternal fasting serum glucose level was below 105 mg/dl. A randomized trial[73] of induction vs. expectant management at 38 weeks' gestation in women with insulin-treated gestational diabetes demonstrated similar Cesarean section rates, but fewer large-for-dates infants and shoulder dystocias with induction of labor.

As mentioned early in this chapter, gestational diabetes is clearly a risk factor for the subsequent development of diabetes. For this reason it is important that each patient with gestational diabetes be counselled to undergo a 75-g, 2-h glucose tolerance test for the diagnosis of diabetes in the non-pregnant state at around the time of the 6-week postpartum check-up and ideally annually thereafter. Such women should attempt to avoid obesity as they age. There is no reason to counsel women with gestational diabetes not to have further pregnancies, although they should be informed of the approximately 50% risk of recurrence.

REFERENCES

1. Buchanan TA. Pregnancy in preexisting diabetes. In Harris ML, *et al*. eds. *Diabetes in America, 2nd edn*, NIH Publication 95–1468. Washington, DC: National Diabetes Data Group, 1995:719–33

2. Coustan DR. Gestational diabetes. In Harris ML, *et al*. eds. *Diabetes in America, 2nd edn*, NIH Publication 95–1468. Washington, DC: National Diabetes Data Group, 1995:703–16

3. Metzger BE, Cho NH. Epidemiology and genetics. In Reece EA, Coustan DR, eds. *Diabetes Mellitus and Pregnancy, 2nd edn*. New York: Churchill Livingstone, 1995:12–26

4. Third International Workshop Conference on Gestational Diabetes Mellitus: summary and recommendations. *Diabetes* 1991;40(suppl 2):197–201

5. O'Sullivan JB. Subsequent morbidity among gestational diabetic women. In Sutherland HW, Stowers JM, eds. *Carbohydrate Metabolism in Pregnancy and the Newborn*. New York: Churchill Livingstone, 1984:174–80

6. Damm P, Hornnes P, Kühl C, Mølsted-Pedersen L. A longitudinal study of plasma insulin and glucagon in women with previous gestational diabetes. *Diabetes Care* 1995;18:654–65

7. Buchanan TA. Metabolic changes during normal and diabetic pregnancies. In Reece EA, Coustan DR, eds. *Diabetes Mellitus and Pregnancy, 2nd edn*. New York: Churchill Livingstone, 1995:59–78

8. Reece EA, Homko CJ. Glucose evaluation and control. In Reece EA, Coustan DR, eds. *Diabetes Mellitus and Pregnancy, 2nd edn*. New York: Churchill Livingstone, 1995:155–72

9. Rudolf MCJ, Coustan DR, Sherwin RS, *et al*. Efficacy of the insulin pump in the home treatement of pregnant diabetics. *Diabetes* 1981;30:891

10. Coustan DR. Diabetic ketoacidosis. In Berkowitz RL, ed. *Critical Care of the Obstetric Patient*. New York: Churchill Livingstone, 1983:411–29

11. Cousins L. Obstetric complications. In Reece EA, Coustan DR, eds. *Diabetes Mellitus and Pregnancy, 2nd edn*. New York: Churchill Livingstone, 1995:287–302

12. Pedersen J. Pathogenesis of the characteristic features of newborn infants of diabetic women. In *The Pregnant Diabetic and Her Newborn*. Baltimore: Williams and Wilkins, 1967:128–37

13. Freinkel N. Of pregnancy and progeny. *Diabetes* 1980; 29:1023

14. Karlson K, Kjellmer I. The outcome of diabetic pregnancies in relation to the mother's blood sugar level. *Am J Obstet Gynecol* 1972;112:213

15. Coustan DR. Hyperglycemia–hyperinsulinemia: effect on the infant of the diabetic mother. In Jovanovic L, Peterson CM, Fuhrmann K, eds. *Diabetes and Pregnancy: Teratology, Toxicity and Treatment*. New York: Praeger, 1986:131–56

16. Mills JL, Baker L, Goldman AS. Malformations in infants of diabetic mothers occur before the seventh gestational week. *Diabetes* 1979;28:292–3

17. Reece EA, Pinter E, Homko C, *et al*. The yolk sac theory: closing the circle on why diabetes-associated malformations occur. *J Soc Gynecol Invest* 1994;1:3–13

18. Leslie RDG, Pyke DA, John PN, White JM. Haemoglobin A₁ in diabetic pregnancy. *Lancet* 1978;2:958–9

19. Miller E, Hare JW, Cloherty JP, *et al*. Elevated maternal hemoglobin A₁c in early pregnancy and major congenital anomalies in infants of diabetic mothers. *N Engl J Med* 1981;304:1331–4

20. Greene MF, Hare JW, Cloherty JP, *et al*. First-trimester hemoglobin A₁ and risk for major malformation and spontaneous abortion in diabetic pregnancy. *Teratology* 1989;39:225–31

21. Mills JL, Knopp RH, Simpson JL, *et al*. Lack of relation of increased malformation rates in infants of diabetic mothers to glycemic control during organogenesis. *N Engl J Med* 1988;318:671–6

22. Fuhrmann K, Reiher H, Semmler K, Glockner E. The effect of intensified conventional insulin therapy during and before pregnancy on the malformation rate in offspring of diabetic mothers. *Exp Clin Endocrinol* 1984;83:173–7

23. Kitzmiller JL, Gavin LA, Gin GD, *et al*. Preconception care of diabetes: Glycemic control prevents congenital anomalies. *J Am Med Assoc* 1991;265:731–6

24. Mills JL, Simpson JL, Driscoll SG, *et al*. Incidence of spontaneous abortion among normal women and insulin-dependent diabetic women whose pregnancies were identified within 21 days of conception. *N Engl J Med* 1988;319:1617–23

25. Hanson U, Persson B, Thunell S. Relationship between haemoglobin A₁c in early type I (insulin-dependent) diabetic pregnancy and the occurence of spontaneous abortion and fetal malformation in Sweden. *Diabetologia* 1990;33:100–4

26. O'Sullivan JB, Charles D, Mahan CM, Dandrow RV. Gestational diabetes and perinatal mortality rate. *Am J Obstet Gynecol* 1973;116:901–4

27. Pettitt DJ, Knowler WC, Baird HR, Bennett PH. Gestational diabetes: infant and maternal complications of pregnancy in relation to third-trimester glucose tolerance in Pima Indians. *Diabetes Care* 1980;3: 458–64

28. Widness JA, Cowett RM, Coustan DR, *et al*. Neonatal morbidities in infants of mothers with glucose intolerance in pregnancy. *Diabetes* 1985;34(suppl 2):61–5

29. Vohr BR, Lipsitt LP, Oh W. Somatic growth of children of diabetic mothers with reference to birth size. *J Pediatr* 1980;97:196–9

30. Pettitt DJ, Knowler WC, Bennett PH, *et al*. Obesity in offspring of diabetic Pima Indian women despite normal birth weight. *Diabetes Care* 1987;10:76–80

31. Green OC, Winter RJ, Depp R, *et al*. Fuel-mediated teratogenesis: prospective correlations between anthropometric development in childhood and antepartum maternal metabolism. *Clin Res* 1987;35:657A

32. Pettitt DJ, Bennett PH, Saad MF, *et al*. Abnormal glucose tolerance during pregnancy in Pima Indian women: long-term effects on offspring. *Diabetes* 1991;40(suppl 2):126–30

33. O'Sullivan JB, Mahan CM. Criteria for the oral glucose tolerance test in pregnancy. *Diabetes* 1964;13:278–85

34. National Diabetes Data Group. Classification and diagnosis of diabetes mellitus and other categories of glucose intolerance. *Diabetes* 1979;28:1039–57

35. American Diabetes Association. Position statement on gestational diabetes mellitus. *Diabetes Care* 1996;19 (suppl 1):S29

36. American College of Obstetricians and Gynecologists. *Management of Diabetes Mellitus in Pregnancy*, Technical Bulletin no. 92. Washington, DC: ACOG, 1986

37. Carpenter MW, Coustan DR. Criteria for screening tests for gestational diabetes. *Am J Obstet Gynecol* 1982; 144:768–73

38. Sacks DA, Abu-Fadil S, Greenspoon JS, Fotheringham N. Do the current standards for glucose tolerance testing in pregnancy represent a valid conversion of O'Sullivan's original criteria? *Am J Obstet Gynecol* 1989; 161:638–41

39. Magee MS, Walden CE, Benedetti TJ, Knopp RH. Influence of diagnostic criteria on the incidence of gestational diabetes and perinatal morbidity. *J Am Med Assoc* 1993;269:609–15

40. Naylor CD, Sermer M, Chen E, Sykora K. Cesarean delivery in relation to birth weight and gestational glucose tolerance: pathophysiology or practice style? *J Am Med Assoc* 1996;275:1165–70

41. Coustan DR. Management of gestational diabetes: a self-fulfilling prophecy? *J Am Med Assoc* 1996;275: 1199–200

42. Coustan DR, Nelson C, Carpenter MW, *et al*. Maternal age and screening for gestational diabetes: a population-based study. *Obstet Gynecol* 1989;73:557–61

43. American College of Obstetricians and Gynecologists. *Diabetes and Pregnancy*, Technical Bulletin no. 200. Washington, DC: ACOG, 1994

44. American Diabetes Association: Report of the Expert Committee on Diagnosis and Classification of Diabetes Mellitus. *Diabetes Care* 1997;20:1183–97

45. Coustan DR. Pregnancy in diabetic women. *N Engl J Med* 1988;319:1663–5

46. Steel JM. Preconception, conception and contraception. In Reece EA, Coustan DR, eds. *Diabetes Mellitus and Pregnancy: Principles and Practice*. New York: Churchill Livingstone, 1988:601–22

47. American Diabetes Association. *Diabetes & Pregnancy: What to Expect*. 3rd edn. Washington: American Diabetes Association, 1996

48. Elixhauser A, Wechsler JM, Kitzmiller JL, *et al*. Cost–benefit analysis of preconception care for women with established diabetes mellitus. *Diabetes Care* 1993; 16:1146–57

49. American Diabetes Association. Position statement on preconception care of women with diabetes. *Diabetes Care* 1996;19(suppl 1):S25–S28

50. Kitzmiller JL, Buchanan TA, Kjos S, *et al*. Technical review of pre-conception care of diabetes, congenital malformations, and spontaneous abortions. *Diabetes Care* 1996;19:514–41

51. Coustan DR. Management of the pregnant diabetic. In Olefsky JM, Sherwin RS, eds. *Diabetes Mellitus: Management and Complications*. New York: Churchill Livingstone, 1985:311–30

52. Landon MB, Gabbe SG. Insulin treatment. In Reece EA, Coustan DR, eds. *Diabetes Mellitus and Pregnancy*, 2nd edn. New York: Churchill Livingstone, 1995: 173–90

53. Lewis SB, Wallin JD, Kuzuya H, *et al*. Circadian variation of serum glucose, C-peptide immunoreactivity and free insulin in normal and insulin-treated diabetic pregnant subjects. *Diabetologia* 1976;12:343–7

54. Lewis SB, Murray WK, Wallin JD, *et al*. Improved glucose control in non-hospitalized pregnant diabetic patients. *Obstet Gynecol* 1976;48:260–5

55. Coustan DR, Reece EA, Sherwin RS, *et al*. A randomized clinical trial of the insulin pump vs intensive conventional therapy in diabetic pregnancies. *J Am Med Assoc* 1986;255:631–6

56. Luke B, Murtaugh MA. Dietary management. In Reece EA, Coustan DR, eds. *Diabetes Mellitus and Pregnancy*, 2nd edn. New York: Churchill Livingstone, 1995: 191–200

57. Phelps RL, Metzger BE. Caloric restriction in gestational diabetes mellitus: when and how much? *J Am Coll Nutrition* 1992;11:259–62

58. Jovanovic-Peterson L, Peterson CM. Diabetic retinopathy. In Reece EA, Coustan DR, eds. *Diabetes Mellitus and Pregnancy*, 2nd edn. New York: Churchill Livingstone, 1995:303–14

59. Kitzmiller JL, Combs CA. Diabetic nephropathy. In Reece EA, Coustan DR, eds. *Diabetes Mellitus and Pregnancy*, 2nd edn. New York: Churchill Livingstone, 1995:315–44

60. Brown FM, Hare JW. Diabetic neuropathy and coronary heart disease. In Reece EA, Coustan DR, eds. *Diabetes Mellitus and Pregnancy*, 2nd edn. New York: Churchill Livingstone, 1995:345–51

61. Klein BEK, Moss SE, Klein R. Effect of pregnancy on progression of diabetic retinopathy. *Diabetes Care* 1990;13:34–40

62. Reece EA, Coustan DR, Hayslett JP, *et al*. Diabetic nephropathy: pregnancy performance and fetomaternal outcome. *Am J Obstet Gynecol* 1988;159:56–66

63. Cousins L. Obstetric complications. In Reece EA, Coustan DR, eds. *Diabetes Mellitus and Pregnancy, 2nd edn*. New York: Churchill Livingstone, 1995:287–302

64. Coustan DR, Berkowitz RL, Hobbins JC. Tight metabolic control of overt diabetes in pregnancy. *Am J Med* 1980;68:845–52

65. Ojomo EO, Coustan DR. Absence of evidence of pulmonary maturity at amniocentesis in term infants of diabetic mothers. *Am J Obstet Gynecol* 1990;163:954–7

66. Coustan DR. Delivery: timing, mode and management. In Reece EA, Coustan DR, eds. *Diabetes Mellitus and Pregnancy, 2nd edn*. New York: Churchill Livingstone, 1995:353–9

67. Jovanovic-Peterson L, Peterson CM, Reed GF, *et al*. Maternal postprandial glucose levels and infant birth weight: the Diabetes in Early Pregnancy Study. *Am J Obstet Gynecol* 1991;164:103–11

68. Combs CA, Gunderson E, Kitzmiller JL, *et al*. Relationship of fetal macrosomia to maternal postprandial glucose control during pregnancy. *Diabetes Care* 1992;15:1251–7

69. DeVeciana M, Major CA, Morgan MA, *et al*. Postprandial versus preprandial blood glucose monitoring in women with gestational diabetes mellitus requiring insulin therapy. *N Engl J Med* 1995;333:1237–41

70. Landon MB, Gabbe SG. Antepartum fetal surveillance in gestational diabetes mellitus. *Diabetes* 1985;34 (suppl 2):50–4

71. Coustan DR. Maternal insulin to lower the risk of fetal macrosomia in diabetic pregnancy. *Clin Obstet Gynecol* 1991;34:288–95

72. Buchanan TA, Kjos SL, Montoro MN, *et al*. Use of fetal ultrasound to select metabolic therapy for pregnancies complicated by mild gestational diabetes. *Diabetes Care* 1994;17:275–83

73. Kjos S, Henry OA, Montoro M, *et al*. Insulin-requiring diabetes in pregnancy: a randomized trial of active induction of labor and expectant management. *Am J Obstet Gynecol* 1993;169:611–15

36
Endocrine diseases

W.E. Clutter

INTRODUCTION

Pregnancy alters the function of many endocrine systems, and these changes must be taken into account in diagnosis of suspected endocrine disease during pregnancy. Endocrine diseases affect maternal, fetal and neonatal health, and pregnancy may affect the course or therapy of endocrine disease.

THYROID DISEASE

Thyroid disorders are common in women. Although both hypothyroidism and hyperthyroidism impair fertility, these endocrine problems are often encountered in pregnancy[1]. The major hormone secreted by the thyroid is thyroxine (T_4), which is converted in many tissues to triiodothyronine (T_3), a more potent hormone. Both are reversibly bound to plasma proteins, primarily thyroxine-binding globulin (TBG). Only the unbound (free) fraction enters cells and produces biological effects. T_4 secretion is stimulated by thyroid stimulating hormone (TSH). In turn, TSH secretion is inhibited by T_4, forming a sensitive negative feedback loop which keeps free T_4 levels within a narrow normal range.

During the first trimester, plasma levels of TBG double in response to high estrogen levels, causing plasma total T_4 and total T_3 concentrations to increase[2]. Mean free T_4 levels decline slightly after the first trimester, but values usually remain within the non-pregnant reference range. Plasma TSH levels decline slightly in the first trimester owing to thyroid stimulation by the weak thyrotropic activity of chorionic gonadotropin, but also usually remain within the reference range. The elevated glomerular filtration rate leads to increased iodine excretion; where dietary iodine intake is marginal this may cause mild iodine deficiency and goiter during pregnancy[3]. Where iodine intake is ample (as in the USA), pregnancy does not cause clinically detectable thyroid enlargement and goiter should not be attributed to pregnancy[4].

The fetal thyroid takes up iodine and synthesizes T_4 after 10 weeks' gestation. Thereafter, fetal plasma levels of TSH and T_4 rise, while T_3 levels remain low[2]. Only a small amount of maternal thyroid hormone crosses the placenta, but this may nevertheless be important for fetal brain development[5],

especially in fetuses with congenital hypothyroidism[6]. Iodine, antithyroid drugs and thyroid stimulating immunoglobulins cross the placenta readily and may profoundly affect the fetal thyroid. After delivery, neonatal TSH levels rise sharply to a peak of about 30 µU/ml at several hours of life, followed by increases in plasma T_4 and T_3 levels. Plasma TSH levels decrease to the adult reference range within a few days, whereas plasma T_4 and T_3 levels do so over about 1 month.

Plasma TSH is the initial test of choice for suspected thyroid disease in pregnancy[7,8]. Clinically important cross-reaction with chorionic gonadotropin does not occur. TSH levels are elevated in even mild primary hypothyroidism, and suppressed to < 0.1 µU/ml in even subclinical hyperthyroidism (i.e. thyroid hormone excess too mild to cause symptoms). Thus, a normal plasma TSH level excludes both hyperthyroidism and primary hypothyroidism. Because even slight changes in thyroid hormone levels affect TSH secretion, abnormal TSH levels are not entirely specific for clinically important thyroid disease, and the diagnosis may need to be confirmed by plasma thyroid hormone measurement.

The most reliable method of measuring plasma free T_4 in pregnancy is equilibrium dialysis[9], but results are seldom rapidly available. Conventional plasma T_4 assays measure total T_4 levels, which correlate well with free T_4 except when TBG levels are altered, as in pregnancy. T_3 resin uptake (T_3RU) is an index of plasma thyroid hormone binding that is inversely proportional to binding capacity. The pregnancy-induced increase in plasma TBG increases plasma T_4 and lowers T_3RU. The T_4 index (the product of total T_4 and T_3RU) is usually, but not invariably, normal in pregnancy.

Hypothyroidism

This is most often due to Hashimoto's disease (chronic lymphocytic thyroiditis), an autoimmune disorder that may produce euthyroid goiter, or hypothyroidism with or without a goiter. It is often familial, and antithyroid antibodies are present in most cases. Iatrogenic hypothyroidism following radioactive iodine (RAI) therapy or thyroidectomy is also common. Rare conditions include iodine- or lithium-induced hypothyroidism, and transient hypothyroidism following subacute thyroiditis or painless lymphocytic thyroiditis. Secondary hypothyroidism (due to pituitary or hypothalamic disease) is quite rare.

Clinical findings include cold intolerance, mild weight gain, fatigue, somnolence, dry skin, constipation, myalgias, myxedema and delayed relaxation of tendon reflexes. A goiter may or may not be present. Menorrhagia and infertility are common, and thus severe hypothyroidism and pregnancy seldom coexist. Untreated maternal hypothyroidism is associated with increased risk of abortion and stillbirth, and may affect mental development of the fetus. This may occur if there is concomitant fetal hypothyroidism due to placental transfer of maternal thyroid autoantibodies, or insufficient maternal supply of thyroid hormone during early embryogenesis[1].

Plasma TSH is the best initial diagnostic test. A normal value excludes primary hypothyroidism, and a markedly elevated value (> 20 μU/ml) confirms the diagnosis. If plasma TSH is only moderately elevated (< 20 μU/ml), plasma free T_4 should be measured by equilibrium dialysis; a low value confirms clinical hypothyroidism. A clearly normal free T_4 value with a mildly elevated plasma TSH level indicates subclinical hypothyroidism, in which thyroid function is impaired, but increased secretion of TSH maintains serum T_4 levels within the reference range.

Hypothyroidism should be treated with thyroxine[8]. The average dose requirement is increased in pregnancy[10], and therapy of newly diagnosed hypothyroidism should start with 150 μg every day and be adjusted in 12–25 μg increments at 6-week intervals until plasma TSH is normal. In pregnant women with pre-existing hypothyroidism, plasma TSH should be measured during the first and second trimesters, and the dose of thyroxine increased if necessary to keep it within the normal range[10]. Although there is debate about the need to treat subclinical hypothyroidism in non-pregnant patients, this condition should be treated during pregnancy in the same way as more severe hypothyroidism.

Congenital hypothyroidism

This occurs in about 1 in 5000 births, and is usually due to thyroid dysgenesis[11]. Rare causes include genetic defects of hormone synthesis, maternal treatment with antithyroid drugs or iodine, and placental transfer of thyroid inhibitory antibodies. Antithyroid drugs and iodine may also cause fetal goiter large enough to produce dystocia or tracheal obstruction[12]. Although thyroid hormone is critical for fetal neurological development, these infants appear normal at birth, probably because sufficient maternal hormone crosses the placenta during early gestation[6]. However, they develop mental retardation and the syndrome of cretinism unless treated soon after birth. Neonatal screening is essential for early diagnosis and prevention of irreversible neurological damage.

Hyperthyroidism

In pregnant women, hyperthyroidism is most often due to Graves' disease, an autoimmune disorder in which thyroid stimulating immunoglobulins (TSI) promote hormone production[13]. Unusual causes include hyperfunctioning (toxic) thyroid adenoma, toxic multinodular goiter, transient hyperthyroidism due to subacute thyroiditis or painless lymphocytic thyroiditis, and factitious hyperthyroidism. Rarely, trophoblastic tumors cause hyperthyroidism by marked overproduction of abnormally glycosylated chorionic gonadotropin that cross-reacts with the TSH receptor[14,15]. Transient elevation of plasma free T_4 occurs in some patients with hyperemesis gravidarum[16].

Clinical manifestations include heat intolerance, weight loss, anxiety, palpitations, sinus tachycardia, atrial fibrillation, fine tremor, lid lag and stare, proximal muscle weakness, warm smooth skin and brisk reflexes. Oligomenorrhea or amenorrhea and impaired fertility are common in severe hyperthyroidism. Patients with Graves' disease usually have a soft diffuse goiter, and may have proptosis (exophthalmos), a finding not seen in other causes of hyperthyroidism. Hyperthyroidism increases the risk of premature labor, low infant birth weight and fetal death[13].

Plasma TSH is the best initial diagnostic test, since a TSH level of > 0.1 μU/ml excludes clinical hyperthyroidism. If the plasma TSH level is < 0.1 μU/ml, the plasma T_4 index and free T_4 by equilibrium dialysis should be measured to determine the severity of hyperthyroidism and as a baseline for therapy. If free T_4 is elevated (or the T_4 index is markedly elevated), the diagnosis of clinical hyperthyroidism is established.

If the plasma TSH level is < 0.1 μU/ml, but the free T_4 by equilibrium dialysis is normal, the patient may have subclinical hyperthyroidism or, in the first trimester, unusually marked physiological suppression of TSH. Such patients should have TSH and free T_4 measurements repeated to determine whether they return to normal, or whether clinical hyperthyroidism develops.

The therapy of choice in pregnancy is propylthiouracil (PTU), at an initial dose of 100–150 mg orally every 8 h[8,13]. Methimazole at an initial dose of 20–40 mg every day is equally effective[17], but has been associated with congenital aplasia cutis. Although the evidence for a causal relationship is weak, it is prudent to limit its use to patients who are intolerant of PTU or are poorly compliant with multiple daily doses[18]. These drugs inhibit thyroid hormone synthesis and lower plasma T_4 levels only when stored hormone is exhausted, usually after several weeks. At monthly intervals, the maternal plasma T_4 index should be measured and the PTU dose adjusted to maintain this value near the upper limit of the non-pregnant reference range. This practice avoids fetal hypothyroidism and goiter, since PTU crosses the placenta readily, whereas T_4 does not[1].

The dose of PTU can often be decreased in the latter part of pregnancy. Side-effects of PTU include rash, pruritis, fever, arthralgias, hepatitis and vasculitis. About 1 in 200 patients develop life-threatening agranulocytosis, and patients must be warned to stop the drug and contact their physician immediately for symptoms such as fever or sore throat. Routine granulocyte counts are not useful. Propranolol 10–40 mg orally four times a day may be used to alleviate symptoms, but should be stopped when the patient is clinically euthyroid. Concentrations of PTU in breast milk are low, and breastfeeding while taking this drug may not affect neonatal thyroid function[19], but neonatal plasma T_4 and TSH should be monitored every 2–4 weeks.

If PTU causes life-threatening side-effects and severe hyperthyroidism persists, subtotal thyroidectomy is indicated[13]. To minimize the risk of perioperative exacerbation of hyperthyroidism, propranolol should be started and the dose adjusted to control tachycardia before surgery. RAI should never be given during pregnancy, because of fetal irradiation and the potential for fetal hypothyroidism. Iodine should also be avoided, since it can cause fetal hypothyroidism and goiter. Stressful events such as labor, surgery or infection may exacerbate hyperthyroidism, causing fever, marked tachycardia, hypotension and confusion. If this occurs, intravenous fluids should be given to correct dehydration, acetaminophen should be used to reduce fever and maternal vital signs should be closely monitored. Hyperthyroidism should be vigorously treated with PTU 300 mg orally every 6 h[20]. Propranolol 20–40 mg orally every 6 h may be given to alleviate tachycardia, but should be used with great caution if congestive heart failure is present. The dose of medications should be gradually reduced as clinical manifestations improve.

Fetal and neonatal hyperthyroidism

This is caused by placental transfer of TSI from a mother with Graves' disease[21]. Signs of fetal hyperthyroidism include tachycardia (>160/min), hyperactivity, growth retardation, goiter, craniosynostosis and increased perinatal mortality[1]. Fetal hyperthyoidism is usually prevented by treatment of the mother with PTU and is more likely if the mother is euthyroid due to prior radioactive iodine therapy or thyroidectomy. If the mother has a history of Graves' disease, the fetus should be closely monitored for tachycardia, and serial ultrasound examinations should be performed during the second half of pregnancy to assess fetal growth and thyroid size[1]. If there is evidence of fetal hyperthyroidism and the mother is euthyroid, it may be controlled by maternal intake of a small dose of PTU (50–100 mg/day)[21].

Neonatal hyperthyroidism complicates 1–2% of pregnancies in women with Graves' disease[22]. It usually becomes apparent within the first week of life as irritability, tachycardia, failure to gain weight, goiter and, in severe cases, heart failure and death. T_4 and TSH should be measured in cord blood if the mother has a history of Graves' disease. Neonatal hyperthyroidism is treated with PTU, iodine and propranolol, and usually resolves within 1–3 months, as TSI are cleared from plasma.

The role of assays for TSI in maternal plasma is not resolved. Although high titers of these antibodies are associated with increased risk of fetal and neonatal hyperthyroidism, the predictive value of current clinical assays is not great enough to affect the need for careful fetal monitoring and neonatal testing.

Postpartum thyroid disorders

Graves' disease often worsens in the postpartum period, and may first become evident then. However, the most common postpartum thyroid disorder is painless lymphocytic thyroiditis, which affects about 5% of postpartum women[23]. It occurs within the first 3 postpartum months and produces mild or moderate hyperthyroidism that lasts up to 2 months, and may be followed by transient hypothyroidism lasting several months. The disorder is often first recognized in the hypothyroid phase. Most patients have a small nontender goiter. Clinical distinction between the hyperthyroid phase and Graves' disease is possible if proptosis is present, since this occurs only in Graves' disease. Otherwise, RAI uptake should be measured, since it is elevated in Graves' disease, but < 5% in postpartum thyroiditis. Hyperthyroidism due to the latter may be treated with propranolol, and symptomatic hypothyroidism should be treated with thyroxine. Although thyroid function returns to normal in most women, the disorder may recur with subsequent pregnancies, and hypothyroidism persists or recurs in one-third.

Thyroid nodules

Single thyroid nodules may be thyroid carcinomas, and should be evaluated by fine needle biopsy, not thyroid scans[24]. If cytology is diagnostic or suspicious for papillary thyroid carcinoma, the patient should undergo thyroidectomy during the second trimester. If cytology is suspicious for a follicular neoplasm (which may be a follicular adenoma or carcinoma), thyroidectomy may be delayed until the postpartum period. Lesions with benign cytology in euthyroid patients may be observed without therapy.

ANTERIOR PITUITARY DISORDERS

The anterior pituitary produces six hormones: thyrotropin (TSH), corticotropin (ACTH), the gonadotropins luteinizing hormone (LH) and follicle stimulating hormone (FSH), prolactin and growth hormone (GH). With the exception of prolactin, their secretion is stimulated by hypothalamic releasing hormones which reach the pituitary by portal veins in the pituitary stalk. Prolactin secretion is inhibited by hypothalamic secretion of dopamine. Hypothalamic lesions increase prolactin release, but decrease secretion of other pituitary hormones. Gonadotropin deficiency prevents fertility and does not complicate pregnancy. Prolactin promotes lactation and inhibits gonadotropin secretion. Growth hormone promotes growth during childhood. Most of its actions are mediated by somatomedin-C [insulin-like growth factor-1(IGF-1)]. In adults, GH excess produces a characteristic syndrome, acromegaly. Disorders of TSH and ACTH are discussed in other sections of this chapter.

During pregnancy the pituitary progressively enlarges owing to hyperplasia of lactotropes[25,26]. Plasma prolactin levels increase, reaching a plateau of about 200 ng/ml during the third trimester, and pituitary gonadotropin secretion is suppressed[27]. The placenta produces a variant GH which causes plasma somatomedin-C levels to rise by the third trimester while suppressing plasma GH levels[28].

Pituitary tumors

These are classified according to size: microadenomas are < 1 cm in diameter, and macroadenomas are larger. They may be clinically non-functional, or produce prolactin, GH or ACTH excess. Microadenomas cause clinical effects only by producing hormone excess. Macroadenomas may also cause hypopituitarism and other effects due to the tumor mass, including headaches and defects of visual fields or acuity due to compression of the optic chiasm[29].

During pregnancy, the only clinically important pituitary hormone deficiencies are secondary hypothyroidism and adrenal insufficiency; other deficiencies cause no symptoms, although prolactin deficiency prevents lactation. If hypopituitarism or a pituitary mass are suspected during pregnancy, the patient should be evaluated with plasma free T_4 measurement, cosyntropin stimulation testing, and magnetic resonance imaging (MRI) of the pituitary[30]. If MRI shows that a tumor abuts or displaces the optic chiasm, visual fields should be tested. If adenoma resection is required, the vast majority can be removed by a trans-sphenoidal approach[31].

Hyperprolactinemia

Hyperprolactinemia is a common endocrine disorder that causes amenorrhea and infertility, with or without galactorrhea[32]. The most common causes in young women are prolactin secreting microadenomas and idiopathic hyperprolactinemia. Less common are prolactin secreting macrodenomas, hypothalamic lesions or non-functioning pituitary adenomas that prevent dopamine from reaching the pituitary, dopamine antagonist drugs (e.g. phenothiazines, metoclopramide), primary hypothyroidism and renal failure.

Mild hyperprolactinemia should be confirmed by repeat measurement. Drugs and other uncommon causes should be excluded by clinical evaluation and plasma TSH measurement. The hypothalamus and pituitary should be evaluated with MRI. Prolactin levels of > 200 ng/ml in non-pregnant women are almost always due to prolactinomas. Since pregnancy causes hyperprolactinemia indistinguishable from a prolactinoma, this diagnosis is not made during pregnancy.

Bromocriptine is the therapy of choice for infertility due to idiopathic hyperprolactinemia or microprolactinoma[32]. Mechanical contraception is used while therapy is started, and stopped after menses become regular. A pregnancy test is promptly obtained when menses are delayed, and bromocriptine is stopped if the test is positive. During pregnancy, headaches or visual symptoms should be promptly evaluated with visual fields and MRI. If there is evidence of tumor growth, restarting bromocriptine usually reduces the tumor size, and trans-sphenoidal resection is rarely required. The usual dose range is 2.5–10 mg/day. Routine testing of visual fields is not warranted, since the risk of clinically evident enlargement of a microadenoma is < 2%; measurement of prolactin is not useful. Bromocriptine may produce transient nausea or orthostatic hypotension, but other toxicity is rare and there is no evidence of a teratogenic effect[33]. Tumor size should be reassessed 2–3 months after delivery. There is no evidence that breastfeeding affects tumor growth.

The risk of enlargement of macroprolactinomas during pregnancy is about 15%[32], and trans-sphenoidal resection should be performed before these patients attempt to conceive. Hyperprolactinemia is seldom completely corrected by surgery, and bromocriptine is then used to restore fertility as described above. Management during pregnancy is similar to that for microadenomas, except that visual fields should be assessed every 1–2 months.

Acromegaly

Acromegaly is the syndrome of growth hormone excess, usually due to a pituitary adenoma[34]. Manifestations include enlargement of hands, feet and jaw, coarsening of facial features, carpal tunnel syndrome and hypertension. Diabetes mellitus develops in 10–25% of patients. Amenorrhea and infertility are common, so pregnancy rarely occurs. Acromegaly produces no apparent effect on the fetus, except when complicated by diabetes[35]. The tumor may produce headaches or visual field defects.

If acromegaly is suspected in a pregnant woman, plasma IGF-1 should be measured. However, the increase in IGF-1 in late pregnancy may confound the diagnosis, and marginally elevated values should be interpreted cautiously. In non-pregnant patients, suppression of plasma GH by 75 g of oral glucose is a useful confirmatory test[36]. Although the reference range for suppression in pregnancy has not been established, failure of plasma GH to suppress to < 2 ng/ml supports the diagnosis of acromegaly. Once the diagnosis is made, MRI should be used to assess tumor size.

Acromegaly is a chronic disorder and, in most cases, therapy can be delayed till after delivery. Bromocriptine may ameliorate clinical features and decrease GH levels (although seldom to normal), and has been used in some cases during pregnancy without apparent adverse effects[37]. The treatment of choice for severe or progressive mass symptoms is trans-sphenoidal resection of the pituitary tumor. The somatostatin analog octreotide is useful in the medical therapy of non-pregnant patients. It was used during the first trimester in one patient[38], but because it suppresses other hormones, it should be avoided in pregnancy.

Lymphocytic hypophysitis

This is a rare autoimmune disorder that occurs primarily in the third trimester or the postpartum period[39]. It may present with symptoms of a pituitary mass, hypopituitarism, or both. Failure of lactation and postpartum amenorrhea are common, and there may be autoimmune deficiencies of other endocrine glands as well. The natural history is poorly defined, since in many cases the pituitary was resected because of a suspected tumor. MRI typically shows intense homogeneous enhancement of a pituitary mass[40]. Spontaneous resolution of hypopituitarism or pituitary enlargement has been reported in a few cases, so if this diagnosis is suspected in a patient with no visual loss, the patient may be observed, with treatment of hypopituitarism and monitoring of visual fields and MRI. If visual symptoms are severe or progressive, trans-sphenoidal biopsy should be performed, with decompression rather than resection if lymphocytic hypophysitis is found.

Sheehan's syndrome

Sheehan's syndrome (peripartum pituitary necrosis) is rare in modern obstetric practice. Pituitary enlargement in pregnancy predisposes it to infarction if hemorrhagic shock occurs during delivery. Hypopituitarism may present early as failure of lactation and amenorrhea, or up to years later as hypothyroidism or adrenal insufficiency[27]. If the diagnosis is suspected, the patient should be evaluated for hypopituitarism and MRI should be performed to exclude a mass lesion.

POSTERIOR PITUITARY DISORDERS

In normal pregnancy, the osmotic thresholds for antidiuretic hormone (ADH) release and thirst are lowered, resulting in plasma osmolality about 10 mOsm/kg lower than in non-pregnant women[41]. The metabolic clearance of ADH is markedly accelerated by mid-pregnancy, probably owing to circulating placental vasopressinase which degrades ADH.

Diabetes insipidus

Diabetes insipidus is the inability to concentrate urine, owing to ADH deficiency (central or neurogenic diabetes insipidus) or renal tubular resistance to ADH (nephrogenic diabetes insipidus)[42]. Causes of central diabetes insipidus include head trauma and hypothalamic lesions such as tumors; many cases are idiopathic. Transient forms of diabetes insipidus may occur in pregnancy, owing to unmasking of subclinical disease by circulating vasopressinase[43] or to excessive circulating vasopressinase in the setting of hepatic dysfuntion[44]. Other causes of polyuria include diabetes mellitus and primary polydipsia, which may be due to a psychiatric disorder or to abnormal thirst sensation.

Symptoms of diabetes insipidus are polydipsia and polyuria due to increased urine volume, not simply increased frequency. Since thirst sensation is intact, plasma osmolality remains normal if patients are able to drink. Decreased water intake quickly leads to dehydration and hypernatremia, however.

Increased urine volume (more than 3 l/24 h) should be confirmed, and glycosuria excluded. Polyuria should be evaluated with a water deprivation test[42], which includes hourly measurement of urine volume and osmolality, body weight and vital signs, and measurement of plasma sodium every 3–4 h. The patient should be seated or standing during the test, since during pregnancy, urinary concentrating ability is limited in the lateral recumbent position. Water deprivation should be stopped when (1) body weight decreases by more than 3%; (2) urine osmolality changes less than 30 mOsm/kg per hour for 3 h; or (3) plasma sodium level exceeds the reference range. Desmopressin (DDAVP) 0.1 ml intranasally should then be given and urine osmolality measured after 1–2 h. In severe central diabetes insipidus, maximal urine osmolality after water deprivation is less than plasma osmolality, and increases after DDAVP. In nephrogenic diabetes insipidus, maximal urine osmolality is less than for plasma, but does not increase after DDAVP. In primary polydipsia, maximal urine osmolality exceeds plasma osmolality and does not increase further after DDAVP.

The drug of choice is the long-acting ADH analog DDAVP, which is not degraded by vasopressinase. The usual dose is 0.1–0.2 ml (10–20 µg) intranasally at bedtime or twice a day. It may also be given subcutaneously or intravenously (the usual dose is 2 μg once or twice a day). Patients with pre-existing diabetes insipidus may require an increase in the dose of DDAVP during pregnancy. Pregnancy is not affected by adequately treated diabetes insipidus, but fluid balance should be carefully monitored during delivery, especially if the patient cannot drink in response to thirst.

CALCIUM DISORDERS

About 50% of plasma calcium is ionized or free, and the remainder is complexed, primarily to albumin. Routine plasma calcium assays measure total calcium, but free calcium measurements are readily available. Calcium metabolism is regulated by parathyroid hormone (PTH), which raises plasma calcium by stimulating bone resorption, renal calcium reabsorption, and conversion of vitamin D to its active metabolite, 1,25-dihydroxyvitamin D (calcitriol). The latter stimulates intestinal calcium absorption. Plasma calcium regulates PTH secretion by a negative feedback mechanism. Only assays for intact PTH should be used to evaluate calcium disorders in pregnancy.

During pregnancy, maternal total calcium levels gradually decrease in parallel with plasma albumin, with little or no change in plasma free calcium[45]. Maternal plasma PTH levels decrease, while levels of PTH-related peptide (PTHrP) rise. Plasma calcitriol levels rise and intestinal calcium absorption is increased. Fetal plasma calcium levels are higher than maternal levels, due to active placental calcium transport stimulated by PTHrP secreted by the placenta and fetal parathyroid glands. Fetal PTH and calcitriol levels are low. PTHrP plays a critical role in regulating maturation of the fetal skeleton.

Hypercalcemia

Hypercalcemia is most often caused by primary hyperparathyroidism. Rare causes in pregnancy include malignancy, sarcoidosis and drugs (lithium, vitamins D or A, excessive calcium carbonate). Familial benign (or hypocalciuric) hypercalcemia is a rare autosomal disorder due to a defect in calcium-sensing receptors. Heterozygotes have asymptomatic hypercalcemia from birth[46], whereas homozygous infants develop severe neonatal hypercalcemia and skeletal demineralization[47]. A syndrome of maternal hypercalcemia during pregnancy and lactation that resolves postpartum has been attributed to elevated plasma PTHrP levels[48].

Hypercalcemic disorders are often asymptomatic, but may produce gastrointestinal symptoms (nausea, vomiting, constipation, abdominal pain or pancreatitis), renal manifestations (polyuria), nephrolithiasis and renal failure), osteopenia and fractures, or neurological findings (lethargy, stupor and coma). Polyuria combined with vomiting may cause marked dehydration. Maternal hypercalcemia may lead to transient neonatal hypocalcemia with tetany, owing to suppression of fetal parathyroid function by hypercalcemia. Severe maternal hypercalcemia increases the risk of fetal death and premature labor[49].

The decreased plasma calcium of normal pregnancy may mask mild hypercalcemic disorders. For values slightly above the non-pregnant reference range, the test should be repeated, and plasma free calcium measured to confirm hypercalcemia. Malignancy and other unusual causes can usually be excluded by history, physical examination and routine laboratory tests. Hypercalcemia in a patient with no clinical evidence of malignancy or other cause is almost always due to primary hyperparathyroidism, and increased plasma intact PTH levels confirm this diagnosis.

Symptomatic hypercalcemia or plasma calcium level of > 12 mg/dl should be treated urgently with intravenous normal saline solution to restore extracellular fluid volume, followed by saline diuresis at 125–250 ml/h to promote calcium excretion[50]. At least 3–4 l should be given in the first 24 h. Plasma electrolytes, calcium and magnesium should be measured every 6–12 h, and potassium and magnesium replaced. Furosemide 20–40 mg twice to four times a day may be given if heart failure develops, but is rarely necessary. Thiazide diuretics should not be used, because they decrease urinary excretion of calcium. Calcitonin 4–8 IU/kg intramuscularly or subcutaneously every 6–12 h may be given if hypercalcemia is not adequately controlled by saline diuresis, but bisphosphonates or mithramycin are contraindicated in pregnancy.

Symptomatic primary hyperparathyroidism should be treated by parathyroidectomy, preferably in the second trimester[49,51]. In asymptomatic patients surgery can usually be postponed until after delivery if plasma calcium is stable[49]. Neonatal hypocalcemia should be anticipated.

Hypocalcemia

Decreased total plasma calcium in pregnancy is most often simply because of hypoalbuminemia with normal free calcium levels. True hypocalcemia, with decreased free calcium, is most often due to hypoparathyroidism, which may be idiopathic or the result of thyroid or parathyroid surgery. Rare causes include hypomagnesemia, vitamin D deficiency, renal failure and pseudohypoparathyroidism.

Clinical findings vary with the degree and rate of onset; chronic hypocalcemia may be asymptomatic. Symptoms include paresthesias and tetany with carpopedal spasm. Trousseau's and Chvostek's signs may be present. Severe hypocalcemia may cause lethargy, confusion, prolonged QT interval and (rarely) seizures. Maternal hypocalcemia stimulates fetal parathyroid function and leads to neonatal hyperparathyroidism with osteopenia and sometimes hypercalcemia[52].

The presence of true hypocalcemia should be confirmed by plasma free calcium measurement. The history, physical examination and routine laboratory tests often reveal the cause. Levels of plasma PTH, magnesium and 25-hydroxyvitamin D should be measured. Hypocalcemia without elevation of plasma PTH indicates hypoparathyroidism.

Symptomatic hypocalcemia should be treated with 10% calcium gluconate, 20 ml intravenously over 10 min, followed by infusion of 0.5–2 mg/kg per hour, adjusted to keep the plasma calcium level between 8 and 9 mg/dl[50]. Chronic therapy of hypoparathyroidism should be started with calcitriol, 0.25–0.5 µg orally every day, along with calcium carbonate 1–2 g orally three times a day. The dose of calcitriol should be adjusted at 2–4-week intervals to maintain the plasma calcium level between 8 and 9 mg/dl. Typical maintenance doses in non-pregnant patients are 0.5–2 µg four times a day; the dose requirement usually increases during pregnancy.

ADRENAL DISORDERS

The adrenal cortex produces two major hormones, cortisol and aldosterone, as well as weak androgens. The glucocorticoid cortisol has many actions including maintenance of normal glucose metabolism. Cortisol secretion is stimulated by ACTH, which is regulated by three mechanisms: negative feedback by glucocorticoids; diurnal variation, with peak ACTH and cortisol levels at about 0600 h, and very low levels at 2300 h; and stimulation by physical stress. ACTH release is stimulated by hypothalamic corticotropin releasing hormone (CRH). Serum cortisol is bound to cortisol binding globulin (CBG); only free cortisol enters cells and produces biological effects.

The mineralocorticoid aldosterone promotes renal sodium reabsorption and potassium excretion, and maintains extracellular fluid volume. Decreased extracellular fluid volume stimulates renin secretion by the kidney, which leads to increased production of angiotensin II, which in turn stimulates aldosterone secretion. Aldosterone increases the extracellular fluid volume, suppressing renin secretion and completing a negative feedback mechanism.

During pregnancy, CBG levels are increased by high estrogen levels, causing plasma cortisol to rise. Cortisol levels increase further during labor and remain elevated for several days. Free plasma and urine cortisol levels also increase, and feedback suppression of cortisol by dexamethasone is impaired[53]. Despite this, pregnant women do not show evidence of cortisol excess, apparently because tissue sensitivity to cortisol is diminished. The placenta produces both CRH and ACTH, but their regulatory role is not known. Plasma levels of renin and aldosterone are also increased. The fetal adrenal gland is large, consisting primarily of the fetal zone, and produces substantial amounts of dehydroandrosterone sulfate (DHA-S) that are converted by the placenta to estrogens[54].

Adrenal failure

Adrenal failure may be due to disease of the adrenal itself (primary adrenal failure, Addison's disease), in which both cortisol and aldosterone are deficient and ACTH levels are increased because of diminished negative feedback; or to disease of the hypothalamus or pituitary, causing ACTH deficiency (secondary adrenal failure) in which only cortisol is deficient. Addison's disease is most often due to autoimmune adrenal destruction. Rare causes include tuberculosis, other granulomatous diseases and adrenal hemorrhage. Secondary adrenal failure is most often due to ACTH suppression by glucocorticoid therapy, but may be caused by any hypothalamic or pituitary lesion, including lymphocytic hypophysitis[39]. Most of the latter patients also have other pituitary hormone deficiencies, and are usually infertile.

Clinical manifestations of cortisol deficiency include anorexia, nausea and vomiting, weight loss, fatigue, orthostatic hypotension, hyponatremia and hypoglycemia. Adrenal crisis, with shock, abdominal pain and fever, may develop spontaneously or during stress such as labor. Unless rapidly treated, adrenal crisis is fatal. Aldosterone deficiency causes hypovolemia, hyperkalemia and hyponatremia. Hyperpigmentation may develop in Addison's disease, probably because of elevated ACTH levels.

Diagnosis is based on the Cortrosyn stimulation test. Plasma cortisol is measured 30 min after cosyntropin (synthetic ACTH 1-24), 0.25 mg intravenously. The normal response in non-pregnant patients is a stimulated cortisol level of > 20 µg/dl. The elevation of plasma CBG and cortisol in pregnancy may decrease the sensitivity of this test, and borderline values should be interpreted with caution. In primary adrenal failure, plasma ACTH is markedly elevated.

Treatment of Addison's disease includes glucocorticoid replacement with prednisone, 5 mg every morning and 2.5 mg every afternoon, and mineralocorticoid replacement with Florinef, 0.1–0.3 mg every day[20]. The dose of Florinef should be adjusted to maintain blood pressure and plasma potassium within the normal range. During labor, surgery or severe illness, additional glucocorticoid is required to prevent adrenal crisis. Hydrocortisone 100 mg intravenously every 8 h should be given during the period of stress, with a gradual decrease in dose during recovery. If adrenal crisis is suspected in a patient who does not have known adrenal failure, dexamethasone 4–10 mg intravenously should be given and infusion of normal saline with 5% dextrose started. A cosyntropin stimulation test should then be performed, followed by hydrocortisone 100 mg intravenously every 8 h until the test results are known.

Cushing's syndrome

Cushing's syndrome is due to glucocorticoid excess[55]. Although ACTH-producing pituitary microadenomas (Cushing's disease) are the most common cause in non-pregnant women, adrenal tumors (benign or malignant) cause the majority of cases in pregnancy[53]. Cushing's syndrome may also be caused by glucocorticoid therapy or, rarely, ectopic ACTH production.

Clinical manifestations include central obesity, rounded plethoric face, dorsal and supraclavicular fat pads, thin skin with easy bruising and reddish striae, muscle wasting and weakness, osteoporosis and hirsutism. Hypertension and diabetes mellitus are common. Most women have oligomenorrhea and infertility, so that Cushing's syndrome and pregnancy seldom coexist. The risks of abortion, premature labor and stillbirth are increased in untreated maternal disease[53]. Only a small fraction of maternal cortisol reaches the fetus, so neonatal ACTH suppression and adrenal insufficiency are rare. Fetal virilization does not occur.

For the diagnosis[55], baseline 24-h urine cortisol level should be measured twice. The low-dose dexamethasone test consists of two consecutive 24-h urine cortisol measurements while the patient is taking dexamethasone 0.5 mg every 6 h; the normal response in non-pregnant patients is suppression to $< 20\ \mu g/24\ h$. Elevated urinary cortisol and diminished feedback suppression in normal pregnancy may confound diagnosis. Reference ranges have not been established in pregnancy, and marginal values should be interpreted with caution.

Differential diagnosis is based on the high-dose dexamethasone test, which consists of two 24-h urine cortisol measurements while the patient is taking dexamethasone 2 mg every 6 h. In Cushing's disease, some degree of negative feedback regulation persists, and urine cortisol level decreases with high-dose dexamethasone. Although a reference range in pregnancy has not been established, a decrease in urine cortisol to less than 10% of the baseline value establishes the diagnosis of Cushing's disease. There is usually no decrease in cortisol excretion during high-dose dexamethasone testing in Cushing's syndrome owing to adrenal tumors or the ectopic ACTH syndrome and, in this situation, a low level of plasma ACTH indicates an adrenal tumor, while elevated levels indicate ectopic ACTH production. If the high-dose dexamethasone test produces equivocal results, additional testing may be required[55]. If testing indicates Cushing's disease, the pituitary should be evaluated with MRI, although less than half of ACTH-secreting microadenomas are visualized. Adrenal tumors are readily located by MRI.

Adrenal tumors should be resected by flank incision with minimal delay, since about 20% are malignant. Drugs that inhibit cortisol synthesis should be avoided because they may have severe adverse effects on the fetus. There is little experience to guide therapy of Cushing's disease in pregnancy. The treatment of choice in non-pregnant patients is trans-sphenoidal adenoma resection, and this has been reported in pregnancy[56]. In mild or equivocal cases, management of hypertension and hyperglycemia may be sufficient, with delay of definitive therapy until after delivery[53].

Fetal virilizing disorders

Fetal virilization because of maternal androgen excess may be due to maternal congenital adrenal hyperplasia (CAH), ingestion of androgenic drugs, or androgen-producing tumors. The last include luteomas and a variety of other ovarian tumors[57], and less common adrenal tumors[58]. Most reported tumors have been histologically benign. Since hyperandrogenism impairs fertility, these disorders are uncommon in pregnancy. Virilization of the mother or female fetus may occur, but male fetuses are not affected. Most women with adequately treated CAH are fertile, and continued glucocorticoid therapy prevents androgen excess. Androgen excess due to luteoma regresses quickly postpartum, but may recur with subsequent pregnancies[57].

Plasma total testosterone level is increased in pregnancy because of elevated levels of testosterone binding globulin. If hyperandrogenism is suspected, plasma free testosterone and DHA-S should be measured. If confirmed, the maternal ovaries and the fetus should be evaluated by ultrasound, and the maternal adrenal glands by MRI. Removal of an androgen-secreting tumor during pregnancy has not been reported, but should be considered if the fetus is female.

Primary hyperaldosteronism

This is a rare cause of hypertension and hypokalemia, due to adrenal adenoma or bilateral adrenal hyperplasia. The elevated aldosterone levels of normal pregnancy confound evaluation, although very low plasma renin activity is evidence for primary hyperaldosteronism. The prudent course in most suspected cases is medical management, with further evaluation after delivery[59]. Blood pressure can usually be controlled by antihypertensive drugs, and hypokalemia corrected by potassium supplements. Potassium-sparing diuretics such as amiloride or triamterene may be used, but spironolactone should be avoided.

Pheochromocytoma

Pheochromocytoma is a rare tumor of the adrenal medulla or extra-adrenal chromaffin tissue that releases catecholamines, primarily norepinephrine[60]. About

10% are part of multiple endocrine neoplasia or other familial syndromes.

The major clinical manifestation is hypertension, which may be stable or paroxysmal. Episodic symptoms, including headache, palpitations and sweating, often accompany hypertensive paroxysms. About one-third of patients have normal blood pressure between episodes. Rarely hypotension and shock occur. Symptoms may be precipitated by certain drugs, general anesthesia, or labor. The diagnosis may be suspected in pregnancy because of characteristic symptoms, labile hypertension (especially early in pregnancy), or family history[54]. Maternal hypertension may lead to intrauterine growth retardation, and perinatal mortality is high without treatment[61].

The most reliable test is 24-h urinary excretion of norepinephrine and epinephrine. Several measurements should be made, since in some cases levels are only intermittently abnormal. Plasma catecholamine levels measured when blood pressure is elevated are very useful, since plasma norepinephrine is markedly elevated during hypertension caused by pheochromocytoma. Moderate elevations are less specific, since they may occur in any stressful situation. After diagnosis, the tumor should be located by MRI of the abdomen. About 90% are in the adrenal gland and most others in the retroperitoneum. In familial cases, tumors may be bilateral.

For treatment[60,61], α-adrenergic blockade with phenoxybenzamine 10 mg twice a day should be started, and the dose gradually increased until hypertension is controlled or symptomatic orthostatic hypotension develops. β-Adrenergic blockade is occasionally needed to control tachycardia or arrhythmias. Before 24 weeks of gestation, adrenalectomy should be performed by a flank incision when adequate α-blockade is achieved[61]. In the third trimester, phenoxybenzamine should be continued, and surgery delayed until the fetus matures. Labor should be avoided and the fetus delivered by Cesarean section with maternal adrenalectomy at the same operation[61]. Maternal and fetal mortality have improved considerably in recent cases.

REFERENCES

1. Mestman JH, Goodwin TM, Montoro MM. Thyroid disorders of pregnancy. *Endocr Metab Clin North Am* 1995;24:41
2. Burrow GN, Fisher DA, Larsen PR. Maternal and fetal thyroid function. *N Engl J Med* 1994;331:1072
3. Glinoer D, Lemone M. Goiter and pregnancy: new insight into an old problem. *Thyroid* 1992;2:65
4. Berghout A, Endert E, Ross A, *et al.* Thyroid function and thyroid size in normal pregnant women living in an iodine replete area. *Clin Endocrinol* 1994;41:375
5. Vulsma T, Gons MH, de Vijlder JJM. Maternal–fetal transfer of thyroxine in congenital hypothyroidism due to a total organification defect or thyroid agenesis. *N Engl J Med* 1989;321:13
6. De Zegher F, Pernasetti F, Vanhole C, *et al.* The prenatal role of thyroid hormone evidenced by fetomaternal Pit-1 deficiency. *J Clin Endocrinol Metab* 1995;80:3127
7. Klee GG, Hay ID. Role of thyrotropin measurements in diagnosis and management of thyroid disease. *Clin Lab Med* 1993;13:673
8. Roti E, Minelli R, Salvi M. Management of hyperthyroidism and hypothyroidism in the pregnant woman. *J Clin Endocrinol Metab* 1996;81:1679
9. Kaptein EM. Clinical application of free thyroxine determinations. *Clin Lab Med* 1993;13:653
10. Kaplan MM. Monitoring thyroxine treatment during pregnancy. *Thyroid* 1992;2:147
11. Fisher DA. Management of congenital hypothyroidism. *J Clin Endocrinol Metab* 1991;72:523
12. Davidson KM, Richards DS, Schatz DA, Fisher DA. Successful *in utero* treatment of fetal goiter and hypothyroidism. *N Engl J Med* 1991;324:543
13. Burrow GN. Thyroid function and hyperfunction during gestation. *Endocr Rev* 1993;14:194
14. Rajatanavin R, Chailurkit L, Srisupandit S, *et al.* Trophoblastic hyperthyroidism: clinical and biochemical features of five cases. *Am J Med* 1988;85:237
15. Yoshimura M, Hershman JM. Thyrotropic action of human chorionic gonadotropin. *Thyroid* 1995;5:425
16. Goodwin TM, Montoro M, Mestman JH. Transient hyperthyroidism and hyperemesis gravidarum: clinical aspects. *Am J Obstet Gynecol* 1992;167:648
17. Wing DA, Millar LK, Koonings PP, *et al.* A comparison of propylthiouracil versus methimazole in treatment of hyperthyroidism in pregnancy. *Am J Obstet Gynecol* 1994;170:90
18. Mandel SJ, Brent GA, Larsen PR. Review of antithyroid drug use during pregnancy and report of a case of aplasia cutis. *Thyroid* 1994;4:129
19. Momotani N, Yamashita R, Yoshimoto M, *et al.* Recovery from fetal hypothyroidism: evidence for the safety of breast-feeding while taking propylthiouracil. *Clin Endocrinol* 1989;31:591
20. Clutter WE. Endocrine disease. In Ewald GA, Mckenzie CR, eds. *Manual of Medical Therapeutics*, 28th edn. Boston: Little Brown, 1995
21. Cove DH, Johnston P. Fetal hyperthyroidism: experience of treatment of four siblings. *Lancet* 1985; 1:430–2
22. McKenzie JM, Zakarija M. Fetal and neonatal hyperthyroidism and hypothyroidism due to maternal TSH receptor antibodies. *Thyroid* 1992;2:155
23. Learoyd DL, Fung HY, McGregor AM. Postpartum thyroid dysfunction. *Thyroid* 1992;2:73
24. Tan GH, Gharib H, Goellner JR, *et al.* Management of thyroid nodules in pregnancy. *Arch Intern Med* 1996; 156:2317
25. Scheithauer BW, Sano T, Kovacs KT, *et al.* The pituitary gland in pregnancy: a clinicopathologic and immunohistochemical study of 69 cases. *Mayo Clin Proc* 1990; 65:461
26. Elster AD, Sanders TG, Vines FS, Chen MYM. Size and shape of the pituitary gland during pregnancy and postpartum: measurement with MR imaging. *Radiology* 1991;181:531
27. Prager D, Braunstein GD. Pituitary disorders during pregnancy. *Endocr Metab Clin North Am* 1995;24:1

28. Caufriez A, Frankenne F, Hennen G, Copinschi G. Regulation of maternal insulin-like growth factor by placental growth hormone in pregnancy. *Horm Res* 1994;42:62

29. Kupersmith MJ, Rosenberg C, Kleinberg D. Visual loss in pregnant women with pituitary adenomas. *Ann Intern Med* 1994;121:473

30. Vance ML. Hypopituitarism. *N Engl J Med* 1994; 330:1651

31. Laws ER, Thapar K. Surgical management of pituitary adenomas. *Baillière's Clin Endocrinol Metab* 1995;9:391

32. Molitch ME. Pathologic hyperprolactinemia. *Endocr Metab Clin North Am* 1992;21:877

33. Krupp P, Monka C. Bromocriptine in pregnancy: safety aspects. *Klin Wochenschr* 1987;65:823

34. Molitch ME. Clinical manifestations of acromegaly. *Endocr Metab Clin North Am* 1992;21:597

35. Ezzat S. Living with acromegaly. *Endocr Metab Clin North Am* 1992;21:753

36. Melmed S, Ho K, Klibanski A, *et al.* Recent advances in pathogenesis, diagnosis and management of acromegaly. *J Clin Endocrinol Metab* 1995;80:3395

37. Cundy T, Grundy EN, Melville H, Sheldon J. Bromocriptine treatment of acromegaly following spontaneous conception. *Fertil Steril* 1984;42:134–6

38. Landolt AM, Schmid J, Wimpfheimer C, *et al.* Successful pregnancy in a previously infertile woman treated with SMS-201-995 for acromegaly (letter). *N Engl J Med* 1989;320:671

39. Thodou E, Asa SL, Kontogeorgos G, *et al.* Lymphocytic hypophysitis: clinicopathological findings. *J Clin Endocrinol Metab* 1995;80:2302

40. Ahmadi J, Meyers GS, Segal HD, *et al.* Lymphocytic adenohypophysitis: contrast-enhanced MR imaging in five cases. *Radiology* 1995;195:30

41. Lindheimer MD, Barron WM. Water metabolism and vasopressin secretion during pregnancy. *Baillière's Clin Obstet Gynecol* 1994;8:311

42. Robertson GL. Diabetes insipidus. *Endocr Metab Clin North Am* 1995;24:549

43. Williams DJ, Metcalfe KA, Skingle L, *et al.* Pathophysiology of transient cranial diabetes insipidus during pregnancy. *Clin Endocrinol* 1993;38:595

44. Durr JA, Hoggard JG, Hunt JM, Schrier RW. Diabetes insipidus in pregnancy associated with abnormally high circulating vasopressinase activity. *N Engl J Med* 1987;316:1070

45. Hosking DJ. Calcium homeostasis in pregnancy. *Clin Endocrinol* 1996;45:1

46. Heath H. Familial benign hypercalcemia – from clinical description to molecular genetics. *West J Med* 1994;160:554

47. Powell BR, Blank E, Benda G, Buist NR. Neonatal hyperparathyroidism and skeletal demineralization in an infant with familial hypocalciuric hypercalcemia. *Pediatrics* 1993;91:144

48. Lepre F, Grill V, Martin TJ. Hypercalcemia in pregnancy and lactation associated with parathyroid hormone-related protein. *N Engl J Med* 1993;328:666

49. Kohlmeier L, Marcus R. Calcium disorders of pregnancy. *Endocr Metab Clin North Am* 1995;24:15

50. Dagogo-Jack S, Clutter WE. Mineral and metabolic bone disease. In Ewald GA, McKenzie CR, eds. *Manual of Medical Therapeutics*, 28th edn. Boston: Little Brown, 1995

51. Inabnet WB, Baldwin D, Daniel RO, Staren ED. Hyperparathyroidism and pancreatitis during pregnancy. *Surgery* 1996;119:710

52. Loughead JL, Mughal Z, Mimouni F, *et al.* Spectrum and natural history of congenital hyperparathyroidism secondary to maternal hypocalcemia. *Am J Perinatol* 1990;7:350

53. Aron DC, Schnall AM, Sheeler LR. Cushing's syndrome and pregnancy. *Am J Obstet Gynecol* 1990;162:244

54. Hadden DR. Adrenal disorders of pregnancy. *Endocr Metab Clin North Am* 1995;24:139

55. Orth DN. Cushing's syndrome. *N Engl J Med* 1995; 332:791

56. Casson IF, Davis JC, Jeffreys RV, *et al.* Successful management of Cushing's disease during pregnancy by transsphenoidal adenectomy. *Clin Endocrinol* 1987; 27:423

57. Shortle BE, Warren MP, Tsin D. Recurrent androgenicity in pregnancy: a case report and literature review. *Obstet Gynecol* 1987;70:462

58. Kirk JMW, Perry LA, Shand WS, *et al.* Female pseudohermaphroditism due to maternal adrenocortical tumor. *J Clin Endocrinol Metab* 1990;70:1280

59. Hammond TG, Buchanan JD, Scoggins BA, *et al.* Primary hyperaldosteronism in pregnancy. *Aust NZ J Med* 1982;12:537

60. Cryer PE. Pheochromocytoma. *West J Med* 1992; 156:399

61. Harper MA, Murnaghan GA, Kennedy L, *et al.* Pheochromocytoma in pregnancy: five cases and a review of the literature. *Br J Obstet Gynaecol* 1989;96:594

37

Gastrointestinal diseases

D.C. Rubin

INTRODUCTION

Pregnancy has a dramatic effect on the normal physiology of the gastrointestinal tract, and gut-related symptoms are extremely common during gestation. In this chapter, a review is presented of the intestinal disorders which are commonest in pregnancy and/or which present difficult management problems. Despite a wealth of clinical studies, the therapeutic options for enteropancreatic diseases in pregnancy are somewhat limited because the effect of most gastrointestinal drugs on the fetus has not been clarified. The treatment of these disorders in the non-pregnant as well as the pregnant patient is discussed, so that the reader will become familiar with the full range of available medications and interventions.

PHYSIOLOGICAL CHANGES ASSOCIATED WITH PREGNANCY

Gastrointestinal symptoms including nausea, vomiting and heartburn are extremely common during pregnancy, beginning as early as 1 week after the first missed menstrual period. Studies of gut function in pregnancy are limited since invasive or radiological procedures cannot be performed, but they have provided some clues regarding the mechanisms underlying these common complaints. Most human studies have focused on the function of the lower esophageal sphincter and the effects of gestation on gut motility[1].

The lower esophageal sphincter (LES) is a collection of circular smooth muscle fibers located at the distal end of the esophagus which creates a high pressure zone that prevents reflux of food and gastric contents from the stomach. LES pressure and its functional responsiveness to a variety of stimuli have been extensively analyzed in pregnancy to determine their role in the pathogenesis of reflux disease (see Reflux section, below). Pharmacological and physiological substances that increase LES pressure in normal subjects do not produce similar responses in the LES in early gestation[2], and basal LES pressure is decreased in pregnant women both with and without reflux symptoms[3,4]. As pregnancy progresses and progesterone levels rise, the LES basal pressure declines[4].

Normal esophageal motility appears to be altered in pregnancy. Nagler and Spiro[3] showed that non-propulsive motor activity was much more common in pregnant subjects than in controls. Ulmsten and Sundstrom[5] could not confirm this but found that peristaltic wave speed and amplitude were both decreased in late pregnancy. These physiological changes may contribute to the pathogenesis of gastroesophageal reflux disease during gestation.

The influence of pregnancy on gastric emptying is unclear. Because progesterone rises in pregnancy and inhibits smooth muscle contractility, it has been postulated that gastric emptying would be decreased during gestation[6]. However, the results of several studies conflict and demonstrate both normal and delayed emptying. These contradictory findings probably result from the use of several different methods to measure emptying (dye dilution, fluoroscopy and paracetamol absorption), although two studies using the same technique also yielded conflicting results[6,7]. Therefore, it is difficult to draw firm conclusions. Intragastric pressures rise in pregnancy[5,8]; elevated pressures may be found even in early gestation before significant uterine enlargement occurs, and may contribute to the risk of gastroesophageal reflux.

Constipation is frequent in pregnancy[9], affecting 30–35% of all pregnancies. The prevalence of this symptom has prompted studies of gastrointestinal transit time, analyzed by measuring breath hydrogen concentration after lactulose ingestion[10,11]. Transit time is delayed in the second and third but not first trimesters and roughly correlates with serum progesterone levels. This phenomenon is reversible, resolving postpartum[11]. Progesterone is often implicated as the hormone responsible for decreased motility yet the role of other hormones which regulate gut motility has not been adequately examined. Although pregnancy seems to have a primary effect on motility, lack of adequate dietary intake of fiber is probably important since an analysis of pregnant patients in a high fiber-eating population showed a much lower incidence of constipation during gestation[12].

REFLUX ESOPHAGITIS

Gastroesophageal reflux disease (GERD) results from the inappropriate backwash of stomach contents into the esophagus. Although this process occurs frequently in asymptomatic individuals[13], it can also result in heartburn and regurgitation. Reflux esophagitis is defined as the presence of typical symptoms of gastroesophageal reflux in conjunction with endoscopic and pathological changes in the esophagus. Symptoms of reflux disease are extremely common in pregnant women[14,15] and are an important cause of morbidity in pregnancy.

The prevalence of symptoms of gastroesophageal reflux is quite high in the general population. Large-scale surveys have revealed that approximately 33–44% of adult Americans experience reflux symptoms on a twice-weekly to monthly basis[16]. However, the great majority of this group does not seek medical attention. Of those individuals who go to a doctor, 40–70% will show endoscopic evidence of esophagitis. Gastroesophageal reflux symptoms are extremely common during pregnancy; most studies show that more than 50% of pregnant women suffer from symptoms of GERD at some time during gestation[14,17]. The incidence of true reflux esophagitis is difficult to determine, because large-scale endoscopic studies of pregnant women have not been performed.

There are several defense mechanisms which act to limit contact with and damage to the esophagus by gastric contents[13] (Table 1). The LES is probably the major protective structure, preventing food, acid and secretions from entering the esophagus from the stomach. The LES relaxes in response to hormones, foods and drugs. Some patients with reflux esophagitis have decreased resting LES pressures or a completely incompetent LES; reflux events also occur in patients with normal LES pressures, presumably owing to transient LES relaxation[18,19]. Contact of the esophageal mucosa with damaging substances is limited by esophageal peristalsis and gravity which promote clearing. Aperistalsis, as found in scleroderma, contributes substantially to the development of esophagitis in these patients (in addition to an incompetent LES). Saliva has also been shown to neutralize acid. Finally, the esophageal epithelial layer has intrinsic defense systems including cell membrane and intercellular components[13] which prevent influx of hydrogen ions, as well as intracellular proteins which function as buffers.

Table 1   Esophageal mucosal defense mechanisms

	Effect
Lower esophageal sphincter	barrier
Esophageal motility	promotes clearing
Gravity (when upright)	promotes clearing
Saliva	acid neutralization
Intrinsic epithelial defense	cell membrane, inter- and intracellular components

The pathophysiology of GERD and reflux esophagitis in pregnant patients is incompletely understood. Some analyses have shown that resting LES pressure decreases in pregnancy, in both early and late gestation[4,20]. In other studies, LES pressure was normal in early pregnancy but hypofunction of the LES was detected, as measured by decreased responsiveness to drugs that increase sphincter pressure[2]. Decreased LES pressure probably results from elevated serum estrogen and especially progesterone levels during pregnancy[4].

Although increased intra-abdominal pressure has been postulated to produce reflux, a study of men with tense ascites as a model of pregnancy[21] showed an increase in LES pressure and no demonstrable acid reflux. Thus, the contribution of increased abdominal girth in reflux esophagitis is unclear, but the relevance of this model may be questioned. Intragastric pressures appear to be increased even in early pregnancy, and patients with heartburn have lower mean barrier pressures (LES pressure – gastric pressure) than asymptomatic pregnant individuals[8]. Normal esophageal motility, which helps clear potentially damaging material from the esophagus, is also altered; peristaltic wave speed and amplitude are both reduced[5]. Esophageal mucosal defense factors and vascular perfusion have not been examined in pregnancy.

Classic symptoms of gastroesophageal reflux disease include heartburn (retrosternal burning pain) and regurgitation. In patients with longstanding reflux esophagitis, strictures may result, producing dysphagia, or difficulty swallowing. Very severe reflux esophagitis may produce pain upon swallowing (odynophagia), although this is more likely to be associated with infectious causes of esophagitis. Acid reflux may lead to esophageal dysmotility and atypical chest discomfort, with chest pressure and pain that mimic symptoms of cardiac disease. A variety of complications can result from reflux esophagitis, including stricture formation, bleeding and pulmonary aspiration. In addition, chronic esophageal inflammation is thought to lead to Barrett's esophagus, in which the normal squamous esophageal epithelium is replaced by gastric or specialized columnar epithelium. This diagnosis is made by endoscopy with biopsy; routine follow-up with periodic endoscopic examination and repeat biopsy, although controversial, is indicated at present because of an increased risk of esophageal cancer. The precise risk of malignancy in Barrett's esophagus has not been established.

Diagnosis

In the non-pregnant symptomatic adult, the diagnosis of reflux disease may be made in a variety of ways[13,22]. To evaluate the mucosal surface for the presence of esophagitis, a standard barium swallow radiographic examination may be performed and can show mucosal ulcerations or strictures, as well as ruling out carcinoma. This test is less sensitive than upper endoscopy, in which direct visualization of the epithelium is achieved and biopsies can be taken for histological analysis. Endoscopy is generally indicated for those with long-standing atypical/systemic symptoms or with symptoms refractory to a trial of standard medical therapy. In patients with atypical symptoms (chest pain), esophageal motility studies with the intraesophageal acid perfusion (Bernstein) test may be performed. Acid is perfused into the esophagus and patient symptoms are recorded. This test is positive when the patient's symptoms are reproduced by acid and relieved by saline. Also useful is prolonged esophageal pH monitoring, which can detect reflux and be used to correlate symptoms with reflux events.

In the pregnant patient, it is rarely necessary to perform any of the aforementioned tests. A description of symptoms is usually sufficient for diagnostic purposes[23], and an empirical trial of treatment may be initiated. Radiographic studies are of course avoided if at all possible. Upper endoscopy may be indicated for evaluation of symptoms that are refractory to routine therapy, for dysphagia or for upper gastrointestinal bleeding. This procedure appears to be safe in pregnancy, as reported in a recent study that showed no risk of premature labor or congenital malformations in endoscopies performed in 83 pregnancies[24].

Management with maternal–fetal consideration

Changes in daily habits can be useful in the treatment of both pregnant and non-pregnant patients. Avoidance of smoking, late-night meals and substances that decrease LES pressure such as high-fat foods, caffeine, alcohol and chocolate often provide some relief. Patients should remain upright after meals to minimize reflux of acidic contents, allowing gravity to aid esophageal clearance. Elevation of the head of the bed by shock blocks helps maintain the beneficial effect of gravity at night.

Various medications can be used (see Table 2). *Antacids* are generally considered safe in pregnancy[25], although a large retrospective study showed an increased incidence of birth defects in women who used antacids along with many other medications in the first trimester[26]. No particular antacid was specified, and these data have not been verified in another study. However, no survey as extensive as this has ever been attempted again. More recent analyses of pregnant women in both the USA and the Netherlands[27,28] indicate that antacid use is common; although no obvious increase in rare birth defects has been noted, small increases in common abnormalities such as spontaneous abortion, cleft palate or low birth weight

would be difficult to detect[27]. Both aluminum- and magnesium-containing antacids can be absorbed, albeit poorly. The major immediate side-effects of large doses of antacids include constipation induced by aluminum-containing antacids and diarrhea caused by magnesium-based preparations. The use of a combination of these medications will usually resolve bowel-related problems. The use of 30 ml of a high-potency antacid (Table 3) 30 min–1 h and 3 h after meals and at bedtime is usually sufficient for symptomatic relief and may promote healing. Sodium bicarbonate should be avoided, owing to fluid overload[1,15].

Sucralfate, a polysulfated salt of sucrose, binds to exposed proteins found in the base of ulcerated mucosa, and produces a protective coating of the ulcer site. Although it has not been definitively shown to be effective in the treatment of reflux esophagitis[22], some authors recommend its use because of its minimal systemic absorption and lack of carcinogenicity/teratogenicity in rodents[23]. However, there are no published case reports examining the safety or efficacy of sucralfate in gastroesophageal reflux. Despite its lack of systemic absorption, experience with this drug in pregnancy is so limited that it cannot be routinely recommended, but may be useful in patients with symptoms refractory to antacids.

The histamine-2 (H2) receptor blockers, including cimetidine, ranitidine, famotidine and nizatidine, are clearly effective agents in healing reflux esophagitis in the non-pregnant patient. However, 8 or more weeks of therapy are generally required to produce complete healing, and recurrences are frequent when medication is discontinued. Because of the paucity of studies

Table 2 Gastrointestinal drugs in pregnancy. From reference 129

Drug name	FDA category
H2 blockers	
Cimetidine	B
Ranitidine	B
Famotidine	B
Nizatidine	C
Sucralfate	B
Pepto Bismol®	C
Proton pump inhibitors	
Omeprazole	C
Lanosoprazole	B₁
Promotility agents	
Metaclopramide	B
Cisapride	C
5-Aminosalicylic acid compounds	
Sulfasalazine	B₁
Mesalamine	B₁
(Rosawa, Asacol, Pentasa)	

Table 3 Antacid preparations. Adapted from reference 137

Antacid	Buffering capacity (mEq/15 ml)	Buffering capacity (ml/100mEq)	Sodium content (mEq/15 ml)
Al (OH)₃			
Amphogel	30	50	0.30
Basalgel	34.5	43	0.39
Basalgel extra strength	66	23	3.00
Al(OH)₃ + Mg(OH)₂			
Maalox TC	82	18	0.09
Maalox Plus*	40	37.5	0.18
Mylanta*	37.5	40	0.10
Mylanta-II*	75	20	0.15
Riopan	45	33	0.04
Gelusila	36	42	0.10
CaCO₃			
Tums tablets	19.5†		0.125†
Titralac	33	45	0.00
Al(OH)₂ + Mg(OH)₂ + CaCO₃			
Camalox	54	26	0.15

*Contains simethicone; †Per two tablets

in pregnant women, the safety of these agents is unclear, and their routine use in pregnancy for symptoms of gastroesophageal reflux is not recommended[25]. However, for those patients whose symptoms are refractory to antacids or sucralfate, or in whom complications of reflux such as bleeding occur, cimetidine may be prescribed in the second and third trimesters. This drug, the first of the H2 blockers, has been used in pregnant women for the therapy of peptic ulcer disease, and is the best studied of this class of drug in pregnancy (FDA category B). There is a further discussion of cimetidine and other H2 blockers in gestation in the following section under Medical therapy in pregnancy for peptic ulcer disease.

Omeprazole and lansoprazole are very effective inhibitors of parietal cell H⁺/K⁺ ATPase (the proton pump responsible for hydrogen ion secretion) that can completely block gastric acid secretion. These are the drugs of choice in non-pregnant patients for treatment of severe erosive reflux esophagitis and can heal esophageal lesions which are refractory to treatment with H2 blockers. However, they are untested in pregnancy and should at present be avoided.

Metoclopramide and cisapride are prokinetic agents that enhance gastric motility and emptying, and also increase lower esophageal sphincter pressure in the normal population, and in patients with reflux. Metoclopramide has been shown to increase LES pressure in pregnant women[29]. Although metoclopramide has been used in the acute treatment of hyperemesis and for the prevention of aspiration during obstetric anesthesia, there is limited experience in its use in

GERD in pregnancy. It is doubtful that metoclopramide will ever play a significant role in this disease, because of the risk of central nervous system side-effects (including restlessness, fatigue, anxiety and extrapyramidal symptoms) and because the effects of long-term use of metoclopramide in pregnancy are unknown. Cisapride also has not been studied in pregnancy.

PEPTIC ULCER DISEASE
An ulcer is an injury to or interruption of the mucosal lining of the gastrointestinal tract extending through the muscularis mucosa. The pathophysiological mechanisms underlying peptic ulcer disease are quite complex; acid production, disruption of mucosal defense mechanisms and *Helicobacter pylori* all play a role. Although peptic ulcer disease is an important cause of morbidity and mortality in the general population, symptoms of peptic disease rarely worsen during pregnancy and may actually improve, and complications such as perforation and hemorrhage are distinctly uncommon[30–33].

Peptic ulcer had been generally recognized to be more common in men than in women[31]. However, recent surveys indicate that the period prevalence as well as mortality rates from ulcer disease for men and women are approximately equivalent[34], resulting from a rapid decline in duodenal ulcer disease in men as well as an increase in gastric ulcer hospitalizations for women older than 65 years.

The incidence of peptic disease in women is quite low in the childbearing years[33,35]. There are also some data to suggest that, in pregnancy, duodenal ulcer becomes even more unusual. This impression is primarily based on the observation that the number of reported cases of ulcer perforation and hemorrhage is very low[30,36]. However, it is quite difficult to ascertain the true incidence of peptic disease in pregnancy, since diagnostic testing is generally avoided. Also, ulcer symptoms may be attributed to gastroesophageal reflux and then treated with resolution of symptoms, thereby precluding further testing[31,33].

The etiology of peptic ulcer disease is complex and multifactorial. *Helicobacter pylori* has recently been implicated in the pathogenesis of peptic ulcer disease. Patients who are colonized with *H. pylori* all have histological evidence of antral gastritis, and eradication of infection leads to resolution of gastritis. Virtually 100% of patients with duodenal ulcer, and gastric ulcer unassociated with the use of non-steroidal anti-inflammatory drugs (NSAIDs), are infected with *H. pylori*. The mechanisms by which *H. pylori* produces ulcer disease has not been completely clarified. However, it is clear that healing of ulcers occurs when *H. pylori* is eradicated, and most importantly, relapse of ulcer disease is prevented[37,38]. A recent NIH Consensus Conference[38] has recommended the use of antibiotics and other medications to eradicate *H. pylori* in patients with peptic ulcer disease.

Other factors that lead to an increased risk of mucosal damage include alcohol consumption, cigarette smoking and, as previously mentioned, use of aspirin and other NSAIDs. Cigarette smoking has been shown to slow ulcer healing and is associated with a higher rate of ulcer recurrence[39] when smokers are compared with non-smokers.

Acid must clearly be present for duodenal ulcer formation. Many, but not all, patients with duodenal ulcer have increased parietal cell mass and, as a group, demonstrate elevated acid secretion. The role of acid in ulcer formation is well illustrated by the Zollinger Ellison syndrome, in which a gastrin-producing tumor leads to marked hypergastrinemia, profuse acid secretion and ulceration throughout the gastrointestinal tract. Other factors include decreased mucosal bicarbonate secretion and elevated nocturnal acid secretion[40], yet the marked degree of overlap of these measurements between normals and patients with duodenal ulcer is indicative of the multifactorial origin of this disease. Unlike duodenal ulcer, acid secretion in patients with gastric ulcers unrelated to aspirin or NSAIDs is either normal or may even be markedly decreased. This suggests that there is a smaller role for acid in this disease than in duodenal ulcer and implies that other factors are more important. Gastric ulcer also differs from duodenal ulcer in that a significant although small percentage of gastric ulcers are malignant. Therefore, upper endoscopy and biopsy of gastric ulcers with follow-up until complete healing is documented is recommended.

Mucosal defense involves those features of the stomach and duodenal epithelium that allow it to resist damage by acid, pepsin and biliary reflux. They include the thick mucous layer that overlies the stomach and duodenal mucosa and the ability of the mucosa to secrete bicarbonate. Increased use of NSAIDs and analysis of the damage that they inflict on the gastroduodenal mucosa has led to recognition of the importance of mucosal defense mechanisms in the pathogenesis of injury. Impairment or disruption of these protective mechanisms occurs because of inhibition of cyclooxygenase, prostaglandin synthesis and mucosal mucus and bicarbonate secretion, leading to superficial gastric mucosal injury or gastric ulcer, predominantly in the gastric antrum.

Studies of pregnant women to determine why ulcer disease is rare during gestation are inconclusive. Gastric acid secretion had been postulated to decrease during pregnancy, yet this suppression is mild at best and recent studies do not confirm this[4]. Interestingly, serum gastrin levels are normal until late pregnancy, and then rise[41]. Although this is controversial, it may explain why ulcer symptoms often recur just prior to delivery. There are no studies addressing the possible role of *H. pylori* in this phenomenon; it is not known how pregnancy affects the infectivity or growth rate of *H. pylori*.

Typical symptoms of peptic ulcer disease include mid-epigastric pain which is relieved by food or antacids. Patients often describe a dull 'gnawing' or burning sensation which may awaken them at night, or may occur in the morning before eating or after meals. Because the abdominal pain is often relieved by eating, patients with ulcer may gain weight. Other symptoms arise when duodenal or gastric ulcer is complicated by hemorrhage, perforation, penetration or obstruction (Table 4). If the ulcer bleeds, the patient may demonstrate black or tarry stools or suffer from hematemesis. Ulcer penetration into even a small arterial blood vessel can lead to massive, brisk bleeding with rapid transit of blood through the gastrointestinal tract and red blood per rectum. Abdominal pain which radiates to the back indicates possible penetration of the ulcer posteriorly through the wall of the stomach or duodenal bulb into surrounding organs. Duodenal bulb ulcers may penetrate into the pancreas, whereas gastric ulcers can erode into the liver or colon. The sudden onset of severe pain in conjunction with physical findings of an acute abdomen (rebound, guarding, absent bowel sounds and distension) are associated with free perforation of the ulcer, which is a surgical emergency. Finally, prolonged nausea and vomiting can result from obstruction caused by edema and inflammation surrounding an ulcer crater located in the prepyloric or pyloric region. It is important to note that complicated ulcer disease may present with no antecedent history of abdominal pain or other symptoms.

In pregnancy, the signs and symptoms of ulcer disease and its complications may be obscured. First, symptoms which are consistent with ulcer disease may also be associated with gastroesophageal reflux, which is quite common in pregnancy. Nausea and vomiting indicating the presence of an obstructing ulcer may be mistakenly considered to be 'normal' pregnancy-related symptoms. Because of the morbidity and mortality associated with complicated peptic disease during gestation, a high index of suspicion for ulcer

Table 4 Complications of peptic ulcer disease

Gastrointestinal bleeding
Perforation
Posterior perforation in duodenal bulb
Perforation in stomach
Obstruction
Intractable pain
Melenic stool, hematemesis
Severe, acute abdominal pain
Pancreatitis
Gastrocolic fistula
Vomiting, early satiety

should be maintained for those patients who develop nausea, vomiting and pain in the second and third trimesters[32]. Finally, in the immediate post-delivery period, signs of perforation such as abdominal rebound or guarding may be absent or decreased due to muscular relaxation, leading to delayed or misdiagnosis.

Diagnosis

In the non-pregnant patient, the diagnosis of peptic ulcer disease may be made by either double-contrast barium upper gastrointestinal radiography or by upper endoscopy. In pregnancy, upper endoscopy is preferable[30,42], since there is no exposure to X-irradiation and patients may be studied with minimal or no anesthesia; local anesthetics applied to the back of the throat as a xylocaine-based spray may be sufficient. In addition, the use of endoscopy permits biopsy as well as detection of lesions, particularly important in the management of gastric ulcers to rule out carcinoma.

In all patients with documented peptic ulcer disease, the presence of *H. pylori* infection should be determined. Upper endoscopy with gastric biopsy and histological detection, or biopsy with detection of urease activity (Clotest), an enzyme produced in abundance by H. pylori, are two common methods. Biopsy and culture of the organism from gastric tissue is technically more difficult and therefore less sensitive. Breath testing (which is not as available as the other methods) and the serological detection of IgG antibodies to *H. pylori* are less invasive methods.

Whereas it is acceptable initially to treat young people (less than age 40) empirically for symptoms of dyspepsia without initial diagnostic testing, it is generally recommended that the following patients be evaluated to make a definitive diagnosis: (1) those aged 50 or older; (2) those with an absent or incomplete response to an adequate treatment trial; (3) those with symptoms of complicated ulcer disease; or (4) those with systemic symptoms such as weight loss. In pregnant patients, it is reasonable to initiate an empirical trial of therapy (see Management, below) and evaluate only those with persistent symptoms, gastrointestinal bleeding or other signs of complicated ulcer disease.

Management with maternal–fetal consideration

Although many effective agents are available to treat peptic ulcers, a lack of adequate clinical trials in pregnant patients often precludes their use in gestation. A general overview of therapy is presented with specific recommendations for pregnancy.

The treatment of peptic ulcer disease focuses on (1) healing of the ulcer crater; and (2) permanently eradicating *H. pylori* if present. To eliminate *H. pylori*, various combinations of antibiotics (including tetracycline,

metronidazole, clarithromycin and amoxicillin) and Pepto Bismol® appear to be effective. Since many of these have teratogenic effects, eradication of *H. pylori* can be delayed until after delivery. Healing of the ulcer crater can be achieved by 4–8 weeks of therapy with antacids (not commonly used now in non-pregnant patients), H2 blockers or proton pump inhibitors. Since duodenal ulcers are benign, follow-up endoscopy to document complete healing is unnecessary. In contrast, resolution of a gastric ulcer may require more than 8 weeks of treatment. Also, unlike duodenal ulcer, it is recommended that gastric ulcers be followed endoscopically with biopsy until they are completely healed, because of the risk of gastric cancer in otherwise benign-appearing ulcers.

Pharmacotherapy in the non-pregnant patient

Acid secretion by the parietal cell is controlled by neural, paracrine and endocrine influences. Receptors for histamine (H2 receptors) and gastrin are present on the surface of the parietal cell; exposure to either histamine or gastrin leads to acid secretion. Cholinergic neural signals interact with muscarinic receptors to produce acid secretion. In response to these and other stimuli, vesicles containing the proton pump, or H^+/K^+ ATPase, fuse to the cell membrane and H^+ ions are secreted into the gastric lumen. Treatment of peptic ulcer disease in the general population is primarily directed at blocking the interaction of histamine with its receptor. First-line drugs include the H2 receptor blockers such as cimetidine, ranitidine, famotidine and nizatidine. These medications are highly effective in reducing acid secretion and generally produce duodenal ulcer healing in the majority of patients within 4–6 weeks. Although these drugs are also effective in the treatment of gastric ulcer, these lesions are generally more resistant and require a longer course of therapy (8–12 weeks).

Although antacids in sufficient quantity can neutralize secreted acid and are as effective as H2 blockers in ulcer healing, the quantity of antacids needed as well as dosage frequency makes this therapy too cumbersome for first-line treatment in the general population, particularly since certain H2 blockers are effective in once-daily doses. Therefore, antacids are generally reserved for as-needed relief of symptoms. Sucralfate, a sulfated disaccharide that is complexed to aluminum hydroxide, binds to the base of ulcer craters and may stimulate prostaglandin synthesis and therefore bicarbonate and mucus secretion. It is effective in healing duodenal ulcers and has the advantage of not being systemically absorbed. A dose of 1 g four times daily is usually adequate.

Omeprazole and lansoprazole, irreversible inhibitors of the proton pump H^+/K^+ ATPase, very effectively block acid secretion and are frequently used to treat duodenal or gastric ulcer, particularly in complicated patients with multiple ulcers or in those with gastrointestinal bleeding.

Medical therapy in pregnancy

Antacids are preferred as the first line of therapy for peptic ulcer disease during gestation. A high-potency antacid (see Table 3) is ingested 1 and 3 h after meals and at night. The dosage should be sufficient to neutralize approximately 100–150 mEq of acid per dose.

Sucralfate may be a good second-line agent in the treatment of peptic disease in pregnancy since it is not absorbed and has not been shown to be teratogenic in rodents[25]. However, its safe use in pregnancy has not been established by clinical trials in humans and so it cannot be routinely recommended.

Although H2 blockers are highly effective in the treatment of peptic ulcer, their use in pregnancy is presently recommended in only the second or third trimesters for refractory peptic disease that does not respond to antacids or for complicated ulcer disease (e.g. gastrointestinal bleeding, obstruction). There are insufficient numbers of clinical trials documenting their safety in human pregnancy. Cimetidine crosses the placenta and is excreted into breast milk[43], but it is approved for use during lactation[44]. There are several reports of small numbers of pregnant women who have been treated with cimetidine for peptic ulcer disease associated with gastrointestinal bleeding without adverse effect[24,45], but one report described a newborn who was jaundiced and showed evidence of decreased hepatic function; this gradually resolved[46]. Cimetidine has also been used without adverse fetal effects during delivery[44] for acute reduction of the risk of gastric aspiration (Mendelson's syndrome).

Very few data are available regarding the safe use of ranitidine or other H2 blockers in pregnancy and so none can be recommended at present. Ranitidine has been used during labor to reduce gastric acidity and in this acute setting did not adversely affect the newborn. Omeprazole or lansoprazole have not been adequately evaluated in pregnancy and cannot be recommended at this time.

Patients with peptic ulcer disease should avoid smoking and ingestion of alcohol and NSAIDs/aspirin. Patients are also advised to eliminate foods which cause abdominal discomfort (for example, highly spiced foods or citrus fruit and drinks).

HYPEREMESIS GRAVIDARUM

Nausea is a common symptom occurring in 80–90% of pregnancies; epidemiological surveys have shown that nausea with vomiting is found in up to 55–70% of pregnant women[47,48]. Hyperemesis gravidarum is a much rarer disorder, occurring in approximately 5 per 1000 pregnancies in the USA[49]. One of the most widely quoted definitions of hyperemesis gravidarum is that proposed by Fairweather[49] in 1968, who described this syndrome as 'vomiting occurring in pregnancy, appearing for the first time before the twentieth week of gestation, and of such severity as to require the patient's admission to the hospital, the vomiting being unassociated with such coincidental conditions as appendicitis, pyelitis, etc.'. In more recent literature, the definition has been expanded to require that the vomiting must be severe enough to interfere with the nutritional and metabolic status of the patient, leading to dehydration, weight loss and electrolyte imbalances. Although nausea and vomiting in pregnancy and hyperemesis have been studied for many years, the etiology of these disorders remains obscure. Whereas uncomplicated nausea and vomiting can usually be tolerated without treatment, the complications which may result from hyperemesis require specific therapy, and successful management is often challenging.

In his extensive review, Fairweather[49] analyzed the worldwide incidence of hyperemesis gravidarum. Hyperemesis much more commonly afflicts women living in Western countries compared to African and Eskimo populations. The incidence in the industrialized West ranges between 1.25 and 9.9 per 1000 pregnancies, with the average of 2–5 per 1000. Several epidemiological risk factors for hyperemesis have been identified (Table 5). High body weight (greater than 170 lb; 76.5 kg), and young age (less than 20 years)[50] seem to be clearly associated with an increased risk of hyperemesis; prior nulliparity may also be a predisposing factor[49–51]. Multiple gestations or molar pregnancy increases the risk of hyperemesis[47,49] and patients who are hyperemetic in their first pregnancy are likely to suffer recurrent symptoms in subsequent gestations[52].

A variety of pathophysiological mechanisms have been proposed to underlie emesis and hyperemesis during pregnancy. Because of its presentation early in the first trimester, a hormonal etiology has been suggested. Serum and urinary human chorionic gonadotrophin (hCG) levels have been compared in emetic, hyperemetic and non-emetic pregnancies; the results of these studies are inconsistent. Some groups have found no correlation between hCG levels and nausea and vomiting[50,53], whereas others report higher levels

Table 5 Epidemiologic factors and associated conditions in hyperemesis

High body weight (> 170 lb; 76.5 kg)
Young age (< 20 years)
Multiple gestations
Molar pregnancy
Prior history of hyperemesis
Prior nulliparity

in emetic vs. non-emetic patients[54,55]. Even in the latter studies serum hCG levels overlap between normal and hyperemetic patients. However, increased free β-subunit of hCG has been found in the sera of hyperemetic patients compared to normal pregnant controls[56].

Analyses of serum estradiol levels also conflict. Depue and co-workers[50] found that estradiol levels and sex hormone binding globulin capacity were elevated in hyperemetic patients in the first trimester. Others[54] did not show a correlation between estradiol levels and nausea and vomiting, but these analyses did not include many hyperemetic patients. The role of estrogens in nausea and vomiting is also suggested by epidemiological data indicating that nulliparous women, heavy women and non-smokers demonstrate a higher incidence of nausea and vomiting; these groups also have higher levels of serum estrogens[50].

Transient hyperthyroidism is frequently observed in hyperemetic patients[57,58]. In one series[58], 73% of hyperemetic pregnant patients (who had severe vomiting associated with weight loss) showed an increased free thyroxine (T_4) index. Hyperthyroxinemic patients demonstrated tachycardia (and weight loss) but no other symptoms of Graves' disease. Triiodothyronine (T_3) concentrations were not elevated, probably owing to decreased peripheral conversion of T_4 to T_3, yet thyroid stimulating hormone (TSH) response to thyrotropin releasing hormone (TRH) was absent, indicating true hyperthyroidism. The hyperthyroidism tends to be short-lived[58], resolving by the third trimester, and usually does not require treatment. The mechanisms underlying transient hyperthyroidism in patients with hyperemesis are unknown. Chorionic gonadotropin has been implicated, since patients with molar pregnancies have high hCG levels and are frequently thyrotoxic. Some studies have shown that hCG acts as a thyroid stimulator, but others indicate that a non-hCG serum activity is responsible[59]. Although many patients with hyperemesis gravidarum demonstrate thyroid abnormalities, a significant percentage do not, suggesting that thyroid dysfunction is not a cause of hyperemesis. In addition, a recent report[60] showed that hyperemesis did not resolve in a patient successfully treated for hyperthyroidism. Recognition of thyrotoxicosis is important, since these patients may be at risk for decreased neonatal birth weight[58] and for preterm labor and spontaneous abortion if hyperthyroidism persists into the second trimester[61].

A right-sided corpus luteum may be instrumental in the pathogenesis of hyperemesis[62] but other studies have refuted this[63]. Measurement of gastric myoelectric activity in women with and without nausea in pregnancy revealed a much higher incidence of abnormal electrical patterns in nauseated patients compared to non-nauseated pregnant women[64]; the physiological significance of these findings is unclear.

Psychological factors have been considered for many years in the pathogenesis of hyperemesis. Analyses of the maternal relationships of pregnant hyperemetic women have revealed a variety of disturbances including over-strong maternal attachments[52] or negative maternal relationships[65]. Persistence of hyperemesis into the third trimester was significantly associated with psychiatric symptoms[65]. These data indicate that hyperemesis is probably of multifactorial origin, with both physiological and psychological components.

Diagnosis

The diagnosis of hyperemesis gravidarum is based on the patient's report of symptoms of intractable nausea and vomiting and the presence of any of several indicators of severity, including weight loss of more than 5% of body weight, ketonuria, signs of dehydration and serum electrolyte imbalances. Evidence of major organ dysfunction may be present in more severe cases, including neurological symptoms (Wernicke's encephalopathy[66], and peripheral neuropathy[67]), renal failure, liver dysfunction or retinal hemorrhage.

Although vomiting may begin even before the first missed menstrual period, persistent vomiting requiring hospitalization usually peaks between 8 and 12 weeks of gestation[49,52]. Vomiting may persist through the second trimester, but most commonly abates by the third trimester. Patients usually describe typical 'morning sickness' which then becomes more severe and persists throughout the day. Physical examination may reveal signs of dehydration with poor skin turgor and tachycardia. Jaundice is occasionally present and the odor of ketones may be noted in the patient's breath. Neurological symptoms include changes in mental status ranging from drowsiness to coma, and evidence of peripheral neuropathy due to vitamin B_6 or B_{12} deficiency. Elevated levels of blood urea nitrogen and creatinine, abnormal liver function tests, ketosis and ketonuria, hyponatremia, hypochloremia and hypokalemia are common laboratory abnormalities.

Before a diagnosis of hyperemesis can be entertained, it is critical to rule out other causes of nausea and vomiting such as appendicitis, cholecystitis or other acute intra-abdominal conditions, and pyelonephritis or gastroenteritis[52].

Management

Because of reluctance to use medications, especially in the first trimester, patients with uncomplicated nausea and vomiting are generally advised simply to eat small meals and avoid ingesting large amounts of liquid; specific therapy is usually not required. In contrast, the management of hyperemesis gravidarum is challenging and often frustrating. Recurrent admissions are common and occur more often in nulliparous women[68]. Initial therapy should focus on repletion of fluids, usually by an intravenous route, and resolution of electrolyte imbalances. Chronic or severe hyponatremia must be corrected slowly and cautiously to avoid the complication of cerebral pontine myelinolysis[67,69]. An increase in serum sodium of no more than 12 mmol/l per day is recommended.

Repletion of vitamin deficiencies including thiamine is critical since prolonged vomiting may lead to severe depletion; patients should be routinely treated with vitamin supplements upon hospital admission. Thiamine deficiency resulting in Wernicke's encephalopathy should be considered in pregnant patients with mental status changes and other neurological symptoms[60]. Antiemetic medications are occasionally used in the acute in-hospital setting and include antihistamines, phenothiazines and pyridoxine. In general, antihistamines are considered to have the lowest teratogenic risk[70] (Table 6). However, there is reluctance to use any medication in the first trimester; in addition to teratogenicity, their efficacy in hyperemesis is unclear and they may act simply as sedatives. When nausea and vomiting have resolved after treatment with intravenous fluids, oral hydration is begun slowly and diet is advanced from liquid to solid as tolerated[52,71]. The cessation of vomiting and commencement of normal weight gain are the therapeutic endpoints to be achieved. In severe cases, in-hospital and even home-based parenteral hyperalimentation can be used if nutrition cannot be maintained orally[72]. Psychological support is offered by nursing staff and physicians depending upon the needs of the patient. Intervention by a psychiatrist is recommended if there is evidence of an obvious psychiatric disorder[52] or occasionally for patients with third-trimester vomiting, which may indicate more serious psychological problems[65].

In the past, hyperemesis was regarded as a dread complication of pregnancy. Maternal mortality was high and primarily caused by severe metabolic disturbances. Improvements in fluid and electrolyte management have dramatically reduced the pregnant woman's mortality rate from hyperemesis to virtually zero[52].

Although uncomplicated nausea and vomiting in pregnancy may be an indicator of a favorable fetal outcome[51], the effects of hyperemesis on the fetus are unclear. A study of hyperemetic pregnancies associated with abnormal thyroid function indicated a higher than expected rate of premature labor[61] and an increased incidence of low birth weight[58]. Whether these effects were due to hyperemesis or hyperthyroxinemia is unclear. Analyses of the birth weights of babies born to hyperemetic mothers have been confounded by a varied patient population. Fairweather[49] found no change in birth weight when he reviewed birth records of a large group of women with hyperemesis. However, others[51,73] have subclassified hyperemetic patients into mild vs. severe disease based on maternal weight loss, heavy ketonuria, elevated urea nitrogen or creatinine and electrolyte disturbances; those with severe hyperemesis gave birth to babies with significantly lower weights. Also, more growth-retarded babies were found in the groups of mothers with hyperemesis and weight loss, or hyperemesis requiring multiple admissions[68]. The risk of congenital anomalies may also be increased. One study suggested an increase in minor integumentary defects including webbed toes and an extra finger, and skin tags. However, the number of patients was small, the possible influence of antiemetic medication was not clarified and other analyses are not confirmatory.

Table 6 Antiemetics used in nausea and vomiting of pregnancy. Adapted from reference 70

Generic name	Dosage	Teratogenicity in animals
Dimenhydrinate	50–100 mg orally every 4 h or 50 mg i.m. or i.v. every 3–4 h	no
Diphenhydramine	50 mg orally 3–4 times daily or 20–50 mg i.m. or i.v. every 2–3 h	yes/no
Meclizine	25–50 mg daily, orally	yes
Metoclopramide	5–10 mg orally three times daily or 5–20 mg i.m. or i.v. three times daily	no
Promethazine	12.5–25 mg i.m. or orally 2–4 times daily	no
Prochlorperazine	5–10 mg i.m. or orally 3–4 times daily	yes
Thiethylperazine	10–20 mg i.m. or orally 1–3 times daily	yes

i.m., intramuscularly; i.v., intravenously

INFLAMMATORY BOWEL DISEASE

The inflammatory bowel diseases (IBD) include two disorders, Crohn's disease (also known as regional enteritis or granulomatous colitis) and ulcerative colitis. Both illnesses are characterized by inflammation of the gastrointestinal tract. Clinical manifestations commonly include diarrhea and abdominal pain and patients may suffer multiple exacerbations and remissions. In Crohn's disease a transmural inflammatory process occurs which can affect any part of the gastrointestinal tract from mouth to anus, whereas the inflammatory lesion of ulcerative colitis is mucosal and is limited to the colon and rectum. Because the peak age of onset of inflammatory bowel disease is in the childbearing years (ages 15–25), problems in management of these disorders in pregnancy are frequently encountered by both the obstetrician and the gastroenterologist. In this section, the effect of IBD on fertility and pregnancy outcome and the impact that pregnancy has on the course of IBD is discussed, and an approach to the management of these disorders in pregnancy presented.

The worldwide incidence of inflammatory bowel disease is 3–20 new cases per 100 000 population[74,75]. There is marked geographic variation in the incidence of inflammatory bowel disease; the regions with the highest incidence of ulcerative colitis include the USA, Northern Europe and Israel. Within the USA there is racial and ethnic variation. Incidence rates are increased in Jews and in white vs. non-white populations, although the incidence in black populations may in fact be increasing[76].

The peak age of onset is 15–25 years; a second peak at ages 55–65 has also been reported but has not been definitively established[77,78]. Most studies indicate a female predominance but these ratios may be changing as well[75–77]. A higher risk for inflammatory bowel disease is found in urban compared to rural communities[75,78].

The etiology of inflammatory bowel disease is at present unknown, but is thought to be multifactorial[78,79]. A number of infectious agents have been postulated to be pathogenic; a recently favored organism was a bacterium similar to *Mycobacterium paratuberculosis* which was isolated from the intestine of patients who underwent surgical resection for active Crohn's disease, yet in the majority of patients, this organism cannot be cultured. Other potential agents involved in eliciting an immune response have been postulated to include cow's milk proteins, other foods, water, viruses and smoking, yet none has been definitively linked to either disease.

Although the antigen that triggers the gut's immunological response is unknown, there is active research directed at understanding the intestinal mucosal immune system in normal and affected individuals.

The contribution of autoimmunity, cytokines, mucosal B and T cell as well as neutrophil function is being actively examined in IBD. The inflammatory process is also being dissected; the role of arachidonic acid metabolites has received much attention lately with the discovery that leukotriene B_4 levels are increased in ulcerative colitis patients. Genetic factors play an important role as indicated by family studies which demonstrate a 30- to 100-fold increased risk of IBD in first-degree relatives when compared to the general population[78]. A stronger familial association has been shown for Crohn's disease than for ulcerative colitis. Twin studies showing disease concordance in monozygotic but not dizygotic twins further strengthen the evidence that genetic influences play a role in the pathogenesis of Crohn's disease. Intestinal permeability has been shown to be altered in Crohn's disease; a 'leaky bowel' may allow translocation of antigens which elicit an immune response.

The inflammatory process of ulcerative colitis is confined to the colon. This disease may affect the rectum alone, the rectum plus the left colon, or it may be pancolonic. In contrast, in Crohn's disease, inflammation can be found anywhere throughout the gastrointestinal tract, from mouth to anus. The commonest sites of involvement are small bowel alone (predominantly distal ileum) (30%), colon alone (15–25%) or ileocolon (40–55%). Perianal and perirectal disease is commonly encountered, manifested by fissures, fistulae and abscesses.

In ulcerative colitis, mucosal lesions predominate; the muscularis propria is rarely involved. Crypt abscesses, in which collections of neutrophils invade crypt epithelium and may even be present in the crypt lumen, are characteristic of ulcerative colitis, yet may also be seen in Crohn's disease. Evidence of chronic inflammation is also apparent, with lymphocytic, plasma cell and eosinophilic involvement of the lamina propria. Marked edema, hemorrhage and pseudopolyps are often found in active ulcerative colitis. In contrast, the presence of granulomas and transmural inflammation with deep ulcerations that extend to the muscularis propria are more characteristic of Crohn's disease. 'Skip areas' (intervening normal mucosa) or rectal sparing are consistent with Crohn's disease. Granulomata may be found in mesenteric lymph nodes, mesentery and peritoneum.

Clinical signs and symptoms

There are both similarities and differences in the presentation of ulcerative colitis and Crohn's disease. Patients afflicted with either disorder may present with abdominal pain, diarrhea, weight loss, fevers and malaise. Multiple extraintestinal manifestations accompany both illnesses.

Ulcerative colitis

The inflammatory process characteristic of ulcerative colitis is confined to the colon. Some patients initially present with inflammation confined to the rectum (ulcerative proctitis); the disease may progress during subsequent exacerbations to other areas of the colon or may remain in the rectum. Other patients suffer from more extensive colitis and may have disease up to and including the cecum. Due to rectal involvement, patients often complain of urgency and frequency of bowel movements as well as tenesmus. Rectal bleeding and diarrhea are the hallmarks of this disease. Abdominal pain is usually mild but may be severe in fulminant colitis. In mild cases, physical examination may be unremarkable, whereas patients with more active disease develop fevers, tachycardia, diffuse abdominal tenderness and occasionally distension. A serious complication of acute ulcerative colitis which may be heralded by the appearance of abdominal distension is toxic megacolon. Massive dilatation of the inflamed colon may progress to perforation; this is a surgical emergency and requires immediate colectomy. A significant long-term complication of ulcerative colitis is the development of colon cancer. Patients with pancolitis are at increased risk for carcinoma after 10–15 years of disease and are screened with yearly colonoscopy.

Crohn's disease

Crohn's disease is a chronic indolent disorder characterized by multiple remissions and exacerbations. Patients commonly present with abdominal pain, diarrhea, weight loss, anal pain and drainage, often accompanied by fevers and malaise. Joint pains, skin lesions and ocular symptoms (see below) may also be present. On physical examination, abdominal tenderness and inflammatory masses particularly in the right lower quadrant and pelvis can be palpated. Because the inflammatory lesion is transmural, perianal fissures, internal fistulae between the bowel and skin, bladder or vagina as well as free perforation with abscess formation are common complications.

Extraintestinal manifestations

Both ulcerative colitis and Crohn's disease are associated with a wide variety of extraintestinal manifestations. The 'colitis-related' manifestations include skin, eye and joint diseases which present in parallel with recrudescent disease activity. Skin manifestations such as erythema nodosum and pyoderma gangrenosum, and oral lesions including diffuse aphthous ulceration may be severe enough to require treatment with corticosteroids. Arthritic complaints include ankylosing spondylitis, sacroileitis and peripheral large joint arthritis. Ocular diseases such as uveitis, iritis and episcleritis may be present in approximately 15–20% of patients and may be the initial symptom that prompts a visit to a physician. Non-specific complications of Crohn's disease include a variety of liver diseases such as fatty liver, pericholangitis, primary sclerosing cholangitis, hepatic granulomas and abscesses. In patients who have had extensive small bowel resection, malabsorption may result in deficiency of vitamin D and calcium, leading to osteoporosis. Increased absorption of oxalate from the gut lumen may lead to enhanced urinary excretion and the development of oxalate stones. The incidence of uric acid stones is also increased in these patients.

Diagnosis in the non-pregnant patient

In the non-pregnant patient, the diagnosis of inflammatory bowel disease usually involves a combination of radiological and endoscopic techniques. An air contrast barium enema often shows loss of haustrations, colonic shortening and narrowing, consistent with ulcerative colitis. In Crohn's disease, aphthous ulcerations, cobblestoning, and mucosal nodularity may be seen. Small bowel barium radiograms may demonstrate terminal ileal narrowing and ulceration as well as the presence of enteric fistulae and strictures.

Endoscopic evaluation including upper endoscopy (for patients who have upper abdominal symptoms suggestive of Crohn's disease), flexible sigmoidoscopy and colonoscopy provides direct visualization of the gut's mucosa. Characteristic findings of ulcerative and Crohn's colitis include erythema, edema, granularity, ulceration and friability of the colonic epithelium. Strictures may result from chronic inflammation. However, it is important to emphasize that these findings, while consistent with inflammatory bowel disease, are not diagnostic, since they may also be found in a variety of infectious and other colitides. Abnormalities such as aphthous ulceration and erythema are also found in the upper gastrointestinal tract in Crohn's disease. Biopsies taken during endoscopy may show the presence of granulomas or crypt abscesses and may help confirm the clinical impression.

Diagnosis in pregnancy

There is a paucity of data regarding the safety of endoscopic procedures during pregnancy (already discussed under Peptic ulcer disease). In those patients with undiagnosed abdominal pain, diarrhea or rectal bleeding in whom IBD is suspected, flexible sigmoidoscopy under either minimal or no sedation appears to be safe[42,80]. A recent multicenter study documented the safety of flexible sigmoidoscopy in 24 pregnancies, and recommended maternal vital sign monitoring with pulse oximetry and electrocardiography, which are now standard procedures in most endoscopy facilities[81]. Complete colonoscopy usually requires a greater degree of anesthesia and is avoided when possible, although it is probably safe with appropriate monitoring of vital signs and oxygenation. In the pregnant patient, all efforts should of course be made to avoid fetal exposure to X-irradiation, and radiological procedures are not recommended. However, in emergent situations (when bowel perforation, abscess or toxic megacolon are being considered), radiological examinations may be necessary; there is some evidence to suggest that a very low dose of irradiation may have no long-term harmful effects[80,82].

Stool cultures for routine bacterial pathogens and ova and parasites are extremely important in the initial evaluation of a patient in whom inflammatory bowel disease is suspected. Infectious colitides such as those caused by salmonella, shigella, yersinia, *Campylobacter fetus*, *ss jejuni* and ameba may present with an identical picture and demonstrate similar endoscopic findings. Chronic infections caused by *Giardia lamblia*, amebae and intestinal tuberculosis should also be ruled out. In patients infected with human immunodeficiency virus, organisms such as *Mycobacterium avium-intracellulare*, cryptosporidiosis, isospora and cytomegalovirus can be ruled out with stool cultures and histological examination of biopsies.

Management with maternal–fetal consideration

Critical issues in the management of inflammatory bowel disease during pregnancy include (1) the effects of pregnancy on the course of IBD; and (2) the impact of IBD and its therapy on fertility, pregnancy and fetal outcome.

Effects of pregnancy on the course of inflammatory bowel disease

Early studies in the 1950s and 1960s indicated that pregnancy had an adverse effect on the course of ulcerative colitis, yet more recent studies dispute these findings. Part of the reason for this discrepancy is the realization that the spontaneous risk of exacerbation of ulcerative colitis in the non-pregnant patient is 30–50%, in agreement with the rate of relapse reported for pregnant patients with this illness. With the advent of more effective medical therapy for ulcerative colitis, it has become apparent that pregnancy does not adversely affect the course of this disease[80]. Those patients with quiescent disease will usually remain inactive[83,84], whereas those with active colitis will demonstrate persistent disease or worsen during pregnancy[85].

Patients with quiescent Crohn's disease are probably not at increased risk for precipitating active disease when pregnant[86,87]. Again, in those patients who are already active, approximately two out of three will continue to be ill or will worsen during pregnancy[85,87,88]. Therefore, patients with inflammatory bowel disease are usually counselled to avoid pregnancy when in a phase of moderate to severe disease activity.

Effects of inflammatory bowel disease on fertility, pregnancy and fetal outcome

Most studies agree that patients afflicted with ulcerative colitis demonstrate fertility rates that are comparable to those of the general population[86,88], although there are few case–control studies. In considering Crohn's disease, there are conflicting reports; some groups have shown that as many as 50% of women of child-bearing age are subfertile, correlating with disease activity, whereas others have shown no difference in fertility rates when compared to the general population[86,89–91]. Many studies did not account for disease activity, the patient's desire to become pregnant, or other risk factors which could decrease fertility. In fact, a recent report revealed that fertility may not be impaired in women who wished to conceive; there was a voluntary decrease in the number of pregnancies, arising from a desire to avoid pregnancy because of illness[89]. Men with IBD who take sulfasalazine may show diminished fertility due to direct toxic effects on sperm[92].

The risk of spontaneous abortion in patients with quiescent Crohn's disease or ulcerative colitis is probably no higher than in the general population[85] but in several studies it has been shown to be increased as much as two-fold in those patients with active disease[80,93–95]. Recent reports indicate that IBD predisposes patients to a significant risk of preterm delivery[89], as defined by birth before 37 weeks of gestation. Therefore, vigilant monitoring of patients in the third trimester is recommended. Fortunately, once pregnancy occurs, the likelihood of a normal fetal outcome is identical to that in the general population; in almost all studies, the incidence of small-for-gestational-age babies and congenital defects is not increased, even in those patients on multiple medications such as steroids and sulfasalazine (see below).

Management of inflammatory bowel disease in pregnancy

To improve the likelihood of a favorable outcome, patients are generally encouraged to avoid pregnancy during periods of disease activity if this is at all possible. Medications should be reduced to the minimal amount required (see Table 2).

Numerous retrospective analyses have ascertained that patients with IBD can be successfully treated without adverse effect to the mother or fetus. In reports in which low birth weight or congenital anomalies were detected, it was often difficult to ascertain whether the severity of the bowel disease or the medications used were the major contributor.

Sulfasalazine, one of the cornerstones of medical therapy of IBD, contains a sulfapyridine residue linked to 5-aminosalicylic acid, the active moiety. It is effective in the acute treatment of both ulcerative and Crohn's colitis and in maintaining remission in ulcerative colitis, but is generally not recommended for the management of small bowel disease. Its mechanism of action is unknown, but it has been shown to inhibit production of leukotriene B_4, an important mediator of inflammation, block prostaglandin production and inhibit immunoglobulin secretion by mononuclear cells. Sulfasalazine crosses the placenta[96] and is found in breast milk, although in low concentrations. The sulfapyridine moiety is similarly transported and its concentration in breast milk reaches up to 50% of serum levels. Serum levels of sulfasalazine in newborns are the same as in the mother[97]. This drug is thought to be safe during pregnancy[25,98]. There are a few reports of congenital defects in infants of treated patients, yet it is unclear whether these effects were related to therapy, the disease itself or other unknown factors. Its efficacy in maintaining remission in ulcerative colitis makes its continuation during pregnancy an important consideration. Patients are usually tapered to the lowest dose that is effective in suppressing disease activity.

Because of multiple side-effects associated with the presumably inactive sulfapyridine moiety, both topical and oral agents which contain only 5-aminosalicylic acid have been developed. Topical therapy with 5-aminosalicylic acid enemas (mesalamine) is an effective treatment for acute proctitis or proctitis with left-sided colitis. In addition, several oral forms of 5-aminosalicylic acid (Pentasa®, Asacol®, and Dipentum®) have been released for treatment of both Crohn's disease and ulcerative colitis. These drugs contain 5-aminosalicylic acid in formulations that prevent their premature absorption from the gastrointestinal tract. There are at present few data available regarding the safety of any of these drugs in pregnancy, but a recent study of 17 pregnant patients (19 pregnancies) treated with oral 5-aminosalicylic acid revealed no maternal or fetal side-effects[99]. These data and the documented safety of sulfasalazine suggest that oral 5-aminosalicylic acid is safe in pregnancy.

Corticosteroid therapy is another cornerstone in the treatment of IBD. Oral corticosteroids such as prednisone are frequently used in the treatment of active ulcerative colitis and in colonic and small bowel Crohn's disease. In severely ill, hospitalized patients, high doses of intravenous prednisolone are employed to control bowel inflammation. Corticosteroid enemas are important topical agents for the treatment of proctitis and left-sided colitis. The major side-effects associated with acute or long-term corticosteroid therapy (such as cataracts, osteoporosis, diabetes and hypertension) make it imperative that patients be tapered off this medication as soon as possible. Unfortunately, some patients with Crohn's disease require long-term corticosteroid use to treat persistently active disease; in these patients, a trial of an immunosuppressive agent such as 6-mercaptopurine or azathioprine may be used to facilitate steroid tapering (see below). In high doses, these medications can cause a variety of congenital defects in mice. However, corticosteroids have been used to treat a number of inflammatory illnesses (including IBD) and in transplant patients without adverse fetal outcome[44,98,100]. The placenta presumably protects the fetus from maternal usage of prednisone or prednisolone by metabolizing it into the inactive 11-keto metabolites. On the other hand, placental conversion of betamethasone or dexamethasone into the 11-keto metabolites is minimal[101]. As in their non-pregnant counterparts, pregnant patients should be taken off steroids if at all possible, yet treatment during pregnancy can be safely initiated or continued as needed to control disease activity.

Immunosuppressive agents such as 6-mercaptopurine and azathioprine are primarily used in the treatment of Crohn's disease. These agents are effective in the closure of fistulas, and are often used to facilitate discontinuation or dose reduction of steroids needed to treat active colitis or small bowel disease. Few data exist regarding the long-term side-effects that may result from the use of these medications in IBD; the doses used for treatment of ulcerative colitis and Crohn's disease are much lower than in transplant patients (e.g. 1–1.5 mg/kg). Regarding usage in pregnancy, there is a large body of data emerging from the transplant population which indicates that treatment with these agents is surprisingly well tolerated; a few reports also indicate their relative safety in pregnant IBD patients[102]. However, because substitution of less toxic medication is usually possible, discontinuation of immunosuppressives prior to pregnancy is recommended unless their use is absolutely necessary.

Antibiotics are often used in the treatment of Crohn's disease. Particularly, metronidazole is active in the treatment of perianal complications such as ulcerations, fistulae, or abscesses. However, due to its teratogenic and carcinogenic potential, its use is contraindicated in the first trimester of pregnancy[44]. It can be used with caution for severe disease in the second and third trimesters, although safer alternatives should be sought. In patients with suspected abscess or small bowel bacterial overgrowth resulting from stasis in small bowel strictures, broad-spectrum antibiotics which are considered safe in pregnancy can be employed.

The use of *total parenteral nutrition* (TPN) plays an important role in the management of IBD. In patients with Crohn's disease, TPN may help heal fistulae and provide crucial nutritional support when enteral alimentation is not tolerated. The safety of TPN during pregnancy is still being evaluated. Only a small number of patients have been reported and potential effects on the fetus are difficult to assess[103]. Complications including catheter sepsis and thrombosis are similar to those in the non-pregnant patient[44,103]. Theoretical considerations about the use of lipids and risk of fat emboli, ketonemia and premature uterine contractions have thus far not been borne out clinically[44]. The use of ultrasonography to monitor fetal growth and involvement of nutritional support teams is recommended[103].

Special considerations – surgical management, pregnancy with ileostomy or ileoanal anastomosis

Despite advances in the medical management of IBD and improved therapy during pregnancy, surgical treatment is occasionally necessary. Emergent colectomy may be indicated for fulminant colitis unresponsive to medical therapy or for complications of ulcerative colitis such as toxic megacolon and colonic perforation. Morbidity and mortality rates for both fetus and mother are unknown; although there are scattered case studies of successful surgical intervention, fetal deaths have been reported.

The presence of an ileostomy or ileoanal anastomosis in women who have undergone colectomy for ulcerative colitis does not appear adversely to affect fertility, pregnancy or delivery[80,104–106]. Ileostomy may predispose to intestinal obstruction, which may be difficult to recognize, since abdominal pain may be mistakenly attributed to uterine contractions. An increased frequency of nocturnal stooling was noted in patients with ileoanal pouches[105]. Patients may undergo vaginal or Cesarean delivery and fetal outcome seems unaffected by the presence of an ileostomy or ileoanal anastomosis.

PANCREATITIS

Acute inflammation of the pancreas, or pancreatitis, is rare in pregnancy, ranging in incidence from 1 case per 1000 to 10 000 pregnancies[107–109]. However, significant fetal and maternal morbidity and mortality may result, including premature delivery, shock, sepsis and pulmonary and other systemic complications. Management of this disorder in pregnancy is often complicated and requires careful monitoring of mother and fetus.

Many factors have been shown to be associated with acute pancreatitis (Table 7). Depending upon the population surveyed, the presence of gallstones or ethanol abuse is the primary etiology of pancreatitis[110]. Acute pancreatitis may be precipitated when gallstones

Table 7 Etiologies of pancreatitis

Gallstones
Alcohol
Drugs
Trauma
Viruses
Hyperlipidemia
Obstruction – tumors, strictures
Hyperparathyroidism
Idiopathic causes

become impacted in the ampulla of Vater, or pass into the duodenum. Alcohol most probably has a direct toxic effect. Pancreatitis may also be precipitated by exposure to a variety of drugs such as thiazide diuretics, azathioprine and antibiotics such as sulfonamides and tetracycline. Traumatic injury to the pancreas resulting from accidents or surgical procedures can also lead to acute inflammation. Viral illnesses that may lead to pancreatitis include mumps and coxsackie. Obstruction of the pancreatic duct by tumors or strictures may also play a causative role. An association with types I, IV and V hyperlipidemias has also been established.

In pregnancy, pancreatitis is most often associated with gallstones[111,112]. Changes in serum hormonal levels are thought to lead to bile stasis and elevation of serum cholesterol/triglyceride levels which in turn favor stone development (see Chapter 36). In women with types I, IV and V hyperlipidemias, further elevation of serum lipid levels in pregnancy lead to an even more pronounced risk of pancreatitis. There is also some debate as to whether pregnancy predisposes to pancreatitis independent of other factors[109,111], postulated because hormonal alterations lead to stasis of pancreatic secretions in animals, and because early reviews[113] indicated that almost 50% of patients with pancreatitis present in the third trimester, when hormonal levels are highest. However, many of the earlier studies suggesting this relationship did not attempt to detect other underlying etiologies, and advanced ultrasonographic equipment was not available for gallstone visualization. A number of reports describe pregnant patients with both hyperparathyroidism and pancreatitis[114], although there is some question as to whether hyperparathyroidism is in fact associated with pancreatitis in the normal population. Pre-eclampsia is an uncommon cause of pancreatitis in pregnancy[115].

Release of activated digestive enzymes into the pancreatic parenchyma may result in autodigestion and injury. Thus, patients who have pancreatic duct obstruction from strictures, tumors or other lesions may develop pancreatitis because of backflow of pancreatic juice into the gland, although the mechanism of enzyme activation in the pancreas is unclear. In gallstone pancreatitis, passage of a stone may cause inflammation of the distal pancreatic duct, leading to obstruction, ductal hypertension and rupture, with release of destructive enzymes[110]. Alcohol is thought to have a direct toxic effect, or may cause contraction of the sphincter of Oddi, resulting in ductal obstruction[110]. In patients with hypertriglyceridemia, it is postulated that pancreatic lipase becomes activated and releases fatty acids into the pancreas, producing inflammation, or that vascular obstruction results from blockage of vessels by fat globules[116].

The presenting signs and symptoms in pregnant patients with pancreatitis are similar to those in the non-pregnant population. The commonest presentation includes nausea, vomiting and upper abdominal pain which often radiates to the back. It is important to remember that patients may also be pain free[107]. Abdominal pain may worsen while lying flat, or improve after assuming a forward or fetal position. Obstruction of the common bile duct as it courses through the head of the pancreas can lead to jaundice. Fever, pleuritic pain and shock may result from peripancreatic fluid collection and pancreatic parenchymal hemorrhage. Physical examination often reveals epigastric tenderness, guarding and rebound, decreased or absent bowel sounds, ecchymosis of the flank (Grey–Turner's sign) or periumbilical region (Cullen's sign) and ascites. In patients who are severely ill, hypotension may result.

Diagnosis

Typical symptoms of nausea, vomiting and abdominal pain in conjunction with elevated serum amylase and/or lipase strongly suggest the diagnosis of pancreatitis. Serum amylase levels are usually within the normal range during pregnancy; in pregnant patients with mild elevations, amylase is of non-pancreatic origin[117]. This enzyme can therefore function as a useful indicator of pancreatitis in the gravid state, especially if it is elevated to more than 1000 IU/l. However, there are many other pathological states in which these enzymes may be elevated, since organs other than the pancreas synthesize and release amylase. Bowel ischemia, obstruction or a perforated viscus, ovarian/tubal diseases such as salpingitis or ruptured ectopic pregnancy, cholecystitis and a variety of salivary gland and pulmonary diseases (mumps, pneumonia) may also lead to elevations in serum amylase and/or lipase. In macroamylasemia, amylase is bound to an abnormal serum protein and cannot be cleared by the kidney, leading to elevated serum levels. Measurement of the amylase/creatinine clearance ratio has limited usefulness since this may also be elevated in toxemia and hyperemesis gravidarum[118]. It is also important to note that serum amylase is occasionally normal in the face of acute pancreatitis[119].

Many less specific laboratory abnormalities are found in acute pancreatitis. Inflammation of the head of the pancreas may lead to common bile duct obstruction with elevation of alkaline phosphatase, direct bilirubin and transaminases. Glucose homeostasis may be deranged with resultant hyperglycemia. Hypocalcemia and hypomagnesemia may be severe (see below).

The severity of pancreatitis can be predicted to a certain extent by using Ranson's criteria, a series of biochemical parameters[120]. Poor prognostic signs include (at presentation): age greater than 55 years, white blood cell count greater than 16 000/mm³, glucose concentration greater than 200 mg/dl, lactate dehydrogenase (LDH) level greater than 350 IU/l, and serum glutamic–oxaloacetic transaminase (SGOT) level greater than 250. Within 48 h, a decrease in hematocrit of more than 10%, a drop in serum Ca^{++} level below 8 mg/dl, arterial oxygen pressure less than 60 mmHg, base deficit greater than 4 mEq/l, rise in blood urea nitrogen level of greater than 5 mg/dl, or positive fluid balance of more than 6.0 l, may also indicate more severe disease.

Complications

Maternal complications

Patients with pancreatitis may develop hypovolemia and shock due to fluid sequestration and prolonged nausea and vomiting. Hypocalcemia may occur, possibly owing to entrapment of calcium in necrotic pancreatic tissue. Other metabolic abnormalities include hypochloremic alkalosis resulting from vomiting. Severe pancreatitis may result in disseminated intravascular coagulation and adult respiratory distress syndrome.

Should fever and leukocytosis develop, pancreatic abscess must be considered. A computed tomography (CT) scan or ultrasonogram (the latter is preferable in the pregnant patient) may reveal the presence of fluid and necrosis in the pancreas, but cannot determine whether or not there is concomitant infection. The diagnosis of abscess is therefore usually made on clinical grounds. Pancreatic pseudocyst is a collection of pancreatic fluid within a fibrous cavity; its presence may be heralded by persistent abdominal pain or chronically elevated amylase levels. Hemorrhagic pancreatitis due to necrosis and blood vessel rupture may lead to massive bleeding. Pancreatic ascites results from rupture of pancreatic ducts with leakage of amylase-rich fluid into the peritoneum.

Maternal mortality rates have undoubtedly decreased with the advent of better recognition and management of pancreatitis[121]. An early analysis by Wilkinson[113] reported a very high overall rate of 37% but later studies are much more optimistic, with few if any fatalities[107,122]. True mortality rates are difficult to assess, owing to the small numbers of patients.

Fetal complications

Premature labor is the main cause of adverse fetal outcome in pancreatitis in late pregnancy[109,113]. Intrauterine growth retardation has also been reported but may in part be avoided by the use of total parenteral nutrition.

Management with maternal–fetal consideration

The treatment of acute pancreatitis in pregnancy follows the same guidelines as in the non-pregnant patient and is primarily supportive. Close observation is imperative, keeping in mind that multiple organ systems may be affected. The treatment of gallstone and hypertrigleridemic pancreatitis in pregnancy deserves special consideration and is discussed separately.

Volume depletion is frequently encountered due to vomiting and fluid sequestration into the retroperitoneum and is treated with intravenous fluid replacement. Patients are given nothing by mouth. Fluid and electrolyte balance is closely observed; in particular, correction of hypocalcemia and hypomagnesemia may be necessary. Since pain is a prominent feature in this illness and may be severe, the cautious use of analgesics is often instituted. There is some controversy regarding the role of nasogastric suctioning for decompression and reduction of pancreatic secretions. While some authors routinely recommend it, others point out that there are no data demonstrating its efficacy in pancreatitis[109,110,121]. Generally, nasogastric suction is reserved for patients who are actively vomiting and who are at risk for aspiration.

Patients with a prolonged course due to severe pancreatitis or its complications are often unable to be nourished by mouth, even after several days of hospitalization. To ensure adequate fetal growth and maintenance of maternal nutrition, TPN can be instituted[123–125]. Most of the reported complications of TPN in pregnancy are the same as those found in the non-pregnant patient and are mainly catheter-related, including sepsis and thrombosis. Monitoring fetal growth with serial ultrasonograms is generally recommended[123] to ensure that caloric demands are met. There are no reports of adverse fetal outcome related to TPN in these patients.

The patient's cardiopulmonary and hematological status should be closely observed to detect the onset of serious systemic complications of pancreatitis, such as hypoxemia associated with adult respiratory distress syndrome or congestive heart failure, as well as disseminated intravascular coagulation. Monitoring in an intensive care unit may be necessary.

Although therapeutic delivery has been considered in the past, recent literature suggests that termination of pregnancy does not in fact affect the outcome of acute pancreatitis, and is not recommended[121].

A variety of drugs which either reduce pancreatic or gastric secretions or act as antiprotease agents have been used without consistent success in pancreatitis. Antibiotics are not routinely recommended in uncomplicated pancreatitis, since they do not appear to alter the course of the disease[110].

Pancreatic abscess is a highly morbid complication of pancreatitis and is suspected when fever, leukocytosis and signs of sepsis evolve in conjunction with a CT scan which reveals necrosis in the pancreas. Surgical intervention is almost always needed for débridement and drainage of infected necrotic areas of the pancreas; aggressive antibiotic therapy with surgery has proven effective and has led to decreased morbidity and mortality from this complication.

Pancreatic pseudocyst may be heralded by persistent abdominal pain and hyperamylasemia. Small pseudocysts may resolve spontaneously, but in general, cysts larger than 5.0 cm may spontaneously rupture with serious consequences. Therefore, these patients should be closely monitored with serial ultrasonograms (or CT scans in the non-pregnant patient) to document resolution of the cysts. Persistence of a pseudocyst beyond 6 weeks after the initial episode of pancreatitis usually indicates that spontaneous resolution will not occur, and surgical intervention for drainage is generally recommended.

Although it is clear that conservative, supportive management of *gallstone-induced pancreatitis* is indicated, the issue of when to perform a cholecystectomy and common bile duct exploration in pregnancy is still being examined. Because of the risk of recurrent pancreatitis due to repeated passage of gallstones, some authors recommend that indications for cholecystectomy should be the same as in the non-pregnant patient. Specifically, if pancreatitis occurs in the first or second trimester, removal of the gallbladder in the second trimester seems to be safe for mother and fetus, after the initial symptoms of pancreatitis resolve[112,121]. In those patients with pancreatitis in the third trimester, postpartum cholecystectomy may be performed. Some authors still recommend conservative management with no operative intervention during pregnancy, but this is generally based on earlier experience; there are no controlled trials to support the choice of one approach over another. The use of endoscopic retrograde cholangiopancreatography with sphincterotomy in pregnancy is useful in very ill patients and has been successfully performed in pregnancy with fetal shielding without maternal or fetal compromise[24,115].

The management of *hypertrigleridemic pancreatitis* poses a challenging problem. In those patients with types I, IV and V hypertriglyceridemia, the underlying lipid abnormalities may worsen during pregnancy[125], due to a physiological increase in lipid levels and a decrease in lipoprotein lipase levels. Attempts at refeeding patients after symptoms of pancreatitis subside may be difficult since even low fat diets may lead to elevation of triglycerides and recurrent symptomatology[124]. In these situations, particularly in patients who are not near term, adequate nutrition must be maintained. Total parenteral nutrition has proven to be an efficacious method for delivering an appropriate calorie load without supplementation with fats, leading to improved regulation of triglyceride levels. Planned delivery of patients at term who have pancreatitis due to hyperlipidemia is recommended by some authors[125], and preterm delivery may be needed in patients whose clinical status severely deteriorates, since lipid abnormalities are clearly worsened by pregnancy. However, therapeutic preterm delivery is generally not recommended for pancreatitis of any other etiology, since it is not clear that this will lead to resolution of pancreatic inflammation and may actually place both mother and fetus at greater risk.

GASTROINTESTINAL BYPASS SURGERY

A variety of intestinal bypass surgeries has been developed for the treatment of morbid obesity. Some, such as the jejunoileal bypass procedure, have been discarded, owing to serious side-effects resulting from malabsorption. More modern procedures such as vertical-banded gastroplasty and Roux-en-Y gastric bypass are presently being evaluated. Recently, an NIH Consensus Statement was issued which identified a subset of obese patients who should be considered for surgical therapy[126]. Since as many as 80% of the surgically treated patients are young women, it has become important to consider the effects of operative management of obesity on fertility and pregnancy outcome. In particular, nutritional management to ensure adequate fetal growth may be challenging. Although some data are available regarding pregnancy outcome in patients treated with the newer procedures, further consideration of these issues must continue before firm recommendations can be made.

Jejunoileal bypass surgery

The jejunoileal bypass operation became popular in the 1960s and 1970s and consisted of creating an anastomosis between a short length of jejunum to the ileum, thereby bypassing the entire remaining small bowel. This operation led to a great deal of morbidity from malabsorption and malnutrition. Severe water- and fat-soluble vitamin deficiencies, hypocalcemia, hypomagnesemia, hypokalemia, hypoglycemia, metabolic acidosis and hypoproteinemia may last up to 2 years or more postoperatively. Fatty liver disease may occur, manifested by elevations of SGOT, alkaline

phosphatase and prothrombin time[127]. A comprehensive review of pregnancies in these patients[128] showed that infants suffered from an increased rate of low birth weight, short gestation and growth retardation. Nutritional and metabolic deficiencies are common[129]. As a result of complications in both pregnant and non-pregnant women, this surgical procedure is no longer performed, and reversal of the bypass is often undertaken, because of intractable complications.

Gastric bypass and vertical banded gastroplasty

The two weight-loss procedures which are most commonly performed today are the Roux-en-Y gastric bypass and the vertical banded gastroplasty. The present recommendations presented at the NIH Consensus Development Conference on Gastrointestinal Surgery for Severe Obesity[126] are that these procedures should be considered in morbidly obese patients who have tried non-surgical approaches to weight loss such as low-calorie diets, behavioral modification, exercise and pharmacological agents. Adults whose body mass index [weight (kilograms)]/[height (meters)]^2 exceeds 40 kg/m^2 or is 35–40 kg/m^2 and who are diabetic, have sleep apnea or obesity-related cardiomyopathy qualify for consideration for surgery.

The purpose of the gastric operations is to create a small reservoir for food which empties slowly[130], producing early satiety. A gastric capacity of approximately 10% of normal is achieved. Although both operations are effective in producing initial weight loss, some weight gain may occur after 2–5 years. The Roux-en-Y bypass seems to produce greater weight loss than does vertical banding, but may also lead to greater nutritional deficiency[131,132]. Postoperative morbidity includes a significant risk for wound infections and dehiscence, thrombophlebitis and stomal obstruction. Although the metabolic and nutritional complications are much less severe in these patients compared to jejunoileal bypass recipients, there is a significant risk of folate, iron and vitamin B$_{12}$ deficiency, as well as persistent hypokalemia[133]. The long-term efficacy and side-effects of these operations have yet to be determined.

Assessments of fertility and pregnancy outcome in women who have undergone gastric bypass are still at a preliminary stage. Fertility rates after bypass have not been analyzed. An uncontrolled study of 38 pregnancies in which complete birth data were available showed that seven were either premature or had low birth weight[130]. A more recent questionnaire-based study showed that bypass patients had a lower risk of producing large-for-gestational-age babies as compared to the weights of babies who were born to these same patients pre-bypass[134]; however, no difference in the incidence of small-for-gestational-age babies was found. Neonatal deaths were not increased in pregnancies of gastric bypass patients, but a possible increase in the incidence of neural tube defects has been reported[135]. Maternal morbidity and mortality during pregnancy seems to be unaffected by bypass. The numbers of patients in all these analyses are quite small and the lack of well controlled trials precludes the drawing of any firm conclusions.

At present, it is recommended that patients who have undergone gastric bypass should avoid pregnancy within the first 12 months after surgery, during the period of rapid weight loss. Bypass patients consume only approximately 500 kcal/day in the initial postoperative months and are generally unable to tolerate protein[134]; the recommended oral intake in pregnancy is at least 2000 kcal/day and 70–90 g of protein. Severe vitamin and nutrient deficiencies can result, as well as persistent ketonemia. When pregnancy is achieved, close monitoring for metabolic abnormalities and vitamin deficiencies (particularly B_{12}, folate and iron) and close follow-up with dietetic support teams throughout gestation[136] is recommended.

REFERENCES

1. Baron TH, Ramirez B, Richter JE. Gastrointestinal motility disorders during pregnancy. *Ann Intern Med* 1993;118:366–75
2. Fisher, RS, Roberts GS, Grabowski CJ, Cohen S. Altered lower esophageal sphincter function during early pregnancy. *Gastroenterology* 1978;74:1233–7
3. Nagler R, Spiro HM. Heartburn in late pregnancy. Manometric studies of esophageal motor function. *J Clin Invest* 1961;40:954–70
4. Van Thiel DH, Gavaler JS, Joshi SN, *et al.* Heartburn of pregnancy. *Gastroenterology* 1977;72:666–8
5. Ulmsten U, Sundstrom G. Esophageal manometry in pregnant and nonpregnant women. *Am J Obstet Gynecol* 1978;132:260–4
6. Macfie AG, Magides AD, Richmond MN, Reilly CS. Gastric emptying in pregnancy. *Br J Anaesth* 1991;67:54–7
7. Simpson KH, Stakes AF, Miller M. Pregnancy delays paracetamol absorption and gastric emptying in patients undergoing surgery. *Br J Anaesth* 1988;60:24–7
8. Brock-Utne JG, Dow TGB, Dimopoulos GE, *et al.* Gastric and lower oesophageal sphincter (LOS) pressures in early pregnancy. *Br J Anaesth* 1981;53:381–4
9. Anderson AS. Dietary factors in the aetiology and treatment of constipation during pregnancy. *Br J Obstet Gynaecol* 1986;93:245–9
10. Lawson M, Kern F Jr, Everson GT. Gastrointestinal transit time in human pregnancy: prolongation in the second and third trimesters followed by postpartum normalization. *Gastroenterology* 1985;89:996–9
11. Braverman DZ, Herbet D, Goldstein R, *et al.* Postpartum restoration of pregnancy-induced cholecystoparesis and prolonged intestinal transit time. *J Clin Gastroenterol* 1988;10:642–6
12. Levy N, Lemberg E, Sharf M. Bowel habit in pregnancy. *Digestion* 1971;4:216–22
13. Orlando RC. Reflux esophagitis. In Yamada T, ed. *Textbook of Gastroenterology*. Philadelphia, PA: JP Lippincott, 1991
14. Atlay RD, Weekes ARL. The treatment of gastrointestinal disease in pregnancy. *Clin Obstet Gynecol* 1986;13:335–47
15. Loans LB, Wolf JL. Gastroesophageal reflux in pregnancy. *Gastrointest Endo Clin North Am* 1994;4:699–712
16. Sontag SJ. The medical management of reflux esophagitis: role of antacids and acid inhibition. *Gastrointest Clin North Am* 1990;19:683–712
17. Nebel OT, Forbes MF, Castell DO. Symptomatic gastroesophageal reflux: incidence and precipitating factors. *Am J Dig Dis* 1976;21:953–6
18. Dodds WJ, Dent J, Hogan WJ. Pregnancy and the lower esophageal sphincter. *Gastroenterology* 1978;74:1334–6
19. Mittal RK, McCallum RW. Characteristic and frequency of transient relaxations of the lower esophageal sphincter in patients with reflux esophagitis. *Gastroenterology* 1988;95:593–9
20. Bainbridge ET, Nicholas SD, Newton JR, Temple JG. Gastro-oesophageal reflux in pregnancy: altered function of the barrier to reflux in asymptomatic women during early pregnancy. *Scand J Gastroenterol* 1984;19:85–9
21. Van Thiel DH, Wald A. Evidence refuting a role for increased abdominal pressure in the pathogenesis of the heartburn associated with pregnancy. *Am J Obstet Gynecol* 1981;140:420–2
22. Ogorek CP, Fisher RS. Detection and treatment of gastroesophageal reflux disease. *Gastrointest Clin North Am* 1989;18:293–313
23. Day JP, Richter JE. Medical and surgical conditions predisposing to gastroesophageal reflux disease. *Gastrointest Clin North Am* 1990;19:587–607
24. Cappell MS, Colon VJ, Sidhom OA. A study of eight medical centers of the safety and clinical efficacy of esophagogastroduodenoscopy in 83 pregnant females with follow-up of fetal outcome with comparison to control groups. *Am J Gastroenterol* 1996;91:348–54
25. Lewis JH, Weingold AB. The use of gastrointestinal drugs during pregnancy and lactation. *Am J Gastroenterol* 1985;80:912–23
26. Nelson MM, Forfar JO. Associations between drugs administered during pregnancy and congenital abnormalities of the fetus. *Br Med J* 1971;1:523–7
27. deJong PCM, Nijdam WS, Zielhuis GA, Eskes TKAB. Medication during low-risk pregnancy. *Eur J Obstet Gynecol Reprod Biol* 1991;41:191–6
28. Buitendijk S, Bracken MB. Medication in early pregnancy: prevalence of use and relationship to maternal characteristics. *Am J Obstet Gynecol* 1991;165:33–40
29. Hey VMF. Gastro-oesophageal reflux in pregnancy: a review article. *J Int Med Res* 1978;6(suppl 1):18–25
30. Singer AJ, Brandt LJ. Pathophysiology of the gastrointestinal tract during pregnancy. *Am J Gastroenterol* 1991;86:1695–712
31. Clark DH. Peptic ulcer in women. *Br Med J* 1953;1:1254–7

32. Sandweiss DJ, Podolsky HM, Saltzstein HC, Farbman AA. Deaths from perforation and hemorrhage of gastroduodenal ulcer during pregnancy and puerperium: a review of the literature and a report of one case. *Am J Obstet Gynecol* 1943;45:131–6

33. Baird RM. Peptic ulceration in pregnancy: report of a case with perforation. *Can Med Assoc J* 1966;94:861–2

34. Kurata JH, Haile BM, Elashoff JD. Sex differences in peptic ulcer disease. *Gastroenterology* 1985;88:96–100

35. Becker-Anderson H, Husfeldt V. Case reports: peptic ulcer in pregnancy. *Acta Obstet Gynecol Scand* 1971;50: 391–5

36. DeVore GR. Acute abdominal pain in the pregnant patient due to pancreatitis, acute appendicitis, cholecystitis, or peptic ulcer disease. *Clin Perinat* 1980;7: 349–69

37. Graham DY, Lew GM, Klein PD, *et al*. Effect of treatment of *Helicobacter pylori* infection on the long term recurrence of gastric or duodenal ulcers: a randomized controlled study. *Ann Intern Med* 1992;116:705–8

38. NIH Consensus Development Panel on *Helicobacter pylori* in peptic ulcer disease. NIH Consensus Conference on *Helicobacter pylori* in Peptic Ulcer Disease. *J Am Med Assoc* 1994;272:65–9

39. Sontag S, Graham DY, Belsito A, *et al*. Cimetidine, cigarette smoking, and recurrence of duodenal ulcer. *N Engl J Med* 1984;311:689–93

40. Isenberg JI, McQuaid KR, Laine L, Rubin D. Acid peptic disorders. In Yamada T, ed. *Textbook of Gastroenterology*. Philadelphia, PA: JP Lippincott, 1991

41. Rooney PJ, Dow TGB, Brooks PM, *et al*. Immunoreactive gastrin and gestation. *Am J Obstet Gynecol* 1975;122:834–6

42. Cunningham JT. Upper gastrointestinal tract disease. In Gleicher N, Elkayam U, eds. *Principles and Practice of Medical Therapy in Pregnancy*, 2nd edn. Norwalk, CT: Appleton & Lange, 1992

43. Somogyi A, Gugler R. Cimetidine excretion into breast milk. *Br J Clin Pharmacol* 1979;7:627–9

44. Briggs GG, Freeman RK, Yaffe JJ. *Drugs in Pregnancy and Lactation*, 3rd edn. Baltimore, MD: Williams and Wilkins, 1990

45. Zulli P, Di Nisio Q. Cimetidine treatment during pregnancy. *Lancet* 1978;2:945–6

46. Glade G, Saccar CL, Pereira GR. Cimetidine in pregnancy: apparent transient liver impairment in the newborn. *Am J Dis Child* 1980;134:87–8

47. Klebanoff MA, Koslowe PA, Kaslow R, Rhoads CG. Epidemiology of vomiting in early pregnancy. *Obstet Gynecol* 1985;66:612–16

48. Jarnfelt-Samsioe A, Samsioe G, Velinder GM. Nausea and vomiting in pregnancy – a contribution to its epidemiology. *Gynecol Obstet Invest* 1983;16:221–9

49. Fairweather DVI. Nausea and vomiting in pregnancy. *Am J Obstet Gynecol* 1968;102:135–75

50. Depue RH, Bernstein L, Ross RK, *et al*. Hyperemesis gravidarum in relation to estradiol levels, pregnancy outcome, and other maternal factors: a seroepidemiologic study. *Am J Obstet Gynecol* 1987;156:1137–41

51. Gross S, Librach C, Cecutti A. Maternal weight loss associated with hyperemesis gravidarum: a predictor of fetal outcome. *Am J Obstet Gynecol* 1989;160:906–9

52. Fairweather DVI. Nausea and vomiting during pregnancy. *Obstet Gynecol Annu* 1978;7:91–105

53. Soules MR, Hughes CL, Garcia JA, *et al*. Nausea and vomiting of pregnancy: role of human chorionic gonadotropin and 17-hydroxyprogesterone. *Obstet Gynecol* 1980;55:696–700

54. Masson GM, Anthony F, Chau E. Serum chorionic gonadotrophin (hCG), schwangerschaftsprotein 1 (SP1), progesterone and oestradiol levels in patients with nausea and vomiting in early pregnancy. *Br J Obstet Gynaecol* 1985;92:211–15

55. Kauppilla A, Huhtaniemi I, Ylikorkala O. Raised serum human chorionic gonadotrophin concentrations in hyperemesis gravidarum. *Br Med J* 1979;1: 1670–1

56. Goodwin TM, Hershman JM, Cole L. Increased concentration of the free β-subunit of human chorionic gonadotropin in hyperemesis gravidarum. *Acta Obstet Gynecol Scand* 1994;73:770–2

57. Bruun T, Kristoffersen K. Thyroid function during pregnancy with special reference to hydatidiform mole and hyperemesis. *Acta Endocrinol* 1978;88:383–9

58. Bouillon R, Naesens M, Van Assche FA, *et al*. Thyroid function in patients with hyperemesis gravidarum. *Am J Obstet Gynecol* 1982;143:922–6

59. Kennedy RL, Darne J, Davies R, Price A. Thyrotoxicosis and hyperemesis gravidarum associated with a serum activity which stimulates human thyroid cells *in vitro*. *Clin Endocrinol* 1992;36:83–9

60. Kirshon B, Lee W, Cotton DB. Prompt resolution of hyperthyroidism and hyperemesis gravidarum after delivery. *Obstet Gynecol* 1988;71:1032–4

61. Chin RKH, Lao TTH. Thyroxine concentration and outcome of hyperemetic pregnancies. *Br J Obstet Gynaecol* 1988;95:507–9

62. Samsioe G, Grona N, Enk L, Jarnfelt-Samsioe A. Does position and size of corpus luteum have any effect on nausea of pregnancy? *Acta Obstet Gynecol Scand* 1986; 65:427–9

63. Thorp JM, Watson WJ, Katz VL. Effect of corpus luteum position on hyperemesis gravidarum. *J Reprod Med* 1991;36:761–2

64. Koch KL, Stern RM, Vasey M, *et al*. Gastric dysrhythmias and nausea of pregnancy. *Dig Dis Sci* 1990;35: 961–8

65. Fitzgerald CM. Nausea and vomiting in pregnancy. *Br J Med Psychol* 1984;57:159–65

66. Mumford CJ. Papilloedema delaying diagnosis of Wernicke's encephalopathy in a comatose patient. *Postgrad Med J* 1989;65:371–3

67. Fraser D. Central pontine myelinolysis as a result of treatment of hyperemesis gravidarum. Case report. *Br J Obstet Gynaecol* 1988;95:621–3

68. Godsey RK, Newman RB. Hyperemesis gravidarum: a comparison of single and multiple admissions. *J Reprod Med* 1991;36:287–90

69. Castillo RA, Ray RA, Yaghmai F. Central pontine myelinolysis and pregnancy. *Obstet Gynecol* 1989;73: 459–61

70. Leathem AM. Safety and efficacy of antiemetics used to treat nausea and vomiting in pregnancy. *Clin Pharm* 1986;5:660–8

71. Schulman PK. Hyperemesis gravidarum: an approach to the nutritional aspects of care. *J Am Diet Assoc* 1982;80:577–8

72. Levine MG, Esser, D. Total parenteral nutrition for the treatment of severe hyperemesis gravidarum: maternal nutritional effects and fetal outcome. *Obstet Gynecol* 1988;72:102–7

73. Chin RKH, Lao TT. Low birth weight and hyperemesis gravidarum. *Eur J Obstet Gynecol Reprod Biol* 1988;28:179–83

74. Whelan G. Epidemiology of inflammatory bowel disease. *Med Clin North Am* 1990;74:1–19

75. Gollop JH, Phillips SF, Melton LJ, Zinsmeister AR. Epidemiologic aspects of Crohn's disease: a population based study in Olmsted County, Minnesota, 1943–1982. *Gut* 1988;29:49–56

76. Calkins BM, Lilienfeld AM, Garland CF, Mendeloff AI. Trends in incidence rates of ulcerative colitis and Crohn's disease. *Dig Dis Sci* 1984;29:913–20

77. Ekbom A, Helmick C, Zack M, Adami HO. The epidemiology of inflammatory bowel disease: a large, population-based study in Sweden. *Gastroenterology* 1991;100:350–8

78. Stenson WF, MacDermott RP. Inflammatory bowel disease. In Yamada T, ed. *Textbook of Gastroenterology*. Philadelphia, PA: JP Lippincott, 1991

79. Gitnick G. Etiology of inflammatory bowel diseases: where have we been? Where are we going? *Scand J Gastroenterol* 1990;25(suppl 175):93–6

80. Donaldson RM. Current concepts: management of medical problems in pregnancy – inflammatory bowel disease. *N Engl J Med* 1980;312:1616–19

81. Cappell MS, Sidhom O. Multicenter, multiyear study of safety and efficacy of flexible sigmoidoscopy during pregnancy in 24 females with follow-up of fetal outcome. *Dig Dis Sci* 1995;40:472–9

82. Hanan MI, Kirsner JB. Inflammatory bowel disease in the pregnant woman. *Clin Perinat* 1985;12:669–81

83. Korelitz BI. Pregnancy, fertility, and inflammatory bowel disease. *Am J Gastroenterol* 1985;80:365–70

84. Willoughby CP, Truelove SC. Ulcerative colitis and pregnancy. *Gut* 1980;21:469–74

85. Mogadam M, Korelitz BI, Ahmed SW, *et al.* The course of inflammatory bowel disease during pregnancy and postpartum. *Am J Gastroenterol* 1981;75:265–9

86. Vender RJ, Spiro HM. Inflammatory bowel disease and pregnancy. *J Clin Gastroenterol* 1982;4:231–49

87. Miller JP. Inflammatory bowel disease in pregnancy: a review. *J R Soc Med* 1986;79:221–5

88. Weterman IT. Fertility and pregnancy in inflammatory bowel disease. *Neth J Med* 1989;35:S67–S75

89. Baird DD, Narendranathan M, Sandler RS. Increased risk of preterm birth for women with inflammatory bowel disease. *Gastroenterology* 1990;99:987–94

90. Khosla R, Willoughby CP, Jewell DP. Crohn's disease and pregnancy. *Gut* 1984;25:52–6

91. Mayberry JF, Weterman IT. European survey of fertility and pregnancy in women with Crohn's disease: a case control study by European collaborative group. *Gut* 1986;27:821–5

92. Toovey S, Hudson E, Hendry WF, Levi AJ. Suphasalazine and male infertility: reversibility and possible mechanism. *Gut* 1981;22:445–51

93. Nielsen OH, Andreasson B, Bondesen S, *et al.* Pregnancy in Crohn's disease. *Scand J Gastroenterol* 1984;19:724–32

94. Woolfson K, Cohen Z, McLeod RS. Crohn's disease and pregnancy. *Dis Colon Rectum* 1990;33:869–73

95. Nielsen OH, Andreasson B, Bondesen S, Jarnum S. Pregnancy in ulcerative colitis. *Scand J Gastroenterol* 1988;18:735

96. Azad Khan AK, Truelove SC. Placental and mammary transfer of sulphasalazine. *Br Med J* 1979;2:1553

97. Jarnerot G, Into-Malmberg MB, Esbjorner E. Placental transfer of sulphasalazine and sulphapyridine and some of its metabolites. *Scand J Gastroenterol* 1981;16:693–7

98. Mogadam M, Dobbins WO, Korelitz BI, Ahmed SW. Pregnancy in inflammatory bowel disease: effect of sulfasalazine and corticosteroids on fetal outcome. *Gastroenterology* 1981;80:72–6

99. Habal FM, Hui G, Greenberg GR. Oral 5-aminosalicylic acid for inflammatory bowel disease in pregnancy: safety and clinical course. *Gastroenterology* 1993;105:1057–60

100. Roubenoff R, Hoyt J, Petri M, *et al.* Effects of antiinflammatory and immunosuppressive drugs on pregnancy and fertility. *Arth Rheum* 1988;18:88–110

101. Blanford AT, Murphy BEP. *In vitro* metabolism of prednisolone, dexamethasone, betamethasone, and cortisol by the human placenta. *Am J Obstet Gynecol* 1977;127:264–7

102. Alstead EM, Ritchie JK, Lennard-Jones JE, *et al.* Safety of azathioprine in pregnancy in inflammatory bowel disease. *Gastroenterology* 1990;99:443–6

103. Kirby DF, Fiorenza V, Craig RM. Intravenous nutritional support during pregnancy. *J Parenter Enter Nutr* 1988;12:72–80

104. Ojerskog B, Kock NG, Philipson BM, Philipson M. Pregnancy and delivery in patients with a continent ileostomy. *Surg Gynecol Obstet* 1988;167:61–4

105. Nestor H, Dozois RR, Kelly KA, *et al.* The effect of pregnancy and delivery on the ileal pouch–anal anastomosis functions. *Dis Colon Rectum* 1989;32:384–8

106. Scott HJ, McLeod RS, Blair J, *et al.* Ileal pouch–anal anastomosis: pregnancy, delivery and pouch function. *Int J Colorect Dis* 1996;11:84–7

107. Corlett RC, Mishell DR. Pancreatitis in pregnancy. *Am J Obstet Gynecol* 1972;113:281–90

108. Hasselgren PO. Acute pancreatitis in pregnancy. *Acta Chir Scand* 1980;146:297–9

109. Ellsbury KE. Abdominal pain in pregnancy. *J Fam Pract* 1986;22:365–71

110. Steer ML. Acute pancreatitis. In Yamada T, ed. *Textbook of Gastroenterology*. Philadelphia, PA: JP Lippincott, 1991

111. McKay AJ, O'Neill J, Imrie CW. Pancreatitis, pregnancy and gallstones. *Br J Obstet Gynaecol* 1980;87:47–50

112. Block P, Kelly TR. Management of gallstone pancreatitis during pregnancy and the postpartum period. *Surg Gynecol Obstet* 1989;168:426–8

113. Wilkinson EJ. Acute pancreatitis in pregnancy: a review of 98 cases and a report of 8 new cases. *Obstet Gynecol Surv* 1973;28:281–303

114. Fabrin B, Eldon K. Pregnancy complicated by concurrent hyperparathyroidism and pancreatitis. *Acta Obstet Gynecol Scand* 1986;65:651–2

115. Hyder SA, Barkin JS. Pancreatic disease. In Gleicher N, Elkayam U, eds. *Principles and Practice of Medical Therapy in Pregnancy*. Norwalk, CT: Appleton & Lange, 1992

116. Lykkesfeldt G, Bock JE, Pedersen FD, *et al.* Excessive hypertriglyceridemia and pancreatitis in pregnancy: association with deficiency of lipoprotein lipase. *Acta Obstet Gynecol Scand* 1980;60:79–82

117. Strickland DM, Hauth JC, Widisch J, *et al.* Amylase and isoamylase activities in serum of pregnant women. *Obstet Gynecol* 1984;63:389–91

118. DeVore GR, Bracken M, Berkowitz RL. The amylase/creatinine clearance ratio in normal pregnancy and pregnancies complicated by pancreatitis, hyperemesis gravidarum, and toxemia. *Am J Obstet Gynecol* 1980;136:747–54

119. Bartelink AKM, Gimbrere JSF, Schoots F, Dony JMJ. Maternal survival after acute haemorrhagic pancreatitis complicating late pregnancy. *Eur J Obstet Gynecol Reprod Biol* 1988;29:41–50

120. Ranson JHC, Rikind KM, Turner JW. Prognostic signs and non-operative peritoneal lavage in acute pancreatitis. *Surg Gynecol Obstet* 1976;143:209–19

121. Young KR. Acute pancreatitis in pregnancy: Two case reports. *Obstet Gynecol* 1982;5:653–7

122. Jouppila P, Mokka R, Larmi TKI. Acute pancreatitis in pregnancy. *Surg Gynecol Obstet* 1979;139:879–82

123. Gineston JL, Capron JP, Delcenserie R, *et al.* Prolonged total parenteral nutrition in a pregnant woman with acute pancreatitis. *J Clin Gastroenterol* 1984;6:249–52

124. Weinberg RB, Sitrin MD, Adkins GM, Lin CC. Treatment of hyperlipidemic pancreatitis in pregnancy with total parenteral nutrition. *Gastroenterology* 1982;83:1300–5

125. Nies BM, Dreiss RJ. Hyperlipidemic pancreatitis in pregnancy: a case report and review of the literature. *Am J Perinatol* 1990;7:166–9

126. NIH Consensus Development Panel. Gastrointestinal surgery for severe obesity. *NIH Consensus Development Conference Consensus Statement* 1991;Mar 25–27:9

127. Woods JR, Brinkman CR. The jejunoileal bypass and pregnancy. *Obstet Gynecol Surv* 1978;33:697–705

128. Knudsen LB, Kallen B. Intestinal bypass operation and pregnancy outcome. *Acta Obstet Gynecol Scand* 1986;65:831–4

129. Hey N, Niebuhr-Jorgensen U. Jejuno-ileal bypass surgery in obesity. *Acta Obstet Gynecol Scand* 1981;60:135–40

130. Printen KJ, Scott D. Pregnancy following gastric bypass for the treatment of morbid obesity. *Am Surg* 1981;48:363–5

131. Naslund I. Gastric bypass vs. gastroplasty. Prospective study of differences in two surgical procedures for morbid obesity. *Acta Chir Scand* (suppl) 1987;536:1–60

132. Sugerman HJ, Starkey JV, Birenhauer R. A randomized prospective trial of gastric bypass vs. vertical banded gastroplasty for morbid obesity and their effects on sweets vs. non-sweets eaters. *Ann Surg* 1987;205:613–24

133. Halverson JD. Micronutrient deficiencies after gastric bypass for morbid obesity. *Am Surg* 1986;52:594–8

134. Richards DS, Miller DK, Goodman GN. Pregnancy after gastric bypass for morbid obesity. *J Reprod Med* 1987;32:172–6

135. Haddow JE, Hill LE, Kloza EM, Thanhauser D. Neural tube defects after gastric bypass. *Lancet* 1986;1:1330

136. Boyce RA, O'Donnell SZ. Dietetic implications of pregnancy following gastric partitioning surgery. *J Hum Nutr Diet* 1992;5:107–12

137. Rubin D. Gastroenterologic diseases. In Woodley M, Whelan A, eds. *Manual of Medical Therapeutics*, 27th edn. Boston, MA: Little, Brown, 1992

38
Hematological diseases

M.A. Blinder

INTRODUCTION

Striking alterations in both the cellular elements of blood and the coagulation factors occur in normal pregnancy. These changes, along with the increased metabolic demands of pregnancy, place women at an increased risk for a number of hematological disorders. Furthermore, therapeutic interventions in many hematological diseases have implications for the developing fetus. Under some circumstances, the approach to treatment remains unchanged from that of the non-gravid state, but the risks of therapy are increased. At other times, the therapeutic approach must be altered because of the pregnancy. This chapter will focus on the diagnosis and treatment of hematological diseases occurring during pregnancy.

HEMATOLOGICAL CHANGES ASSOCIATED WITH NORMAL PREGNANCY

Red cells and plasma volume

The physiological expansion of blood volume during pregnancy is dramatic. The plasma volume expands by 40–60%, while the red cell mass increases by 20–50% so that the net effect is a dilution of the red cells and a drop in the hematocrit. At full term, the maternal hematocrit is 28–39%[1,2]. During pregnancy, the red cells demonstrate more variability in size and shape than in non-pregnant women[3]. Serum erythropoietin levels steadily increase from a normal non-gravid level of 16 ± 4 mU/ml to 35 ± 18 mU/ml during the third trimester[4]. The role of the expanded maternal blood volume is to provide for the metabolic and perfusion needs of the growing fetus and to buffer the potential blood loss during delivery of the infant.

White blood cells

The neutrophil count increases during pregnancy and circulating immature neutrophils may occasionally be identified. However, the elevated neutrophil count rarely leads to difficulties in the diagnosis of leukemia or serious infection. The neutrophil morphology is generally unremarkable, but small, pale-blue inclusions known as 'Döhle bodies' may be present in the cytoplasm. Lymphocyte and eosinophil counts fall modestly during pregnancy[3].

Platelets and coagulation factors

In uncomplicated pregnancy the platelet count usually remains normal, although mild thrombocytopenia occasionally occurs. Platelet production is driven in part by thrombopoietin, a recently identified protein that promotes the proliferation and maturation of megakaryocytes[5]. In normal non-pregnant individuals, the circulating levels are below 0.16 ng/ml, but significantly higher levels are detected in conditions with decreased megakaryocytes, such as in patients receiving ablative chemotherapy[6]. In contrast, patients with thrombocytopenia from peripheral destruction of platelets have increased numbers of megakaryocytes and a low thrombopoietin level. During pregnancy, most cases of thrombocytopenia are the result of peripheral destruction, suggesting that the level would be low. Clinical trials are under way to assess the efficacy of thrombopoietin infusions in a variety of disorders with thrombocytopenia.

Levels of many coagulation factors change during pregnancy. Most striking is the progressive elevation of factor VIII and von Willebrand factor throughout pregnancy; by full term, these levels may reach 200–300%. In general, procoagulant clotting factors increase during pregnancy, while factors responsible for natural anticoagulant and fibrinolytic activity decrease, so that the balance favors increased clotting. These changes are thought to occur to help prepare for the added stress of bleeding during delivery. Normal hemostasis is further altered by the presence of placental-derived factors within the maternal circulation. One such factor, placental plasminogen activator inhibitor, rises to very high levels during pregnancy, decreasing the fibrinolytic capacity of the blood[7]. On the other hand, dermatan sulfate, presumably derived from the placenta, is detected only in the maternal circulation and functions as an antithrombotic agent similar to heparin.

DISORDERS OF RED BLOOD CELLS
Iron deficiency anemia

Iron is absorbed from the proximal small intestine where it enters the circulation and binds to its carrier protein, transferrin. The iron–transferrin complex binds to the transferrin receptor that is present on the membrane of cells that utilize iron, allowing for internalization of the iron. Excess iron is stored predominantly in the liver where it is complexed to ferritin. Total body iron in a non-pregnant woman is about 3000 mg, most of which is in hemoglobin in red cells, myoglobin in muscle or as a component of other enzymes. In women 18–44 years of age, stored iron accounts for only approximately 300 mg of the total[8]. During development, a fetus requires about 500 mg of iron which consumes the maternal storage pool; therefore, unless supplemental iron is provided, iron deficiency is likely to occur[9].

Iron deficiency anemia should be suspected in pregnant women with a microcytic anemia. The diagnosis is usually made by detecting a low serum ferritin, confirming that iron stores have been depleted. In addition, the serum transferrin receptor level may be increased, reflecting increased receptor synthesis in cells that are starved of iron. Women with low ferritin but normal serum transferrin receptor levels probably have a less severe iron deficiency, reflecting depleted iron stores but adequate erythropoiesis[10].

Almost all pregnant women require supplemental iron to avoid iron deficiency anemia. The usual prenatal multivitamin contains 36–65 mg of elemental iron. In most pregnant women and in those with overt iron deficiency in particular, additional oral iron, given as ferrous sulfate, fumarate or gluconate is also necessary. Despite the tenuous iron stores of most pregnant women, neonatal red cell production is rarely iron deficient[9].

Megaloblastic anemia

Folate and vitamin B_{12} are required for normal DNA synthesis in all cells, but deficiencies first appear in rapidly dividing cells, such as those involved in hematopoiesis. In most cases, the diagnosis is suspected by finding a macrocytic anemia or pancytopenia and confirmed by detecting low levels of red cell folate or serum vitamin B_{12}.

Since folate is not adequately stored in humans and is rapidly consumed in pregnancy, a diet rich in folate as well as supplementation is frequently needed to avoid a deficiency. Folate requirements increase in proportion to the size of the fetus and consequently by the third trimester, they are increased approximately fivefold from the non-pregnant state. Folate deficiency is most common in women of lower socioeconomic status or with poor eating habits, and in pregnancies complicated by chronic anorexia, vomiting, infection or alcohol consumption. Less commonly, women with hemolytic anemia or those on anticonvulsant medication are at risk for folate deficiency. Maternal folate deficiency leading to megaloblastic anemia in the newborn

is rare, but it may lead to premature, low-birth-weight infants[11]. Furthermore, folate supplementation after conception reduces the incidence of neural tube defects including spina bifida, meningocele, and anencephalopathy[12]. Supplementation with 1 mg of folate daily, usually as a component of a prenatal multivitamin, is generally recommended. Lactation also consumes maternal folate so that in women who breastfeed, folate supplementation may be required beyond the time of delivery.

Ingested vitamin B_{12} binds to intrinsic factor that is synthesized in the stomach. Absorption of the intrinsic factor–vitamin B_{12} complex occurs in the terminal ileum. Therefore, vitamin B_{12} deficiency occurs most commonly in individuals with disorders of either the stomach or the terminal ileum. Typically, the vitamin B_{12} level is low during pregnancy because of hemodilution and increased uptake by the fetus, but deficiencies that lead to clinical abnormalities are rare[13]. Though uncommon, breastfed infants of women who have subclinical deficiency (e.g. strict vegetarians or patients with sprue) are at risk of developing vitamin B_{12} deficiency[14,15]. Most prenatal vitamin preparations contain vitamin B_{12}.

Hemoglobinopathies and thalassemias

The major form of normal adult hemoglobin (hemoglobin A) is composed of a tetramer consisting of two α- and two β-globin chains. Each of the globin chains binds a heme molecule and the intact hemoglobin carries oxygen to all tissues. Disorders of hemoglobin are classified as a 'hemoglobinopathy' if a structural abnormality is present in the α- or β-globin chain or as a 'thalassemia' if there is insufficient globin chain production.

Sickle cell anemia

The most frequently identified abnormal hemoglobin in North America is hemoglobin S, which is the result of a mutation of the sixth amino acid in the β-globin gene (β6 Glu→Val). About 8% of Afro-Americans have sickle cell trait, in which one β-globin gene is normal and the other encodes the hemoglobin S mutation. Sickle cell trait is not associated with any significant risk during pregnancy, but in women known to carry the mutant gene, the opportunity for paternal and prenatal testing and counselling should be available if requested[16].

Sickle cell anemia is inherited in an autosomal recessive manner so that about one in 600 Afro-Americans is afflicted with this disorder. Variants of this disease also occur, in which the hemoglobin S mutation occurs along with a second mutation on the other β-globin gene. A common variant, hemoglobin SC disease, has similar, although less severe, findings than sickle cell anemia and consequently the outcome of pregnancy is favorable[17,18]. The incidence of complications in patients with sickle cell anemia during pregnancy is not well defined, but seems to be increased when compared to non-pregnant patients and, therefore, prenatal care is best administered by an obstetrician with experience in the management of this disease. The most common complication is vaso-occlusive pain, the result of obstructed blood flow from 'sickled' red cells in the microcirculation. In many patients, narcotic analgesics are needed for adequate pain control. All of the widely used opioid analgesics are considered 'class C' for use in pregnancy and can generally be used at doses similar to those in non-pregnant patients[19]. Other complications of sickle cell disease, including the acute chest syndrome, sickle cell hepatopathy, neurological events and infection, should be managed in a similar manner to that in non-pregnant patients[19,20].

Complications of pregnancy, such as placenta previa, placental abruption, eclampsia, amnionitis and preterm delivery, have all been reported to be higher in patients with sickle cell anemia in comparison to patients without a hemoglobinopathy[19,20]. In general, treatment of these disorders is similar to that in patients who do not have sickle cell anemia. Intrauterine growth retardation has been reported to occur in about 15% of pregnancies complicated by sickle cell anemia[19]. One explanation for this complication is that recurrent vaso-occulsive episodes lead to placental hypoperfusion and fetal hypoxia.

In the non-pregnant patient, red cell transfusions are indicated in a limited number of well-defined clinical circumstances, such as the acute chest syndrome, stroke, red-cell aplasia and preoperative management[21]. When indicated, automated red cell exchange can be accomplished within a few hours[22]. Red cell transfusions in pregnancy do not affect the obstetric or infant outcome, although there may be some decrease in the incidence of vaso-occlusive painful events[23,24]. Because there is no proven benefit to transfusions in pregnancy, they are not routinely recommended and must be used with caution in women of reproductive age, since they are associated with the development of neonatal alloimmune hemolytic anemia[25].

Recently, hydroxyurea has been advocated for the prevention of vaso-occlusive pain in sickle cell anemia. Studies show a decrease in the frequency of painful episodes by about one-half[26]. The response appears to be mediated by an increased production of hemoglobin F, diluting the hemoglobin S within the red cell. The toxicity of hydroxyurea is not well defined during pregnancy and consequently its use in women without contraception is discouraged. Nevertheless, anecdotal data are available on hydroxyurea in other clinical settings, suggesting that it may be successfully used in pregnancy without fetopathic effects.

Infants born with sickle cell anemia are usually in good health, because they are protected by high levels of hemoglobin F. Although clinical symptoms leading to the diagnosis of sickle cell anemia develop between 9 and 12 months of age, many infants are now identified during neonatal screening programs which allow for the early institution of prophylactic antibiotics to decrease the incidence of infection[27].

All methods of contraception that are available to other individuals may be considered in patients with sickle cell disease[19]. There is no evidence that estrogen-containing oral contraceptive agents pose added thromboembolic risk to women with sickle cell disease. Nevertheless, many patients favor long-acting intramuscular medroxyprogesterone acetate (Depo-Provera®) for contraception.

Thalassemia

There are four α- and two β-globin genes in the normal cell and production of the α- and β-chains is nearly equal. Thalassemias are a heterogeneous group of inherited disorders characterized by underproduction of either α- or β-chains. These disorders usually occur in persons of Mediterranean, African, Middle Eastern, Indian or Asian descent.

In β-thalassemia, there is reduced production of β-globin with normal amounts of α-globin. The excess α-globin chains form insoluble tetramers in the red cells, leading to membrane damage, ineffective erythropoiesis and hemolytic anemia. Classification of this disease is based on the severity of the anemia and is divided into thalassemia minor, intermedia and major. Thalassemia minor (β-thalassemia trait) is caused by diminished or absent β-globin chain synthesis from one gene. Patients are usually asymptomatic, but have a mild, microcytic anemia. Thalassemia intermedia is typically associated with moderate dysfunction of both β-globin genes and is associated with a more severe anemia (hemoglobin 7–10 g/dl), but the patient is not usually transfusion-dependent. Pregnancy poses no special problems in thalassemia minor or intermedia, but a serum ferritin should be measured because many patients have very high levels of iron stores and require no additional iron[28]. Paternal hemoglobin testing and prenatal counselling may be appropriate, especially in areas of the world with a high incidence of β-thalassemia. Thalassemia major causes a severe, transfusion-dependent anemia which frequently results in infertility because of iron overload and, therefore, pregnancy is uncommon. Successful pregnancy may require aggressive red cell transfusion support to avoid heart failure[29].

α-Thalassemia occurs when one or more of the α-genes is inactive. Individuals with the loss of one of the four α-globin genes may have only mild microcytosis; the loss of two α-globin genes is associated with a mild microcytic hypochromic anemia which poses a potential problem in pregnancy. If both α-genes from the same chromosome are abnormal, the offspring is at risk of losing three or four α-genes, depending on the α-globin genes from the other parent. Loss of three α-globin genes causes hemoglobin H disease, a moderately severe microcytic anemia that is associated with splenomegaly. The loss of all four α-globin genes causes hydrops fetalis and is incompatible with life. This occurs most frequently in persons of south-east Asian ancestry.

Red cell aplasia

Human parvovirus B19 was discovered in 1975 and remains the only member of the parvoviridae family known to cause human disease. Parvovirus B19 has been shown to be the causative agent of erythema infectiosum, or 'fifth disease' of childhood, which results in a coryzal prodrome, followed by a low-grade fever, bright erythema of the face and a reticular rash elsewhere on the body. Adults with acute parvoviral infection may by asymptomatic or may develop polyarthralgias with less pronounced skin manifestations[30].

The diagnosis of a parvoviral infection is established by measuring IgG and IgM antiparvovirus antibodies in serum. Detection of IgM in the presence or absence of IgG indicates a recent infection, whereas the presence of IgG antibody alone is indicative of a past infection and presumed immunity. About one-half of the adults in the USA have serological evidence of antiparvovirus antibodies. In immunocompromised adults or in fetal or neonatal samples, an antibody response may not be detected, but viral DNA can be detected from serum or tissue.

Parvovirus B19 replicates in erythroid progenitor cells, causing a transient arrest of red cell production for 7–14 days. In patients with an underlying hemolytic anemia, such as sickle cell disease, a severe anemia requiring transfusions may result. With the resolution of the acute infection, erythropoiesis recovers over 1–2 weeks. Patients with a known hemolytic anemia admitted with a febrile illness and a low reticulocyte count should be suspected as having a parvovirus B19 infection. It is recommended that these patients be placed in respiratory and contact isolation to avoid nosocomial infection of hospital workers[31]. Furthermore, it is recommended that these patients should not be cared for by staff who may be pregnant.

In pregnant women who become infected, fetal death and non-immune hydrops fetalis occur in one-quarter of pregnancies within 12 weeks of the infection[32]. The use of intrauterine red cell transfusions for hydrops fetalis has resulted in healthy infants whose red cell production has recovered. Neonates with hydrops fetalis or congenital red cell aplasia should be tested for parvovirus infection in their sera and bone marrow. Infants who survive may suffer with a lifelong transfusion-dependent anemia[33]. In cases of suspected parvovirus infection, treatment of either the mother or fetus with intravenous immunoglobulin for passive immunity is unproven.

Pure red cell aplasia of pregnancy in the absence of an underlying hemolytic disease has rarely been described. This disorder occurs in the first or second trimester and the treatment includes red cell transfusions. Erythroid recovery within 3 months of delivery is the rule and the infants are unaffected[34].

Immune hemolytic anemias

Alloimmune hemolytic anemia

Red cell alloimmunization is the result of maternal sensitization to red cell antigens which occurs during a transfusion or from a prior pregnancy. All pregnant women should be screened for the presence of alloantibodies with an indirect antiglobulin test (indirect Coombs'). Despite the widespread use of Rh(D) immune globulin prophylaxis, alloimmunization against Rh(D) occurs in 0.1–0.2% of women and remains a common cause of immune hemolytic disease in the newborn[35]. Other antigens, including Kell, E and C, account for the majority of antibodies that are currently detected, suggesting that, in women of reproductive age who require transfusions, an expanded cross-match to include additional antigens besides rhesus factor should be performed. Incompatibility against the ABO blood system also occurs in mothers of blood type O who give birth to infants with blood type A or B. In this case, the hemolytic anemia is independent of birth order and occurs in the absence of previous red cell sensitization.

There are no direct maternal consequences to red cell alloimmunization, but this disorder may lead to fetal death, hydrops fetalis or hemolytic disease of the newborn. The outlook for an affected fetus has improved dramatically with fetal blood sampling and intrauterine blood transfusion. In infancy, complications include hyperbilirubinemia, which is treated with phototherapy, and anemia, which may require red cell transfusions. The hemolysis resolves over 3 months. In contrast to alloimmunization by minor red cell antigens, ABO incompatibility is less severe.

Autoimmune hemolytic anemia

Most cases are caused by an IgG autoantibody that interacts best with red cells at 37 °C. The target antigens are found on all red cells and consequently transfused red cells are destroyed at a rate similar to that of the native cells. In about one-half of cases, no underlying disorder is found, but the disease may be triggered by medication or may be associated with malignancy or collagen vascular disease. Although this disorder is not rare, cases occurring in pregnancy have been described infrequently. Hemolysis in pregnant women may be severe, but the disorder typically responds to glucocorticoids[36]. Placental transfer of antibodies may occur, causing a neonatal hemolytic anemia. Treatment is usually supportive, but occasionally a severe anemia may require additional therapy similar to that administered in alloimmune hemolytic anemia[37].

HEMATOLOGICAL MALIGNANCY, MYELOPROLIFERATIVE DISEASES AND STEM-CELL DISORDERS

Acute leukemia

The diagnosis of acute leukemia has dramatic consequences for the patient and her family. Patients typically present with cytopenias, lymphadenopathy or splenomegaly. The two categories of acute leukemia include acute myelocytic leukemia and acute lymphocytic leukemia. A bone marrow examination is usually needed to establish the diagnosis.

The majority of cases of acute leukemia diagnosed in adulthood are acute myelocytic leukemia. Chemotherapy with cytosine arabinoside (Ara-C) is usually used in induction chemotherapy and is administered with daunorubicin or idarubicin to achieve a remission. After complete remission, additional chemotherapy or a bone marrow transplantation is used as consolidation and the result is an overall cure rate of 30–50%. Acute myelocytic leukemia diagnosed in pregnancy is an uncommon event, but complete remission rates of 77% have been reported which is a similar response to non-pregnant patients of the same age. In patients diagnosed and treated for acute myelocytic leukemia in the first or second trimester, the risk of miscarriage, fetal death and premature birth is high[38]. Although many chemotherapeutic agents, including Ara-C, cross the placenta, the incidence of fetal malformation appears to be low[39,40]. In general, if acute myelocytic leukemia is in complete remission at the time of delivery, there is decreased maternal and fetal morbidity when compared with uncontrolled or untreated leukemia so that, despite the pregnancy, induction chemotherapy should be inititated.

Acute lymphocytic leukemia is the most common leukemia of childhood, but when it occurs in adults, it is considerably more difficult to cure. Treatment usually consists of vincristine, prednisone and L-asparaginase, and craniospinal prophylaxis is necessary. After achieving a complete remission, additional consolidation chemotherapy followed by maintenance chemotherapy for at least 1 year is recommended. In most cases, young girls who are successfully treated for acute lymphocytic leukemia have normal reproductive function[41]. Furthermore, there does not appear to be an increased incidence of birth defects in the offspring of

adult survivors of childhood acute lymphocytic leukemia[42]. As in women with acute myelocytic leukemia treated during pregnancy, the risk of miscarriage, fetal death and premature delivery in acute lymphocytic leukemia is high[38].

Hodgkin's disease and non-Hodgkin's lymphoma

Hodgkin's disease usually presents with cervical adenopathy and spreads in a predictable manner along lymph node groups. Treatment is based on the presenting stage of the disease; the cell type is relatively unimportant in the natural history and prognosis. In the non-pregnant state, disease that is limited to a single lymph node group (Stage I), or to more than one lymph node group but confined to one side of the diaphragm (Stage II), is usually treated with radiation therapy. When a large mediastinal mass exceeding one-third the diameter of the chest width is present, chemotherapy is added. More advanced disease [Stage III (disease occurring on both sides of the diaphragm) or Stage IV (liver or bone marrow involvement)] or any stage that includes B symptoms (fever above 38.5 °C, night sweats or a 10% weight loss) generally requires combination chemotherapy.

Treatment of Hodgkin's disease with chemotherapy frequently leads to amenorrhea, but in women who continue to menstruate there does not appear to be any effect on fertility, pregnancy or offspring[43]. Treatment during pregnancy seems to be associated with an increased risk of miscarriage or fetal death, but, in successful pregnancy, the children appear to be normal[44]. Radiation therapy has been associated with an increased number of fetal malformations and is generally not recommended during pregnancy.

Non-Hodgkin's lymphoma is classified as low-, intermediate- or high-grade, based on the histological type. Staging evaluation is the same as for Hodgkin's disease, but non-Hodgkin's lymphoma has a less predictable pattern of spread. Most patients have advanced-stage disease (Stage III or IV) at the time of diagnosis. Low-grade lymphomas often have an indolent course and do not require immediate therapy, since there is no impact on survival. Intermediate- and high-grade lymphomas are more aggressive and therefore combination chemotherapy is frequently used, leading to a cure in some patients. In general, when indicated for the cure of a patient, chemotherapy may be given during pregnancy and the risk to the developing fetus appears to be small[44].

Chronic myeloid leukemia

The earliest finding in this disorder is an asymptomatic elevation of the neutrophil count. In most cases, the diagnosis of chronic myeloid leukemia is confirmed on cytogenetic analysis of blood or bone marrow by the presence of the Philadelphia chromosome, representing a translocation between chromosomes 9 and 22. Symptoms from an anemia or discomfort related to splenomegaly may occur. Although the disease remains quiescent for a period of 3–5 years, known as the 'chronic phase', chronic myeloid leukemia generally terminates as a 'blast crisis' which is similar to acute myelocytic leukemia, but more difficult to treat successfully. Treatment of the chronic phase involves control of the neutrophil count with hydroxyurea or α-interferon; younger patients may have successful long-term control of the disease with a bone marrow transplant[45].

Chronic myeloid leukemia diagnosed during pregnancy is a rare occurrence in which the woman typically presents with an asymptomatic increase in neutrophils noted on routine prenatal blood testing. Pregnancy can usually be completed successfully and treatment with intermittent leukopheresis to control the neutrophil count is generally recommended[46,47]. Nevertheless, conception and full-term pregnancies have also been successful in patients treated with α-interferon or hydroxyurea[46,48–51].

Polycythemia vera

This disorder is characterized by unregulated production of red cells, resulting in a high hemoglobin and hematocrit. Elevated platelet and white blood cell counts frequently occur and splenomegaly is common. The clinical course is indolent, but the disease is frequently complicated by venous and arterial thromboembolism over the long term[52]. Treatment usually includes phlebotomy or hydroxyurea which is directed at controlling the peripheral blood counts[53].

Pregnancy has infrequently been reported in patients with polycythemia vera and the maternal outcome is usually good. The incidence of preterm delivery, miscarriage and fetal death has been reported to be high, but the results are improved when the hematocrit is controlled[54]. Therefore, treatment should be directed at controlling the hematocrit and a target level of 40% is reasonable. While phlebotomy has been the standard therapy, use of hydroxyurea or α-interferon might also be helpful in controlling the platelet count to decrease the risk of thromboembolism in patients with thrombocytosis. Pregnant patients with polycythemia vera probably do not need supplemental iron.

Essential thrombocytosis

Persistent elevations in the platelet count above 600 000/µl and a proliferation of the megakaryocytes in the bone marrow unrelated to other causes is a type of myeloproliferative disease known as 'essential thrombocytosis' (also termed 'primary' or 'essential' thrombocythemia). The clinical manifestations of this disease commonly include thromboembolic events in the cerebrovascular circulation, the microcirculation of the extremities, and in the peripheral and mesenteric venous and arterial circulations. Less commonly, bleeding of mucosal surfaces, such as the gastrointestinal tract, may occur[55,56]. The disease generally occurs in older adults, but an increased incidence in women of reproductive age has also been observed. Treatment of the disease to control the platelet count is generally recommended in patients with thrombotic or hemorrhagic complications or in asymptomatic patients with cardiovascular risk factors. The usual agents include hydroxyurea, α-interferon or the recently approved agent, anagrelide[55].

A number of cases of essential thrombocytosis in pregnancy have been described and the outcome is variable. The overall incidence of successful pregnancy is about 60%, with first-trimester miscarriages being the most common complication[57]. In many pregnancies, a progressive decline in the platelet count of about 20%, beginning in the 10th week of gestation, has been observed, followed by a rapid recurrence of the thrombocytosis postpartum[58,59].

In asymptomatic pregnant patients, no specific therapeutic intervention is generally needed and the outcome is likely to be successful[57,60]. In symptomatic patients, or those with poor outcomes from prior pregnancies, it is reasonable to consider platelet-reductive therapy. In patients with prior miscarriages or other thrombotic complications, institution of α-interferon prior to pregnancy and continuation through the pregnancy has resulted in successful outcomes[61,62]. This suggests that normalization of the platelet count during pregnancy is helpful in avoiding fetal and maternal complications. The safety of anagrelide in pregnancy is not yet established.

Aplastic anemia

The diagnosis of aplastic anemia during pregnancy is rare and the causal association between the two is not well established. Nevertheless, in a few cases, a temporal association exists between the onset of pancytopenia during pregnancy and resolution after delivery of the infant or termination of the pregnancy[63]. Life-threatening complications are usually the result of neutropenic infections and, therefore, the decision to terminate a pregnancy should be based on the severity of the aplasia as judged by the difficulty in supporting the peripheral blood counts. Since the mechanism remains unknown, women with a history of aplastic anemia should be advised of the potential risk of future pregnancies. The blood counts of infants delivered from women with aplastic anemia appear to be unaffected[64].

Paroxysmal nocturnal hemoglobinuria

Paroxysmal nocturnal hemoglobinuria (PNH) is a clonal disorder of hematopoietic stem cells caused by the absence of an entire family of membrane-linked proteins[65]. The diagnosis is usually established by flow cytometry of peripheral blood cells that lack a member of this family known as 'decay accelerating factor' or CD55. The clinical manifestations of PNH include both a hemolytic anemia and impaired production of red cells, neutrophils and platelets. A common complication of this disorder is venous thrombosis, which may occur in the cerebral, mesenteric or hepatic veins[66]. Because of this thrombotic risk, most patients with PNH require long-term anticoagulation therapy.

Pregnancy in patients with PNH is hazardous. Some patients develop worsening bone marrow aplasia or increased hemolysis that requires red cell transfusions. Venous thromboses may occur during pregnancy and are more likely in patients with previous thrombotic episodes; therefore, preventative anticoagulation administration is generally recommended throughout pregnancy[67]. Patients with prior thrombotic episodes are urged to avoid pregnancy.

DISORDERS OF PLATELETS

Thrombocytopenia during pregnancy is a frequently encountered clinical problem. Although thrombocytopenia may be caused by either insufficient bone marrow production or increased peripheral destruction of platelets, most cases occurring in pregnancy are the result of platelet destruction and consequently a bone marrow examination is not usually necessary. Evaluation of thrombocytopenia should always include a morphological review of a peripheral blood smear to help exclude the possibility of ethylenediaminetetraacetic acid-induced platelet agglutination or enlarged platelets which may not be appropriately detected by an automated counter[68]. In addition, identification of red cell abnormalities on the peripheral smear may help define the cause of the disorder. Common causes of maternal thrombocytopenia are summarized in Table 1.

Gestational thrombocytopenia

About 10% of pregnancies are associated with an incidentally detected thrombocytopenia that ranges from 70 000–150 000/μl. In individuals with gestational thrombocytopenia, there is no antecedent history of autoimmune disease or other identifiable cause of thrombocytopenia and the platelet count prior to pregnancy is normal. Gestational thrombocytopenia is not associated with an adverse outcome in the mother or newborn[69–71]. Women with gestational thrombocytopenia are likely to have similar courses in subsequent pregnancies. In the past, many of these patients were felt to have an immune-mediated thrombocytopenia that led to a more aggressive therapeutic approach, especially during delivery. At present, it is recommended that in uncomplicated pregnancies with incidental thrombocytopenia, vaginal delivery can be completed without special precautions[69,70].

Immune thrombocytopenic purpura

Immune destruction of platelets by antibodies that react with the platelet surface may cause thrombocytopenia

Table 1 Thrombocytopenia in pregnancy

Etiology	Diagnosis	Severity	Associated clinical findings	Coagulopathy	Effect on neonatal platelet count
Gestational	second or third trimester	mild	none	none	none
ITP	any time	moderate–severe	none	none	none–severe
Pre-eclampsia	third trimester	mild–moderate	hypertension	none	none–mild
HELLP	third trimester or postpartum	moderate–severe	MAHA, renal insufficiency, hepatic dysfunction	none	none–mild
TTP	second trimester	moderate–severe	MAHA, CNS disease, renal insufficiency	none	none
HUS	Postpartum	moderate–severe	MAHA, renal insufficiency	none	none
AFLP	third trimester	mild	hepatic dysfunction	severe DIC	none–mild

ITP, immune thrombocytopenic purpura; HELLP, hemolysis, elevated liver enzymes, low platelets; TTP, thrombotic thrombocytopenic purpura; HUS, hemolytic uremic syndrome; AFLP, acute fatty liver of pregnancy; MAHA, microangiopathic hemolytic anemia; CNS, central nervous system; DIC, disseminated intravascular coagulation that is occasionally severe. The disorder may be unrelated to other diseases or may be the result of medications, viral infections (including human immunodeficiency virus), lymphoproliferative disorders or autoimmune disease.

When compared to gestational thrombocytopenia, immune thrombocytopenic purpura (ITP) is a relatively uncommon cause of thrombocytopenia of pregnancy[72]. It is important to attempt to distinguish gestational thrombocytopenia from ITP, since the diagnosis has major implications. The diagnosis is established, in part, by the severity of the thrombocytopenia. Laboratory testing for antiplatelet antibodies is rarely helpful[73]. However, clinical and laboratory evaluation should include careful monitoring of blood pressure, liver function testing and human immunodeficiency virus antibody testing in patients with risk factors to assess for other causes of thrombocytopenia. Unless otherwise clinically indicated, routine evaluation for systemic lupus erythematosis or the antiphospholipid antibody syndrome is not generally required.

The treatment of ITP during pregnancy is based on the severity of the thrombocytopenia and the presence or absence of bleeding. No specific therapy is recommended if the platelet count is greater than 50 000/µl or greater than 30 000/µl in the first or second trimester[73]. Initial therapy for more severe thrombocytopenias, or when bleeding occurs, is controversial. Some authorities advocate glucocorticoids, similar to treatment in non-pregnant patients with ITP. However, the toxicity from this approach is substantial and includes gestational diabetes mellitus[74]. Many other investigators recommend intravenous immunoglobulin for the initial therapy, particularly in patients with a platelet count of less than 10 000/µl in the third trimester. Splenectomy is appropriate for severe thrombocytopenia and is best used in the second trimester, since splenectomy in the first trimester is associated with increased preterm labor and in the third trimester is technically difficult[73]. Other cytotoxic or immunosuppressive agents are generally not recommended during pregnancy.

Fetal and neonatal thrombocytopenia may occur with passive transfer of antiplatelet antibodies to the placental circulation. A large number of studies have shown that no maternal characteristic, including the platelet count, reliably correlates with the fetal platelet count. The incidence of neonatal thrombocytopenia (platelet count < 50 000/µl) is estimated to be less than 10%, but varies considerably among studies, suggesting that the diagnosis of maternal ITP is not always well established[73,75,76]. Percutaneous umbilical blood sampling is the most reliable means of obtaining an accurate fetal platelet count, but it is associated with some fetal complications and this test should therefore be performed with caution[77,78]. The platelet count may fall in the first few days of life and continued monitoring is therefore recommended[79,80]. In infants with thrombocytopenia, the risk of bleeding appears to be low, although a small number of infants may develop intracranial hemorrhage. Because of this risk, an imaging study of the brain is recommended if the platelet count is below 20 000/µl[73]. Neonatal thrombocytopenia is generally treated with intravenous immunoglobulin or glucocorticoids[73,79].

Pre-eclampsia and the HELLP syndrome

Pre-eclampsia is defined by the presence of hypertension and proteinuria, which occur in approximately 10% of pregnancies during the third trimester. Up to one-half of patients with pre-eclampsia will have thrombocytopenia, although the decrease in platelet count is usually mild and bleeding is uncommon[72,81]. Although the pathogenesis of this disorder is uncertain, the thrombocytopenia is the result of increased platelet destruction and, therefore, persistent thrombocytopenia should be considered a marker of ongoing disease[72]. Microangiopathic hemolytic anemia is rare and the lack of liver, renal and neurological complications help to make the distinction from other causes of thrombocytopenia. However, laboratory findings of disseminated intravascular coagulation may be present[72,82,83].

Resolution of pre-eclampsia is facilitated by delivery of the infant and consequently the clinical manifestations, including thrombocytopenia, resolve in about 2 days. Neonatal thrombocytopenia may occur, but this is usually related to other intervening illnesses, such as sepsis. The role of antiplatelet agents, such as aspirin, for the prevention and treatment of pre-eclampsia is unproven.

A related syndrome to pre-eclampsia is known as HELLP (hemolysis, elevated liver enzymes, low platelet count). Since proteinuria and hypertension frequently occur, the overlap may make these two disorders difficult to distinguish. Thrombocytopenia is a prominent finding in this disorder and many patients have platelet counts < 50 000/µl. Although elevated transaminase levels occur, severe liver dysfunction is uncommon, allowing distinction from the acute fatty liver of pregnancy. Microangiopathic hemolytic anemia is common and consequently distinction from thrombotic thrombocytopenic purpura may be difficult[82].

Treatment of HELLP generally includes prompt delivery of the infant. Strategies to extend the pregnancy for several days to allow for fetal maturation are occasionally used[82]. The use of glucocorticoids or plasmapheresis remains of uncertain benefit. Thrombocytopenia that persists longer than 5–6 days postpartum suggests an alternative diagnosis, such as thrombotic thrombocytopenic purpura.

Thrombotic thrombocytopenic purpura and the hemolytic uremic syndrome

Thrombotic thrombocytopenic purpura (TTP) and the hemolytic uremic syndrome (HUS) are related disorders that are characterized by microangiopathic hemolytic anemia causing fragmented red cells (schistocytes) and thrombocytopenia. TTP is characterized by the clinical findings of neurological abnormalities, fever and renal dysfunction, along with the laboratory findings of a microangiopathic hemolytic anemia, thrombocytopenia and an increased serum lactate dehydrogenase. Most patients will not demonstrate all of the clinical findings[81,83]. The pathogenesis remains uncertain, but the end result is widespread thrombotic occlusion within the microvasculature. Although this disorder may occur anytime during pregnancy or the postpartum, most cases occur before 24 weeks of gestation. When presenting in the third trimester or postpartum, the distinction between TTP and pre-eclampsia or HELLP is particularly difficult[82]. Serial reviews of the peripheral blood smear to observe for schistocytes may be helpful in identifying patients with TTP.

Treatment of TTP in pregnancy is similar to that of non-pregnant patients. The use of daily plasmapheresis has markedly improved the outlook for this disease for both the mother and the infant[82,84,85]. Although not well defined, the risk of recurrence with subsequent pregnancies seems to be high[84].

HUS is similar to TTP, although the clinical manifestations are usually limited to acute renal disease and the disorder typically occurs in the postpartum period. Treatment of HUS is poorly defined and the prognosis is poor, with mortality rates as high as 46%[83,86]. Success with plasmapheresis has been reported, but the results are less satisfying than with TTP. Anecdotal therapy with platelet function inhibitors, glucocorticoids, heparin, vincristine and splenectomy have also been reported[83]. Long-term dialysis or renal transplantation may be required in patients who survive.

Acute fatty liver of pregnancy

The typical findings in acute fatty liver of pregnancy include a 1–2-week history of nausea, vomiting, malaise, abdominal pain and jaundice in the third trimester. Most patients develop thrombocytopenia and the laboratory findings of disseminated intravascular coagulation. Liver biopsy shows lipid accumulation within the hepatocytes. The etiology of this disorder is uncertain, but a defect in fatty acid metabolism recently has been proposed[87]. The distinction from pre-eclampsia may be difficult at times. Treatment includes rapid delivery, which improves fetal and maternal mortality, and complete hepatic recovery is typical[82].

Neonatal alloimmune thrombocytopenia

Most cases are diagnosed after birth in which an infant develops purpura or other signs of hemorrhage. Clinically significant neonatal alloimmune thrombocytopenia has been estimated to occur in one in 2000 to one in 10 000 births. Most cases are caused by maternal sensitization to the PL[A1] antigen from either a prior pregnancy or a transfusion and the resulting antibodies cross-react with platelets from the infant. The disease may be severe and intracranial hemorrhage *in utero* or in the neonatal period may occur. Treatment with compatible platelets (including maternal platelets that have been washed and irradiated) may be needed. Intravenous immunoglobulin has also been used successfully. Subsequent pregnancies may also be affected and, therefore, fetal blood sampling and *in utero* platelet transfusions should be considered[72]. Screening of all pregnant women for PL[A1] antigen status has been proposed, but is not routinely performed[88].

Congenital thrombocytopenia

Non-immune congenital thrombocytopenia is an uncommon cause of low platelet counts in infants. In some cases, megakaryocytes are absent on bone marrow examination and this may progress to widespread bone marrow failure. In addition, several clinical syndromes have been described, including thrombocytopenia with absent radii (TAR) and the Wiskott–Aldrich syndrome. In other cases, thrombocytopenia that is associated with renal disease, albinism or intrinsic platelet defects (Bernard–Soulier syndrome) may occur[89]. Treatment of these disorders usually involves platelet transfusions, but, because the bleeding is usually mild, the diagnosis may be delayed into adulthood.

VENOUS THROMBOEMBOLISM
Diagnosis of venous thromboembolism

Lower extremity venous stasis, caused by compression of the pelvic veins from an enlarging uterus, is a significant risk factor for thrombosis. Changes in the coagulation and fibrinolytic factors that favor procoagulant activity provide a second thrombotic risk factor. The postpartum period represents a time of continued high risk for venous thromboembolism that accounts for about 25% of the thromboses associated with pregnancy[90].

Because of the therapeutic implications of a venous thromboembolism in pregnancy, care should be taken to ensure that the diagnosis is correct. The clinical features of a deep venous thrombosis in the leg include pain, swelling, warmth and erythema. There is also a striking predilection for thrombosis in the left leg during pregnancy, but these are unreliable indicators of the disease[90]. The diagnosis is usually confirmed by either duplex ultrasonography or impedance plethysmography, both of which have been proven reliable so that contrast venography is rarely needed[90,91]. In the absence of a clinical deep venous thrombosis, signs and symptoms of a pulmonary embolism, such as chest pain, dyspnea and tachypnea, are unreliable and the diagnosis therefore requires objective confirmation. To avoid radiation exposure during pregnancy, one approach is to perform a non-invasive study of the legs for the diagnosis of a deep venous thrombosis and a positive study would be adequate evidence of thromboembolism. However, this approach may not be helpful if the thrombosis originates in the pelvic veins and, therefore, ventilation–perfusion scanning or pulmonary angiography may need to be performed[90].

Treatment of venous thromboembolism

Women diagnosed with venous thromboembolism during pregnancy should receive heparin for the initial management. Typically, this is given as an intravenous bolus followed by a continuous infusion adjusted to achieve an activated partial thromboplastin time of 1.5–2.5 times the laboratory control value. Heparin anticoagulation should be continued throughout pregnancy and this is usually administered as an adjusted-dose subcutaneous injection every 12 h[90]. Some investigators recommend that heparin be discontinued about 24 h prior to the planned delivery to allow adequate time for clearance of the drug[92]. Using this approach, regional anesthesia or a Cesarean section may be safely undertaken. About 6 h postpartum, heparin should be restarted and warfarin initiated for at least 6 weeks or to complete a 3-month course of therapy[90].

Complications of this approach include the risk of clinically significant bleeding that is estimated to occur in approximately 2% of patients. Decreased bone density is a frequent finding in women treated with heparin throughout pregnancy, although clinically significant osteoporosis leading to a fracture is uncommon. Bone loss is reversible when the heparin is discontinued[90,93]. Thrombocytopenia is a rare, but life-threatening, complication of heparin use in which antibody-mediated platelet thrombi are formed. When diagnosed, heparin must be discontinued and an alternative anticoagulant utilized, since further heparin use may lead to arterial or venous thromboembolism[94].

Recently, several preparations of low-molecular-weight heparin have become available and will probably prove adequate alternatives to standard heparin in many settings. These agents are administered subcutaneously once or twice daily and do not appear to cross the placenta[95,96]. Furthermore, they appear to have a lower risk of thrombocytopenia and osteoporosis than standard heparin. To date, the published experience with low-molecular-weight heparin for the treatment of venous thromboembolism in pregnancy is limited and, therefore, until sufficient experience is developed, these agents cannot be routinely recommended in this setting.

Prevention of venous thromboembolism

Prophylaxis against venous thrombosis should be considered during pregnancy in patients with a history of a prior thrombosis, a history of an inherited or acquired hypercoagulable state, or any other condition that requires long-term anticoagulation therapy, such as prosthetic heart valves. Patients with a history of mechanical valves, antithrombin III deficiency or antiphospholipid antibodies with thrombosis are at the highest risk; therefore, by current standards, they should receive full-dose heparin throughout pregnancy. The use of low-molecular-weight heparin for these conditions may be considered, but is not yet well established[97,98]. The risk of thrombosis in other situations does not appear as high and prophylaxis with low-molecular-weight heparin therefore appears to be adequate[90,95,98].

Inherited coagulation disorders and pregnancy

Women of reproductive age who develop a venous thromboembolism should be considered for testing of known hypercoagulable risk factors including deficiencies in antithrombin III, protein C and protein S, as well as a resistance to activated protein C (APC). When a known hypercoagulable state is identified in patients with a thromboembolism, patients are at risk of a recurrence during pregnancy and should receive prophylaxis against further thrombosis. In women with recurrent miscarriage or fetal loss, there appears to be a modest risk (approximately two-fold) of identifying an inherited hypercoagulable state[99–101]. Whether these women would benefit from prophylactic anticoagulation has yet to be defined.

Antithrombin III deficiency

Antithrombin III is a naturally occurring anticoagulant that inhibits proteases of the coagulation pathway. This reaction is increased approximately 1000-fold in the presence of heparin[102]. The incidence of thrombosis during pregnancy in women with antithrombin III deficiency is reported to be as high as 70% and, therefore, anticoagulation with heparin is indicated throughout pregnancy and warfarin is indicated in the postpartum state[90]. Although its role is not well defined, daily administration of antithrombin III concentrate during the peripartum period may also be used[103].

Protein C and protein S deficiencies

Protein C and protein S are naturally occurring anticoagulants that act together to inactivate factor Va and factor VIIIa in the coagulation pathway. Protein C is activated by thrombin in the presence of thrombomodulin on the endothelial surface. The activated form of protein C combines with protein S to cleave factors Va and VIIIa so that these molecules no longer accelerate hemostasis (Figure 1).

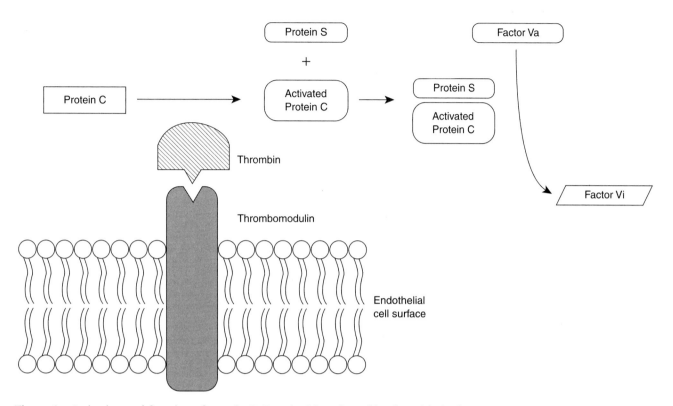

Figure 1   Activation and function of protein C. Protein C is activated by thrombin in the presence of thrombomodulin on the endothelial surface. Activated protein C (APC) combines with protein S to cleave factor Va and factor VIIIa (not shown) so that the inactive form of these molecules (factor Vi and VIIIi) no longer accelerates hemostasis. An inherited mutation in factor V (factor V Leiden) renders the factor Va molecule resistant to breakdown by APC, which leads to increased hemostatic activity and a risk of venous thromboembolism

Women with deficiency in protein C or protein S are at risk of venous thromboembolism, although the risk is not as high as in antithrombin III deficiency[90,104]. Patients with these deficiencies have been successfully treated with heparin or low-molecular-weight heparin for prophylaxis during pregnancy followed by warfarin postpartum. Anticoagulant treatment of individuals with a deficiency who have never had a thrombotic event is of uncertain benefit.

Resistance to activated protein C

Beginning in 1993, the understanding of hypercoagulable states changed dramatically with the identification of resistance to activated protein C (APC)[105]. In this study, the activated partial thromboplastin time was measured with and without the addition of exogenous APC and the ratio between the two was determined. In most healthy individuals, the addition of APC to plasma leads to a prolongation of the clotting time. This is the expected result, since factors Va and VIIIa are essential for the rapid formation of a fibrin clot. In contrast, the addition of APC does not affect the clotting time nearly as much in some patients, suggesting a 'resistance'. The cause of this resistance has been determined to be a mutation in the gene for factor V,

known as 'factor V Leiden', rendering the protein resistant to breakdown by APC[106]. Persons with this mutation have persistent factor Va activity, leading to increased clotting. APC resistance is found in 2–7% of Europeans and about 3% of Americans, but is much less common in persons of other ethnic backgrounds. Resistance to APC appears to be the most prevalent hereditary risk for venous thrombosis identified to date.

Pregnant women with resistance to APC (or factor V Leiden) seem to be at increased risk of thrombosis. For example, in selected women with thrombosis, as many as one-half of patients have this mutation[107]. However, in women with factor V Leiden, but without prior venous thromboembolism, the incidence of a pregnancy-related thrombosis is undefined. Until larger studies are completed, the question of whether all pregnant women should be tested for the mutation remains unanswered.

Antiphospholipid antibody syndrome

Antiphospholipid antibodies are associated with arterial or venous thrombosis, thrombocytopenia and recurrent miscarriage or fetal loss. One-third to one-half of patients with systemic lupus erythematosus will have detectable antiphospholipid antibodies, but the syndrome frequently occurs in the absence of other autoimmune diseases[108].

Because the antiphospholipid antibody syndrome is associated with a variety of adverse events in pregnancy, testing in women of reproductive age has become common practice. These antibodies may be defined as either a lupus anticoagulant or as anticardiolipin antibodies. The diagnosis of a lupus anticoagulant depends on demonstrating an abnormal clotting time in a phospholipid-dependent assay, usually measured as a dilute Russell viper venom time. This result is usually confirmed by a phospholipid neutralization procedure. The activated partial thromboplastin time is prolonged in about 70% of patients with a lupus anticoagulant, but this is an unreliable screening test. Anticardiolipin antibodies are detected immunologically and classified as either IgG or IgM antibodies[109]. When the antiphospholipid antibody syndrome is suspected, tests for both the lupus anticoagulant and anticardiolipin antibodies should be performed.

Pregnancy-related thrombosis associated with antiphospholipid antibodies should be treated with full-dose heparin throughout pregnancy and with warfarin for 6–8 weeks postpartum[90]. Low-molecular-weight heparin has also been used successfully in a smaller number of patients[98]. It has been recommended that women with antiphospholipid antibody syndrome, but without previous thrombosis, be treated with lower doses of heparin, but the optimal dose is undefined.

Recurrent first-trimester miscarriage or an unexplained second- or third-trimester fetal death are associated with women with antiphospholipid antibodies[109]. In comparison, a large case–control study found no difference in the incidence of antiphospholipid antibodies in patients experiencing a single miscarriage or fetal death[110]. Prevention of further miscarriages and fetal loss in pregnant women with antiphospholipid antibodies remains controversial and poorly defined. Prednisone, heparin and low-dose aspirin are frequently used alone or in combination, with apparently similar results[109].

Prosthetic heart valves

Women of reproductive age who require heart-valve replacement generally receive mechanical valves, because of a concern that bioprosthetic valves deteriorate at an accelerated rate during pregnancy[111]. In women with mechanical valves, anticoagulation throughout pregnancy is recommended, but the most appropriate regimen has not been defined, primarily because of the concern of warfarin embryopathy during the first trimester. Heparin given throughout pregnancy to achieve an activated partial thromboplastin time greater than two times the control is commonly employed, but the use of warfarin in the second and third trimesters (switching to heparin prior to delivery)

has also been used successfully[112]. Low-molecular-weight heparin may prove an acceptable approach, although data remain scant[95,113].

Hormonal therapy and thrombosis

Early studies on the use of oral contraceptives identified high doses of estrogen as a risk factor for venous thrombosis[114]. Because of this, the current generation of oral contraceptive agents contain lower estrogen doses (less than 50 µg of ethinyl estradiol per day) and the relative risk is about 16/100 000 women-years, considerably lower than the thromboembolic risk of pregnancy[115]. Recent data have also suggested that there is an increased venous thromboembolic risk of the newer progestin agents gestodene and desogesteral when compared to earlier products[116,117].

In women with a personal or family history of venous thromboembolic disease, evaluation of other risk factors should be considered prior to the start of oral contraceptives. In particular, the identification of factor V Leiden appears to be an independent risk factor for venous thromboembolism in women on oral contraceptives[118,119].

The use of postmenopausal hormone replacement therapy with estrogen is widespread and of proven benefit. Although some observers consider these agents to be of thrombogenic potential, similar to early oral contraceptives containing high doses of estrogen, this remains unproven. No increased thromboembolic risk has been identified in individuals without other risk factors[120]. Whether patients with an additional acquired or hereditary risk for venous thrombosis may safely use postmenopausal hormone replacement is undetermined.

BLEEDING DISORDERS
von Willebrand disease

The most common inherited bleeding disorder in women is von Willebrand disease, which occurs in about one in 10 000 individuals. The normal function of von Willebrand factor includes binding to factor VIII to increase its plasma half-life and acting as an aggregating agent that links platelets to subendothelium during vascular injury. Levels of von Willebrand factor normally change by about 10% during the menstrual cycle and are lowest during menses[121]. Oral contraceptives and pregnancy increase von Willebrand factor by two- to three-fold, making the diagnosis of von Willebrand disease difficult in these settings.

The classification of von Willebrand disease has recently been updated and simplified to include three broad categories[122]. Type 1 von Willebrand disease is a quantitative decrease in the circulating amount of von Willebrand factor and this type accounts for 80–90% of all patients with the disease. Type 2 von Willebrand disease is a qualitative deficiency in von Willebrand factor so that some of the circulating factor (usually about one-half of the total level) is dysfunctional. Several subtypes of type 2 disease are recognized. Type 3 von Willebrand disease is a rare form of the disease in which there is a complete absence of von Willebrand factor.

The diagnosis of von Willebrand disease requires a careful personal and family history and appropriate laboratory testing. In patients with a bleeding history suggestive of von Willebrand disease, the activated partial thromboplastin time and bleeding time may be measured, but neither is sensitive or specific for this disorder. Determination of von Willebrand factor antigen and von Willebrand factor activity (or ristocetin cofactor activity) are necessary to establish the diagnosis and type[122].

Treatment of von Willebrand disease varies, depending on the type and severity of bleeding. Women with type 1 disease rarely require therapy during pregnancy, since the plasma levels normalize in most patients, particularly in the third trimester. However, factor levels decline rapidly in the postpartum period and patients are therefore at risk of hemorrhage during that time. When appropriate, most patients with type 1 disease can be treated with 1-desamino-8-D-arginine vasopressin (DDAVP), a synthetic analog of vasopressin that has little pressor effect. The medication causes a release of pre-formed von Willebrand factor from the endothelium into the plasma so that normal levels are usually achieved. After several days of therapy, some patients develop tachyphylaxis to this agent, limiting its usefulness in the treatment of severe bleeding[123]. Two preparations of DDAVP are widely available. The intravenous form is administered once or twice daily and is usually well tolerated, although hypotension, flushing and hyponatremia may develop. An intranasal form of DDAVP is particularly useful for women with von Willebrand disease and heavy menstrual bleeding[124]. DDAVP is useful in some patients with type 2 disease, but is of no benefit in type 3 disease.

Patients with type 1 disease and severe bleeding, some patients with type 2 disease and all patients with type 3 disease require replacement therapy of von Willebrand factor. In the past, cryoprecipitate was the standard treatment, but, at present, several preparations of factor VIII are available that contain sufficient von Willebrand factor to be reliably used for von Willebrand factor replacement. These products offer a potential advantage over cryoprecipitate in that they have undergone virucidal treatment[125].

Type 2B von Willebrand disease represents a unique subtype in which the von Willebrand factor has increased platelet affinity, resulting in spontaneous platelet aggregation and mild thrombocytopenia[126]. The use of DDAVP is generally not recommended, because the increased levels may lead to the development of thrombocytopenia. In pregnancy, the von Willebrand factor levels are increased and worsening thrombocytopenia, leading to hemorrhage, may occur[127].

Hemophilia and other inherited clotting factor disorders

Deficiencies of factor VIII and factor IX cause hemophilia A and B, respectively. Since the genes for these factors occur on the X chromosome, hemophilia A and B are inherited in a sex-linked recessive pattern and, consequently, it is rare for women to be afflicted with the disease. During pregnancy, factor VIII levels increase in proportion to von Willebrand factor. Approximately 50% of the affected factor circulates in female carriers of hemophilia A or B, although some women have significantly lower levels[128]. Peripartum hemorrhage may occur in either hemophilia A or B and replacement with either DDAVP (for low levels of factor VIII) or a purified factor preparation should be used.

Other inherited clotting factor deficiencies, including factors XI and VII, do not pose a significant risk of bleeding unless the level is below 25% of normal. In these cases, treatment with fresh frozen plasma to supplement the deficient factor for several days postpartum should prevent hemorrhage.

Factor XIII deficiency is a rare cause of bleeding, but poses a special problem because of its association with miscarriages in affected individuals. Replacement with fresh frozen plasma throughout pregnancy has been used successfully. Since the half-life of factor XIII is long and only approximately 5% of the normal levels is required, replacement therapy is not difficult. In patients with prior spontaneous abortions, prophylactic plasma infusion has led to an uncomplicated pregnancy[129].

Acquired factor VIII inhibitor

Autoantibodies to factor VIII are an uncommon cause of serious bleeding[130]. Approximately 10% of cases occur in the postpartum setting and most cases occur within 3 months of delivery. Postpartum inhibitors occur spontaneously after the first or any subsequent pregnancy. Sites of bleeding are similar to those found in hemophilia and include soft tissue, intramuscular, intra-articular and the genitourinary tract[131].

Treatment of this disorder has not been well defined, but is based primarily on the strength of the inhibitor [as measured in Bethesda Units (BU)] and the severity of bleeding. Patients with low titer inhibitors (< 5 BU) may be treated with infusions of factor VIII for bleeding episodes. High-titer inhibitors that are associated with serious bleeding are usually treated with immunosuppressive therapy to eradicate the antibody and replacement products to control the bleeding[132]. Since a high antibody titer is difficult to overcome with the usual human factor VIII preparation, porcine factor VIII or factor IX concentrate is usually needed for the treatment of bleeding[133,134]. Plasmapheresis or intravenous immunoglobulin may be of benefit for some patients. Although the average time to resolution is 11 months, a complete recovery occurs in over 90% of patients[131]. A small number of patients have had subsequent pregnancies after resolution of an acquired factor VIII inhibitor and no recurrences have been reported[135,136]. However, subsequent pregnancy while the inhibitor is still detectable may pose a significant risk of bleeding to the fetus and, therefore, pregnancy should be avoided during that time.

Disseminated intravascular coagulation

Activation of blood coagulation factors in the absence of a distinct clot leads to formation of fibrin within the circulation. The procoagulants that lead to fibrinogen activation may either be exogenous or endogenous to the vasculature, but, during pregnancy, they frequently arise from fetal or placental tissue. Fibrin formation within the circulation may lead to microthrombi in the small blood vessels of the lung, liver, kidney or other tissues. In addition, fibrinolysis occurs simultaneously and consequently the identification of fibrin(ogen) degradation products in serum is common. Along with the consumption of fibrinogen, platelet activation may occur; therefore, thrombocytopenia is commonly found in this syndrome.

Disseminated intravascular coagulation (DIC) is a clinical diagnosis that is a manifestation of an underlying disorder[137]. In pregnancy, DIC may occur in placental abruption, amniotic fluid embolism, saline-induced abortions, or dead fetus syndrome. Other causes of DIC, including shock or sepsis, may also occur during pregnancy.

Placental abruption results in DIC and hypofibrinogenemia that may develop within 8 h. In this setting, the major complication is hemorrhage. Treatment includes blood component support followed by delivery of the infant. Replacement of fibrinogen is not typically necessary and this will usually correct within 12 h[138,139].

Amniotic fluid emboli is a rare event that is thought to occur more often in older, multiparous women or in the setting of a difficult delivery. The presence of amniotic fluid in the maternal circulation is the result of injury or rupture of the uterus. The immediate consequence of this syndrome is sudden circulatory and pulmonary failure; treatment therefore entails correction of the circulatory collapse and mechanical ventilation. Procoagulants released into the circulation from the amniotic fluid lead to rapid and severe DIC. The use of cryoprecipitate to correct hypofibrinogenemia may also be of benefit[140–142]. Despite aggressive therapy, the mortality of this syndrome is greater than 80%.

Fetal death *in utero* is an uncommon cause of DIC, since it is easily recognized by ultrasound and can be treated with evacuation of the uterus. In saline-induced abortions, laboratory evidence of DIC may be present, but this is usually transient and does not require therapy. However, cases of amniotic fluid embolism and severe DIC complicating therapeutic abortion have also been described[143]. DIC associated with a hydatidiform mole resolves quickly with the emptying of the uterus.

REFERENCES

1. Balloch AJ, Cauchi MN. Reference ranges for haematology parameters in pregnancy derived from patient populations. *Clin Lab Haematol* 1993;15:7–14
2. Hytten F. Blood volume changes in normal pregnancy. *Clin Hematol* 1985;14:601–12
3. Bain BJ. *Blood Cells: A Practical Guide.* London: Blackwell Science, 1995
4. Beguin Y, Lipscei G, Oris R, et al. Serum immunoreactive erythropoietin during pregnancy and in the early postpartum. *Br J Haematol* 1990;76:545–9
5. Kaushansky K. Thrombopoietin: the primary regulator of platelet production. *Blood* 1995;86:419–31
6. Meng YG, Martin TG, Peterson ML, et al. Circulating thrombopoietin concentrations in thrombocytopenic patients, including cancer patients following chemotherapy, with or without peripheral blood progenitor cell transplantation. *Br J Haematol* 1996;95:535–41
7. Lecander I, Astedt B. Isolation of a new specific plasminogen activator inhibitor from pregnancy plasma. *Br J Haematol* 1986;62:221–8
8. Cook JD, Skikne BS, Lynch SR, Reusser ME. Estimates of iron sufficiency in the US population. *Blood* 1986;68:726–31
9. Bentley DP. Iron metabolism and anaemia in pregnancy. *Clin Haematol* 1985;14:613–28
10. Carriaga MT, Skikne BS, Finley B, et al. Serum transferrin receptor for the detection of iron deficiency in pregnancy. *Am J Clin Nutr* 1991;54:1077–81
11. Iyengar L, Rajalakshmi K. Effect of folic acid supplement on birth weights of infants. *Am J Obstet Gynecol* 1975;122:332–6
12. Czeizel AE, Dudas I. Prevention of the first occurrence of neural-tube defects by periconceptional vitamin supplementation. *N Engl J Med* 1992;327:1832–5
13. Chanarin I. Diagnosis of cobalamin deficiency: the old and the new. *Br J Haematol* 1997;97:695–700
14. Higginbottom MC, Sweetman L, Nyhan WL. A syndrome of methylmalonic aciduria, homocystinuria, megaloblastic anemia and neurologic abnormalities in a vitamin B_{12}-deficient breast-fed infant of a strict vegetarian. *N Engl J Med* 1978;299:317–23
15. Johnson PR, Roloff JS. Vitamin B_{12} deficiency in an infant strictly breast-fed by a mother with latent pernicious anemia. *J Pediatr* 1982;100:917–19
16. Armbruster DA. Neonatal hemoglobinopathy screening. *Lab Med* 1990;21:815–22
17. Milner PF, Jones BR, Dobler J. Outcome of pregnancy in sickle cell anemia and sickle cell-hemoglobin C disease. *Am J Obstet Gynecol* 1980;138:239–45

18. Powars DR, Sandhu M, Niland-Weiss JJ, *et al.* Pregnancy in sickle cell disease. *Obstet Gynecol* 1986;67:217–28

19. Reid CD, Charache S, Lubin B, *et al.* Contraception and pregnancy. In *Management and Therapy of Sickle Cell Disease.* Bethesda: National Institutes of Health, 1995:75–8

20. Koshy M, Burd L, Wallace D, *et al.* Prophylactic red-cell transfusions in pregnant patients with sickle cell disease. *N Engl J Med* 1988;319:1447–52

21. Wayne AS, Kevy SV, Nathan DG. Transfusion management of sickle cell disease. *Blood* 1993;81:1109–23

22. Janes SL, Pocock M, Bishop E, Bevan DH. Automated red cell exchange in sickle cell disease. *Br J Haematol* 1997;97:256–8

23. Charache S, Scott J, Niebyl J, Bonds D. Management of sickle cell disease in pregnant patients. *Obstet Gynecol* 1980;55:407–10

24. Koshy M. Sickle cell disease and pregnancy. *Blood Rev* 1994;8:157–64

25. Rosse WF, Gallagher D, Kinney TR, *et al.* Transfusion and alloimmunization in sickle cell disease. *Blood* 1990; 76:1431–7

26. Charache S, Terrin ML, Moore RD, *et al.* Effect of hydroxyurea on the frequency of painful crises in sickle cell anemia. *N Engl J Med* 1995;332:1317–22

27. Gaston MH, Verter JI, Woods G, *et al.* Prophylaxis with oral penicillin in children with sickle cell anemia. *N Engl J Med* 1986;314:1593–9

28. Van der Weyden MB, Fong H, Hallam LJ, Harrison C. Red cell ferritin and iron overload in heterozygous β-thalassemia. *Am J Haematol* 1989;30:201–5

29. Mordel N, Birkenfeld A, Goldfarb AN, Rachmilewitz EA. Successful full-term pregnancy in homozygous β-thalassemia major: case report and review of the literature. *Obstet Gynecol* 1989;73:837–40

30. Harris JW. Parvovirus B19 for the hematologist. *Am J Hematol* 1992;39:119–30

31. Bell LM, Naides SJ, Stoffman P, *et al.* Human parvovirus B19 infection among hospital staff members after contact with infected patients. *N Engl J Med* 1989;321:485–90

32. Levy M, Read SE. Erythema infectiosum and pregnancy-related complications. *Can Med Assoc J* 1990;143: 849–58

33. Brown KE, Green SW, de Mayolo JA, *et al.* Congenital anaemia after transplacental B19 parvovirus infection. *Lancet* 1994;343:895–6

34. Baker RI, Manoharan A, De Luca E, Begley CG. Pure red cell aplasia of pregnancy: a distinct clinical entity. *Br J Haematol* 1993;85:619–22

35. Geifman-Holtzman O, Wojtowycz M, Kosmas E, Artal R. Female alloimmunization with antibodies known to cause hemolytic disease. *Obstet Gynecol* 1997;89:272–5

36. Chaplin H Jr, Cohen R, Bloomberg G, *et al.* Pregnancy and idiopathic autoimmune haemolytic anaemia: a prospective study during 6 months gestation and 3 months post-partum. *Br J Haematol* 1973;24:219–29

37. Fanaroff AA, Martin RJ. *Neonatal–Perinatal Medicine. Diseases of the Fetus and Infant,* vol.2. St. Louis: Mosby-Yearbook, 1997

38. Reynoso EE, Shepherd FA, Messner HA, *et al.* Acute leukemia during pregnancy: the Toronto Leukemia Study Group experience with long-term follow-up of

children exposed *in utero* to chemotherapeutic agents. *J Clin Oncol* 1987;5:1098–106

39. Tannirandorn Y, Rodeck CH. Management of immune haemolytic disease in the fetus. *Blood Rev* 1991;5:1–14

40. Zuazu J, Julia A, Sierra J, *et al.* Pregnancy outcome in hematologic malignancies. *Cancer* 1991;67:703–9

41. Siris ES, Leventhal BG, Vaitukaitis JL. Effects of childhood leukemia and chemotherapy on puberty and reproductive function in girls. *N Engl J Med* 1976;294: 1143–6

42. Kenney LB, Nicholson HS, Brasseux C, *et al.* Birth defects in offspring of adult survivors of childhood acute lymphoblastic leukemia. *Cancer* 1996;78:169–76

43. Andrieu JM, Ochoa-Molina ME. Menstrual cycle, pregnancies and offspring before and after MOPP therapy for Hodgkin's disease. *Cancer* 1983;52:435–8

44. Aviles A, Diaz-Maqueo JC, Talavera A, *et al.* Growth and development of children of mothers treated with chemotherapy during pregnancy: current status of 43 children. *Am J Hematol* 1991;36:243–8

45. Kantarjian HM, Deisseroth A, Kurzrock R, *et al.* Chronic myelogenous leukemia: a concise update. *Blood* 1993;82:691–703

46. Arthur CK, Mijovic A, Dannie E, *et al.* Management of chronic myeloid leukaemia in pregnancy. *J Obstet Gynaecol* 1991;11:396–9

47. Fitzgerald D, Rowe JM, Heal J. Leukapheresis for control of chronic myelogenous leukemia during pregnancy. *Am J Hematol* 1986;22:213–18

48. Baer MR, Ozer H, Foon KA. Interferon-α therapy during pregnancy in chronic myelogenous leukaemia and hairy cell leukaemia. *Br J Haematol* 1992;81:167–9

49. Delmer A, Rio B, Bauduer F, *et al.* Pregnancy during myelosuppressive treatment for chronic myelogenous leukaemia. *Br J Haematol* 1992;82:783–4

50. Patel M, Dukes IAF, Hull JC. Use of hydroxyurea in chronic myeloid leukemia during pregnancy: a case report. *Am J Obstet Gynecol* 1991;165:565–6

51. Reichel RP, Linkesch W, Schetitska D. Therapy with recombinant interferon α-2c during unexpected pregnancy in a patient with chronic myeloid leukaemia. *Br J Haematol* 1992;82:472–3

52. Marchioli R. Polycythemia vera: the natural history of 1213 patients followed for 20 years. *Ann Intern Med* 1995;123:656–64

53. Berk PD, Goldberg JD, Donovan PB, *et al.* Therapeutic recommendations in polycythemia vera based on polycythemia vera study group protocols. *Semin Hematol* 1986;23:132–43

54. Ferguson JE II, Ueland K, Aronson WJ. Polycythemia rubra vera and pregnancy. *Obstet Gynecol* 1983;62: 16S–20S

55. Schafer A. Management of thrombocythemia. *Curr Opin Hematol* 1996;3:341–6

56. Tefferi A, Hoagland HC. Issues in the diagnosis and management of essential thrombocythemia. *Mayo Clin Proc* 1994;69:651–5

57. Beressi AH, Tefferi A, Silverstein MN, *et al.* Outcome analysis of 34 pregnancies in women with essential thrombocythemia. *Arch Intern Med* 1995;155:1217–22

58. Beard J, Hillmen P, Anderson CC, *et al.* Primary thrombocythaemia in pregnancy. *Br J Haematol* 1991; 77:371–4

59. Chow EY, Haley LP, Vickars LM. Essential thrombocythemia in pregnancy: platelet count and pregnancy outcome. *Am J Hematol* 1992;41:249–51

60. Randi ML, Barbone E, Rossi C, Girolami A. Essential thrombocythemia and pregnancy: a report of six normal pregnancies in five untreated patients. *Obstet Gynecol* 1994;83:915–17

61. Diez-Martin JL, Banas MH, Fernandez MN. Childbearing age patients with essential thrombocythemia: should they be placed on interferon? *Am J Hematol* 1996;52:331–2

62. Williams JM, Schlesinger PE, Gray AG. Successful treatment of essential thrombocythaemia and recurrent abortion with α-interferon. *Br J Haematol* 1994; 88:647–8

63. Aitchison RGM, Marsh JCW, Hows JM, *et al*. Pregnancy associated aplastic anaemia: a report of five cases and review of current management. *Br J Haematol* 1989; 73:541–5

64. Gordon-Smith EC. Acquired aplastic anemia. In Hoffman R, Benz EJ Jr, Shattil SJ, *et al*. eds. In *Hematology. Basic Principles and Practice*. New York: Churchill Livingstone, 1995:337–49

65. Rosse WF, Ware RE. The molecular basis of paroxysmal nocturnal hemoglobinuria. *Blood* 1995;86: 3277–86

66. Hillmen P, Lewis SM, Bessler M, *et al*. Natural history of paroxysmal nocturnal hemoglobinuria. *N Engl J Med* 1995;333:1253–8

67. Solal-Celigny P, Tertian G, Fernandez H, *et al*. Pregnancy and paroxysmal nocturnal hemoglobinuria. *Arch Intern Med* 1988;148:593–5

68. Altes A, Pujol-Moix N, Muniz-Diaz E, *et al*. Hereditary macrothrombocytopenia and pregnancy. *Thromb Haemost* 1996;76:29–33

69. Aster RH. 'Gestational' thrombocytopenia: a plea for conservative management. *N Engl J Med* 1990;323: 264–6

70. Burrows RF, Kelton JG. Thrombocytopenia at delivery: a prospective survey of 6715 deliveries. *Am J Obstet Gynecol* 1990;162:731–4

71. Samuels P, Bussel JB, Braitman LE, *et al*. Estimation of the risk of thrombocytopenia in the offspring of pregnant women with presumed immune thrombocytopenic purpura. *N Engl J Med* 1990;323:229–35

72. Letsky EA, Greaves M. Guidelines on the investigation and management of thrombocytopenia in pregnancy and neonatal alloimmune thrombocytopenia. *Br J Haematol* 1996;95:21–6

73. George JN, Woolf SH, Raskob GE, *et al*. Idiopathic thrombocytopenic purpura: a practice guideline developed by explicit methods for The American Society of Hematology. *Blood* 1996;88:3–40

74. Rayburn WF. Glucocorticoid therapy for rheumatic diseases: maternal, fetal, and breast-feeding considerations. *Am J Reprod Immunol* 1992;28:138–40

75. Burrows RF, Kelton JG. Low fetal risks in pregnancies associated with idiopathic thrombocytopenic purpura. *Am J Obstet Gynecol* 1990;163:1147–50

76. Dreyfus M, Kaplan C, Verdy E, *et al*. Frequency of immune thrombocytopenia in newborns: a prospective study. *Blood* 1997;89:4402–6

77. Moise KJ Jr, Carpenter RJ Jr, Cotton DB, *et al*. Percutaneous umbilical cord blood sampling in the evaluation of fetal platelet counts in pregnant patients with autoimmune thrombocytopenia purpura. *Obstet Gynecol* 1988;72:346–50

78. Scioscia AL, Grannum PAT, Copel JA, Hobbins JC. The use of percutaneous umbilical blood sampling in immune thrombocytopenic purpura. *Am J Obstet Gynecol* 1988;159:1066–8

79. Blanchette VS, Sacher RA, Ballem PJ, *et al*. Commentary on the management of autoimmune thrombocytopenia during pregnancy and in the neonatal period. *Blut* 1989;59:121–3

80. Burrows RF, Kelton JG. Fetal thrombocytopenia and its relation to maternal thrombocytopenia. *N Engl J Med* 1993;329:1463–6

81. McCrae KR, Samuels P, Schreiber AD. Pregnancy-associated thrombocytopenia: pathogenesis and management. *Blood* 1992;88:2697–714

82. McCrae KR, Cines DB. Thrombotic microangiopathy during pregnancy. *Semin Hematol* 1997;34:148–58

83. Weiner CP. Thrombotic microangiopathy in pregnancy and the postpartum period. *Semin Hematol* 1987;24:119–29

84. Ezra Y, Rose M, Eldor A. Therapy and prevention of thrombotic thrombocytopenic purpura during pregnancy: a clinical study of 16 pregnancies. *Am J Hematol* 1996;51:1–6

85. Rock GA, Shumak KH, Buskard NA, *et al*. and the Canadian Apheresis Study Group Comparison of plasma exchange with plasma infusion in the treatment of thrombotic thrombocytopenic purpura. *N Engl J Med* 1991;325:393–7

86. Li PKT, Lai F, Tam JSL, Lai KN. Acute renal failure due to postpartum haemolytic uraemic syndrome. *Aust NZ J Obstet Gynaecol* 1988;28:228–30

87. Sims HF, Brackett JC, Powell CK. The molecular basis of pediatric long chain 3-hydroxyacyl-CoA dehydrogenase deficiency associated with maternal acute fatty liver of pregnancy. *Proc Natl Acad Sci USA* 1995;92: 841–5

88. Flug F, Karpatkin M, Karpatkin S. Should all pregnant women be tested for their platelet PLA (Zw, HPA-1) phenotype? *Br J Haematol* 1994;86:1–5

89. Warrier I, Lusher JM. Congenital thrombocytopenias. *Curr Opin Hematol* 1995;2:395–401

90. Toglia MR, Weg JG. Venous thromboembolism during pregnancy. *N Engl J Med* 1996;335:108–14

91. Hull RD, Raskob GE, Carter CJ. Serial impedance plethysmography in pregnant patients with clinically suspected deep-vein thrombosis. *Ann Intern Med* 1990; 112:663–7

92. Anderson DR, Ginsberg JS, Burrows R, Brill-Edwards P. Subcutaneous heparin therapy during pregnancy: a need for concern at the time of delivery. *Thromb Haemost* 1991;65:248–50

93. Douketis JD, Ginsberg JS, Burrows RF, *et al*. The effects of long-term heparin therapy during pregnancy on bone density: a prospective matched cohort study. *Thromb Haemost* 1996;75:254–7

94. Ginsberg JS, Hirsh J. Use of antithrombotic agents during pregnancy. *Chest* 1995;108:305s–11s

95. Fejgin MD, Lourwood DL. Low molecular weight heparins and their use in obstetrics and gynecology. *Obstet Gynecol Surv* 1994;49:424–31

96. Rasmussen C, Wadt J, Jacobsen B. Thromboembolic prophylaxis with low molecular weight heparin during pregnancy. *Int J Gynecol Obstet* 1994;47:121–5

97. Dulitzki M, Pauzner R, Langevitz P, *et al.* Low-molecular-weight heparin during pregnancy and delivery: preliminary experience with 41 pregnancies. *Obstet Gynecol* 1996;87:380–3

98. Hunt BJ, Doughty H-A, Majumdar G, *et al.* Thrombo-prophylaxis with low molecular weight heparin (Fragmin) in high risk pregnancies. *Thromb Haemost* 1997;77:39–43

99. Brenner B, Mandel H, Lanir N, *et al.* Activated protein C resistance can be associated with recurrent fetal loss. *Br J Haematol* 1997;97:551–4

100. Preston FE, Rosendaal FR, Walker ID, *et al.* Increased fetal loss in women with heritable thrombophilia. *Lancet* 1996;348:913–16

101. Sanson B-J, Friederich PW, Simioni P, *et al.* The risk of abortion and stillbirth in antithrombin-, protein C-, and protein S-deficient women. *Thromb Haemost* 1996; 75:387–8

102. Pratt CW, Church FC. Antithrombin: structure and function. *Semin Hematol* 1991;28:3–9

103. Owen J. Antithrombin III replacement therapy in pregnancy. *Semin Hematol* 1991;28:46–52

104. Trauscht-Van Horn JJ, Capeless EL, Easterling TR, Bovill EG. Pregnancy loss and thrombosis with protein C deficiency. *Am J Obstet Gynecol* 1992;167:968–72

105. Dahlback B, Carlsson M, Svensson PJ. Familial thrombophilia due to a previously unrecognized mechanism characterized by poor anticoagulant response to activated protein C: prediction of a cofactor to activated protein C. *Proc Natl Acad Sci USA* 1993;90:1004–8

106. Bertina RM, Koeleman BPC, Koster T, *et al.* Mutation in blood coagulation factor V associated with resistance to activated protein C. *Nature (London)* 1994; 369:64–7

107. Bokarewa MI, Bremme K, Blomback M. Arg506–Gln mutation in factor V and risk of thrombosis during pregnancy. *Br J Haematol* 1996;92:473–8

108. Love PE, Santoro SA. Antiphospholipid antibodies: anticardiolipin and the lupus anticoagulant in systemic lupus erythematosus (SLE) and in non-SLE disorders. *Ann Intern Med* 1990;112:682–98

109. Danilenko-Dixon DR, Van Winter JT, Homburger HA. Clinical implications of antiphospholipid antibodies in obstetrics. *Mayo Clin Proc* 1996;71:1118–20

110. Infante-Rivard C, David M, Gauthier R, Rivard G-E. Lupus anticoagulants, anticardiolipin antibodies, and fetal loss. *N Engl J Med* 1991;325:1063–6

111. Oakley CM. Anticoagulants in pregnancy. *Br Heart J* 1995;74:107–11

112. Iturbe-Alessio I, Fonseca MDC, Mutchinik O, *et al.* Risks of anticoagulant therapy in pregnant women with artificial heart valves. *N Engl J Med* 1986;315:1390–3

113. Lee LH, Liauw PCY, Ng ASH. Low molecular weight heparin for thromboprophylaxis during pregnancy in 2 patients with mechanical mitral valve replacement. *Thromb Haemost* 1996;76:627–31

114. Stadel BV. Oral contraceptives and cardiovascular disease. *N Engl J Med* 1981;305:612–18

115. Hull R, Pineo GF. *Disorders of Thrombosis.* Philadelphia: WB Saunders Company, 1996

116. Jick H, Jick SS, Gurewich V, *et al.* Risk of idiopathic cardiovascular death and nonfetal venous thromboembolism in women using oral contraceptives with differing progestagen components. *Lancet* 1995;346: 1589–93

117. Spitzer WO, Lewis MA, Heinemann LAJ, *et al.* Third generation oral contraceptives and risk of venous thromboembolic disorders: an international case–control study. *Br Med J* 1996;312:83–8

118. Bloemenkamp KWM, Rosendaal FR, Helmerhorst FM, *et al.* Enhancement by Factor V Leiden mutation of risk of deep-vein thrombosis associated with oral contraceptives containing a third-generation progestagen. *Lancet* 1995;346:1593–6

119. Vandenbroucke JP, Koster T, Briet E, *et al.* Increased risk of venous thrombosis in oral-contraceptive users who are carriers of factor V Leiden mutation. *Lancet* 1994;344:1453–7

120. Devor M, Barrett-Connor E, Renvall M, *et al.* Estrogen replacement therapy and the risk of venous thrombosis. *Am J Med* 1992;92:275–82

121. Kouides PA, Phatak PD, Sham RL, *et al.* von Willebrand factor and factor VIIIC levels change in relation to the menstrual cycle. *Blood* 1996;88:41a

122. Sadler JE. A revised classification of von Willebrand disease. *Thromb Haemost* 1994;71:520–5

123. Rodeghiero F, Castaman G, Mannucci P. Clinical indications for desmopressin (DDAVP) in congenital and acquired von Willebrand disease. *Blood Rev* 1991; 5:155–61

124. Rose EH, Aledort LM. Nasal spray desmopressin (DDAVP) for mild hemophilia A and von Willebrand disease. *Ann Intern Med* 1991;114:563–8

125. Mannucci PM, Tenconi PM, Gastaman G, Rodeghiero F. Comparison of four virus-inactivated plasma concentrates for treatment of severe von Willebrand disease: a cross-over randomized trial. *Blood* 1992;79:3130–7

126. Ruggeri ZM, Pareit FI, Mannucci PM, *et al.* Heightened interaction between platelets and factor VIII/von Willebrand factor in a new subtype of von Willebrand's disease. *N Engl J Med* 1980;302: 1047–51

127. Giles AR, Hoogendoorn H, Benford K. Type IIB von Willebrand's disease presenting as thrombocytopenia during pregnancy. *Br J Haematol* 1987;67:349–53

128. Greer IA, Lowe GDO, Walker JJ, Forbes CD. Haemorrhagic problems in obstetrics and gynaecology in patients with congenital coagulopathies. *Br J Obstet Gynaecol* 1991;98:909–18

129. Rodeghiero F, Castaman GC, Di Bona E, *et al.* Successful pregnancy in a woman with congenital factor XIII deficiency treated with substitutive therapy: report of a second case. *Blut* 1987;55:45–8

130. Green D, Lechner K. A survey of 215 non-hemophilic patients with inhibitors to factor VIII. *Thromb Haemost* 1981;45:200–3

131. Hauser I, Schneider B, Lechner K. Post-partum factor VIII inhibitors: a review of the literature with special

reference to the value of steroid and immunosuppressive treatment. *Thromb Haemost* 1995;73:1–5

132. Lian EC-Y, Larcada AF, Chiu AY-Z. Combination immunosuppressive therapy after factor VIII infusion for acquired factor VIII inhibitor. *Ann Intern Med* 1989;110:774–8

133. Lusher JM. Prediction and management of adverse events associated with the use of factor IX complex concentrates. *Semin Hematol* 1993;30:36–40

134. Morrison AE, Ludlam CA, Kessler C. Use of porcine factor VIII in the treatment of patients with acquired hemophilia. *Blood* 1993;81:1513–20

135. Coller BS, Hultin MB, Hoyer LW. Normal pregnancy in a patient with a prior postpartum factor VIII inhibitor: with observations on pathogenesis and prognosis. *Blood* 1981;58:619–24

136. Vicente V, Alberca I, Gonzalez R, Alegre A. Normal pregnancy in a patient with a postpartum factor VIII inhibitor. *Am J Hematol* 1987;24:107–9

137. Kitchens CS. Disseminated intravascular coagulation. *Curr Opin Hematol* 1995;2:402–6

138. Lowe TW, Cunningham FG. Placental abruption. *Clin Obstet Gynecol* 1990;33:406

139. Pritchard JA, Brekken AL. Clinical and laboratory studies on severe abruptio placentae. *Am J Obstet Gynecol* 1967;97:681–95

140. Morgan M. Amniotic fluid embolism. *Anaesthesia* 1979;34:20–32

141. Rodgers GP, Heymach GJ III. Cryoprecipitate therapy in amniotic fluid embolism. *Am J Med* 1984;76:916–20

142. Sprung J, Cheng EY, Patel S. Understanding and management of amniotic fluid embolism. *J Clin Anesth* 1992;4:235

143. Guidotti RJ, Grimes DA, Cates W Jr. Fatal amniotic fluid embolism during legally induced abortion, United States, 1972–1978. *Am J Obstet Gynecol* 1981;141:257–61

39

Hepatic diseases

H.M. White and M.G. Peters

A variety of hepatic disorders occur during pregnancy. Jaundice is observed in 1 in 1500 gestations, and is thus uncommon[1]. Accurate diagnosis is essential, as patient management and therapy are dependent upon the specific disorder. This chapter focuses on normal liver function during pregnancy and reviews various hepatic disorders which may occur during pregnancy. The hepatic diseases are subdivided into disorders incidental to pregnancy, chronic liver disease coexistent with pregnancy and hepatic disorders unique to pregnancy.

NORMAL LIVER FUNCTION IN PREGNANCY

Anatomically, hepatic morphology and histology remain unaltered during pregnancy. Physiological changes including an increase in circulating plasma volume do occur. Plasma volume is most affected during the second trimester and this results in falling albumin and hemoglobin levels. Elevations in estrogen and progesterone levels alter cholesterol metabolism and cause cholestasis, the production of lithogenic bile and a decrease in gallbladder contractility. Under normal circumstances, serum aminotransferases are not altered by pregnancy. Conjugated hyperbilirubinemia as a result of physiological cholestasis occurs in approximately 20% of patients[2]. The serum alkaline phosphatase level may rise, but the enzyme is primarily of placental origin[3]. α-Fetoprotein levels are also elevated, owing to fetal growth, and these do not reflect intrinsic hepatic disease. Physical examination during a normal pregnancy may reveal several spider angiomata (up to five in 67% of patients), palmar erythema and displacement of the liver by an enlarging uterus[4].

LIVER DISEASE INCIDENTAL TO PREGNANCY

Infectious hepatitis

Viral hepatitis is the most common cause of jaundice in pregnancy. The hepatotrophic viruses (hepatitis A, B, C, D, E and non-A, non-B) are responsible for the majority of these infections. The course and outcome of viral hepatitis is no different in pregnant patients than in other individuals except in the case of hepatitis

E, which has been associated with a higher morbidity and mortality in pregnant women[4]. The diagnosis of viral hepatitis is usually made on the basis of serological testing (Table 1). Although viral hepatitis is not associated with teratogenicity, transmission of viral infection to the fetus may ensue and prematurity is a common consequence[4]. Transmission of infection is believed to occur primarily during the peripartum[3]. For some infections, measures can be taken to prevent or lessen the severity of hepatitis in the newborn.

Hepatitis A (HAV) infection is caused by an RNA virus and is usually associated with a self-limited clinical course. The virus is transmitted by the fecal–oral route. Outbreaks have been described in contaminated food and water supplies occurring frequently with inadequate sanitation. Population groups most commonly affected include homosexuals, children in day-care centers and individuals in institutions or crowded living conditions. Household contacts are at high risk of infection. Fecal shedding occurs for about 2 weeks after infection. Serological diagnosis of acute HAV is made by the presence of anti-HAV IgM antibody; antibody is typically present for several weeks but may be present for up to 1 year. The presence of anti-HAV IgG antibody denotes prior infection and immunity. The HAV does not cause chronic infection; prolonged intrahepatic cholestasis and relapsing episodes occurring 30–90 days after the primary episode have been described[5]. Neonates of mothers who acquire HAV in the last trimester should receive immune serum globulin (ISG) at the dosage of 0.02 ml/kg intramuscularly at the time of delivery[6,7]. Pregnant women who travel to an endemic area should receive ISG prophylactically at 0.06 ml/kg intramuscularly every 5 months. Individuals who are exposed to acute HAV should receive ISG within 10 days of exposure. Adult dosage is 0.06 ml/kg and infant/child dosage is 0.02 ml/kg intramuscularly. Studies show that post-exposure prophylaxis can prevent infection or lessen its severity in those who become infected. Children and adults who continue to be exposed to HAV should be vaccinated with HAVRIX at doses of 360 and 720 elisa units respectively[8]. Children should receive two doses 1 month apart and adults one dose intramuscularly. A booster is given after 6–12 months. There are no data on the safety of HAVRIX in pregnancy.

Table 1 Serological diagnosis of viral hepatis

Organism	Acute	Chronic	Recovered	Vaccinated
Hepatitis A	anti-HAV IgM	not applicable	anti-HAV IgG	anti-HAV total
Hepatitis B	anti-HBc IgM HBsAg HBeAg	anti-HBc total HBsAg HBeAg[†] or HBeAb[†]	anti-HBc total anti-HBsAg	anti-HBsAg
Hepatitis C	all tests may be negative anti-HCV Ab HCV RNA	anti-HCV Ab HCV RNA	anti-HCV Ab	not applicable
Hepatitis D	anti-HDV IgM HD Ag[‡]	anti-HDV total HD Ag[‡]	anti-HDV total[‡]	not applicable[**]
Hepatitis E	available from CDC only	not applicable	available from CDC only	not applicable
Hepatitis non-A, non-B	all tests negative	all tests negative	all tests negative	not available

[†]HBeAg will be present during periods of high replication. HBeAb will be present during periods of low replication; [‡]markers of hepatitis B infection will also be present because HDV cannot replicate without HBV; [**]although no specific vaccine for hepatitis D exists, individuals vaccinated for HBV will be protected from infection with HDV. CDC, Centers for Disease Control

Hepatitis B (HBV) infection is caused by a DNA virus which can result in both acute and chronic infections. The virus is transmitted horizontally by sexual and parenteral routes and vertically by transmission from infected mothers to their infants perinatally. HBV is endemic to certain parts of the world, especially southeast Asia and sub-Saharan Africa; in the USA the major risk groups for this infection include homosexuals, promiscuous heterosexuals, intravenous drug abusers, hemodialysis patients, hemophiliacs, native Asians and health care workers. Typical incubation periods range from 2 to 26 weeks. Acute infection is diagnosed by the presence of hepatitis B surface antigen (HBsAg) and the IgM fraction of antibody to hepatitis B core (anti-HBcIgM) (Figure 1). During periods of high replication, especially with either acute infection or reactivation in chronic hepatitis B, hepatitis B e antigen (HBeAg) and HBV DNA will be detectable in the serum. This has been generally accepted to connote high infectivity. Patients with lower levels of replication may have low levels of HBV DNA and antibody to hepatitis B e antigen (anti-HBeAg). Extrahepatic manifestations of this disease including arthritis, glomerulonephritis, vasculitis and angioedema are known to occur because of circulating immune complexes. The majority of adults who acquire HBV infection do not develop chronic disease, as > 90% will recover without sequelae.

The risk of transmission of HBV during pregnancy is related primarily to the replicative status of the mother, the trimester in which infection occurs and whether

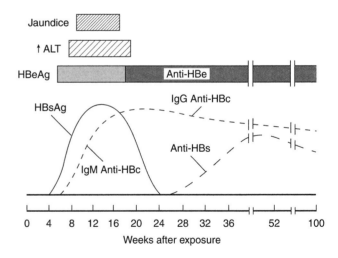

Figure 1 Diagnosis of hepatitis B (HB) infection by the assessment of the presence of the surface antigen (HBs Ag) and the IgG or IgM antibody to the HB core (Anti-HBc). ALT, alanine aminotransferase

the mother has acute or chronic disease[9]. Perinatal infection is particularly common if the mother is HBeAg seropositive and is associated with a > 90% chronicity rate[10]. Currently, universal prenatal screening for HBsAg is recommended. Neonatal acquisition occurs at the time of delivery when there is a mixing of the maternal and fetal circulations. Data would suggest that Cesarean section does not decrease the risk of transmission[9]. Transmission of acute HBV does not occur in the first or second trimester. However, if the

Table 2 Vaccination for hepatitis B

Group	Recombivax HB*		Engerix-B*	
	Dose (μg)	Dose (ml)	Dose (μg)	Dose (ml)
Infants of HBsAg-negative mothers and children < 11 years	2.5	0.25	10	0.5
Infants of HBsAg-positive mothers; prevention of perinatal infection	5	0.5	10	0.5
Children and adolescents 11–19 years	5	0.5	20	1.0
Adults > 20 years	10	1.0	20	1.0
Dialysis patients and other immunocompromised persons	40	1.0[†]	40	2.0[‡]

*Vaccines administered in a three-dose series at 0, 1 and 6 months. Engerix-B has also been licensed for a four-dose series administered at 1, 1, 2 and 12 months; [†]special formulation; [‡] two 1.0 ml doses administered at one site, in a four-dose schedule at 0, 1, 2 and 6 months

mother develops chronic HBV as a sequela of acute HBV in the first or second trimester, the infant is at risk for perinatal infection. If the mother acquires acute HBV in the third trimester, transmission from the mother to the infant is likely to occur unless immunoprophylaxis is given perinatally. The Centers for Disease Control (CDC) recommended universal HBV vaccination for all infants and children[11] (Table 2). One such immunization schedule includes three intramuscular injections, the first one given between the time of birth and before the hospital discharge, and the second and third injections given at 1 month and 6 months of age, respectively. It should be noted, however, that if the mother is HBsAg positive, the infant should receive the first HBV vaccine dose and 0.5 ml of hepatitis B immunoglobulin (HBIG) within 12 h of life. Similarly, if the maternal HBV status is unknown, the infant should receive the first HBV vaccine within 12 h of life and 0.5 ml of HBIG as soon as the maternal HBsAg positivity is known, preferably within 1 week of birth. HBIG is given intramuscularly and at a different site from that used for vaccination[11]. HBV vaccination is also recommended for individuals who have sexual or household contact with a chronic HBV carrier or have percutaneous or permucosal exposure to HBV-containing products. The vaccine is safe for use in pregnancy.

Although HBV may be found in breast milk, a study comparing breastfed vs. non-breastfed babies of seropositive mothers demonstrated no difference in the infection rate[12].

Hepatitis C (HCV) infection is caused by an RNA virus and accounts for the majority of non-A, non-B viral hepatitis infections. Both non-A, non-B and hepatitis C are primarily transmitted by the parenteral route by transfusion and intravenous drug usage. However percutaneous transmission with tattoos and snorting cocaine can occur. Sexual and intra-familial transmission is unusual (< 5%). The virus can be detected most readily by HCV RNA in the blood and rarely in other bodily secretions[13].

There are two tests available for HCV – an enzyme-linked immunosorbent assay (ELISA: HCVAb) and a radioimmunoblot assay (RIBA-3). Both of these test the host immune response to the virus to antibodies against the core and non-structural regions of the virus. They may not become positive until 3–6 months after acquisition of infection. Therefore diagnosis of acute infection, which is rare, should include HCV RNA by PCR. The RIBA-3 is used to rule out false positive tests in those with positive HCVAb and no risk factors. A positive test indicates exposure to the virus; the presence of antibody does not confer immunity.

The diagnosis of HCV infection at the present time is still largely clinical, in the setting of appropriate serology and risk factors. The majority of patients with this infection are anicteric and asymptomatic. The chronicity rate is > 85%. Transmission from mother to fetus is < 5%[14–17], with HCV RNA detected in infants born to mothers with chronic hepatitis C infection[16,18]. Transmission appears to be more likely when maternal HIV infection coexists[15]. In one study, 44% of infants born to mothers with both HIV and HCV infection developed HCVAb positivity at 6–12 months[15]. ISG administration does not prevent HCV infection.

Hepatitis D (HDV) infection is caused by an RNA virion which requires the presence of HBV to replicate. HDV occurs either as a coinfection in a patient with acute HBV or as a superinfection in a patient with chronic HBV. Superinfection with HDV carries a significant morbidity with a high rate of chronic HDV infection frequently leading to cirrhosis and liver failure[19–21]. HDV is an infrequent cause of hepatitis is pregnancy; the major risk groups for hepatitis D in the USA are intravenous drug abusers and hemophiliacs. Serological diagnosis of acute hepatitis D infection is made by the presence of hepatitis D antigen (HD Ag) and anti-HDV IgM antibody. Prevention of transmission of hepatitis B with HBIG and vaccination will prevent neonatal hepatitis D infection[6].

Hepatitis E (HEV) is an RNA virus which has been described as the causative agent of waterborne epidemic viral hepatitis in countries of the Indian subcontinent and Mexico but has not been reported in the USA except in travelers to endemic areas. The transmission and clinical presentation are similar to those of HAV. Unlike the other hepatotrophic viruses, HEV results in significant maternal morbidity and, despite supportive care, mortality rates have been reported up to 30%[22]. Testing for HEV is not commercially available in the USA but can be arranged through the Hepatitis Branch of the CDC. Clinicians should consider this disease in the differential diagnosis of patients returning from an endemic area in whom more common etiologies have been excluded. No immunoprophylaxis is effective in preventing this infection, as ISG from the USA does not contain protective antibody to this virus.

The management of viral hepatitis from any of the hepatotrophic viruses in pregnancy is supportive. Patients with acute viral hepatitis should be followed for clinical signs of fulminant hepatic failure such as encephalopathy, and laboratory tests should include the prothrombin time, transaminases and bilirubin. Clinicians should avoid hepatotoxic drugs and eliminate any non-essential medications. Diagnostic testing should be limited to serological evaluation and monitoring of hepatocellular function using pediatric collection tubes. After an initial ultrasound evaluation, radiographic studies should be avoided. Liver biopsies are unnecessary and pose potential risks to the fetus and mother. Invasive procedures such as amniocentesis, fetal scalp blood sampling and funicentesis could potentially transmit HBV or HCV infection to the fetus by introducing the virus directly into the fetal circulation from the maternal infectious blood. Breastfeeding has not been shown to be a mode of transmission[10]. Appropriate immunoprophylaxis for infants is essential.

Some pregnant patients may develop fulminant hepatic failure (FHF) due to viral hepatitis. The incidence of FHF in pregnant women is < 1% with HAV, < 5% with HBV, HCV and HDV, and up to 30% with HEV. These patients will need aggressive supportive care and monitoring. Individuals who develop prolongation of prothrombin time in association with altered mental status and acute hepatic dysfunction should receive gastroenterological consultation and transfer to a center capable of performing liver transplantation. Liver transplantation for FHF due to viral hepatitis has been successfully accomplished during pregnancy[23], but there is only one reported case of intrapartum transplantation with survival of the fetus and mother[24]. Pregnant patients require the same intensive pre-transplantation assessment as other individuals being evaluated for transplantation. To minimize the risk of radiation exposure to the fetus, the primary imaging modality utilized is ultrasound.

Among the other infectious agents that can produce hepatitis during pregnancy are herpes virus, cytomegalovirus, toxoplasmosis and syphilis. These agents are usually associated with extrahepatic manifestations. Infections can result in significant morbidity/mortality for the fetus. Diagnosis is made by an index of clinical suspicion and the appropriate serological testing.

CHRONIC LIVER DISEASE WITH COEXISTENT PREGNANCY

Chronic liver disease is associated with impaired fertility, anovulatory cycles and amenorrhea. Patients with advanced cirrhosis rarely conceive. However, if underlying liver disease is treated, fertility may improve[25]. Patients with chronic liver disease appear to have a higher incidence of premature delivery and fetal wastage[1,26]. Management of the underlying liver disease may require adjustment during pregnancy.

Wilson's disease is an autosomal recessive disorder of hepatic metabolism of copper, resulting in abnormal accumulation of copper in many tissues such as liver, nervous system and eyes. Clinical manifestations depend on the affected organs and include acute or chronic hepatitis, chorea, tremors, spasticity and psychiatric changes. A Kayser–Fleisher ring is often observed once neurological or psychiatric sypmtoms develop. A diagnosis is made by a low serum level of ceruloplasmin, a plasma copper-carrying protein, and an elevated concentration of copper in the liver tissue obtained by a liver biopsy. The main therapy is penicillamine, a copper-chelating agent. This agent has been used in pregnancy without teratogenic effect[27,28]. Patients with Wilson's disease should continue on copper chelation therapy (D-penicillamine or trientene) during pregnancy[27]. Cessation of therapy can lead to fulminant liver failure and death[27]. It remains advisable to use the lowest dosage during the pregnancy to minimize any potential fetal effects. Since penicillamine has an antipyridoxine effect, supplementation with vitamin B_6 is recommended.

Autoimmune chronic active hepatitis (AIH) is a rare liver disorder accounting for about 1% of all liver disease. AIH occurs at two age peaks, one in adolescence and young adulthood and the other in the 6th or 7th decade. About 70% of cases involve females, and there is a frequent association with other autoimmune disorders such as thyroiditis. Generally, classic AIH is diagnosed by the presence of a positive antinuclear antibody, an elevated sedimentation rate and elevated immunoglobulins in conjunction with a liver biopsy that is consistent with the diagnosis. However, several subtypes of AIH are now being described and are summarized elsewhere[29,30]. Patients with autoimmune hepatitis usually respond to immunotherapy such as prednisone alone or in combination with azathioprine[29]. Corticosteroids should be continued throughout the pregnancy.

Owing to teratogenic effects in animals, most clinicians discontinue azathioprine in patients becoming or attempting to become pregnant[1]. Individuals with autoimmune chronic active hepatitis have reduced fertility, a higher frequency of stillbirths, with prematurity and low birth weight contributing to neonatal mortality. Patients may be at risk for preterm labor, intrauterine fetal demise and pre-eclampsia[26].

A variety of cholestatic liver diseases exist, but the most common ones in the reproductive age group are drug-induced liver disease, primary biliary cirrhosis and primary sclerosing cholangitis. Patients may experience severe pruritus requiring pharmacological intervention. Safe agents during pregnancy include cholestyramine, a non-absorbable bile acid binding resin at 4 g/dose orally up to 6 doses/day, or phenobarbital, which stimulates bile flow at 15–60 mg orally. These medications have been used during pregnancy without apparent significant adverse fetal effects[31].

Extrahepatic portal vein obstruction (EHPVO) typically occurs after either congenital injury or perinatal infection of the umbilical vein resulting in extrahepatic portal hypertension. These patients have normal liver function tests and liver biopsies are normal. Patients may be asymptomatic from portal hypertension until the plasma volume is expanded, resulting in distended collaterals and varices. EHPVO presents a significant risk of variceal hemorrhage in the last two trimesters. In one series of 58 patients, 43% had variceal bleeding and 7% of the mothers died. An increase in spontaneous abortions and neonatal mortality was also observed[32].

In general, for patients with chronic liver disease of any origin, lower fertility and higher fetal wastage has been observed. Maternal morbidity is related to the underlying liver disease and the severity of portal hypertension. Women with chronic liver disease should be counseled regarding the potential impact of pregnancy on their disease. They should receive concurrent care by obstetricians and gastroenterologists during pregnancy. If life-threatening complications ensue during pregnancy (such as variceal hemorrhage, portosystemic encephalopathy, or marked hepatocellular dysfunction with coagulopathy), termination of the pregnancy should be considered[1]. It is of special note that the pregnant patient with chronic liver disease may develop peripartum hemorrhage[1] related to coagulopathy from synthetic dysfunction or to thrombocytopenia from splenic sequestration.

LIVER DISEASES UNIQUE TO PREGNANCY

Hyperemesis gravidarum

During pregnancy, nausea and vomiting is common; however, in some instances the entity is protracted and may result in hospitalization. Although the liver is usually normal, some laboratory abnormalities have been observed. These include mild elevations in serum bilirubin and serum aminotransferases. In a small study of 12 patients with hyperemesis gravidarum, elevated serum transaminases were observed in 50% of patients, with a few patients having enzyme levels up to 800 IU/l[33]. Although the older literature suggested that the histology was normal[34], patients in a more recent study with liver biopsy demonstrated cholestasis, central-zone vacuolization and cell dropout[33]. Treatment is supportive and directed at symptomatic relief. Hyperemesis with hepatic abnormalities has been reported to occur in consecutive pregnancies with resolution[35].

Intrahepatic cholestasis of pregnancy

Intrahepatic cholestasis of pregnancy (benign jaundice of pregnancy, sex hormone-induced jaundice) is characterized by pruritus and biochemical cholestasis typically presenting in the second or third trimester. This condition accounts for approximately 20% of jaundice during pregnancy[36]. Although this is an uncommon disorder, it frequently recurs with subsequent pregnancies or the administration of synthetic estrogen compounds. Pruritus gravidarum is a term applied to patients with pruritus and biochemical cholestasis, whereas cholestasis of pregnancy is generally reserved for those patients with jaundice. Although the exact etiology is unknown, genetic and hormonal factors play a role. Genetic factors have been implicated owing to the frequent history of cholestasis in female family members of index patients[36]. Estrogens produce lithogenic bile because estrogens decrease bile salt independent flow and increase diffusion of water from bile to plasma[37]. Patients have pruritus and resultant excoriations. Jaundice may or may not be present. Some patients will have subclinical steatorrhea that may affect nutritional status[38]. Laboratory abnormalities are cholestatic with elevations in alkaline phosphatase up to ten-fold and modest hyperbilirubinemia, typically less than 5 mg/dl[1,36]. Maternal outcome is favorable with prompt resolution of symptoms postpartum. However, these patients do have an increased incidence of gallstones due to lithogenic bile[36]. Generally, maternal laboratory abnormalities resolve quickly postpartum, but alkaline phosphatase may take up to 3 months to normalize[36]. If maternal symptoms or jaundice persist for more than 1 week postpartum, the diagnosis of intrahepatic cholestasis should be reconsidered, as this is atypical for the disorder[38]. Liver biopsy is unnecessary for diagnosis. In those patients in whom biopsy was performed, findings included canalicular bile plugs with centrilobular cholestasis[1,36] and intact parenchymal architecture[1]. Intrahepatic cholestasis of pregnancy recurs in about 70% of patients[39,40]. Fetal outcome is not so favorable. Premature delivery occurs in 10–20%, meconium staining in 35–60% and fetal distress in 19–60%[36,37].

Treatment of intrahepatic cholestasis of pregnancy is largely symptomatic. Pruritus is usually responsive to the administration of cholestyramine in doses of 4–20 g/day[1,36,37] and antihistamines[37]. Neither cholestyramine nor antihistamines affect laboratory values[38]. Phenobarbital has also been used in refractory cases; clinicians should exercise caution in the administration of phenobarbital, owing to the potential risk of neonatal respiratory depression[41–43]. Experimentally, ursodeoxycholic acid at 15 mg/kg per day was successful in alleviating pruritus and reducing biochemical abnormalities[44]. However, controlled clinical trials have not yet been performed to evaluate the effects of ursodeoxycholic acid in pregnancy and thus the drug is not approved by the US Food and Drug Administration for this purpose. Occasionally, prothrombin time may become prolonged due to malabsorption of vitamin K which may accompany cholestasis[1,36]. Patients should receive parenteral vitamin K if coagulation abnormalities are evident, as cases of severe postpartum hemorrhage have been reported[36]. The absorption of other fat-soluble vitamins – A, D and E – may be affected by mild steatorrhea. Ultimately, intrahepatic cholestasis of pregnancy resolves with interruption of pregnancy. Since maternal sequelae of this disorder are minimal, the timing of delivery is determined by the condition and age of the fetus in order to ensure optimal fetal survival.

Eclampsia and pre-eclampsia

Five per cent of pregnant women experience pre-eclampsia characterized by the triad of proteinuria, edema and hypertension. If the central nervous system becomes involved, e.g. seizures or coma, the disorder is termed eclampsia. Typically, hepatic abnormalities are a sign of advanced pre-eclampsia/eclampsia and are not the primary manifestation. Of those patients with symptoms referrable to liver disease, major symptoms included right upper quadrant pain, nausea, vomiting and a tender enlarged liver[2]. Levels of transaminases range from 300 to 3000 IU/l and serum bilirubin is usually less than 5 mg/dl, but higher values have been reported. Hepatic parenchymal injury results from microangiopathic hemolytic anemia, thrombocytopenia and localized segmental vasospasm, and may lead to hepatic infarction, hematoma and rupture resulting in maternal death[2,4]. Liver biopsies or autopsy specimens show periportal fibrin deposition and hemorrhage; portal tracts are usually involved but in some cases lesions may be focal[2]. More recently, hepatic mircrovesicular fat similar to that seen in acute fatty liver of pregnancy (AFLP) has been observed in histological specimens, leading to speculation that pre-eclampsia and AFLP may be different presentations of the same process[45,46]. Although initial therapy is directed at control of hypertension and prevention of seizures, optimal management includes prompt delivery[4,36]. Eclampsia accounts for 8% of maternal deaths, and may recur in subsequent pregnancies[36]. HELLP (hemolysis, elevated liver enzymes, and low platelets) was first described by Weinstein in 1982 as a syndrome occurring in pre-eclamptic/eclamptic patients[47]. If hepatic parenchymal injury is severe, hypoglycemia may be observed[48]. Patients should have frequent monitoring of serum glucose (every 30 min) and intravenous dextrose solutions (10, 20, or 50%) administered as needed[4]. In the scenario of this diagnosis, fetal lung maturation or a duration of gestation of 34 weeks or more may be an indication for delivery[49]. Maternal outcomes are generally favorable with mortality ranges from 2 to 4% in reported cases. Rarely, women may have persistent life-threatening microangiopathy > 72 h postpartum. These patients should be considered for plasma exchange with fresh frozen plasma[49]. Recurrent HELLP has been reported to occur at rates of 3.4–27%[36,50,51].

Acute fatty liver of pregnancy

AFLP is a rare disorder (1 per 13 000 deliveries) occurring in the third trimester or peripartum and characterized by a microvesicular fatty infiltration[36]. Although the disease was previously associated with a very poor prognosis and high maternal/fetal morbidity and mortality, recent series suggest that more benign presentations may occur, perhaps owing to earlier diagnosis and prompt management. AFLP is more common in primagravidas, twin gestations and those with a male fetus[36,52]. Previously, the use of intravenous tetracycline was associated with the development of AFLP[53]. Defects in fatty acid oxidation have been recently associated with this condition in mothers and infants[54]. Typically patients present with nausea and vomiting for several days, followed by jaundice and then progressive encephalopathy. Hepatic failure ensues[52]. Approximately 20% of patients may also have features of pre-eclampsia/eclampsia[36]. Laboratory abnormalities include elevated serum aminotransferases usually 300–500 IU/l, increased serum bilirubin 3–25 mg/dl[52], and variable degrees of leukocytosis, disseminated intravascular coagulation, hypoglycemia, hyperuricemia and bacteremia[4]. Patients may develop gastrointestinal hemorrhage, pancreatitis and renal failure[36]. Radiographic evaluations may suggest the diagnosis from steatosis seen by ultrasound, computerized tomography, or magnetic resonance imaging. However, this finding may not be universally present and normal studies do not exclude the diagnosis[4]. Histological findings in AFLP include pericentral microvesicular steatosis, intrahepatic cholestasis and diffuse cytoplasmic ballooning. Gross inspection usually demonstrates a small, greasy, yellow liver[52]. Because early AFLP may be difficult to distinguish from viral hepatitis histologically, fresh specimens should always be stained with oil-red-O for fat. Enlarged needle-shaped mitochondria that contain crystalline inclusions and dilated smooth endoplasmic reticulum can by seen by electron microscopy[36,52].

Successful management of AFLP is dependent upon prompt delivery and supportive care. Overall reported maternal and fetal mortality is around 50%, but more recent series suggest improving maternal and fetal mortality to 22% and 42%, respectively[36]. Fetal mortality is believed to occur as a result of rapid maternal decompensation[36], a high rate of premature delivery[36,55] and the maternal disseminated intravascular coagulation resulting in fibrin deposition in the placenta, culminating in uteroplacental insufficiency, infarct and fetal asphyxia[55]. AFLP occurs in the third trimester and often late in pregnancy. Immediate delivery would therefore be expected to improve fetal outcome, since basic organ systems are developed. Although no specific therapy for AFLP exists, delivery of the fetus is usually successful in ameliorating the disease. There are no cases of spontaneous resolution without delivery. One case of persistent maternal clinical decompensation postpartum was managed with successful orthotopic liver transplantation[56]. Several women with a history of AFLP have had subsequent pregnancies without sequelae or recurrence[36]. A recent report suggested that AFLP may recur; interestingly, this recurrence was associated with a fatty-acid oxidation defect in the offspring[57].

MISCELLANEOUS HEPATIC DISORDERS

Hepatic rupture

Hepatic hemorrhage and rupture have been primarily associated with pre-eclampsia/eclampsia during pregnancy. Rupture is estimated to occur in 1–2% of patients with pre-eclampsia[36]. However, rupture/hemorrhage may also occur in women who have benign liver adenomas, liver cell cancer, or hepatic abscess. Hemorrhage or rupture associated with toxemia typically develops late in pregnancy. Herald symptoms include sudden onset of right upper quadrant pain and tenderness, followed by diffuse abdominal pain and peritoneal signs. Typically, bleeding is massive and shock occurs in 50% of patients, and is accompanied by a rapid fall in hematocrit[36]. Accurate diagnosis requires a high index of clinical suspicion; radiographic studies usually demonstrate hematomas or overt blood. Survival of rupture without treatment has not been reported. Successful therapies include hemodynamic support, immediate laparotomy with packing, sutures or lobectomy. Angiographic embolization has been performed in only a limited number of patients, with variable results[58]. If the hematoma is contained and hemodynamic stability is achieved, conservative observation may be all that is required. Maternal mortality is approximately 50%, and recurrence in subsequent pregnancies has not been reported[36].

Hepatic adenoma

Hepatic adenomas are benign hepatocellular tumors. Growth of adenomas has been linked to both natural and synthetic estrogens. Since enlargement of tumors with associated complications may occur during pregnancy, surgical excision is recommended for large symptomatic tumors that do not decrease after discontinuing estrogen-containing oral contraceptives or for those patients contemplating pregnancy. Other options for managing these tumors are ethanol injection or arterial embolization. Pregnancy *per se* is not linked with the development of adenomas. Adenomas may be associated with serious complications including acute hemorrhage, pain, mass effects, cell necrosis and hepatic rupture[36].

Focal nodular hyperplasia

Focal nodular hyperplasia is a benign tumor occurring almost exclusively in women. The lesion may be associated with oral contraceptives, and these lesions may increase in size during pregnancy. As for hepatic adenomas, surgery should be considered for symptomatic patients and for patients who desire pregnancy. Other options include ethanol injection or arterial embolization.

Budd–Chiari syndrome

Budd–Chiari syndrome is the development of hepatic vein thrombosis. Many associated diseases predispose patients to Budd–Chiari syndrome; the use of oral contraceptives and pregnancy are among the examples. Predisposition during pregnancy is presumed to be related to increases in circulating estrogens and decreases in levels of antithrombin III[36]. The disorder is characterized by acute onset of ascites and hepatomegaly. Abdominal pain is usually present.

Malignant tumors

Patients with metastatic disease occasionally experience rupture of hepatic metastases[59]; however, pregnancy among these patients is rare. Choriocarcinoma is associated with pregnancy and occurs in the USA in 1/24 000 pregnancies[59]. The source of the tumor, the placental trophoblast, is frequently associated with an antecedent pregnancy such as hydatidaform mole, abortion, normal delivery or ectopic pregnancy.

The liver is the site of about 10% of metastases. Hepatic metastases are associated with a poorer prognosis[59].

Hepatocellular carcinoma has been reported in only a few pregnant patients. Diagnosis may be confounded by high serum α–fetoprotein levels normally found during pregnancy. Patients have generally had underlying liver disease or familial incidence of hepatocellular carcinoma. The prognosis is poor[60].

Drug-induced hepatotoxicity in pregnancy

In general, medication use during pregnancy is restricted due to the known or unknown potential risks to the fetus. A large number of drugs may cause hepatotoxicity; for further reading on drug hepatotoxicity see Zimmerman[61]. Hydralazine merits special mention because of its frequent use in attempts to control pregnancy-induced hypertension. Hydralazine may be associated with hepatotoxicity. In patients who have HELLP syndrome or who are pre-eclamptic/eclamptic, it may be difficult to distinguish drug-induced toxicity from the pregnancy-associated disorder[62].

Liver transplantation and pregnancy

Given the improving success of liver transplantation over the past two decades and decreasing levels of immunosuppression, most organ transplant recipients lead happy and healthy lives with an average 1-year survival rate of > 85% at better transplant programs[63]. The ability of these patients to lead normal lives and to conceive is not surprising. Approximately 27 cases of pregnancy subsequent to liver transplantation have been reported[23], although there are believed to be many unreported cases. Pregnancy has been reported as early as 3 weeks post-transplantation. Prenatal planning is highly recommended for these patients. The majority of transplantation literature relates to renal transplantation and these patients do have an increased frequency of pre-eclampsia, preterm delivery and fetal wastage. The use of immunosuppressive drugs has been associated with small-for-gestational-age babies in 8–45% of births[64]. Hepatic transplantation *per se* probably does not predispose patients to pre-eclampsia, but the use of cyclosporin and pre-existing hypertension clearly do contribute.

Every effort should be made to minimize potentially teratogenic medications. Immunosuppression regimens typically include cyclosporin or FK506, and prednisone with or without azathioprine. Additional medications for liver transplant recipients may include prophylaxis for *Pneumocystis carinii* infection with trimethoprim/sulfamethoxasole or pentamidine; and for herpes virus infection with acyclovir. Although neither cyclosporin nor FK506 is recommended for use during pregnancy, patients will not be able to maintain graft function without one of these two agents; both cross the placenta and reach maternal serum concentrations in breast milk[64,65]. For this reason, patients taking cyclosporin and FK506 should not breastfeed[65]. Prednisone is considered safe in pregnancy and during breastfeeding[65]. Controlled studies of azathioprine have not been performed in pregnancy. Azathioprine may be associated with fetal immunosuppression, bone marrow toxicity and growth retardation[66–68]. The use of azathioprine for transplant immunosuppression during pregnancy should be limited to selected situations where other immunosuppressives do not control graft rejection. Insufficient data exist to determine whether continued use of azathioprine is safe during breastfeeding. Trimethoprim/sulfamethoxasole therapy may be continued during pregnancy and during breastfeeding[65]. Although bactrim crosses the placenta, it presents no known risks to human fetuses except at term, when hyperbilirubinemia may develop in some neonates. Insufficient data exist to evaluate the use of pentamidine in pregnancy or lactation. Pentamidine is classified as having animal teratogenic effects but no controlled studies have been performed in pregnant women. Acyclovir is considered safe during breastfeeding but is concentrated in breast milk[65].

The development of abnormal liver enzymes in the pregnant transplant recipient should prompt a search for infection and rejection. Typical infections in transplant recipients include cytomegalovirus and occasionally herpes. These infections are potentially lethal to the mother and teratogenic to the fetus. Graft rejection may complicate pregnancy or the puerperium. One might expect the relative immunotolerance of pregnancy to decrease the risk of rejection. Only small numbers of patients with pregnancy after liver transplantation have been reported, but episodes of rejection have been documented[69]. Pregnancies in transplant patients should be managed with input from the transplant hepatologist or surgeon.

SUMMARY

This chapter discusses a variety of chronic hepatic disorders which may render patients anovulatory and infertile or may occur during pregnancy. Although liver disease is uncommon in pregnancy, prompt management with early involvement of a gastroenterologist or hepatologist will ensure optimal care and the highest likelihood of a successful maternal and fetal outcome.

REFERENCES

1. Yip DM, Baker AL. Liver diseases in pregnancy. *Clin Perinatol* 1985;12:683–92
2. Rolfes DB, Ishak KG. Liver disease in pregnancy. *Histopathology* 1986;10:555–61

3. Bynum TE. Hepatic and gastrointestinal disorders in pregnancy. *Med Clin North Am* 1977;61:129–35

4. White H, Peters M. Severe liver disease in pregnancy. *J Intensive Care Med* 1990;5:104–8

5. Sjogren MH, Tanno H, Fay O, *et al*. Hepatitis A virus in stool during clinical relapse. *Ann Intern Med* 1987; 106:221–3

6. Rustgi VK, Hoofnagle JH. Viral hepatitis in pregnancy. *Sem Liv Dis* 1987;7:40–6

7. CDC. Protection against viral hepatitis. Recommendations of the Immunization Practices Advisory Committee (ACIP). *Morbid Mortal Weekly Rep* 1990; 39(RR-2):1–2

8. Werzberger A, Mensch B, Kuter B, *et al*. A controlled trial of formalin-inactivated hepatitis A vaccine in healthy children. *N Engl J Med* 1992;327:453–8

9. Mishra L, Seeff LB. Viral hepatitis, A through E, complicating pregnancy. *Gastro Clin North Am* 1992; 21:873–9

10. Beasley RP, Trepo C, Stevens CE, Szmuness W. The e antigen and vertical transmission of hepatitis B surface antigen. *Am J Epidemiol* 1977;105:94–8

11. CDC. Hepatitis B virus: a comprehensive strategy for eliminating transmission in the United States through universal vaccination: recommendations of the immunization practices advisory committee (ACIP). *Morbid Mortal Weekly Rep* 1991;40(44–13):1–4

12. Beasley RP, Stevens CE. Vertical transmission of HBV and interruption with globulin. In Vyas GN, Cohen SN, Schmid R, eds. *Viral Hepatitis: a Contemporary Assessment of Etiology, Pathogenesis, and Prevention*. Philadelphia: Franklin Institute Press, 1978:333–6

13. Hsu HH, Wright TL, Luba D, *et al*. Failure to detect hepatitis C virus genome in human secretions with the polymerase chain reaction. *Hepatology* 1991;14:763–7

14. Wejstal R, Hermodsson S, Iwarson S, Norkrans G. Mother to infant transmission of hepatitis C virus infection. *J Med Virol* 1990;30:178–81

15. Giovannini M, Tagger A, Ribero ML, *et al*. Maternal–infant transmission of hepatitis C virus and HIV infections: a possible interaction. *Lancet* 1990;2:1166–9

16. Thaler MM, Park C-K, Landers DV, *et al*. Vertical transmission of heaptitis C virus. *Lancet* 1991;338:17–22

17. Tong MJ, Thrusby M, Rakela J, *et al*. Studies on the maternal–infant transmission of the viruses which cause acute hepatitis. *Gastroenterology* 1981;80: 999–1002

18. Joung MK, Park CK, Buskell-Bales Z, *et al*. Transmission of HCV from infected mother to infant. Presented at the *Third International HCV Conference*, Paris, September 1991

19. Hoofnagle JH. Type D (delta) hepatitis. *J Am Med Assoc* 1989;261:1321–5 (Erratum to *J Am Med Assoc* 1989; 261:3552–5)

20. Jacobson IM, Dienstag JL, Werner BG, *et al*. Epidemiology and clinical impact of hepatitis D virus (delta) infection. *Hepatology* 1985;5:188–91

21. Shattock AG, Irwin FM, Morgan BM, *et al*. Increased severity and morbidity of acute hepatitis in drug abusers with simultaneously acquired heaptitis B and hepatitis D virus infections. *Br Med J* 1985; 290:1377–80

22. Belabbes EH, Bougermouth A, Bentallah A, Illoul G. Epidemic non-A, non-B viral hepatitis in Algeria: strong evidence for its spreading by water. *J Med Virol* 1985;16:257–60

23. Laifer SA, Darby MJ, Scantlebury VP, *et al*. Pregnancy and liver transplantation. *Obstet Gynecol* 1990; 76:1083–7

24. Fair J, Klein AS, Feng T, *et al*. Intrapartum orthotopic liver transplantation with successful outcome of pregnancy. *Transplantation* 1990;50:534–6

25. Varma RR. Course and prognosis of pregnancy in women with liver disease. *Sem Liv Dis* 1987;7:59–66

26. Steven MM, Buckley JD, Mackay IR. Pregnancy in chronic active hepatitis. *Q J Med* 1979;48:519–23

27. Scheinberg IH, Jaffe ME, Sternlieb I. The use of trientine in preventing the effects of interrupting penicillamine therapy in Wilson's disease. *N Engl J Med* 1987;317:209–12

28. Walsh FB, Hoyt WF. *Clinical Neuro-opthalmology*, 3rd edn. Baltimore: Williams & Wilkins, 1969

29. Czaja AJ. Autoimmune hepatitis: current approaches. *Contemp Gastroenterol* 1992;2:11–21

30. Johnson PJ, McFarlane IG. Meeting report: International Autoimmune Hepatitis Group. *Hepatology* 1993;18:998–1002

31. Landon MB, Soloway RD, Freedman LJ, Gabbe SJ. Primary sclerosing cholangitis and pregnancy. *Obstet Gynecol* 1987;69:457–60

32. Varma RR, Michelsohn NH, Borkowf HI, Lewis JD. Pregnancy in cirrhotic and noncirrhotic portal hypertension. *Obstet Gynecol* 1977;50:217–21

33. Wallstedt A, Riely CA, Shaver D, *et al*. Prevalence and characteristics of liver dysfunction in hyperemesis gravidarum. *Clin Res* 1990;38:970–3

34. Adams RH, Gordon J, Combes B. Hyperemesis gravidarum. *Obstet Gynecol* 1968;31:659–63

35. Larrey D, Rueff B, Feldman G, *et al*. Recurrent jaundice caused by recurrent hyperemesis gravidarum. *Gut* 1984;25:1414–18

36. Van Dyke RW. The liver in pregnancy. In Zakim D, Boyer TD, eds. *Hepatology: a Textbook of Liver Disease*, 3rd edn. Philadelphia, PA: W.B. Saunders, 1990:1734

37. Kreek MJ, Kerrins JF. Recurrent idiopathic jaundice of pregnancy. *N Engl J Med* 1963;268:1180–6

38. Reyes H. The spectrum of liver and gastrointestinal disease seen in cholestasis of pregnancy. *Gastro Clin North Am* 1992;21:905–21

39. Haemmerli UP, Wyss HI. Recurrent intrahepatic cholestasis of pregnancy: report of six cases and review of the literature. *Medicine* 1967;46:299–308

40. Johnston WG, Baskett TF. Obstetric cholestasis: a 14 year review. *Am J Obstet Gynecol* 1979;133:299–303

41. Espinoza J, Barnafi L, Schnaidt E. The effect of phenobarbital on intrahepatic cholestasis of pregnancy. *Am J Obstet Gynecol* 1974;119:234–40

42. Heikkinen J, Maentausta O, Ylostalo P, *et al*. Serum bile acid levels in intrahepatic cholestasis of pregnancy during treatment with phenobarbital or cholestyramine. *Eur J Obstet Gynecol Reprod Biol* 1982;14:153–61

43. Laatikainen T. Effect of cholestyramine and phenobarbital on pruritus and serum bile acid levels in cholestasis of pregnancy. *Am J Obstet Gynecol* 1978;132:501–9

44. Palma J, Reyes H, Ribalta J, *et al.* Effects of ursode-oxycholic acid in patients with intrahepatic cholestasis of pregnancy (preliminary report). *Revista Medica de Chile* 1991;119:169–76

45. Minakami H, Oka N, Sato T, *et al.* Preeclampsia: a microvesicular fat disease of the liver? *Am J Obstet Gynecol* 1988;159:1043–9

46. Reily CA, Latham PS, Romero R, *et al.* Acute fatty liver of pregnancy. *Ann Intern Med* 1987;106:703–11

47. Weinstein L. Syndrome of hemolysis, elevated liver enzymes, and low platelet counts: a severe consequence of hypertension in pregnancy. *Am J Obstet Gynecol* 1982;142:159–68

48. Egley CC, Gutliph J, Bowes WA. Severe hypoglycemia associated with HELLP syndrome. *Am J Obstet Gynecol* 1985;152:576–81

49. Barton JR, Sibai BM. Care of the pregnancy complicated by HELLP syndrome. *Gastro Clin North Am* 1992;21:937–43

50. Martin JN Jr, Perry KG Jr, Blake PG, *et al.* The recurrence risk of the syndrome of hemolysis, elevated liver enzymes, and low platelets (HELLP) in subsequent gestations. *Semin Perinatol* 1999;23:100–12

51. Sibai BM. The HELLP syndrome (hemolysis, elevated liver enzymes, and low platelets): much ado about nothing? *Am J Obstet Gynecol* 1990;162:311–19

52. Rolfes DB, Ishak KG. Acute fatty liver of pregnancy: a clinicopathologic study of 35 cases. *Hepatology* 1985;5:1149–56

53. Kunelis CT, Peters JL, Edmondson HA. Fatty liver of pregnancy and its relationship to tetracycline therapy. *Am J Med* 1965;38:359–66

54. Strauss AW, Bennett AJ, Rinaldo P, *et al.* Inherited long-chain 3-hydroxyacyl-CoA dehydrogenase deficiency and a fetal–maternal interaction cause maternal liver disease and other pregnancy complications. *Am J Obstet Gynecol* 1994;171:940–3

55. Moise KJ, Shah DM. Acute fatty liver of pregnancy: etiology of fetal distress and fetal wastage. *Obstet Gynecol* 1987;69:482–89

56. Ockner SA, Brunt EM, Cohn SM, *et al.* Fulminant hepatic failure due to acute fatty liver of pregnancy treated by orthotopic liver transplantation. *Hepatology* 1990;11:59–64

57. Schoeman MN, Batey RG, Wilcken B. Recurrent acute fatty liver of pregnancy associated with a fatty-acid oxidation defect in the offspring. *Gastroenterology* 1991;100:544–50

58. Terasaki KK, Quinn MF, Lundell CJ. Spontaneous hepatic hemorrhage in preeclampsia: treatment with hepatic arterial embolization. *Radiology* 1990;174:1039

59. Erb RE, Gibler WB. Massive hemoperitoneum following rupture of hepatic metastases from unsuspected choriocarcinoma. *Am J Emerg Med* 1989;7:196

60. Seaward PGR, Koch MAT, Mitchell RW, *et al.* Primary hepatocellular carcinoma in pregnancy. *South African Med J* 1986;69:700–7

61. Zimmerman HJ. *Hepatotoxicity: the Adverse Effects of Drugs and other Chemicals on the Liver.* New York: Appleton-Century-Crofts, 1978

62. Hod M, Friedman S, Schoenfeld A, *et al.* Hydralazine-induced hepatitis in pregnancy. *Int J Fertil* 1986;31:352–9

63. Health Resources and Services Administration, Bureau of Health Resources Development, Division of Organ Transplantation. *Annual Report on the US Scientific Registry for Organ Transplantation and the Organ Procurement and Transplantation Network.* Rockville, MD: US Department of Health and Human Services, 1990

64. Kossoy LR, Herbert CM, Wentz AC. Management of heart transplant recipients: guidelines for the obstetrician–gynecologist. *Am J Obstet Gynecol* 1988;159:490–9

65. American Academy of Pediatrics Committee on Drugs. Transfer of drugs and other chemicals into human milk. *Pediatrics* 1989;84:924–31

66. Schardein JL. *Chemically Induced Birth Defects.* New York: Marcel Dekker, 1985:495–502

67. Cote CJ, Muewissen HJ, Pickering RJ. Effects on the neonate of prednisone and azathioprine administered to the mother during pregnancy. *J Pediatr* 1974;85:324–30

68. DeWitte DB, Buick MK, Cyran SE, *et al.* Neonatal pancytopenia and severe combined immunodeficiency associated with antenatal administration of azathioprine and prednisone. *J Pediatr* 1984;105:625–32

69. Grow DR, Simon NV, Liss J, *et al.* Twin pregnancy after orthotopic liver transplantation, with exacerbation of chronic graft rejection. *Am J Perinatol* 1991;8:135–41

40

Hypertension

W.F. Rayburn

INTRODUCTION

Pregnancy is known sometimes to induce or aggravate hypertension, and the incidence and severity of the condition are highly variable. Chronic hypertension may be defined as any sustained blood pressure elevation to 140/90 mmHg or greater, either before pregnancy or earlier than 20 weeks of the present pregnancy[1]. A number of factors appear to be related to hypertensive vascular disease in pregnancy. The condition is more common among older women, obese mothers, diabetics and black people. Often many members of a single family are hypertensive.

Although hypertension is a common complication of pregnancy, guidelines for management are somewhat unclear. The pregnant woman usually tolerates chronic hypertension if her diastolic pressures remain below 100 mmHg. However, complications such as mid-trimester loss, growth restriction and abruptio placentae may occur.

HYPERTENSION IN REPRODUCTIVE-AGE WOMEN

Young hypertensive women who are not pregnant are generally active individuals with increased sympathetic tone and elevated plasma renin activity. Extracellular fluid volumes are usually normal or decreased. More than 90% of hypertensive adults have hypertension of unknown etiology, which is an elevation of blood pressure without an identifiable cause[2]. Nearly 80% of these adults have mild hypertension, defined as a diastolic blood pressure of 90–104 mmHg.

It is difficult to specify an elevated blood pressure that is truly risk free. Arguments have been made both for and against treating mild elevations of diastolic pressure[3]. Antihypertensive therapy reduces morbidity and mortality from stroke, coronary artery disease, heart failure and renal failure for all degrees of hypertension. However, this effect is modest for mild hypertension and is concentrated primarily on those with hypercholesterolemia, glucose intolerance, left ventricular hypertrophy and cigarette smoking[4].

In the USA, patients with diastolic pressures of 90 mmHg or greater are considered candidates for drug intervention. The World Health Organization and the International Society of Hypertension recommend that, after 3–6 months of observation, a diastolic recording of 95 mmHg or greater should be used as the level to begin drug therapy[5]. A 2–4-month trial of non-pharmacological therapy may be appropriate for young adults with mild hypertension who show no evidence of end-organ damage. Drug therapy may be added when the patient does not respond to non-drug modalities alone or has major risk factors for coronary vascular disease (family history, hypercholesterolemia, diabetes, cigarette smoking).

The traditional 'step-care' approach to pharmacological treatment of mild to moderate hypertension has been called into question. In this approach, the patient is first given a diuretic or β-blocking drug, and other drugs are added if necessary to reduce blood pressure to the desired level. However, many large trials employing the step-care approach in mild hypertension have shown no significant reduction in mortality and morbidity from coronary artery disease[6,7]. Therefore, several authorities have advocated a 'tailored-substitution' approach[8]. Here, initial drug screen selection is based on the patient's demographic, hemodynamic and clinical profile, and her propensity for certain side-effects. The intention is to use the fewest possible medications and minimize side-effects.

Most reproductive-age women with mild hypertension can attain adequate blood pressure control with a single drug. If control is not achieved, another agent within the same class is unlikely to be any more effective, although such a substitution may be useful in reducing side-effects. α/β-Blockers, $α_1$-selective blockers, calcium antagonists and angiotensin converting enzyme (ACE) inhibitors are all regarded as first-step agents. Only one or two daily doses are necessary, and fatigue is less common with these relatively new drugs. β-Blockers alone are also effective, but may elevate cholesterol levels, reduce cardiac output, impede athletic performance and cause sexual dysfunction. Diuretics and β-blockers have numerous liabilities in the diabetic with nephropathy, and calcium antagonists may adversely affect insulin secretions. Centrally acting adrenergic inhibitors (e.g. methyldopa, clonidine), hydralazine and reserpine are reserved as second choices.

PRECONCEPTION COUNSELING AND EARLY PRENATAL CARE

Generally, elevated blood pressure is the only sign in women with chronic hypertension, but a few face complications that threaten their lives as well as any pregnancy. Among such complications are hypertensive heart disease, ischemic heart disease, renal insufficiency and retinal hemorrhages and exudates.

Ideally, hypertensive women considering pregnancy should be counseled before conception so that they understand both the high likelihood of a favorable outcome with mild to moderate (diastolic blood pressure 105–120 mmHg) essential hypertension and the potential difficulties[1]. They should be informed of the potential for superimposed pre-eclampsia and worsening of renal disease or systemic illness. Lifestyle changes, such as activity restriction, bed rest and hospitalization may be necessary if the blood pressure becomes elevated.

Valuable reference data are provided by laboratory tests performed when high-risk patients are first seen before conception or in early pregnancy. An exhaustive search for secondary causes of hypertension (renovascular hypertension, primary aldosteronism, Cushing's syndrome, pheochromocytoma) is warranted in most cases[2,9]. Tests are usually performed on an outpatient basis, but, if the blood pressure is elevated, hospitalization may be necessary.

The preliminary investigation should include a urinalysis and urine culture, electrocardiogram and measurement of serum electrolytes. Baseline determination of renal function (24-h proteinuria and creatinine clearance) and platelet count are useful for comparison with values in later pregnancy, to help determine whether increases in blood pressure during pregnancy are the usual physiological increases or the onset of pre-eclampsia. Because of the high risk of fetal growth restriction, an early sonogram for dating and fetal size should be performed.

Normotensive patients with intrinsic renal disease but minimal renal dysfunction usually do well in pregnancy[10]. Those with azotemia (serum creatinine > 2 mg/dl) and hypertension should be advised of a high incidence of superimposed pre-eclampsia, perinatal morbidity and mortality, and deteriorating renal function[10–12]. Women with renal transplants are of particular concern, and should undertake pregnancy only after consultation with a nephrologist expert in this area.

NON-PHARMACOLOGICAL THERAPY

Most authorities agree that blood pressure can often be controlled without antihypertensive medications. Diastolic blood pressures from 90 to 99 mmHg are not difficult to attain, because blood pressure falls during the first and second trimesters in most pregnant women[1].

Some standard methods of treating hypertension must be changed in pregnancy. For example, weight reduction and vigorous exercise are not encouraged during pregnancy. Although exercise has not been studied, theoretical concerns exist about the role of uteroplacental blood flow in the pathogenesis of pre-eclampsia.

Weight reduction is advisable before pregnancy for those who weigh more than 115% of their ideal body weight[2,13]. Saturated fat intake should be reduced[14]. Alcohol and smoking should be avoided. Data are insufficient for routine recommendation of additional dietary calcium supplementation for treatment of pregnant women with chronic hypertension.

Research suggests that the severity of hypertension correlates with the extent of plasma volume contraction, and that pregnant women with chronic hypertension have lower plasma volumes than normotensive women[15]. Therefore, sodium is generally not restricted during pregnancy. Restriction is advisable for the rare pregnant woman with chronic hypertension who is salt-sensitive and for those whose creatinine clearance is reduced.

Regular dynamic exercise (walking, swimming) should not be discouraged if blood pressures are not elevated[16]. Rest during pregnancy in a lateral reclining position helps to maximize uteroplacental blood flow. Despite the lack of formal research on the subject, management should include bed rest to lower blood pressure and promote diuresis[17]. Strict bed rest is seldom necessary, but the patient should limit activities and set aside time each day for rest. Adjustments may be necessary in child care and the employment situation.

Patients should be encouraged to take their blood pressures outside the physician's office and keep a record of readings[18]. Candidates for monitoring should have formal instruction on the correct technique for applying the cuff and measuring blood pressure. Medical personnel should be available if the blood pressure rises significantly before the next scheduled visit. Self-monitoring of blood pressure is often helpful in determining whether borderline or mildly elevated blood pressures remain elevated at home or in the work setting and whether limitation of activity is necessary for better control of blood pressure. Also, adjustment of drug therapy or withdrawal are more plausible with knowledge of frequent blood pressure recordings.

DRUG THERAPY

The goal of treating a pregnant woman with chronic hypertension is to reduce the short-term cardiovascular risks to the mother while avoiding compromise of fetal well-being. Since most pregnant women with chronic hypertension have only borderline or mild elevations in blood pressure, the risk of acute cardiovascular complication is extremely low. Non-pharmacological treatment is urged when the diastolic blood pressure is 90 mmHg or higher.

Treatment of hypertension at diastolic levels of 90–99 mmHg must be undertaken cautiously because of the possibilities that medication may reduce placental blood flow or cross the placenta to affect the fetus directly[1]. Although the literature is conflicting, many obstetricians do not prescribe drugs for chronic hypertension in pregnancy unless the mother's blood pressure is above 150/100 mmHg or her hypertension had been well controlled by medication before the pregnancy. Clinical trials and experience have not shown whether long-term treatment of chronic hypertension prevents pre-eclampsia. Trials of antihypertensive drugs have evaluated treatment begun in the third trimester, but little information is available regarding treatment begun in the first half of pregnancy[19,20].

Research has suggested, but not conclusively demonstrated, that treatment of mild to moderate hypertension results in improved fetal well-being. In the largest clinical trial, which demonstrated a reduction in perinatal deaths, most patients began taking methyldopa during the second trimester, and a significant proportion began earlier[21]. Adjusting or withdrawing any drug therapy should be undertaken cautiously. A conservative approach is necessary to avoid excessive reductions or rises in blood pressure.

Table 1 lists drugs commonly used to treat chronic hypertension before or during pregnancy, their standard oral dose regimens, and adverse effects to mother and fetus. The prescribing clinicians should know the efficacy of these drugs and their acute and long-range effects on fetal well-being. At present, only methyldopa meets the criteria of efficacy and safety.

The vast majority of non-pregnant women can achieve adequate blood pressure control with many agents. Considerations of safety during pregnancy are as important as the patient's hemodynamic status. Experience has shown that, except for the ACE inhibitors, the drugs currently used pose no increased risk of perinatal morbidity or mortality. A detailed description of the different classes of antihypertensive drugs is presented elsewhere[2], but experience with their use during pregnancy is summarized below.

Centrally acting adrenergic inhibitors

Methyldopa was the first antihypertensive used during pregnancy and remains the most commonly prescribed central adrenergic antagonist for pregnant women. Because of its long-term safety, methyldopa is considered by many authorities to be the initial drug of choice for pregnant women with chronic hypertension and the standard by which other drugs must be measured[22]. The number of mid-trimester abortions has been reduced with the use of methyldopa without fetal growth or neonatal survival being affected[23]. Reports of smaller head circumferences in male infants exposed to the drug between 16 and 20 weeks' gestation have raised some questions[24]. However, long-term follow-up evaluations by the same investigators have been reassuring, and other studies of children exposed *in utero* to methyldopa have found normal mental and physical development at 10 years of age[23].

Clonidine, another drug which inhibits sympathetic output from the central nervous system, may be used in the postpartum period. An acute withdrawal syndrome with reported rebound hypertension may occur when the drug is discontinued.

β-Adrenergic blocking agents

The safest second-line antihypertensive is disputed. Many women with chronic hypertension are treated with labetalol or a β_1-adrenergic blocker (atenolol, metoprolol). Labetalol causes a decrease in maternal blood pressure without diminishing blood flow through the fetal aorta, umbilical vein, or intervillous space[25,26]. Use with another agent was required less often with labetalol than methyldopa and may have improved renal function[27,28]. In randomized trials comparing oral atenolol with metoprolol, no adverse fetal effects were demonstrated with either drug[29]. Unlike earlier reports using propranolol, several studies have not found labetolol to be associated with intrauterine growth retardation, fetal bradycardia, or neonatal hypoglycemia[27,30–34]. Neonatal apnea and bradycardia have been associated with maternal labetolol treatment late in pregnancy[35–37].

Most studies of these drugs have included relatively small numbers of cases with gestational ages at entry usually being at 29 to 33 weeks[38,39]. β-Blocking agents cross the placenta easily; they may interfere with interpretation of the fetal heart rate pattern, and, in theory, may compromise the fetus's ability to withstand hypoxic stress. A search for intrauterine growth restriction is recommended after long-term exposure to β-Blockers.

Calcium channel blockers

The most experience with calcium channel blockers has been during the second half of pregnancy in the treatment of women with either hypertension or cardiac disease[40–43] or for tocolysis[44–49]. Nifedipine, the best known and perhaps most promising calcium channel blocker, exerts a greater effect on vascular smooth muscle than on the myocardium[50,51]. A review of 102 women who received oral nifedipine for tocolysis concluded that therapy appeared to be safe for the mother and fetus[52]. A human investigation that utilized the Doppler ultrasound technique to assess fetal

Table 1   Standard oral doses and maternal and fetal adverse effects of antihypertensive drugs

Drug	Daily dosage(mg)	Maternal adverse effects*	Fetal adverse effects
Central adrenergic antagonists			
Methyldopa	500–4000	sedation, decreased mental acuity, fatigue, sodium retention, hepatic dysfunction, drug fever, positive antinuclear antibody Cooms test, hemolytic anemia, galactorrhea, postural hypotension	sedation, decreased mental acuity fatigue, sodium retention, hepatic dysfunction, drug fever, positive antinuclear antibody Cooms test, hemolytic anemia, galactorrhea, postural hypotension
Clonidine	0.2–2.4	dry mouth, drowsiness, orthostatic hypotension, acute withdrawal syndrome	unknown, embryotoxic in animals; none reported on humans
β-Adrenergic agents			
Metoprolol	50–100	sodium retention, aggravation of heart failure, bradycardia, depression, aggravation of bronchoconstrictor disease, vivid dreams, interference of diabetic control, CNS disturbances	intrauterine growth retardation, hypoglycemia, respiratory depression, bradycardia
Atenolol	25–50		
Labetalol	200–1200		
Vasodilators			
Hydralazine	30–300	tachycardia, palpitations, flushing, headache, sodium retention, aggravation of angina, lupus syndrome, neuropathy, dizziness	none reported on long-term use; fetal heart rate changes when given acutely at term
Calcium channel blockers			
Nifedipine	20–80	palpitations, flushing, headache	none reported but chance for reduced placental perfusion

*Maternal adverse effects are usually dose dependent, and low doses are most commonly employed during pregnancy

and uteroplacental circulation did not uncover any significant effects after short-term nifedipine therapy[53]. Oral nifedipine is rapid acting and has been used without complications; however, long-term trials of calcium channel blockers during pregnancy are necessary[49]. A comparison of nifedipine and atenolol reported no differences with either agent. Fetoplacental hemodynamics, birth weights and Apgar scores were similar between the two groups.

Vasodilators

Hydralazine, a peripheral vasodilator, is relatively ineffective when used orally and alone. In pregnant women with chronic hypertension, it should be limited to use as a second- or third-line drug. When hydralazine is combined with a β-adrenergic blocking agent, reflex tachycardia is lessened and blood pressures are reduced. Hydralazine is most often prescribed with methyldopa in treating pre-existing hypertension in pregnancy. It is considered to be safe for both mother and fetus, although one survey in Scandinavia has reported fetal thrombocytopenia[54].

Angiotensin converting enzyme inhibitors

ACE inhibitors, such as captopril and enalapril, are commonly prescribed to reproductive-age women.

Side-effects are minimal, and the drugs have considerable appeal for patients with renal disease. Their use during pregnancy is to be discouraged, however, because of multiple impairments in the fetus[55]. A patent ductus could be more common in the presence of these drugs owing to their inhibitory effect on kinase II which could eventually induce the release of vasodilatory prostaglandins. A persistent inhibition of the renin–angiotensin system may explain the fetal oligohydramnios and neonatal anuria. Any hypoplasia of the fetal calvarium may result from uterine pressure on the head, from oligohydramnios, or from decreased perfusion to the developing head. In March 1992 the US Food and Drug Administration issued a warning about ACE inhibitors. It is now recommended that women in the second and third trimesters avoid taking these drugs.

Diuretics

Diuretics reduce intravascular volume, thereby worsening fetal outcome in women with chronic hypertension who do not have an expanded plasma volume[56]. Women who use diuretics from early in pregnancy do not develop the expanded blood volume normal in pregnancy[57]. Little is known about the use of diuretics in pregnant women with essential hypertension. A meta-analysis of nine randomized trials involving more than 7000 patients revealed a tendency towards less edema or hypertension with no increase in adverse fetal effects[58].

Diuretics are not routinely prescribed during pregnancy. In the absence of pulmonary edema or congestive heart failure, such medication, and especially a loop diuretic, is best avoided because of electrolyte and rare thrombocytopenic disturbance in the mother and fetus[59,60].

Aspirin

Several studies have indicated that small doses of aspirin (60–100 mg) in women at high risk of pre-eclampsia may significantly reduce the incidence of pregnancy-induced hypertension[61]. Conclusions from a multinational study of more than 9000 women indicated that low-dose aspirin begun before 20 weeks reduced fetal morbidity in a select population[62]. These women had pre-existing disorders, such as chronic hypertension or renal disease, or had developed pre-eclampsia before 32 weeks of gestation in a previous pregnancy. No fetal complications attributable to the aspirin were identified. Studies have confirmed that low-dose aspirin therapy during pregnancy does not alter fetal cardiovascular waveforms, decrease fetal urine excretion, or increase neonatal bleeding complications[63–65].

WORSENING HYPERTENSION

Risks to women with diastolic blood pressures of 100 mmHg or greater are sufficient to warrant drug therapy. If blood pressures cannot be maintained at less than 160/110 mmHg, hospitalization is necessary[66]. Methyldopa is currently the initial drug of choice. If methyldopa is not successful or the patient does not tolerate it, reasonable additions are β-adrenergic blockers or perhaps calcium channel blockers.

No evidence exists to show that antihypertensive therapy improves fetal well-being or reduces risks of placental abruption, disseminated intravascular coagulation, seizures, or other maternal complications[67]. Therefore, both fetus and mother should receive frequent assessments, with special alertness for signs of renal disease or superimposed pre-eclampsia.

The prevalence of superimposed pre-eclampsia averages 15–25% among women with chronic hypertension. Some studies have shown that infants of chronically hypertensive women who do not develop superimposed pre-eclampsia do as well as those born to normotensive women[1]. However, other studies have reported higher perinatal loss rates in otherwise uncomplicated hypertensive pregnancies than among those without hypertension. Also affecting perinatal loss are coexisting renal disease, diabetes and obesity.

The diagnosis of superimposed pre-eclampsia is especially difficult in women with chronic hypertension.

Signs of pre-eclampsia may mimic worsening primary renal disease. Conversely, pre-eclampsia may be disguised by pre-existing proteinuria or antihypertensive medications. Some investigators have suggested that diagnosis can be improved by monitoring for decreasing platelet counts and increasing serum uric acid levels. A sudden rise in blood pressure complicated by proteinuria and central nervous system irritability should raise a strong suspicion of superimposed severe pre-eclampsia. With either superimposed pre-eclampsia or eclampsia, the outlook for both infant and mother is grave, unless the pregnancy is terminated.

In the presence of severe hypertension (diastolic blood pressure > 120 mmHg) near term or during labor, the degree to which blood pressure should be decreased has been disputed. Attempts to reduce levels down to 90 and 104 mmHg diastolic are generally recommended. Intravenous hydralazine is the drug of choice, beginning with a 5-mg dose every 20–30 min. Tachycardia and headache are side-effects. Intravenous labetolol (10 mg to 20 mg every 15–30 min) may be used as the second-line drug. Calcium channel blockers are not currently recommended if magnesium sulfate is being infused, since the magnesium ion may accentuate the effect of calcium channel blockers and precipitate hypotension[1]. Diazoxide is recommended for the very uncommon patient whose hypertension is refractory to hydralazine. Repeated miniboluses (30 mg) are safer than the customary 300-mg dose.

INDICATIONS FOR DELIVERY AND INTRAPARTUM CARE

Delivery is recommended, even early in gestation, if severe superimposed pre-eclampsia is evidenced, i.e. if blood pressures increase rapidly above 110 mmHg diastolic, significant proteinurea develops, renal function deteriorates, severe fetal growth retardation is confirmed, or biophysical assessment reveals fetal compromise. The most common techniques of antepartum fetal surveillance are fetal movement counting, non-stress testing, oxytocin challenge testing and biophysical profiles. Daily fetal movement charting should begin early in the third trimester. Weekly or semi-weekly fetal heart rate testing is recommended to begin by the 30th gestational week if antihypertensive medications are used or if the hypertension worsens[68].

Serial ultrasound examinations to assess fetal growth and amniotic fluid are recommended every 2–3 weeks during the third trimester. As long as the fetus continues to grow appropriately and the quantity of amniotic fluid is adequate, it can be inferred that placental function and uterine blood flow are appropriate. A reduction in the quantity of amniotic fluid may be associated with the umbilical cord compression before and during labor.

Hospitalization is indicated when systolic and diastolic values are persistently above 170 mmHg and

100 mmHg respectively, in spite of increasing dosage of medications, or there are other signs of superimposed pre-eclampsia, fetal growth restriction, or fetal distress. If the maternal condition deteriorates rapidly or fetal compromise is present, delivery is recommended. The predictive value of fetal surveillance testing may be invalidated by rapid changes in maternal health. Progressively reduced perfusion of brain, kidneys and such target organs as the liver and placenta should be watched for.

Fetal considerations often dictate the timing of delivery. The physician should reconsider delivery as soon as fetal lungs are mature if control of blood pressure has been problematic or fetal growth is suboptimal, or at term if maternal blood pressures have been well controlled and fetal growth has been normal. When delivery is anticipated before 34 weeks, glucocorticoids may be given to enhance fetal lung maturity if the mother's condition is stable, and delivery can be delayed at least 24 h[69]. Amniocentesis is often performed if determination of pulmonary maturity would influence decision-making.

Whether these plans of action decrease perinatal morbidity and mortality is unclear. Despite good intentions, the approach towards delivering a very immature but surviving fetus who requires intensive care and faces the attendant risk of long-range developmental disability is open to debate. Such an approach should ideally be attempted in well-equipped health centers staffed with specialized personnel.

Vaginal delivery is preferable to Cesarean delivery. If the condition permits, induction should be attempted regardless of cervical condition. A clear endpoint is encouraged for the onset, with delivery usually being expedited within 72 h after the decision to induce labor. Induction of labor should be expeditious, with an amniotomy being performed early. If vaginal delivery cannot be effected within a reasonable time, Cesarean delivery should be considered.

Although intrapartum analgesia with narcotics may be used, attempting to manage or prevent eclampsia with profound maternal sedation is dangerous and ineffective. A regional anesthetic such as epidural analgesia can be utilized for both vaginal and Cesarean delivery. Epidural anesthesia is permissible when an experienced anesthesiologist is available and no coagulopathies are present. Hazards include the possibility of extensive sympatholysis with resultant decreased cardiac output, hypotension and impairment of an already compromised uteroplacental perfusion. Bearing-down efforts should probably be avoided, and forceps may be necessary at times to shorten the second stage of labor.

POSTPARTUM CONSIDERATIONS

Acute hypertensive changes usually dissipate within the first few days after delivery. If severe hypertension persists, intravenous hydralazine or sublingual or oral nifedipine may be used repeatedly until blood pressures regress to near normal. The likelihood of underlying chronic hypertension is greatly increased if hypertension persists for more than 3 days after delivery. In such cases, oral antihypertensive therapy is begun before discharge and the woman is evaluated in 1 or 2 weeks. Oral nifedipine, clonidine, or labetalol has been favored, at the lower doses shown in Table 1.

Reinstituting pre-pregnancy treatment is likely to be necessary for women who were already hypertensive. Self blood pressure monitoring at home or work is helpful in determining the need to continue any antihypertensive agent. If pre-pregnancy blood pressures were normal or unknown, it is reasonable to stop the oral medications after 3 or 4 weeks and observe for any changes in recording at semiweekly intervals for 1 month and at monthly intervals for 1 year[70].

Many chronically hypertensive women wish to breastfeed. When hypertension is mild, the medication may be withheld, and the blood pressure should be observed closely. For breastfeeding mothers with elevated recordings, the clinician should continue drug therapy at the lowest effective dose. All agents have measurable amounts in the milk, and no clinical trials have studied the cardiovascular effects of an antihypertensive agent on the breastfed infant[71]. If the mother requires multiple agents to control the hypertension, breastfeeding is probably inadvisable.

Oral contraceptives and depot medroxyprogesterone acetate (Depo-Provera®) are not absolutely contraindicated in chronically hypertensive patients. The risk of the 'pill' is less than that of an unplanned pregnancy. Any low-dose preparation may be prescribed as long as the hypertension is controlled by non-pharmacological therapy and if other non-permanent forms of contraception cannot be used. Self blood pressure monitoring is encouraged. Persistent elevations in blood pressures would warrant consideration of discontinuing the pill.

REFERENCES

1. Chelsey LC. *Hypertensive Disorders in Pregnancy*. New York: Appleton-Century-Crofts, 1978
2. Mckenzie CR. Hypertension. In Carey C, Lee H, Woeltje K, eds. *The Washington Manual of Medical Therapeutics*, 29th edn. Philadelphia: Lippincott-Raven, 1998:61
3. MCR trial of treatment of mild hypertension: principal results. *Br Med J* 1985;291:97–104
4. Kannel WB. Hypertension and other risk factors in coronary disease. *Am Heart J* 1987;114:918
5. 1986 guidelines for the treatment of mild hypertension: memorandum from a WHO/ISH meeting. *Bull WHO* 1986;64:31–5
6. Roberts J. Pregnancy-related hypertension. In Creasy R, Resnik R, eds. *Maternal–Fetal Medicine: Principles and Practice*, 2nd edn. Philadelphia: WB Saunders, 1990:814–17

7. Leren P, Helgeland A. Oslo Hypertension Study. *Drugs* 1986;64:31–5

8. The 1988 Report of the Joint National Committee on Detection, Evaluation, and Treatment of High Blood Pressure. *Arch Intern Med* 1988;148:1023–38

9. Ellison GT, Mansberger AR Jr. Malignant recurrent pheochromocytoma during pregnancy: case report and review of the literature. *Surgery* 1988;103:484–9

10. Packham DK, Fairley KF, Ihle BU, *et al*. Comparison of pregnancy outcome between normotensive and hypertensive women with primary glomerulonephritis. *Clin Exp Hypertens* 1987–1988;B6:387–99

11. Hou SH, Grossman SD, Madias NE. Pregnancy in women with renal disease and moderate renal insufficiency. *Am J Med* 1985;78:185–94

12. Lindheimer MD, Katz AI. Gestation in women with kidney disease: prognosis and management. *Clin Obstet Gynecol* 1987;1:921–37

13. MacMahon SW, MacDonald GJ, Bernstein L, *et al*. Comparison of weight reduction with metoprolol in treatment of hypertension in young overweight patients. *Lancet* 1985;1:1233–9

14. Puska PO, Ianoco J, Nissinen A, *et al*. Dietary fat and blood pressure: an intervention study on the effects of a low fat diet with low levels of polyunsaturated fat. *Prevent Med* 1985;14:573–84

15. Gallery ED, Hunyor SN, Gyory AZ. Plasma volume contraction: a significant factor in both pregnancy-associated hypertension (pre-eclampsia) and chronic hypertension in pregnancy. *Q J Med* 1979;48:593–602

16. Nelson L, Jennings GL, Esler MD, Korner PI. Effect of changing levels of physical activity on blood-pressure and hemodynamics in essential hypertension. *Lancet* 1986;2:473–6

17. Rapiernik E, Kaminski M. Multifactorial study of the risk of prematurity at thirty-two weeks of gestation. I.A. Study of the frequency of thirty predictive characteristics. *J Perinat Med* 1974;2:30–6

18. Zuspan F, Rayburn W. Self blood pressure monitoring during pregnancy: practical considerations. *Am J Obstet Gynecol* 1990;164:2–6

19. Leather HM, Humphreys DM, Baker P, Chadd MA. A controlled trial of hypotensive agents in hypertension in pregnancy. *Lancet* 1968;2:488–90

20. Rubin PC, Buuters L, Clark DM, *et al*. Placebo-controlled trial of atenolol in treatment of pregnancy-associated hypertension. *Lancet* 1983;1:431–4

21. Wichman K, Ryden G, Karlberg BE. A placebo-controlled trial of metoprolol in the treatment of hypertension in pregnancy. *Scand J Clin Invest* (suppl) 1984;169:90–5

22. Redman CW, Beilin LJ, Bonnar J, Ounsted MK. Fetal outcome in trial of antihypertensive treatment in pregnancy. *Lancet* 1976;2:753–6

23. Ounsted M, Cockburn J, Moar VA, Redman CW. Maternal hypertension with superimposed pre-eclampsia: effects of child development at 7 1/2 years. *Br J Obstet Gynaecol* 1983;90:644–9

24. Redman CW. Treatment of hypertension in pregnancy. *Kidney Int* 1980;18:267–78

25. Nylund L, Lunell R, Lewander R, *et al*. Labetolol: pharmacokinetics and effects on *in utero* placental blood flow. *Acta Obstet Gynecol Scand* (suppl) 1984;118:71–3

26. Jouppila P, Kirkinen P, Koivula A, Ylikorkala O. Labetalol does not alter the placental and fetal blood flow or maternal prostanoids in pre-eclampsia. *Br J Obstet Gynaecol* 1986;93:543–7

27. Plouin PF, Breat G, Maillard F, *et al*. Maternal effects and perinatal safety of labetalol in the treatment of hypertension in pregnancy. Comparison with methyl-dopa in a randomized cooperative trial. *Arch Ms Coeur* 1987;80:952–5

28. Lamming GD, Pipkin FB, Symonds EM. Comparison of the alpha and beta blocking drug, labetalol, and methyl dopa in the treatment of moderate and severe pregnancy-induced hypertension. *Clin Exp Hypertens* 1980;2:865–95

29. Wichman K, Ryden G, Karlberg B. A placebo controlled trial of metoprolol in the treatment of hypertension in pregnancy. *Scand J Clin Lab Invest* 1984;169:80–7

30. Lardoux H, Bazquez G, Leperlier E, Gerald J. Randomized, comparative study on the treatment of moderate arterial hypertension during pregnancy: methyldopa, acebutolol, labetalol. *Arch Mal Coeur* 1988;81:137–40

31. Ashe RG, Moodley J, Richards A, Philpott R. Comparison of labetalol and dihydralazine in hypertensive emergencies of pregnancy. *S Afr Med J* 1987;71:354–6

32. Ramanathan J, Sibai B, Mabie W, *et al*. The use of labetalol for attenuation of the hypertensive response to endotracheal intubation in pre-eclampsia. *Am J Obstet Gynecol* 1988;159:650–4

33. Macpherson M, Pipkin F, Rutter N. The effect of maternal labetalol on the newborn infant. *Br J Obstet Gynaecol* 1986;93:539–42

34. Pickles CJ, Symonds EM, Pipkin F. The fetal outcome in a randomized double-blind controlled trial of labetalol versus placebo in pregnancy-induced hypertension. *Br J Obstet Gynaecol* 1986;96:38–43

35. Garden A, Davey DA, Donmisse J. Intravenous labetalol and intravenous dihydralazine in severe hypertension in pregnancy. *Clin Exp Hypertens (B)* 1982;1:37–83

36. Haraldsson A, Geven W. Severe adverse effects of maternal labetalol administration in preeclampsia. *Act Obstet Gynecol Scand* 1989;78:956–8

37. Olsen KS, Beier-Holgerson R. Fetal death following labetalol administration in preeclampsia. *Acta Obstet Gynecol Scand* 1992;71:145–7

38. Sibai BM, Gonzalez AP, Mabie WC, Moretti M. A comparison of labetalol plus hospitalization versus hospitalization alone in the management of pre-eclampsia remote from term. *Obstet Gynecol* 1987;70:323–7

39. Butters L, Kennedy S, Rubin P. Atenolol and fetal weight in chronic hypertension (abstr). *Clin Exp Hypertens (A)* 1989;B8:468

40. Walters BNJ, Redman CWG. Treatment of severe pregnancy-associated hypertension with the calcium antagonist nifedipine. *Br J Obstet Gynaecol* 1984;91:330–6

41. Constantine G, Beevers DG, Reynolds AL, Luesley DM. Nifedipine as a second line antihypertensive drug in pregnancy. *Br J Obstet Gynaecol* 1987;94:1136–42

42. Klein V, Repke JT. Supraventricular tachycardia in pregnancy: cardioversion with verapamil. *Obstet Gynecol* 1984;63(suppl):16S–18S

43. Rotmensch HH, Elkaya U, Frishman W. Antiarrhythmic drug therapy during pregnancy. *Ann Intern Med* 1983;98:487–97

44. Ulmsten U. Treatment of premature labor with the calcium antagonist nifedipine. *Arch Gynecol* 1980;229:1–5

45. Kaul AF, Osathanondh AR, Safon L, *et al*. The management of preterm labor with the calcium channel-blocking agent nifedipine combined with the betamimetic terbutaline. *Drug Intell Clin Pharm* 1985; 19:369–71

46. Read MD, Wellby DE. The use of calcium antagonist (nifedipine) to suppress preterm labor. *Br J Obstet Gynaecol* 1986;93:933–7

47. Ferguson JE, Dyson D, Holbrook H, *et al*. Cardiovascular and metabolic effects associated with nifedipine and ritodrine tocolysis. *Am J Obstet Gynecol* 1989; 161:788–95

48. Childress CH, Katz VL. Nifedipine and its indications in obstetrics and gynecology. *Obstet Gynecol* 1994;83: 616–24

49. Magee L, Schick B, Donnerfeld A, *et al*. The safety of calcium channel blockers in human pregnancy: a prospective, multi-center cohort study. *Am J Obstet Gynecol* 1996;174:823–8

51. Constantine G, Beevers DG, Reynolds AL, Luesley DM. Nifedipine as a second-line antihypertensive drug in pregnancy. *Br J Obstet Gynaecol* 1987;94:1136–42

52. Waisman G, Mayorga L, Amera M, *et al*. Magnesium plus nifedipine: potentiation of hypertensive effect in pre-eclampsia? *Am J Obstet Gynecol* 1989;159:308–9

52. Ulmsted U. Treatment of normotensive and hypertensive patients with preterm labor using oral nifedipine, a calcium antagonist. *Arch Gynecol* 1984;236:69–72

53. Chernoff EA, Hilfer SR. Calcium dependence and contraction in somite fromation. *Tissue Cell* 1982;14: 435–49

54. Widerlov E, Karlman I, Storsater J. Hydralazine-induced neonatal thrombocytopenia (letter). *N Engl J Med* 1980;301:1235

55. Hanssens M, Keirse M, Vankelecom F, Van Assche F. Fetal and neonatal effects of treatment with angiotensin-converting enzyme inhibitors. *Obstet Gynecol* 1991;78: 128–33

56. Arias F, Zamora J. Antihypertensive treatment and pregnancy outcome in patients with mild chronic hypertension. *Obstet Gynecol* 1979;53:489

57. Sibai BM, Grossman RA, Grossman HG. Effects of diuretics on plasma in pregnancies with long-term hypertension. *Am J Obstet Gynecol* 1984;150:831–5

58. Collins R, Yusuf S, Peto R. Overview of randomized trials of diuretics in pregnancy. *Br Med J* 1985;290:17–23

61. Sibai BM, Caritis SN, Thom E, *et al*. Prevention of pre-eclampsia with low dose aspirin in healthy, nulliparous pregnant women. *N Engl J Med* 1993;329:1213–18

62. CLASP Collaborative Group. CLASP: a randomized trial of low-dose aspirin for the prevention and treatment of pre-eclampsia among 9364 pregnant women. *Lancet* 1994;343:619–29

63. Veille J-C, Hanson R, Sivakoff M, *et al*. Effects of maternal ingestion of low-dose aspirin on the fetal cardiovascular system. *Am J Obstet Gynecol* 1993;168:1430–7

64. DiSessa TG, Moretti ML, Khoury A, *et al*. Cardiac function in fetuses and newborns exposed to low-dose aspirin during pregnancy. *Am J Obstet Gynecol* 1994;171: 892–900

65. Maher JE, Owen J, Goldenberg R, *et al*. The effect of low-dose aspirin on fetal urine output and amniotic fluid volume. *Am J Obstet Gynecol* 1993;169:885–8

66. Sibai BM, Mabie WC, Shamsa F, *et al*. A comparison of no medication versus methyldopa or labetalol in chronic hypertension during pregnancy. *Am J Obstet Gynecol* 1990;162:960–6

67. National High Blood Pressure Education Program Working Group. Report on high blood pressure in pregnancy. *Am J Obstet Gynecol* 1990;163:1689–712

68. Pircon RA, Lagrew DC, Towers CV, *et al*. Antepartum testing in the hypertensive patient: when to begin. *Am J Obstet Gynecol* 1991;164:1563–70

69. Allbert J, Morrison J. Glucocorticoid and fetal pulmonary maturity. In Rayburn W, Zuspan F, eds. *Drug Therapy in Obstetrics and Gynecology*, 3rd edn. St Louis: Mosby, 1992:90–102

70. Zuspan F, Zuspan K. Hypertensive therapy during pregnancy. In Rayburn W, Zuspan F. eds. *Drug Therapy in Obstetrics and Gynecology*, 3rd edn. St Louis: Mosby, 1992:105–26

71. White WB. Management of hypertension during lactation. *Hypertension* 1984;6:297–300

41

Neurologic diseases

D.B. Clifford

HEADACHE

Headache is perhaps the most common neurological complaint, and no stranger to young women in the childbearing years. Fortunately, the vast majority of headaches are benign and their etiology remains unknown in most cases. The challenge in confronting headaches is first, safely to rule out serious neurological pathology requiring direct treatment, and then to provide symptomatic relief.

As in all of neurology, the history is of paramount importance. Severe headaches associated with fever, stiff neck or change in mental status require emergency evaluation for meningeal infection or subarachnoid blood. Similarly, new headaches associated with focal neurological findings, or evidence of increasing intracranial pressure (nausea, vomiting, increase while sleeping, papilledema, bradycardia) require immediate structural brain studies. However, these situations are rare, and the majority of headaches fall into the categories of muscle tension/stress headaches or migrainous headaches. Tension headaches typically build up during the day and are characterized by pressure or squeezing sensation in the head and neck. Migraine headaches typically have pounding pain related to the pulse and thus have been called vascular headaches. There is often a family history of such headaches, and they frequently start rather early in life. In the classical migraine, the headaches occur with an aura often involving the vision, followed by the headache, which is very often associated with nausea. While some migraineurs can identify dietary triggers for their headaches (cheese, chocolate, red wine), most occur with no particular trigger. Whereas migraines are often unilateral, they need not be so, and common migraine is practically identified as a 'sick headache' requiring the sufferer to alter normal activities.

Treatment for headache generally starts with simple analgesic medications. Acetaminophen is probably the safest of these agents and has been in use for many years without apparent association with birth defects. Aspirin and ibuprofen are reasonable alternatives but should be avoided late in the pregnancy, as their inhibition of prostaglandins may be associated with difficulties with labor and increased blood loss. When additional therapy is required for acute headache,

codeine may be added to these medications to increase the analgesic potential. If headaches are frequent, prophylactic therapy is warranted. The two most commonly useful prophylactic treatments are the daily use of either an antidepressant or a β-adrenergic blocking medication. The choice between them is best made on the grounds of which would have the most useful or least troublesome side-effects. The most clearly useful antidepressants are amitriptyline and imipramine. Fortunately, the dose required for treatment of pain is smaller than is generally needed for depression, so side-effects from these medications tend to be tolerable. However, patients must be warned about sedation, particularly in the first few weeks of use, as well as the dry mouth almost universally noted with these tertiary tricyclic medications. Propranolol in doses of 40–160 mg/day is similarly effective and may be particularly useful if the blood pressure is at all elevated, or if sedation will be poorly tolerated. Both of these treatments may be used during pregnancy. Most authorities suggest that the use of ergotamine-containing preparations which are also useful in treatment of migraine should be avoided in pregnant patients, because these may hyperstimulate uterine contractions[1]. Fortunately, pregnancy appears to have an inhibitory effect on migraine with about three-quarters of migraineurs improving during pregnancy[2].

PSEUDOTUMOR CEREBRI

Pseudotumor cerebri, or benign intracranial hypertension, is the syndrome in which elevated intracranial pressure develops without mass lesions. It typically presents with headaches in young, obese women and may occur during pregnancy. The neurological examination is normal, save for the occasional development of sixth nerve palsies or visual field deficits accompanying the elevated intracranial pressure. Papilledema is routinely seen. Evaluation includes brain scanning (magnetic resonance imaging (MRI) or computerized tomography (CT)), which rules out significant mass lesions and shows normal or small cerebral ventricles. Spinal tap is then carried out to document the elevated intracranial pressure and otherwise grossly unremarkable cerebrospinal fluid (CSF) studies. When this condition develops during pregnancy, it may be expected to clear in 1–3 months. It may recur in subsequent pregnancies. When a subject has pseudotumor cerebri in the non-gravid state, pregnancy may exacerbate the condition.

Treatment is controversial and includes acetazolamide, corticosteroids, optic nerve fenestration and lumboperitoneal shunt[3]. The lumboperitoneal shunt may markedly improve vision in patients who fail medical therapy. As in the case of the ventriculoperitoneal shunt, vaginal delivery can be attempted in patients with the lumboperitoneal shunt without adverse impacts on the shunts[3,4]. For some cases developing during pregnancy, delivery of the child results in remission[5]. Close monitoring of visual fields is imperative to avoid the serious complication of permanent visual loss. In general, the condition does not threaten the fetus, and pregnancy proceeds without complication.

EPILEPSY

Preconceptual counselling

The epileptic woman should be counselled about the relationship between epilepsy and pregnancy. The best possible seizure control, preferably with monotherapy, should be established prior to considering pregnancy. If multidrug therapy is necessary, the lowest number and doses of anticonvulsants for full control is desirable. Furthermore, the serum drug level required to maintain a seizure-free state should be determined before pregnancy, so that doses may be adjusted during the pregnancy for effective control of seizures.

Epileptic mothers should be informed of their increased risk of having a child with a fetal malformation. Although the statistics on this vary, a large Norwegian study with more than 3000 pregnancies of epileptics indicated a risk for major malformation of 4.4% for children of epileptic mothers, compared to a risk of 3.5% for controls[6]. Other studies also revealed that mothers who received anticonvulsant medications had an increased risk of fetal malformations compared to those who did not take the medications[7–10]. Unfortunately, there has been no adequate population study that separates the impact of epilepsy alone from that of anticonvulsant medications on the development of fetal anomalies. It remains unsettled whether fetal facial clefting or congenital heart diseases are associated with epilepsy or anticonvulsant medications[11–13]. The overall increased risk of fetal malformations in epileptic patients probably arises from both the inherent risk of epilepsy and the medications. Fetal abnormalities can be detected with a maternal triple screen test at 14–16 weeks of gestation and level II ultrasound examinations at 18–20 weeks of gestation.

The choice of anticonvulsant medications should not be inordinately directed by the potential impact of the specific drugs on pregnancy, since no medication is absolutely safe for the fetus. Rather, the most effective medication for controlling seizures for a given patient should be the primary determinant in selecting the medication. It is important to emphasize to the patient that the medications should be taken faithfully to prevent seizures, because maternal injury, fetal injury and possible fetal demise from hypoxia may occur as a result of a maternal seizure. Mechanisms of teratogenicity in epileptics appear multifactorial, with the anticonvulsants being one driving force, along with genetic susceptibility, other environmental factors (other teratogens such as alcohol, folate deficiency in part due to anticonvulsants, toxicity of metabolites of the drugs) and associated demographic features such as poverty, malnutrition and drug use.

Effect of pregnancy on seizure control

Pregnancy exerts an unpredictable effect on seizure control, but more often makes control more difficult. This may partly result from the decreased serum drug levels during pregnancy for a variety of reasons such as nausea, vomiting, higher volume of distribution, decreased protein binding, increased hepatic metabolism and renal excretion of drugs[14]. In addition, fears of potential teratogenicity may encourage noncompliance with medications. Failure to adjust doses by measuring serum levels would cause deteriorated control during pregnancy in about 50% of epileptic women. This incidence may be decreased to 5–15% if previously therapeutic levels are maintained by dose adjustment during pregnancy[15,16].

Anticonvulsant use during pregnancy

Phenytoin

As perhaps the most widely used adult anticonvulsant, phenytoin has several advantages, such as efficacy against many partial and generalized motor seizures, relatively low cost, availability of a parenteral formulation, lack of marked sedation and cognitive toxicity and convenient, rapid loading administration. Consequently, it is the appropriate therapy for many childbearing women. During the course of pregnancy, serum levels of phenytoin consistently fall on a constant dose, exposing the mother to the threat of recurrent seizures. The loading dose is 18–20 mg/kg which can be administered intravenously in a glucose-free solution. The daily maintenance dose is 4–8 mg/kg or 300–500 mg which can be given as a single dose or in divided doses. The doses can be adjusted to maintain a serum therapeutic level of 10–20 µg/ml. Rapid intravenous infusion of phenytoin may cause maternal transient hypotension and heart block. Regular monitoring of the therapeutic level (10–20 µg/ml) and adjustment of the dose is recommended. Because of the widespread use of phenytoin, it has received close scrutiny for adverse effects. Although a 'fetal hydantoin syndrome' has been described[17], the literature remains contradictory concerning the degree of risk incurred by the use of phenytoin. The fetal hydantoin syndrome consists of hypoplasia of the distal phalanges, fetal growth retardation and craniofacial abnormalities such as microcephaly and cleft lip or palate[18,19].

Carbamazepine

This anticonvulsant is enjoying increasing use as its advantages are recognized. It has a broad therapeutic spectrum similar to that of phenytoin, but it does not have some of the cosmetic side-effects of phenytoin, such as gingival hyperplasia and hirsutism, and marked cognitive blunting or sedation. Aplastic anemia is a very rare but serious complication of carbamazepine. Mild to moderate leukopenia, which is usually not clinically significant, is more common. Overall, carbamazepine is a well tolerated and effective anticonvulsant.

The major effect of pregnancy on carbamazepine metabolism is increasing the hepatic clearance. The drug rapidly crosses the placenta, and the fetal concentration is about 40% of the maternal value. While carbamazepine has enjoyed a relatively good review of its teratogenic profile, it may be associated with less favorable fetal outcomes[20]. Maternal ingestion of carbamazepine has been associated with a 1% risk of fetal neural tube defects[21].

Valproic acid

This anticonvulsant is most effective against generalized absence seizures and is also effective in certain other generalized motor seizure disorders and myoclonic seizures. Although it has been associated with fatal hepatic failure, this complication is almost exclusively encountered in relatively young children, generally with severe seizure disorders, who are receiving multiple medications. It appears that this complication does not occur in adults[22]. For partial seizures it may sometimes be useful as a second drug. A special risk (1.5%) of neural tube defects has been associated with maternal use of valproic acid[23,24]. When this drug is clearly indicated, parents should be counselled about the special associated risk and should consider prenatal diagnostic evaluation including genetic counselling, detailed ultrasound examination by an expert and measurement of maternal serum α-fetoprotein (MSAFP).

Phenobarbital

This anticonvulsant is still widely used. Its advantages include efficacy against a broad spectrum of seizures, low cost, oral and parenteral formulation, low number of serious complications and long half-life. The disadvantages, such as its generalized depressant characteristic and somewhat lower efficacy against focal seizure disorders, make it less favorable for chronic use. This drug is generally a second-line therapy. Clearance of phenobarbital by the kidneys increases during pregnancy. The drug readily crosses the placenta, but the neonate has reduced drug clearance. Neonatal intoxication may delay recovery. Contributions of the drug from maternal milk may compound the problem, and therefore breastfeeding mothers should be cautioned to watch for neonatal sedation. In some epileptic mothers who require high doses, or who are addicted to barbiturates, the children may suffer withdrawal syndromes manifested as excitability, tremor, or feeding problems that start about 1 week after delivery. While enjoying a reputation as a relatively safe anticonvulsant, phenobarbital shares the same risks as the major anticonvulsants with associated increased risk of fetal malformations. It therefore appears to be unwarranted specifically to switch to this drug as far as teratogenicity is concerned.

Other drugs

Several newer anticonvulsant medications have been introduced in recent years, including gabapentin, lamotrigene and topiramate. Although these drugs have provided clinicians with significant new options for the treatment of refractory epilepsy, the human experience with them is limited, particularly in pregnant women. Some of the drugs have been associated with increased fetal malformations in animals. Use of these newer agents in pregnancy should be undertaken only if the benefits appear to outweigh the unknown risks of increased malformations or other unfavorable outcomes. In cases in which these agents dramatically improve seizure control, this risk may be deemed to be acceptable.

Trimethadione, which is rarely used in current neurological practice in the USA, is also associated with a wide range of fetal anomalies called fetal trimethadione syndrome[25-27]. The maintenance dose is 90–180 mg in two or three divided doses and the therapeutic total serum level is 15–20 mg/l.

Interaction of drugs and vitamin metabolism

Folic acid

Anticonvulsants commonly interfere with folic acid metabolism and may increase the requirement for folic acid. The Centers for Disease Control suggests that all women capable of conception supplement their diet with 0.4 mg of folic acid per day[28].

Vitamin K

At least phenytoin and phenobarbital are associated with vitamin K-induced defective coagulation in babies exposed during pregnancy. This may also be true of other anticonvulsants. Currently, there is no consensus on the prophylaxis of neonatal coagulopathy secondary to maternal use of anticonvulsants. One approach is to supplement the maternal diet with vitamin K_1 20 mg/day over the final month of the pregnancy. Alternatively, at least 4 h before delivery 10 mg of vitamin K_1 parenterally may be used. Infants at risk should receive phytonadione 1 mg intramuscularly.

CEREBROVASCULAR DISEASE

Subarachnoid hemorrhage

Arteriovenous malformations (AVM) and cerebral aneurysms are the most common causes of subarachnoid hemorrhage (SAH) in pregnancy. The presentation of SAH is most commonly associated with severe headache ('the worst of my life') and with a stiff neck. Very early or in the presence of markedly depressed mental status, the neck may not be stiff, but active testing of neck flexion is helpful in suspicion of meningeal irritation associated with SAH. Mental status changes will vary from none to profound, depending on the extent of the hemorrhage. The risk of first hemorrhage from AVM during pregnancy is about 3.5% which is not significantly different from that of nonpregnant patients and not influenced by gestational age or the mode of delivery[29]. Aneurysms may also bleed throughout gestation with a peak of hemorrhage occurring at 30–34 weeks of gestation[30].

Diagnosis of SAH is often made on CT scans. However, it is important to do a lumbar puncture if there is any doubt about the diagnosis radiographically. In general, once SAH is diagnosed, further evaluation and treatment of the causative condition must proceed regardless of the risk to the fetus. Management of AVMs will be highly dependent on their size and location. If possible, excision is the preferable treatment. In the case of aneurysm, angiographic localization of lesions and clipping of the one which has bled is generally recommended during the pregnancy, while other aneurysms discovered in the evaluation serendipitously may be dealt with following delivery. Surgical intervention for cerebral aneurysm is associated with lower maternal and perinatal mortality. This may not be true with AVM[30]. The mode of delivery of patients with intracranial hemorrhage during pregnancy should depend on obstetric indications until further data are available[29,30].

Ischemic cerebrovascular disease

Studies indicate that risk of stroke may be as much as ten times higher during pregnancy than it would be otherwise[31]. Some of the increased risk is probably shared by people taking oral contraceptive pills (OCPs). In general, other risk factors seem to combine with risks of OCP use or pregnancy; particularly notable (and modifiable) is the additional risk of smoking. The increased risk of diabetes, hypertension or pathological hypercholesterolemia cannot be ignored. The location of the strokes will vary, but there is evidence for an increase in middle cerebral occlusions in pregnancy-associated strokes, and for vertebrobasal strokes with OCPs.

Sometimes cerebrovascular disease, even in young patients, is heralded by transient ischemic attacks (TIAs). These events are transient (generally a few hours or less, but by definition less than 24 h) losses of cerebral function which could be understood by occlusion of a vascular distribution of brain function. In the case of a TIA or a small stroke, a rather extensive evaluation is indicated in a young person, searching for conditions requiring more directed management. It must be recognized that the major alternative diagnoses, both of which are relatively common in younger people, are 'migraine equivalent' and a seizure. The history should be directed at these differential issues and pursued as necessary. Evaluation for a TIA after a complete physical examination with particular attention to the cardiac and neurological examinations should include blood counts with examination of smears, platelet studies, coagulation studies (PT and PTT), urinalysis, blood chemistries, sedimentation rate and antinuclear antibody (ANA), serology for syphilis, electrocardiogram and echocardiogram, particularly if there is any doubt of the complete normalcy of the cardiac examination. Clearly, neurological structural work-up should include a CT or MRI scan of the brain. Spinal fluid examination is required if fever is present, suggesting possible central nervous system infection, if the neck is stiff or if there is evidence of increased intracranial pressure without mass lesion on brain scan. Finally, a decision as to the use of cerebral arteriography must be made on consideration of the entire case.

Therapy is highly dependent on the evaluation. Any risk factors for stroke should be addressed as thoroughly as possible. Hypertension should be controlled, though care must be exercised in reducing chronically elevated pressure in the face of recent ischemia. Rapid reductions in pressure or hypotension may cause extension of the stroke. Diabetes must be optimally treated and controlled. If there are cardiac arrhythmias, cardiomyopathy, or valvular disease, anticoagulation is probably indicated. During pregnancy, heparin is generally used because of teratogenic effects of warfarin early in gestation, and the potential for hemorrhage at delivery. Some authors advocate use of coumarin derivatives during the second and third trimesters[32]. The place of surgery in ischemic cerebrovascular disease is controversial. Practices for operating on carotid plaques or occlusions vary between countries and within different parts of the same country. However, when substantial occlusive disease is present and symptomatic, it is particularly in young patients who are otherwise good surgical risks that consideration of carotid surgery remains reasonable.

Venous thrombosis

Venous thrombosis is a complication commonly associated with pregnancy, the puerperium or oral contraceptive use[33]. A hypercoagulable state present in these situations is suspected to be the cause. The venous thrombosis may affect any part of the venous system, but the most common syndromes are cortical vein thrombosis, in which a syndrome of headache and seizures may develop, and sagittal sinus thrombosis, in which increased intracranial pressure, headache, seizures and infarcts are present in various combinations with lesions on either or both sides of the midline. The development of venous thrombosis may occur at any time, but the highest prevalence (80%) occurs in the second and third postpartum weeks[34]. Repeated cases have rarely been reported.

Evaluation with appropriate ruling out of septic causes (now rare), lumbar puncture to evaluate infection and determine any degree of intracranial hypertension, electroencephalogram to evaluate the epileptic processes often accompanying the cortical thrombosis and radiological evaluations are appropriate. On contrasted CT scans, a clot in the sagittal sinus will produce an 'empty delta sign' in some cases, highly suggestive of a sagittal venous thrombosis. Alternatively, cerebral angiography with attention to the venous stage may be required to make this diagnosis.

Treatment is directed at precipitating causes (dehydration, infection) and symptomatic. Anticonvulsant drugs should certainly be used in the face of seizures. The place of anticoagulants remains controversial. Some investigators believe that use of heparin, aiming at preventing propagation of the clot, is reasonable, but convincing evidence that the potential benefits of anticoagulation outweigh the real risks is lacking[35].

PITUITARY APOPLEXY

The pituitary gland enlarges during pregnancy because of stimulation of prolactin-secreting chromophobe cells. The gland is then vulnerable to ischemia in the face of hypotension in the peripartum period. Sometimes hemorrhage occurs into the pituitary, resulting in precipitous loss of function. As anterior pituitary function can be rapidly lost, replacement with corticosteroids and thyroid hormone are required on a permanent basis.

CHOREA GRAVIDARUM

Chorea gravidarum involves involuntary movements starting during pregnancy. One of the important historical causes of this movement disorder has been pregnancy. At one time it was said to occur as often as one case per 3000 deliveries, but the present incidence is very much lower, about one case per 139 000 pregnancies[36]. It is thought that many of the cases were associated with rheumatic disease and akin to Sydenham's chorea. In any case, the hormonal changes associated with pregnancy are capable of inducing or activating a predisposed brain to generate choreic movements[33]. A similar mechanism may well underlie more recently described cases of chorea associated with OCPs. These choreic disorders generally remit with discontinuation of the oral contraceptive or termination of the pregnancy, and may be symptomatically treated with neuroleptic drugs such as haloperidol. It is important to consider the differential diagnoses when confronted with chorea. These include acute rheumatic fever, Wilson's disease, Tay–Sachs disease, Hungtington's disease, systemic lupus erythematosus, antiphospholipid syndrome, hyperthyroidism, hypoparathyroidism, tardive dyskinesia and basal ganglia tumor or infarction. Tardive dyskinesia is most commonly associated with prior neuroleptic use. Appropriate evaluation, including a magnetic resonance scan of the head, for these diagnoses should be taken before the movement disorders are attributed to chorea gravidarum.

PERIPHERAL NERVE DISEASE

Carpal tunnel

The most common compression neuropathy, and a leading cause of hand pain, results from compression of the median nerve at the wrist. Curiously, symptoms often extend beyond the distribution of the affected nerve and include the entire hand, and frequently extend up the arm. Presumably, increased edema during pregnancy is the cause of this frequently encountered problem. Typically, a rather sudden onset of painful, burning or tingling sensations occur in the hands; this may be intermittent. Although classical signs such as Tinel's sign (dysesthesia produced by percussion over the carpal tunnel) are suggestive if present, they are often absent. With advanced cases, wasting is seen in the thenar eminence, but this is rarely present during pregnancy. Diagnosis is made with nerve conduction studies, the median sensory conduction studies being the most sensitive. The differential diagnosis should include ruling out arthritic involvement, hypothyroidism, amyloidosis and acromegaly, all of which are rare causes. If significant wasting and weakness are absent, conservative therapy with dorsal splinting particularly at night, avoidance of wrist trauma and repetitive wrist flexion/extension (as seen in various occupations, particularly typists), and sometimes brief use of diuretics will often result in symptomatic relief. After pregnancy, it may be anticipated that the condition will reverse. When weakness develops or conservative therapy fails, surgery to release the carpal tunnel is generally very effective.

Meralgia paresthetica

This results from compression of the lateral femoral cutaneous nerve, an entirely sensory nerve innervating the lateral thigh. It is commonly compressed in situations of obesity and weight gain. These clearly occur during pregnancy. In general, when the condition is recognized and the patient's concerns over dangerous implications of the symptoms are allayed, no other treatment is required.

Brachial neuritis

Brachial neuritis is an idiopathic disorder associated with pregnancy as well as the situation after surgery, immunization or viral illnesses. It typically presents with marked shoulder pain followed by rapid onset of wasting and weakness in the brachial musculature. No specific therapy is of value, and spontaneous improvement generally occurs. The condition may be bilateral in some cases.

Bell's palsy

Bell's palsy is a common mononeuropathy of the peripheral facial nerve. It is generally of idiopathic origin and occurs more commonly in pregnancy and the puerperium. The experience of Adour and Wingerd[37] demonstrated an increased incidence of approximately ten-fold for the third trimester and two puerperal weeks compared with the incidence in the general population. The clinical findings are those of peripheral facial weakness (involving the forehead as well as the lower face) sometimes associated with loss of taste on the anterior two-thirds of the tongue and hyperacusis. Recovery from the condition with good cosmetic outcomes is usual, although the most severe cases may retain variable degrees of weakness. Protection of the eye is the most important therapeutic task. Neurologists often use a 10-day course of prednisone 40–60 mg/day which is believed to increase the chance of full recovery if started early, although the long-term prognosis may be similar without steroid therapy[38]. If contraindication to the use of steroids exists, they need not be employed.

Guillain–Barré syndrome

Although pregnancy does not increase the incidence of this neurological problem, it does occur during pregnancy, as at all stages of life. The subacute onset of ascending weakness, accompanied by decreased to absent reflexes and eventual elevation of cerebrospinal fluid (CSF) protein levels, characterize this inflammatory peripheral neuropathy. It often occurs several weeks after otherwise nondescript viral illnesses. A notable increase in the incidence of this condition in patients with human immunodeficiency virus (HIV) infection has been noted, and Guillain–Barré syndrome may be the presenting complaint, as it typically occurs in earlier stages of HIV infection. It is critical that the complaints not be ignored, as the weakness may well progress rapidly enough to threaten the life of the patient, due to respiratory compromise. Autonomic instability and variable sensory loss and dysesthetic pains are not infrequently encountered in these patients and add to the challenge of caring for them. Supportive care and very close monitoring of the respiratory status until the condition stabilizes are the essentials of care. If walking is threatened, recent studies support the use of plasmapheresis or intravenous immunoglobulins, which may be accomplished during pregnancy with reasonable safety. Steroids have not benefitted these patients, and the risks of their use appear to outweigh the benefits. Improvement usually begins after 3–4 weeks and may take many months to reach plateau. In general, a good functional recovery can be anticipated in patients with Guillain–Barré syndrome.

Maternal obstetric palsies

Nerves traversing the pelvis are subject to injury and compression during pregnancy and delivery. Among the most common nerve injuries are those involving the lumbosacral cord carrying fibers from L4–5. Injury produces a footdrop. Femoral neuropathies also occur during vaginal childbirth, or during Cesarean or other lower abdominal surgery. Less commonly the obturator nerve may be injured. Therapy for all of the conditions should be supportive. Splints accompanied by range of motion exercise directed by physical therapy should be employed. Generally recovery may be expected over a period of several months.

Myasthenia gravis

Myasthenia gravis (MG) is an important autoimmune disease affecting neuromuscular transmission which has a peak occurrence during childbearing years in women. Rapid fatiguing weakness of muscles, sometimes generalized, sometimes restricted to the eyelids, or pharyngeal musculature, is the hallmark of this disease. Antibodies to the muscular acetylcholine receptor play an important role in this disease. Modern management techniques have markedly improved the prognosis for the formerly grave condition. Management is individualized according to the degree of involvement, but current practice is to perform thymectomy early in generalized myasthenia. Various methods of corticosteroid and immunosuppressive therapy are generally used to put the disease into remission. Symptomatic relief of weakness can generally be achieved with anticholinesterase drugs such as pyridostigmine. In acute exacerbations, plasmapheresis in conjunction with immunosuppression has been demonstrated to be efficacious, and may be used during pregnancy. Many drugs such as aminoglycoside antibiotics, lidocaine, quinidine, procainamide, phenytoin, magnesium sulfate and penicillamine can exacerbate the MG.

In general, pregnancy has an unpredictable effect on the clinical course of MG[39]. However, one large study found that most pregnant women had exacerbation of the symptoms of MG within 6 months of delivery[40]. MG does not affect labor and delivery, because the uterus is composed of smooth muscles.

It must also be remembered that the child born to a myasthenic mother may be affected and require additional support for neonatal myasthenia. This appears to be due to transfer of the acetylcholine receptor antibody from the mother[41,42]. The occurrence of neonatal MG correlates with the maternal serum level of autoantibodies against the acetylcholine receptor. These autoantibodies are directed against the acetylcholine receptors of both maternal and embryonic skeletal muscles; the latter appear to play a major role in the pathogenesis of neonatal MG[41]. The child's condition may not parallel the severity of the mother's condition, as some children have been born with myasthenic symptoms when their mother's disease was in remission. The affected fetus may present with severe polyhydramnios[42]. With supportive care, the neonatal myasthenic syndrome may be expected to clear on its own, as the antireceptor antibody titer clears, but this may take several months. Curiously, the onset of the neonatal myasthenic syndrome may be delayed several days after delivery.

DEMYELINATING DISEASE

Multiple sclerosis

Multiple sclerosis is the most common of the demyelinating conditions. Areas of demyelination called plaques occur in multiple regions of the brain and spinal cord, resulting in a wide variety of symptoms. The typically involved systems, from the substantial demyelination, include the corticospinal tracts (resulting in spastic weakness), dorsal columns (resulting in vibratory and proprioceptive deficits), cerebellar systems (resulting in ataxia and sometimes tremors), the visual system (resulting in optic neuritis with visual loss) and spinal pathways (resulting in bladder dysfunction). The disease typically involves relatively young women, and thus is not an infrequent neurological factor in the care of childbearing women.

Multiple sclerosis is diagnosed by the appearance of a typical clinical pattern, exclusion of other diagnoses and presence of typical test findings. The disease follows either a pattern of relapsing and remitting activity with neurological deficits referable to white matter disease with acute onset (over 24 h to a few days) and gradual recovery over several weeks, or a steadily progressive course. Other causes for dysfunction must be sought. Confirmatory tests often showing abnormalities compatible with multiple sclerosis include spinal fluid studies (few mononuclear cells, normal glucose and near-normal protein, elevated gamma globulins with 'oligoclonal' pattern, myelin basic protein (during exacerbation), MRI abnormalities in the white matter and delayed visual, auditory and somatosensory evoked potentials suggesting lesions in these pathways.

The decision as to whether a subject with multiple sclerosis should attempt to have children must be based on several factors including the severity of the individual case, social support and the effects of pregnancy on multiple sclerosis in the short and long term.

The decision about whether to become pregnant is an individual one. The disease does not appear to affect fertility, or cause adverse perinatal outcomes. Parents are often concerned about passing the disease on to their children. There is a slightly increased risk for multiple sclerosis in the siblings of affected parents.

TUMORS

Brain tumors are complications rarely discovered in pregnancy. When a brain tumor is discovered, coordination of neurological, neurosurgical and obstetric evaluation is required to determine the most satisfactory management of the problem. In general, optimal care for the mother with the brain tumor will take precedence in decision-making discussions. Tumors may become symptomatic during pregnancy because of growth experienced coincident with the pregnancy. In some reported cases, tumors have grown during pregnancy and regressed after delivery[34,43,44].

Tumors can be assessed radiographically (CT scanning or angiography when required for surgical planning) with appropriate shielding of the abdomen or with MRI. Neurosurgery can often be performed without interruption of a pregnancy. In some centers hypothermia is used during pregnancy. Because many tumors show at least temporary regression after parturition[41], interruption of the pregnancy or the earliest possible delivery is often considered in the face of an aggressive tumor. Similar considerations may apply early in pregnancy when seizures are uncontrolled or intracranial pressure threatens vision or herniation.

INFECTIOUS DISEASE OF THE CENTRAL NERVOUS SYSTEM

Bacterial infections of particular importance include meningitis, epidural and intraparencyhmal abscesses.

The most important organisms in adult meningitis are *Streptococcus pneumoniae*, *Neisseria meningitidis*, and much less frequently *Haemophilus influenzae* and *Listeria monocytogenes*. Key to successful management of these infections is early suspicion leading to prompt high-dose antibiotic therapy. Fever, mental status changes, seizures and nuchal rigidity in any combinations should make the physician consider the possibility of meningitis. Prompt lumbar puncture is advised so that etiological diagnosis is most directly determined. However, if lumbar puncture is delayed for more than an hour (for such potentially worthwhile efforts as ruling out mass lesions in patients with focal deficits or evidence of intracranial hypertension) empirical broad-spectrum therapy should be initiated. Blood cultures drawn before the start of antibiotic therapy, and counterimmunoelectrophoresis (CIE) on spinal fluid allow hope for etiological diagnosis even when therapy had begun before the spinal fluid can be sampled. Therapy for meningitis should include a third-generation cephalosporin such as ceftriaxone or cefotaxime, plus vancomycin with or without rifampin to cover resistant pneumococci. The latter agents may be stopped if organisms susceptible to cephalosporins are isolated.

Tuberculosis

Mycobacterium tuberculosis (TBC) infections may also be exacerbated by pregnancy, although treated patients have little to fear from pregnancy. The most common neurological presentation of TBC is as a subacute meningitis. This life-threatening infection is suspected when subacute meningitis occurs in a subject with TBC (whether symptomatic or not in the past). The spinal fluid has a variable lymphocytic pleocytosis, and variable degrees of elevated protein and lowered glucose levels. Organisms are difficult to identify but should be sought in smears of CSF. Culturing takes many weeks, and treatment must be undertaken before positive cultures can be documented. Development of polymerase chain reaction (PCR) methods of identifying TBC genetic material may make earlier diagnosis possible in the future. Normal therapy consists of isoniazid, rifampin and ethambutol, which appear to be safe during pregnancy[45].

Syphilis

Syphilis is another important infectious disease of increasing incidence in sexually active young people. Diagnosis is made by typical clinical characteristics with serological evidence of infection, and with appropriate response to penicillin therapy. Neurosyphilis occurs after a latent period of at least several years, but may be accelerated by immunodeficiency. Non-treponemal tests such as the VDRL and RPR are often used to screen for syphilis. Biological false-positive reactions are more common in pregnancy than at other times. The specific treponemal tests are used to verify infection. Neurosyphilis may present as an aseptic meningitis, as a vascular disease (cerebrovascular), as degenerative disease (general paresis or dementia paralytica), or tabetic disease (with pain and ataxia)[46]. The spinal fluid shows at least some degree of pleocytosis and protein elevation, although these changes may be modest. Elevated CSF VDRL titers when present are a reliable indicator of active central nervous system syphilis, but recent studies suggest that they are quite insensitive. It has been suggested that the CSF FTAABS test is more sensitive, and should be used to rule out central nervous system syphilis when it is a consideration[47]. Therapy consists of high doses of penicillin. A 10–14 day intravenous penicillin course (2–4 million units every 4 h) is often used when central nervous system syphilis is encountered[48]. Alternatively, high doses of procaine penicillin intramuscularly 2–4 million units daily with oral probenecid 500 mg four times a day have been suggested, both for 10–14 days[48]. In the non-pregnant patient who is allergic to penicillin, tetracycline is recommended. Tetracycline is contraindicated in pregnancy because of its fetal toxicity; currently, the US Public Health Service recommends penicillin desensitization in this situation. Ceftriaxone 1–2 g intramuscularly or intravenously for 14 days may be a viable alternative, although the presence of cross allergic reactions remains possible with this approach.

Viral infections

Viral infections are most common during pregnancy and fortunately rarely cause serious problems for the mother or the child. Herpes encephalitis, the most common non-seasonal serious form of encephalitis encountered, has occurred in pregnant subjects. Suspicion of this infection when fever, seizures and mental status changes occur should rapidly lead to appropriate investigation and treatment. Acyclovir is the treatment of choice and should be used as promptly as the diagnosis is made, as the final outcome for the patient rests on early institution of therapy. Cytomegalovirus is another common DNA virus with a high occurrence rate in pregnant patients. Fortunately, it rarely causes serious disease in immunocompetent subjects. In cases of immune-incompetent subjects, ganciclovir has been demonstrated to be efficacious at least for ocular cytomegalovirus.

The most important RNA virus to consider in sexually active populations is HIV. In Africa HIV spread has usually been through heterosexual contact, but in the USA the largest cohort of patients has been in the male gay and bisexual population. However, growth in the population of infected women is occurring, particularly those who abuse drugs or have sexual partners who do so. Recommendations for antiviral therapy and prophylaxis from the many opportunistic infections that occur in the HIV population are dependent on the stage of immunosuppression, and are still under study. The incidence of perinatal infection appears to depend on the maternal viral load, maternal CD4 count and prolonged rupture of membranes, and occurs in approximately 13–40% of cases[49-51]. Prenatal and intrapartum treatment with zidovudine reduces the risk of perinatal transmission to 8.3%[52].

Toxoplasmosis

Another important pathogen for pregnant women is *Toxoplasma gondii*. Normally an innocuous organism, it is a frequent cause of brain lesions in immunosuppressed subjects. More important, when the maternal infection occurs just prior to or during pregnancy, even without immunosuppression, the fetus may be infected and develop such problems as microphthalmia, microcephaly, seizures, cerebral calcifications, retinochoroiditis and hydrocephalus. Avoidance of exposure to *Toxoplasma*, most practically by avoiding exposure to cat feces, soil where cats defecate and raw meat, is an important precaution for pregnant women.

Fungal infections

Systemic fungal infections occur rarely during pregnancy. There is no evidence that the incidence is any more frequent during pregnancy, and the treatment of these serious infections is not modified by pregnancy.

REFERENCES

1. Au KL, Woo JSK, Wong VCW. Intrauterine death from ergotamine overdosage. *Eur J Obstet Gynecol* 1985;19: 313–15
2. Sommerville BW. A study of migraine in pregnancy. *Neurology* 1972;22:824–8
3. Shapiro S, Yee R, Brown H. Surgical management of pseudotumor cerebri in pregnancy: case report. *Neurosurgery* 1995;37:829–31
4. Landwehr JN, Isada NB, Pryde PG, *et al*. Maternal neurosurgical shunts and pregnancy outcome. *Obstet Gynecol* 1994;83:134–7
5. Foley J. Benign forms of intracranial hypertension – 'toxic' and 'otitic' hydrocephalus. *Brain* 1955;78:1–41
6. Bjerkedahl T. Outcome of pregnancy in women with epilepsy, Norway, 1967–1978; gestational age, birth weight, and survival of the newborn. In Janz D, Dam M, Richens A, *et al.*, eds. *Epilepsy, Pregnancy and the Child*. New York: Raven Press, 1982:175–8
7. Dalessio DJ. Seizure disorders and pregnancy. *N Engl J Med* 1985;312:559–63
8. Nakane Y, Okuma T, Takashi R, *et al*. Multi-institutional study on the teratogenicity and fetal toxicity of antiepileptic drugs: a report of a collaborative study group in Japan. *Epilepsia* 1980;21:663–80
9. Kaneko S, Otani K, Fukushima Y, *et al*. Teratogenicity of antiepileptic drugs: analysis of possible risk factors. *Epilepsia* 1988;29:459–67
10. Koch S, Lösche G, Jager-Romän E, *et al*. Major and minor birth malformations and antiepileptic drugs. *Neurology* 1992;42(suppl 5):83–8
11. Friis ML, Hauge M. Congenital heart defects in liveborn children of epileptic parents. *Arch Neurol* 1985;42: 374–6
12. Friis ML, Holm NV, Sindrup EH, *et al*. Facial clefts in sibs and children of epileptic patients. *Neurology* 1986; 36:346–50
13. Hecht JT, Annegers JF, Kurland LT. Epilepsy and clefting disorders: lack of evidence of a familial association. *Am J Med Genet* 1989;33:244–7
14. Hopkins A. Epilepsy and anticonvulsant drugs. *Br Med J* 1987;294:497–501
15. Schmidt D, Canger R, Ayanzini G, *et al*. Change of seizure frequency in pregnant epileptic women. *J Neurol Neurosurg Psychiatr* 1983;46:751–5
16. Robertson IG. Epilepsy in pregnancy. *Clin Obstet Gynecol* 1986;7:175–9
17. Bodendorfer TW. Fetal effects of anticonvulsant drugs and seizure disorders. *Drug Intell Clin Pharm* 1978; 12:14–21
18. Hanson JW, Buehler BA. Fetal hydantoin syndrome: current status. *J Pediatr* 1982;101:816–18
19. Meadow SR. Anticonvulsant drugs and congenital abnormalities. *Lancet* 1968;2:1296
20. Jones KJ, Lacro RV, Johnson KA, Adams J. Pattern of malformations in children of women treated with carbamazepine during pregnancy. *N Engl J Med* 1989; 320:1661–6
21. Rosa FW. Spina bifida in infants of women treated with carbamazapine during pregnancy. *N Engl J Med* 1991; 324:674–7
22. Dreifuss FE, Langer DH, Moline KA, Maxwell JE. Valproic acid hepatic fatalities. II. US experience since 1984. *Neurology* 1989;39:201–7
23. Lindhout D, Schmidt D. *In utero* exposure to valproate and neural tube defects. *Lancet* 1986;2:1392–3
24. Robert E, Guibaud P. Maternal valproic acid and congenital neural tube defects. *Lancet* 1982;2:937
25. Zackae EH, Mellman WJ, Neiderer B, Hanson JW. The fetal trimethadione syndrome. *J Pediatr* 1975;87:280–4
26. Rosen RC, Lightner ES. Phenotypic malformation in association with maternal trimethadione therapy. *J Pediatr* 1978;92:240–4
27. National Institutes of Health. Anticonvulsants found to have teratogenic potential. *J Am Med Assoc* 1981; 245:36
28. Centers for Disease Control and Prevention. Recommendations for use of folic acid to reduce number of spina bifida cases and other neural tube defects. *J Am Med Assoc* 1993;269:1233
29. Horton JC, Chambers WA, Lyons SL, *et al*. Pregnancy and the risk of hemorrhage from cerebral arteriovenous malformations. *Neurosurgery* 1990;27:867–72
30. Dias MS, Sekhar LN. Intracranial hemorrhage from aneurysms and arteriovenous malformations during pregnancy and the puerperium. *Neurosurgery* 1990;27: 855–66

31. Wiebers DO, Whisnant JP. The incidence of stroke among pregnant women in Rochester, Minnesota, 1955 through 1979. *J Am Med Assoc* 1985;254:3055–7

32. Iturbe-Alessio I, Fonseca M, Mutchinik O, *et al*. Risks of anticoagulant therapy in pregnant women with artificial heart valves. *N Engl J Med* 1986;315:1390–3

33. Schipper HM. Neurology of sex steroids and oral contraception. *Neurol Clin* 1986;4:721–51

34. Donaldson JO. *Neurology of Pregnancy*. London: Saunders, 1989

35. Gettelfinger DM, Kokmen E. Superior sagittal sinus thrombosis. *Arch Neurol* 1977;34:2–6

36. Golbe LI. Pregnancy and movement disorders. Neurologic complications of pregnancy. *Neurol Clin* 1994;12:497–508

37. Adour K, Wingerd J. Idiopathic facial paralysis (Bell's palsy): factors affecting severity and outcome in 446 patients. *Neurology* 1974;24:1112–16

38. May M, Hardin WB, Sullivan J, Wette R. Natural history of Bell's palsy: the salivary flow test and other prognostic indicators. *Laryngoscope* 1976;86:704–12

39. Parry G, Heimann-Patterson TD. Pregnancy and autoimmune neuromuscular disease. *Semin Neurol* 1988;8:197

40. Simpson JF, Westerberg MR, Magee KR. Myasthenia gravis: an analysis of 295 cases. *Acta Neurol Scand* 1966;42(suppl 23):1–27

41. Vernet-der Garabedian B, Lacokova M, Eymard B, *et al*. Association of neonatal myasthenia gravis with antibodies against the fetal acetylcholine receptor. *J Clin Invest* 1994;94:555–9

42. Verspycj E, Mandelbrot L, Dommergues M, *et al*. Myasthenia gravis with polyhydramnios in the fetus of an asymptomatic mother. *Prenat Diagn* 1993;13:539–42

43. Fujimoto M, Yoshino E, Mizukawa N, *et al*. Spontaneous reduction in size of prolactin-producing adenoma after delivery. *J Neurosurg* 1985;63:973–4

44. Leiba S, Schindel B, Weinstein R, *et al*. Spontaneous postpartum regression of pituitary mass with return of function. *J Am Med Assoc* 1986;255:230–2

45. Briggs GG, Freeman RK, Yaffe SJ. *A Reference Guide to Fetal and Neonatal Risk: Drugs in Pregnancy and Lactation* 3rd edn. Baltimore, MD: Wilkins and Wilkins, 1990

46. Simon RP. Neurosyphilis. *Arch Neurol* 1985;42:606–13

47. Davis LE, Schmitt JW. Clinical significance of cerebrospinal fluid tests for neurosyphilis. *Ann Neurol* 1989;25:50–5

48. Sexually transmitted diseases treatment guidelines. *Morbid Mortal Weekly Rep* 1993;42(RR-14):1–102

49. Minkoff H, Burns DN, Landesman S, *et al*. The relationship of the duration of ruptured membranes to vertical transmission of human immunodeficiency virus. *Am J Obstet Gynecol* 1995;173:585–9

50. Dickover RE, Garratty EM, Herman SA, *et al*. Identification of levels of maternal HIV-1 RNA associated with risk of perinatal transmission: effect of maternal zidovudine treatment on viral load. *J Am Med Assoc* 1996;275:599–605

51. Centers for Disease Control and Prevention. U.S. Public Health Service recommendations for human immunodeficiency virus counseling and voluntary testing for pregnant women. *Morbid Mortal Weekly Rep* 1995;44(RR-7):1–15

52. Connor EM, Sperling RS, Gelber R, *et al*. Reduction of maternal–infant transmission of human immunodeficiency virus type 1 with zidovudine treatment. *N Engl J Med* 1994;331:1173–80

42
Psychiatric diseases

M. Artal

Pregnancy and childbirth are naturally occurring life events accompanied by momentous neuroendocrine and psychosocial changes. The myriad interactions of the biopsychosocial variables and their effects on mental disorders are insufficiently understood and remain one of the most challenging areas of modern psychiatry. Growing data suggest potential neurobiological mechanisms by which psychological experiences, particularly early life stress, may produce persistent neural alterations in the central nervous system and in the pituitary. These alterations may be associated with altered behavioral responses and may contribute to adult psychopathology[1,2].

Research methodology and the interpretation of the findings must overcome several formidable obstacles: the enormous complexity of the subject; the plasticity and individual variability of human responses even to similar stressors; the need to consider multifactorial causation; the degree to which personal experience and socio-cultural attitudes may interact with biological variables; the temptation to overcome or reduce complexity by oversimplification and by offering reductionistic explanatory models; the tendency to connect events which may not be related especially in retrospective questionnaires; and the possible effect of unconscious positive and negative attitudes toward female procreative processes by either idealizing fertility or attributing to it negative qualities.

One of the most unique aspects of perinatal medicine is its subject matter: it addresses the life and well-being of both the mother and her offspring. Likewise perinatal psychiatry must address the suffering of the individual pregnant woman and her safety while being mindful of the significant potential effects of maternal mental illness on early child development[3–8].

Pregnancy has been depicted as a time of well being, calm and inner peace for women[9]. The elevated gonadotropin levels, the sense of fulfillment, and the responsibility of caring for the young have been suggested to confer protection from mental disorders[10]. Recent studies, however, found no such decrease in incidence[1,11–15]. Events in women's reproductive cycles such as menstruation, pregnancy, childbirth and menopause are increasingly being seen as biological risk factors for mood disorders[16] even though the great majority of women experience such natural events without any significant psychiatric impairment. The comparison of pregnant women to matched non-childbearing women shows no difference in the rates of depression[17]. This chapter provides a current overview of the most common psychiatric disorders during pregnancy and the postpartum period.

ANXIETY DISORDER IN PREGNANCY

The course of anxiety and panic disorders in pregnancy is variable. Symptoms may decrease in some women while persist in others[11,12,18]. Treatment options include psychotherapy and medication. Psychotherapy may allow the patients to avoid using medications during the critical period of embryogenesis during the first trimester when the risk of fetal malformations is maximal[18,19]. Patients who can most benefit from psychotherapy are those who are: (1) worried about the potential risk of medication; (2) psychologically minded and curious about 'what makes them tick'; and (3) willing and able to engage in psychotherapy. Anxiety disorders and panic disorder are frequently associated with interpersonal difficulties such as fears of expressing anger, and excessive concern of being judged by others. Psychotherapy may be effective for the anxiety and for the interpersonal difficulties these patients have, while the benefit of medication is mostly limited to symptomatic relief[18,20–22].

Medication may be necessary if severe symptoms interfere significantly with daily functions and psychotherapy is not feasible. Selective serotonin re-uptake inhibitor (SSRI) antidepressants such as sertraline, paroxetine, fluoxetine or the tricyclic antidepressants, such as desipramine, may be helpful. The latter group may cause orthostatic hypotension and constipation.

OBSESSIVE–COMPULSIVE DISORDER IN PREGNANCY

Clinically, obsessive–compulsive disorder (OCD) presents with obsessions (intrusive thoughts) and/or compulsions (actions and rituals that the individual feels compelled to perform to reduce intense anxiety).

These patients frequently report a fear of: (1) harming the baby by stabbing, which may result in a fear of knives or of entering the kitchen; (2) dropping the baby, which may lead to a fear of holding the baby; or (3) germs, which may lead to rituals of excessive washing. These behaviors may seriously interfere with the patient's ability to carry out daily functions. The clinician should keep in mind that some patients may feel guilty because of their strange and frightening thoughts and may not report them spontaneously. It is helpful, therefore, for the clinician to inquire in a tactful and nonjudgmental way if the mother has any of the above fears. Obsessive–compulsive disorders are associated with a higher risk of a major depression.

The incidences of onset and of exacerbation of OCD during pregnancy vary widely in the literature, mainly due to the retrospective nature of the published studies[13,14,23]. Most epidemiological studies use questionnaires specifically asking women about the connection between reproductive events such as pregnancy, miscarriage, abortions or childbirth and the onset or exacerbation of their OCD symptoms[14,23]. The major drawback of these studies is inadequate or incorrect recall of many life events, which occurred years earlier. Wide variations in the risk of onset and of exacerbation of OCD during pregnancy are reported in the literature[14,23]. One study reports that 69%, 17% and 13%, respectively, of pregnant patients experience no change, worsening or improvement of symptoms during pregnancy[23]. Some women may be well during one pregnancy, yet develop OCD in subsequent pregnancies[13,23].

The onset of OCD may be neurohormonally modulated. Research into the possible role of estrogen, progesterone, oxytocin and the serotonergic system is underway[23–28]. Biological and/or psychological concomitants of puberty may play a role in the pathogenesis of OCD because the ratio of OCD incidences in boys and girls before puberty is 7 : 1 and 1 : 1.5 after puberty[29]. Heredity may also contribute to the etiology of OCD as shown by the higher incidence of OCD in homozygotic twins than in heterozygous twins[30].

Women with a history of OCD who plan to conceive may be informed of the variable course and the potential treatments. A psychiatrist can help the patient identify and address the psychosocial stresses in her life prior to pregnancy. Psychotherapy and selective medications (preferably taken after the first trimester) may be indicated. The SSRI antidepressants or clomipramine are the drugs of first choice for OCD in non-pregnant women[13]. Fluoxetine given in the first trimester does not appear to increase the risk of congenital malformation[31]. Since clomipramine taken in the weeks prior to labor may be associated with infant hypothermia, respiratory acidosis and seizures, it may need to be tapered off during the last trimester, especially during the few weeks prior to labor[32].

MOOD DISORDERS IN PREGNANCY AND THE PUERPERIUM

Depressed or sad mood is a normal reaction to the disappointments, setbacks and losses inherent in everyday life. It is usually transient and not associated with a significantly functional impairment. Depressed mood, however, may be a part of a serious, potentially disabling disorder such as major depressive disorder (MDD), bipolar disorder (depressive episodes alternate with periods of abnormally elevated, or irritable mood), and dysthymic disorder (characterized by low-grade, more persistent depressive mood that has been present for at least 2 years and usually longer). Epidemiological data from around the world show that MDD is twice as common in women as in men[33–35].

The incidence of major and minor depression during pregnancy is approximately 10%, which is similar to the non-pregnant female population[17,36,37]. The course of major depressive disorder may be limited to a single episode or show recurrences. The onset of MDD is variable; it may occur prior to pregnancy, during pregnancy or in the postpartum period. If the onset occurs within 3 months after childbirth, the specifier 'with postpartum onset' is added to the diagnosis[38]. The disease could be mild or seriously disabling. Depression may contribute to non-compliance with prenatal care and an increased risk of alcohol and drug abuse. Severe depression may lead to suicide, to other self-destructive behaviors, and to infanticide.

The detection rate of depression remains low; only a small proportion of depressed women are identified as depressed by health professionals[39,40]. Depression in pregnant and recently delivered women may be under-diagnosed because of the common presence of symptoms such as fatigue, insomnia, weight change, constipation and worrying in these groups[41,42].

The *Diagnostic and Statistical Manual of Mental Disorders*[38] (DSM–IV) requires the presence of depressed mood or loss of interest and at least four of the following symptoms over the same 2 week period to diagnose major depression: weight loss or gain, insomnia or hypersomnia nearly every day, psychomotor agitation or retardation, fatigue or loss of energy, difficulties with concentration and memory, and guilt or suicidal thoughts.

While approximately 15% of depressed individuals in the general population end their lives by suicide[43], having living children seems to offer some protection from suicide in the postpartum period[10]. Risk factors for suicide include past psychiatric history of depression, schizophrenia or prior suicide attempts, and several psychosocial risk factors such as living alone, lack of family or social support, and feelings of guilt and hopelessness. Obstetricians should be aware of the risk and ask women about depression and suicide with such questions as: "Have you been feeling like life is not worthwhile?", or: "Have you been feeling like giving up hope?". When suicidal ideation is present, emergent psychiatric consultation is warranted[44]. Because depressed/sad mood may be normally experienced, it is important for the clinician to be familiar with the diagnostic criteria for clinical depression, a serious condition requiring treatment and usually successfully resolved with treatment[40].

The treatment and the therapeutic responses for depression are similar during pregnancy or postpartum period and the non-pregnant condition[45]. The treatments of choice are psychotherapy and antidepressant medications[20–22]. A review of the treatments is presented below.

POSTPARTUM MOOD DISORDERS

Traditionally, the spectrum of postpartum mood disorders includes postpartum blues, postpartum depression, and postpartum psychosis.

Postpartum blues

Postpartum blues is most frequently a transient episode characterized by insomnia, anxiety, irritability, tearfulness and overwhelmed feeling within the first 2 weeks after delivery. It occurs in more than 30% of pregnant women and peaks between the third and seventh postpartum day[15,41,46]. It has a minor functional impact and usually resolves spontaneously within 2 weeks to 3 months. Management is limited to reassurance and support without medications.

Postpartum depression (PPD)

Postpartum depression is most likely to be a heterogeneous disorder[47,48,49]. The estimated rate is 6.8–13% of pregnant women[18,36,37,39,42,50,51] and up to 26% among adolescent mothers[52]. Twenty-five per cent of women with postpartum blues may go on to have postpartum depression[15,53]. Clinical manifestations include persistent (for at least 2 weeks) negative mood states (sadness, loss of interest, loss of pleasure in activities that used to be a source of pleasure, anxiety and irritability), appetite and sleep disturbances, psychomotor agitation or retardation, fatigue, decreased energy, impaired concentration and memory, feelings of worthlessness, guilt or suicidal thoughts. Risk factors for PPD include:

(1) Positive personal and family history of depression is associated with an increased risk for PPD[15,42]. It should be noted that the majority of women with PPD have no such prior history[42,54]. Women with a prior history of bipolar affective disorder show an even a higher relapse rate (40–60%)[55,56,57].

(2) Psychosocial factors such as marital conflict, being a single mother, lack of social/family support, the stress of caring for the infant (disrupted sleep and sleep deprivation), multiple births, complications during pregnancy (especially if necessitating prolonged bed rest), and other stressful life events during the year preceding the birth also contribute to the development of PPD[58,59,60].

The onset of postpartum depression occurs in most patients (> 60%) within 6 weeks postpartum. The depressive episode may last from 3 months to 14 months and the severity may range from mild to severe depression[61]. The clinical picture of PPD is similar to that of major depression occurring in the non-puerperal period[41,48,53]. Suicide and infanticide are the most serious complications. Unrecognized or untreated depression may impair function and adversely affect the new mother's ability to care for her infant. This is likely to increase her guilt, helplessness, and hopelessness and worsen her depression. This may also interfere with and limit the new mother's ability to respond optimally to the infant and consequently may have adverse effects on early child development[3–8,62].

The pathogenesis of PPD remains undetermined. The belief that hormonal factors contribute to the etiology of PPD persists even though there has been no empirical support[16]. Likewise, there has been no clear evidence to support the hypothesis that a rapid decline of gonadal hormones and cortisol and/or the effect of their withdrawal on neurotransmitter activity trigger PPD[15,49,53,59]. Several investigators[41,46,63] have looked at the potential role serotonin might play in PPD since it may play a role in the pathophysiology of depression. However, treatment with tryptophan (a serotonin precursor) did not prevent the onset of PPD[46]. In addition, there is no significant difference in platelet serotonin transporter binding sites (a model for presynaptic nerve terminals of the central nervous system) between women with PPD and non-depressed postpartum controls[41]. Sichel and colleagues[49] suggested that estrogen withdrawal after birth may initiate PPD in a subset of women who had no history of non-puerperal affective illness. The authors proposed administering high doses of estrogen immediately after delivery for 4 weeks to prevent relapse of PPD in subsequent births in this subset of patients. Such a treatment is still preliminary and is not considered a standard preventive treatment. Reports on good results in PPD patients receiving transdermal estradiol patches[64] have not been confirmed.

Postpartum psychosis (PPP)

The incidence of psychotic disorder during the first 4 weeks postpartum is 0.1–0.2% or 1–2 per 1000 births[50]. In most cases the onset occurs a few days after delivery, usually during the first 2 weeks postpartum. It is frequently heralded by 1–2 nights of insomnia and irritability[16]. The most characteristic clinical presentation consists of confusion and of delirium-like psychosis with bizarre behaviors and hallucinations. In most cases the differential diagnoses include bipolar disorder presenting as a manic episode, schizoaffective disorder, and major depression with psychotic features. A personal or family history of bipolar disease increases the risk of PPP. Relapse rates are estimated to be 40–60%[55–58]. Patients with a prior history of postpartum psychosis are most vulnerable to relapse[49].

The mainstay of treatment and prevention of relapse in bipolar disorder is a mood stabilizer such as lithium carbonate, valproic acid or carbamazepine[65]. An antidepressant or an antipsychotic medication may be necessary during an acute depressive or manic episode. Sleep hygiene in bipolar patients has been shown to be a very important therapeutic modality and sleep deprivation may trigger relapse[66].

SCHIZOPHRENIA AND OTHER PSYCHOSES

The incidence of schizophrenia in the USA is between 0.3–0.6 per 1000. The lifetime prevalence is about 1.5% spread equally across both genders. Given that its peak age of onset is between 15 and 35 years of age, it is of significant clinical importance during women's reproductive years.

Schizophrenia and other psychotic disorders manifest a variable course ranging from acute and discrete episodes to a protracted disturbance of thought and behavior leading to residual decline. Clinical course and prognosis are significantly improved by the availability of family and social support and psychiatric care. Patients may show eccentric thinking and behavior or acute psychotic manifestations with the potential for significant risks to both mother and fetus. Any new onset psychosis during pregnancy should be promptly evaluated for differential diagnosis of possibly identifiable medical cause (drug induced psychosis, temporal lobe epilepsy, stroke, systemic lupus erythematosus, acute intermittent porphyria) or psychiatric (brief reactive psychosis, manic or depressive phase of bipolar disorder). Treatment includes control of the symptoms of disorganized thought and behavior through the administration of the lowest possible dose of antipsychotic medication (preferably from the high potency subgroup, such as haloperidol or trifluoperazine), and by addressing the psychosocial stressors identified by supportive psychotherapy.

Schizophrenia may have an extremely disorganizing effect on patients' thinking, judgment and behavior. The potential for suicide and other self-destructive behaviors is significant.

MEDICATIONS

All psychotropic medications cross the placenta and their potential effects on the developing fetus must be considered[18,19,29,30,31,67]. Three potential fetal impacts of medications given during pregnancy are teratogenicity, if the medication is administered during the period of organogenesis; neonatal toxicity or withdrawal if the medication is given close to the time of birth, and potential later behavioral sequelae[18].

Depression during pregnancy, postpartum depression (PPD) and psychosis are potentially severe and disabling. Untreated they may carry a significant risk to both the mother and to her offspring. The clinician needs to carefully weigh both the maternal benefits from the medications and the potential fetal risks[18,19,31,32,67]. Medications during the first trimester might be avoided if the depression is not severe and psychotherapy could be undertaken[21]. Determination of gestational age might be helpful in timing the initiation of antidepressant medications, especially if psychotherapy alone is insufficient to alleviate the depression, to avoid the critical periods of organogenesis.

Antidepressants

Tricyclic antidepressants are the oldest agents and have been available in the USA since 1963. Extensive cumulative experience with their use has revealed no increased risk of major congenital malformations in the first trimester[67]. Most investigators recommend the use of the secondary amine tricyclic antidepressants (nortriptyline and desipramine) over the tertiary amines (amitriptyline). While the SSRI antidepressants have been used for a shorter period of time, they have significant advantages over the tricyclic antidepressants. They have a more benign side-effect profile, lacking cardiac toxicity or anticholinergic side-effects, and have a much better safety profile compared with the tricyclics in cases of overdose[67]. First-trimester exposure to fluoxetine did not result in an increased incidence of fetal anomalies[31]. The SSRIs are frequently the first-choice antidepressants. The shorter half-life medications, such as sertraline and paroxetine, are preferred over longer half-life agents such as fluoxetine because of the potential accumulation of active metabolites[67].

Given the risk of recurrence, psychiatric follow-up and maintenance treatment is considered the standard of care[20]. Women with a previous history of major depression who take antidepressants immediately after birth have a significantly lower rate of recurrence[68]. A reasonable therapeutic goal for treating depression or PPD during pregnancy is to control symptoms and to recover the function at a minimum effective dose of medication[67]. To minimize the risk of neonatal toxicity and withdrawal after delivery, the maternal dose of medication should be reduced during the 2 weeks prior to delivery[67]. Since several reports associated clomipramine during pregnancy with neonatal problems immediately after birth, it is advisable to taper it off prior to delivery[32]. Hepatic immaturity in the newborn may affect the metabolism of psychotropic medications, thus potentially raising their levels in blood[67]. The infant's pediatrician should informed of maternal medications to prevent possible adverse drug interactions with other medications which may be prescribed for the infant.

All psychotropic medications are found in the breast milk at various concentrations. Infants' absorption rates vary and significant drug levels are rarely detected in infants' serum. The long-term effects of trace levels of medications in the neonatal serum are unknown[69]. The following antidepressants appear to be safe for women who breastfeed: sertraline, nortriptyline, desipramine, amitriptyline, and clomipramine. These medications are not found in quantifiable amounts in breast milk and have not caused any adverse neonatal effect[71]. Fluoxetine is not recommended for use in nursing mothers because it has high neonatal serum levels and may cause colic symptoms[70]. Prescription of an antidepressant for a breast-feeding woman is a case specific, risk–benefit decision[70].

Mood stabilizers in pregnancy

The following mood stabilizers have been used in the management and prevention of relapse in bipolar disorder: lithium carbonate, carbamazepine and valproic acid[56]. The association of cardiac malformations with lithium exposure in the first trimester is widely documented by the Lithium Baby Register. The risks of major congenital anomalies, cardiovascular abnormalities and Ebstein's anomaly in fetuses who were exposed to lithium during the first trimester are about 11% (20/183), 8% (15/183) and 3%, respectively[71–73]. The risk seems to be smaller than initially reported and is estimated to be 1.5–3.5[19]. Women who are on lithium maintenance and contemplate pregnancy should have preconception counseling. In patients who have had a single episode of mood disorder, lithium could be gradually tapered before conception and restarted if necessary after the first trimester. Since the half-life of lithium is 20 hours it should be tapered 48 hours before delivery to avoid toxicity in the newborn[67]. Patients with bipolar disorder who have had multiple episodes run a high risk of relapse without the medication. The maternal risk from recurrence may outweigh the fetal risk from exposure to lithium[29,67]. Lithium is contraindicated during breast-feeding because its concentration in breast milk is about 40% of maternal serum[74,75]. Both valproic acid and carbamazepine are compatible with breast-feeding[67,69]. Both should be avoided during pregnancy if possible because of their association with neural tube defects[19,67,76,77]. An ultrasound examination of the fetal anatomy including fetal echocardiogram at 18–20 weeks is advisable.

Antipsychotics

All antipsychotic medications (neuroleptics) cross the placenta and are secreted in breast milk. Several of the typical antipsychotics (chlorpromazine, haloperidol) have been previously prescribed during pregnancy for hyperemesis. The newly added atypical antipsychotics (clozapine, olanzapine and resperidone) lack sufficient data in respect to potential teratogenic effects. The high potency antipsychotics (haloperidol, trifluoperazine) are preferable to the low potency drugs (chlorpromazine, thioridazine), because the former cause only minimal autonomic effects and significantly less sedation, hypotension, and tachycardia than the latter.

REFERENCES

1. Coplan JD, Andrews MW, Rosenbaum LA, *et al.* Persistent elevations of cerebrospinal fluid concentrations of corticotropin-releasing factor in adult non-human primates exposed to early-life stressors: implications for the pathophysiology of mood and anxiety disorders. *Proc Nat Acad Sci USA* 1996;93:1619–23
2. Ladd CO, Owens MJ, Nemeroff CB. Persistent changes in corticotropin-releasing factor neuronal systems induced by maternal deprivation. *Endocrinology* 1996;137:1212–18
3. Beck CT. The effects of postpartum depression on child development: a meta-analysis. *Arch Psychiatr Nurs* 1998;12:12–20
4. Beck CT. The effects of postpartum depression on maternal-infant interaction: a meta-analysis. *Nurs Res* 1995;44:298–304
5. Murray L. Postpartum depression and child development. *Psychol Med* 1997;27:253–60
6. Murray L, Hipwell A, Hooper R, *et al.* The cognitive development of 5-year-old children of postnatally depressed mothers. *J Child Psychol Psychiatry Allied Discip* 1996;37:927–35
7. Murray L, Fiori-Cowley A, Hooper R, *et al.* The impact of postnatal depression and associated adversity on early mother-infant interactions and later infant outcome. *Child Develop* 1996;67:2512–26
8. Philipps LH, O'Hara MW. Prospective study of postpartum depression: 4 1/2-year follow-up of women and children. *J Abnorm Psychol* 1991;100:151–5
9. Zajicek E. Psychiatric problems during pregnancy. In Wolkind S, Zajicek E, eds. *Pregnancy: A Psychological and Social Study.* London: Academic Press, 1981:57–73
10. Appleby L. Suicidal behavior in childbearing women. *Intl Rev Psychiatry* 1996;8:107–15
11. Cohen LS, Sichel DA, Dimmock JA, *et al.* Impact of pregnancy on panic disorder: a case series. *J Clin Psychiatry* 1994;55:284–8
12. Cohen LS, Sichel DA, Faraone SV, *et al.* Course of panic disorder during pregnancy and the puerperium: a preliminary study. *Biol Psychiatry* 1996;39:950–4
13. Diaz SE, Grush LR, Sichel DA, *et al.* Obsessive-compulsive disorder in pregnancy and the puerperium. In Dickstein LJ, Riba MB, Oldham JM, eds. *Review of Psychiatry*, vol. 16. Washington, DC: American Psychiatric Press, 1997:97–111

14. Neziroglu F, Anemone R, Yaryura TJA. Onset of OCD in pregnancy. *Am J Psychiatry* 1992;149:947–50

15. O'Hara MW, Schlecte JA, Lewis DA, *et al*. Prospective study of postpartum blues. Biologic and psychosocial factors. *Arch Gen Psychiatry* 1991;48:801

16. Wisner KL, Zachary NS. Psychobiology of postpartum mood disorders. *Semin Reprod Endocrinol* 1997; 15:77–89

17. O'Hara MW, Zekoski EM, Philipps LH, *et al*. Controlled prospective study of postpartum mood disorders: comparison of childbearing and non childbearing women. *J Abnorm Psychol* 1990;99:3–15

18. Altshuler LL, Cohen L, Szuba MP, *et al*. Pharmacologic management of psychiatric illness in pregnancy; dilemmas and guidelines. *Am J Psychiatry* 1996;153:592–606

19. Miller LJ. Psychiatric medication during pregnancy: understanding and minimizing the risks. *Psychiatr Ann* 1994;24:69–75

20. Practice guideline for major depressive disorder in adults. *Am J Psychiatry* 1993;150(Suppl.):1

21. Spinelli MG. Interpersonal psychotherapy for depressed antepartum women: a pilot study. *Am J Psychiatry* 1997; 154:1028–30

22. Stuart S, O'Hara MW. Interpersonal psychotherapy for postpartum depression: a treatment program. *J Psychother Pract Res* 1995;4:18–29

23. Williams KE, Koran LM. Obsessive compulsive disorder in pregnancy, the puerperium, and the menstruum. *J Clin Psychiatry* 1997;58:330–4

24. Biegor A, Reches A, Snyder L. Serotonergic and noradrenergic hormones. *Life Sci* 1983;32:2015–21

25. Ehrenkranz JRL. Effects of sex steroids on serotonin uptake in blood platelets. *Acta Endocrinol (Copenh)* 1976;83:420–8

26. Leckman JF, Goodman WK, North WG, *et al*. Elevated CSF levels of oxytocin in obsessive compulsive disorder. *Arch Gen Psychiatry* 1994;51:782–92

27. Murphy DL, Zohar J, Benkelfat MT, *et al*. Obsessive compulsive disorder as a 5-HT subsystem-related behavioral disorder. *Br J Psychiatry* 1989;155:15–24

28. Swedo SE, Leonard HL, Kruesi MJP, *et al*. CSF neurochemistry in children and adolescents with obsessive compulsive disorder. *Arch Gen Psychiatry* 1992;49: 29–36

29. Swedo SE, Rapoport JL, Leonard H, *et al*. Obsessive compulsive disorder in children and adolescents: clinical phenomenology of 70 consecutive cases. *Arch Gen Psychiatry* 1989;46:335–41

30. MacDonald AM, Murray RM, Clifford CA. The contribution of heredity to obsessional disorder and personality: a review of family and twin study evidence. In Tsuang MT, Kendler KS, Lyons MJ, eds. *Genetic Issues in Psychosocial Epidemiology*, vol 8. New Brunswick, NJ: Rutgers University Press, 1991:191–212

31. Pastuszak A, Schick-Boschetto B, Zuber C, *et al*. Pregnancy outcome following first trimester exposure to fluoxetine. *J Am Med Assoc* 1993;269:2246–8

32. Schimmell MS, Katz EZ, Shaag Y, *et al*. Toxic neonatal effects following maternal clomipramine therapy. *Clin Toxicol* 1991;29:479–84

33. Blazer DG, Kessler RC, McGonagle KA, *et al*. The prevalence and distribution of major depression in a national community sample: the National Comorbidity Survey. *Am J Psychiatry* 1994;15:979–86

34. Weissman MM, Olfson M. Depression in women: implications for health care research. *Science* 1995;269: 799–801

35. Weissman MM, Bland R, Joyce PR, *et al*. Sex differences in rates of depression: cross-national perspectives. *J Affect Dis* 1993;29:77–84

36. Gotlib IH, Whiffen VE, Mount JH, *et al*. Prevalence rates and demographic characteristics associated with depression in pregnancy and the postpartum. *J Consult Clin Psychol* 1989;57:269–74

37. Kumar R, Robson KM. A prospective study of emotional disorders in childbearing women. *Br J Psychiatry* 1984;144:35–47

38. *DSM-IV: Diagnostic and Statistical Manual of Mental Disorders*, 4th edn. (DSM-IV-R) Washington, DC: American Psychiatric Association, 1994

39. Beck CT. Screening methods for postpartum depression. *J Obstet Gynecol Neonatal Nurs* 1995;24:308–12

40. Keller MB, Hanks DL. The natural history and heterogeneity of depressive disorders: implications for rational antidepressant therapy. *J Clin Psychiatry* 1994; 9(Suppl A):25

41. Affonso DD, Lovett S, Paul SM, *et al*. A standardized interview that differentiates pregnancy and postpartum symptoms from perinatal clinical depression. *Birth* 1990;17:21

42. Stowe ZN, Nemeroff CB. Women at risk for postpartum onset major depression. *Am J Obstet Gynecol* 1995; 173:639–45

43. Gotlib IH, Whiffen VE, Wallace P, *et al*. A prospective investigation of postpartum depression: factors involved in onset and recovery. *J Abnorm Psychol* 1991; 100:122–32

44. Pariser SF, Nasrallah HA, Gardner DK. Postpartum mood disorders: clinical perspectives. *J Women Health* 1997;6:421–34

45. Dean C, Kendell RE. The symptomatology of puerperal illness. *Br J Psychiatry* 1981;139:128–35

46. Harris B, Lovett L, Newcombe RG, *et al*. Maternity blues and major endocrine changes: Cardiff puerperal mood and hormone study II. *Br Med J* 1994;308:949

47. Bell AJ, Land NM, Milne S, *et al*. Long-term outcome of postpartum psychiatric illness requiring admission. *J Affect Disord* 1994;31:67

48. Purdy D, Frank E. Should postpartum mood disorders be given a more prominent or distinct place in the DSM–IV? *Depression* 1993;1:59–70

49. Sichel DA, Cohen LS, Robertson LM, *et al*. Prophylactic estrogen in recurrent postpartum affective disorder. *Biol Psychiatry* 1995;38:814–18

50. Kendell RE, Chalmers JC, Platz C. Epidemiology of puerperal psychoses. *Br J Psychiatry* 1987;150:662–73

51. O'Hara MW, Swain AM. Rates and risk of postpartum depression: a meta-analysis. *Int Rev Psychiatry* 1996; 8:37–54

52. Troutman B, Cutrona C. Non psychotic postpartum depression among adolescent mothers. *J Abnorm Psychol* 1990;99:69

53. O'Hara MW. Postpartum "blues", depression, and psychosis: a review. Special issue: maternal development

during reproduction. *J Psychosom Obstet Gynecol* 1987; 7:205–27

54. Stowe ZN, Casarella J, Landry JC, *et al*. Sertraline in the treatment of women with postpartum major depression. *Depression* 1999;(in press)

55. Bratfos O, Hang JO. Puerperal mental disorder in manic depressive females. *Acta Psychiatr Scand* 1966;42: 285–94

56. Cohen LS, Sichel DA, Robertson LM, *et al*. Postpartum prophylaxis for women with bipolar disorder. *Am J Psychiatry* 1995;152:1641–5

57. Reich T, Winokur G. Postpartum psychosis in patients with manic depressive disease. *J Nerve Ment Dis* 1970; 151:60–8

58. Marks MN, Wieck A, Checkley SA, *et al*. Life stress and postpartum psychosis: a preliminary report. *Br J Psychiatry* 1991;158:45

59. O'Hara MW, Schlecte JA, Lewis DA, *et al*. Controlled prospective study of postpartum mood disorders: psychological, environmental, and hormonal variables. *J Abnorm Psychol* 1991;100:63–73

60. O'Hara MW. Social support, life events, and depression during pregnancy and the puerperium. *Arch Gen Psychiatry* 1986;43:569–73

61. Cox JL, Rooney A, Thomas PF. How accurately do mothers recall postnatal depression? Further data from a 3-year follow-up study. *J Psychosom Obstet Gynecol* 1984;3:185–7

62. Zekoski EM, O'Hara MW, Wills KE. The effects of maternal mood on mother-infant interaction. *J Abnorm Child Psychol* 1987;15:361–78

63. Owens MJ, Nemeroff CB. The role of serotonin in the pathophysiology of depression: focus on the serotonin transporter. *Clin Chem* 1994;40:288–95

64. Henderson AF, Gregoire AJP, Kumar RC, *et al*. Treatment of severe postnatal depression with estradiol skin patches. *Lancet* 1991;338:816–17

65. American Psychiatric Association. Practice guidelines for the treatment of patients with bipolar disorder. *Am J Psychiatry* 1994;151(Suppl. 12):1

66. Wehr TA. Sleep loss: a preventable cause of mania and other excited states. *J Clin Psychiatry* 1989;50(Suppl.):8

67. Stowe ZN, Nemeroff CB. Psychopharmacology during pregnancy and lactation. In Schatzberg AF, Nemeroff CB, eds. *Textbook of Psychopharmacology*. Washington, DC: American Psychiatric Press, 1995: 823–37

68. Wisner KL, Wheeler SB. Prevention of recurrent postpartum major depression. *Hosp Comm Psychiatry* 1994; 45:1191–6

69. Committee on Drugs, American Academy of Pediatrics. The transfer of drugs and other chemicals into human milk. *Pediatrics* 1994;93:137

70. Wisner KL, Perel JM, Findling RL. Antidepressant treatment during breast feeding. *Am J Psychiatry* 1996; 153:9

71. Weinstein MR. Recent advances in clinical psychopharmacology. I. Lithium carbonate. *Hosp Form* 1977; 12:759–62

72. Rane A, Tomson G, Bjarke B. Effects of maternal lithium therapy in a newborn infant. *J Pediatr* 1978;93:296–7

73. Arnon RG, Marin-Garcia J, Peeden JN. Tricuspid valve regurgitation and lithium carbonate toxicity in a newborn infant. *Am J Dis Child* 1981;135:941–3

74. Schou M, Amdisen A. Lithium and pregnancy. III. Lithium ingestion by children breast-fed by women on lithium treatment. *Br Med J* 1973;2:138

75. Committee on Drugs, American Academy of Pediatrics. Transfer of drugs and other chemicals into human milk. *Pediatrics* 1989;84:924–36

76. Centers For Disease Control, US Department of Health and Human Services. Valproic acid and spina bifida: a preliminary report – France. *MMWR* 1982;31:565–6

77. Lammer EJ, Sever LE, Oakley GP Jr. Teratogen update: valproic acid. *Teratology* 1987;35:465–73

43
Pulmonary diseases

D. Schuller and D.P. Schuster

RESPIRATORY PHYSIOLOGY DURING PREGNANCY

The most consistent physiological change in lung function during pregnancy is an increase in resting ventilation (V_E), primarily via an increase in tidal volume from about 500 to 700 ml[1,2]. The increase in V_E is out of proportion to the 20% increase in oxygen consumption (VO_2) which also occurs during pregnancy. Minute ventilation increases during the first trimester, and remains elevated during the rest of pregnancy. These changes result in a characteristic increase in the ventilatory equivalent (V_E/VO_2), a fall in $PaCO_2$ to a plateau of 27–32 mmHg and a resultant mild chronic respiratory alkalosis[1].

The increase in V_E has been attributed to increased circulating progesterone during pregnancy, which may increase the sensitivity of the respiratory center to CO_2[3,4]. Progesterone may also act as a primary respiratory center stimulant[5].

Pregnancy also changes lung volumes and respiratory mechanics, probably owing to changes in thoracic cage configuration and diaphragmatic elevation. Most studies have not found any significant change in vital capacity (VC), total lung capacity (TLC), forced expiratory volume in 1 s (FEV_1) or maximal expiratory flow rates early in pregnancy. However, after the 5th month, a consistent finding is a progressive decrease in expiratory reserve volume (ERV) and residual volume (RV), causing a 9–25% reduction in functional residual capacity (FRC). Despite the reduction in FRC which would tend to result in airway closure and worsened ventilation–perfusion matching, oxygenation usually changes little because of the increase in alveolar ventilation[6–8].

SMOKING DURING PREGNANCY

The incidences of cigarette smoking during pregnancy vary geographically and ethnically. In California, about 6% of pregnant women are cigarette smokers with the highest smoking rate among black women and the lowest among Asian and Hispanic women[9]. In Wisconsin and Oklahoma the overall incidence of cigarette smoking among pregnant women is about 22%[10,11]. Smoking is associated with an increased risk of uterine bleeding as a result of abruptio placenta or placenta previa[12–15]. Cigarette smoking is also associated with a two-fold increased risk of fetal growth retardation[10,11]. The cause of fetal growth retardation is probably placental dysfunction. Furthermore, fetal exposure to maternal cigarette smoking also affects postnatal development such as in reduced respiratory function, a higher risk of sudden infant death syndrome and attention deficit hyperactive disorders[16–19].

Aggressive smoking cessation intervention programs during the prenatal period are effective in helping the pregnant women to stop smoking[20]. Therefore, all pregnant patients should be counseled about the hazards of smoking at their first prenatal visit and this information should be frequently reinforced thereafter. The local chapters of the American Lung Association and the American Cancer Society are excellent resources for educational material.

ASTHMA

Asthma is the most common respiratory disorder complicating pregnancy, reported in 0.4–1.3% of pregnant women[21]. Approximately 15% of asthmatics will require hospitalization during their pregnancy.

The hallmark of asthma is the non-specific hyperirritability of the tracheobronchial tree, which causes a decrease in airway diameter due to smooth muscle contraction, thick and tenacious secretions and, most importantly, bronchial wall edema and inflammation.

The effects of pregnancy on asthma are unpredictable. Turner and colleagues[21] reviewed studies involving 1059 pregnancies and found that 49% of the patients had no change in their asthma during pregnancy, 29% improved and 22% deteriorated. Furthermore, patients did not necessarily change in the same way during different pregnancies. A more recent prospective study revealed that asthmatic symptoms improved during the last 4 weeks of pregnancy and rarely occurred during labor and delivery[22].

The effect of asthma on pregnancy depends upon maternal oxygenation or the degree of asthmatic control. Well controlled asthma even in patients taking steroids does not adversely affect the natural course of pregnancy, and suboptimal control of asthma as reflected by the decreased FEV_1 may be associated with fetal growth retardation[23–25]. Thus, adequate control of asthma and close monitoring of the fetus can improve maternal and fetal outcomes.

The clinical presentation of asthma may vary from an isolated cough to severe chest tightness and fulminant respiratory failure. Most patients present with non-productive cough and wheezing, often accompanied by chest tightness and dyspnea.

The initial examination should include a search for a precipitating factor, as this not only helps in managing the acute episode, but also helps prevent future exacerbations. Common precipitating events include: upper respiratory infections, allergies, exercise, non-compliance with treatment, hypersensitivity to aspirin or other non-steroidal anti-inflammatory agents, sinusitis and gastroesophageal reflux. Allergic bronchopulmonary aspergillosis can also occur during pregnancy, and its presence should be excluded in the appropriate setting (wheezing, fleeting radiographic infiltrates and eosinophilia).

During an attack, physical examination usually reveals tachycardia and tachypnea with varying degrees of respiratory distress, chest hyperinflation, and widespread rhonchi. The use of accessory respiratory muscles and pulsus paradoxus (i.e. a decrease in systolic blood pressure during inspiration) greater than 10 mmHg usually indicates that the FEV_1 is reduced to 20–40% of the predicted value (i.e. usually less than 1 l). If the patient can perform a forced expiration, the peak expiratory flow rate (PEFR) or the FEV_1 can be used to assess severity and to follow progress. In general, a patient with an acute flare of asthma will require hospitalization if, despite intensive treatment, the FEV_1 remains less than 35–40% of the predicted value. With an FEV_1 less than 25% of the predicted value, the patient is at risk for respiratory failure. Peak flows greater than 200 l/min (50% predicted) are virtually never associated with significant hypoxemia or hypercapnia[26].

Equally important, however, are the arterial blood gases, which typically reveal mild hypocapnia and moderate hypoxemia during an acute asthma attack. Thus, a pH of < 7.35 despite a 'normal' $PaCO_2$ of 35–40 mmHg in the midst of an exacerbation represents 'pseudonormalization', and signals respiratory muscle fatigue and impending respiratory failure. An additional concern during an acute attack is that persistent hypocapnia and respiratory alkalosis may cause uterine artery vasoconstriction and decreased fetal perfusion[27].

The goal of therapy is to achieve maximum control of the disease with minimum toxicity to mother and fetus. However, in general, the care of the pregnant asthmatic patient differs little from that of the non-pregnant woman.

The National Asthma Education Program recommends four steps in the management of asthma in pregnancy. The first step involves objective assessment of maternal pulmonary function and monitoring of fetal well-being. The second step is to identify, to avoid and to control the precipitating factors. The third step is pharmacological therapy. The fourth step involves education of patients about the disease, the interaction between pregnancy and asthma and vice versa, and the medications[28].

β-Adrenergic agonists are the most commonly used bronchodilators. They are effective both for treating and for preventing asthma attacks. Importantly, they do not prevent the late asthmatic response to allergens nor do they decrease bronchial hyper-responsiveness[29]. $β_2$-Selective agonists are preferred because they are usually associated with fewer side-effects.

β-Adrenoceptor agonists are available for intravenous and oral use. However, the preferred mode of delivery is by inhalation since this achieves an adequate clinical response with the fewest systemic side-effects. Various methods for aerosol administration are available, including spacers, rotocaps, metered-dose inhalers (MDI) and nebulizers.

Albuterol, pirbuterol, terbutaline and metoproterenol MDIs offer the best combination of $β_2$ selectivity and long duration of action. Large dosages and frequent administration may be beneficial in seriously ill patients. Two to four initial puffs may be followed by 1–2 puffs every 10–20 min until improvement is obtained or toxicity is noted. Thereafter, two puffs every 4 h may be given until the patient becomes stable. The addition at night of a long-acting inhaled β-agonist (salmeterol two puffs at bedtime) might be considered to control nocturnal symptoms. Inhalation technique is important to achieve adequate drug delivery to the distal airway. Therefore, patient education is a critical aspect of asthma management during pregnancy.

Side-effects with the β-agonists, although infrequent, can be important. The side-effects of particular concern in obstetric practice include pulmonary edema, hypertension, hypokalemia and hyperglycemia. Hyperglycemia is rarely a problem except in the pregnant diabetic patient with asthma, in which case an adjustment of insulin requirements may be needed.

Pulmonary edema has occurred when these drugs have been given at normal infusion rates, for the management of premature labor. The pulmonary edema occurs during current or recent (< 24 h) usage. Worsening dyspnea, chest pain and cough associated with pink, frothy sputum in addition to widening of the alveolar–arterial oxygen gradient and bilateral alveolar infiltrates on the chest film are suggestive of this complication. Interestingly, it has not been a common problem while treating asthma.

Theophylline is another bronchodilator and has been used widely during pregnancy without untoward effects[30,31]. However, it is a less effective bronchodilator than β-adrenergic agonists. Thus, theophylline has recently moved from being a first-choice therapy in asthma to a more restricted use in difficult management cases, especially since the margin of safety is so much greater with inhaled β-agonists.

Theophylline dosing in pregnancy is similar to the usual adult dosing: an intravenous loading dose of 5.6 mg/kg up to a maximum of 400 mg given over 20–30 min, followed by a maintenance infusion of 0.5 mg/kg per hour. In adolescents and smokers, a maintenance dose of 0.7 mg/kg per hour is usually needed to achieve therapeutic levels, whereas patients currently taking cimetidine, erythromycin, or with liver or cardiac disease require a downward adjustment of 0.3 mg/kg per hour. The theophylline dosage must be modified to maintain the therapeutic level of 8–12 µg/ml. Recent studies have shown that theophylline clearance is affected particularly during the third trimester[32,33]. Frequent dose adjustments are necessary to avoid toxicity to both the mother and the fetus[34].

Although theophylline is assumed to cross the placenta and is secreted in breast milk, it is usually well tolerated and its use is free of long-term sequelae[35,36]. However, neonatal theophylline toxicity can occur and is characterized by tachycardia and transient jitteriness. The maternal and newborn (umbilical cord and heelstick) theophylline concentrations have a good correlation, and the newborn seems to tolerate theophylline concentrations within the usual therapeutic range without serious side-effects[37].

Steroids can be used during pregnancy to treat asthma by suppressing inflammation[38]. When given by inhalation, they are effective in reducing airway hyperresponsiveness, while not producing the systemic side-effects of adrenal suppression[39]. Inhaled steroids are now considered a first-line therapy for chronic asthma. In contrast, during acute exacerbations, short courses of systemic steroids are indicated (prednisone 30–50 mg daily for 4–7 days). Prednisone and prednisolone cross the placenta poorly, and few if any fetal side-effects can be attributed to steroid administration.

Exacerbations of asthma are an unusual complication of labor. Perhaps this is because of an even greater secretion of glucocorticoids and catecholamines from the adrenal gland. Increased prostaglandin secretion during labor may also cause bronchodilatation. When an exacerbation does occur, aggressive conventional therapy to reverse bronchospasm and early use of intravenous steroids are indicated. In patients who were controlled on chronic corticosteroids, 100 mg intravenous hydrocortisone should be given upon admission to the hospital, and repeated every 8 h for 24 h.

Asthmatic patients can have induction of labor with intravenous oxytocin or cervical ripening with prostaglandin E$_2$ (PGE$_2$); the latter has a bronchodilatory effect. Similarly, these medications can be used to treat postpartum hemorrhage from uterine atony. Prostaglandin PGF$_{2\alpha}$, however, is contraindicated in asthmatic patients because it is a bronchoconstrictor.

If a Cesarean section is required, epidural or spinal anesthesia is preferred. If general anesthesia is necessary, intubation should be carried out orally with a small endotracheal tube[7], with direct visualization of the vocal cords, to avoid trauma to the upper airway, which is often edematous during pregnancy. Halothane is an anesthetic that has bronchodilating properties, but it is not usually used in most obstetric situations because of the risk of postpartum hemorrhage secondary to relaxation of the uterus. Opiates are avoided, because they may worsen bronchoconstriction and cause respiratory depression in the fetus.

Little alteration of the patient's medication is required during lactation. A negligible amount of inhaled β-agonists or oral steroids are secreted into milk, and therefore these are unlikely to harm the infant. Tetracycline (sometimes used for upper airway infections during asthma) and iodine-containing medication (used in some expectorants) should be avoided during pregnancy and lactation.

CYSTIC FIBROSIS

Cystic fibrosis (CF) is the most common life-threatening genetic disorder in Caucasians. The gene frequency in white Americans is estimated to be 1 in 20 with the disease occurring in 1/1600 to 1/2000 live births. It is an autosomal recessive disease with a median survival of approximately 30 years; nearly 35% of persons with CF are 18 years old or older.

Prenatal diagnosis of this condition can be achieved by DNA analysis of fetal cells obtained from amniocentesis or chorionic villus sampling. Direct polymerase chain reaction amplification of the mutation gene F508 can facilitate this process and can be used in preimplantation diagnosis and possible screening of fetal CF from harvested fetal cells in the maternal blood[40]. Genetic counseling and testing should be offered to couples at risk for CF.

An increased life expectancy has led to a greater frequency of pregnancy among women with CF. Women with CF can conceive and deliver healthy infants, but the maternal and fetal risks are a function of the extent of pulmonary disease and its complications.

Cystic fibrosis does not appear to be associated with an increased rate of spontaneous abortion (4.6%). However, it is associated with an increased rate of preterm delivery (24.3%), mainly from preterm labor (88% of the cases) and maternal complications of CF. Preterm delivery seems to be related to pancreatic insufficiency and the degree of impaired pulmonary function[41,42]. Normalization of pancreatic function by pancreatic enzyme replacement reduces the risk of preterm delivery[41]. A prepregnancy FEV$_1$ of less than 60% of predicted value is associated with a higher rate of preterm delivery, increased loss of lung function and higher maternal mortality compared to that associated with mildly impaired pulmonary function[42]. It should be emphasized that normal pregnancy outcomes can occur in patients with forced vital capacity (FVC) of less than 50% of the predicted value[43]. Overall, pregnancy does not increase maternal mortality[41]. Thus, CF with moderately or severely impaired pulmonary function *per se* is not a contraindication to pregnancy.

The inflammatory and structural changes in the airway and lung parenchyma lead to airway obstruction, hyperinflation and ventilation perfusion imbalance.

The airways of patients with CF are chronically colonized with bacteria. *Staphylococcus aureus* and *Haemophilus influenzae* remain the most frequent isolates, but *Pseudomonas aeruginosa*, especially the mucoid forms, is detected in more than 90% of patients. Once *P. aeruginosa* is recovered from the sputum, it is rarely, if ever, eradicated. Other species of *Pseudomonas* are recovered with increasing frequency in patients with CF. *Burkholoeria cepacia* and *Stenotrophomonas maltophilia* are particularly difficult to treat because of their resistance to multiple antibiotics. In addition, *B. cepacia* has been linked to an unfavorable short-term prognosis.

The clinical manifestations of CF are variable, and mainly due to chronic pulmonary disease and pancreatic insufficiency. Respiratory manifestations include sinusitis, nasal polyps, purulent sputum, atelectasis, hemoptysis and pneumothorax. The diagnosis of CF is based on defined clinical criteria and analysis of sweat chloride levels. A sweat chloride level of more than 60 mEq/l in children or more than 80 mEq/l in adults in association with the typical pulmonary and/or gastrointestinal manifestation are acceptable as sufficient criteria to establish the diagnosis. Measurement of nasal potential difference and CF gene mutation analysis are useful adjuncts to diagnosis.

In addition, not only is mutation analysis helpful for screening purposes, but it will undoubtedly be helpful in a variety of difficult clinical circumstances, such as a course suggestive of CF in a deceased newborn, the presence of echogenic masses suggestive of meconium ileus on prenatal evaluation, or the difficulty of diagnosis in a patient with borderline sweat test results. Although no specific therapy exists for CF, the therapeutic goals are focused on the control of infection, the clearance of respiratory secretions, reduction in the viscoelasticity of sputum and the replacement of pancreatic enzymes and nutrients. In addition, these patients should receive immunizations against *Streptococcus pneumoniae* and influenza.

During labor, attention should be given to keeping an adequate fluid balance, since patients with CF are susceptible to salt depletion and hypovolemia on the one hand, while on the other hand, they can be very sensitive to fluid overload, particularly in the presence of cor pulmonale.

Breast milk from patients with CF can have a very high sodium content[44]. However, a more recent report found normal electrolyte concentrations in milk from patients with CF, suggesting that the initial report was abnormally high, owing to the way the milk was obtained[45]. It is therefore recommended that the sodium content of breast milk be checked prior to initiating breastfeeding.

PNEUMONIA

The incidence of pneumonia during pregnancy is similar to that in the general population (0.04–1%). With very few exceptions, the major infectious diseases that affect the lung during pregnancy are the same as those in the non-pregnant population. However, reduced maternal immune responses, particularly decreased cell-mediated immunity, probably accounts for the increased morbidity and mortality associated with respiratory infections[46–48].

The pathogens, clinical manifestations and diagnostic approach to respiratory infection during pregnancy are not different from those seen and used in the general population. The unique aspects of pneumonia during pregnancy are related to its impact on the fetus and the rapid identification and selection of specific therapy that is effective and without toxicity.

Community-acquired pneumonia complicates 1 in 2300 deliveries and is responsible for 8% of all maternal deaths[49,50]. Historically, pneumonia during pregnancy was associated with a 70% incidence of preterm labor and 20% mortality. More recently with the use of effective antibiotics, mortality is significantly lower, and preterm labor has decreased to approximately 8%[51].

The usual presentation is unchanged by pregnancy: fever, cough productive of purulent sputum and chest pain. Likewise, the most common agents are *Streptococcus pneumoniae* and *Mycoplasma pneumoniae*. *Legionella* and *Haemophilus influenzae* are other bacteria frequently isolated[51].

For community-acquired pneumonia in pregnancy, the penicillins, cephalosporins and erythromycin (excluding estolate, which is associated with cholestatic jaundice in pregnancy) are considered to be safe. The aminoglycosides have the potential of causing renal and ototoxicity in the fetus and should only be used when strongly indicated, with close monitoring of serum drug levels. Tetracycline is contraindicated in pregnancy because it is both teratogenic and hepatotoxic[52].

Viral pneumonia during pregnancy appears to carry a higher risk of complications than in the general population. Maternal mortality due to influenza during epidemics has been reported to be between 30 and 50%[53,54]. Women in their third trimester appear to be at the highest risk. The virus can generally be cultured from nasopharyngeal secretions and may be identified by immunofluorescence.

Patients may present with symptoms of headache, fever, myalgia, malaise, coughing and sore throat.

Physical findings may be minimal or include injected pharynx, rhonchi, wheezes or rales in the lungs. Influenza pneumonia can lead to respiratory failure.

Prevention is the most effective means of reducing the complications of influenza pneumonia. Vaccination during the second trimester is recommended if the second or third trimesters are likely to coincide with the influenza season. Pregnant women with high-risk medical conditions (e.g. chronic lung or cardiovascular disease, diabetes, renal disease, hemoglobinopathy or immunosuppression) should be vaccinated; the vaccine is considered safe during pregnancy[55]. The vaccine should preferably be administered after the first trimester, unless the influenza season begins during that time.

Amantadine taken orally within 48 h of the onset of the symptoms may alleviate the course of the disease[56]. The use of amantadine in pregnancy has not been well studied in humans. Therefore, its use should probably be limited to unvaccinated patients with clinical evidence of pneumonia and positive cultures for influenza-A pneumonia[26]. The virus does not appear to cause fetal infection or congenital anomalies.

Varicella pneumonia is another potentially devastating disease during pregnancy and is associated with significant mortality. Symptoms of cough (89%), dyspnea (70%), hemoptysis (38%) and pleuritic pain (21%) usually begin 3–6 days after the vesicular exanthem, and can progress rapidly to respiratory failure[57]. Acyclovir has been reported to be safe and effective[58]. It therefore seems reasonable to initiate acyclovir given intravenously at the first evidence of respiratory system involvement in a pregnant patient with cutaneous varicella infection. The doses range from 5 to 10 mg/kg every 8 h. In addition, infants born to mothers who developed varicella within 4 days preceding delivery should receive zoster immunoglobulin because of the risk of disseminated varicella neonatal infection. Infection during the first trimester may be associated with congenital varicella syndrome characterized by limb hypoplasia, cutaneous scar, cortical atrophy and seizure[59–61]. Maternal therapy with immune globulin has not been shown to be effective in preventing fetal varicella infection.

Fungal pneumonia during pregnancy can present as chronic, unresolved, community-acquired pneumonia. With the exception of coccidioidomycosis, such pneumonias are rare. The clinical course appears to be similar to that in the non-pregnant host.

Coccidioidomycosis during pregnancy is a potentially fatal disease if left untreated. Although early reports suggested a very high incidence of dissemination (20%) compared to that in non-pregnant patients (0.2%) and a poor outcome, the incidence of coccidioidomycosis during pregnancy in endemic areas is only 1 per 1000 pregnancies, and with treatment maternal mortality is extremely rare[48,62]. This 'higher risk' for dissemination may be related to the effects of 17β-estradiol, progesterone and estrogen on the fungus, promoting fungal growth. Treatment with amphotericin-B has been used successfully during pregnancy, although it crosses the placenta and is present in the umbilical cord serum at concentrations one-third that of maternal serum. However, amphotericin-B does not appear to have an adverse effect on the fetus[26,62].

TUBERCULOSIS

There is no evidence that pregnancy has any effect on the course of tuberculosis. Furthermore, antituberculosis therapy is as effective in pregnant women as in their non-pregnant counterparts[1,63,64]. Pregnancy does not appear to increase the risk of developing active tuberculosis in patients asymptomatically harboring *Mycobacterium tuberculosis* regardless of HIV status[65]. On the other hand, HIV-positive status adversely affects the natural course of tuberculosis by rapid and fulminant progression of active infection, reactivation of latent infection, and reinfection[66–68]. The problem of tuberculosis during pregnancy focuses on the risk for the fetus, from either acquiring the infection itself or from the toxicity of chemotherapeutic agents.

Fetal infection is rare and may occur if infected amniotic fluid is swallowed, or it may be acquired hematogenously via the umbilical vein. Although congenital infection occurs, neonatal acquisition by postpartum maternal contact is the most common means of transmission. Fetal infection may result in fetal demise or neonatal infection. Untreated maternal tuberculosis results in a high perinatal mortality, up to 30–40%. However, excellent maternal and fetal prognosis can be obtained with adequate treatment of maternal tuberculosis[69–71].

Pulmonary tuberculosis during pregnancy may present with non-specific symptoms of pneumonia: fever and cough (with or without sputum production), hemoptysis, weight loss, or pleuritic pain from a pleural effusion. Alternatively the diagnosis may be considered after an incidental finding during a chest X-ray taken for a different reason.

A definitive diagnosis of tuberculosis requires the demonstration of *Mycobacterium tuberculosis* by culture. In many cases, the diagnosis is made on the basis of a compatible clinical picture with a positive tuberculin test or by demonstrating acid-fast bacilli in appropriately stained material. However, cultures should always be performed, not only to confirm the diagnosis but also to determine drug sensitivity.

Although the validity of tuberculin testing during pregnancy has been questioned, available evidence supports its value through the course of pregnancy[72]. The threshold for performing purified protein derivative (PPD) skin testing during pregnancy should be low and should be offered to populations at risk for tuberculosis: those who have been exposed to known cases, persons who live in crowded or impoverished conditions, health workers and the chronically ill. The skin test is performed by intradermal injection of 0.1 ml of PPD and the skin induration is measured at 48–72 h afterwards. The American Thoracic Society defines the following criteria for a positive skin reaction depending on the risk of tuberculosis infection[64]. An induration of ≥ 5 mm is considered positive in patients with HIV infection, close contacts of infectious patients or those having fibrotic lesions on the chest radiograph. An induration of ≥ 10 mm is considered positive in other at-risk patients including children younger than 4 years of age. A cut-off induration of ≥ 15 mm is considered positive if the test is performed in patients who are not exposed to a high-risk environment.

A chest roentgenogram should be performed in recent tuberculin convertors, in patients in whom the time of conversion is unknown, or in those with a suggestive history or physical examination, regardless of the skin test result. Multinodular infiltration in the apical and posterior segments of the upper lobes and superior segments of the lower lobes is the most typical lesion of pulmonary tuberculosis. Cavitation is frequently present, and is usually associated with an area of infiltrate.

With the exception of 'newly infected' women, or exposure to high-risk environments, especially HIV infection, chemoprophylaxis should be withheld until after delivery if the PPD is positive and no active disease is found[64]. In those cases in which it is thought that infection has occurred within the previous 2 years and has not been adequately treated, the risk of developing active disease is high enough that isoniazid prophylaxis should be given. Preferably, prophylaxis should be started after the first trimester. Prophylaxis consists of isoniazid 300 mg orally once daily for 6 months. When isoniazid is used, pyridoxine 50 mg daily should be given to prevent peripheral neuropathy[64].

Active tuberculosis requires prompt treatment. Without treatment, tuberculosis is a great hazard to the mother and the fetus. The recommended initial therapeutic regimen consists of isoniazid 300 mg/day, rifampin 600 mg/day and ethambutol 15 mg/kg per day for 8 weeks, and then isoniazid and rifampin to complete 6 months. Pyrazinamide should be avoided in pregnancy[64]. All patients should be placed on directly observed multidrug chemotherapy and reported appropriately to the health department agencies.

Special attention should be paid to the management of the mother–infant pair. Since the perinatal acquisition of tuberculosis is a definite risk, the neonate born to a mother with active tuberculosis needs to be treated with isoniazid for 2–3 months, or at least until the mother is smear- and culture-negative and compliant with therapy. If, after 3 months of therapy, the mother is sputum-negative and the infant is tuberculin-negative and has a normal chest roentgenogram, then the isoniazid may be stopped and skin testing surveillance kept at 3-monthly intervals.

If the infants' tuberculin reaction is significant at 3 months or clinical signs or symptoms of tuberculosis exist, then one should treat with additional drugs. There is no need to isolate the infant from the mother as long as the mother has been on effective chemotherapy for at least 2 weeks. Similarly, there is no contraindication to breastfeeding. Small concentrations of antituberculous drugs are secreted in breast milk, but do not produce toxicity in the infant[64].

Rifampin is known to impair the efficacy of oral contraceptives. Numerous pregnancies have been described in women taking rifampin while using oral contraceptives. The patient should therefore be informed and a barrier method be prescribed if pregnancy is to be avoided.

SARCOIDOSIS

Sarcoidosis is a multisystem disease of unknown etiology characterized by the formation of non-caseating granulomas in multiple organs. Because it is a disease that predominantly affects young females, it is not rare among pregnant women. In the USA, sarcoidosis is ten times more common in blacks, in whom it tends to follow a more chronic course and carry a worse prognosis[73,74].

Usually, sarcoidosis becomes clinically evident because of pulmonary manifestations, most frequently, dyspnea, cough, chest pains or typical findings on the chest roentgenogram (including bilateral hilar lymphadenopathy or diffuse interstitial infiltrates). General symptoms, such as fever, weight loss, anorexia or arthralgia occur in about 25% of patients. Less than 10% of patients will present with complaints from extrapulmonary involvement, such as the central nervous system, heart, or liver.

Radiographically, patients with sarcoidosis are frequently divided into three groups depending on the following characteristics:

(1) Stage I shows the presence of hilar adenopathy alone;

(2) Stage II is characterized by hilar adenopathy and parenchymal infiltrates; and

(3) Stage III includes parenchymal abnormalities alone[75].

Pulmonary function tests reveal a restrictive abnormality with reduced diffusing capacity. A definitive diagnosis of sarcoidosis requires demonstration of non-caseating granulomas in a biopsy specimen.

Several studies have investigated the effects of sarcoidosis on pregnancy. There is no evidence that sarcoidosis has any adverse effect on either fertility or the course of pregnancy. The obstetric management of pregnancy, labor and delivery does not differ from that for a normal patient. Although sarcoid granulomata have been reported in the placenta, there is no current evidence that it affects the fetus.

The overall effect of pregnancy on sarcoidosis is believed by many authors to be beneficial. The improvement is presumed to be secondary to an increase in circulating cortisol levels. However, during the puerperium, corticosteroid levels drop, resulting in an exacerbation of symptoms[76].

The major treatment of sarcoidosis is through the use of steroids. Because of the waxing and waning nature of the illness, it has been difficult to prove that steroids improve outcome. The indications for treatment of sarcoidosis with corticosteroids during pregnancy are the same as in the non-pregnant state (Table 1).

ASPIRATION SYNDROMES

It has been estimated that 2% of maternal deaths in the USA result from aspiration of gastric contents[77]. Aspiration is of particular concern at the time of labor and delivery.

The factors that make the pregnant woman particularly susceptible to aspiration include:

(1) Increased intragastric pressure caused by the gravid uterus;

(2) Decreased tone of the lower esophageal sphincter caused by progesterone;

(3) Delayed gastric emptying; and

(4) Impaired laryngeal sensation/reflex and decreased level of consciousness following sedation, induction or emergence from general anesthesia, often administered in emergency cases.

Multiple clinical syndromes can develop after aspiration of gastric contents (Table 2). The development of

Table 1 Indications for treatment of sarcoidosis with corticosteriods

---

Extrapulmonary sarcoidosis
Cardiac involvement (heart block or arrhythmias)
Central nervous system involvement
Hypercalcemia and hypercalciuria
Acute iridocyclitis or uveitis
Disfiguring skin lesions
Hypersplenism
Progressive liver disease
Xerophthalmia or xerostomia
Persistent systemic disease (fever, weight loss)

Pulmonary sarcoidosis
Stage I disease should be left untreated unless there is severe ventilatory impairment
Stage II or III treated when symptomatic (dyspnea), or when there is no objective evidence of improvement by chest roentgenogram or pulmonary function tests

---

Table 2 Pulmonary syndromes associated with aspiration of gastric contents. From reference 79, with permission

---

Irritant/toxic injury (liquids containing acid or fine particulate material)
Acute pneumonitis
Acute recurrent pneumonitis
Chronic pneumonitis
Granulomatous interstitial pneumonitis
Pulmonary fibrosis
Chronic respiratory symptoms (cough, dyspnea, hemoptysis, hoarseness)
Bronchial hyper-reactivity
Laryngospasm
Laryngitis
Apnea
Tracheobronchitis
Bronchiectasis

Inert/non-toxic injury with airway obstruction (large volumes of liquid or large particulate material)
Sudden death ('cafe coronary')
Atelectasis
Bronchiectasis
Chronic respiratory symptoms (cough, wheezing, dyspnea, hemoptysis)

Infectious injury (liquid contaminated with bacteria)
Mixed aerobic–anaerobic bronchopneumonia
Lung abscess
Necrotizing pneumonia
Empyema
Ventilator-associated pneumonia

---

a particular syndrome depends on many factors including the nature and volume of the aspirated material, the frequency of aspiration and the underlying host response[78]. Respiratory distress may develop as a result of aspiration, depending upon the amount, pH and type of gastric contents. More than 25 ml at a pH of less than 2.5 regularly provokes a chemical pneumonitis[79]. However, liquids containing fine particulate matter may also produce a chemical pneumonitis, and inert liquids or foreign bodies may cause airway obstruction. Material contaminated by bacteria will give rise to mixed aerobic–anaerobic pleuropulmonary infections.

The clinical manifestations of gastric acid aspiration include tachycardia, tachypnea, bronchospasm, cyanosis and perhaps hypotension or cardiopulmonary arrest. The more serious manifestations are usually associated with diffuse infiltrates on chest roentgenogram. The clinical course may follow one of three patterns:

(1) Rapid improvement over the next few days;

(2) Initial improvement, followed by supervening bacterial pneumonia; or

(3) Development of the adult respiratory distress syndrome[80].

Treatment during the initial phase is supportive, with maintenance of adequate oxygenation by supplemental oxygen and, if necessary, intubation and mechanical ventilation. Recent studies have not shown any benefit for corticosteroids in the treatment of aspiration pneumonitis[81–83]. Although there have been no controlled trials, most authors now agree that empirical antibiotic treatment should be withheld until there is clinical microbiological or radiographic evidence of superinfection[79,84]. An exception to this rule is made when aspiration is associated with severe gingivitis or intestinal obstruction[79].

Recently, more attention has been given to the prophylaxis of aspiration[85,86]. Particulate antacids containing $Mg(OH)_2$ and $Al(OH)_3$ can increase gastric volume and, if aspirated, can produce injury despite an elevated pH, and so should be avoided. On the other hand, soluble antacids such as sodium citrate are effective if they are given 15–20 min prior to induction of general anesthesia. Regimens containing H_2-blockers (cimetidine or ranitidine) have been equally effective in raising gastric pH above 2.5[85,87]. If used intravenously, they should be given 45–60 min prior to induction of anesthesia.

Metoclopramide represents a different approach to aspiration prophylaxis in that it does not increase pH, but speeds gastric emptying, increases lower esophageal sphincter tone and has antiemetic properties. To date, when given to parturients, metoclopramide has been shown to be safe, does not impede the progression of labor and does not adversely affect Apgar scores[85]. Cricoid pressure upon endotracheal intubation is another beneficial maneuver in preventing aspiration.

THROMBOEMBOLIC DISEASE

Pulmonary embolism is the second leading cause of maternal mortality with a death rate of 0.1 to 0.7 for every 100 000 deliveries[88]. Amniotic fluid embolism, venous air embolism and thromboembolism account for approximately 20% of maternal deaths[49].

The risk of symptomatic thromboembolic disease in pregnancy is approximately six times greater than in the non-pregnant state, presumably because of the increase in clotting factors VII, VIII and X, as well as an increased fibrinogen level and decreased fibrinolytic activity[89]. Venous stasis caused by uterine pressure on the inferior vena cava may also be a contributing factor. The risk of thromboembolism is highest during the puerperium, with two-thirds of the cases occurring postpartum. Contributing factors that further increase the risk for thromboembolism are: (1) Cesarean section, which has a 10 times greater risk of fatal pulmonary embolism compared to vaginal delivery; (2) maternal age more than 40 years; (3) obesity; (4) bed rest; (5) suppression of lactation with estrogens; (6) surgical procedures during pregnancy and early puerperium; (7) hypercoaguable state, e.g. lupus

anticoagulant, anticardiolipin antibodies, protein C or S deficiency, decreased antithrombin-III; (8) history of previous thromboembolic disease; (9) blood group type other than type O; and (10) pelvic infection[89,90].

Dyspnea and tachypnea are the most common clinical findings that suggest a pulmonary embolism. Other symptoms include cough, pleuritic chest pain and hemoptysis. The physical findings also depend on the extent to which the pulmonary circulation has been obstructed, and include hypotension, tachycardia, cyanosis, an accentuated second heart sound, and signs of right-sided congestive heart failure. The arterial blood gases usually reveal an increased alveolar–arterial oxygen gradient and frequently an acute respiratory alkalosis. The most common electrocardiographic finding is sinus tachycardia. A right axis shift with an $S_1Q_3T_3$ pattern may be observed with large emboli.

The chest film is abnormal in 70% of patients. The most common abnormalities are atelectasis, pleural effusion, an elevated hemidiaphragm and focal oligemia.

The clinical features of deep vein thrombosis are notoriously unreliable. Therefore, for diagnosis one usually resorts to more specific diagnostic techniques, especially impedance plethysmography and vascular Doppler ultrasound. Thrombi that remain confined to the calf appear to pose only a limited risk for pulmonary embolism, whereas deep vein thromboses that extend into, or originate at, the level of the popliteal veins and above pose a significant risk. In fact, untreated calf vein thrombi have an excellent clinical outcome – although it is important to document the fact that there is no extension to more proximal veins with serial examinations[91]. Traditionally, there has been some concern that all the non-invasive approaches have the potential to be falsely positive during the third trimester of pregnancy because they may be unable to differentiate extrinsic venous compression from obstruction caused by an intraluminal thrombus[92]. However, a recent large prospective study established the safety of withholding anticoagulant therapy in pregnant patients who have negative results after serial impedance plethysmography[93]. Although the use of duplex ultrasound appears to be very accurate in detecting acute proximal deep vein thrombosis in the non-pregnant population it has not been formally evaluated in the pregnant population[94–96].

As with deep vein thrombosis, the clinical features of pulmonary embolism are also non-specific and unreliable. Thus, ventilation/perfusion (V/Q) lung scans are very useful in diagnosing acute pulmonary embolism, and should be obtained in suspected cases. Perfusion lung scans are highly sensitive and provide definitive information on the presence or absence of pulmonary embolism; a normal study virtually excludes a clinically significant pulmonary embolism. The diagnostic reliability of V/Q scans for pulmonary embolism in combination with non-invasive testing for deep vein thrombosis is approximately 90%[95]. V/Q scans are usually interpreted as showing high, intermediate or low probability for pulmonary embolism. When a scan is intermediate or indeterminate, and especially if it does not correlate with the clinical suspicion, a pulmonary arteriogram should be considered to establish the diagnosis[97]. Because of the risks involved in using anticoagulant therapy during pregnancy (see below), a firm diagnosis or exclusion of pulmonary embolism is mandatory. We agree with the approach of obtaining pulmonary angiography in all 'non-diagnostic' scans, unless this is obviated by venous studies indicating the presence of venous thrombosis which would require therapy, regardless of whether pulmonary embolism is present or not.

Heparin does not cross the placenta and therefore is not expected to provoke fetal complications, whereas oral anticoagulants cross the placenta and have the potential to produce adverse fetal effects. The risk of oral anticoagulants during pregnancy include not only teratogenicity, but also the fact that the anticoagulant effect cannot be rapidly reversed. The fetopathic effects reported with warfarin include: (1) chondroplasia puctata, a condition characterized by abnormal bone and cartilage formation; (2) microcephaly, with optic atrophy and mental retardation, which has been attributed to repeated small cerebral hemorrhage in the baby; (3) dorsal midline dysplasia, characterized by agenesis of the corpus callosum, Dandy–Walker malformations and midline cerebellar atrophy; (4) ventral midline dysplasia, characterized by optic atrophy; (5) asplenia syndrome; and (6) fetal bleeding, both retroplacental and intracerebral[89,98,99].

In patients who develop venous thromboembolism during pregnancy, full doses of heparin should be given intravenously. Once baseline laboratory data have been obtained, full anticoagulation can be achieved with a weight-based bolus of heparin, 80 U/kg or 5000 to 10 000 U. A continuous heparin infusion is then started at a dose of 18 U/kg per hour or 1000 U/h, while the activated partial thromboplastin time (aPTT) is followed closely to achieve a therapeutic range of 1.5 to 2.5 times control. A minimum of 5 days of intravenous therapy is suggested[95,100,101]. Afterwards, in the stable patient, conversion to a subcutaneous heparin regimen is reasonable. To calculate the approximate subcutaneous dose, the total daily intravenous dose is divided by two or three to estimate the every-12-h or every-8-h dosing schedule, respectively. This approach usually provides adequate anticoagulation. An aPTT from blood drawn at midpoint intervals should be kept at a therapeutic range of 1.5 to 2 times control[95].

Low molecular weight heparin (LMWH) has been used and well-tolerated during pregnancy. Advantages of LMWH over unfractionated heparin include its longer half-life following subcutaneous injection, potential for once daily dosing, lower incidence of heparin-induced thrombocytopenia, lower risk of osteoporosis and decreased need for blood sampling to follow therapeutic levels.

The duration of anticoagulant therapy depends on when the thromboembolic event occurs. If it occurs during the pregnancy, therapeutic anticoagulation is recommended for the duration of pregnancy and 6 weeks postpartum. A postpartum thromboembolus requires at least 3 months of anticoagulation. In pregnant patients with extensive deep vein thrombosis of the lower extremities which is not responsive to anticoagulation therapy, insertion of an inferior vena cava filter for prophylaxis of pulmonary embolism is a reasonable alternative[102].

In pregnant women with a history of previous venous thromboembolic disease, the risk of recurrence has been estimated at 4–12%. Therefore, some form of prophylaxis should be considered. Because the risk of heparin-induced osteoporosis is dose-related and the risk of recurrent thrombosis is highest during the third trimester, a reasonable approach is to use low-dose heparin (5000 U every 12 h subcutaneously) for the first 28–36 weeks and to increase the dose of heparin during the third trimester[95]. In addition, calcium supplements (500 mg daily) are recommended to minimize the risk for osteoporosis.

Heparin should be stopped within 4 h before delivery and then both heparin and warfarin can be started postpartum. Operative intervention in the anticoagulated patient necessitates heparin discontinuation and reversal with protamine sulfate. Protamine is administered as a 2-mg/ml solution in saline. Protamine sulfate should be administered slowly, no faster than 50 mg over a 10-min period or 200 mg over 2 h. The dose of protamine is based on the amount of heparin estimated as still being present. Immediately after a bolus injection of heparin, about 1 mg of protamine is required to neutralize 100 U heparin; if given 30 min later, about 0.5 mg of protamine/100 U of heparin is required. During a continuous infusion of heparin, approximately half of the preceding hourly dose of heparin must be neutralized. The neutralizing effect should be monitored by determining the APTT immediately after administration of protamine[95].

For the nursing mother, either heparin or warfarin is safe. At least two studies have documented the finding that warfarin does not induce an anticoagulant effect in the breastfed infant[103,104]. The experience with thrombolytics during pregnancy is limited to a few case reports. Streptokinase and urokinase have been used successfully to treat massive pulmonary embolism or deep vein thrombosis without adverse fetal effects[105–109].

PULMONARY EDEMA ASSOCIATED WITH TOCOLYTIC THERAPY

Pulmonary edema resulting from tocolytics is estimated to occur in 4.4% of pregnant women who receive these agents[110]. The most frequent tocolytic agent involved is terbutaline (40%), followed by isoxsuprine (33%), ritodrine (17%) and salbutamol (10%)[111]. Pulmonary edema has been reported with the use of β-sympathomimetic agents alone at normal infusion rates, or in combination with high-dose steroids or magnesium sulfate (MgSO₄)[111,112]. In addition, pulmonary edema has been described in patients treated with MgSO₄ alone for preterm labor. This complication, however, is rare: 4/355 in one study[113] and 0/75 in another[114].

Although the pathophysiology of pulmonary edema in this setting is controversial, the available clinical data support the opinion that the combination of the following factors unique to pregnancy result in a syndrome of 'hypotonic fluid overload', which then leads to pulmonary edema: (1) a large volume of fluid infused; (2) decreased colloid-oncotic pressure; and (3) physiological alterations caused by pregnancy and β-adrenergic agents (e.g. decreased water and sodium excretion, increased aldosterone and antidiuretic hormone, intravascular volume expansion, etc.). There is little to no evidence supporting cardiac dysfunction or increased pulmonary capillary permeability as a mechanism for increased lung water in these patients[112]. However, any condition that produces even a small 'pulmonary capillary leak' will be further intensified with the concurrent use of β-agonist therapy.

Twin gestation appears to be a common risk factor, occurring in 24% of cases in one series[112]. Patients with twin gestations are at increased risk for premature labor, and thus are more likely to encounter the complications of β-sympathomimetic agents. Thus, the association may simply reflect a patient selection bias. Alternatively, the increased volume expansion associated with multiple gestation may be of primary importance.

Symptoms frequently occur before delivery and consist of dyspnea (76%), chest pain (24%) and cough (17%), frequently productive of pink, frothy sputum. However, these symptoms can also develop after therapy when β-agonists have been discontinued. The physical examination usually reveals respiratory distress, tachypnea and tachycardia. Cardiac examination typically fails to show a gallop and crackles are heard in the lung bases. Arterial blood gases typically show respiratory alkalosis and hypoxemia. The chest roentgenogram shows diffuse, bilateral alveolar infiltrates.

The management protocol for a patient with sympathomimetic associated pulmonary edema should start with the discontinuation of the sympathomimetic agent. Supplemental oxygen by mask in addition to intravenous furosemide (20–40 mg) is all that is necessary for the majority of patients. Additional hemodynamic monitoring, intubation and mechanical ventilation are rarely necessary[112]. Evidence of hemodilution (i.e. decreased hematocrit or hypokalemia) and rapid clinical response to treatment with oxygen and diuresis support the hypothesis that the pulmonary edema is related to tocolytic therapy. In contrast, the picture of non-cardiogenic pulmonary edema associated with amniotic fluid embolus or other obstetric disasters is quite different, as described elsewhere in this text.

PNEUMOMEDIASTINUM AND PNEUMOTHORAX

The presence of free air in the mediastinal space is rare during pregnancy, with an estimated incidence of 1 in every 2000 to 100 000 patients[115]. Prolonged, dysfunctional labor seems to be a predisposing factor. It generally occurs during the second stage of labor when very high intra-alveolar pressures are generated by the Valsalva maneuver associated with 'bearing down'. Under most circumstances, air leaks from the alveolar space, to the perivascular tissue toward the hilum and mediastinum, subsequently tracking through the fascial planes in the neck, finally resulting in subcutaneous emphysema. Pneumothorax will develop if the alveoli rupture into the pleural space.

The symptoms associated with pneumomediastinum include acute chest pain, frequently radiating to the shoulder and associated with dyspnea. Physical examination may reveal the presence of subcutaneous emphysema, and on auscultation a crunching or crackling sound synchronous with the heartbeat may be heard over the precordium (Hamman's sign)[116]. The diagnosis can be confirmed radiographically by observing a radiolucent stripe outlining the heart border.

The natural course of pneumomediastinum during labor in the spontaneously breathing patient is benign in the majority of cases, with spontaneous resorption of air usually occurring over several days. Small pneumothoraces also tend to resolve spontaneously. Supplemental oxygen can hasten the reabsorption of the air by replacing nitrogen for oxygen. Larger pneumothoraces may require the placement of a small drainage catheter connected to suction, underwater seal or a Heimlich valve.

ADULT RESPIRATORY DISTRESS SYNDROME

Adult respiratory distress syndrome (ARDS) during pregnancy has been reported to occur in association with the same common causes of ARDS in the non-pregnant patient, such as sepsis, shock or pneumonia. In addition, it can occur in association with conditions that are either more common or unique to the pregnant state, such as aspiration of gastric contents, amniotic fluid emboli, pre-eclampsia, eclampsia, abruptio placentae, dead fetus syndrome, chorioamnionitis or hydatidiform mole. The main causes in pregnancy are hemorrhage, infection and severe pre-eclampsia[117,118].

Pathophysiologically, there is increased pulmonary capillary permeability due to acute alveolar injury leading to pulmonary edema. The consequences of this lung injury include a decrease in lung volume and pulmonary compliance, and marked arterial hypoxemia secondary to intrapulmonary shunting of blood.

The clinical picture is characterized by acute hypoxemic respiratory failure in association with diffuse bilateral pulmonary infiltrates on the chest roentgenogram. If hemodynamic monitoring is performed, the typical patient will show a low pulmonary artery occlusion pressure (PAOP < 18 mmHg) and pulmonary hypertension.

The therapy of patients with ARDS should include identifying and eliminating (if possible) the causal agent or agents, maximizing oxygen delivery to peripheral tissues and preventing or minimizing the risk for complications (e.g. barotrauma, oxygen toxicity, fluid overload, nosocomial infections, stress ulcers, deep venous thrombosis, etc.).

The guidelines for instituting, optimizing and withdrawing mechanical ventilation have recently been reviewed elsewhere[119] and are beyond the scope of this chapter.

Frequently, pregnant patients in acute hypoxemic respiratory failure enter into spontaneous premature labor. The use of a β-sympathomimetic tocolytic agent in the setting of increased permeability pulmonary edema is not advised, since its tendency to retain water and to develop higher pulmonary capillary pressures would worsen the accumulation of extravascular lung water. Magnesium sulfate can be used for tocolysis in this setting.

There are no studies specifically addressing the mortality of ARDS during pregnancy. However, in the non-pregnant population, it averages 40–60%, despite early recognition and modern supportive therapy.

KYPHOSCOLIOSIS

The reported incidence of kyphoscoliosis is 0.1–0.7% of pregnancies. However, this may be an overestimation since it includes mild cases with no clinical impact[120].

Since the incidence of progressive idiopathic scoliosis is approximately eight times higher in female patients than in male patients, the possibility exists that pregnancy and scoliosis are related.

Pregnancy may increase the risk of increasing the spinal curve, but reports are scanty and contain small numbers of patients. Recently, however, a large retrospective study concluded that pregnancy does not increase the risk of increasing the scoliotic curve in patients whose spinal curvature is not severe. Not the age of the patient, nor the time of the first pregnancy,

nor the number of pregnancies, nor the stability of the curve affected the overall rate of change in the spinal curve. In addition, mild to moderate scoliosis did not appear to have a deleterious effect on pregnancy or delivery. However, the incidence and severity of back pain during pregnancy is higher in scoliosis patients who have not had a spinal fusion[121].

REFERENCES

1. Weinberger SE, Weiss ST, Cohen WR, *et al.* Pregnancy and the lung. *Am Rev Respir Dis* 1980;121:559–81
2. Cugell DW, Frank NR, Gaensler EA, Badger IL. Pulmonary function in pregnancy. Serial observations in normal women. *Am Rev Tuberc* 1953;67:568–97
3. Pemoll ML, Metcalfe J, Kovach PA, *et al.* Ventilation during rest and exercise in pregnancy and postpartum. *Respir Physiol* 1975;25:295
4. Prowse CM, Gaensler EA. Respiratory and acid base changes during pregnancy. *Anesthesiology* 1965;26:381
5. Skatrud JB, Dempsey JA, Kaiser DG. Ventilatory response to medroxyprogesterone acetate in normal subjects: time, course and mechanism. *J Appl Physiol: Respir Environ Exercise Physiol* 1978;44:939–44
6. Awe RJ, Nicotra MB, Newsome ID, Viles R. Arterial oxygenation and alveolar–arterial gradients in term pregnancy. *Obstet Gynecol* 1979;53:182
7. Andersen GJ, James GB, Mathers NP, *et al.* The maternal oxygen tension and acid–base status during pregnancy. *J Obstet Gynecol Br Commonw* 1969;76:16
8. Templeton A, Kelman GR. Maternal blood gases (PAO_2-PaO_2), physiological shunt and V_D/V_T in normal pregnancy. *Br J Anaesth* 1976;48:1001
9. Castro LC, Azen C, Hobel CJ, Platt LD. Maternal tobacco use and substance abuse: reported prevalence rates and associations with the delivery of small for gestational age neonates. *Obstet Gynecol* 1993;81:396–401
10. Ramsey AM, Blose D, Lorenz D, *et al.* Cigarette smoking among women in Oklahoma: before, during, and after pregnancy. *J Oklahoma State Med Assoc* 1993;86:231–6
11. Aronson RA, Uttech S, Soref M. The effect of maternal cigarette smoking on low birth weight and preterm birth in Wisconsin, 1991. *Wisconsin Med J* 1993;92:613–17
12. Williams MA, Mittendorf R, Lieberman E, *et al.* Cigarette smoking during pregnancy in relation to placenta previa. *Am J Obstet Gynecol* 1991;165:28–32
13. Handler AS, Mason ED, Rosenberg DL, Davis FG. The relationship between exposure during pregnancy to cigarette smoking and cocaine use and placenta previa. *Am J Obstet Gynecol* 1994;140:884–9
14. Chelmow D, Andrew DE, Baker ER. Maternal cigarette smoking and placenta previa. *Obstet Gynecol* 1996;87:703–6
15. Ananth CV, Savitz DA, Luther ER. Maternal cigarette smoking as a risk factor for placental abruption, placenta previa, and uterine bleeding in pregnancy. *Am J Epidemiol* 1996;144:881–9
16. Stick SM, Burton PR, Gurrin L, *et al.* Effects of maternal smoking during pregnancy and a family history of asthma on respiratory function in newborn infants. *Lancet* 1996;348:1060–4

17. Poets CF, Schlaud M, Kleeman WJ, *et al*. Sudden infant death and maternal cigarette smoking: results from the Lower Saxony Perinatal Working Group. *Eur J Pediatr* 1995;154:326–9

18. DiFranza JR, Lew RA. Effect of maternal cigarette smoking on pregnancy complications and sudden infant death syndrome. *J Fam Pract* 1995;40:385–94

19. Milberger S, Biederman J, Faraone SV, *et al*. Is maternal smoking during pregnancy a risk factor for attention deficit hyperactivity disorder in children? *Am J Psychiatry* 1996;153:1138–42

20. Dolen-Mullen P, Ramirez G, Groff JY. A meta-analysis of randomized trials of prenatal smoking cessation interventions. *Am J Obstet Gynecol* 1994;171:1328–34

21. Turner ES, Greenberger JA, Patterson R. Management of the pregnant asthmatic patient. *Ann Intern Med* 1980;93:905

22. Schatz M, Harden K, Forsythe A, *et al*. The course of asthma during pregnancy, postpartum, and with successive prenancies: a prospective analysis. *J Allergy Clin Immunol* 1988;81:509–17

23. Schatz M, Patterson R, Zeitz S, *et al*. Corticosteroid therapy for the pregnancy asthmatic patient. *J Am Med Assoc* 1975;233:804

24. Stenius-Aarniala N, Piirlä P, Teramo K. Asthma and pregnancy: a prospective study of 198 pregnancies. *Thorax* 1988;43:12–18

25. Schatz M, Zeigler RS, Hoffman CP. Intrauterine growth is related to gestational pulmonary function in pregnant asthmatic women. *Chest* 1990;98:389–92

26. Hollingsworth HM, Pratter MR, Irwin RS. Acute respiratory failure in pregnancy. *J Intensive Care Med* 1989;4:11–34

27. Novy MJ, Edwards MJ. Respiratory problems in pregnancy. *Am J Obstet Gynecol* 1967;99:1024

28. National Asthma Education Program. Report of the Working Group on Asthma in Pregnancy. *Management of Asthma during Pregnancy*, NIH publication no. 93–3279. Bethesda, MD: Department of Health and Human Services, 1993

29. Cockcroft DW, Murdock KY. Comparative effects of inhaled salbutamol, sodium cromoglycate and beclomethasone on allergenic-induced early asthmatic responses and increased bronchial responsiveness to histamine. *J Allergy Clin Immunol* 1987;79:734–40

30. Greenberger P, Patterson R. Safety of therapy for allergic symptoms during pregnancy. *Ann Intern Med* 1978;89:234–7

31. Stenius-Aarniala BS, Riikonen S, Teramo K. Slow-release theophylline in pregnant asthmatics. *Chest* 1995;107:642–7

32. Rubin PC. Prescribing in pregnancy. General principles. *Br Med J* 1986;293:1415–17

33. Carter BL, Criscoll CE, Smith GD. Theophylline clearance during pregnancy. *Obstet Gynecol* 1986;68:555

34. Gardner MJ, Schatz M, Cousius L, *et al*. Longitudinal effects of pregnancy on the pharmacokinetics of theophylline. *Eur J Clin Pharmacol* 1987;31:289

35. Weinstein AM, Dubin BD, Podleski WK, *et al*. Asthma and pregnancy. *J Am Med Assoc* 1979;241:1161

36. Yurchak AM, Jusko WJ. Theophylline secretion in breast milk. *Pediatrics* 1976;75:518–20

37. Mawhinney H, Spector SL. Optimum management of asthma in pregnancy. *Drugs* 1986;32:178–87

38. Greenberger PA, Patterson R. Beclomethasone diproprionate for severe asthma during pregnancy. *Ann Intern Med* 1983;98:478

39. Jenkins PF, Benfield GFA, Smith AP. Predicting recovery from acute severe asthma. *Thorax* 1981;36:835–41

40. Cui K-H, Haan EA, Wang L-J, Matthews CD. Optimal polymerase chain reaction amplification for preimplantation diagnosis in cystic fibrosis (ΔF508). *Br Med J* 1995;311:536–40

41. Kent NE, Farquharson DF. Cystic fibrosis in pregnancy. *Can Med Assoc J* 1993;149:809–13.

42. Edenborough FP, Stableforth DE, Webb AK, *et al*. Outcome of pregnancy in women with cystic fibrosis. *Thorax* 1995;50:170–4

43. Canny GJ, Corey M, Livingstone RA, *et al*. Pregnancy and cystic fibrosis. *Obstet Gynecol* 1991;77:850–3

44. Whitelaw A, Butterfield A. High breast milk sodium in cystic fibrosis. *Lancet* 1977;2:1288

45. Alpert SE, Cormier AD. Normal electrolyte and protein content in milk from mothers with cystic fibrosis: an explanation for the initial report of elevated milk sodium concentration. *J Pediatr* 1983;102:77–80

46. Sridana V, Pacini F, Yang SL, *et al*. Decreased level of helper T cells: a possible because of immunodeficiency in pregnancy. *N Engl J Med* 1982;307:352–6

47. Lederman MM. Cell mediated immunity and pregnancy. *Chest* 1984;86:6S–9S

48. Barbee RA, Hicks MJ, Grosso D, Sandel C. The maternal immune response in coccidioidomycosis. Is pregnancy a risk factor for serious infection? *Chest* 1991;100:709–15

49. Kaunitz AM, Hughes JM, Grimes DA, *et al*. Causes of maternal mortality in the United States. *Obstet Gynecol* 1985;65:605

50. Hughes CH, Popovich J. Pinpointing the cause of respiratory crisis in pregnancy. *J Crit Illness* 1990;5:559–76

51. Benedetti TJ, Valle R, Ledger WJ. Antepartum pneumonia in pregnancy. *Obstet Gynecol* 1982;144:413–17

52. Chow AW, Jewesson RJ. Pharmacokinetics and safety of antimicrobial agents in pregnancy. *Rev Infect Dis* 1985;7:278–313

53. Kort BA, Cefalo RC, Baker VV. Fatal influenza A pneumonia in pregnancy. *Am J Perinatol* 1986;3:179–82

54. Maccato ML. Pneumonia in pregnancy. In Gilstrap LC, ed. *Infections in Pregnancy*. New York: Wiley-Liss, 1990:255–66

55. Mostow SR, Cate TR, Ruben FL. Prevention of influenza and pneumonia. *Am Rev Respir Dis* 1990;142:487–8

56. Mostow SR. Prevention, management, and control of influenza: role of amantadine. *Am J Med* (suppl 6A) 1987;82:35

57. Triebwasser JH, Harris RE, Bryand RE, *et al*. Varicella pneumonia in adults. *Medicine* 1967;46:409

58. Smego RA, Asperilla MO. Use of acyclovir for varicella pneumonia during pregnancy. *Obstet Gynecol* 1991;78:1112–16

59. Balducci J, Rodis JF, Rosengreen S, *et al.* Pregnancy outcome following first-trimester varicella infection. *Obstet Gynecol* 1992;79:5–6

60. Paryani SG, Arvin AM. Intrauterine infection with varicella-zoster virus after maternal varicella. *N Engl J Med* 1986;314:1542–6

61. Siegel M. Congenital malformations following chickenpox, measles, mumps, and hepatitis: results of a cohort study. *J Am Med Assoc* 1973;226:1521–4

62. Cantazaro A. Pulmonary mycosis in pregnant women. *Chest* 1984;86:14S

63. Hedvall E. Pregnancy and tuberculosis. *Acta Med Scan* 1953;286:1–101

64. American Thoracic Society. Treatment of tuberculosis and tuberculosis infection in adults and children. *Am J Respir Crit Care Med* 1994;149:1359–74

65. Espinal MA, Reingold AL, Lavandera M. Effect of pregnancy on the risk of developing active tuberculosis. *J Infect Dis* 1996;173:488–91

66. Barnes PF, Bloch AB, Davidson PT, *et al.* Tuberculosis in patients with HIV infection. *N Engl J Med* 1991; 324:1644

67. Small PM, Schechter GF, Goodman PC, *et al.* Treatment of tuberculosis in patients with advanced HIV infection. *N Engl J Med* 1991;324:289

68. Small PM, Shafer RW, Hopewell PC, *et al.* Exogenous reinfection with multidrug-resistant *Mycobacterium tuberculosis* in patients with advanced HIV infection. *N Engl J Med* 1993;328:1137

69. Snider D. Pregnancy and tuberculosis. *Chest* 1984; 86S:10S

70. Hamadeh MA, Glassroth J. Tuberculosis and pregnancy. *Chest* l992;101:1114

71. Vallejo JG, Starke JR. Tuberculosis and pregnancy. *Clin Chest Med* 1992;13:693

72. Present PA, Comstock GW. Tuberculin sensitivity in pregnancy. *Am Rev Respir Dis* 1975;112:413

73. Sartwell PE. Racial differences in sarcoidosis. *Ann NY Acad Sci* 1976;278:368–70

74. Siltzbach LE, James DG, Neville E, *et al.* Course and prognosis of sarcoidosis around the world. *Am J Med* 1974;57:847–52

75. DeRemee RA. The roentgenographic staging of sarcoidosis: historic and contemporary perspectives. *Chest* 1983;83:128–32

76. O'Learly JA. Ten year study of sarcoidosis and pregnancy. *Am J Obstet Gynecol* 1962;84:462

77. Baggish MS, Hooper S. Aspiration a cause of maternal death. *Obstet Gynecol* 1974;43:327

78. Bartlett JG, Gorbach SI. The triple threat of aspiration. *Chest* 1975;68:560–6

79. DePaso WJ. Aspiration pneumonia. *Clin Chest Med* 1991;12:269–84

80. Bynum LJ, Pierce AK. Pulmonary aspiration of gastric contents. *Am Rev Respir Dis* 1976;114:1129–36

81. Bernard GR, Luce JM, Sprung CL, *et al.* High-dose corticosteroids in patients with the adult respiratory distress syndrome. *N Engl J Med* 1987;317: 1565–70

82. Wolfe JE, Bone RC, Ruth WE. The effect of corticosteroids in the treatment of patients with gastric aspiration. *Am J Med* 1977;63:719–22

83. Downs JB, Chapman RL Jr, Modell JH, *et al.* An evaluation of steroid therapy in aspiration pneumonitis. *Anesthesiology* 1974;40:129–35

84. Murray HW. Antimicrobial therapy in pulmonary aspiration. *Am J Med* 1979;66:188–90

85. McCammon RL. Prophylaxis for aspiration pneumonitis. *Can Anaesth Soc J* 1986;33:S47–S53

86. Gipson SL, Stovall TG, Elkins TE, *et al.* Pharmacologic reduction of the risk of aspiration. *South Med J* 1986;70:1356

87. Hoyt J. Aspiration pneumonitis: patient risk factors, prevention, and management. *J Intensive Care Med* 1990;5:52–9

88. Bonnar J. Venous thromboembolism and pregnancy. *Clin Obstet Gynecol* 1981;8:455

89. de Sweit M. Thromboembolism. *Clin Hematol* 1985; 14:643–60

90. Treffers PE, Huidekoper BL, Weenik GH, Kloosterman GJ. Epidemiological observations of thrombo-embolic disease during pregnancy and in the puerperium, in 52,022 women. *Int J Gynecol Obstet* 1983;21:327–31

91. Moser KM. Venous thromboembolism. *Am Rev Respir Dis* 1990;141:235–49

92. Clarke-Pearson DL, Jelovsek FR. Alterations of occlusive cuff impedance plethysmography results in obstetric patients. *Surgery* 1981;89:594–8

93. Hull RD, Raskob GE, Carter CJ. Serial impedance plethysmography in pregnant patients with clinically suspected deep-vein thrombosis. *Ann Intern Med* 1990; 112:663–7

94. White RH, McGahan JP, Daschbach MM, Harting RP. Diagnosis of deep-vein thrombosis using duplex ultrasound. *Ann Intern Med* 1989;111:297–304

95. Rutherford SE, Phelan JP. Clinical management of thromboembolic disorders in pregnancy. *Crit Care Clin* 1991;7:809–28

96. Greer IA, Barry J, Mackon N, Allan PL. Diagnosis of deep venous thrombosis in pregnancy: a new role for diagnostic ultrasound. *Br J Obstet Gynaecol* 1990; 97:53–7

97. The PIOPED Investigators. Value of the ventilation/ perfusion scan in acute pulmonary embolism: results of the Prospective Investigation of Pulmonary Embolism Diagnosis (PIOPED). *J Am Med Assoc* 1990; 263:2753–9

98. Howie PW. Anticoagulants in pregnancy. *Clin Obstet Gynecol* 1986;13:349–63

99. Ginsberg JS, Hirsh J, Turner C, *et al.* Risk to the fetus of anticoagulant therapy during pregnancy. *Thromb Hemost* 1989;61:197

100. Doyle DJ, Turpie GG, Hirsh J, *et al.* Adjusted subcutaneous heparin or continuous intravenous heparin in patients with acute deep vein thrombosis. *Ann Intern Med* 1987;107:441–5

101. Hull RD, Raskob GE, Hirsh J, *et al.* Continuous intravenous heparin compared with intermittent subcutaneous heparin in the initial treatment of proximal-vein thrombosis. *N Engl J Med* 1986;315: 1109–14

102. Narayan H, Cullimore J, Krarup K, *et al.* Experience with the Cardial inferior vena cava filter as prophylaxis against pulmonary embolism in pregnant women with

extensive deep venous thrombosis. *Br J Obstet Gynaecol* 1992;99:637–40

103. Orme MLE, Lewis PJ, de Sweit M, *et al*. May mothers given warfarin breast-feed their infant? *Br Med J* 1977; 1:1564–5

104. McKenna R, Cale ER, Vasan U. Is warfarin sodium contra-indicated in the lactating mother? *J Pediatr* 1983;103:325–7

105. Kramer WB, Belfort M, Saade S, Moise KJ. Successful urokinase treatment of massive pulmonary embolism in pregnancy. *Obstet Gynecol* 1995;86:660–2

106. Hall RJC, Young C, Sutton GC, *et al*. Treatment of acute massive pulmonary embolism by streptokinase during labor and delivery. *Br Med J* 1972;4:647–9

107. McTaggert DR, Ingram TG. Massive pulmonary embolism during pregnancy treated with streptokinase. *Med J Aust* 1977;1:18–20

108. Ludwig H. Results of streptokinase therapy in deep venous thrombosis during pregnancy. *Postgrad Med J* 1973;49 (suppl 5):65–7

109. Witchitz S, Veyrat C, Moisson P, *et al*. Fibrinolytic treatment of thrombus on prosthetic heart valves. *Br Heart J* 1980;44:545–54

110. Ingemarson I, Bengtsson B. A five year experience with terbutaline for preterm labor: low rate of severe side effects. *Obstet Gynecol* 1985;66:176–80

111. Pisani RJ, Rosenow EC III. Pulmonary edema associated with tocolytic therapy. *Ann Intern Med* 1989; 110:714–18

112. Nimrod C, Rambihar V, Fallen E, *et al*. Pulmonary edema associated with isoxsuprine therapy. *Am J Obstet Gynecol* 1984;148:625–9

113. Elliot JP. Magnesium sulfate as a tocolytic agent. *Am J Obstet Gynecol* 1983;147:277–84

114. Beall NM, Edgar BW, Paul RH, Smith-Wallace T. A comparison of ritodrine, terbutaline, and magnesium sulfate for the suppression of preterm labor. *Am J Obstet Gynecol* 1985;153:854–9

115. Karson EM, Saltzman D, Davis NR. Pneumomediastinum in pregnancy: two case reports and a review of the literature, pathophysiology, and management. *Obstet Gynecol* 1984;64(suppl):39S

116. Munsell WP. Pneumomediastinum: a report of 28 cases and review of the literature. *J Am Med Assoc* 1967; 202:689

117. Mabie WC, Barton JR, Sibai BM. Adult respiratory distress syndrome in pregnancy. *Am J Obstet Gynecol* 1992;167:950–7

118. Deblieux PM, Summer WR. Acute respiratory failure in pregnancy. *Clin Obstet Gynecol* 1996;39:143–52

119. Schuster DP. A physiologic approach to initiating, maintaining, and withdrawing mechanical ventilatory support during acute respiratory failure. *Am J Med* 1990;88:268–78

120. Kopenhagen T. A review of 50 pregnant patients with kyphoscoliosis. *Br J Obstet Gynaecol* 1977;84:585

121. Betz RR, Bunnell WP, Lambrecht-Mulier E, *et al*. Scoliosis and pregnancy. *J Bone Joint Surg* 1987; 69-A:90–6

44

Renal diseases

F. Horvath

INTRODUCTION

The combination of renal disease and pregnancy has for years generated great concern among clinicians with respect to maternal and perinatal morbidity and mortality. This chapter will address the following issues: pregnancy-induced changes in renal hemodynamics and physiology; the influence of underlying chronic renal diseases and hypertension on pregnancy; the effect of pregnancy on the natural course of pre-existing chronic renal disease; acute renal failure; and renal dialysis and transplantation.

Pregnancy and chronic renal insufficiency are states of persistent renal vasodilatation. Theoretically, systemic hypertension during pregnancy may be easily transmitted to the glomeruli, producing higher glomerular capillary pressures and further renal injury. Therefore, severe systemic hypertension in pregnant women with chronic renal disease must be aggressively treated. However, treatment of mild to moderate primary hypertension in pregnancy is controversial.

If there is no maternal hypertension and only mild renal insufficiency, then the underlying renal disease process, regardless of type, is unlikely to affect the pregnancy adversely. Moreover, a large majority of pregnancies in women with chronic renal disease are successful. Fetal loss correlates directly with the degree of hypertension during pregnancy and is related in a large part to premature delivery.

Acute renal failure during pregnancy is usually secondary to volume depletion or acute tubular necrosis. Severe pre-eclampsia, postpartum hemolytic–uremic syndrome and other causes unique to pregnancy may occur in the third trimester and postpartum, presenting diagnostic and therapeutic challenges.

RENAL ANATOMY AND PHYSIOLOGY DURING PREGNANCY

The anatomy of the renal urinary system during pregnancy is similar to the non-pregnant state except for dilatation. Early in the second trimester, the renal collecting system dilates by as much as 1 cm, due predominantly to relaxation of the smooth musculature of the ureter and bladder. The dilatation usually is greater on the right. This 'hydronephrosis of pregnancy' may persist for up to 12 weeks postpartum. The mechanism for the dilatation is not understood, although hormonal effects of prostaglandin E (PGE), estrogen and progesterone on smooth muscle have all been postulated as contributory. How much of the dilatation is secondary to mechanical obstruction from the gravid uterus and other pelvic structures (e.g. iliac or ovarian vessels) is unclear.

There are three important consequences of this physiologic dilatation. Twenty-four hour urine collections for creatinine clearance may underestimate glomerular filtration rate (GFR), due to a portion of the timed urine remaining in the collecting system. This effect can be minimized by hydration of the patient before the collection begins and by obtaining the last few hours of the collection in the left lateral recumbent position. Secondly, vesico-ureteral reflux is more likely to occur or be aggravated during pregnancy. Thirdly, the reflux and/or stasis leads to a significantly increased predisposition for acute pyelonephritis when bacteriuria is present.

Renal plasma flow (RPF) and GFR increase during pregnancy by as much as 50% above normal (Figure 1). This change begins early in the first trimester and is sustained until 36 weeks of gestation when both begin

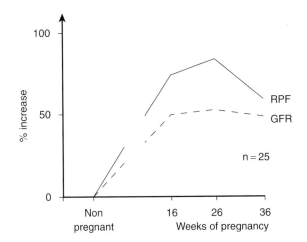

Figure 1 Relative changes in renal hemodynamics during normal human pregnancy. RPF, renal plasma flow; GFR, glomerular filtration rate. Reproduced with permission from Davison JM. Overview: Kidney function in pregnant women. *Am J Kidney Dis* 1987;9:248–52

505

to decline towards pre-pregnancy values[1]. Maternal extracellular volume increases by 4–6 l during pregnancy, with the plasma volume accounting for 1.2 l. Plasma volume expansion is responsible for some of the increase in RPF, GFR and cardiac output. However, most of the RPF change is due to a pregnancy-induced decrease in renal vascular resistance, possibly prostaglandin-mediated[2].

Some of the consequences of the rise in RPF and GFR are predictable. Since there is little increase in the generation of creatinine, urea, or urate during pregnancy, the increase in RPF and GFR produces lower serum values of these substances via increased clearance (increased filtration in the case of urea and creatinine and increased tubular secretion for urate). The average creatinine level falls from 0.67 mg/dl pre-pregnancy to 0.46 mg/dl during pregnancy; the blood urea nitrogen (BUN) from 13 mg/dl to 9 mg/dl; and urate from 6.0 mg/dl to 4.0 mg/dl. Therefore, a serum creatinine value greater than 0.8 mg/dl in pregnancy may well represent a substantial decline in GFR and should be evaluated further[3]. Other consequences of a rise in RPF and GFR are less predictable, such as the relatively stable glomerular capillary hydrostatic pressure (P_{GC}) in the face of a rising RPF. One would expect that as the afferent arteriolar resistance decreases and RPF increases, this flow would be transmitted to the glomerular capillary in such a way as to increase the capillary hydrostatic pressure. However, micropuncture studies in pregnant rats show that despite significant increases in GFR and RPF, the P_{GC} remains unchanged due to parallel and proportionally similar reductions in preglomerular and postglomerular arteriolar resistances. This 'protected' P_{GC} may explain why, in animals, there appears to be no adverse effects of serial pregnancies on renal function or glomerular histology[4]. As will be discussed later in this chapter, the occurrence of systemic hypertension in pregnant women with chronic renal disease changes the relationship between RPF, mean systemic arterial pressure and P_{GC} to the detriment of the kidney.

Renal function is usually assessed by 24-h urine collection to determine creatinine clearance and total proteinuria. Alternatively, one can use the random urine protein to creatinine ratio (P/C) to estimate protein excretion. The GFR or creatinine can also be estimated from the following formula:

$$\frac{[140 - \text{age (years)}] \times \text{pre-pregnancy weight (kg)} \times 0.85}{72 \times \text{serum creatinine (mg/dl)}}$$

There is an excellent correlation between estimated values and those from 24-h urine collection, even during pregnancies. A random urine P/C ratio of < 0.3 correlates with a 24-h urine protein excretion of less than 300 mg with a positive predictive value (PPV) of 88% and negative predictive value (NPV) of 93.9%.

Table 1   Summary of physiologic changes in the pregnant state

Net sodium retention	900 mEq
Extracellular volume	Increased 4–6 l
Plasma volume	Increased 1.2 l
Cardiac output	Mild increase
GFR and RPF	Increased 50%
Systemic vascular resistance	Decreased
Renal vascular resistance	Decreased
Systemic blood pressure	Decreased
systolic	15 mmHg
diastolic	10 mmHg
Glomerular capillary pressure	No change
Serum osmolality	Decreased 10 mOsm
Urine concentration and dilution	No change
T_{Max} for glucose reabsorption	Decreased
T_{Max} for amino acid reabsorption	Decreased (for some amino acids)
Acid–base balance	Compensated respiratory alkalosis
Serum creatinine, BUN, urate concentrations	Decreased

GFR, glomerular filtration rate; RPF, renal plasma flow

Similarly, a random urine P/C ratio > 3 corresponds to 24-h protein excretion of > 3.5 g with a PPV of 72.7% and NPV of 100%[5].

SODIUM AND WATER METABOLISM

Although there is a net total body gain of sodium during a normal gestation, the renal tubules handle a salt load normally (Table 1). The balance between glomerular filtration of sodium (which increases with the rise in GFR) and tubular reabsorption of sodium is maintained. Aldosterone levels are increased in pregnancy; however this does not explain the avid reabsorption of sodium needed to balance the GFR. Other factors such as peritubular Starling's forces and natriuretic peptide regulation are believed to be operative. The kidneys' abilities to maximally dilute and concentrate urine are intact. The serum sodium concentration and serum osmolality concentration are about 5 mEq/l and 10 mOsm/kg respectively, lower throughout most of gestation than in the non-pregnant state due to a decrease in osmotic threshold for thirst and arginine vasopressin (AVP) release[6]. There is a transient increase in AVP clearance during mid-gestation that may produce a diuresis, sometimes known as 'transient diabetes insipidus of pregnancy'.

TUBULAR FUNCTION

Glucosuria seen in some pregnancies is more a reflection of altered renal function than of abnormal carbohydrate metabolism. Both the proximal and distal tubule appear to have a decreased capacity to reabsorb filtered glucose (i.e. decreased T_{Max} for glucose reabsorption). This tubular defect persists in the non-pregnant state in these women. The exact mechanism for the altered glucose handling by the tubule is not known. The marked increases in plasma volume and GFR that occur during pregnancy probably have a greater contribution to the glucosuria than does any tubular defect. Plasma volume and GFR affect sodium handling by the tubule, and sodium and glucose reabsorption are linked[1]. Altered tubular maxima for amino acids also occur in pregnancy. Certain amino acids, such as histidine and alanine, are excreted in large amounts due to decreased reabsorptive capacity, while other amino acids, such as glutamic acid and methionine, are not affected.

ACID–BASE BALANCE

In pregnancy, there is a compensatory respiratory alkalosis which begins early in gestation and continues to term. The P_{CO_2} decreases from 39 to 31 mmHg, the serum bicarbonate ranges from 18 to 22 mEq/l, and the arterial pH is about 7.44[3]. The respiratory alkalosis may be due to progesterone-induced hyperventilation. There is no apparent defect in renal handling of acid.

PREGNANCY IN WOMEN WITH UNDERLYING CHRONIC RENAL DISEASE

Pre-existing maternal renal disease during pregnancy raises three issues: maternal health, the effect of the pregnancy on the natural progression of the renal disease and fetal outcome. Available literature suggests the following:

(1) The risk to the mother is related to hypertension and pre-eclampsia;

(2) The natural course of most chronic renal disease is not adversely affected by pregnancy as long as there is only mild renal insufficiency and no hypertension;

(3) Perinatal mortality is related to prematurity and retarded fetal growth; the overall mortality rate is approximately 10%[7];

(4) Pre-existing proteinuria is worsened in pregnancy, sometimes to the nephrotic degree, but it is generally well tolerated by the fetus and mother;

(5) Worsening of proteinuria, hypertension and GFR late in pregnancy may be due to superimposed pre-eclampsia; and

(6) Pregnancy in patients with mildly impaired renal disease, a serum creatinine at conception < 1.4 mg/dl, is usually uneventful if there is no significant hypertension and absence of nephrotic proteinuria.

Recent remnant kidney models in animals and humans have shown that as nephrons are lost, remaining nephrons adapt by increasing their single nephron glomerular filtration rate (SNGFR). The increase in SNGFR is accomplished predominantly through a rise in P_{GC}. This elevation in P_{GC} is caused by afferent arteriolar vasodilatation and efferent arteriolar vasoconstriction. PGE_2, thromboxane A_2, PGI_2 and angiotensin-II appear to be mediators of these vascular alterations[8]. Adaptive changes that elevate P_{GC} result in a temporary advantage of increased GFR but in the long term produce a sclerosing effect on remaining glomeruli. High protein dietary intake produces changes in renal hemodynamics similar to those seen in the remnant kidney model and those induced by pregnancy[9]. Therefore, physicians are concerned about the potential deleterious effects of pregnancy on the natural course of various renal diseases. The increase in proteinuria as seen in some pregnancies may have a sclerosing effect via mesangial cell overload. Although pregnancy produces a state of chronic renal vasodilatation, there is no evidence that P_{GC} increases in normotensive women, probably because of a proportional reduction in afferent and efferent arteriolar tone. If, however, systemic hypertension is superimposed on a state of reduced nephron mass, the dilated preglomerular vasculature of pregnancy may allow the systemic pressure to be transmitted to the glomerular capillaries, affecting glomerular hydrostatic pressure (P_{GC}). The potentially damaging effect of chronic renal disease in pregnant women, therefore, is its tendency to cause systemic hypertension, which may well lead to increase in P_{GC} (an important final pathway for glomerular injury and nephron loss). In this regard, angiotensin-converting enzyme inhibitors would seem to be ideal antihypertensive agents in pregnant women with chronic renal disease because of their effects on decreasing efferent arteriolar tone, which leads to a fall in P_{GC}. This effect has been well demonstrated in diabetic renal disease. Unfortunately, their use has been associated with increased incidence of stillbirth in animal studies[10] and a few cases of neonatal acute renal failure[11,12]. Avoidance of angiotensin-converting enzyme inhibitors during pregnancy is prudent.

CHRONIC PRIMARY GLOMERULAR RENAL DISEASE

Several clinical studies reveal that the proteinuria of chronic renal disease increases in approximately one-half of women during pregnancy and that hypertension develops or worsens in 25% to 60%[7,13,14]. In the study by Katz and co-workers[7], 29% of women with increased proteinuria during pregnancy had persistent proteinuria after a 5-year follow-up, and 6% had a persistent loss of GFR. The studies did not reveal to what degree the proteinuria or renal insufficiency was a result of a natural progression of the renal disease or to what degree these changes could be attributed to the pregnancy.

There is no evidence to suggest that the immunological injury of various types of glomerulonephritis is aggravated by pregnancy. It appears, rather, that injury during pregnancy (manifested by increased proteinuria and fall in GFR) is mediated by an increase in P_{GC}, by superimposed pre-eclampsia, or by a natural progression of the disease process. A large retrospective study showed that pregnancy in patients with renal disease was usually uneventful if there was no significant hypertension, proteinuria was not in the nephrotic range, and renal function was reasonably good at conception (serum creatinine < 1.8 mg/dl)[15]. Jungers and colleagues looked at long-term renal survival in 320 women with biopsy-proven primary chronic glomerulonephritis[15]. Almost half, or 148 women, had been pregnant at least once after the onset of the renal disease, and most had near-normal renal function at conception. The clinical courses of these women were compared to 172 women who did not conceive. He found no significant difference between the two groups in the eventual development of end-stage renal disease (Figure 2). On the other hand, significantly impaired renal function (serum creatinine > 1.8 mg/dl) and uncontrolled hypertension at conception frequently led to accelerated deterioration of renal function during pregnancy. Considering the various histological types of chronic glomerulonephritis, membranoproliferative glomerulonephritis appears to have the worst prognosis during and following pregnancy[16] (Figure 3).

A recent report of 67 pregnant patients with moderate or severe renal insufficiency revealed that 43% of patients had pregnancy-related loss of renal function and 10% of patients had rapid deterioration in renal function. Accelerated decline in GFR developed in 2% of patients with the initial serum creatinine of less than 2.0 mg/dl and in 33% of patients with the serum creatinine of 2.0 mg/dl or greater. In addition, the percentages of patients having hypertension (mean arterial pressure above 105 mmHg) and high-grade proteinuria (> 3000 mg/l) rise from 28% and 23% during the first prenatal visit to 48% and 41% during the third trimester, respectively. Moderate and severe renal insufficiency are defined as having serum creatinine ranges of 1.4–2.4 mg/dl and above 2.4 mg/dl respectively[17].

Perinatal outcomes depend on the degree of renal impairment, and the development of hypertension and pre-eclampsia. Perinatal complications include fetal growth retardation, fetal death and preterm delivery, the latter because of fetal distress, rapidly worsening renal function or pre-eclampsia. The frequencies of preterm delivery and fetal growth retardation are 55% and 31% respectively in patients with moderate renal insufficiency, and 73% and 57%

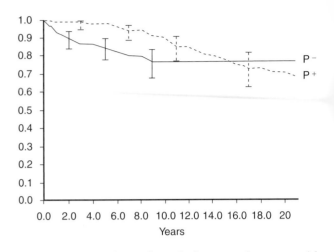

Figure 2 Actuarial renal survival curve of women with primary glomerulonephritis having been pregnant (P⁺) or not (P⁻) after the clinical onset of glomerulonephritis. Reproduced with permission from reference 15

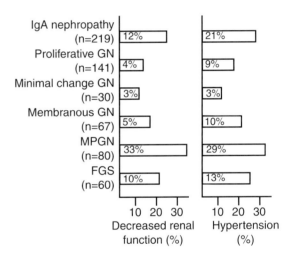

Figure 3 Effect of pregnancy on underlying glomerulonephritis determined during final follow-up. Reproduced with permission from reference 16

respectively in patients with severe renal insufficiency[17]. The overall perinatal survival rate is 90% or greater[15–18].

LUPUS NEPHRITIS

Early studies suggest that pregnant women with systemic lupus erythematosus (SLE) clinically flare their disease three times more frequently during pregnancy and seven times more frequently postpartum compared to non-pregnant controls[19]. This observation has not been corroborated in more recent studies. Hayslett[20] correlated the incidence of SLE flares with activity of the disease prior to conception. If the disease was quiescent for 6 months prior to conception, there was a 30% chance of increased activity during pregnancy. Activity at conception increased the chance of a flare to 62%, and was correlated with a 90–100% live birth rate if SLE was quiescent and 50–86% if SLE was active.

The presence of circulating anticardiolipin antibodies and lupus anticoagulant factors appears to worsen the perinatal outcomes. Fetal loss rate increases from 25% to about 60%, and the risk of maternal thromboembolism increases to about 50%[21–24].

It is currently believed that aggressive immunosuppressive therapy (steroids, etc.) is warranted for clinical evidence of active SLE during pregnancy in light of improved maternal and perinatal outcomes associated with disease remission.

DIABETIC RENAL DISEASE

The majority of women who have insulin-dependent diabetes mellitus and become pregnant already have microvascular changes of diabetes, notably retinal and glomerular injury. In the non-pregnant patient, hypertension accelerates the glomerular sclerosis of diabetic nephropathy. There is, however, no evidence that pregnancy worsens diabetic nephropathy beyond the normal progression to injury, despite a high incidence of hypertension in this group. This might be explained by the short duration over which the hypertension is operative. The incidence of chronic hypertension and superimposed pre-eclampsia in 'Classes B and C' and 'Classes D, F and R' diabetic patients increases to 8% and 16%, respectively, when compared to non-diabetic pregnant patients[25].

NEPHROTIC SYNDROME

The most common cause of the nephrotic syndrome in pregnancy is pre-eclampsia. Other causes are: diabetic nephropathy; one of the primary glomerulopathies such as membranous, focal segmental glomerulonephritis or membranoproliferative glomerulonephritis; amyloidosis; lupus nephritis; and renal vein thrombosis. Twenty-five per cent of mothers with mild to moderate proteinuria can be expected to develop the nephrotic syndrome during pregnancy[26]. If not accompanied by hypertension or severe renal insufficiency, the nephrotic state is tolerated well by the fetus and mother, though one study did show a correlation between severely depressed serum albumin levels and low birth weight infants[27]. In patients with primary glomerular disease, the presence of significant proteinuria (> 3.0 g/day) either before pregnancy or during pregnancy is associated with accelerated deterioration of renal function after pregnancy[28].

AUTOSOMAL DOMINANT POLYCYSTIC KIDNEY DISEASE (ADPKD)

Pregnant patients with polycystic kidney disease generally have not reached the point in their disease where renal insufficiency and hypertension are a problem; therefore, uneventful pregnancies are the rule. In patients with hypertension antedating the pregnancy, there is a somewhat higher incidence of pre-eclampsia and worsening hypertension usually in the third trimester of gestation. Episodes of acute pyelonephritis, when they occur, are usually severe. The following risk factors are associated with worse renal function at a given age: the PKD1 gene, younger age at diagnosis, hypertension, hepatic cysts, and three or more pregnancies[29].

MANAGEMENT

Women with chronic renal disease require frequent measurements (e.g. monthly) of serum creatinine, blood pressure and urinalysis. Patients should be instructed in self home blood pressure monitoring. Although there is a considerable debate regarding whether to treat mild primary hypertension during pregnancy, a patient with chronic renal disease should have hypertension treated aggressively. Renal biopsy is occasionally needed when an unexplained nephrotic syndrome suddenly appears and renal function dramatically declines, particularly when associated with a nephritic urine (proteinuria, hematuria, red cell casts). The histologic information obtained by biopsy may be helpful in therapeutic decisions. It appears that pregnancy does not increase the risk of renal biopsy[30]. During the third trimester, serial ultrasound examinations to assess fetal growth and close surveillance of fetal well-being with non-stress tests and/or biophysical profile are recommended.

ACUTE RENAL FAILURE IN PREGNANCY

Acute renal failure (ARF) is defined as an abrupt deterioration in GFR with a subsequent rise in BUN and serum creatinine, often accompanied by oliguria (urine output < 400 ml/day). Currently, 1–3% of all episodes of ARF occur during pregnancy. Realizing that some mild cases are not detected, acute renal failure is an unusual complication of pregnancy, occurring in less than 0.01% of all pregnancies in Western industrialized countries[31–34]. This is a marked decrease from that seen in 1950s and 1960s when septic abortions were common.

Acute renal failure in pregnancy occurs in a context of unique physiologic alterations discussed earlier. Serum creatinine, BUN, urate and blood pressure levels are lower in pregnancy than in the non-pregnant

Table 2   Disorders causing acute renal failure in pregnancy

Prerenal (underperfusion)
  volume depletion from hemorrhage
  volume depletion from hyperemesis or diuretics
  edema-related diseases (e.g. nephrotic syndrome)

Postrenal (obstruction)
  urolithiasis
  ureteropelvic junction obstruction (pre-existing)
  polyhydramnios

Intrinsic renal disease
  acute glomerulonephritis
  acute interstitial nephritis
    acute pyelonephritis
    non-steroidal anti-inflammatory drugs
    penicillin and sulfa hypersensitivity
  acute tubular necrosis
    nephrotoxic drugs
    myoglobinuria
    shock
    radiographic contrast

Pregnancy-related acute renal failure
  pre-eclampsia
  HELLP syndrome
  acute fatty liver of pregnancy
  postpartum hemolytic-uremic syndrome

state. The usual causes of ARF include acute tubular necrosis (ATN) and a group of diseases unique to pregnancy such as pre-eclampsia. The clinical problem can also be complicated by an acute deterioration of an underlying chronic renal disease, such as lupus nephritis and primary glomerulopathy (e.g. focal segmental glomerulonephritis). Clinically, it is helpful to divide ARF into etiologies that occur in the first and second trimesters and those that occur late in pregnancy and postpartum. It is also helpful to divide further the etiologies of ARF into those related to underperfusion of the kidneys (prerenal), obstruction of urine flow (postrenal) and injury intrinsic to the kidneys (Table 2).

Most cases of renal underperfusion during pregnancy are secondary to volume depletion. Demonstration of a marked reduction in systolic blood pressure (> 20 mmHg) and pulse increase (> 10 bpm) from the supine to the upright position is an important diagnostic clue to volume depletion. Direct measurements of central venous pressure may be necessary. Urine sodium concentration is low (< 10 mEq/1), the fractional excretion of sodium is low (< 1%) and urinalysis is normal. The fractional excretion of sodium (FE_{Na^+}) can be calculated from random urine and serum tests according to the following formula:

$$FE_{Na^+} = \frac{\text{Urine Na}}{} \times \frac{\text{Serum creatinine}}{} \times 100$$

Usual causes of hypovolemia are hyperemesis gravidarum and obstetrical hemorrhage. If the plasma protein concentration becomes low enough due to the nephrotic syndrome, the kidney may behave in a prerenal fashion. This usually occurs at plasma albumin levels < 2.0 g/dl.

Obstruction of the urine flow in pregnancy is generally secondary to urolithiasis or pregnancy-aggravated ureteropelvic junction (UPJ) obstruction. If the obstruction is acute (measured in days), the urinalysis is generally normal. Symptoms, types of stone and clinical course are the same as in the non-pregnant state. Diagnosis of clinically significant obstruction is often difficult because dilatation of the upper ureter and pelvis may be normally present during pregnancy beyond 20 weeks' gestation. An intravenous urogram may be necessary to define the cause and level of obstruction. Dilatation of the ureters below the pelvic rim is very suggestive of obstruction[35]. To minimize fetal radiation exposure, an abbreviated intravenous pyelogram (IVP) can be done, i.e. a scout film followed by an additional film at 20 minutes. Obstruction of the urine flow associated with infection is a medical emergency and requires immediate decompression in addition to antibiotic therapy. Ureteral stents can be placed retrograde or percutaneously antegrade to provide relief of the obstruction during pregnancy.

Cortical necrosis can be considered a severe form of ATN, often associated with disseminated coagulopathy and usually occurring in a setting of septic shock, septic abortion, or severe abruptio placentae. Acute pyelonephritis is the most common infection in pregnancy and may lead to acute renal failure[36]. The clinical presentation of acute pyelonephritis is the same as in the non-pregnant state. Flank tenderness, bacteriuria and leukocyte casts are important findings.

Acute glomerulonephritis would be suggested by hypertension, proteinuria, hematuria and particularly red blood cell casts. Acute interstitial nephritis may be secondary to pyelonephritis, adverse reactions to non-steroidal anti-inflammatory drugs and allergic reactions to penicillin, sulfa or other drugs. Demonstrating eosinophils in the urine (using a Wright's stain or Hansel stain) is helpful in making the diagnosis of allergic interstitial nephritis. Non-steroidal anti-inflammatory drugs do not cause interstitial eosinophilic infiltration and eosinophiluria, but rather a plasma cell and lymphocyte infiltration (similar to acute renal transplant rejection) and sterile pyuria on urinalysis. Renal biopsy may sometimes be required for diagnosis.

Acute renal failure late in pregnancy and postpartum may be due to any of the preceding causes or diseases specific to pregnancy, i.e. pre-eclampsia, postpartum hemolytic–uremic syndrome or acute fatty liver of pregnancy. These pregnancy-associated illnesses can present clinically with proteinuria, hematuria, edema, hypertension and thrombocytopenia. Acute renal failure associated with pre-eclampsia is usually due to acute tubular necrosis. Intravascular volume contraction and intense vasoconstriction leads to renal blood flow and hence to ischemic tubular injury[36]. Tubular reabsorption of sodium is abnormal and hence the FE_{Na^+} is high ($> 3\%$). Urinalysis is quite abnormal with white cells, red cells, tubular epithelial cells and casts present.

Pre-eclampsia appears to be a disease of endothelial dysfunction in part related to prostaglandin imbalance (a reduced PGI_2/thromboxane A_2 (T_xA_2) ratio)[37–39]. PGI_2 is a potent vasodilator, decreases platelet aggregation and increases uterine placental blood flow, while T_xA_2 causes the opposite effects. The renal histopathology includes swollen glomerular endothelial cells (glomeruloendotheliosis), enlarged glomerular tufts, reduction of capillary lumen size and fibrinoid subendothelial deposits[40,41]. The diagnosis is essentially clinical, however, and rarely requires a renal biopsy. The disease usually occurs in primigravidas who present in the third trimester with proteinuria, edema and hypertension. Most multiparas with similar signs and symptoms, on the other hand, are more likely to have chronic hypertension with underlying renal disease and/or superimposed pre-eclampsia. The hemolysis, elevated liver enzyme, low platelet syndrome (HELLP) appears to be a manifestation of severe pre-eclampsia.

Acute fatty liver of pregnancy is a rare disease occurring during the third trimester. Presentation includes abdominal pain, jaundice, abnormal liver enzyme profile and ARF. Serum transaminases are generally not as severely elevated as they are in hepatitis. Disseminated intravascular coagulopathy is usually present. Liver biopsy shows microvesicular fat in swollen hepatocytes. The distribution is centrilobular and there are no inflammatory cell infiltrates or hepatocellular necrosis. Prompt delivery is mandatory to reduce the very high maternal and fetal mortality[42].

Postpartum renal failure is clinically indistinguishable from adult hemolytic–uremic syndrome. The pathophysiology is related to vascular endothelial injury with deposition of platelet thrombi and occlusion of capillaries and arterioles (a thrombotic microangiopathy). This condition usually presents with severe hypertension in 2–30 days following an unremarkable prenatal course and delivery, thrombocytopenia, microangiopathic hemolysis and anuric ARF. The prothrombin time (PT), partial thromboplastin time (PTT) and fibrinogen are characteristically normal. Many researchers have postulated that endothelial damage leads to the deposition of platelets in microvessels, and that this enothelial damage may be related to deficiencies of PGE_2 or of a plasma PGI_2-stimulating factor as in the case of severe pre-eclampsia[32].

Plasma exchange and antiplatelet therapy are becoming the mainstays of therapy despite the lack of large controlled studies to verify the efficacy of this therapeutic program.

DIALYSIS AND TRANSPLANTATION IN PREGNANCY

Pregnancy in the dialysis population is uncommon due to diminished fertility. The chances of a successful pregnancy are low, and maternal risk is high. In the transplant population, pregnancy is not uncommon, and the prospects for the pregnancy are encouraging.

To superimpose pregnancy upon the clinical problems associated with maintenance dialysis or transplantation adds a significant layer of complexity. Fortunately, fertility in the chronic dialysis population is low enough that pregnancy is uncommon (in the order of one pregnancy in 200 women of childbearing age). The chance of a live birth from a pregnancy while on chronic dialysis is approximately one in five[43]. Maternal risks are related to a significant increase in the likelihood of hypertension, intravascular volume overload and pre-eclampsia. There have been a few reports of successful outcome with hemodialysis (HD) and continuous ambulatory peritoneal dialysis (CAPD)[44–46]. The usual hemodialysis prescription of three times weekly dialysis treatments for non-pregnant patients is typically intensified to daily or five times weekly sessions. This change is made empirically to accomplish better clearance of toxins such as urea and to gain better blood pressure control via improved intravascular volume control. Fetal monitoring during hemodialysis has shown that the procedure is fairly well tolerated by the fetus if hypotension is avoided[47]. CAPD appears to have some advantages over HD, particularly in diabetics where intraperitoneal insulin administration provides better blood sugar control, and anticoagulation required during hemodialysis can be eliminated. There are less frequent hypotensive episodes with CAPD than with hemodialysis, in part because intravascular fluid is removed gradually over each 24-h period[43]. This tighter control of intravascular volume also accounts for improved hypertension management compared with hemodialysis.

In contrast to dialysis, transplantation restores fertility to near normal, and pregnancy is more common (one pregnancy in 50 women of childbearing age). Davison[43] recently summarized the experience with 2300 pregnancies in 1600 women with renal transplants. Forty per cent of the pregnancies did not go beyond the first trimester due to therapeutic abortions (27%) and spontaneous abortions (13%). Of pregnancies that went beyond the first trimester, 92% were successful. Approximately 50% of infants were born prematurely and 25% had intrauterine growth retardation.

The anatomic location of the transplant generally does not prevent a vaginal delivery. Cesarean section should be employed only for obstetrical indications. A permanent decline in transplant graft function occurred in 15% of these pregnancies while the chance of maternal hypertension or pre-eclampsia increased by 30%. Patients with good transplant function at conception (serum creatinine < 1.4 mg/dl) fared better. The mechanism for a transient fall in GFR near the end of gestation in most patients and for a permanent loss of GFR in some is not well understood. Moreover, it is not clear whether pregnancy *per se* plays a role in permanent functional loss.

Deterioration of transplant graft function during pregnancy must be considered a serious problem that requires the immediate attention of the transplant team. Manifestations of acute transplant rejection include fever, decreased renal function and renal transplant graft tenderness or enlargement. Transplant biopsy may be necessary to distinguish between such possibilities as acute allograft rejection, cyclosporine toxicity, acute pyelonephritis, or pre-eclampsia. There appears to be no increase in the frequency of acute renal rejection during pregnancy. Renal biopsy is indicated before beginning anti-rejection therapy[43].

Most pregnant patients with renal allograft have immunosuppression with azathioprine and prednisone. Hemopoiesis depression with leukopenia and thrombocytopenia has been observed with maternal azathioprine therapy. While there is a correlation between maternal leukocyte counts and fetal leukocyte counts, there is no correlation between maternal platelet counts and fetal ones[48]. The risk of fetal hemopoiesis suppression can be minimized or eliminated by maintaining maternal leukocyte counts in the normal range. No significant birth defects can be attributed to maternal azathioprine administration. Cyclosporin A has not been used for immunosuppression during pregnancy as widely as azathioprine. Limited experience suggests that fetal bone marrow suppression may occur as a result of maternal cyclophosphamide therapy[49]. Since chromosomal abnormalities have been associated with cyclophosphamide usage[50], extreme caution should be taken when using this medication during pregnancy, especially during the time of conception and during the first trimester.

Given the current experience with renal transplantation and pregnancy, it would seem prudent to recommend pregnancy only for those women who are 1–2 years post-transplant, have good graft function (serum creatinine < 1.5 mg/dl) and have excellent blood pressure control. Satisfying these three criteria markedly increases the chances of a successful pregnancy.

REFERENCES

1. Davison JM, Dunlop W. Renal hemodynamics and tubular function in normal human pregnancy. *Kidney Int* 1980;18:152–161
2. Bay WH, Ferris TF. Factors controlling plasma renin and aldosterone during pregnancy. *Hypertension* 1979;1:410–15
3. Lindheimer MD, Katz AI. The kidney and hypertension in pregnancy. In Brenner BM, Rector FC, eds. *The Kidney*, 4th edn. Philadelphia: WB Saunders Co., 1991:1551–95
4. Baylis C, Rennke HG. Renal hemodynamics and glomerular morphology in repetitively pregnant aging rats. *Kidney Int* 1985;28:140–45
5. Quadri KHM, Bernardi J, Greenberg A, *et al.* Assessment of renal function during pregnancy using a random urine protein to creatinine ratio and cockcroft-gault formula. *Am J Kidney Dis* 1994;24:416–20
6. Lindheimer MD, Barron WM. Osmotic and volume control of vasopressin release in pregnancy. *Am J Kidney Dis* 1991;17:105–14
7. Katz AI, Davison JM, Hayslett JP, *et al.* Pregnancy in women with kidney disease. *Kidney Int* 1980;18:192–206
8. Meyer TW, Scholey JW, Brenner BM. Nephron adaptation to renal injury. In Brenner BM, Rector FC, eds. *The Kidney*, 4th edn. Philadelphia: WB Saunders Co., 1991:1551–95
9. Brenner BM, Meyer TW, Hostetter TH. Dietary protein intake and the progressive nature of kidney disease: the role of hemodynamically mediated glomerular injury in the pathogenesis of glomerular sclerosis in aging, renal ablation, and intrinsic renal disease. *N Engl J Med* 1982;307:652–9
10. Pipkin FB, Turner SR, Symonds EM. Possible risk with captopril in pregnancy: some animal data *Lancet* 1980;1:1256
11. Rosa FW, Bosco LA, Graham CF, *et al.* Neonatal anuria with maternal angiotensin-converting enzyme inhibition. *Obstet Gynecol* 1989;74:371–4
12. Schubiger G, Flury G, Nussberger J. Enalapril for pregnancy-induced hypertension: acute renal failure in a neonate. *Ann Int Med* 1988;108:215–16
13. Hayslett JP. Interaction of renal disease and pregnancy. *Kidney Int* 1984;25:579–87
14. Hou SH, Grossman SD, Madias NE. Pregnancy in women with renal disease and moderate renal insufficiency. *Am J Med* 1985;78:185–94
15. Jungers P, Houiller P, Forget D, *et al.* Specific controversies concerning the natural history of renal disease in pregnancy. *Am J Kidney Dis* 1991;17:116–22
16. Abe S. An overview of pregnancy in women with underlying renal disease. *Am J Kidney Dis* 1991;17:112–15
17. Jones DC, Hayslett JP. Outcome of pregnancy in women with moderate or severe renal insufficiency. *N Engl J Med* 1996;335:226–32
18. Jungers P, Forget D, Henry-Amar M, *et al.* Chronic kidney disease and pregnancy. *Adv Nephrol* 1986;15:103–41
19. Garsenstein M, Pollak VE, Kark RM. Systemic lupus erythematosus and pregnancy. *N Engl J Med* 1962;267:165–9
20. Hayslett JP. Maternal and fetal complications in pregnant women with systemic lupus erythematosus. *Am J Kidney Dis* 1991;17:123–6
21. Kincaid-Smith P, Fairley KF, Kloss M. Lupus anticoagulant associated with renal thrombotic microangiopathy and pregnancy-related renal failure. *Q J Med* 1988;258:795–815

22. Loizons S, Byron MA, Englest HJ, *et al*. Associations of quantitative anticardiolipin antibody levels with fetal loss and time of loss in systemic lupus erythematosus. *Quart J Med* 1988;68:525–31

23. Lubbe WF, Bulter WS, Palmer SJ, *et al*. Lupus anticoagulant in pregnancy. *Br J Obstet Gynaecol* 1984;91:357–63

24. Alarcon-Segovia D, Deleze M, Oria CV, *et al*. Antiphospholipid antibodies and the antiphospholipid syndrome in systemic lupus erythematosus. *Medicine* 1989;68:353–65

25. Cousins L. Pregnancy complications among diabetic women: review 1965–1985. *Obstet Gynecol Surv* 1987; 42:140–9

26. Hou S. Chronic renal disease in pregnancy. In Decker BC, ed. *Current Therapy in Neonatal-Perinatal Medicine* Philadelphia: CV Mosley, 1990;2:41–7

27. Studd JW, Blainey JD. Pregnancy and the nephrotic syndrome. *Br Med J* 1969;1:276–80

28. Hemmelder MH, de Zeeuw D, Fidler V, *et al*. Proteinuria: a risk factor for pregnancy-related renal function decline in primary glomerular disease? *Am J Kidney Dis* 1995;26:187–92

29. Gabow PA, Johnson AM, Kaehny WD, *et al*. Factors affecting the progression of renal disease in autosomal-dominant polycystic kidney disease. *Kidney Int* 1992; 41:1311–19

30. Lindheimer MD, Davison JM, Renal biopsy during pregnancy: To b... or not to b...? *Br J Obstet Gynaecol* 1987;94:932–4

31. Krane NK. Acute renal failure in pregnancy. *Arch Intern Med* 1988;148:2347–57

32. Grunfeld JP, Pertuiset N. Acute renal failure in pregnancy: 1987. *Am J Kidney Dis* 1987;9:359–62

33. Stratta P, Canavese C, Dogliani M, *et al*. Pregnancy-related acute renal failure. *Clin Nephrol* 1989;32:14–20

34. Klein EA. Urologic problems of pregnancy. *Obstet Gynecol Surv* 1984;39:605–15

35. Lindheimer MD, Katz AI, Ganeval D, *et al*. Acute renal failure in pregnancy. In Brenner BM, Lazaras JM, eds. *Acute Renal Failure*, 2nd edn. New York, NY: Churchill Livingstone, 1987

36. Lindheimer MD, Katz AI, Ganeval D, *et al*. Acute renal failure in pregnancy. In Lazarus JM, Brenner BM, eds. *Acute Renal Failure*, 3rd edn. New York: Churchill Livingstone, 1993:417–33

37. Wang Y, Walsh SW, Guo J, *et al*. The imbalance between thromboxane and prostacyclin in pre-eclampsia is associated with an imbalance between lipid peroxides and vitamin E in maternal blood. *Am J Obstet Gynecol* 1991; 165:1695–700

38. Rodgers GM, Taylor RN, Roberts JM. Pre-eclampsia is associated with serum factor cytotoxic to human endothelial cells. *Am J Obstet Gynecol* 1988;159:908–14

39. Hubel CA, Roberts JM, Taylor RN, *et al*. Lipid peroxidation in pregnancy: new perspectives on pre-eclampsia. *Am J Obstet Gynecol* 1989;161:1024–34

40. Fisher KA, Luger H, Spargo BH, *et al*. Hypertension in pregnancy: clinical pathological correlations and remote prognosis. *Medicine* 1981;60:267–76

41. Kincaid-Smith P. The renal lesion of pre-eclampsia revisited. *Am J Kidney Dis* 1991;17:144–8

42. Burroughs AK, Seong NG, Dojcino DM, *et al*. Idiopathic acute fatty liver of pregnancy in 12 patients. *Q J Med* 1982;204:481–97

43. Davison JM. Dialysis, transplantation and pregnancy. *Am J Kidney Dis* 1991;17:127–32

44. Hou S. Peritoneal dialysis and hemodialysis in pregnancy. *Clin Obstet Gynaecol (Ballières)* 1987;1:1009–25

45. Kioko EM, Shaw KM, Clarke HD, *et al*. Successful pregnancy in a diabetic patient treated with continuous ambulatory peritoneal dialysis. *Diabetes Care* 1983;6: 298–300

46. Melendez R, Franquero C, Gill P, *et al*. Successful pregnancy with CAPD. American Nephrology Nurses Association *Journal* 1988;15:280–2

47. Hou S. Pregnancy in women requiring dialysis for renal failure. *Am J Kidney Dis* 1987;9:368–73

48. Davison JM, Dellagrammatikas H, Parkin JM. Maternal azathioprine therapy and depressed haemopoiesis in the babies of renal allograft patients. *Br J Obstet Gynaecol* 1985;92:233–9

49. Pizzento J, Aviles H, Noriega L, *et al*. Treatment of acute leukemia during pregnancy: presentation of nine cases. *Cancer Treat Rep* 1980;64:679–83

50. Tolchin SF, Winkelstein H, Rodnan GP, *et al*. Chromosome abnormalities from cyclophosphamide therapy in rheumatoid arthritis and progressive systemic sclerosis. *Arthritis Rheum* 1974;17:375–82

45

Rheumatological diseases and antiphospholipid syndrome

A.T. Masi, S.L. Feigenbaum and M.D. Lockshin

Rheumatic diseases and associated autoimmune phenomena occur frequently in women of childbearing age[1]. Many of these disorders occur in women who are pregnant or desire to become so. Problems of pregnancy are common and varied among these conditions[2–5]. Collectively, they may range from minor exacerbations of low back pain in women with HLA-B27-related spondyloarthropathy syndromes to life-threatening complications, e.g. progressive glomerulonephropathy, in patients with renal involvement from systemic lupus erythematosus (SLE) or systemic sclerosis (SSc), or to serious pregnancy-related thromboembolic events in patients with antiphospholipid (aPL) syndromes.

GENERAL CONSIDERATIONS

Strategies for managing some of these patients are controversial. Although all pregnancies in women with diffuse connective tissue disorders (CTD), e.g. SLE or SSc, should be considered high risk, little effect from pregnancy may occur in such patients with remitted or mild disease. The obstetrician and internist or rheumatologist team should construct a well-planned assessment and management strategy in anticipation of pregnancy. The plan should be aimed at:

(1) Surveillance for disease activity;
(2) Provision of fully adequate therapy for maternal disease; and
(3) Assessment of fetal growth and well-being.

Diligent search for indications of maternal or fetal compromise is required if prompt and effective therapy is to be provided.

Management decisions should consider both the effects of pregnancy on maternal disease and of the disease on the developing fetus. Active management of the pregnancy might include:

(1) Monitored progression to delivery[6];
(2) Interruption by early delivery and immediate specialized neonatal care[7]; or
(3) Therapeutic abortion, if maternal survival is jeopardized[8].

The optimal goal is to attain a healthy term outcome for both mother and baby.

RHEUMATOID ARTHRITIS (RA) AND PREGNANCY

Clinical profile of RA

Rheumatoid arthritis is a systemic inflammatory and often destructive, symmetrical, polyarticular disorder which primarily affects the smaller joints of hands and wrists as well as feet, rather than the larger proximal extremity joints or the spinal column[1]. The disease occurs at any age, but the incidence increases with aging[1,9]. The overall female to male (F : M) sex ratio is about 3 : 1, but is increased to 5 : 1 during the childbearing years[9]. Familial factors and HLA types, e.g. HLA-DR4/DR1, are believed to increase the risk of developing this disease[1]. Diagnosis is usually based upon the pattern of joint involvement, presence of rheumatoid factor and typical bony erosive changes on X-ray. Criteria sets for classification have been formulated[1].

Course of RA in pregnancy

A high proportion (75%) of RA patients substantially improve during pregnancy. Improvement starts during the first trimester[2,10–15]. After the end of the pregnancy, the disease exacerbates within several weeks to months to the pre-pregnancy status[2,10]. Extension of the pregnancy-amelioration effect into the postpartum period may occur and be related to breast-feeding[10]. However, this question is unsettled[15]. One report indicates that RA is more likely to develop within 1 year following a first pregnancy, if breast-feeding occurred[15]. About a quarter of patients do not improve or worsen during the course of pregnancy[2]. Patterns of improvement or non-improvement in individuals tend to recur with subsequent pregnancies[2,13]. An increased onset frequency of RA, within 6[11] or 12[15,16] months postpartum, has been reported. The effects of pregnancy on RA and on autoimmune disorders has been recently reviewed[17].

Theories of pregnancy-amelioration of RA

Multiple hypotheses have been advanced to explain gestational improvement in RA[10–15,17–20]. Pregnancy-induced generalized immunosuppression[13] does not explain why gestation might dramatically improve RA[2,10–15,21], but not ankylosing spondylitis[21], SLE[5,17] or other CTD (*vide infra*). Uniform or marked depression of humoral immunity is not evident during pregnancy[13]. However, cell-mediated immunity (CMI) is depressed in the mother[13,17]. Pregnancy increases susceptibility, recurrence, or virulence of certain infections[22]. Depression of CMI may be due to decreased levels of T-helper cells[23] or to effects of immunosuppressive mediators[13]. A down-regulation of T-helper 1 (T_H1) cytokines by T-helper 2 (T_H2) cytokines[24], as well as suppression of polymorphonuclear[25,26] and macrophage[27] functions, have been reported in pregnancy. An interaction of these mechanisms with hormone-mediated immunomodulatory processes[28–30] may contribute collectively to CMI depression in pregnancy.

Pregnancy-associated α2-glycoprotein (PAG) synthesis by mononuclear leukocytes in the maternal decidua was inversely correlated with RA activity during pregnancy in one study[31], but not in another[32]. Increased disease activity in the puerperium correlated with a postpartum decline in PAG and a rise in immunoglobulin M (IgM) rheumatoid factor (RF) titer[33].

Elevated serum free cortisol[19] and reproductive steroid hormone[20,28–30] levels may also ameliorate RA. However, oral contraceptives (estrogen–progestogen) do not seem to affect the risk of developing RA[34,35]. Maternal–fetal disparities for HLA class II antigens occurred significantly ($p = 0.003$) more frequently in pregnancies in which RA remitted or improved [26 of 34 (76%)] compared to pregnancies in which RA remained active [3 of 12 (25%)][14]. The basis for such an effect is unknown. It may be due to immunological[14,36], hormonal[28–30], or other mechanisms.

Effects of RA on fertility

Whether RA influences biological fertility is unknown[37]. Women with RA have lessened sexual desire and a substantial reduction of coital frequency after onset of disease[38]. Decreased fecundity occurs long before the onset of RA[39]. Subfertility, both before and after development of RA[40], may be related to lessened frequency of intercourse. Constitutionally lower androgenicity may contribute to both RA[9,30,41,42] and decreased sexual activity[42].

Fetal outcome in RA patients

Increased fetal morbidity or mortality is not generally observed in RA[2,13]. However, few data are available on women with severe disease, especially those with systemic manifestations.

Effects of pregnancy on risk of developing RA

A question has been raised whether pregnancy[43] or breast-feeding[15] are risk factors for developing RA. There is an association of multiparity, particularly more than four childbirths, and either RA[44] or more severe disease[2]. Maternal serum dehydroepiandrosterone sulfate (DHEAS) decreases significantly after a first pregnancy for at least 12 years[45]. This long-term decrease in a maternal androgen may affect risk of subsequently developing RA[9,30,41,42].

Familial predisposition to RA and counseling

Although the overall chances that a person with a positive family history will develop RA are rather low, genetic factors contribute to its risk[1,46–48]. Susceptibilities are increased in individuals with HLA-DR4 or -DR1[46–48], particularly HLA DRB1 *0401/0404 (QKRAA and QRRAA)[48]. However, HLA testing is not recommended for counseling on such risk issues.

Effects of antirheumatic medications on the fetus and pregnancy

Major concerns are the effects of antirheumatic medications on the fetus and on pregnancy outcome[2–5,8,37,49–51]. When needed, anti-inflammatory agents should be administered in the lowest possible dosages[2–5,13,51]. Actively inflamed joints may be treated effectively with local intra-articular depocorticosteroids at essentially no maternal or fetal risk. Acetaminophen may be used if necessary.

Many mild cases of RA improve during the course of pregnancy[2,10–15,21]. Stopping all systemic medication, including salicylates and non-steroidal anti-inflammatory drugs (NSAID) is optimal[51], but often not practical. For those who do not improve, appropriate treatment should be given, with due considerations of risks and benefits[2–5,18,49–51].

Salicylates and NSAID

Aspirin crosses the placenta. When used at anti-inflammatory dosage, aspirin can reach significant concentrations in the fetus[49]. Low doses, e.g. 60–80 mg of aspirin daily, given not as treatment for RA but to prevent pre-eclampsia, selectively inhibit maternal platelet cyclo-oxygenase without affecting neonatal platelet aggregation or the pulmonary circulation[52]. Low-dose aspirin significantly decreases production of thromboxane, but not prostacyclin, in human placental arteries *in vitro*[53].

Whether first-trimester aspirin use can cause fetal malformations is generally but not universally believed to be of low-risk potential[50,51,54–57]. A large-scale, case–control study suggests no association of aspirin with an increased risk of cardiac defects[57].

High-dose aspirin, administered within the 8 weeks prior to expected delivery, has potential effects on: prolonging labor; enhancing maternal and fetal bleeding tendencies; premature closure of the ductus, and other side-effects[49,51,56]. The US Food and Drug Administration issued a warning label on such risks[58]. There are similar concerns about use of NSAID[13,49–51,56]. Because of greater experience with aspirin[51,54–56], it may be preferred to NSAID for anti-inflammatory therapy in pregnancy. If possible, it is best to stop these drugs at least 2 weeks[58] to 2 months[51] before delivery.

Glucocorticoids

The placental enzyme, ll-β-hydroxysteroid dehydrogenase, inactivates cortisol, prednisone and certain other corticosteroid analogs, allowing relative protection of the fetus[59]. Prednisone in low oral dosage appears to be safe in pregnancy[4,13,18,51,56,59]. Dexamethasone is not effectively inactivated by the placenta[59] and should not be used for treatment of RA in the pregnant woman.

Slow acting antirheumatic drugs (SAARD)

Sulfasalazine   The combined molecule of sulfapyridine and 5-aminosalicylic acid (mesalamine), sulfasalazine is an effective agent in the treatment of RA[60]. It has low potential to cause teratogenic effects; it may have advantages as a SAARD in pregnant women[60].

Antimalarial drugs   Chloroquine phosphate or hydroxychloroquine sulfate cross the placental barrier and deposit in fetal tissue such as the uveal tract[56,61]. Early intrauterine exposure to these agents may not cause congenital abnormalities or clinical visual loss[62]. Nerve deafness has been reported in children exposed to chloroquine phosphate during pregnancy[63]. Because of slow excretion, it is prudent to discontinue antimalarial drugs 3–6 months before conception as well as during pregnancy and lactation[56], if possible.

D-penicillamine   This drug traverses the placental barrier and can probably decrease molecular cross-linking of collagen in the fetus. Two reports describe congenital cutis laxa and associated connective tissue birth defects, probably due to D-penicillamine treatment during pregnancy[64,65]. Discontinuation of this drug is recommended in RA prior to conception as well as during pregnancy and lactation[56,66].

Gold compounds   Therapy with intramuscular gold salts or the oral gold compound, auranofin, have not been well studied in humans[2,56]. It is not known if there is an increased risk of teratogenicity. Gold transfers across the placenta[56] and corneal deposits may occur[67]. Excretion is very slow. It is generally not recommended

to initiate or continue gold therapy for RA during pregnancy or lactation[2,56]. Sulfasalazine may be a better choice[60]. If patients have been treated within a year of pregnancy, some exposure of the fetus is likely. Optimally, these agents should be stopped 3–6 months before conception in order to minimize fetal exposure to these drugs.

Cytotoxic agents   Although congenital abnormalities have been reported to occur in association with use of cytotoxic agents, such as azathioprine (and its more active metabolite, 6-mercaptopurine), methotrexate, and cyclophosphamide or chlorambucil[2,4,56,59,68], solid evidence linking congenital abnormalities to azathioprine does not exist[51,59,68]. Chlorambucil and methotrexate are abortifacients[59]. Methotrexate and misoprostol are used to terminate early pregnancy[69].

Unless these drugs are absolutely medically necessary, it is prudent to avoid or discontinue their use prior to conception and during pregnancy, especially in the first trimester, as well as during lactation[51,59,68]. Increased dosage of glucocorticoids may be needed in their place. Therapeutic termination should be considered if there has been fetal exposure to methotrexate or alkylating agents.

Drugs during lactation (reviewed in ref. 68)   Effects of NSAID on the infant are generally unknown. Aspirin is generally considered safe for nursing mothers. However, the American Academy of Pediatrics recommends that aspirin should be used cautiously by the mother during lactation because of potential adverse effects in the nursing infant[68]. Breast-feeding considerations of glucocorticoid therapy are mentioned under SLE. The SAARD and particularly cytotoxic agents are not recommended during lactation[49,59,68].

ANKYLOSING SPONDYLITIS (AS) AND PREGNANCY

Clinical profile of AS

Ankylosing spondylitis, like Reiter's syndrome and other spondyloarthropathies, is significantly associated with the cell surface marker, HLA-B27[1]. Unlike RA[1,9], AS occurs predominantly in males and has disease onset mainly during adolescence or early adulthood[1,70]. It affects mainly the spine, sacroiliac and large proximal girdle joints and has more limited internal organ and systemic involvement than does RA. Pain and restricted motion of the spine and hips are typical of AS, rather than inflammatory, erosive involvement of small joints, as seen in RA[1]. Prevalence among Scandinavian women may be as high as 0.3%[71], but varies with the frequency of HLA-B27 in the population[1,70]. The condition is believed to be milder in women than men[70–74], at least radiographically[75]. Fertility is not adversely affected by AS[21,76,77].

Course of AS during pregnancy

Pregnancy does not improve manifestations of AS[21,76–78]. In a prospective study, only six of 22 women (27 pregnancies) with mild AS (radiographic sacroiliitis, but without spinal ankylosing deformity) improved during pregnancy[77]. All six had AS associated with ulcerative colitis or psoriasis[77], i.e. 'secondary' AS, rather than 'primary' or 'idiopathic' disease[1]. The 16 patients with 'primary' AS had persisting symptoms and required NSAID through pregnancy[77].

Ankylosing spondylitis during pregnancy usually manifests as chronic low back or sacroiliac area pain. Anterior uveitis, cervical spine, symphysis pubis, or peripheral arthritis manifestations may be present[75–78]. Available data suggest that AS does not adversely affect pregnancy[21,76,77]. Mechanical hindrance to normal vaginal delivery is also rare, even in women with advanced disease[77]. Postpartum flare of AS may occur during the first 6 months after delivery in about 50% of cases[21,77,78]; it causes no substantial change in the overall course of disease.

Management of women with AS

Worsening of spinal symptoms or peripheral arthritis during pregnancy may require additional rest, physical therapy[77,79], or use of NSAID[51,80]. The lowest effective dose is advised for limited periods of time, until the last month of pregnancy[51,77,80]. As delivery approaches, acetaminophen may be used[80].

Reiter's syndrome and other HLA-B27-related seronegative spondyloarthropathy disorders are less common than AS[1] but are similar to AS with regard to pregnancy issues.

SYSTEMIC LUPUS ERYTHEMATOSUS (SLE) AND PREGNANCY

Clinical profile of SLE

Systemic lupus erythematosus (SLE or lupus) is distinguished from other diffuse CTD by its characteristic multiple organ system and serological abnormalities[1,5,37]. Erythematosus malar rash, discoid skin lesions, photosensitivity and painless oral or nasopharyngeal ulcers are characteristic mucocutaneous features. The arthritis of SLE is non-erosive, but may show deformities, such as ulnar deviation of the fingers. Pleuritis, pericarditis, renal (proteinuria or cellular casts), neurologic (seizures or psychosis) and hematologic (hemolytic anemia, leukopenia or thrombopenia) abnormalities are also clinically typical of SLE and contribute to its classification criteria[1].

Lupus predominantly affects younger adult women, having an F : M sex ratio in the child-bearing ages of about 8 : 1; the disease is more common in non-Caucasians[1]. The clinical presentation, degree of severity cind course of disease are all highly variable[5].

Diagnosis depends upon characteristic clinical manifestations together with confirmation by typical laboratory abnormalities[1–5,37]. The antinuclear antibody (ANA) test is positive in essentially all SLE patients. However, it also occurs frequently in other CTD. The ANA has greater diagnostic import when either absent (tending to exclude SLE) or when present in high titers, especially with homogeneous or peripheral-staining nuclear patterns (typical of SLE). An isolated low titer ANA lacks association with SLE or adverse pregnancy outcome, compared with high titer ANA or the more specific antibodies which correlate with this disorder. Specific and confirmatory immunological abnormalities of SLE include anti-native (double-stranded) DNA or anti-Sm antibody. Positive lupus erythematosus (LE) cell preparation or chronic (at least 6 months) biologic false-positive test for syphilis support, but are not specific for SLE[1]. The LE test is rarely done today.

Course of SLE in pregnancy

Few data are available on the untreated course of SLE in pregnancy on the mother[81,82] or fetus[81,83]. Some early and recent reviews state that pregnancy exacerbates disease in up to one-third or more of patients[2–5,81,82]. A recent British study estimated that the rate of lupus flares during pregnancy, especially in the second and third trimesters and during the puerperium, was about twice the control experience[84]. Investigators from Johns Hopkins[85] found an annual frequency of flares per lupus patient of 1.6 during pregnancy versus 0.64 after delivery and 0.65 among non-pregnant women. A flare occurred in 24 (60%) of 40 completed pregnancies. Renal involvement was twice as common in the flares of pregnant (43%) than non-pregnant (22%) lupus patients[85].

Other studies state that pregnancy may not increase the risk of lupus flares in the inactive or well-controlled patient[5,86–93]. The frequency of flares may not be greater during pregnancy in the well-controlled lupus patient than in the non-pregnant state[5,92,93]. Differences in patient populations and criteria (for patient entry and flares) may account for different conclusions. Whether pregnancy predisposes to flare of lupus is unknown[5,84,85,92,93].

In controlled experience from New York City[87,88], flares occurred in 13–25% (conservative and liberal definitions) of 80 pregnant SLE patients. With inactive SLE at onset of gestation, flares tend to be mild and occur about equally in each trimester and postpartum[2,91].

Mucocutaneous involvement, synovitis or hematological abnormalities are the most common clinical features seen during flares[2,89]. However, nephritis[85,89] and central nervous system deficits[5,84,93] can also occur and be more serious for both mother and fetus. In retrospective analysis of 213 pregnancies among 73 SLE patients, observed from 1962 to 1985, severe renal flares occurred in six patients, five with active disease at conception[89]. The severity of flares during pregnancy does not seem different from those in the general lupus patient population[2,86], except for the possibility of increased risk of renal flares[85]. Overall prognosis for maternal survival of carefully managed SLE patients is now considered to be excellent, especially if disease is inactive at the onset of pregnancy[2,86,91].

Although apparent, activity of SLE at onset of gestation is related to its subsequent course[89] and provides a rational basis for preconception counseling. The managing internist and obstetrician team can emphasize contraception and preconception disease control measures, as appropriate.

Fetal outcome in SLE patients

Fetal loss and prematurity are increased in SLE[2-5,81,83]. The fetus, not the mother, has the greater risk of death in SLE pregnancies.

Reported frequencies

Heterogeneity among patients hinders precise prediction about fetal outcome in SLE patients[2-5,81,83]. SLE patients have a higher prevalence of spontaneous abortions and stillborns, ranging from 10% to 41%[2-5,81,83], than normal women. In a retrospective review of fetal wastage reported from 1950 to 1980[2], the level remained constant at 27–28%. Maternal mortality and perinatal deaths decreased from 5.4% in 1950–1959 reports to essentially none in 1970–1980 reports[2].

At least two schools of thought exist on predictive factors for adverse outcome of pregnancy in lupus. One school believes that adverse fetal outcome may be anticipated in patients with new onset SLE during pregnancy (or postpartum) and in those with active disease or nephritis[4] (reviewed in refs. 82, 83). Another school believes that severity or activity of maternal disease has little influence on fetal outcome, provided that the mother is well enough to maintain pregnancy[5,86,93]. Most American physicians do not believe that routine 'prophylactic' steroid therapy to suppress disease activity during pregnancy reduces risk for maternal flare or decreases fetal wastage.

In the Mexico City study of 102 prophylactically treated pregnancies[86], active and inactive SLE patients had similar spontaneous abortion rates. Prematurity occurred in 58.8% of deliveries and was more frequent in patients with clinically active disease. Among term deliveries in SLE patients, an excess frequency of small for gestational age (SGA) infants and those with features of symmetric and asymmetric intrauterine growth restriction (IUGR) occurred[86]. High rates of Cesarean section are attributable to fetal distress.

Placental insufficiency hypothesis for fetal problems in SLE

Excess early fetal deaths in SLE pregnancies are associated with persistently positive, high-titer IgG anticardiolipin (aCL) antibody[94-96] as well as an obstetrical history of at least two previously unexplained pregnancy failures[94-96].

Decidual vasculopathy with necrotizing inflammatory lesions and 'acute atherosis' occurs in placentas from lupus patients[97,98] as well as those with the aPL syndrome[98,99], whether the pregnancies resulted in fetal deaths[98] or in liveborn SGA infants[100]. Placental size is reduced in SLE patients compared to both healthy and diabetic controls[101]. Most later pregnancy losses may be attributable to placental dysfunction[97-99,101].

Disordered placental endothelial cell and microvascular function, including villous infarction, results in 'decidual or placental insufficiency'. Placental insufficiency may contribute to fetal growth restriction[100] and to fetal compromise in SLE[97-99,101]. The 'placental insufficiency' concept provides a rationale for active fetal surveillance, starting in the late second trimester[6,7]. Other experimental evidence suggests that IgG fractions from lupus subjects can be toxic to whole rat embryos[102].

Neonatal lupus syndrome and congenital heart block

Neonatal lupus (transient hematologic and cutaneous disorders; permanent incomplete or complete congenital heart block) occurs rarely in the offspring of SLE patients[4,5,83,103-105]. Heart block is estimated to occur in less than 1% of infants of lupus mothers[4,83]. In one prospective study of sequential pregnancies, none of 38 infants of lupus mothers with anti-SSA (Ro) (i.e. Sjögren's syndrome A) antibody had children with heart block[105]. Most infants with this syndrome are born to asymptomatic mothers[106,107]. A few may develop a lupus-like disorder at a later time[104,106,107]. Neonatal lupus occurs only in pregnancies associated with maternal SSA/Ro or SSB/La (i.e. Sjögren's syndrome B) antibodies[106], which occur in 25–32% of SLE pregnancies[105].

Congenital complete heart block (CCHB)

This rare, potentially fatal complication[103-108] is more problematic than the non-cardiac transient abnormalities in the neonatal lupus syndrome. The CCHB is associated with myocarditis and with simultaneously present maternal anti-Ro (SSA) and anti-La (SSB) antibodies[103-108]. If cardiac conduction defects are detected by antepartum fetal heart rate monitoring, a fetal echocardiogram should be obtained for detection of other cardiac anomalies[103-105,109]. Appropriate fetal monitoring and management procedures should be employed[109].

Effects of SLE on fertility

Fertility is not impaired in women with SLE[81,108], except in those with severe renal disease[4,82] or those exposed to cyclophosphamide or chlorambucil.

Management of pregnant women with SLE

Careful monitoring

A team approach and individualized management are optimal. On diagnosis of pregnancy, the following maternal studies should be obtained: complete blood count including platelet count, blood urea nitrogen, creatinine and uric acid, complement 3, complement 4, anti-dsDNA, aCL antibodies, lupus anticoagulant (LAC), anti-SSA(Ro) and anti-SSB(LA), 24-h urine protein, creatinine clearance and microscopic urinalysis. The complete blood count, complement 3, anti-dsDNA, creatinine clearance and urinalysis should be repeated at 1–2 month intervals, as appropriate, during pregnancy and for 3 months postpartum. Anticardiolipin antibody should be retested, if initially negative, each trimester. Both clinical and laboratory indicators of disease activity are used to distinguish kidney involvement from superimposed pre-eclampsia. This approach emphasizes early detection and aggressive management of lupus activity. Determination of lupus activity during pregnancy can be complex[88].

Maternal effects of steroid administration

Prednisone is the first-line and the mainstay of therapy in pregnant patients with active SLE[5,81,82,84–90]. Osteoporosis can be an important adverse effect of prednisone treatment. Gastrointestinal side-effects and gestational diabetes are further risks when steroids are administered to pregnant patients.

Additional parenteral hydrocortisone or methylprednisolone should be administered to cover the physiological stresses during labor, delivery and the immediate postpartum period[89]. Parenteral administration should continue in the recovering Cesarean section patient until oral medication can be taken. Breast-feeding considerations are mentioned below.

Fetal complications from prednisone

Rare fetal complications have been attributed to prednisone or prednisolone therapy[55,56,59,86]. However, risk is low, and inadequately controlled disease is a greater risk. Fetal concentrations of methylprednisolone are 10% of maternal blood levels[110]. Insignificant levels of prednisone metabolites are found in the fetal circulation[59,110]. Rarely does fetal adrenal hypoplasia occur following long-term maternal corticosteroid use during gestation[111]. Dexamethasone is only partially metabolized by the placenta, in contrast to analogs of naturally occurring glucocorticoids[59], and its concentration is equal in the fetal and maternal circulations[59,86]. Therefore, treatment of SLE with dexamethasone is not recommended during pregnancy[83,86].

Cytotoxic agents

Ordinarily, cytotoxic agents are withheld during pregnancy, unless high-dose glucocorticoids do not control active disease[5,56,59,82]. Under such circumstances, addition of cytotoxic drugs is usually delayed until after the first trimester[2]. When informed risk–benefit analysis warrants cytotoxic drug use, normal pregnancies have resulted after both azathioprine and cyclophosphamide administration[59]. However, one azathioprine-treated infant showed immunosuppression; the mother also received 30 mg prednisone daily throughout pregnancy[112]. Some pregnancies have been associated with fetal growth retardation[113].

Renal considerations

Because renal involvement is a common, potentially life-threatening manifestation of SLE, particular attention must be paid to controlling such activity in pregnant women[5,82,85,89,90].

Among 102 pregnancies reported in the Mexico City study[86], renal disease developed *de novo* during three (6.8%) of the 44 gestations in which kidney disease was not previously present and worsened in six (10.3%) of the 58 pregnancies in which kidney disease was previously known. Exacerbations developed after 2–5 years inactivity of renal involvement prior to gestation. All nine episodes of kidney disease in pregnancy were controlled with prednisone therapy within several months.

Similar data were reported by a large Paris nephrology referral group[89]. In 35 women with previously diagnosed SLE, severe renal flares occurred during or following pregnancy in six (11%) of 53 gestations, including one in a patient who was in remission at conception. Corticosteroid therapy failed to reverse renal failure in four patients. In 14 women who first developed SLE during pregnancy, the postpartum, or post-abortum period, high-dose corticosteroids improved lupus nephritis in all but one, including two with renal failure. However, one woman progressed to renal failure within 3 years. These authors concluded that in patients with severe, pre-existing nephritis, the course of lupus nephropathy cannot be accurately predicted, even considering the remission or activity status at conception[89].

No patient received cytotoxic drugs during gestation in either the series from Mexico City[86] or that from Paris[89]. However, such therapy may rarely be required if a severe renal flare fails to respond to high-dose prednisone.

Pre-eclampsia or lupus flare?

In pregnant SLE patients, a difficult challenge is to determine whether the development of new or increasing proteinuria and hypertension might be due to either pre-eclampsia or a lupus flare[2,4,5,93]. The former complication requires aggressive management of fluid volume and hypertension, without excessive glucocorticosteroids. In contrast, prednisone is the mainstay of therapy, plus supportive management, for active lupus. Antecedent decreases in glucocorticoids or hydroxychloroquine sulfate[114] may suggest a lupus flare.

Changes that may reflect SLE activity rather than pre-eclampsia include synovitis, fever, pleuritis, lymphadenopathy active urinary sediment, decreasing serum complement, and increasing anti-dsDNA[5,86–88]. Authors disagree whether decreases in serum complement alone do[115] or do not[88] predict flare. Microscopic urine findings of significant hematuria and cellular casts as well as clinical findings of extrarenal disease can help distinguish between lupus flare[5,87,88] and pre-eclampsia.

A mild normocytic anemia is non-specific and not necessarily suggestive of a lupus flare. Pre-eclampsia may be associated with a gradually increasing hematocrit, secondary to a reduction in plasma volume. Proteinuria, low serum complement, increased serum uric acid, elevated liver enzymes and thrombocytopenia may occur in both SLE and pre-eclampsia[5,88].

Currently, scant data exist in SLE patients followed prospectively to determine confidently those variables which predict a flare or distinguish between lupus nephritis and pre-eclampsia.

Lupus brain involvement This is usually preceded by deteriorating and labile mental function; anticonvulsant therapy may be necessary. Magnesium sulfate, the treatment for both prevention of seizures and for seizure activity in association with eclampsia, has been often given but not formally studied in lupus patients.

Treatment of acute hypertension Doppler studies of umbilical blood flow may be required to evaluate safe maternal blood pressures and to maintain adequate uteroplacental perfusion. Angiotensin-converting enzyme (ACE) inhibitors, when used in the second and third trimesters of pregnancy, can cause injury and even death to the developing fetus (FDA Mailgram, March 1992). Some beta-blockers may depress fetal reflexes. Calcium-channel blockers and hydralazine may be used in pregnancy[68].

Fetal risks and surveillance

Fetal surveillance This is mandatory[2,5,7,83,93] and should be instituted early and continuously[6,7]. The presence of high-titer IgG aCL antibodies[94,98], especially in the setting of prior unexplained pregnancy losses[95,96], appears to be most important for identifying patients at risk for mid-trimester fetal deaths. Active lupus and corticosteroid therapy are risk factors for premature delivery[2,86]. Antiphospholipid antibody and active SLE may affect the fetus[94–96,98] through placental abnormalities[97–101], as indicated above.

Presence of nephropathy This did not significantly alter fetal outcome overall among patients in the Mexico City study[86]. Spontaneous abortions were somewhat higher among those with (20.6%) than without (11.3%) renal involvement.

Ultrasound studies These should include first-trimester confirmation of menstrual dates, serial fetal growth measurements, including growth-adjusted sonographic age, and a mid-gestational study for detection of cardiac anomalies. Should IUGR be detected, appropriate surveillance should be initiated[6,7].

Fetal heart rate monitoring It is recommended that monitoring, with non-stress tests, be started as early as 25 weeks, with follow-up of abnormalities by contraction stress test or biophysical profile. In centers that start antepartum fetal heart rate testing at 25 weeks, several infants have been delivered before 30 weeks. IUGR, decreasing amniotic fluid and abnormal fetal heart rate patterns are ominous and may mandate both aggressive treatment of the mother and preparation for emergency delivery[7]. Second-trimester occurrence of non-periodic decelerations and fetal bradycardia suggest impending fetal death[7]. Infants delivered after 29 weeks and weighing more than 1500 g generally do well in experienced nurseries equipped for care of premature deliveries.

Route and timing of delivery For SLE patients these should be based upon results of fetal studies with attention to the maternal condition, especially renal and blood pressure status. The need for neonatologist attendance should be determined prior to labor by both maternal and fetal status. If necessary, transport may be arranged to a facility equipped for care of complicated premature infants.

Breast-feeding and antirheumatic drug therapy

A paucity of good data on guidelines for anti-rheumatic drug therapy during breast-feeding are available[49,59,80,83,116,117] (reviewed in ref. 68). SLE patients on steroids, particularly 30 mg or greater, should consider refraining from breast-feeding, if they can produce milk at all.

The American Academy of Pediatrics considers prednisone and prednisolone therapy compatible with breast-feeding[117]. Potential exists for active steroids to be secreted into breast milk. However, at 80 mg/day maternal consumption of prednisolone, the infant would ingest < 0.1% of the dose which would correspond to < 10% of the infant's endogenous cortisol production[116]. The infant's exposure can be reduced by avoiding nursing during the first 2[116] to 4[59] hours after the steroid dose. Lactating mothers should avoid alkylating agents, as well as methotrexate, if at all possible[59,68,117].

ANTIPHOSPHOLIPID (APL) ANTIBODIES AND SYNDROMES

Definition of aPL syndrome

Antibodies to anionic (negatively charged) phospholipids are associated with recurrent, usually midtrimester, spontaneous abortions, 'autoimmune' thrombocytopenia, arterial and deep venous thromboses, and livedo reticularis[118–123]. The definition of recurrent miscarriage has varied in the literature, with implications as to prognosis of the untreated pregnancy. The standard obstetrical definition is three or more consecutive losses. However, the definition used for most rheumatologic patients has been two or more losses (sometimes even one). Incidence of pregnancy loss increases with greater number of preceding miscarriages, which has implications in evaluating efficacy of one or another therapeutic approach.

Laboratory tests

The aPL antibodies may vary in titer over the course of follow-up. Lupus anticoagulants (LAC)[124,125] are antibodies that interfere with phospholipid-dependent coagulation reactions *in vitro*. [The Venereal Disease Research Laboratories test (VDRL) may be falsely positive in the aPL syndromes, but the fluorescent treponemal antibody (FTA) test is negative[126]. It is not a reliable indicator of clinically important aPL syndrome.]

The anticardiolipin (aCL) test[119,120] uses the enzyme-linked immunosorbent assay method to determine IgG, IgM and IgA reactivity to chemically pure cardiolipin, a phospholipid. The aPL antibodies are heterogeneous and polyclonal. The 'pathogenic' antibodies are directed against a complex antigen that includes a lipid-binding inhibitor of coagulation, apolipoprotein H or β_2-glycoprotein I[127], which binds to cardiolipin and other negatively charged phospholipids. The exact relationship among these antibody systems and their association with clinical aPL syndromes is complex and evolving[120–125]. Both LAC and high titer IgG aCL do appear to predict fetal compromise[94–96,123–125], with or without an association to lupus.

Primary and secondary aPL syndromes

Antiphospholipid antibodies without clinical symptoms may be found in otherwise healthy persons[121]. Persons with symptoms who do not have SLE or previously recognized clinical disorders are designated as 'primary' aPL syndrome[128]. Persons with SLE or other rheumatic disorders[120–123,129] are designated as 'secondary' aPL syndrome. In lupus, aPL syndrome seems to be part of the disease, rather than a separate, associated condition[129], but it does seem to correlate with increased fetal loss[94–96,98]. There may be a negative correlation of aPL antibodies with active lupus[98], nephrotic syndrome and certain cutaneous forms of lupus[129]. Secondary (lupus) and primary aPL syndrome patients have similar overall clinical and laboratory profiles[130]. Lupus patients have more hemolytic anemia, endocardial valve disease, neutropenia and low C4 levels[130].

In pregnancy, lupus and aPL syndrome are independent. A patient with remitted lupus and secondary aPL syndrome behaves like one with primary aPL syndrome. A patient with active lupus and aPL syndrome develops complications of, and needs treatment for, both diseases.

Are aPL antibodies etiologic factors or disease markers?

Complex relationships

The *in vitro* antibody assay systems are complex and their relationships to the different clinical manifestations are incompletely understood[120–125,128–134]. The assays vary considerably in sensitivity, specificity and repeatability[135,136]. Furthermore, titers may vary with activity of disease, as in SLE[129], or over the course of pregnancy[132]. Clinical correlations are influenced by the specific testing system[120,121,125,126,134,135], the degree of titer elevation (compared to the normal range)[94,119,120,132], and immunoglobulin type of the antibody[119,120,122]. Recent studies of monoclonal antibodies derived from patients with aPL syndromes demonstrate that 'antiphospholipid' antibody is actually an antibody to a phospholipid-binding protein, β_2-glycoprotein I (β_2GPI), while infection (syphilis)-induced aPL is directed against a lipid antigen[127,133]. The β_2-GPI-dependent aCL antibody, but not β_2-GPI-independent aCL antibodies, correlated with adverse pregnancy outcomes in healthy pregnant women[134].

Significant interlaboratory variation exists in aPL measurements, and particularly aCL testing[135,136], which might lead to unnecessary therapeutic interventions. The test should be repeated several times before a clear diagnosis is made. In the future, differentiation of β_2-GPI-dependent from β_2-GPI-independent aCL antibodies will improve this assay. Some patients appear to have antibody directed against β_2-GPI (or other phospholipid-binding protein) that is not identified in the standard aPL assay. It requires research laboratory technology to identify the abnormality in these patients.

Experimental studies

The LAC behaves as an anticoagulant *in vitro*, by virtue of its inhibition of procoagulant phospholipid-containing factors[124,125]. However, *in vivo*, it is associated with procoagulation states[118,120,125,137,138]. Perturbations of membranes of circulating platelets[131] or vascular endothelial cells[139] may contribute to either aPL antibody formation[125,127,131,140–144] or thrombosis[137,138,145–148]. LAC and aPL antibodies from SLE patients do not react with intact platelets, but do react with freeze-thawed or activated platelets[125,131], suggesting exposure of hidden antigenic sites.

The aPL antibodies have been demonstrated in[149] and eluted from[150] affected maternal placentas. Also, IgG fractions from sera of lupus patients induced fetal resorptions in experimental mice[102]. However, aPL antibodies may not be 'pathogenic' *per se*, but may result secondarily from an immunological reaction to otherwise-damaged membranes of platelets[131,147,148], apoptotic cells[145], abnormal placental vessels[97–101,118,124], or other endothelial cell damage[139,141,142,144]. Under this hypothesis, aPL antibodies would be markers of platelet activation[131,146–148] and thrombosis, as well as of placental insufficiency leading to fetal loss[97–99,101,118,124] or IUGR[100]. Alternatively, aPL antibodies may act as 'pathogenic' procoagulant factors[120,140,143,151,152].

Anticoagulant therapy for recurrent fetal loss

On the assumption that aPL either contribute to or correlate with procoagulant states[137,138,151,152], low-dose aspirin has been used as a treatment[153–158]. It may be administered either alone[154,158], for women considered to be at low risk for fetal loss, or in conjunction with heparin[155–157]. Subcutaneous heparin plus aspirin is the preferred treatment for women with three recurrent fetal losses and high antibody titers[155–157]. Although formal dosing studies remain to be done, most authorities begin treatment with 5000–10 000 units twice daily, and adjust dose up to 1.5 times the baseline activated partial thromboplastin time (aPTT) at 6 hours after injection (in patients whose baseline aPTT is normal)[155]. In a recent study[156], equally good outcomes were obtained when the aPTT was kept within the high normal range (low-dose heparin) as when the higher dose was used[155].

Do aPL antibodies predispose to fetal wastage?

A literature review concluded that the available data support an association between the prevalence of aPL antibodies in women with SLE and history of fetal loss (60%), but are inconclusive in women without SLE (4–13% losses)[121]. Most studies do find an association between high-level aPL antibodies and repeated, but not a first, fetal loss[5,94–96,123–125]. In one study, aCL titers remained high in the aborting patients[159], which is a commnon finding[94,119,160]. Antiphospholipid antibodies have been detected in 5–15% of otherwise healthy women with a history of unexplained recurrent abortions[121].

Frequencies of aCL antibodies are low (< 5%) in consecutive samples of healthy pregnant women without prior pregnancy losses; and there is no significant correlation with fetal or maternal complications[161]. Moderate to high levels of aCL antibodies, of the IgG isotype, do correlate with fetal wastage, in referral, high-risk[94,119] and general obstetric[160,162] populations.

Antibodies to β_2-GPI–CL complex were significantly associated with fetal complications in a large cohort of apparently healthy pregnant women followed prospectively in Japan[134]. It is not known if women with positive titers have other primary risk factors for increased fetal wastage, for instance, clinically inactive lupus[97–99,101,124].

To complicate further the interpretation of fetal relationships with aPL antibodies[160,162–167], women with aCL antibodies and a history of fetal loss may have antitrophoblast antibodies, which may be serologically distinct from the aCL system and may contribute to fetal loss[168].

Fetal complications reported with aPL antibodies

Recurrent fetal losses due to intrauterine death at any stage of pregnancy, but particularly in the second and third trimesters of gestation, and fetal growth restriction, are characteristic complications associated with aPL antibodies[160,162–166]. Recurrent, late first-trimester fetal loss after detection of fetal heart activity has also been associated with aPL antibodies[167]. No fetal pathology explains the spontaneous abortions and stillbirths. Instead, the placentas invariably show scattered areas of infarction, intervillous thrombosis and fibrin deposition[97–101,163].

Few published data are available on the aPL antibody status of live-born infants of mothers positive for these antibodies. Most of those in whom antibody can be detected are normal. A 1000 g female infant was reported[169] who was delivered at 24 weeks by Cesarean section because of spontaneous abnormal fetal heart rate patterns. She was found to be positive for LAC and subsequently developed neonatal aortic thrombosis. Other unusual problems reported in infants of mothers with aPL antibodies include protracted adrenal insufficiency, frontal lobe hypoplasia and delayed neuromuscular development[165]. It is not known if some of these disorders can be attributed to high dosages of corticosteroid therapy used in the mother during pregnancy. Most live-born infants are well except for the effects of prematurity and IUGR.

Maternal complications reported with aPL syndromes

Over half of women presenting with such aPL syndrome obstetrical problems have not had prior recognized autoimmune disease[124]; some do go on to develop SLE, but more experience thrombotic vascular complications of aPL syndrome[130,166]. Maternal complications of pregnancies associated with aPL syndromes can be life-threatening or fatal from severe pre-eclampsia[170], arterial or venous thromboses[164,165,171,172]. Severe pre-eclampsia prior to 34 weeks' gestation and transient monocular blindness have been associated with aPL antibody[170]. Maternal deaths resulting from disseminated small-vessel thromboses (in a woman with sickle cell trait) and myocardial infarction (in a woman with prior pulmonary embolism) have also been reported[171,172]. There may also be an increased risk of stroke in the postpartum period[170].

Severe postpartum idiopathic pleuropulmonary syndromes have been reported in women with aPL antibodies, consisting of pleural effusion, pulmonary infiltrates and fever, with or without cardiomyopathy[173] or pulmonary embolism[174], but not attributable to either documented infection or SLE. It is not established that this syndrome is attributed to aPL antibodies.

Dilemmas in interpreting complications reported with aPL antibodies

In an analysis of 129 SLE patients with aPL antibodies, a significant ($p < 0.001$) association was found between the number of blood samples tested and the titer of antibody[129]. The data suggest that aPL titers fluctuate during pregnancy and that higher titers are more likely to be found with more frequent testing. High titer tests are also more often repeated than low titer tests when aPL syndrome is clinically suspected.

Further confusion is engendered by seemingly healthy people and patients with lupus who appear to coexist happily with aPL antibodies[175]. In these patients, there is a weak correlation of aCL antibodies with adverse pregnancy outcomes[160]. Thus, the diagnosis or treatment of aPL syndromes should not be based upon a single test titer. History of multiple previous vascular insults[175] or an obstetrical history of at least two previously unexplained pregnancy failures[95] correlates with the presence of aPL antibodies and increased future risk of complications, whatever may be the underlying pathogenesis[162,166].

Treatment of pregnancy-related complications associated with aPL antibodies

Controlled clinical trials[155–158] suggest that heparin and aspirin are the preferred treatments for repeated fetal losses associated with aPL antibodies.

Patients with positive aPL antibodies should have consultations with a maternal–fetal specialized physician, either on a preconception basis or immediately following verification of pregnancy. Patients with prior complicated aPL-related gestations should be managed by a maternal–fetal medicine team familiar with the illness and skilled in critical care. Infants of such gestations should be delivered in facilities experienced in the care of premature small infants (500–1500 gm birthweight). Careful monitoring of fetal growth, uteroplacental

function[6], and fetal monitoring[7], beginning as early as the second trimester, may detect impending fetal compromise and necessitate early delivery[7].

Prednisone suppression of maternal LAC

The first papers in the 1980s[124,163] suggested that high-dose prednisone therapy (e.g., 40–60 mg per day, orally) promotes fetal survival in pregnancies of women with recurrent abortions associated with LAC. However, with evolving understanding of the pathogenesis of aPL-associated fetal losses and its procoagulant phenomena, most recent experience argues against such 'prophylactic' glucocorticoid approach[5,95,153] in favor of anticoagulation therapies[154–158]. Importantly, lupus patients must also be treated with sufficient prednisone for suppression of disease activity in pregnancy. However, higher dosages intended for immunosuppression of aPL antibodies *per se* may not be beneficial and increase the risk of long-term complications, especially osteonecrosis and osteoporosis.

Anticoagulation with heparin

In an earlier, uncontrolled study, fetal wastage was prevented with heparin therapy in most women with aCL and LAC antibodies who had recurrent losses or previous abnormal outcomes[176]. However, successful pregnancy may occur in SLE with untreated LAC[177]. A subsequent, small-scale, randomized, controlled trial[157] suggested that corticosteroids and heparin were equally efficacious, but that moderate-dose heparin was associated with less fetal and maternal morbidity. A recent trial[155] found that full-dose heparin plus low-dose aspirin provided significantly better pregnancy outcome than low-dose aspirin alone in women who had at least three consecutive pregnancy losses, without causing increased complications. Ongoing studies[156] indicate that treatment of aPL antibody-associated pregnancy loss with lower dose heparin and aspirin is equivalent to full-dose anticoagulation[155]. The latter has been implicated in maternal gestational stroke in unpublished reports. Heparin, in addition to its anticoagulant effects, may act by directly binding aPL antibodies *in vivo*[178].

Intravenous gammaglobulin therapy

A small number of patients have been reported to have improved pregnancy outcomes with experimental gammaglobulin therapy[179,180]. However, the Pregnancy Loss Study Group reported a double-blinded randomized trial of IVIG which was negative[181].

Low-dose aspirin

Mini-dose aspirin (e.g. 60–100 mg daily) has been recommended for treatment in pregnant women with primary aPL syndrome and history of recurrent abortion[154]. Recent studies suggest it is not sufficient in high-risk pregnancies[155].

Pre-eclampsia considerations in therapy

Since pre-eclampsia may be associated with the presence of LAC[124] and may be severe[170], the induction of fluid retention and hypertension are reasons not to use high-dose prednisone[153]. High-dose prednisone therapy is not indicated to suppress aPL antibodies. It may be needed to suppress disease activity in the active lupus patient with predisposition to pre-eclampsia. Treatment with prophylactic doses of heparin, with consideration of combined low-dose aspirin (e.g. 80–100 mg daily), seems to be helpful in such patients[155,156,170].

Postpartum surveillance

Reports of patients with aPL antibodies having cardio-pulmonary complications associated with delivery[171–174] necessitate careful postpartum monitoring. Deaths due to embolic disease have occurred as late as 4 weeks following delivery and after a symptom-free interval in such patients. Severe pre-eclampsia associated with postpartum cerebral infarction, deep venous thrombosis, pulmonary embolism and transient blindness have also been described in patients with aPL antibodies[170], requiring close monitoring and expectant therapy.

POLYMYOSITIS–DERMATOMYOSITIS (PM–DM) AND PREGNANCY

Clinical profile of PM–DM

Polymyositis (PM) and dermatomyositis (DM) are acquired degenerative and inflammatory diseases of striated muscles belonging to the spectrum of diffuse connective tissue disorders[1,182,183]. Clinically, PM and DM are similar; PM does not have the evident skin involvement[183]. These disorders may occur at all ages, with peaks in the juvenile and later middle years[1]. It is likely that some patients diagnosed as PM have other disorders.

Because of the low incidence of PM–DM, i.e. about one-tenth of SLE over all ages, and its relative paucity in younger adults[1], the active condition is rarely seen in association with pregnancy. However, some remitted patients with a prior history of juvenile-onset PM–DM may present for pre-pregnancy counseling or already be pregnant. Less common are patients with either prior adult-onset PM–DM who have become pregnant or those few who develop PM during pregnancy. Overall, the prognosis is good for the mother, but fetal risk of morbidity and mortality is increased[184–193]. The pregnancy should be considered high-risk, with careful monitoring of the mother for disease activity and the fetus for growth and well-being[184–187].

Onset of PM–DM in pregnancy

Onset of PM–DM during pregnancy is reported to have the poorest prognosis for the fetus. The eight adult- and one juvenile-onset cases reported[184–193] mainly occurred in the prefetal monitoring era and may not represent modern expectations. Fetal outcome has been variable. Active PM–DM seems to improve following delivery. Of nine cases reviewed[187], six had onset of PM–DM in the first trimester. Two healthy, term spontaneous deliveries occurred in this group of pregnancies[187]. Five of the ten neonates (one set of twins) survived[187], including the twin set and the juvenile delivery[187].

PM–DM antedating pregnancy

Pregnancy in patients with a preceding history of PM–DM has been reviewed[185–187] and summarized, both in total[185,187] and stratified according to juvenile-versus adult-onset[186].

Pregnancy in juvenile-onset PM–DM

Six juvenile-onset PM–DM women with 10 pregnancies[186] conceived during a period of remission of some months to 4 years duration. Exacerbation of PM–DM occurred in four pregnancies, two of which were post-abortion (one spontaneous, one elective). The other two pregnancies resulted in live births. All six pregnancies without exacerbation of PM–DM resulted in live, term births[186].

Pregnancy in adult-onset PM–DM

Of 10 adult-onset PM–DM cases with 13 pregnancies (one twin set)[184–193], four patients conceived with active disease and all delivered healthy infants[186,187]. Nine conceptions occurred during a time of inactive disease[184,186–188], one neonatal death occurred secondary to extreme prematurity and two spontaneous abortions occurred. Only one postpartum maternal death was reported in gestational PM–DM[193].

These experiences suggest that pregnancy outcome is generally less favorable in patients with adult- than juvenile-onset PM–DM and more favorable in remitted disease which does not exacerbate during gestation[187,188]. No neonatal effects of PM–DM have been reported in surviving children nor have placental abnormalities been reported[186].

Management of pregnancy in PM–DM

Planning for pregnancy during a period of inactive disease is desirable. During pregnancy, close monitoring both for disease flares and fetal well-being are indicated, extending into the postpartum period[185,186,193]. When PM–DM is first diagnosed during pregnancy, patients should have early sonographic confirmation of menstrual dates, serial growth studies and early institution of electronic fetal heart rate monitoring.

Prednisone therapy is recommended for disease activity in the same doses sufficient for control as in non-pregnant patients[185,186]. Cytotoxic agents are not recommended, particularly in the first trimester[185,186]. However, when the disease is unresponsive to corticosteroids, more aggressive therapy may be considered, especially in gestational PM–DM, which has high reported fetal mortality. Experimental therapy in such circumstances may include intravenous immunoglobulins, plasmapheresis and even azathioprine. Methotrexate, commonly used in PM–DM, is contraindicated in pregnancy.

SYSTEMIC SCLEROSIS (SCLERODERMA) AND PREGNANCY

Clinical profile of systemic sclerosis

Systemic sclerosis (SSc) or scleroderma is a relatively uncommon, multisystem CTD which encompasses a broad spectrum of clinical entities[1,194,195]. The SSc spectrum of disorders ranges from diffuse scleroderma, affecting extremities and truncal skin, to more limited forms, affecting mainly the distal extremities[1,194,195]. An example of the later syndrome is CREST (i.e., calcinosis cutis, Raynaud's phenomenon[194], esophageal dysmotility, sclerodactyly and telangiectasias). Vascular changes are prominent in these disorders which affect women more frequently than men, especially during the reproductive ages[1,195]. The incidence of SSc increases with age and overall is about one-fifth of SLE and twice that of PM–DM[1], making pregnancy in SSc relatively uncommon.

The severity of SSc spectrum disorders varies considerably. Only digital or distal extremity skin may be affected (the CREST variant) or widespread skin and vital organs may be involved (diffuse scleroderma)[1,195]. Advanced cases may have important cardiorespiratory and renal sequelae[195] as well as significant impairment of fertility and fetal outcome[196–203].

Raynaud's phenomenon, which is an almost universal manifestation of SSc in women, also occurs in a 'primary' form without associated systemic disease[194]. The latter not infrequently occurs in pregnancy[204]. No serious outcomes were noted in pregnancies which occurred after onset of primary Raynaud's[204]. However, premature births were more common than among controls[9% vs. 1%]. Also, mean weights of full-term babies were less than babies born to control mothers[204], findings similar to pregnancy outcomes in women with limited SSc[199].

Review of individual case reports

A review of individual case reports[200] included 21 women with SSc who had 27 pregnancies, between the ages of 18 and 40 years (median 25½ years). Duration of SSc at the time of pregnancy ranged from a few months to 10 years (median 3½ years) and all but four patients had diffuse cutaneous sclerosis, suggesting a bias toward more advanced cases having been reported, as might be expected.

Effect of pregnancy on SSc

Among the 21 patients reviewed[200], nine (43%) died of complications of pregnancy, six with pre-eclampsia. Postpartum renal failure was the cause of death in five of the six. All had biopsy-proven renal scleroderma. Among the 12 surviving mothers, three (25%) also experienced pre-eclampsia. Among the nine maternal deaths, all but one (89%) had progression of disease during pregnancy, compared with four (33%) who progressed among the 12 survivors. In contrast, regression of SSc occurred in only one patient during two pregnancies, but progression occurred in a third pregnancy. As with PM–DM case reports[184–193], one must be wary that the most severe patients are more likely to be reported and may not represent current general experience.

Effect of SSc on pregnancy Twenty (74%) of the 27 pregnancies progressed to live-births, two (7.4%) were electively aborted and five (18.5%) resulted in perinatal deaths (one intrauterine death undelivered, one still-born and three early neonatal deaths)[200]. Perinatal death did not correlate with either pre-eclampsia or maternal death (or both combined); two occurred in nine surviving mothers without eclampsia and three in the remaining 12 who either had pre-eclampsia or succumbed. Among the nine pre-eclamptic pregnancies, two resulted in both maternal and perinatal deaths, four in maternal death alone and three in survival of mother and child.

Review of reported series

In contradistinction to individual case reports, review of available series[200] yields a more favorable impression of the frequency of pre-eclampsia, as well as maternal and perinatal survival, although abortions were relatively more common. Among 101 pregnancies (most in patients with limited scleroderma involvement), two maternal deaths were noted and only six patients experienced pre-eclampsia. Only five (5%) pregnancies resulted in perinatal death. However, spontaneous abortions occurred in 24 (24%) of the pregnancies.

Onset of scleroderma occurred during nine pregnancies. Among the remaining 92 pregnancies, SSc progressed in 30, regressed in 11, was stable in 34 and was unspecified in 17. Progression was significantly more common than regression, as described in the review of individual case reports[200].

Spontaneous abortion in case–control studies

In a retrospective study of 86 SSc patients and 86 healthy controls[201], spontaneous abortion occurred in 50 (16.7%) of the 299 case pregnancies compared with 32 (9.6%) of the 332 control pregnancies (*p* < 0.05). The rate was not separately analyzed before or after onset of scleroderma.

In a nationwide case–control, paired study conducted in Britain, using a postal questionnaire[202], the relative risk of abortion prior to a diagnosis of scleroderma (28.7%) was twice (2.1 : 1) that of the controls (17.4%), 95% confidence interval, 1.0–4.3. This result was supported by a small-sample, controlled study (14 SSc patients) from Bath, England[203].

Case–control studies of pregnancy outcome in SSc and Raynaud's phenomenon (RP):

No statistically significant increase was found in the rate of miscarriages, fetal deaths, maternal morbidity or mortality among 48 women with a history of scleroderma and a concomitant pregnancy compared with neighborhood and rheumatoid arthritis controls, all of whom had been pregnant at least once[199]. This study did not show significantly increased deterioration of scleroderma in pregnancy compared to the non-pregnant state. Significantly more small full-term infants were born to women with scleroderma. Also, preterm births occurred slightly more frequently among the scleroderma than control women.

In women with RP selected by attendance at a referral rheumatology clinic, no difference in fetal loss rates were found compared to healthy women[204]. The patient group had a higher proportion of premature births than controls (9% versus 1%, respectively) and lower mean weight full-term babies[204].

Close monitoring for premature labor and IUGR was advised[199]. Overall, in the absence of major systemic disease, risks to mother and child should not preclude pregnancy. Patients with progressive, diffuse scleroderma should avoid becoming pregnant because of their intrinsically higher risk of developing renal crisis[199].

Reproductive function prior to SSc disease onset

A subsequent case–control study from the UK employed a self-administered postal questionnaire to survey reproductive history in a national sample of women with SSc, RP and a control group from a general practitioner register local to the West Middlesex Hospital[205]. The rates of spontaneous abortions (defined as fetal loss before 28 weeks of pregnancy) for first pregnancies were similar in the three groups: SSc (11.6%); RP (15.6%) and controls (12.5%). The rates for subsequent pregnancies were higher in the patient groups, i.e. SSc

(16.8%); RP (21.3%) and controls (12.8%). Authors indicated that the SSc women were older, the RP women may have included some with lupus and that it is difficult to determine exact onset of disease[205]. Low birth weight for all pregnancies also tended to be more frequent in the SSc (10.6%) and RP (8.1%) than control (3.7%) women. Perinatal deaths for all pregnancies were non-significantly higher in the SSc (2.4%) and RP (2.0%) than the control (0.9%) groups. Also, these figures were not adjusted for sociodemographic factors[205].

Management of pregnancy in scleroderma

In women with significant pulmonary, cardiac, or renal involvement from SSc, pregnancy may not be medically advised. Should pregnancy result from a failure of contraception, in an advanced case, the patient will be confronted with the choice of high-risk pregnancy or therapeutic abortion[8,199,200]. As with SLE or PM–DM pregnancies, close monitoring of both the gravida and fetus is required in the scleroderma pregnancy. In patients with renal involvement, a scleroderma renal crisis (SRC) may be difficult to distinguish from pre-eclampsia. Plasma renin activity is likely to be elevated in SRC. Episodes occurring during the first half of a viable pregnancy are more likely due to SRC, whereas pre-eclampsia is more likely to occur in later pregnancy. If severe maternal, life-threatening complications develop, the options of prompt delivery or even termination of pregnancy arise[8]. Special attention must be given to the possible fetal effects of medications which may be necessary to control maternal disease[8,55], especially D-penicillamine[64–66], or cytotoxic agents[59,68]. Close monitoring of fetal growth and fetal well-being should be initiated.

ACKNOWLEDGEMENTS

We wish to express sincere appreciation to Debbie Harper for her extended contributions in preparation of this manuscript; to research assistant, Bobbi Vanover, for her generous help with literature searches and documentation; and to secretary, Margaret Walsh, for her generous assistance. Also, we would like to thank Drs Robert T. Chatterton and Robert H. Persellin for their critical reviews of the manuscript and helpful suggestions.

REFERENCES

1. Masi AT, Medsger TA, Jr. Epidemiology of the rheumatic diseases. In McCarty, DJ, ed. *Arthritis and Allied Conditions*, edn 11. Philadelphia: Lea & Febiger, 1989; 16–54

2. Cecere FA, Persellin RH. The interaction of pregnancy and the rheumatic diseases. *Clin Rheum Dis* 1981; 7:747–68

3. Zurier RB. Pregnancy in patients with rheumatic diseases. *Rheum Dis Clin North Am* 1989;15:193–405

4. Dombroski RA. Autoimmune disease in pregnancy. *Med Clin North Am* 1989;73:605–21

5. Lockshin MD, Druzin ML. Rheumatic disease. In Barron WM, Lindheimer MD, eds. *Medical Disorders During Pregnancy* 2nd edn. St Louis, MO: Mosby-Year Book, Inc., 1995:307–37

6. Trudinger BJ, Stewart GJ, Cook CM, *et al*. Monitoring lupus anticoagulant – positive pregnancies with umbilical artery flow velocity waveforms. *Obstet Gynecol* 1988;72:215–18

7. Druzin ML, Lockshin M, Edersheim TG, *et al*. Second-trimester fetal monitoring and preterm delivery in pregnancies with systemic lupus erythematosus and/or circulating anticoagulant. *Am J Obstet Gynecol* 1987; 157:1503–10

8. Maymon R, Fejgin M: Scleroderma in pregnancy. *Obstet Gynecol Surv* 1989;44:530–34

9. Masi AT. Incidence of rheumatoid arthritis: do the observed age-sex interaction patterns support a role of androgenic-anabolic (AA) steroid deficiency in its pathogenesis? *Br J Rheumatol* 1994;33:697–9

10. Hench PS. The ameliorating effect of pregnancy on chronic atrophic (infectious rheumatoid) arthritis, fibrositis, and intermittent hydrarthrosis. *Proc Staff Meet Mayo Clin* 1938;13:161–7

11. Oka M. Effect of pregnancy on the onset and course of rheumatoid arthritis. *Ann Rheum Dis* 1953;12:227–9

12. Østensen M, Aune B, Husby G. Effect of pregnancy and hormonal changes on the activity of rheumatoid arthritis. *Scand J Rheumatol* 1983;12:69–72

13. Klipple GL, Cecere FA. Rheumatoid arthritis and pregnancy. *Rheum Dis Clin North Am* 1989;15:213–39

14. Nelson JL, Hughes KA, Smith AG, *et al*. Maternal-fetal disparity in HLA class II alloantigens and the pregnancy-induced amelioration of rheumatoid arthritis. *N Engl J Med* 1993;329:466–71

15. Brennan P, Silman A. Breast-feeding and the onset of rheumatoid arthritis. *Arthritis Rheum* 1994;37:808–13

16. Felbo M, Snorrason E. Pregnancy and the place of therapeutic abortion in rheumatoid arthritis. *Acta Obstet Gynecol Scand* 1961;40:116–26

17. Buyon JP, Nelson JL, Lockshin MD. The effects of pregnancy on autoimmune diseases (Short Analytical Review). *Clin Immunol Immunopathol* 1996;78:99–104

18. Bulmash JM. Rheumatoid arthritis and pregnancy. *Obstet Gynecol Annu* 1979;8:223–76

19. Nolten WE, Rueckert PA. Elevated free cortisol index in pregnancy: possible regulatory mechanisms. *Am J Obstet Gynecol* 1981;139:492–8

20. Ansar S, Penhale WJ, Talal N. Sex hormones, immune responses, and autoimmune diseases: mechanisms of sex hormone action. *Am J Pathol* 1985;121:531–59

21. Østensen M, Husby G. A prospective clinical study of the effect of pregnancy on rheumatoid arthritis and ankylosing spondylitis. *Arthritis Rheum* 1983;26:1155–9

22. Brabin BJ. Epidemiology of infection in pregnancy. *Rev Infect Dis* 1985;7:579–603

23. Sridama V, Pacini F, Yang SL, *et al*. Decreased levels of helper T cells: a possible cause of immunodeficiency in pregnancy. *N Engl J Med* 1982;307:352–6

24. Wegmann TG, Lin H, Guilbert L, *et al*. Bidirectional cytokine interactions in the maternal-fetal relationship: is successful pregnancy a TH2 phenomenon? *Immunol Today* 1993;14:353–6

25. Krause PJ, Ingardia CJ, Pontius LT, *et al*. Host defense during pregnancy: neutrophil chemotaxis and adherence. *Am J Obstet Gynecol* 1987;157:274–80

26. Crouch SPM, Crocker IP, Fletcher J. The effect of pregnancy on polymorphonuclear function. *J Immunol* 1995;155:5436–43

27. Østensen M, Revhaug A, Volden G, *et al*. The effect of pregnancy on functions of inflammatory cells in healthy women and in patients with rheumatic disease. *Acta Obstet Gynecol Scand* 1987;66:247–53

28. Sites DP, Siiteri PK. Steroids as immunosuppressants in pregnancy. *Immunol Rev* 1983;75:117–38

29. Szekeres-Bartho J, Faust Zs, Varga P. The expression of a progesterone-induced immunomodulatory protein in pregnancy lymphocytes. *Am J Reprod Immunol* 1995; 34:342–8

30. Masi AT, Feigenbaum SL, Chatterton RT. Hormonal and pregnancy relationships to rheumatoid arthritis: convergent effects with immunologic and microvascular systems. *Semin Arthritis Rheum* 1995;25:1–27

31. Unger A, Kay A, Griffin AJ, *et al*. Disease activity and pregnancy associated alpha 2-glycoprotein in rheumatoid arthritis during pregnancy. *Br Med J (Clin Res Ed)* 1983;286:750–2

32. Østensen M, von Schoultz B, Husby G. Comparison between serum alpha 2-pregnancy-associated globulin and activity of rheumatoid arthritis and ankylosing spondylitis during pregnancy. *Scand J Rheumatol* 1983; 12:315–8

33. Quinn C, Mulpeter K, Casey EB, *et al*. Changes in levels of IgM RF and alpha 2 PAG correlate with increased disease activity in rheumatoid arthritis during the puerperium. *Scand J Rheumatol* 1993;22:273–9

34. Hernandez-Avila M, Liang MH, Willett WC, *et al*. Exogenous sex hormones and the risk of rheumatoid arthritis. *Arthritis Rheum* 1990;33:947–53

35. Pladevall-Villa M, Delclos GL, Varas C, *et al*. Controversy of oral contraceptives and risk of rheumatoid arthritis: meta-analysis of conflicting studies and review of conflicting meta-analyses with special emphasis on analysis of heterogeneity. *Am J Epidemiol* 1996;144:1–14

36. Nelson JL. Maternal-fetal immunology and autoimmune disease: is some autoimmune disease auto-alloimmune or allo-autoimmune? *Arthritis Rheum* 1996;39:191–4

37. Peaceman AM, Ramsey-Goldman R. Autoimmune connective tissue disease in pregnancy. In Sciarra JJ, ed. *Gynecology and Obstetrics*, Vol. 3. Philadelphia: Lippincott-Raven Publishers, 1998:1–12

38. Yoshino S, Uchida S. Sexual problems of women with rheumatoid arthritis. *Arch Phys Med Rehabil* 1981; 62:122–3

39. Nelson JL, Koepsell TD, Dugowson CE, *et al*. Fecundity before disease onset in women with rheumatoid arthritis. *Arthritis Rheum* 1993;36:7–14

40. Kay A, Bach F. Subfertility before and after the development of rheumatoid arthritis in women. *Ann Rheum Dis* 1965;24:169–73

41. Masi AT, Josipovic DB, Jefferson WE. Low adrenal androgenic-anabolic steroids in women with rheumatoid

arthritis (RA): gas-liquid chromatographic studies of RA patients and matched normal control women indicating decreased 11-deoxy-17-ketosteroid excretion. *Semin Arthritis Rheum* 1984;14:1–23

42. Masi AT, DaSilva JAP, Cutolo M. Perturbations of hypothalamic-pituitary-gonadal (HPG) axis and adrenal androgen (AA) functions in rheumatoid arthritis. *Bailières Clin Rheumatol* 1996;10:295–332

43. Silman AJ. Is pregnancy a risk factor in the causation of rheumatoid arthritis? *Ann Rheum Dis* 1986; 45:1031–4

44. Engel A. Rheumatoid arthritis in U.S. adults 1960–1962. In Bennet PH, Wood PHN, eds. *Population Studies in the Rheumatic Diseases*. Amsterdam: Excerpta Medica Foundation, 1968:83–89

45. Musey VC, Collins DC, Brogan DR, *et al*. Long term effects of a first pregnancy on the hormonal environment: estrogens and androgens. *J Clin Endocrinol Metab* 1987;64:111–8

46. Gao X, Olsen NJ, Pincus T, *et al*. HLA-DR alleles with naturally occurring amino acid substitutions and risk for development of rheumatoid arthritis. *Arthritis Rheum* 1990;33:939–46

47. Nelson JL, Dugowson CE, Koepsell TD, *et al*. Rheumatoid factor, HLA-DR4, and allelic variants of DRB1 in women with recent-onset rheumatoid arthritis. *Arthritis Rheum* 1995;38:290–300

48. Jawaheer D, Thomson W, MacGregor AJ, *et al*. Homozygosity for the HLA-DR shared epitope contributes the highest risk for rheumatoid arthritis concordance in identical twins. *Arthritis Rheum* 1994; 37:681–6

49. Lee P. Anti-inflammatory therapy during pregnancy and lactation. *Clin Invest Med* 1985;8:328–32

50. Witter FR. Clinical pharmacokinetics in the treatment of rheumatoid arthritis in pregnancy. *Clin Pharmacokinet* 1993;25:444–9

51. Østensen M. Optimization of antirheumatic drug treatment in pregnancy. *Clin Pharmacokinet* 1994; 27:486–503

52. Sibai BM, Mirro R, Chesney CM, *et al*. Low-dose aspirin in pregnancy. *Obstet Gynecol* 1989;74:551–7

53. Thorp JA, Walsh SW, Brath PC. Low-dose aspirin inhibits thromboxane, but not prostacyclin, production by human placental arteries. *Am J Obstet Gynecol* 1988;159:1381–4

54. Slone D, Heinonen OP, Siskind V, *et al*. Aspirin and congenital malformations. *Lancet* 1976;1:1373–6

55. Heinonen OP, Slone D, Shapiro S. *Birth Defects and Drugs in Pregnancy*. Littleton, USA: Publishing Sciences Group, 1977:516

56. Roubenoff R, Hoyt J, Petri M, *et al*. Effects of anti-inflammatory and immunosuppressive drugs on pregnancy and fertility. *Semin Arthritis Rheum* 1988; 18:88–110

57. Werler MM, Mitchell AA, Shapiro S. The relation of aspirin use during the first trimester of pregnancy to congenital cardiac defects. *N Engl J Med* 1989; 321:1639–42

58. FDA: Labeling for oral and rectal over-the-counter aspirin and aspirin-containing drug products; final rule. *Fed Regist* 1990;55(120):27776–84

59. Bermas BL, Hill JA. Effects of immunosuppressive drugs during pregnancy. *Arthritis Rheum* 1995; 38:1722–32

60. Rains CP, Noble S, Faulds D. Sulfasalazine. A review of its pharmacological properties and therapeutic efficacy in the treatment of rheumatoid arthritis. *Drugs* 1995; 50:137–56

61. Ullberg S, Lindquist NG, Sjöstrand SE. Accumulation of chorio-retinotoxic drugs in the foetal eye. *Nature* 1970;227:1257–8

62. Buchanan NMM, Toubi E, Khamashta MA, *et al*. Hydroxychloroquine and lupus pregnancy: review of a series of 36 cases. *Ann Rheum Dis* 1996;55:486–8

63. Hart CW, Naunton RF. The ototoxicity of chloroquine phosphate. *Arch Otolaryngol* 1964;80:407–12

64. Mjølnerød OK, Rasmussen K, Dommerud SA, *et al*. Congenital connective-tissue defect probably due to D-penicillamine treatment in pregnancy. *Lancet* 1971; 1:673–5

65. Solomon L, Abram G, Dinner M, *et al*. Neonatal abnormalities associated with D-penicilliamine treatment during pregnancy (Letter). *N Engl J Med* 1977; 296:54–5

66. Endres W. D-Penicillamine in pregnancy: To ban or not to ban? *Klin Wochenschr* 1981;59:535–7

67. Gabbe SG. Drug therapy in autoimmune diseases. *Clin Obstet Gynecol* 1983;26:635–41

68. Briggs GG, Freeman RK, Yaffe SJ, eds. *A Reference Guide to Fetal and Neonatal Risk. Drugs in Pregnancy and Lactation*, 4th edn. Baltimore: Williams & Wilkins, 1995

69. Hausknecht RU. Methotrexate and misoprostol to terminate early pregnancy. *N Engl J Med* 1995; 333:537–40

70. Masi AT. Do sex hormones play a role in ankylosing spondylitis? *Rheum Dis Clin North Am* 1992;18:153–76

71. Gran JT, Husby G, Hordvik M. Prevalence of ankylosing spondylitis in males and females in a young middle-aged population of Tromsø, northern Norway. *Ann Rheum Dis* 1985;44:359–67

72. Hart FD. Bechterew's syndrome in women: is it different from that in men? *Scand J Rheumatol* 1980; 32:38–40

73. Goodman CE, Lange RK, Waxman J, *et al*. Ankylosing spondylitis in women. *Arch Phys Med Rehab* 1980; 61:167–70

74. Gran JT, Østensen M, Husby G. A clinical comparison between males and females with ankylosing spondylitis. *J Rheumatol* 1985;12:126–9

75. Gran JT, Husby G. Ankylosing spondylitis in women. *Semin Arthritis Rheum* 1990;19:303–12

76. Østensen M, Husby G. Pregnancy and rheumatic disease. A review of recent studies in rheumatoid arthritis and ankylosing spondylitis. *Klin Wochenschr* 1984;62:891–5

77. Østensen M, Husby G. Ankylosing spondylitis and pregnancy. *Rheum Dis Clin North Am* 1989;15:241–54

78. Østensen M, Romberg Ø, Husby G. Ankylosing spondylitis and motherhood. *Arthritis Rheum* 1982; 25:140–3

79. Veille JC, Hohimer AR, Burry K, *et al*. The effect of exercise on uterine activity in the last eight weeks of pregnancy. *Am J Obstet Gynecol* 1985;151:727–30

80. Østensen M, Husby G. Antirheumatic drug treatment during pregnancy and lactation. *Scand J Rheum* 1985;14:1–7

81. Fraga A, Mintz G, Orozco J, et al. Sterility and fertility rates, fetal wastage and maternal morbidity in systemic lupus erythematosus. *J Rheumatol* 1974;1:293–8

82. Kitridou RC, Mintz G. The mother in systemic lupus erythematosus. In Wallace DJ and Hahn BH, eds. *Dubois' Lupus Erythematosus*, 5th edn. Baltimore, MD: Williams & Wilkins, 1997:967–1002

83. Kitridou RC, Mintz G. Pregnancy in lupus: The fetus in systemic lupus erythematosus. In Wallace DJ and Hahn BH, eds. *Dubois' Lupus Erythematosus*, 5th edn. Baltimore, MD: Williams & Wilkins, 1997:1003–21

84. Ruizirastorza G, Lima F, Alves J, et al. Increased rate of lupus flare during pregnancy and the puerperium: a prospective study of 78 pregnancies. *Br J Rheumatol* 1996;35:133–8

85. Petrie M, Howard D, Repke J. Frequency of lupus flare in pregnancy: The Johns Hopkins Lupus Pregnancy Center experience. *Arthritis Rheum* 1991;34:1538–45

86. Mintz G, Rodriguez-Alvarez E. Systemic lupus erythematosus. *Rheum Dis Clin North Am* 1989;15:255–74

87. Lockshin MD, Reinitz E, Druzin ML, et al. Lupus pregnancy. Case-control prospective study demonstrating absence of lupus exacerbation during pregnancy. *Am J Med* 1984;77:893–8

88. Lockshin MD. Pregnancy does not cause systemic lupus erythematosus to worsen. *Arthritis Rheum* 1989;32:667–70

89. Bobrie G, Liote F, Houillier P, et al. Pregnancy in lupus nephritis and related disorders. *Am J Kidney Dis* 1987;9:339–43

90. Fine LG, Barnett EV, Danovitch GM, et al. Systemic lupus erythematosus in pregnancy. UCLA conference. *Ann Intern Med* 1981;94:667–77

91. Urowitz MB, Gladman DD, Farewell VT, et al. Lupus and pregnancy studies. *Arthritis Rheum* 1993;36:1392–7

92. Lockshin MD. Does lupus flare during pregnancy? *Lupus* 1993;2:1–2

93. Lockshin MD, Druzin ML. Rheumatic disease. In Barron WM, Lindheimer MD, eds. *Medical Disorders During Pregnancy*, St. Louis, MO: Mosby-Year Book, Inc., 1991:366–99

94. Lockshin MD, Druzin ML, Goei S, et al. Antibody to cardiolipin as a predictor of fetal distress or death in pregnant patients with systemic lupus erythematosus. *N Engl J Med* 1985;313:152–6

95. Englert HJ, Derue GM, Loizou S, et al. Pregnancy and lupus: prognostic indicators and response to treatment. *Q J Med* 1988;66:125–36

96. Kutteh WH, Lyda EC, Abraham SM, et al. Association of anticardiolipin antibodies and pregnancy loss in women with systemic lupus erythematosus. *Fertil Steril* 1993;60:449–55

97. Abramowsky CR, Vegas ME, Swinehart G, et al. Decidual vasculopathy of the placenta in lupus erythematosus. *New Engl J Med* 1980;303:668–72

98. Samaritano L, Magid M, Kaplan C, et al. A prospective study of clinical features and placental pathology in systemic lupus erythematosus (SLE) with and without antiphospholipid antibodies (aPL). *Arthritis Rheum* 1995;38:S218(abst)

99. Nayar R, Lage JM. Placental changes in a first-trimester missed abortion in maternal systemic lupus erythematosus with antiphospholipid syndrome. A case report and review of the literature. *Hum Pathol* 1996;27:201–6

100. Althabe O, Labarrere C, Telenta M. Maternal vascular lesions in placentae of small-for-gestational-age infants. *Placenta* 1985;6:265–76

101. Hanly JG, Gladman DD, Rose TH, et al. Lupus pregnancy: a prospective study of placental changes. *Arthritis Rheum* 1988;31:358–66

102. Nadler DM, Klein NW, Aramli LA, et al. The direct embryotoxicity of immunoglobulin G fractions from patients with systemic lupus erythematosus. *Am J Reprod Immunol* 1995;34:349–55

103. Watson RM, Lane AT, Barnett NK, et al. Neonatal lupus erythematosus: A clinical, serological and immunogenetic study with review of the literature. *Medicine (Baltimore)* 1984;63:362–78

104. Buyon J, Szer I. Passively acquired autoimmunity and the maternal fetal dyad in systemic lupus erythematosus. *Springer Semin Immunopathol* 1986;9:283–304

105. Lockshin MD, Bonfa E, Elkon K, et al. Neonatal lupus risk to newborns of mothers with systemic lupus erythematosus. *Arthritis Rheum* 1988;31:697–701

106. Waltuck J, Buyon JP. Autoantibody-associated congenital heart block: outcome in mothers and children. *Ann Intern Med* 1994;120:544–51

107. Press J, Uziel Y, Laxer RM, et al. Long-term outcome of mothers of children with complete congenital heart block. *Am J Med* 1996;100:328–32

108. Boumpas DT, Austin HA III, Fessler BJ, et al. Systemic lupus erythematosus: emerging concepts. Part II. Dermatologic and joint disease, the antiphospholipid antibody syndrome, pregnancy and hormonal therapy, morbidity and mortality, and pathogenesis. *Ann Intern Med* 1995;123:42–53

109. Copel J, Buyon JP, Kleinman CS. Successful in utero therapy of fetal heart block. *Am J Obstet Gynecol* 1995;173:728–32

110. Levitz M, Jansen V, Dancis J. The transfer and metabolism of corticosteroids in the perfused human placenta. *Am J Obstet Gynecol* 1978;132:363–6

111. Walsh SD, Clark FR. Pregnancy in patients on long-term corticosteroid therapy. *Scott Med J* 1967;12:302–6

112. Cote CJ, Meuwissen HJ, Pickering RJ. Effects on the neonate of prednisone and azathioprine administered to the mother during pregnancy. *J Pediatr* 1974;85:324–8

113. Pirson Y, Van Lierde M, Ghysen J, et al. Retardation of fetal growth in patients receiving immunosuppressive therapy. *N Engl J Med* 1985;313:328

114. The Canadian Hydroxychloroquine Study Group. A randomized study of the effect of withdrawing hydroxychloroquine sulfate in systemic lupus erythematosus. *N Engl J Med* 1991;324:150–4

115. Shibata S, Sasaki T, Hirabashi Y, et al. Risk factors in the pregnancy of patients with systemic lupus erythematosus: association of hypocomplementemia with poor prognosis. *Ann Rheum Dis* 1992;51:619–23

116. Ost L, Wettrell G, Bjorkhem I, *et al*. Prednisolone excretion in human milk. *J Pediatr* 1985;106:1008–11

117. Committee on Drugs, American Academy of Pediatrics. The transfer of drugs and other chemicals into human breast milk. *Pediatrics* 1994;93:137–50

118. Nilsson IM, Astedt B, Hedner U, *et al*. Intrauterine death and circulating anticoagulant, "Antithromboplastin". *Acta Med Scand* 1975;197:153–9

119. Harris EN, Chan JKH, Asherson RA, *et al*. Thrombosis, recurrent fetal loss, and thrombocytopenia. Predictive value of the anticardiolipin antibody test. *Arch Intern Med* 1986;146:2153–6

120. Harris EN, Pierangeli SS. Antiphospholipid antibodies and the antiphospholipid syndrome. *Springer Semin Immunopathol* 1994;16:223–45

121. Love PE, Santoro SA. Antiphospholipid antibodies: anticardiolipin and the lupus anticoagulant in systemic lupus erythematosus (SLE) and in non-SLE disorders. Prevalence and clinical significance. *Ann Intern Med* 1990;112:682–98

122. Sammaritano LR, Gharavi AE, Lockshin MD. Antiphospholipid antibody syndrome: immunologic and clinical aspects. *Semin Arthritis Rheum* 1990; 20:81–96

123. Lockshin MD. New perspectives in the study and treatment of the antiphospholipid syndrome. In Asherson RA, Cervera R, Piette J-C, Shoenfeld Y, eds. *The Antiphospholipid Syndrome*. CRC Press: Boca Raton, 1996:323–9

124. Branch DW, Scott JR, Kochenour NK, *et al*. Obstetric complications associated with the lupus anticoagulant. *N Engl J Med* 1985;313:1322–6

125. Triplett DA, Brandt JT, Musgrave KA, *et al*. The relationship between lupus anticoagulants and antibodies to phospholipid. *J Am Med Assoc* 1988;259:550–4

126. Koskela P, Vaarala O, Mäkitalo R, *et al*. Significance of false positive syphilis reactions and anticardiolipin antibodies in a nationwide series of pregnant women. *J Rheumatol* 1988;15:70–3

127. McNeil HP, Simpson RJ, Chesterman CN, *et al*. Antiphospholipid antibodies are directed against a complex antigen that includes a lipid-binding inhibitor of coagulation: β2-glycoprotein I (apolipoprotein H). *Proc Natl Acad Sci USA* 1990;87:4120–4

128. Asherson RA, Khamashta MA, Ordi-Ros J, *et al*. The "primary" antiphospholipid syndrome: major clinical and serological features. *Medicine (Baltimore)* 1989; 68:366–74

129. Alarcón-Segovia D, Pérez-Vázquez ME, Villa AR, *et al*. Preliminary classification criteria for the antiphospholipid syndrome within systemic lupus erythematosus. *Semin Arthritis Rheum* 1992;21:275–86

130. Vianna JL, Khamashta MA, Ordi-Ros J, *et al*. Comparison of the primary and secondary antiphospholipid syndrome: A European Multicenter Study of 114 patients. *Am J Med* 1994;96:3–9

131. Khamashta MA, Harris EN, Gharavi AE, *et al*. Immune mediated mechanism for thrombosis: antiphospholipid antibody binding to platelet membranes. *Ann Rheum Dis* 1988;47:849–54

132. Qamar T, Levy RA, Sammaritano L, *et al*. Characteristics of high-titer IgG antiphospholipid antibody in systemic lupus erythematosus patients with and without fetal death. *Arthritis Rheum* 1990;33:501–4

133. Wang M-X, Kandiah DA, Ichikawa K, *et al*. Epitope specificity of monoclonal anti-β₂-glycoprotein I antibodies derived from patients with the antiphospholipid syndrome. *J Immunol* 1995;155:1629–36

134. Katano K, Aoki K, Sasa H, *et al*. β₂-glycoprotein I-dependent anticardiolipin antibodies as a predictor of adverse pregnancy outcomes in healthy pregnant women. *Hum Reprod* 1996;11:509–12

135. Peaceman AM, Silver RK, MacGregor SN, *et al*. Interlaboratory variation in antiphospholipid testing. *Am J Obstet Gynecol* 1992;166:1780–7

136. Reber G, Arvieux J, Comby E, *et al*. Multicenter evaluation of nine commercial kits for the quantitation of anticardiolipin antibodies. *Thromb Haemost* 1995; 73:444–52

137. Mueh JR, Herbst KD, Rapaport SI. Thrombosis in patients with the lupus anticoagulant. *Ann Intern Med* 1980;92:156–9

138. Boey ML, Colaco CB, Gharavi AE, *et al*. Thrombosis in systemic lupus erythematosus: striking association with the presence of circulating lupus anticoagulant. *Br Med J* 1983;287:1021–3

139. Angles-Cano E, Sultan Y, Clauvel JP. Predisposing factors to thrombosis in systemic lupus erythematosus: possible relation to endothelial cell damage. *J Lab Clin Med* 1979;94:312–23

140. Nakamura N, Shidara Y, Kawaguchi N, *et al*. Lupus anticoagulant autoantibody induces apoptosis in umbilical vein endothelial cells: involvement of annexin V. *Biochem Biophys Res Commun* 1994;205:1488–93

141. Meroni PL, Del Papa N, Gambini D, *et al*. Antiphospholipid antibodies and endothelial cells: an unending story. *Lupus* 1995;4:169–71

142. Le Tonquèze M, Salozhin K, Dueymes M, *et al*. Role of ß₂-glycoprotein I in the antiphospholipid antibody binding to endothelial cells. *Lupus* 1995;4:179–86

143. Simantov R, La Sala JM, Lo SK, *et al*. Activation of cultured vascular endothelial cells by antiphospholipid antibodies. *J Clin Invest* 1995;96:2211–9

144. Del Papa N, Guidali L, Spatola L, *et al*. Relationship between antiphospholipid and antiendothelial cell antibodies. III. ß₂-glycoprotein I mediates the antibody binding to endothelial membranes and induces the expression of adhesion molecules. *Clin Exp Rheumatol* 1995;13:179–85

145. Casiola-Rosen L, Rosen A, Petri M, Schlissel M. Surface blebs on apoptotic cells are sites of enhanced procoagulant activity: implications for coagulation events and antigenic spread in systemic lupus erythematosus. *Proc Natl Acad Sci USA* 1996;93:1624–9

146. Barquinero J, Ordiros J, Selva A, *et al*. Antibodies against platelet-activating factor in patients with antiphospholipid antibodies. *Lupus* 1994;3:55–8

147. Vazquez-Mellado J, Llorente L, Richaud-Patin Y, *et al*. Exposure of anionic phospholipids upon platelet activation permits binding of beta-2 glycoprotein I and through it that of IgG antiphospholipid antibodies: studies in platelets from patients with antiphospholipid antibody syndrome and normal subjects. *J Autoimmunol* 1994;7:335–48

148. Tokita S, Arai M, Yamamoto N, *et al*. Specific cross-reaction of IgG antiphospholipid antibody with platelet glycoprotein IIIA. *Thromb Haemostasis* 1996; 75:168–74

149. La Rosa L, Meroni PL, Tincani A, *et al*. Beta2 glyco-protein I and placental anticoagulant protein I in placentae from patients with antiphospholipid syndrome. *J Rheumatol* 1994;21:1684–93

150. Katano K, Aoki K, Ogasawara M, *et al*. Specific antiphospholipid antibodies (aPL) eluted from placentae of pregnant women with aPL-positive sera. *Lupus* 1995;4:304–8

151. Carreras LO, Defreyn G, Machin SJ, *et al*. Arterial thrombosis, intrauterine death and "lupus" anticoagulant: detection of immunoglobulin interfering with prostacyclin formation. *Lancet* 1981;1:244–6

152. Cariou R, Tobelem G, Soria C, *et al*. Inhibition of protein C activation by endothelial cells in the presence of lupus anticoagulant. *N Engl J Med* 1986;314:1193–4

153. Lockshin MD, Druzin ML, Qamar T. Prednisone does not prevent recurrent fetal death in women with antiphospholipid antibody. *Am J Obstet Gynecol* 1989; 160:439–43

154. Balasch J, Carmona F, López-Soto A, *et al*. Low-dose aspirin for prevention of pregnancy losses in women with primary antiphospholipid syndrome. *Hum Reprod* 1993;8:2234–9

155. Kutteh WH. Antiphospholipid antibody-associated recurrent pregnancy loss: Treatment with heparin and low-dose aspirin is superior to low-dose aspirin alone. *Am J Obstet Gynecol* 1996;174:1584–9

156. Kutteh WH, Ermel LD. A clinical-trial for the treatment of antiphospholipid antibody-associated recurrent pregnancy loss with lower dose heparin and aspirin. *Am J Reprod Immunol* 1996;35:402–7

157. Cowchock FS, Reece EA, Balaban D, *et al*. Repeated fetal losses associated with antiphospholipid antibodies: a collaborative randomized trial comparing prednisone with low-dose heparin treatment. *Am J Obstet Gynecol* 1992;166:1318–23

158. Silver RK, MacGregor SN, Sholl JS, *et al*. Comparative trial of prednisone plus aspirin versus aspirin alone in the treatment of anticardiolipin antibody-positive obstetric patients. *Am J Obstet Gynecol* 1993;169:1411–17

159. Melk A, Mueller-Eckhardt G, Polten B, *et al*. Diagnostic and prognostic significance of anticardiolipin antibodies in patients with recurrent spontaneous abortions. *Am J Reprod Immunol* 1995;33:228–33

160. Lockwood CJ, Romero R, Feinberg RF, *et al*. The prevalence and biologic significance of lupus anticoagulant and anticardiolipin antibodies in a general obstetric population. *Am J Obstet Gynecol* 1989;161:369–73

161. Harris EN, Spinnato J. Should sera of healthy pregnant women be screened for anticardiolipin antibodies? *Arthritis Rheum* 1990;33:S28(Abstr)

162. Silver RM, Porter TF, van Leeuwen I, *et al*. Anticardiolipin antibodies: clinical consequences of "low titers". *Obstet Gynecol* 1996;87:494–500

163. Lubbe WF, Butler WS, Palmer SJ, *et al*. Lupus anticoagulant in pregnancy. *Br J Obstet Gynaecol* 1984;91: 357–63

164. Reece EA, Gambrielli S, Cullen MT, *et al*. Recurrent adverse pregnancy outcome and antiphospholipid antibodies. *Am J Obstet Gynecol* 1990;163:162–9

165. Makar A Ph, Vanderhayden JS, Verheyen A. Maternal and fetal complications associating lupus anticoagulant and its management; three case reports. *Eur J Obstet Gynecol Reprod Biol* 1990;36:185–95

166. Silver RM, Draper ML, Scott JR, *et al*. Clinical consequences of antiphospholipid antibodies: an historic cohort study. *Obstet Gynecol* 1994;83:372–77

167. Rai RS, Clifford K, Cohen H, *et al*. High prospective fetal loss rate in untreated pregnancies of women with recurrent miscarriage and antiphospholipid antibodies. *Hum Reprod* 1995;10:3301–4

168. McCrae KR, DeMichele AM, Pandhi P, *et al*. Detection of antitrophoblast antibodies in the sera of patients with anticardiolipin antibodies and fetal loss. *Blood* 1993;82:2730–41

169. Sheridan-Pereira M, Porreco RP, Hays T, *et al*. Neonatal aortic thrombosis associated with lupus anticoagulant. *Obstet Gynecol* 1988;71:1016–18

170. Branch DW, Andres R, Digre KB, *et al*. The association of antiphospholipid antibodies with severe preeclampsia. *Obstet Gynecol* 1989;73:541–5

171. Bendon RW, Wilson J, Getahun B, *et al*. A maternal death due to thrombotic disease associated with anticardiolipin antibody. *Arch Pathol Lab Med* 1987;111:370–3

172. Rallings P, Exner T, Abraham R. Coronary artery vasculitis and myocardial infarction associated with antiphospholipid antibodies in a pregnant woman. *Aust N Z J Med* 1989;19:347–50

173. Kochenour NK, Branch DW, Rote NS, *et al*. A new postpartum syndrome associated with antiphospholipid antibodies. *Obstet Gynecol* 1987;69:460–8

174. Ayres MA, Sulak PJ. Pregnancy complicated by antiphospholipid antibodies. *So Med J* 1991;84:266–9

175. Petrie M. The clinical syndrome associated with anti-phospholipid antibodies. *J Rheumatol* 1992; 19:505–7

176. Rosove MH, Tabsh K, Wasserstrum N, *et al*. Heparin therapy for pregnant women with lupus anticoagulant or anticardiolipin antibodies. *Obstet Gynecol* 1990; 75:630–4

177. Stafford-Brady FJ, Gladman DD, Urowitz MB. Successful pregnancy in systemic lupus erythematosus with an untreated lupus anticoagulant. *Arch Int Med* 1988;148:1647–8

178. Ermel LD, Marshburn PB, Kutteh WH. Interaction of heparin with antiphospholipid antibodies (APA) from the sera of women with recurrent pregnancy loss (RPL). *Am J Reprod Immunol* 1995;33:14–20

179. Scott JR, Branch DW, Kochenour NK, *et al*. Intravenous immunoglobulin treatment of pregnant patients with recurrent pregnancy loss caused by antiphospholipid antibodies and Rh immunization. *Am J Obstet Gynecol* 1988;159:1055–6

180. Spinatto JA, Clark AL, Pierangelli SS, *et al*. Intravenous immunoglobulin therapy for the antiphospholipid syndrome in pregnancy. *Am J Obstet Gynecol* 1995;172: 690–4

181. The Pregnancy Loss Study Group. A multi-center randomized double blind pilot study of IVIG therapy

during pregnancy in women with antiphospholipid syndrome. *Lupus* 1998;7(suppl. 2):S196(Abstract)

182. Plotz PH, Dalakas M, Leff RL, *et al*. Current concepts in the idiopathic inflammatory myopathies: polymyositis, dermatomyositis, and related disease. NIHD Conference. *Ann Intern Med* 1989;111:143–57

183. Bunch TW: Polymyositis: A case history approach to the differential diagnosis and treatment. *Mayo Clin Proc* 1990;65:1480–97

184. Gutierrez G, Dagnino R, Mintz G. Polymyositis/dermatomyositis and pregnancy. *Arthritis Rheum* 1984;27:291–4

185. Rosenzweig BA, Rotmensch S, Binette SP, *et al*. Primary idiopathic polymyositis and dermatomyositis complicating pregnancy: diagnosis and management. *Obstet Gynecol Surv* 1989;44:162–70

186. Mintz G. Dermatomyositis. *Rheum Dis Clin North Am* 1989;15:375–82

187. Pinheiro GDC, Goldenberg J, Atra E, *et al*. Juvenile dermatomyositis and pregnancy: report and literature review. *J Rheumatol* 1992;19:1798–801

188. Ohno T, Imai A, Tamaya T. Successful outcomes of pregnancy complicated with dermatomyositis: case reports. *Gynecol Obstet Invest* 1992;33:187–9

189. Tsai A, Lindheimer MD, Lamberg SI. Dermatomyositis complicating pregnancy. *Obstet Gynecol* 1973;41:570–3

190. Bauer KA, Siegler M, Lindheimer MA. Polymyositis complicating pregnancy. *Arch Intern Med* 1979;139:449

191. Katz AL. Another case of polymyositis in pregnancy (Letter). *Arch Intern Med* 1980;140:1123

192. Ditzian-Kadanoff R, Reinhard JD, Thomas C, *et al*. Polymyositis with myoglobinuria in pregnancy: a report and review of the literature. *J Rheumatol* 1988;15:513–4

193. England MJ, Perlmann T, Veriava Y. Dermatomyositis in pregnancy. A case report. *J Reprod Med* 1986;31:633–6

194. Luggen M, Belhorn L, Evans T, *et al*. The evolution of Raynaud's phenomenon: A longterm prospective study. *J Rheumatol* 1995;22:2226–32

195. Masi AT. Clinical-epidemiologic perspective of systemic sclerosis (scleroderma). In Jayson MIV, Black CM, eds. *Systemic Sclerosis-Scleroderma*. Sussex, England: John Wiley and Sons Ltd, 1988:7–31

196. Ballou SP, Morley JJ, Kushner I. Pregnancy and systemic sclerosis. *Arthritis Rheum* 1984;27:295–8

197. Kitridou RC. Pregnancy in mixed connective tissue disease, poly/dermatomysitis and scleroderma. *Clin Exp Rheumatol* 1988;6:173–8

198. Siamopoulou-Mavridou A, Manoussakis MN, Mavridis AK, *et al*. Outcome of pregnancy in patients with autoimmune rheumatic disease before the disease onset. *Ann Rheum Dis* 1988;47:982–7

199. Steen VD, Conte C, Day N, *et al*. Pregnancy in women with systemic sclerosis. *Arthritis Rheum* 1989;32:151–7

200. Black CM, Stevens WM. Scleroderma. *Rheum Dis Clin North Am* 1989;15:193–212

201. Giordano M, Valentini G, Lupoli S, *et al*. Pregnancy and systemic sclerosis (Letter). *Arthritis Rheum* 1985;28:237–8

202. Silman AJ, Black C. Increased incidence of spontaneous abortion and infertility in women with scleroderma before disease onset: a controlled study. *Ann Rheum Dis* 1988;47:441–4

203. McHugh NJ, Reilly PA, McHugh LA. Pregnancy outcome and autoantibodies in connective tissue disease. *J Rheumatol* 1989;16:42–6

204. Kahl LE, Blair C, Ramsey-Goldman R, *et al*. Pregnancy outcomes in women with primary Raynaud's phenomenon. *Arthritis Rheum* 1990;33:1249–55

205. Englert H, Brennan P, McNeil D, *et al*. Reproductive function prior to disease onset in women with scleroderma. *J Rheumatol* 1992;19:1575–9

Section V

Maternal surgical disorders

46

Acute abdomen in pregnancy

W.L. Holcomb, Jr

INTRODUCTION

The obstetrician must often evaluate acute abdominal pain during pregnancy. It is known that about one in 500 pregnancies is complicated by a laparotomy for non-obstetric reasons[1,2]. Many other patients receive non-operative treatment or are observed. Care for the pregnant patient with abdominal pain presents three particular challenges: diagnostic findings may be altered by pregnancy; conditions unique to pregnancy may be present; and the effects of the disease and the therapy on the fetus must be considered.

In general, the recommended treatment for conditions causing acute abdominal pain is the same during pregnancy as it is in the non-gravid state. The major effect of pregnancy is to obscure the diagnosis. Care of the pregnant woman should not be compromised for fear of harm to the fetus. With rare exception, the fetus is best served by prompt diagnosis and treatment for the mother. An approach to the patient with acute abdominal pain will be discussed, followed by consideration of selected diseases in which prompt diagnosis may be life-saving. Pregnancy-associated conditions that are well known to obstetricians (e.g. ectopic pregnancy, placental abruption, uterine rupture) will not be considered in this chapter.

GENERAL APPROACH TO THE PATIENT

'Acute abdominal pain' specifies a clinical situation and not a distinct pathophysiological entity. Distinguishing the multitude of possible causes, often associated with overlapping signs and symptoms, is difficult. It has been shown that physicians adopt a small set of hypotheses early in the process of evaluating a patient's complaint. Subsequent history-taking, physical examination and test ordering proceed in a manner to test the chosen hypotheses[3]. The causes of acute abdominal pain are legion. A potential pitfall is failure to consider a sufficiently broad differential diagnosis.

A helpful method for developing diagnostic hypotheses in patients with abdominal pain is to categorize diseases according to anatomical sites (Table 1). Some conditions do not lend themselves to anatomical assignment and are called 'non-anatomical'. A further pathophysiological subclassification may also be useful.

Table 1 Causes of acute abdominal pain in pregnancy

Bowel	Spleen
appendicitis	rupture
colonic perforation	Pancreas
colonic pseudo-obstruction	pancreatitis
duodenal perforation	pseudocyst
duodenal ulcer	Urinary tract
gastroenteritis	pyelonephritis
herniation	rupture of renal pelvis
intussusception	ureteral calculus
Meckel's diverticulitis	ureteral obstruction
obstruction (small or	Adnexae
large bowel)	abscess
superior mesenteric	adnexal torsion
artery syndrome	ectopic pregnancy
thrombosis/infarction	ovarian rupture
toxic megacolon	salpingitis
Stomach	Uterus/placenta
gastritis	chorioamnionitis
ulcer	placenta percreta
Lungs	placental abruption
pneumonia	preterm labor
pulmonary embolism	uterine myomata
Liver	uterine rupture
acute fatty liver	Non-anatomic
hepatitis	acute intermittent
rupture	porphyria
subcapsular hemorrhage	diabetic ketoacidosis
Gallbladder	pre-eclampsia
cholecystitis	sickle cell disease
cholelithiasis	
empyema	
perforation	

Pain may be due to inflammation (e.g. perforated viscus, cholecystitis), distension (e.g. bowel obstruction, ureteral calculus), hemorrhage (e.g. ruptured tubal pregnancy, ruptured spleen), ischemia (e.g. adnexal torsion, mesenteric thrombosis) or a metabolic disorder (e.g. porphyria, diabetic ketoacidosis). In some conditions, more than one mechanism applies.

A thorough history should include questions about the onset, character, duration, progression and severity of the pain, as well as query about any associated symptoms. Nausea, vomiting, anorexia, constipation, abdominal discomfort and urinary frequency are common symptoms in pregnancy. In effect, they constitute background noise in which the diagnostic signal must be detected. It is helpful to focus on any recent change in symptoms, or the sudden appearance of symptoms at an unexpected stage in pregnancy. For instance, nausea and vomiting are primarily first-trimester problems for pregnant women; they should be viewed warily when appearing later in gestation.

Pregnant patients may have less prominent physical findings than those who are non-pregnant with the same disease process[4,5]. For example, direct tenderness, rebound tenderness and rigidity of the abdominal muscles are important signs of appendicitis. Unfortunately, peritoneal signs are often absent in pregnancy, despite obvious pathology at laparotomy. The psoas sign (internal rotation of the flexed hip) and rectal examination may be informative in the diagnosis of appendicitis during pregnancy, especially in the first trimester. Later in pregnancy, the gravid uterus often displaces the appendix superiorly, eliminating these signs. In the third trimester, direct tenderness may be elicited instead in the right upper quadrant. Examination of the patient in the left or right lateral decubitus position may help to distinguish uterine from extrauterine tenderness. Such shifts in position can separate the uterus from the surrounding structures. Pressure on the left side of the gravid uterus may cause right-sided pain in a patient with appendicitis (modified Rovsing's sign).

Laboratory tests commonly ordered for patients with acute abdominal pain, and any changes in results normally expected during pregnancy, are listed in Table 2. For some conditions, such as pyelonephritis, hepatitis or pancreatitis, the results of laboratory tests may be diagnostic. Most conditions, however, are associated with changes in laboratory values that are too insensitive or non-specific to aid substantially in diagnosis.

Electronic fetal heart-rate and uterine-contraction monitoring are important in the care of patients with acute abdominal pain during the third trimester. The fetal heart-monitor pattern is a sensitive guide to fetal well-being and to maternal organ perfusion. An abnormal tracing may be the first clue to an obstetric cause for the symptoms, such as placental abruption. Preterm labor may complicate any of the conditions causing acute abdominal pain. Early detection of abnormal preterm uterine contractions allows for appropriate preparedness or intervention. The increased risk of preterm labor is present for at least several days following emergency laparotomy.

Information gained from obstetric ultrasonography may be helpful in the management of a patient with acute abdominal pain. Fetal measurements aid in estimating gestational age. Major fetal structural abnormalities or malpresentations may be diagnosed. Such knowledge will influence decisions about the timing or mode of delivery should labor begin. Uterine

Table 2 Changes in laboratory test results expected in pregnancy

Test	Result
Hemoglobin	decreased
Hematocrit	decreased
White-blood-cell count	increased
Differential white-blood-cell count	increased neutrophils
Platelet count	unchanged
Electrolytes (serum)	decreased CO_2
Glucose (fasting)	decreased
Creatinine (serum)	decreased
Amylase	slightly increased
Aspartate aminotransferase	unchanged
Alanine aminotransferase	unchanged
Alkaline phosphatase	increased
γ-Glutamyl transpeptidase	unchanged
Urinalysis	unchanged
Arterial blood gas	decreased P_{CO_2}; slightly increased pH

leiomyomata, a possible source of acute pain and localized tenderness, or adnexal masses may be identified.

Sonographic examination of the maternal gallbladder, pancreas and kidneys may aid in differential diagnosis[6]. In non-pregnant patients, ultrasound with graded compression has been used for the diagnosis of appendicitis[7]. The superior displacement of the appendix and reluctance to compress the gravid abdomen limit this approach during pregnancy, though some have reported excellent diagnostic accuracy[8]. Therapeutic options are expanded by the availability of ultrasound-directed percutaneous urinary and biliary tract drainage procedures, as well as appendiceal abscess drainage in selected patients[9]. The use of ultrasound guidance enhances the safety of diagnostic amniocentesis. Information about fetal lung maturity and evidence of intrauterine infection may be critical for the management of some patients.

Abdominal plain films and chest films are useful for the evaluation of pneumonic processes, intestinal obstruction and the presence of free intraperitoneal air. Intravenous pyelography may be essential to assess ureteral obstruction in occasional cases. If necessary, diagnostic radiography should not be avoided for fear of fetal exposure. Fetal effects have not been conclusively proven at less than 5–10 rad, well in excess of the absorbed dose with standard diagnostic procedures. However, there are lingering concerns about the association between prenatal radiation exposure and childhood cancers; therefore, all else being equal, it is best to minimize the use of ionizing radiation[10]. Often, alternative diagnostic methods may be used (e.g. ultrasound or magnetic resonance imaging), or radiation may be limited by shielding the uterus and planning exposures carefully. The value of abdominal computed tomography for the pregnant patient with acute abdominal pain is uncertain. It may be useful in selected cases; the radiation dose (about 1 rad) is not prohibitive.

Appropriate therapy depends on a specific diagnosis, but a few generalizations are possible. Indications for emergency laparotomy are no different for the pregnant patient than for other patients. Elective procedures (e.g. cholecystectomy for uncomplicated gallstones) should be deferred until after the pregnancy unless there is a clear benefit from earlier intervention. The second trimester appears to be the best time for elective procedures that need be performed during pregnancy. The decision to perform a Cesarean delivery is separate from the decision to perform an exploratory laparotomy. Usually, a successful vaginal delivery can be accomplished, even when labor begins in the early postoperative period. Abdominal delivery is warranted only if obstetrically indicated or if essential for adequate surgical exposure.

The greatest threat to the fetus associated with acute intra-abdominal disease seems to be that of preterm labor and delivery. Quantification of this risk is difficult, given the retrospective and incomplete data available for analysis. There is evidence that severity of disease is the major determinant of risk[1,2,11]. The use of tocolytic agents for patients with abdominal emergencies in pregnancy has not been studied prospectively. Benefits of such therapy must be weighed against the risks in each case. In one study, administration of tocolytic agents was associated with an increased risk of pulmonary injury among pregnant women with appendicitis[12]. It should be certain that contraindications, such as a large placental abruption or intrauterine infection, are not present before tocolytic therapy is instituted. Magnesium sulfate has less cardiovascular effect than β-mimetic adrenergic agents and may be a better choice for patients with uncertain diagnoses. The efficacy of prophylactic therapy with tocolytic agents remains unproven. If preterm delivery appears likely, glucocorticoid administration may be considered in order to decrease the risk of neonatal complications. Glucocorticoids should not be given for this purpose if the mother is at high risk for infectious complications (e.g. if she has appendicitis). Some items to consider before proceeding with operative intervention during pregnancy are summarized in Table 3.

SOME SPECIFIC DISORDERS

Appendicitis

Occurrence

Appendicitis is the most common non-obstetric surgical emergency in pregnancy with case : delivery ratios ranging from approximately 1 : 2000 to approximately

Table 3 Preoperative checklist for the pregnant patient

Adequate preoperative stabilization
Differential diagnosis
Positioning of the patient
Type of anesthesia
Antibiotics, if indicated
Availability of blood products
Rh immunoglobulin, if indicated
Availability of consultants (e.g. surgical, pediatric)
Tocolytic agent, if indicated
Fetal monitoring, if appropriate
Concomitant delivery, if indicated
Special needs (e.g. insulin, corticosteroids)

1 : 6000[4,13–15]. Pregnancy has no apparent effect on the overall incidence of disease, although the severity may be increased. Cases have been reported throughout gestation and in the puerperium. Occurrence in the mid-trimester seems to be more common for reasons that are unclear[5,13–21].

Symptoms

During pregnancy, as in the non-pregnant state, the symptoms of appendicitis are abdominal pain, nausea, vomiting and anorexia. Pain is almost always present. In early gestation, the pain is usually in the right lower quadrant. As pregnancy advances beyond 20 weeks, the appendix rises above the level of the umbilicus. In later gestation, pain is likely to be diffuse or located in the right upper quadrant[5,13,14,16,17]. Confusion with renal disease or gallbladder disease is possible. About two-thirds of pregnant patients with appendicitis complain of vomiting at presentation[13,16,17,20]. Those without vomiting will frequently, but not always, have nausea[5,13,14]. Anorexia is often considered a *sine qua non* for appendicitis outside of pregnancy. During pregnancy, between one-third and two-thirds of patients with appendicitis lack this symptom[5,13,14,21].

Signs

Direct abdominal tenderness is the most constant physical finding among pregnant patients with appendicitis. Only rarely is this finding absent[5,16]. In the first trimester, tenderness is usually well localized in the right lower quadrant. With advancing gestation, it is common to find tenderness in the right periumbilical area or right upper quadrant, or more diffuse tenderness. About 55–75% of patients have demonstrable rebound tenderness[5,13,14,16,20]. One-half to two-thirds of patients have abdominal muscle rigidity[5,13,14,16,17,20]. Rovsing's sign is present approximately equally in pregnant as in non-pregnant patients with appendicitis. Psoas irritation is less frequently observed in pregnancy[21]. Rectal examination is often overlooked in the pregnant patient with appendicitis, but one group has found that tenderness is usually present, especially in the first trimester[5]. Fever and tachycardia are variably present and are not sensitive signs for appendicitis in pregnancy.

Diagnostic aids

The physiological leukocytosis (as high as 15 000/mm³) during pregnancy and the wide range of normal values limit the usefulness of the leukocyte count for the diagnosis of appendicitis[13]. Severe disease may be present when the leukocyte count is normal[20]. Greater than 80% polymorphonuclear leukocytes are often present when appendicitis complicates pregnancy[5,13]. Again, however, the test is not sufficiently sensitive to rule out disease and it discriminates poorly between those patients with and those without appendicitis. Ten to twenty per cent of pregnant patients with appendicitis have an abnormal urinalysis, usually showing pyuria alone[5,14]. Bacteriuria indicates a urinary tract infection. Asymptomatic bacteriuria is common enough in pregnancy that it may well occur coincidentally with appendicitis[4]. Imaging techniques have not been shown to be of help in ruling out appendicitis during pregnancy, with the possible exception of sonography in some centers[8]. With severe disease, an upright abdominal film may show a right-sided mass or intraperitoneal free air.

Treatment

The treatment of appendicitis is surgical and should be undertaken as soon as the diagnosis is seriously suspected. In most patients the appendix is removed, but simple drainage may be appropriate for some patients with abscesses. If the appendix appears normal at laparotomy, there is a solid rationale for removing it. First, early disease may be present despite the grossly normal appearance[22]. Second, diagnostic confusion may be avoided should the symptoms recur. Broad-spectrum antibiotic coverage is warranted if the appendix is perforated. Some surgeons leave the wound open above the fascia to prevent wound infection in such cases.

In choosing an incision, the surgeon must consider the variable location of the appendix, the possibility of other unsuspected pathology and the need for adequate exposure. A guide to the location of the appendix is the point of maximal tenderness. Most authors recommend a right mid-tranverse incision directly over this point[4]. Cunningham and McCubbin[5] advocate a low abdominal midline incision to accommodate unexpected surgical findings and Cesarean delivery, if indicated. An approach tailored to the clinical situation may be preferable to a rigid policy. Tilting the operating table 30° to the patient's left will help bring the uterus away from the surgical site and will improve maternal venous cardiac return as well. Laparoscopic appendectomy has been performed in pregnancy at up to 25 weeks' gestation[23]. Experience with this approach is, as yet, quite limited.

Course

Perforation and abscess formation are more likely to complicate appendicitis in the pregnant patient[20]. Some investigators have found a trend toward increasing severity of disease in the third trimester[5]; others have not[13,14]. Any effect may be due to difficulty of diagnosis and delay in therapy. The frequency of generalized peritonitis is directly related to the interval from the time of onset of symptoms to the time of operation[18]. Risks of fetal and maternal mortality and morbidity are increased once perforation has occurred[16].

Acute cholecystitis

Occurrence

Gallbladder disease is four times as common among women of reproductive age as it is among men of the same age. Estimates of the occurrence of acute cholecystitis in pregnancy vary widely, with case : delivery ratios lying between 1 : 1130 and 1 : 12 890[24,25]. Asymptomatic disease is much more common, since about 3–4% of pregnant women have demonstrable gallstones[26]. The mean weight among a series of 20 gravid patients undergoing cholecystectomy was 71 kg, suggesting that obesity is not strongly related to symptomatic disease in pregnancy[24]. Chronic hemolytic conditions, such as sickle cell disease, increase the risk of gallstone formation.

Symptoms and signs

As in the non-pregnant patient, the most reliable symptom is right upper quadrant pain. About half of the patients have vomiting and a minority are febrile[25]. Patients will often give a history of previous similar episodes. Right upper quadrant direct tenderness is usually present, but, in the absence of complications, rebound tenderness is rare. The pain may radiate to the back. In the occasional patient there is a palpable gallbladder.

Cholecystitis may be confused with appendicitis, particularly in the third trimester. Landers and colleagues[25] reported a woman at 30 weeks' gestation who underwent laparotomy to rule out appendicitis. The appendix was normal, but she developed *Salmonella* sepsis postoperatively. The gallbladder was found to be the source of the organism when she subsequently returned to the operating room for cholecystectomy.

Diagnostic aids

Gallstones are present in more than 95% of patients with cholecystitis. Ultrasonography has been found to be extremely accurate in the diagnosis of cholelithiasis.

Since this modality does not require ionizing radiation, it is preferred in pregnancy. If additional diagnostic information is needed for clinical management, the radiation dose of a radionucleatide scan of the gall-bladder is not prohibitive.

Blood tests are of limited diagnostic value for the patient suspected to have cholecystitis. Leukocytosis may be present, but it is neither a sensitive nor a specific marker. Serum alkaline phosphatase is normally elevated in pregnancy. A high value should not be taken as evidence of cholestasis. Other hepatic enzymes, such as aspartate transferase and alanine transferase, may be helpful in distinguishing cholecystitis from hepatitis. Transient elevation of the serum amylase level may be seen in up to one-third of patients[27,28]. A markedly elevated serum amylase level suggests pancreatitis, which may complicate the course of gallbladder disease. Occasionally, a patient may be jaundiced with an elevated bilirubin level. If the patient has had persistent vomiting, evaluation of electrolyte status is essential.

Treatment

Initial treatment for the pregnant patient with uncomplicated acute cholecystitis is supportive. Intravenous fluids should be given to prevent dehydration. Nasogastric suction is appropriate if there has been significant vomiting. Analgesia may be given as needed. Meperidine is preferred to morphine, as the latter may produce spasm of the sphincter of Oddi. Since early cholecystitis is a sterile process, antibiotics are often unnecessary. If symptoms are persistent, or if systemic or local signs are prominent, broad-spectrum antibiotic coverage is warranted[29]. Patients who fail to respond to conservative measures, or who have recurrent bouts of illness, are candidates for surgery. Selected patients may be considered for a percutaneous drainage procedure in order to defer definitive therapy[30].

The patient who responds promptly to supportive therapy may be observed, with hope of avoiding an operation during pregnancy, or may be scheduled for an elective cholecystectomy. A prospective comparison of these treatment strategies is unavailable. Many authors favor the former approach, but the latter has proponents[31,32]. Medical therapy is associated with a high risk of relapse, often requiring hospitalization prior to delivery[32]. If there is choice about the timing of cholecystectomy, the second trimester seems to be the interval when fetal complications are minimized.

Though once considered contraindicated, there is a growing body of literature supporting the safety of laparoscopic cholecystectomy during pregnancy[33,34]. The procedure is usually performed in the second trimester, but a few cases have been reported in the first and third trimesters. Endoscopic retrograde cholangiopancreatography with papillotomy and stone extraction may also be performed during pregnancy[35–37]. Candidates for this procedure would be those with known or suspected calculous obstruction of the biliary duct. Fetal irradiation can be minimized by uterine shielding and limitation of fluoroscopy time.

Course

Acute cholecystitis may be complicated by empyema, perforation, pancreatitis or failure to respond to medical management. Among patients managed conservatively during pregnancy, 62–84% may be carried through to delivery without operation[25,27,28]. In the series reported by Landers and co-workers[25], medical therapy was deemed to have failed if symptoms persisted beyond the 4th day in the hospital, or if there were more than three recurrences in the same trimester. Pleading against excessive conservatism, Dixon and colleagues[31] cited two cases in which patients required total parenteral nutrition for 27 and 30 days, respectively. One of these patients developed pancreatitis. Fifteen of 26 patients in their series had recurrent episodes of biliary colic during pregnancy[31]. Data from published series are often incomplete, but perinatal outcome appears to be favorable if disease is uncomplicated or if surgical treatment is effected in the second trimester[24,27,28,31].

Pancreatitis

Occurrence

Pancreatitis is an unusual, but potentially devastating, complication of pregnancy that may present with acute abdominal pain. In more recent series, case : delivery ratios range from 1 : 1289 to 1 : 3333[38–41]. Pregnancy may predispose women to the development of pancreatitis, but this notion is poorly substantiated and controversial[38,39,42,43]. Recognized risk factors for pancreatitis include cholelithiasis, alcohol use, hyperlipidemia, hyperparathyroidism, abdominal trauma, viral infections and certain drugs (particularly diuretics). The presence of gallstones is the most common etiology among pregnant patients; they are found in up to 90% of cases[40–42,44].

Symptoms and signs

The presentation of pancreatitis is similar in the pregnant and the non-pregnant patient. Among cases reviewed by Wilkinson[40], 75% presented with acute abdominal pain. Typically, the pain is of sudden onset and located in the epigastrium. Nausea and vomiting are usually present and may be severe. Very ill patients may present in shock. Generally, the patient is in acute distress. There may be a low-grade fever and a few patients are jaundiced. Epigastric tenderness is the most reliable physical finding. Peritoneal signs are absent or minimal. Bowel sounds are diminished. With severe hemorrhagic pancreatitis, blood may infiltrate the flanks (Grey Turner's sign) or the umbilicus (Cullen's sign).

Laboratory aids

The serum amylase level is the most useful aid for the diagnosis of pancreatitis. Serum concentration rises rapidly following the onset of disease and often declines into the normal range after about 48 h. The enzyme is rapidly excreted by the kidneys. Elevated levels may be detected in a 24-hour urine specimen after the serum peak is past. There have been conflicting reports about the behavior of amylase levels in normal pregnancy. Levels seem to be increased in pregnancy, but not more than twice the upper limit of normal[45,46]. Slight elevations, therefore, must be interpreted with caution. Elevations of serum amylase also may be seen with intestinal perforation, infarction or obstruction, and a variety of other conditions.

Other laboratory findings may be hypoglycemia (sometimes severe), hyperglycemia, hyperbilirubinemia, hypocalcemia, hemoconcentration and electrolyte derangements. Imaging procedures are of limited usefulness for the patient with suspected pancreatitis in pregnancy. Upper abdominal ultrasonography may yield information about concomitant gallbladder disease, but the pancreas is often not well seen. Computed tomography or magnetic resonance imaging may be of benefit in severely ill patients with a doubtful diagnosis.

Treatment

The initial treatment of pancreatitis in pregnancy is supportive and does not differ from treatment for the non-pregnant patient. Correction of hypovolemia, as well as the electrolyte, glucose and calcium disturbances, are necessary. Oral intake is withheld. If the patient has moderate or severe disease, continuous nasogatric suctioning is often instituted. Total parenteral nutrition may be used if the course of disease is prolonged[47]. If gallbladder disease is causative, cholecystectomy or endoscopic papillotomy may be considered once the patient's condition is stable[35].

Course

The mean duration of acute symptoms is about 6 days, but recovery may be prolonged and complicated[40]. Estimates of maternal mortality vary widely from 0 to 37%, probably reflecting bias in case selection and improvements in diagnosis and therapy[38,40–42,44]. In one compilation of reported cases, the perinatal mortality associated with maternal pancreatitis was estimated to be 38%[40]. More recent series indicate a better outlook with perinatal mortality of 11% or less[38,42,44]. In a recent review of 43 pregnant patients at one institution from 1983 to 1993, there were no maternal deaths, two stillbirths and one neonatal death due to prematurity[41]. As expected, the risk of perinatal death increased with severity of maternal disease.

Intestinal obstruction

Occurrence

An increasing frequency of intestinal obstruction during pregnancy has been attributed to a higher rate of intra-abdominal operations, with subsequent adhesions, among women of reproductive age. The case : delivery ratio is estimated to be between 1 : 3600 and 1 : 5700[48–50]. Cases rarely occur during the first 4 months of pregnancy, but are fairly evenly distributed thereafter and into the puerperium. A previous laparotomy, most often appendectomy or an adnexal operation, seems to be the most important risk factor. About one-half of simple intestinal obstruction during pregnancy is due to postoperative adhesions. Volvulus is the next most common condition and it, too, may be caused by adhesions. Intussusception is less common. Incarcerated inguinal or femoral hernias, or obstruction resulting from carcinoma, are exceedingly rare among pregnant patients[51].

Symptoms and signs

Abdominal pain, vomiting and constipation are symptoms expected with intestinal obstruction. Almost 90% of affected pregnant patients will have abdominal pain[50]. The pain may be constant or periodic. In the third trimester, it may be confused with the pain of labor or placental abruption. Pain may sometimes radiate to the flank, imitating that of pyelonephritis[51]. The severity of the pain may not reflect the severity of the disease[52]. Patients are often anxious and apprehensive[48]. Emesis is a highly variable symptom among patients with intestinal obstruction during pregnancy. With more proximal obstruction, vomiting appears earlier in the course of disease and is more frequent. There may be considerable delay in resumption of emesis after the first episode. Severe obstruction may be present without any vomiting[50]. Whereas constipation is a common symptom in pregnancy, complete cessation of stool and flatus is not. Such a report should strengthen suspicion for the diagnosis. With proximal obstruction, bowel movements may continue for a time following the onset of disease.

Early in the course of disease, physical findings may be subtle. The classic picture of direct abdominal tenderness, distension and high-pitched tinkling bowel sounds is the exception rather than the rule. Abdominal tenderness may be entirely absent[52]. Pressure on the uterus may cause pain when transmitted to distended bowel, misleading the clinician to suspect a uterine process. Abdominal distension is difficult to assess in late pregnancy when the risk for bowel obstruction is greatest. At presentation, bowel sounds are often described as normal[50]. In some cases, particularly with cecal volvulus, a tender cystic mass may be palpable[53,54]. Rebound tenderness, fever, tachycardia and shock are late findings[52].

Diagnostic aids

Leukocytosis may occur, but is of little help in the diagnosis of intestinal obstruction. Electrolyte abnormalities and hemoconcentration may be present if there has been prolonged emesis or if fluid has accumulated within distended bowel. There may be an elevation of serum amylase levels. Radiographic studies are often essential for diagnosis and should not be avoided out of concern for fetal effects. An upright plain film of the abdomen is the best initial study. Other studies, with or without contrast media, may also be appropriate. Sequential films may be necessary for proper evaluation of initially normal or equivocal radiological findings[52].

Treatment and course

Treatment of intestinal obstruction in pregnancy is the same as that for the non-pregnant patient. Clinical management includes correction of fluid and electrolyte deficits, decompression of bowel, relief of obstruction and resection of non-viable tissue. Prompt fluid resuscitation is especially important in pregnancy, since uterine blood flow depends upon a normal maternal blood volume. Adequate operative exposure and thorough inspection of the full length of the bowel should not be compromised. Usually, a midline abdominal incision is optimal. In some cases, it may be necessary to empty the uterus to accomplish satisfactory surgical therapy. However, this can most often be avoided[55]. As a rule, the treatment of intestinal obstruction is surgical. Selected cases of early sigmoid volvulus have been successfully treated with long-tube and rectal-tube decompression alone[56].

The obstetrician should be aware of the entity called colonic pseudo-obstruction, or Ogilvie's syndrome, which tends to occur following Cesarean section[57]. The clinical presentation is that of large bowel obstruction, but no mechanical stricture or volvulus is present. Radiographs will show marked gaseous distension of the cecum that usually extends to involve the ascending colon and transverse colon. The distal colon and rectum are gasless. Typically, there is little, if any, fluid in the distended bowel and contrast studies reveal no site of mechanical obstruction. If massive distension goes unrelieved, cecal perforation, a life-threatening complication, may occur. Treatment consists of bowel decompression by either colonoscopy or operative cecostomy[58].

Intestinal obstruction is a serious complication of pregnancy associated with maternal mortality in 10–20% and perinatal mortality in 20–30% of cases[48,55,59]. There are several recent reviews of the topic[60–62]. Intrauterine fetal death and preterm delivery are the most common perinatal complications. Diagnostic vigilance and timely therapy afford the best prospects for a favorable outcome.

Ureteral calculi

A case : delivery ratio of approximately 1 : 1600 has been estimated for symptomatic urolithiasis in pregnancy[63,64]. Stone passage seems to occur as often during pregnancy as outside of pregnancy. The causes for urolithiasis are varied. Among 78 women of reproductive age who were evaluated for urolithiasis, 42% had idiopathic hypercalciuria, 13% had hyperuricuria, 10% had primary hyperparathyroidism, 13% had infection stone, 3% had cystinuria and 19% had idiopathic lithiasis[65].

Pain, usually in the flank but sometimes in the abdomen, is almost always the presenting complaint. Nausea, vomiting, dysuria, urgency, fever or gross hematuria may be associated. About one patient in four will give a past history of urolithiasis[63,64]. Costovertebral angle tenderness is almost always present. In one series, abdominal tenderness was elicited in six of 20 patients[63]. Concomitant urinary tract infection may obscure the diagnosis of ureteral calculi.

Microscopic hematuria is found in about 75% of cases. The absence of hematuria at presentation does not rule out a stone. The patient suspected of urolithiasis should be instructed to strain her urine in search of a stone until the diagnosis is clarified. Ultrasonographic imaging of the urinary tract may be helpful in evaluation of the patient with suspected urinary calculi; the stone, or evidence of ureteral obstruction, may be apparent. Transvaginal ultrasound examination may reveal a distal ureteral calculus[66].

The urinary collecting system, particularly the right side, is often physiologically dilated in the latter half of pregnancy[67]. This effect should not be confused with ureteral obstruction. Duplex Doppler waveforms of the intrarenal arteries may help distinguish obstructed from non-obstructed collecting systems, obstruction being associated with a high resistivity index[68]. Intrarenal resistivity in pregnancy appears to be no different from that outside of pregnancy, even in the presence of physiological pelvicaliectasis[69]. Radiographic evaluation, if needed, may be accomplished with minimal radiation exposure by obtaining a plain abdominal film and a film 20–30 min after injection of contrast dye. Additional delayed films may be necessary in some cases. If urolithiasis is confirmed, a metabolic evaluation is warranted.

In planning treatment, relevant factors include the size and location of the stone, the degree of obstruction, the severity of symptoms and the presence of infection. Most calculi will pass spontaneously with hydration. If necessary, minimally invasive treatment options, such as ureteral stent placement, ureteroscopic retrieval or percutaneous nephrostomy, may be considered[70]. These procedures have been safely performed throughout pregnancy[71–73]. Open ureterolithotomy is rarely required. Extracorporeal shock-wave lithotripsy has not been approved for use during pregnancy. Unless severe infection complicates the course of urolithiasis, a good perinatal outcome is expected.

Adnexal torsion

Among women requiring laparotomy for adnexal torsion, about 20% are pregnant[74,75]. About one-half of the cases of adnexal torsion are associated with an ovarian neoplasm, most often a dermoid cyst. In the reproductive age group, approximately 2% of cases are associated with ovarian malignancy[74]. Gonadotropin-induced ovarian hyperstimulation is a risk factor for torsion and about 16% of affected pregnancies are complicated by adnexal torsion[76]. Symptomatic torsion occurs usually in the first, sometimes in the second, but rarely in the third trimester. The right side is involved more frequently than the left[74].

Pain is almost always the presenting symptom, but the nature of the pain is highly variable. The onset may be sudden or gradual. The character may be sharp and intermittent, or dull and constant. In about two-thirds of cases, the pain is unilateral in the lower abdomen. It may be generalized or, uncommonly, it may radiate to the back or flank. Nausea and/or vomiting are present in about half of the patients. Various urinary symptoms are less often reported[75,76]. Abdominal tenderness is the most constant physical finding. Peritoneal signs are variably present. There may be adnexal tenderness or a mass. Leukocytosis may be present, but a normal white-blood-cell count does not rule out the diagnosis. Ultrasonographic imaging may aid in the identification and characterization of an adnexal mass. Color Doppler sonography may show absent arterial flow in the central ovarian parenchyma. Absent central ovarian venous flow may be a more sensitive finding in cases of adnexal torsion[77]. Given the non-specific clinical presentation, it is not surprising that the preoperative diagnosis is often erroneous[74,75].

Torsion of the ovary and/or the Fallopian tube leads to venous congestion, edema and, ultimately, arterial compromise. The course may be complicated by ovarian rupture or hemorrhage. Some patients report previous episodes of transient pain, indicating that spontaneous reversal of torsion may, at times, occur. The conventional surgical therapy of adnexal torsion is extirpation of the involved tissues, particularly if they appear ischemic or necrotic. If it is necessary to remove the corpus luteum prior to 10 weeks' gestation, there is justification for progesterone supplementation in an effort to maintain the pregnancy. If tissue distal to the site of torsion appears viable, unwinding of the adnexa is an alternative therapy. One group has advocated unwinding, regardless of the appearance of the adnexa, in cases of ovarian hyperstimulation syndrome[78]. If the ovary is conserved, the surgeon must be assured that it does not contain a neoplasm. There is little information available to quantify the fetal risk following adnexal torsion. Generally, the pregnancy outcome is good[76].

CONCLUSION

Proper evaluation of acute abdominal pain in the pregnant patient requires awareness of conditions that may be unfamiliar to many obstetricians. In addition, knowledge of the influence of pregnancy on the course of disease is essential. For many of the conditions discussed or alluded to in Table 1, collaboration among specialists is needed for optimal patient care. It is important for responsibilities to be well demarcated and understood so that procrastination and oversight are avoided. There should be a set endpoint and plan for any period of observation. If the course of disease takes an unexpected turn, diagnostic hypotheses must be reassessed.

REFERENCES

1. Allen J, Helling T, Langenfeld M. Intraabdominal surgery during pregnancy. *Am J Surg* 1989;158:567–9
2. Saunders P, Milton P. Laparotomy during pregnancy: an assessment of diagnostic accuracy and fetal wastage. *Br Med J* 1973;3:165
3. Sox H Jr, Blatt M, Higgins M, Marton K. *Medical Decision Making*. Boston: Butterworths, 1988
4. McGee T. Acute appendicitis in pregnancy. *Aust NZ J Obstet Gynaecol* 1989;29:378–85
5. Cunningham F, McCubbin J. Appendicitis complicating pregnancy. *Obstet Gynecol* 1975;45:415–20
6. Kuuliala I, Niemi L. Sonograph as an adjunct to plain film in the evaluation of acute abdominal pain. *Ann Clin Res* 1987;19:355–8
7. Puylaert J, Rutgers P, Lalisang R, *et al*. A prospective study of ultrasonography in the diagnosis of appendicitis. *N Engl J Med* 1987;317:666–9
8. Lim H, Bae S, Seo G. Diagnosis of acute appendicitis in pregnant women: value of sonography. *Am J Radiol* 1992;159:539–42
9. Mueller P, vanSonnenberg E. Interventional radiology in the chest and abdomen. *N Engl J Med* 1990;322:1364–73
10. Harvey E, Boice JJ, Honeyman M, Flannery J. Prenatal X-ray exposure and childhood cancer in twins. *N Engl J Med* 1985;312:541–5
11. Kammerer W. Nonobstetric surgery during pregnancy. *Med Clin North Am* 1979;63:1157–64

12. de Veciana M, Towers CV, Major C, *et al*. Pulmonary injury associated with appendicitis in pregnancy: who is at risk? *Am J Obstet Gynecol* 1994;171:1008–13

13. Bailey L, Finley RJ, Miller S, Jones L. Acute appendicitis during pregnancy. *Am Surg* 1986;52:218–21

14. Gomez A, MacDonald W. Acute appendicitis during pregnancy. *Am J Surg* 1979;137:180–3

15. Horowitz M, Gomez G, Santiesteban R, Burkett G. Acute appendicitis during pregnancy. *Arch Surg* 1985; 120:1362–7

16. Babaknia A, Hossein P, Woodruff J. Appendicitis during pregnancy. *Obstet Gynecol* 1977;50:40–4

17. Brant H. Acute appendicitis in pregnancy. *Obstet Gynecol* 1967;29:130–8

18. Bronstein E, Friedman M. Acute appendicitis in pregnancy. *Am J Obstet Gynecol* 1963;86:514–16

19. Doberneck R. Appendectomy during pregnancy. *Am Surg* 1985;51:265–8

20. Finch D, Lee E. Acute appendicitis complicating pregnancy in the Oxford region. *Br J Surg* 1974;61:129–32

21. Richards C, Daya S. Diagnosis of acute appendicitis in pregnancy. *Can J Surg* 1989;32:358–60

22. Lau W, Fan S, Yiu T, *et al*. The clinical significance of routine histopathologic study of the resected appendix and safety of appendiceal inversion. *Surg Gynecol Obstet* 1986;162:256–8

23. Schreiber J. Laparoscopic appendectomy in pregnancy. *Surg Endosc* 1990;4:100–2

24. Hill L, Johnson C, Lee R. Cholecystecomy in pregnancy. *Obstet Gynecol* 1975;46:291–3

25. Landers D, Carmona R, Crombleholme W, Lim R. Acute cholecystitis in pregnancy. *Obstet Gynecol* 1987; 69:131–3

26. Stauffer R, Adams A, Wygal J, Lavery J. Gallbladder disease in pregnancy. *Am J Obstet Gynecol* 1982;144:661–4

27. Hiatt J, Hiatt J, Williams R, Klein S. Biliary disease in pregnancy: strategy for surgical management. *Am J Surg* 1986;151:263–5

28. Friley M, Douglas G. Acute cholecystitis in pregnancy and the puerperium. *Am Surg* 1972;38:314–17

29. Malet P, Soloway R. Diseases of the gallbladder and bile ducts. In Wyngaarden J, Smith LJ, eds. *Cecil Textbook of Medicine*, 18th edn. Philadelphia: WB Saunders, 1988: 859–72

30. Allmendinger N, Hallisey M, Ohki S, Straub J. Percutaneous cholecystostomy treatment of acute cholecystitis in pregnancy. *Obstet Gynecol* 1995;86:653–4

31. Dixon N, Faddis D, Silberman H. Aggressive management of cholecystitis during pregnancy. *Am J Surg* 1987;154:292–4

32. Swisher S, Schmit P, Hunt K, *et al*. Biliary disease during pregnancy. *Am J Surg* 1994;168:576–9

33. Lanzafame R. Laparoscopic cholecystectomy during pregnancy. *Surgery* 1995;118:627–33

34. Soper N, Hunter J, Petrie R. Laparoscopic cholecystectomy during pregnancy. *Surg Endosc* 1992;6:115–16

35. Nesbitt T, Kay H, McCoy M, Herbert W. Endoscopic management of biliary disease during pregnancy. *Obstet Gynecol* 1996;87:806–9

36. Friedman R, Friedman I. Acute cholecystitis with calculous biliary duct obstruction in the gravid patient. *Surg Endosc* 1995;9:910–3

37. Jamidar P, Beck G, Hoffman B, *et al*. Endoscopic retrograde cholangiopancreatography in pregnancy. *Am J Gastroenterol* 1995;90:1263–7

38. Corlett R, Mishell D. Pancreatitis in pregnancy. *Am J Obstet Gynecol* 1972;113:281–90

39. Jouppila P, Mokka R, Larmi T. Acute pancreatitis in pregnancy. *Surg Gynecol Obstet* 1974;139:879–82

40. Wilkinson E. Acute pancreatitis in pregnancy: a review of 98 cases and a report of 8 new cases. *Obstet Gynecol Surv* 1973;28:281–300

41. Ramin K, Ramin S, Richey S, Cunningham F. Acute pancreatitis in pregnancy. *Am J Obstet Gynecol* 1995; 173:187–91

42. Block P, Kelly T. Management of gallstone pancreatitis during pregnancy and the postpartum period. *Surg Gynecol Obstet* 1989;168:426–8

43. DeVore G. Acute abdominal pain in the pregnant patient due to pancreatitis, acute appendicitis, cholecystitis, or peptic ulcer disease. *Clin Perinatol* 1980;7:349–69

44. McKay A, O'Neill J, Imrie C. Pancreatitis, pregnancy and gallstones. *Br J Obstet Gynaecol* 1980;87:47–50

45. Kaiser R, Berk J, Fridhandler L, *et al*. Serum amylase changes during pregnancy. *Am J Obstet Gynecol* 1975; 122:283–6

46. Strickland D, Hauth J, Widish J, *et al*. Amylase and isoamylase activities in serum of pregnant women. *Obstet Gynecol* 1984;63:389–91

47. Kirby D, Fiorenza V, Craig R. Intravenous nutritional support during pregnancy. *J Parenter Enter Nutr* 1988;12:72–80

48. Goldthorp W. Intestinal obstruction during pregnancy and the puerperium. *Br J Clin Pract* 1966;20: 367–76

49. Harer W. Intestinal obstruction associated with pregnancy. *Obstet Gynecol* 1962;19:11–15

50. Morris E. Intestinal obstruction and pregnancy. *J Obstet Gynaecol Br Commonw* 1965;72:36–44

51. Hill L, Symmnonds R. Small bowel obstruction in pregnancy: a review and report of four cases. *Obstet Gynecol* 1976;49:170–3

52. Davis M, Bohon C. Intestinal obstruction in pregnancy. *Clin Obstet Gynecol* 1983;26:832–42

53. Pratt A, Donaldson R, Evertson L, Yon J. Cecal volvulus in pregnancy. *Obstet Gynecol* 1981;57:37S–40S

54. Fanning J, Cross C. Post-Cesarean cecal volvulus. *Am J Obstet Gynecol* 1988;158:1200–2

55. Harer W, Harer W. Volvulus complicating pregnancy and puerperium. *Obstet Gynecol* 1958;12:399–406

56. Malkasian G, Welch J, Hallenbeck G. Volvulus associated with pregnancy: a review and report of 3 cases. *Am J Obstet Gynecol* 1959;78:112

57. Reece E, Petrie R, Hutcherson H. Ogilvie's syndrome in the post-Cesarean section patient. *Am J Obstet Gynecol* 1982;144:849–50

58. Rodriguez-Ballesteros R, Torres-Bautista A, Torres-Valdez F, Ruiz-Moreno J. Ogilvie's syndrome in the post-Cesarean section patient. *Int J Gynecol Obstet* 1989; 28:185–7

59. Beck W. Intestinal obstruction in pregnancy. *Obstet Gynecol* 1974;43:374–8

60. Connolly M, Unti J, Nora P. Bowel obstruction in pregnancy. *Surg Clin North Am* 1995;75:101–13

61. Meyerson S, Holtz T, Ehrinpreis M, Dhar R. Small bowel obstruction in pregnancy. *Am J Gastroenterol* 1995;90:299–302

62. Perdue P, Johnson H, Stafford P. Intestinal obstruction complicating pregnancy. *Am J Surg* 1992;164:384–8

63. Jones W, Correa R, Ansell J. Urolithiasis associated with pregnancy. *J Urol* 1979;122:333–5

64. Strong D, Murchison R, Lynch D. The management of ureteral calculi during pregnancy. *Surg Gynecol Obstet* 1978;146:604–8

65. Coe F, Parks J, Lindheimer M. Nephrolithiasis during pregnancy. *N Engl J Med* 1978;298:324–6

66. Loughlin K. Management of urologic problems during pregnancy. *Urology* 1994;44:159–69

67. Schulman A, Herlinger H. Urinary tract dilation in pregnancy. *Br J Radiol* 1975;48:638–45

68. Platt J, Rubin J, Ellis J, DiPietro M. Duplex Doppler US of the kidney: differentiation of the obstructive from nonobstructive dilation. *Radiology* 1989;171:515–17

69. Hertzberg B, Carroll B, Bowie J, *et al*. Doppler US assessment of maternal kidneys: analysis of intrarenal resistivity indexes in normal pregnancy and physiologic pelvicaliectasis. *Radiology* 1993;186:689–92

70. Hendricks S, Ross S, Krieger J. An algorithm for diagnosis and therapy of management and complication of urolithiasis during pregnancy. *Surg Gynecol Obstet* 1991; 172:49–54

71. Peer A, Strauss S, Witz E, *et al*. Use of percutaneous nephrostomy in hydronephrosis of pregnancy. *Eur J Radiol* 1992;15:220–3

72. Scarpa R, de Lisa A, Usai E. Diagnosis and treatment of ureteral calculi during pregnancy with rigid ureteroscopes. *J Urol* 1996;155:875–7

73. Ulvik N, Bakke A, Hoisaeter P. Ureteroscopy in pregnancy. *J Urol* 1995;154:1660–3

74. Hibbard L. Adnexal torsion. *Am J Obstet Gynecol* 1985; 152:456–61

75. Lomano J, Trelford J, Ullery J. Torsion of the uterine adnexa causing an acute abdomen. *Obstet Gynecol* 1970; 35:221–5

76. Mashiach S, Goldenberg M, Bider D, *et al*. Adnexal torsion of hyperstimulated ovaries in pregnancies after gonadotropin therapy. *Fertil Steril* 1990;53:76–80

77. Fleischer A, Stein S, Cullinan J, Warner M. Color Doppler sonography of adnexal torsion. *J Ultrasound Med* 1995;14:523–8

78. Bider D, Ben-Rafael Z, Godenberg M, *et al*. Pregnancy outcome after unwinding of twisted ischaemic–haemorrhagic adnexa. *Br J Obstet Gynaecol* 1989;96: 428–30

47

Non-obstetrical surgery during pregnancy: medical evaluation and management

M. Pietrantoni, S. Sawai and R.A. Knuppel

FUNDAMENTAL CONSIDERATIONS

The approach to the pregnant patient undergoing emergent or elective non-obstetrical surgery is first and foremost to perform a thorough, but concise, history and physical examination, and appropriate initial laboratory tests. Particular attention should be directed to the antenatal history, with elaboration if there is a pre-existing disease, and documentation of estimated date of confinement.

Pregnant women are susceptible to all the surgical diseases of the non-pregnant patient. Major medical complications are observed in approximately 15–20% of pregnancies, but surgical complications are relatively uncommon (1–2%)[1]. Medical and surgical evaluation calls for prompt diagnosis and appropriate surgical referral for possible emergent operative intervention. The operating surgeon should evaluate the pregnant woman not as a single patient but as two. Fundamental operative maternal–fetal considerations regarding surgical risks are related to those of the altered maternal physiology, i.e. circulatory system: 45% and 33% increase in plasma volume and erythrocytes respectively, 10–20% increase in heart volume, a 30% increase in resting stroke volume and cardiac output, as well as a 15–20% increase in heart rate[2,3]; respiratory system: increase in tidal volume, minute ventilatory volume and minute oxygen uptake[4,5]; gastrointestinal system: most important being delayed gastric emptying time, decreased esophageal tone and incompetence of the esophageal–stomach sphincter[6]; and including hormonal (estrogen and progesterone), chemical, anatomical alterations and fetal viability. Table 1 summarizes the changes in hemodynamic parameters.

PREOPERATIVE FETAL/MATERNAL MANAGEMENT

The initial management for an acute perioperative event should include stabilization of vital signs (blood pressure, pulse, temperature and respiration rates), placement of an intravenous line with a No. 16 gauge needle, transcutaneous oximeter, complete blood count (CBC), type & cross-match if blood products are needed

Table 1 Central hemodynamic parameters in non-pregnant and pregnant women

	Non-pregnant	*Pregnant*
Central venous pressure (mmHg)	1–10	1–10
Pulmonary artery pressure (mmHg)	9–16	9–16
Pulmonary capillary wedge pressure (mmHg)	3–10	3–10
Pulmonary vascular resistance (Dyne × Sec × cm^{-5})	20–120	78 (decreased)
Systemic vascular resistance (Dyne × Sec × cm^{-5})	770–1500	1210 (decreased)
Cardiac output (l/Min)	4–7	6.2 (increased)

(otherwise a Type & screen), serum electrolytes, liver enzymes, electrocardiogram, urinalysis and culture, clotting profiles and documentation of fetal age, viability, and anomalies by Doppler ultrasonography. Table 2 outlines the basic electrolyte values during pregnancy. The hemoglobin and hematocrit should be kept at or above 10 mg/dl and 30% respectively in order to maintain sufficient oxygenation, hemostasis and adequate perfusion. Prophylactic broad spectrum antibiotics should be given to those patients at high risk for infection (diabetes, cardiac surgery and cardiac valvular disease). In addition, prophylactic low-dose heparin (8000 IU) should be provided for the morbidly obese patient, or those with previously documented pulmonary embolism and thromboembolism[7]. Patients receiving glucocorticoid therapy should be treated with hydrocortisone (100 mg intravenously at 8-hour intervals for 24 hours) during any surgical procedures in order to avoid a crisis. Only in the area in which the skin incision will be made is a preoperative clipping preferable[8]. A Kleihauer–Betke test is useful even in cases with minor trauma to evaluate fetal–maternal transfusion[9].

In general, if non-emergent operations have to be performed during pregnancy, the optimal time for

Table 2　Hematologic alterations in pregnancy

Laboratory tests	Normal values	
	Non-pregnant	*Pregnant*
Total protein (g/dl)	6.5–8.5	6.8
Serum albumin (g/dl)	3.5–5.0	2.5–4.5
Blood urea nitrogen (mg/dl)	10–25	5–15
Glucose (mg/dl)	70–110	65–100
Serum calcium (mEq/l)	4.6–5.5	4.2–5.2
Serum phosphate (mg/dl)	2.5–4.8	2.3–4.6
Alkaline phosphatase (IU/l)	35–48	35–150
Cholesterol (mg/dl)	120–290	177–345
Triglycerides (mg/dl)	33–166	130–400
Hemoglobin (g/dl)	12	> 11
Hematocrit (%)	36	33
Platelets (Plt/l)	$140\text{–}440 \times 10^9$	Unchanged
Fibrinogen (mg/dl)	150–300	250–600
Serum creatinine (mg/dl)	0.6	0.8

surgery is the early second trimester because there is a much higher risk of spontaneous abortion during the first trimester, and the risk of preterm labor increases as gestational age advances starting in the late second trimester. In addition, surgery during the first trimester would subject the embryo to medications which may be teratogenic during the crucial period of organogenesis. Prophylactic tocolysis with magnesium sulfate, betamimetics (terbutaline, ritodrine), or calcium channel blockers (nifedipine), is often used perioperatively. If time and the patient's condition permit, autologous blood donation may be offered to the patient. Acute penetrating injuries to the abdomen with high-velocity projectiles, e.g. bullets and shrapnel, are to be observed closely with selective exploration[10]. Surgical intervention is suggested by peritoneal irritation, a positive abdominal tap, persistent unexplained shock, proctorrhagia, hematemesis, or free air on a roentgenogram[11]. Traumatic uterine rupture and/or fetal injuries should prompt immediate abdominal delivery. Uterine evacuation leads to decompression of the abdominal vessels, raising the cardiac output which may improve maternal resuscitation[12].

General anesthesia is considered for any obstetrical emergency and/or prolonged operative procedures. General anesthesia must be taken with the greatest possible caution and attention, because it may cause fetal anomalies early in gestation[13]. General anesthesia involves a rapid sequence induction of anesthesia with sodium thiopental, followed by inhalation of isofluorane which is the most commonly used anesthetic in obstetric anesthesia. Halothane is less commonly used due to its association with an increased incidence of hepatitis and cardiac arrhythmias secondary to an increase in catecholamine[14]. These adverse effects, though rarely serious, argue for preferably the administration of a regional anesthetic, such as an epidural

and spinal or a combination[15]. Hypotension (systolic blood pressure less than 100 mmHg) has been reported to occur with an incidence from as low as 1.4% to 10% following regional anesthesia[16].

The stomach should be emptied before any emergency procedures. An in-dwelling urinary catheter is also recommended for it provides useful information regarding vascular perfusion and blood volume. Because there is an increased risk of aspiration in pregnant women, liberal usage of nasogastric suction is advised. Administering antacids shortly before induction of anesthesia has dramatically decreased mortality[17]. The use of non-particulate antacids like 30 ml of 0.3 mol/l sodium citrate with citric acid (Bicitra) is suggested to neutralize the acidity (pH of 1.0) of the gastric contents. Gibbs and Banner[18] reported that Bicitra neutralizes about 70 ml of gastric acid in nearly 90% of women undergoing Cesarean section when prescribed 45 min preoperatively. Magnesium hydrochloride is also effective in neutralizing gastric juice, but it has a short duration, and due to the particulate matter, it has been shown to cause pneumonitis. Cimetidine is often given but it requires a 60-min interval to decrease gastric acidity when parenterally administered. With abdominal surgery the nasogastric tubes should not be removed until there is evidence of normal bowel function.

During surgery it is imperative that provisions for adequate fetal oxygenation be maintained with maternal oxygen saturation above 90% in order to meet fetal oxygenation demands. In the critically ill patient oxygen transport can be impaired by one of three processes: decreased hemoglobin concentration (anemic hypoxia), decreased hemoglobin oxygen saturation (hypoxic hypoxia), and reduced cardiac output (stagnant hypoxia)[19]. Demand should be minimized by eliminating factors that increase the metabolic work of the cell, e.g. fever, pain, activity, labored breathing, malnutrition and infection. The younger fetuses can tolerate the decreased oxygen levels better than the older fetuses[20]. Oxygen requirements of the preterm fetus are minimized by decreasing 'non-essential' metabolism.

POSTOPERATIVE FETAL/MATERNAL MANAGEMENT

Continuous fetal heart rate monitoring is advocated postoperatively as is monitoring for preterm labor through the use of a tocodynamometer. Attempts to arrest premature contractions, in addition to bed rest and left lateral position, may be with either intravenous magnesium sulfate, subcutaneous terbutaline, or oral nifedipine. The use of progesterone supplementation to decrease postoperative fetal loss in gestations < 20 weeks is controversial, although a stronger argument can be made if the corpus luteum is excised prior to the luteal–placental shift in progesterone production. Fetal loss rates of 0–7.6% have been reported after adjustment for non-procedure-related losses[21]. Analgesic relief for minor aches and pains may be controlled with plain acetaminophen. For pain that exceeds minor pain relievers, acetaminophen and codeine, plain codeine, is recommended since both are relatively safe. Narcotics may cause neonatal depression if given within 1–2 h of delivery.

NERVOUS SYSTEM

The nature and timing of therapy directed at a brain tumor is affected by the existence of the pregnancy. In the USA, approximately 89 pregnant women per year have a primary brain tumor[22]. Decisions about whether to continue the pregnancy and the selection of the best means of delivery are critically influenced by the nature and prognosis of the mother's intracranial lesion. Proteinuric hypertension during pregnancy often produces symptoms similar to those of a brain tumor, i.e. convulsions, coma, scotomata, headaches and edema[23].

Diagnostic evaluation

Early diagnosis hinges on a high index of suspicion in patients with headaches, visual disturbances, or other cerebral symptoms that do not subside. The signs and symptomatology of those with 'tumors of the brain' hinge on whether they are inside the brain or outside the brain matter (Table 3), the size and rate of growth. Intracranial tumors are either benign or malignant, chronic inflammatory (tuberculoma, toruloma, sarcoidosis, cysticercosis, toxoplasmosis), and granulomatous or congenital (craniopharyngioma, chordoma, dermoid, teratoma). Intracranial tumors may be gliomas, neurofibromas, or tumors of blood vessels (hemangiomas, meningiomas). Neoplasms outside the brain substance are usually meningiomas, acoustic neuromas, pineal or pituitary tumors[24]. Malignant tumors may be found intra- and/or extracranially or both, especially carcinomas, sarcomas, melanocarcinoma, embryonal carcinoma, renal cell carcinoma and choriocarcinoma. Excluding pituitary tumors, the incidence of intracranial tumors is not increased during pregnancy. Also, extracranial tumors except for choriocarcinoma are not likely to metastasize. The prognosis with malignant tumors is poor and patients appear to have an accelerated downhill course once diagnosed.

The literature concerning pregnancy and intracranial neoplasms consists largely of case reports, case series and reviews of previously collected data. Disregarding tumor type and malignancy, maternal prognosis is greatly influenced by the location and size of the neoplasm. Otherwise a tissue diagnosis is necessary for optimal management. Benign or malignant supratentorial neoplasms without increased intracranial pressure

Table 3 Intracranial tumors inside and outside the brain substance

Inside	*Outside*
Glial cell origin	*Arachnoid cell origin*
Astrocytomas	Meningiomas
Oligodendroglioma	(meningotheliomatous,
Ependymoma	psammomatous,
Medulloblastoma	fibroblastic)
1° Reticulum cell sarcoma	*Schwannoma cell origin*
(microglioma)	Acoustic Schwannoma
Polar spongioblastoma	(neurilemoma, neuroma)
Gangliogliaoma	Trigeminal neurilemoma
Ganglioneuroma	Neurofibroma
Anaplastic astrocytoma	
Glioblastoma multiforme	*Chromophobic, acidophilic*
	or basophilic cell origin
Blood vessel tumors	Adenomas of the pituitary
Hemangioendothelioblastoma	craniopharyngiomas
(angioblastoma or	
hemangioblastoma; von	*Pineal gland tumors*
Hippel-Lindau syndrome)	Pinealomas (germinomas)
Metastatic tumors	Neuroglial tumors
Carcinomas	teratomas
Sarcomas	
Melanocarcinoma	
Embryonal carcinoma	
Renal cell carcinoma	
Choriocarcinoma	

pose little risk to either mother or fetus. Neurologic disorders that are not amenable to neurosurgical approaches include pre-eclampsia, eclampsia, pseudotumor cerebri and stroke. The relative frequency of primary brain tumors of various types becoming symptomatic or showing acceleration of symptoms is similar in pregnant women to non-pregnant women[25].

As always, a reliable and careful history and neurologic examination will guide the physician to the judicious use of investigative procedures and a correct diagnosis. An intracranial lesion should always be considered in any differential diagnosis of chronic unremitting headache in pregnancy. Most brain tumors present non-emergency in pregnancy with either headache, visual disturbances, or nausea and vomiting (Table 4), which may be considered a diagnostic pitfall since these symptoms are also common to pregnancy. Once one makes a diagnosis of an intracranial tumor, management must be individualized. Early consultation with a neurologist and neurosurgeon is necessary once a brain tumor is suspected.

Non-invasive magnetic resonance imaging (MRI) and computed tomography usually provide good visualization and localization of brain tumors with very low risk to either the mother or fetus. If radiologic investigations are used (skull series and tomograms), shielding of the upper torso and abdomen may help protect the fetus from excessive radiation. Injuries sustained from radiation late in fetal life are less harmful than

Table 4   General and focal signs and symptoms of intra-cranial neoplasms

Headache
Headaches are the most common symptom in over 50% of pregnant women[26,27]. Benign headaches often occur for the first time during pregnancy, and are of the migrainous variety. Ominous symptoms are new headaches, worse during morning hours or an increase in severity. Pregnancy is thought to be protective for those headaches that are pregestational in origin. Nausea and vomiting often accompany headaches secondary to increased intracranial pressure.

Sensorial alterations
Mental changes are also common and often associated with headaches (secondary to intracranial pressure). Symptoms include depression, lethargy, stupor, coma, irritability, inertia, dizziness, fatigue, loss of short term memory, unable to focus on routine tasks, visual field disturbances (papilledema; second most common symptom), bitemporal hemianopsia, unilateral scotomas, ptosis, and unilateral optic atrophy[28].

Psychomotor irritability
A third of the patients experience generalized or focal convulsions. Hemiparesis, and respiratory abnormalities are associated with brain-stem compression, pain is also a possibility.

Endocrine abnormalities
Prolactinemia producing amenorrhea and galactorrhea, and diabetes insipidus. Pineal tumors may secrete the beta subunit of human chorionic gonadotropin, and alpha-fetoprotein.

Table 5   Neurologic history and laboratory examination

Medical assessment	Laboratory evaluation
Medical history for; exposure to toxins and drugs, maternal–fetal trauma or infection,	CBC, Serum electrolyte, serology, chemistries, cranial roentenograms, CT scan and MRI evaluation,
Epilepsy, prior vascular disorders, current medications, multiple sclerosis and myasthenia gravis	Cerebrospinal fluid analysis, myelography, angiography, electromyography, VDRL or RPR, hemoglobin and hematocrit, electrophoresis

CBC, complete blood count; CT, computerized tomography; MRI, magnetic resonance imaging; VDRL, Venereal Disease Research Laboratories; RPR, Rapid Plasma Reagin

those sustained during embryogenesis[29,30]. The central nervous system, eyes and mesenchymal tissues appear to be more radiosensitive. In addition, other measures useful in making the diagnosis are electroencephalogram (EEG) and echoencephalography, lumbar puncture and arteriography (with or without contrast). If the benefits outweigh the risks of using contrast medium then it should be used. Both ^{203}Hg and ^{197}Hg chlormerodrin are appropriate, since both have placental impermeability[31].

Management

Neurologic disease in pregnancy is treated similarly to that of the non-pregnant women, and co-managed with a neurologist and neurosurgeon (Table 5). Patients with intracranial neoplasia should be seen on a weekly basis in the office for early detection of intracranial pressure. Unless the pregnancy is considered to be at high risk increased antenatal testing with non-stress tests or biophysical profile is not warranted. Ecumenical management during labor and delivery is based on obstetrical considerations[32]. If an intracranial neoplasm (ICN) is diagnosed, emergency neurosurgical extirpation may be required, especially if the suspected malignancy is potentially operable and is possibly decreasing the overall life expectancy of the patient. If the neoplasm is benign but causes serious symptomatology, like subarachnoid hemorrhage, and

spinal disk disease, surgical extirpation may still be necessary. In either case, regardless of fetal gestational age the neoplasm may need to be removed. Surgery may be deferred if at all possible until near term, especially if diagnosed during late third trimester. Early in pregnancy many factors must be considered, including duration of gestation, the location and severity of the tumor, and the patient's desire to continue the pregnancy. Prophylactic antibiotics are recommended prior to neurosurgery. If cerebral edema presents itself then the use of dexamethasone and/or mannitol intravenously, and tracheal intubation with hyperventilation is suggested. For those tumors that are inoperable, stereotactic radiosurgery holds much promise due to a computer guided grid system which delivers high intensity radiation in the exact shape and size as the tumor[33]. Additionally, the presence of steroid receptors in central nervous system tumors might open therapeutic possibilities. The influence of pregnancy on meningiomas, gliomas, and vascular tumors suggests hormonal sensitivity[34]. Vaginal delivery is preferable and avoidance of Valsalva maneuvers is also desirable. Therefore shortening the second stage of labor with forceps or vacuum extraction may be selected. Because the physiologic changes during labor are potentially hazardous in women with ICN, adequate pain relief during labor with epidural anesthesia provides both pain-free labor and reduces maternal risk[35].

A premature delivery may be considered for deteriorating maternal conditions or if the fetus weighs approximately 1500 g or more. The survival rate of such a fetus in a tertiary care center is greater than 95%[36].

BREAST DISEASE

Approximately three in 10 000 pregnancies are complicated by breast cancer. About 2% of breast cancers are found within 1 year of pregnancy[37]. More than 70% of all breast cancers are accidently detected by the patient. Delayed recognition of breast disease is common in pregnancy because of normal engorgement, enlargement, increased vascularity and lactation. Because breast congestion tends to mask parenchymal masses, physical examination is made more difficult. The lactating breast may grow to as much as two to three times its normal size. This active growth of breast tissue during gestation is due to increasing amounts of estrogen, progesterone, and human placental lactogen (hPL). Early diagnosis is desirable for it improves survival and broadens therapeutic modalities. The obstetrician should be astute enough to examine the breast bilaterally at the first prenatal visit and instruct the patient in self-breast examination (SBE) throughout gestation. Although the presenting complaints are numerous, the vast majority will complain of a 'new mass'.

Benign or non-proliferative lesions are seen just as commonly in the non-pregnant state as well as during pregnancy. Fibrocystic change and fibroadenomas are the most common benign conditions of the breast[38]. Fibrocystic change occurs most frequently in women between the ages of 25 and 50, and occurs in only 10% of patients under 21 years of age. It is surmised that the etiology is due to an imbalance of the ratio of estrogen to progesterone. Benign breast conditions have a diverse array of clinical presentations, and clinical signs of lumpiness have little correlation with histological correlations.

Diagnostic evaluation

Clinically defined, benign breast symptoms are common and have been estimated to occur in 50% of women. Nodularity and cyclic bilateral diffuse pain are the most frequent signs and symptoms of this disease. Fibrocystic disease, a progression of fibrocystic change, is characterized by macrocyst formation usually greater than 3 mm, whereas fibrocystic change consists of many small 1 mm microcysts. Fibrocystic disease is less common during pregnancy than in the non-gestational state. Because of neighboring lobular hyperplasia, areas of fibrocystic disease may actually appear to regress as the pregnancy proceeds. Occasionally, these conditions may be associated with a colorless, watery or grey-green to brownish bilateral nipple discharge. Fibrocystic disease is not associated with an increased risk of breast cancer unless the histologic pattern is of proliferation and atypia (5%)[39]. Women with atypical hyperplasia and a family history of breast cancer have a relative risk of 11. Fibroadenomas are ubiquitous in young females and tend to enlarge during pregnancy. Of the pure adenomas of the breast, only lactating adenomas arise during gestation or lactation.

The incidence of breast cancer in pregnancy is approximately one per 3300–5000 pregnant women[40]. The obstetrician obtaining a history should inquire in all women for a history of breast cancer in family members[41]. The etiology of breast cancer is exceedingly complex but risk is known to be increased by early menarche, late menopause, first pregnancy after age 20, nulliparity, unilateral breast cancer, obesity, benign breast disease with atypical epithelial hyperplasia, mammographic evidence of severe dysplasia and a high fat and protein diet. Early full-term pregnancy and/or multiparity may confer some protection against subsequent development of carcinoma but not if the cancer has already developed. Earlier studies have suggested a rapid spread of the cancer with early patient demise. Anderson's review[42] concluded that the prognosis is the same in pregnancy as it is in the non-pregnant women. However, others have stated that it has a poor prognosis because delay in diagnosis is more likely and therefore the carcinoma is more often advanced than not. Axillary nodes are more likely to be involved because of the increased drainage. Approximately 75% of pregnant patients with breast cancer have positive nodes at the time of diagnosis. The 5-year survival in this group is approximately 17%. Uninvolved bilateral axillary nodes in pregnant patients with breast cancer result in a 5-year survival rate of 87.5% when found during the first trimester[43].

Management

The most important goal of breast disease management in pregnancy is the untimely recognition of a carcinoma so therapeutic decisions are made promptly. During pregnancy, the breast becomes radiodense limiting the sensitivity of mammography. Therefore fine-needle aspiration (No. 22 or 23 Gauge) of any new lump or mass should be performed without delay during gestation[44]. Although it is a simple procedure, needle aspiration is most effective with small cysts and those that are not palpable. A nipple discharge during gestation is more likely to be due to a proliferation of mammary epithelium than to breast cancer; however any nipple discharge, whether serous or bloody, should be sent for cytologic evaluation. Despite the possibility that the Papanicolaou may be misleading because a negative report does not rule out malignancy[45]. The false-negative rate is between 2 to 10% in cases that are diagnosed early[46]. Ultrasonography may be useful in giving additional information regarding whether the mass is cystic or solid.

Breast biopsy should be performed with the patient under local anesthesia in all but the rarest cases if cancer is suspected. Cytologically equivocal lesions should be subjected to excisional biopsy under local anesthesia. Local anesthesia is commonly used because it is well tolerated, and quite safe, although incidental intravenous injections of bupivacaine and lidocaine have been known to cause fetal bradycardia and central nervous system depression in neonates. Tissue should be sampled through a curvilinear incision conforming to the skin lines of the breast. Strict attention to hemostasis and ligation of ductules is necessary to prevent postoperative hematoma and milk leak. Excisional biopsy is also recommended for all presumed fibroadenomas: this procedure may be performed in an outpatient setting whether the patient is pregnant or not[47]. Nevertheless, the obstetrician should not be passive in managing a breast mass in pregnancy. Biopsy should never be delayed without a good reason. Management of breast cancer is essentially the same in pregnancy as is in non-pregnant patients, except that mastectomy is favored over radiotherapy[48]. To date no metastatic spread of breast cancer is known to have spread to the fetus. Pregnancy need not be terminated unless disseminated cancer is present and chemotherapy is necessary. If chemotherapy is needed during the first trimester then termination of pregnancy is recommended.

THORACIC SURGERY IN PREGNANCY

Most thoracic injuries in pregnancy (6–8%) are related to chest trauma[49]. Both maternal and fetal anoxia is the principle threat to survival, for maternal death is the most common cause of fetal mortality. Also, trauma is the most frequent cause of non-obstetric death during pregnancy[50,51].

Diagnostic evaluation

Thoracic injuries during pregnancy are handled the same as if the patient were not pregnant. Therefore the history and physical examination, with the consequence of thoracotomy, forms the foundation of the initial assessment; the initial evaluation of trauma patients is in performing the ABC's (airway maintenance, establish breathing, and circulation)[52]. The most important and initial laboratory assessment needed in the preoperative evaluation of thoracic surgery is an arterial blood-gas measurement. A measurement of Pa_{CO_2} above 55 mmHg indicates hypoventilation and oral intubation may be required. Arterial Pa_{CO_2} does not vary with age (range 35–45 mmHg).

The exact incidence of thoracic wall tumors is not available from the literature and is limited to case reports. Table 6 summarizes common chest wall tumors. The more likely benign and malignant tumors found produce a wide variety of signs and symptoms, the most common being mild pain, palpable mass, prior chest trauma, or an abnormality on a chest roentgenogram. Wide local excisional biopsies are recommended. Any patient with a chest wall mass should have a metastatic work-up with imaging studies like MRI or computer assisted tomographic scans, ultrasonography and pulmonary function; in the pregnant woman diagnostic procedures with radioisotopes are contraindicated. The differential diagnosis of a chest mass includes: actinomycosis, nocardiosis, tuberculosis chondritis, costochondral separation, and

Table 6   Benign and malignant chest wall tumors

Benign tumors	Malignant tumors
Fibrous dysplasia	Fibrosarcoma
Eosinophilic granuloma	Chondrosarcoma
Osteochondroma	Osteogenic sarcoma
Chondroma	Ewings sarcoma
Dermoid tumors	Myeloma

Tietze's syndrome (nonspecific chondritis – most common sites are the 2nd, 3rd, and 4th cartilages), intercostal neuritis, pulmonary hypertension, myocardial ischemia, pulmonary embolism, and pericarditis.

A pleural effusion may be produced by an infectious agent (*Pneumococcus*, *Streptococcus*, *Staphylococcus*, and Gram-negative organisms) which is called empyema. Pneumonia is the most common cause, however the condition may also be an antecedent from trauma, pulmonary infarction, or from an intra-abdominal source. Clinical diagnosis and management includes, a chest X-ray, thoracentesis (closed drainage system), a culture and Gram stain. Effective antibiotic treatment is based on identification of the offending organism and obliteration of the dead space. Use of tetracycline, nitrogen mustard, adriamycin and quinacrine are relatively contraindicated during pregnancy because of concerns for possible immune suppression, carcinogenesis, and unknown effects on growth. The latter drugs are commonly used for the obliteration of the pleural space when malignancy is present.

Spontaneous pneumothorax commonly results from a ruptured bulla or bleb in young adults[53]. They are usually found in the lung apices with a 50% ipsilateral recurrence risk. Out-patient treatment with a small pneumothorax may be done using the one way flutter valve (Heimlich valve), otherwise thoracostomy tube drainage is the most common treatment. Follow-up consists of serial chest X-rays. Patients that are asymptomatic with less than a 30% pneumothorax that has not increased over a short period of time (6–8 h) can safely be observed.

Mediastinal and lung tumors may be either benign or malignant. Benign tumors are infrequent compared with malignant tumors, the most common being hamartoma (chondroadenoma). Table 7 depicts tumors of the lung and mediastinum.

Management

Physical examination of the chest includes assessment and location of the types of wounds, congenital deformity, respiratory rate and effort, skin and nail color for adequate ventilation. Initial wound care in a sucking injury (open pneumothorax) should be to press firmly with a gauze and adhesive tape to prevent airflow. In flail chest injuries either a local pain control with 1%

Table 7   Mediastinal and lung lesions

Benign lung tumors	Malignant lung tumors
Papillomas (squamous)	Carcinoma (squamous)
Adenomas	Adenocarcinoma
Atelectasis	Large cell carcinoma
Emphysema	Carcinoid tumor
Fibromas	Bronchial gland
Lipomas	Malig. mesothelioma
Chondromas	Carcinosarcoma
Mesothelioma	Malignant melanoma
Teratoma	Malignant lymphoma
Hamartomas	Pulmonary blastoma
	Small cell carcinoma
	Clear cell carcinoma
	Non-small cell
	Sarcoma
	Embryoma
	Transitional cell
Benign mediastinal tumors	*Malignant mediastinal tumors*
Neuroma	Lymphoma
Thymomas	Choriocarcinoma
Congenital cysts	Mature teratoma
Fibroma	Fibrosarcoma
Leiomyoma	Liposarcoma
Lipoma	
Hemangioma	
Lymphangioma	
Neurofibroma	
Pericardial cysts	

Table 8   Criteria to facilitate ventilation in pregnancy

Function	Normal values	Abnormal values
Pulmonary		
Respiratory rate (inspiration/min)	16	> 35
Vital capacity (ml/kg)	3310	< 15
Maximum inspiratory force (cmH$_2$O)	97	< 25–35
Oxygenation		
Pao$_2$ (Torr; room air)	76–100	< 65
Alveolar–arterial O$_2$ difference (Torr: 100% oxygen)	30–70	> 350
Pa$_{co2}$ (mmHg)	35–45	55

lidocaine as an intercostal block should be performed, or oral/nasal intubation. Complete bandaging of the chest may be too restrictive and impair respiratory efforts. A chest roentgenogram is of vital importance and should be obtained as soon as possible with the patient in the upright position. Arterial blood gases are crucial and routine in the evaluation of possible anoxia and hypoxia and in the planning of further treatments. Prior to elective thoracic surgery, assessment of pulmonary function is accomplished by measuring the forced expiratory volume (FEV$_1$ = 83% per 1.7 m^2), but this will not appraise small-airway disease. Criteria for assisted ventilation are seen in Table 8.

CARDIAC SURGERY IN PREGNANCY

The incidence of cardiac disease in pregnancy has been variously reported to be 0.5–1.5%[54] with rheumatic heart disease being the most common. Most patients with symptomatic congenital heart disease have undergone corrective surgery prior to pregnancy and the majority of patients with acquired cardiac disease can be managed medically. Therefore, corrective or palliative cardiac surgery during pregnancy is rarely necessary and is recommended in the pre-pregnancy period or postponed until after pregnancy when physiologic conditions are more optimal. When symptoms become refractory to medical management (persistent pulmonary edema, massive hemoptysis) and termination of pregnancy is not an option, then cardiac surgery must be considered.

Diagnostic evaluation

Knowledge of the anatomic and physiologic changes induced by pregnancy are essential in the assessment of cardiac disease in the gravida. The following produce significant hemodynamic changes: 1–1.5 l/min increase in cardiac output, 40% increase in blood volume by term, progressive increase in oxygen consumption due to increased uterine blood flow (500 ml/min at term) and the oxygen demands of the fetus, as well as the potential decreased venous return from inferior vena cava compression by the enlarging uterus. These changes can either mimic symptoms of cardiac disease or exacerbate an already compromised cardiovascular system. Common symptoms of pregnancy such as 'dyspnea of pregnancy' or increased awareness of breathing, orthopnea, easily fatigued, dizzy spells, and syncope must be distinguished from symptoms of cardiac disease such as severe dyspnea, syncope with exertion, hemoptysis, paroxysmal nocturnal dyspnea, and chest pain related to exertion. Physical examination during normal pregnancy may reveal dependent edema, rales in the lower lung fields, visible neck veins, systolic murmurs in over 95% of patients, and mammary flow murmurs and venous hums. Physical findings requiring further investigation are cyanosis, clubbing, diastolic murmurs, cardiac arrhythmias, or loud harsh systolic murmurs, and edema associated with hepatomegaly.

Evaluation of cardiac disease in a pregnant patient should not differ from that of a non-pregnant patient. Table 9 suggests the medical assessment of cardiac disease in pregnancy. The course of the pregnancy should be managed in cooperation with a cardiologist or cardiovascular surgeon, if necessary, assessing the patient's functional status, the condition of an existing prosthetic valve, and cardiovascular reserve capacity. A baseline

Table 9   Medical assessment of cardiac disease in pregnancy

Echocardiogram (12 lead)
Chest roentgenogram
Hemoglobin/hematocrit with differential
Exercise stress test (optional)
Cardiac catheterization
Medical internist consultation (cardiologist)
Surgical consultation (cardiovascular surgeon)

ECG should be obtained to document the patient's pre- or early pregnancy rhythm. Shifts in the electrical axis and non-specific ST-T wave changes may be seen in normal pregnancies. The patient should be instructed on how to take her pulse and look for changes in rate and rhythm, especially atrial fibrillation. A baseline chest X-ray and hematologic exam are advised for reference in cases of future deterioration. Older mechanical valves may produce a destructive anemia, therefore a differential, white blood cell count, platelet count, and iron store indices should be obtained in addition to a hematocrit[55]. An echocardiogram is a non-invasive procedure which can provide information on several aspects of cardiac chambers and valvular function. Knowledge of alterations in cardiac dimensions (e.g. increased left ventricular internal dimension) and function (e.g. stroke volume, cardiac output, ejection fraction) are necessary for accurate interpretation. If indicated and approved by the cardiologist, exercise stress testing may provide an objective assessment of exercise capacity and cardiac functional status. Radiographic diagnostic procedures are best avoided during pregnancy unless they provide essential information for management of the maternal condition.

Management

Medical management should be attempted prior to considering cardiac surgery as listed in Table 10. The underlying philosophy is to take into consideration all factors that constitute 'the total cardiac burden' and to maintain the load within the cardiovascular tolerance of the patient[56].

Due to the physiologic response to pregnancy, some cardiac conditions may worsen as pregnancy progresses, eventually becoming refractory to medical management or life-threatening. Unless termination of pregnancy is an option, cardiac surgery may be medically necessary. The optimal time for open heart procedures is probably during the early second trimester as discussed earlier. The increasing hemodynamic burden on the cardiovascular system peaks at 28–32 weeks.

Surgical management

It has been reported that maternal and fetal outcome after cardiopulmonary bypass are not significantly

Table 10   Medical management of cardiac disease in pregnancy

Activity restriction
Avoid passive standing and supine positions
Avoid excessive heat and humidity
Diet modification
    Avoid excessive weight gain
    Supplemental iron and/or folic acid
Medical team
    Obstetrician (perinatologist)
    Internist (cardiologist)
    Surgeon (cardiovascular)
    Anesthesiologist
    Neonatologist
Infection control
    Pre-pregnancy immunization
    SBE prophylaxis
    Chronic suppressive treatment (rheumatic heart disease)
Interruption of pregnancy
    Cardiomyopathy
    Pulmonary hypertension
    Marfan's syndrome (dilated aortic root)
Persistent marked cardiac enlargement (2° cardiomyopathy)
Cardiovascular drugs (arrhythmias & fluid overload)

SBE, sub-acute bacterial endocarditis

influenced by maternal age, previous obstetrical history or parity. Although pregnancy may contribute to functional cardiac deterioration, it does not increase the risk for further surgical procedures. Maternal mortality does not differ for equivalent procedures performed in the non-pregnant population. Bernal and Miralles[57] reviewed 46 procedures involving cardiopulmonary bypass which resulted in one maternal death (2.2%) and nine fetal deaths (19.6%). When analyzed according to whether the procedure was performed prior to, or after 1969, Zitnik *et al.*[58] initially reviewed pregnant patients undergoing open-heart surgery; the fetal mortality rate was 29.1% and 9.5%, respectively. The latter figure also included a termination of pregnancy for hydrocephalus which if omitted would decrease the incidence of fetal mortality to 4.8%. Becker[59] surveyed members of The Society of Thoracic Surgeons and reported one maternal death (1.5%) and 11 fetal deaths (16%) in his review of 68 procedures using cardiopulmonary bypass in pregnancy.

For patients who will require cardiac surgery, consideration may be given to fetal pulmonary maturity studies. Time allowing, subsequent pulmonary maturation therapy with scheduled Cesarean delivery followed by immediate cardiac surgery in pregnancies greater than 28 weeks may be necessary.

The management of anesthesia during cardiac surgery in pregnancy has been reviewed elsewhere[60]. In general, the objective is to maximize maternal and fetal oxygenation and safety and not to produce adverse effects for the remainder of the pregnancy. Arterial blood pressures and blood gases should be monitored frequently and a pulmonary artery catheter is essential in assessing left ventricular filling pressures and for the treatment of hypovolemia or pulmonary edema.

Because most cardiac surgery proceeds through a median sternotomy with the patient in a supine position, it is important to keep the uterus elevated off the vena cava in order to avoid supine hypotension. The right lateral decubitus position can be used in most closed cardiac techniques, including mitral valvuloplasty through the left atrial appendage, repair of aortic coarctation through a left lateral thoracotomy incision, and ligation and division of a patent ductus arteriosus.

Cardiopulmonary bypass involves cannulation of the venae cavae independently through the right atrium and aorta cannulation for arterial return. The initiation of cardiopulmonary bypass produces a severe decrease in the systemic vascular resistance as blood is diverted from the pulmonary circulation to the pump oxygenator and thus simultaneous systemic vasodilation occurs. The sudden decrease in blood pressure and flow are gradually compensated for by volume transfusion from the oxygenator to the patient and by endogenous catecholamine release. Fetal bradycardia has been described with the onset of cardiopulmonary bypass and was corrected with an increase in perfusion rate[61]. Alterations in the rate of maternal blood flow during cardiopulmonary bypass can be measured by the fetal heart rate response, therefore continuous fetal tocodynometry is pivotal to ensure adequate uterine and placental perfusion.

It has also been noted that the frequency of uterine contractions increases coincident with rewarming from systemic hypothermia which is used to reduce cardiac metabolism as a myocardial protectant. During pregnancy, the patient should be maintained at normothermic or very mild hypothermic temperatures in order to prevent fetal hypothermia and dysrhythmias as well as to decrease the time on cardiopulmonary bypass. Short perfusion time and high flow bypass are recommended for pregnant patients in order to have maximal placental perfusion. Rossouw[62] reported 0% maternal mortality and 14% (one of seven) fetal mortality with high flow, normothermic (mean temperature maintained at 32 °C), high pressure (mean blood pressure > 70 mmHg), perfusion during cardiopulmonary bypass.

The pregnant cardiac surgery patient should be maintained on the ventilator for the first 24 h to provide optimal oxygenation for both the mother and fetus. Also, liberal use of analgesics to prevent acceleration of anxiety and pain and its physiologic consequences is suggested. The pulmonary artery catheter should remain in place to monitor cardiac function and continuous fetal heart rate monitoring should be maintained for at least 48 h. Consideration may be given to the use of prophylactic tocolytic agents which do not increase the cardiac work load. Postoperative management is determined by the appearance, degree of cardiac and vascular residua, uncorrected defects, the effects of ventriculotomy, electrophysiological disturbances, residual valvular aberrations, prosthetic elements, and postoperative residual of myocardial ischemia and increased ventricular size.

Mitral stenosis

Almost all cases of mitral stenosis result from rheumatic fever. Most patients can be managed medically; however, the progressive increase in blood volume throughout the gestation along with the decreased cardiac output from the stenotic valve and shortened filling time from mild tachycardia of pregnancy may worsen the disease. Acute or chronic interstitial pulmonary edema may occur due to a rise in pulmonary artery pressure and capillary wedge pressure. The symptoms include dyspnea on exertion, shortness of breath, orthopnea or hemoptysis. Pulmonary edema refractory to medical management or recurrent despite medical management and persistent massive hemoptysis are indications for surgical treatment.

Mitral valvuloplasty or commissurotomy was first reported in 1948, independently by Harken *et al.*[63] and Bailey[64]. This was accomplished by physically dilating the mitral valve orifice with a finger placed through the left atrial appendage or physically fracturing the commissures. An alternative to surgery during pregnancy is balloon valvotomy; a safe, feasible, and effective method in symptomatic patients refractory to medical therapy which offers good long-term palliation[65]. Fetal bradycardia during balloon inflation should be anticipated and preparation made for possible emergent Cesarean section should fetal distress persist after catheter removal from the maternal heart[66]. Closed valvotomy is safe in all stages of pregnancy, with a mortality rate of 1.8% for fetal death[67]. The obvious advantage of closed mitral commissurotomy is that cardiopulmonary bypass is not necessary, making the procedure safer for the mother and fetus. Valves with fibrotic shortening of the chordae and thickening of the leaflets yield less desirable results than those with mobile cusps.

Nevertheless, the incidence of stenosis recurring again is significant, and despite the greater theoretical safety of a closed procedure, in the long term the surgical results do not compare with those obtained with open mitral valvuloplasty or valve replacement, which is currently the procedure of choice. Mitral valvotomy is felt to be palliative rather than corrective in most cases. Progression of the disease process eventually leads to re-operation with increased morbidity and less satisfactory results. Closed mitral commissurotomy is rarely performed in current surgical practice in the USA. Cardiac compromise severe enough to require surgery is usually treated with valve replacement.

Cardiac valve replacement

Cardiac valve replacement is most common for mitral and aortic valvular disease for the indications mentioned above. The procedure is associated with a low mortality rate in obstetrical and non-obstetrical patients and the use of continuous fetal monitoring during cardiopulmonary bypass has decreased the risk to the fetus. Becker's survey of cardiovascular surgeons[59] revealed a 72.4% fetal survival rate (21 out of 29) with mitral or aortic valve replacement as compared with a 95.7% fetal survival rate with open mitral commissurotomy (22 out of 23). This may reflect the effects of longer duration on cardiopulmonary bypass or greater severity of disease in patients undergoing valve replacement. Larrea *et al.*[55] report a 23% fetal and 2.6% maternal mortality associated with valve replacement.

Morbidity associated with artificial valves in pregnancy is related to which valve is replaced, the type of prosthesis, and the need for further medications in order to maintain valve function. Maternal complications of prosthetic valves include thromboembolism (7–20% risk even on anticoagulants), prosthetic dysfunction, adverse reactions to medications, hemorrhage, and infective endocarditis. Prosthetic valve thrombi may become manifest as systemic embolization, which occurs in 4.2–7% of patients per year despite anticoagulation, or obstruction of valve function, with an incidence of 0.7–1.3% per year. Mitral valve prosthesis obstruction carries a mortality of greater than 85%. Without anticoagulation the incidence of systemic embolization increases three-fold and the incidence of valve obstruction increases to 8.1% per year. Prosthetic valves also carry a risk of tissue overgrowth resulting in valvular stenosis. Fetal risks in pregnancies both requiring and after valve replacement include intrauterine growth retardation, possible congenital anomalies, an increased rate of fetal wastage, and hemorrhage due to maternal anticoagulation, in addition to the risks incurred during cardiopulmonary bypass and the immediate postoperative period[68].

The type of prosthetic valve used in women of reproductive age or in pregnancy is influenced by a variety of factors. A bioprosthesis is indicated if anticoagulation cannot be provided due to lack of compliance, facility, or cost. In the past, the deterioration of tissue valves with time was a major concern. Reports also suggested that there was an acceleration of calcification of tissue valves during pregnancy[69,70] and in younger patients[71,72]. Patients should be advised that a re-operation for replacement of a tissue prosthesis

may be necessary. Those that are contemplating further pregnancies should give consideration to planning them in reasonable succession prior to deterioration of their prosthetic valve and/or cardiac function. The advantage of tissue valves is that anticoagulation and its inherent risks are not a complicating factor during pregnancy, except in the first three postoperative months and perhaps chronically with a large left atrium and/or atrial fibrillation. Glutaraldehyde-preserved porcine valves have been reported to have a 5–8 year survival that is comparable to that of mechanical valves, however the long-term survival is uncertain[73].

Mechanical valves offer the advantage of durability, however they require chronic anticoagulation during pregnancy. Multiple reports in the literature emphasize the danger of discontinuing anticoagulation during pregnancy with resulting thrombosed valves leading to emergency open heart procedures. Mechanical prostheses also require more extensive removal of leaflet tissue, which, in addition to cutting of the chordae, may reduce left ventricular function. Finally, mitral valve reconstruction should be considered when at all feasible as it would eliminate the need for long-term anticoagulation.

Endocarditis

The incidence of bacterial endocarditis in pregnancy has been reported to be 1 : 8000 pregnancies[74]. The maternal mortality with appropriate treatment is 15–25%[75]; however, medical therapy of bacterial endocarditis with moderate to severe congestive heart failure is associated with a maternal mortality of 50–90%. With early valve replacement the 5-year survival is 75%[76]. Valve replacement is indicated in acute bacterial endocarditis when the disease becomes refractory to medical management and cardiac failure is progressive. The hemodynamic status of the patient should be the determining factor in the timing of cardiac valve replacement rather than infection or the duration of antibiotic therapy. Other indications for surgery in the treatment of infective endocarditis are listed in Table 11. Surgery is of no benefit if heart failure is due to myocarditis, embolic coronary artery disease or to microabscesses in the myocardium. Valve replacement within 2 to 7 days of the diagnosis of *Staphylococcus aureus* is recommended due to an associated mortality of 45–73%. Similarly, surgical treatment is required for Gram-negative bacillary infections as they are often resistant to medical management. Fungal endocarditis is associated with a mortality of 80% with medical management, and close to 100% in patients with a prosthetic valve.

Congenital heart disease

The majority of symptomatic congenital heart lesions have undergone repair prior to the reproductive years.

Table 11 Surgical indications in patients with endocarditis

Increasing heart failure (unmanageable)

Infection not responsive to antibiotics

Fungal (e.g., primarily *Candida, Aspergillus*)
Staphylococcus (e.g., *aureus* > adherence to aortic valves)
Coagulase-negative staphylococcus (e.g., usually *epidermidis*)
Gram-negative bacillary (e.g., *Pseudomonas, Serratia, Enterobactor*)

Embolism (recurrent)

Acquired atrio-ventricular heart block

Other
   Acquired intraventricular conduction defects
   Suppurative pericarcarditis
   Mycotic aneurysm of
      Coronary artery
      Sinus of Valsalva
   Rupture of
      Intraventricular septum
      Atrial septum

Cyanotic congenital heart lesions such as tetralogy of Fallot and transposition of the great vessels can become more symptomatic during pregnancy. Progressive shortness of breath, cardiac enlargement, oxygen desaturation, and a rising hematocrit (which can increase the risk of stroke or myocardial infarction) are all indications for surgical correction. With rare exceptions, in most situations surgery can be safely deferred until after delivery.

Left atrial myxoma

There are five reported cases of excision of a left atrial myxoma during pregnancy with subsequent uncomplicated pregnancies and normal full-term deliveries[77-79]. Of the latter, a case was diagnosed as a result of ECG changes reflecting subendocardial ischemia after administration of ritodrine for tocolysis.

Other cardiac lesions

Reports in the literature of uncommon conditions requiring cardiac surgery in pregnancy include heart block[80-82], constrictive pericarditis[83], and coronary artery bypass graft[84]. Becker's survey[59] included three patients who underwent coronary artery bypass grafting for unstable angina and Majdan and colleagues[84] included a triple coronary artery bypass requiring 90 mins of cardiopulmonary bypass with a subsequent normal full-term infant. The chest discomfort produced by coronary artery disease is difficult to diagnose in pregnancy since this symptom is often ascribed to gastrointestinal, musculoskeletal, abdominal, or other non-specific causes. Coronary artery disease in pregnancy will often manifest as an acute myocardial infarction rather than angina.

A more recent report documents the effectiveness of treating aortic stenosis with percutaneous balloon aortic valvuloplasty[85]. The advantages over valvulotomy and valve replacement are the avoidance of cardiopulmonary bypass and its fetal risks, general anesthesia, median sternotomy, prolonged recovery time, and use of anticoagulants or blood products. It can also be conveniently performed at the time of cardiac catheterization. The disadvantages are the significant radiation exposure time for fluoroscopic guidance and the unknown long-term efficacy. It is not recommended for treatment of critical aortic stenosis and cardiomyopathy, moderate to severe aortic insufficiency, or calcified aortic valves; however, for mild to moderate symptomatic disease one may delay surgical intervention until the puerperium. A recent review of reported cases of congenital aortic stenosis in pregnancy without previous valvular replacement reported an 11% maternal and 4% perinatal mortality rate[86].

HEPATIC RUPTURE IN PREGNANCY

Spontaneous hepatic rupture is rare in pregnancy, occurring in 0.4/100 000 pregnancies, and is associated with pre-eclampsia 75–85% of the time[87]. Other etiologies of hepatic hemorrhage in pregnancy are hepatic neoplasms, infectious processes, aneurysms, and biliary disease. The fact that 70% of patients presenting with pre-eclampsia and liver rupture are multiparas may imply a role of previous episodes of pre-eclampsia which impairs the ability of the reticuloendothelial system to remove fibrin deposits in the current pregnancy. With recurrent pre-eclampsia, this leads to larger fibrin deposits, more vascular occlusion, periportal necrosis, and increased areas of hemorrhage, including possible subcapsular hematoma with rupture. Spontaneous hepatic rupture can occur without significant hypertension. Most cases occur near term or immediately postpartum and in 75–90% of cases involve the right lobe of the liver and are limited to the anterior and superior aspects, whereas rupture of the capsule occurs at the inferior margin[88]. Multiple areas of rupture can occur, they are usually shallow and linear and range from a few millimeters to several centimeters in size. Hemorrhage, necrosis, fatty degeneration, or non-specific changes are seen on biopsy.

Diagnostic evaluation

Early hepatic hemorrhage can present as vague epigastric or right upper quadrant discomfort, sometimes radiating to the right shoulder, and mild to severe nausea. Bis and Waxman[89] reported jaundice in nine of 89 cases of hepatic rupture in pregnancy. The pain may precede the onset of rupture by several days and is often incorrectly diagnosed as gastritis, esophageal reflux, or biliary colic. It is unusual for the diagnosis to be made clinically prior to rupture of the subcapsular hematoma. Henny *et al.*[88] describe a biphasic response to hepatic rupture: the first phase presents with epigastric or right upper quadrant pain with or without nausea and vomiting. Hypertension or other signs of pre-eclampsia may be evident and the abdominal examination is unremarkable. The onset of phase two is heralded by the rupture of Glisson's capsule, manifest as a progressive increase in pain followed by sudden vascular collapse which becomes an acute surgical emergency. Other entities which must be considered in the differential diagnosis are uterine rupture, acute cholecystitis, acute pancreatitis, perforated gastric ulcer or appendix, pulmonary embolus, myocardial infarction, pyelonephritis, and placental abruption. The causes of hepatic rupture may be an initiating trauma either from an exogenous source such as transportation of the patient, abdominal palpation, or manual expression of the placenta, or an endogenous source such as the contraction of the diaphragm or abdominal wall, convulsions, emesis, or any inciting event which increases the intra-abdominal pressure.

Laboratory studies can be helpful in the diagnosis of hepatic rupture. Liver function tests are frequently abnormal, but are non-specific. Hematocrit and platelet count should be followed and a high index of suspicion for hepatic rupture maintained should they decline.

Ultrasonography and computerized tomography are helpful in identifying subcapsular hematoma and intraperitoneal hemorrhage. If the latter is suspected, a paracentesis should be performed to confirm the diagnosis. Radionuclide scanning using technetium has also been used in pregnancy with minimal risk of radiation exposure[90].

Management

Previous reports have given patients experiencing hepatic rupture a very poor prognosis with maternal and perinatal mortality rates of 59 and 62%, respectively[85]. For this reason, immediate surgical intervention was advocated. Henny *et al.*[88] reported a maternal mortality of 96% with conservative treatment in contrast to 33% yielded by surgical therapy. More recent reports indicate that hepatic hemorrhage without rupture can be managed medically with successful outcomes. Phase one, as described by Henny, can be managed with blood pressure control, transfusions and correction of any coagulopathy.

Manas and colleagues[91] managed seven patients with hepatic hemorrhage conservatively and obtained a 100% maternal survival rate by closely following the hematocrit and other clotting parameters and maintaining hemodynamic stability. They conclude, however, that surgical intervention is appropriate for hepatic rupture with hemodynamic instability. Goodlin and colleagues[92] also employed medical management in treating two patients with signs of a leaking subcapsular

hematoma in the postpartum period with favorable results. They emphasize that early diagnosis with computed tomography or ultrasonography allows early and aggressive correction of anemia and hypotension and that continued close monitoring may permit avoidance of a prolonged and complicated hospital course which often accompanies surgical repair or drainage of the liver. Hibbard[87] was able to avoid surgical treatment in a patient who was bleeding by using a gravity suit in order to control the hemorrhage.

Failure of surgical management is usually due to inadequate hemostasis of multiple areas of infarction and hematomas, especially with a coinciding coagulopathy. Irregular hemorrhagic areas and marked friability are characteristic of the abnormal liver tissue underlying the hematoma. Percutaneous angiographic embolization of the hepatic artery can be used to achieve liver hemostasis. Terasaki *et al.*[93] infused 1 mm gelfoam particles into the hepatic artery to completely occlude blood flow to the liver. Loevinger *et al.*[94] embolized 2–3 mm gelfoam particles to obstruct intermediate size arterial feeders and reduce the pulse pressure at bleeding sites without producing total ischemia and necrosis. After several weeks, the gelfoam is absorbed and the hepatic vessels become recanalized. This technique is contraindicated in patients with severe portal hypertension since blood flow from the portal system is necessary to perfuse the liver in the absence of hepatic arterial blood flow. Common side-effects of embolization are right upper quadrant pain, nausea, and pyrexia at the time of embolization which may persist for up to one week[95]. Leukocytosis and intrahepatic gas formation are also common. More serious but rare side-effects include hepatic abscess, septicemia, renal failure, and bowel infarction.

Rittenberry *et al.*[96] attempted overseeing and packing ruptured livers as well as hepatic artery ligation in two postpartum patients. When these attempts failed, they resorted to hemostatic wrapping of the liver with 5 mm mersilene strip ligatures in a latticework fashion. Hemorrhaging from multiple hematoma and rupture sites of both hepatic lobes was successfully abated using this technique.

Smith *et al.*[97] in a review of 27 cases in the literature, managed by packing and grainage, report an 82% survival rate as opposed to a 25% survival rate in eight cases managed with hepatic lobectomy. In the case of hepatic hemorrhage with persistent hypotension, they advocate evacuation of the hematoma, packing the liver and drainage of the operative site. Hepatic artery ligation and lobectomy were reserved for refractory cases of life threatening hemorrhage.

In summary, a variety of therapeutic measures have been used to manage hepatic subcapsular hematoma and rupture including: medical management with transfusions and serial liver scans when there is no evidence of rupture, evacuation and drainage, overseeing the damaged liver bed, application of topical hemostatic agents and abdominal packing, hepatic artery ligation, lobectomy, hepatic artery embolization, and hemostatic wrapping.

ADNEXAL MASSES IN PREGNANCY

Adnexal masses are being detected at earlier stages and with greater frequency as increased emphasis is placed on early prenatal care and more routine use of ultrasound examinations. This may carry implications for an increased frequency of surgery in pregnancy; therefore, the significance of ultrasonographic findings, the natural history of adnexal masses, the frequency and distribution of their pathology, and the effect on pregnancy outcome and maternal morbidity and mortality are important to understand.

The incidence of adnexal masses varies with the composition of the study population, the gestational age at the initial examination, the degree of use of ultrasonographic assessments, and the definition of what is considered significant for tumor size. The numbers range from 1 : 81 deliveries[98] to 1 : 6226 with late prenatal care[99]. Ballard[100] reported the incidence of ovarian tumors diagnosed at the time of pregnancy termination as 1 : 594. Sonographic diagnosis of ovarian cysts in pregnancy can be made in 1 : 346 deliveries[101] and the incidental finding of an adnexal mass at Cesarean section is 1 : 197[102].

In a retrospective review of patients undergoing ultrasound examinations before 20 weeks, Lavery's group[103] found that cystic adnexal lesions greater than 2 cm were common in the first 10 weeks of pregnancy. In the first 5 weeks of pregnancy, 8.8% of patients had significant adnexal masses. The numbers dropped to 7.4% of patients at 6–10 weeks, 1.3% of patients at 11–15 weeks, and 0.3% by 16–20 weeks.

In a review of nine major studies of ovarian tumors requiring surgery in pregnancy from 1973–1986, Podratz and Field[21] reported an incidence of 634 lesions in 491 000 deliveries or an overall incidence of 1 : 764. Of these, only 25 (3.9%) were malignant for an incidence of 1 : 19 640 deliveries which is within the range of 2–5% malignant findings in adnexal masses reported in the literature. This compares favorably to the 20% incidence of ovarian malignancies in adnexal masses in non-pregnant women. The low incidence of malignant lesions is obvious in the frequency and distribution of the histological types of the adnexal masses in their review. Table 12 demonstrates the distribution of adnexal masses during pregnancy. Masses that may be considered in the 'other' category include endometriomas, parovarian cysts, and luteomas of pregnancy.

The more favorable histological subtypes among the malignant lesions can be compared with the greater preponderance of epithelial cell carcinomas in older non-pregnant populations. Ovarian cancer is

Table 12 Adnexal masses in pregnancy: distribution and frequency of histologic subtypes

	Frequency (%)
Serous	16
Mucinous	14
Teratoma	29
Functional cyst	21
Other	16
Malignant	4
Epithelial	44
Germ cell	31
Gonadal stromal	18
Other	7

limited to the ovaries in over 70% of the lesions in pregnancy, reflecting not only the natural history of the histological subtypes, but also earlier clinical detection and/or sonographic imaging during prenatal care. The greater frequency of early stage disease and of non-epithelial subtypes yields more favorable survival rates for ovarian cancer in pregnancy. Novak and colleagues[104] report a 5-year survival rate of 76% in a review of his tumor registry from 1942–1972.

Diagnostic evaluation

The natural course of an adnexal mass as assessed by serial bimanual and sonographic evaluations will dictate the course of management. Lavery *et al.*[103] reported significant ovarian enlargement in 7.5% of patients scanned in the first 10 weeks of pregnancy with rapid resolution in the subsequent 10 weeks. Surgical intervention was required in 8.5% of the adnexal masses for diagnosis or therapy or 0.2% of all the patients scanned during pregnancy (*n* = 3918). Most lesions diagnosed during early prenatal care are asymptomatic. Buttery *et al.*[105] report that 30% of 164 masses were detected by a routine pelvic examination in asymptomatic patients. It is important to note that if the opportunity to diagnose an adnexal mass during the first trimester is missed, the progressing gestation will elevate the mass into the abdomen, obscuring its detection and possibly increasing the risk of complications during delivery from labor obstruction, rupture of the cystic mass, or impaction in the pelvis.

The most common presenting symptom is abdominal pain due to ovarian capsule distension, tissue ischemia secondary to torsion of the adnexa, or chemical or inflammatory irritation of the peritoneum from the contents of a ruptured cyst or infection of an intact abdominal mass. Because of its insidious nature, ovarian cancer is usually diagnosed late in pregnancy or during the puerperium and is less frequently associated with symptoms and complications. Twelve per cent of patients with ovarian cancer in pregnancy will present with an acute surgical abdomen while 24% may present with pressure symptoms, usually attributable to the mass or ascites. Obstruction of labor may occur in 9% of patients with ovarian cancer, while 26% of patients may be asymptomatic and remain undiagnosed until labor or delivery or during the puerperium. For this reason, visualization of the ovaries during a Cesarean section or tubal ligation should be mandatory.

Clinical detection of torsion usually occurs at 10 to 15 weeks gestation suggesting that the rapid increase in size and mobility of the gravid uterus and ovaries at this time may predispose the adnexa to rotation. A survey of menotropin-induced pregnancies ($n = 648$) revealed an incidence of torsion of 1 : 162 pregnancies, each as a result of mild ovarian hyperstimulation syndrome. Others have not reported an increased incidence of adnexal torsion in patients with severe ovarian hyperstimulation syndrome[106]. In 201 cycles of ovarian hyperstimulation syndrome, Mashiach and colleagues[107] reported a 16% incidence of adnexal torsion in patients who conceived, and a 2.3% incidence in non-pregnant patients. The combination of lower abdominal pain, ovarian enlargement, nausea, low grade fever, progressive leukocytosis, and sometimes shock-like symptoms is suggestive of adnexal torsion. The sometimes fluctuating pain of a torsed adnexa must also be differentiated from a ureteral calculus. The sudden onset of acute pain with nausea and vomiting may also be indicative of rupture of an adnexal cyst. Rupture of a corpus luteal cyst with hemoperitoneum would be more likely during early gestation, whereas, in late gestation, during labor or delivery, or in the puerperium mature teratomas, cystadenomas, or endometriomas are more likely to rupture. A ruptured adnexal cyst may also simulate the symptoms of an acute appendicitis or, if early in gestation, a ruptured ectopic pregnancy. Other clinical presentations of an adnexal mass in pregnancy may be the obstruction of labor, abdominal distension, palpable abdominal masses, or virilization as in the presence of a hormonally active stromal tumor. Ultrasound evaluation of adnexal masses can assist in delineating the location of the mass, its internal architecture and consistency, and any changes in size over serial scans. Table 13 gives a sonographic differential diagnosis for adnexal masses.

Management

The management of an adnexal mass during pregnancy is dictated by the assessment of the growth pattern, consistency and associated symptoms of the mass. It is generally agreed that any cystic mass > 6 cm which persists into the second trimester requires further surgical evaluation. A cystic adnexal mass diagnosed in the first trimester should be managed expectantly with serial ultrasound examinations. If it is a corpus luteal cyst, most will spontaneously regress by

Table 13   Adnexal masses in pregnancy: sonographic differential diagnosis

Unilocular cysts
    Corpus luteum
    Serous cystadenoma
    Para-ovarian cyst
    Endometrioma
    Hydrosalpinx

Multilocular cysts
    Mucinous cystadenoma
    Theca-lutein cyst
    Multi-cystic ovary
    Hydrosalpinx

Complex masses
    Dermoid cyst (malignant or benign teratoma)
    Granulosa cell tumor
    Ectopic pregnancy
    Hemorrhage cyst
    Cystic tumor necrosis
    Malignant tumor (gross)
    Leiyomyomata "red" degeneration
    Endometrioma
    Tubo-ovarian abscess
    Pelvic kidney
    Congenital uterine anomalies

Solid masses
    Benign (fibroma, thecoma)
    Malignant (sarcoma)

16 weeks. An adnexal cyst > 8 cm or displaying rapid growth is of some concern, although Beisher[108] reports that the frequency of ovarian cancer in a mass > 15 cm is no different from that of cystic masses measuring 6–15 cm. The presence of a solid ovarian mass, ascites, or other evidence of intra-abdominal malignancy, should be surgically explored immediately if distant from term. Non-emergent management of an adnexal mass is determined by the gestational age of the fetus, the risk of developing complications, and the risk of malignancy. Surgical intervention should be considered for any adnexal masses with characteristics listed in Table 14[109]. Expectant management of a lesion detected during the late first or early third trimester, in order to gain greater fetal maturity, can be considered after counseling the patient regarding timing options, her vulnerability, and with the use of periodic sonographic assessments. A suspicious lesion diagnosed in the second trimester can undergo prompt surgical evaluation. Lesions detected during the first or early second trimester can be managed with serial ultrasound exams as spontaneous resolution can be anticipated in a majority of cystic lesions. If possible, surgery is avoided during the first trimester in order to allow resolution of functional cysts, to avoid excision of the corpus luteum, avoid risks of a spontaneous abortion in the first trimester and the possible adverse effects of anesthesia on the fetus. Surgery should not be delayed

Table 14 Adnexal masses in pregnancy: poor prognostic characteristics

Diameter greater than 10 cm
Thick capsule
Vegetative margins
Septaded
Solid or nodular consistency
Increasing size
Cul de sac infiltrates
Pelvic fixation
Ascites

beyond 16 weeks as the expanding uterus makes surgery more difficult with an increased chance of uterine manipulation and subsequent risk of premature labor. Hess *et al.*[110] reviewed 54 cases requiring laparotomy for therapy of adnexal masses and found significantly fewer adverse outcomes in patients who underwent elective laparotomy compared to those who underwent emergency laparotomy. Expectant management is advised with diagnosis of an adnexal mass in the late third trimester. If there is an obstetrical indication for a Cesarean delivery, then simultaneous excision of the mass can be performed. If not, and an uneventful labor and delivery course is anticipated, surgical excision of the mass can be scheduled 48–72 h postpartum.

Preoperative counseling should include a discussion of the possibility of a malignancy, and the possible need for oophorectomy (possibly bilateral) and hysterectomy. The patient's desire for future childbearing should be clarified prior to surgery.

ORTHOPEDIC SURGERY IN PREGNANCY

The metabolic changes inflicted by pregnancy taxes the musculoskeletal system and the extracellular pool in the regulation of calcium and phosphorus[111]. Without supplementation during pregnancy and lactation demineralization may cause maternal osteoporosis and fetal hypocalcemia under abnormal conditions. To provide for the needs of pregnancy, levels of intestinal calcium-binding protein are normally increased. Mechanically there is progressive lordosis and increased joint mobility. This is attributed to the mechanics of shifting the center of gravity over the lower extremities.

Diagnosis

Breaks are classified anatomically as to their location and plane of the bone (epiphyseal, metaphyseal, and diaphyseal). A closed fracture occurs when the skin surface is not broken versus an open fracture where the break communicates with the skin surface. Pathologic fractures are areas of weakness caused by an infectious agent, cancer, and/or a metabolic process. A stress fracture is truly not a fracture but the response of bone to repeated stress. Osteoclastic reabsorption occurs which is followed by periosteal calus. A greenstick fracture is one in which there is an incomplete break through the bone. Fractures of the shoulder are the most common (humerus or clavicle).

Fracture or dislocation of the hip and pelvis (coxea and sacrum) usually ensues after automobile accidents, or falls from great heights. These patients are at increased risk for internal injuries, especially to the bladder, and shock (one out of three die from local hemorrhage). Therefore early diagnosis is needed so reduction may be accomplished as soon as possible to prevent avascular necrosis of the femoral head. Local, diffuse, radicular, or referred pain are all possible. Bone pain is carried by myelinated and unmyelinated nerve fibers from the periosteum through the spinothalamic tract. In addition, one may find swelling, ecchymosis, instability, crepitus and obvious anatomical deformity.

Management

One problem of particular importance is whether to use X-rays when the patient is pregnant. Besides abortion the concerns are damage which may result in microcephaly (most common), skull defects, microphthalmia, micromelia, clubfoot, and cleft palate when fetal exposure is greater and equal to 50 rads[112]. Therefore the health care provider has an obligation to ensure whether women needing orthopedic surgery are or are not pregnant. If at all possible, informed consent is given and X-rays are taken with shielding of the lower abdomen. A calculation of fetal radiation exposure by the radiation physicist is recommended. If the blastocyst is exposed to 10 rads or greater perinatal death is very likely through cell death and mitotic delay[113,114]. Perinatal death of the embryo is increased if the exposure is greater than 25 rads[115]. Fetal exposure to 5 rads or less has not been demonstrated to have an increased risk in major malformations[116]. Although MRI relies on harmless radiofrequency waves, it is not readily available, it is very expensive and requires high maintenance, but is a good alternative if extensive imaging is needed. All in all, at no time are X-rays to be withheld if they are necessary. Orthopedic open and closed reductions are not to be treated any differently during pregnancy. Open wounds should be debrided immediately in order to prevent osteomalacia. If abduction is compromised at the thighs after a hip reduction than future vaginal delivery is relatively contraindicated[117].

REFERENCES

1. Barron WM. The pregnant surgical patient: medical evaluation and management. *Ann Intern Med* 1984; 101:683–91

2. Ueland K. Maternal cardiovascular dynamics: VII. Intrapartum blood volume changes. *Am J Obstet Gynecol* 1976;126:671–7

3. Schrier RW, Durr JA. Pregnancy: an overfill or underfill state. *Am J Kidney Dis* 1987;9:284–9

4. Gilroy RJ, Mangura BT, Laviets MH. Rib cage and abdominal volume displacements during breathing in pregnancy. *Am Rev Resp Dis* 1988;137:668–72

5. Clark SL, Cotton DB, Lee W, *et al.* Central hemodynamic assessment of normal term pregnancy. *Am J Obstet Gynecol* 1989;161:1439–42

6. O'Sullivan GM, Sutton AJ, Thompson SA, *et al.* Noninvasive measurement of gastric emptying in obstetric patients. *Anesth Analg* 1987;66:505–11

7. Hyers TM, Hull RD, Weg JG. Antithrombotic therapy for venous thromboembolic disease. *Chest* 1992; (Suppl 4):408s–25s

8. Alexander JW, Fischer JE, Boyajian M, *et al.* The influence of hair-removal methods on wound infections. *Arch Surg* 1983;118:347–52

9. Virgilio LA, Simon NV. Measurement of fetal cells in the maternal circulation. *Obstet Gynecol* 1977;50: 364–6

10. Awwad JT, Ghassan AB, Muhieddine SA, *et al.* High-velocity penetrating wounds of the gravid uterus: Review of 16 years of civil war. *Obstet Gynecol* 1994;83: 259–64

11. Shaftan GW. Indications for operation in abdominal trauma. *Am J Surg* 1960;99:657–64

12. Lee RV, Rodgers BD, White LM, *et al.* Cardiopulmonary resuscitation of pregnant women. *Am J Med* 1986;81:311–12

13. Knill-Jones RP, Newman BJ, Spence AA. Anaesthetic practice and pregnancy. *Lancet* 1975;2:807–9

14. Farrell G, Prendergrast D, Murray M. Halothane hepatitis: detection of a constitutional susceptibility factor. *N Engl J Med* 1985;313:1310–14

15. Lyons G, MacDonald R, Mikl B. Combined epidural/spinal anaesthesia for Cesarean section: through the needle or in separate spaces?. *J Anaesth* 1992;47:199–201

16. Jouppila R, Jouppila P, Karinen JM, *et al.* Segmental epidural analgesia in labour: related to the progress of labour, fetal malposition and instrumental delivery. *Acta Obstet Gynecol Scand* 1979;58:135–9

17. Roberts RB, Shirley MA. The obstetrician's role in reducing the risk of aspiration pneumonitis, with particular reference to the use of oral antacids. *Am J Obstet Gynecol* 1976;124:611–17

18. Gibbs CP, Banner TC. Effectiveness of Bicitra as a preoperative antacid. *Anesthesiology* 1984;61:97–9

19. Barcroft J. On anoxaemia. *Lancet* 1920;2:485–9

20. Sidi D, Kuipers J, Teital D, *et al.* Developmental changes in oxygenation and circulatory responses to hypoxemia in lambs. *Am J Physiol* 1983;245:H674–82

21. Podratz KC, Field CS. Ovarian tumors during pregnancy. In Cibils LA, ed. *Surgical Diseases in Pregnancy.* New York: Springer-Verlag, 1990:165–77

22. Simon RH. Brain tumors in pregnancy. *Semin Neurol* 1988;8:214–21

23. Aminoff MJ. Neurological disorders and pregnancy. *Am J Obstet Gynecol* 1978;132:325–35

24. Toakley G. Brain tumors in pregnancy. *Aust NZ J Surg* 1965;35:149–54

25. Bailey P, Bucy PC. The origin and nature of meningeal tumors. *Am J Cancer* 1931;15:15–54

26. Sommerville BW. A study of migraine in pregnancy. *Neurology* 1972;22:824–8

27. Carmel WP. Neurologic surgery in pregnancy. In Barber HRK, Graber EA, eds. *Surgical Disease in Pregnancy.* Philadelphia, PA: WB Saunders Company, 1974:203–24

28. Bikerstaff ER, Small JM, Guest IA. The relapsing course of certain meningiomas in relation to pregnancy and menstruation. *J Neurol Neurosurg Psychiatry* 1958;21:89–91

29. Brent RL. Radiation teratogenesis. *Teratology* 1980; 21:281–98

30. Brent RL. The effects of embryonic and fetal exposure to X-ray, microwaves, and ultrasound. *Clin Obstet Gynecol* 1983;26:484–510

31. Sternberg J. Irradiation and radiocontamination during pregnancy. *Am J Obstet Gynecol* 1970;108:490–513

32. Briani S, Cagnoni G, Benvenuti L, *et al.* Neurosurgical indications during pregnancy. *Clin Exp Obstet Gynecol* 1980;7:13–16

33. Friedman AW, LINAC Radiosurgery. *Neurosurg Clin North Am* 1990;1:991–1008

34. Brentani MM, Lopes MTP, Martins VR, *et al.* Steroid receptors in intracranial tumors. *Clin Neuropharmacol* 1984;7:347–50

35. Finfer SR. Management of labour and delivery in patients with intracranial neoplasms. *Br J Anaesth* 1991;67:784–7

36. Goldberg RL, Nelson KG, Hale CD, *et al.* Survival of infants with low birth weight and early gestational age, 1979 to 1981. *Am J Obstet Gynecol* 1984;149:508–11

37. White TT. Prognosis of breast cancer for pregnant and nursing women: analysis of 1,413 cases. *Surg Gynecol Obstet* 1955;100:661–6

38. Ashikari R, Farrow JH, O'Hara J. Fibroadenomas in the breast of juveniles. *Surg Gynecol Obstet* 1971;132: 259–62

39. Dupont WD, Page DL. Risk factors for breast cancer in women with proliferative breast disease. *N Engl J Med* 1985;312:146–51

40. Deemarsky LJ, Neishtadt EL. Breast cancer and pregnancy. *Breast* 1981;7:17–21

41. Dupont WD, Page DL. Breast cancer risk associated with proliferation disease, age at first birth, and a family history of breast cancer. *Am J Epidemiol* 1987; 125:769–79

42. Anderson JM. Mammary cancers and pregnancy. *Br Med J* 1979;1:1124–7

43. Hubay CA, Barry FM, Marr CC. Pregnancy and breast cancer. *Surg Clin North Am* 1978;58:819–31

44. Zinns JS. The association of pregnancy and breast cancer. *J Reprod Med* 1979;22:297–301

45. Holleb AI, Farrow JH. The relationship of carcinoma of the breast and pregnancy in 283 patients. *Surg Gynecol Obstet* 1962;115:65–71

46. Wilkinson EJ, Schuettke CM, Ferrier CM, *et al.* Fine needle aspiration of breast masses: analysis of 276 aspirates. *Acta Cytol* 1989;33:613–19

47. Fudge TL, McKinnon WMP. Fibroadenoma of the breast during pregnancy and lactation: disappearance postpartum. *J La State Med-Soc* 1976;6:157–8

48. Harvey JC, Rosen PP, Ashikari R, *et al*. The effect of pregnancy on the prognosis of carcinoma of the breast following radical mastectomy. *Surg Gynecol Obstet* 1981;153:723–5

49. Pepperill R, Rubinstein E, MacIsaac I. Motor car accidents during pregnancy. *Med J Aust* 1977;1:203–5

50. Rothenberger D, Quattlebaum FW, Perry JF Jr, *et al*. Blunt maternal trauma: a review of 103 cases. *J Trauma* 1978;18:173–9

51. Pearlman MD, Tintinalli JE. Trauma in pregnancy (clinical conference). *Ann Emerg Med* 1988;17:829–34

52. Committee on Trauma American College of Surgeons. *Advanced Trauma Life Support Course*. Chicago: American College of Surgeons, 1984

53. Serementis MG. The management of spontaneous pneumothorax. *Chest* 1970;57:65–8

54. Ueland K. Rheumatic heart disease and pregnancy. In Elkayam U, Gleicher N, eds. *Cardiac Problems in Pregnancy*. New York, NY: Alan R. Liss Inc., 1990

55. Larrea JL, Nunez L, Reque JA, *et al*. Pregnancy and mechanical valve prothesis: a high-risk situation for the mother and the fetus. *Ann Thorac Surg* 1983;36:459–63

56. Benedetti TJ. Cardiopulmonary disorders. In Eden RD, Boehm FH, eds. *Assessment and Care of the Fetus*. Norwalk, CT: Appleton & Lange, 1990

57. Bernal JM, Miralles PJ. Cardiac surgery with cardiopulmonary bypass during pregnancy. *Obstet Gynecol Surv* 1986;41:1–6

58. Zitnik RS, Brandenburg RO, Sheldon R, Wallace RB. Pregnancy and open-heart surgery. *Circulation* 1969;39(suppl 5):I1257–62

59. Becker RM. Intracardiac surgery in pregnant women. *Ann Thorac Surg* 1983;36:453–8

60. Estafanous FG, Buckley S. Management of anaesthesia for open heart surgery during pregnancy. *Cleveland Clin Q* 1976;43:121–4

61. Koh KS, Friesen RM, Livingstone RA, *et al*. Fetal monitoring during maternal cardiac surgery with cardiopulmonary bypass. *Can Med Assoc J* 1975;112:1102–4

62. Rossouw GJ, Knott-Craig CJ, Barnard PM, *et al*. Intracardiac operation in seven pregnant women. *Ann Thorac Surg* 1993;55:1172–4

63. Harken DE, Ellos LB, Ware PF, *et al*. The surgical treatment of mitral stenosis. *N Engl J Med* 1948;239:801

64. Bailey CP. The surgical treatment of mitral stenosis (mitral commissurotomy). *Dis Chest* 1949;15:377

65. Loya YS, Desai DM, Sharma S. Mitral and pulmonary balloon valvotomy in pregnant patients. *Ind Heart J* 1993;45:57–9

66. Glantz JC, Pomerantz RM, Cunningham MJ, *et al*. Percutaneous balloon valvuloplasty for severe mitral stenosis during pregnancy: a review of therapeutic options. *Obstet Gynecol Surv* 1993;48:503–8

67. Stephen SJ. Changing patterns of mitral stenosis in childhood and pregnancy in Sri Lanka. *J Am Coll Cardiol* 1992;19:1276–84

68. Ayhan A, Yapar EG, Kisnisci HA, *et al*. Pregnancy and its complications after cardiac valve replacement. *Int J Gynecol Obstet* 1991;35:117–22

69. Deviuri E, Yechezkel M, Levinsky L, *et al*. Calcification of a porcine valve xenograft during pregnancy: a case report and review of the literature. *Thorac Cardiovasc Surg* 1984;32:266–8

70. Bortolotti U, Milano A, Mazzucco V, *et al*. Pregnancy in patients with a porcine valve bioprosthesis. *Am J Cardiol* 1982;50:1051–4

71. Galioto FM Jr, Midgley FM, Kapur S, *et al*. Early failures of Ionescu-Shiley bioprothesis after mitral valve replacement in children. *Thorac CV Surg* 1982;83:306–10

72. Wagilligan DJ Jr, Lewis JW Jr, Jara FM, *et al*. Spontaneous degeneration of porcine bioprosthetic valves. *Ann Thorac Surg* 1980;30:259–66

73. Cohn LH, Mudge GH, Pratter F, *et al*. Five to eight-year follow-up of patients undergoing porcine heart-valve replacement. *N Engl J Med* 1981;304:258–62

74. Humphry W, Hickman RC. Bacterial endocarditis in pregnancy. *Aust NZ J Obstet Gynaecol* 1971;11:189–91

75. McAnulty JH, Rahimtoola SH. Surgery for infective endocarditis. *J Am Med Assoc* 1979;242:77–9

76. Jung JY, Saab SB, Almond CH. The case for early surgical treatment of left-sided primary infective endocarditis: a collective review. *J Thorac Cardiovasc Surg* 1975;70:509–18

77. Mercer LJ, Aisenbrey G. Atrial myxoma as a complication of tocolytic therapy: a case report. *J Reprod Med* 1985;30:561–2

78. Trimakas AP, Maxwell KD, Berkay S, *et al*. Fetal monitoring during cardiopulmonary bypass for removal of a left atrial myxoma during pregnancy. *Johns Hopkins Med J* 1979;144:156–60

79. Casarotto D, Bortolotti U, Russo R, *et al*. Surgical removal of a left atrial myxoma during pregnancy. *Chest* 1979;75:390–2

80. Schonbrum M, Rowland W, Quiroz AC. Complete heart block in pregnancy. *Obstet Gynecol* 1966;27:243–6

81. Kenmure ACF, Cameron AJV. Congenital complete heart block in pregnancy. *Br Heart J* 1967;29:910–2

82. Ginns HM, Hollinrake K. Complete heart block in pregnancy treated with an internal cardiac pacemaker. *J Obstet Gynaecol Br Commonw* 1970;70:710–2

83. Watson PT, Havelda CJ, Sorosky J, *et al*. Irradiation-induced constrictive pericarditis requiring pericardiectomy during pregnancy. *J Reprod Med* 1980;24:127–30

84. Majdan JF, Walinsky P, Cowchock SF, *et al*. Coronary artery bypass surgery during pregnancy. *Am J Cardiol* 1983;52:1145–6

85. Angel JL, Chapman C, Knuppel RA, *et al*. Percutaneous balloon aortic valvuloplasty in pregnancy. *Obstet Gynecol* 1988;72:438–40

86. Lao TT, Sermer M, MaGee L, *et al*. Congenital aortic stenosis and pregnancy - a reappraisal. *Am J Obstet Gynecol* 1993;169:540–5

87. Hibbard LT. Spontaneous rupture of the liver in pregnancy: a report of eight cases. *Am J Obstet Gynecol* 1976;126:334–8

88. Henny P, Lim AE, Brummelkamp WH, *et al*. A review of the importance of acute multidisciplinary treatment following spontaneous rupture of the liver

capsule during pregnancy. *Surg Gynecol Obstet* 1983; 156:593–8

89. Bis KA, Waxman B. Rupture of the liver associated with pregnancy: a review of the literature and report of 2 cases. *Obstet Gynecol Surv* 1976;31:763–73

90. Marcus CS, Mason GR, Kuperus JW, *et al*. Pulmonary imaging in pregnancy. Maternal risk and fetal dosimetry. *Clin Nucl Med* 1985;10:1–4

91. Manas KJ, Welsh JD, Rankin RA, *et al*. Hepatic hemorrhage without rupture in preeclampsia. *N Engl J Med* 1985;312:424–6

92. Goodlin RC, Anderson JC, Hodgson PE. Conservative treatment of liver hematoma in the postpartum period. A report of two cases. *J Reprod Med* 1985;30: 368–70

93. Terasaki KK, Quinn MF, Lundell CJ, *et al*. Spontaneous hepatic hemorrhage in preeclampsia: treatment with hepatic arterial embolization. *Radiology* 1990; 174:1039–41

94. Loevinger EH, Vujic I, Lee WM, *et al*. Hepatic rupture associated with pregnancy: treatment with transcatherter embolotherapy. *Obstet Gynecol* 1985;65:281–4

95. Allison DJ, Jordan H, Hennessy O. Therapeutic embolization of the hepatic artery: a review of 75 procedures. *Lancet* 1985;8429:595–9

96. Rittenberry AB, Arnold CL, Taslimi MM. Hemostatic wrapping of ruptured liver in two postpartum patients. *Am J Obstet Gynecol* 1991;165:705–7

97. Smith LG, Moise KJ, Dildy GA, *et al*. Spontaneous rupture of liver during pregnancy: current therapy. *Obstet Gynecol* 1991;77:171–5

98. Grimes WH Jr, Bartholomew RA, Colvin ED, *et al*. Ovarian cyst complicating pregnancy. *Am J Obstet Gynecol* 1954;68:594–605

99. Sinnathuray TA. Ovarian tumors in pregnancy: a clinicopathologic study of 19 surgically proven cases in a Southeast Asian hospital. *Int Surg* 1971;55:422–30

100. Ballard CA. Ovarian tumors associated with pregnancy termination patients. *Am J Obstet Gynecol* 1984; 149:384–7

101. Thornton JG, Wells M. Ovarian cysts in pregnancy: does ultrasound make traditional management inappropriate? *Obstet Gynecol* 1987;69:717–21

102. Koonings PP, Platt LD, Wallace R. Incidental adnexal neoplasms at Cesarean section. *Obstet Gynecol* 1988;72: 767–9

103. Lavery JP, Koontz WL, Layman L, *et al*. Sonographic evaluation of the adnexa during early pregnancy. *Surg Gynecol Obstet* 1986;163:319–23

104. Novak ER, Lambrou CD, Woodruff JD. Ovarian tumors in pregnancy. *Obstet Gynecol* 1975;46:401–6

105. Buttery BW, Beischer NA, Fortune DW, *et al*. Ovarian tumours in pregnancy. *Med J Aust* 1973;1:345–9

106. Kemmann E, Ghazi DM, Corsan GH. Adnexal torsion in menotropin-induced pregnancies. *Obstet Gynecol* 1990;76:403–6

107. Mashiach S, Bider D, Moran O, *et al*. Adnexal torsion of hyperstimulated ovaries in pregnancies after gonadotropin therapy. *Fertil Steril* 1990;53:76–80

108. Beischer NA, Buttery BW, Fortune DW, Macafee CA. Growth and malignancy of ovarian tumours in pregnancy. *Aust NZ J Obstet Gynaecol* 1971;11:208–20

109. Bezjian AA. Pelvic masses in pregnancy. *Clin Obstet Gynecol* 1984;27:402–15

110. Hess LW, Peaceman A, O'Brien WF, *et al*. Adnexal mass occurring with intrauterine pregnancy: report of fifty-four patients requiring laparotomy for definitive management. *Am J Obstet Gynecol* 1988;158:1029–34

111. National Academy of Sciences. Recommended Dietary Allowances, Subcommittee on 10th Ed of the RDAs, Food and Nutrition Board, Commission on Life Sciences, National Research Council. National Institute of Health, National Research Council (US). *Committee on Dietary Allowances*. Washington, DC: National Academy Press, 1989

112. National Council on Radiation Protection. *Basic Radiation Protection*. Washington, DC: NCRP, Report No. 39, 1971

113. National Council on Radiation Protection and Measurements. *Medical Radiation Exposure of Pregnant and Potentially Pregnant Women*. Washington, DC: NCRP, Report No. 54, 1977

114. Rugh R. Radiology and the human embryo and fetus. In Dalrymple GW, Gaulden ME, Kollmorgen FM, *et al*. eds. *Medical Radiation Biology*. Philadelphia: WB Saunders Co., 1973:83–96

115. Wagner LK, Lester RG, Saldana LR. *Exposure of the Pregnant Patient to Diagnostic Radiations. A Guide to Medical Management*. Philadelphia: JB Lippincott Co., 1985;7–34:40–78

116. Vos O. Effects and consequences of prenatal irradiation. *Bolletino Soc Ital Biol Sperim* 1989;65:481–500

117. Nichols J. Orthopedic surgery in pregnancy. In Barber HRK, Graber EA, eds. *Surgical Diseases in Pregnancy*. Philadelphia, PA: WB Saunders, 1974;11:169–83

48

Trauma in pregnancy

R. Hayashi

INTRODUCTION

Management of serious trauma occurring during pregnancy nearly always requires the involvement of various medical/surgical subspecialty groups. Co-ordinated and thoughtful care of the victim and her fetus is essential for optimal outcomes of both patients. There is no justification for compartmentalized care of the pregnant trauma patient. A systematic, organized approach is critical. A recent review article states the issues well:

'The pregnant trauma victim presents unique challenges to medical care providers because two lives must be treated concurrently. Physiologic changes, inherent in the normal pregnancy, modify the assessment and treatment routines. Care directed to the mother impacts the fetus. Management of the pregnant trauma victim requires a high index of suspicion. Accurate assessment and timely interventions will enhance the probability of healthy outcomes for both mother and infant'[1].

This chapter will deal with some principles in the approach to the care of the pregnant trauma victim.

INCIDENCE AND EPIDEMIOLOGY

The most frequent cause of death in women 35 years old or less is trauma[2]. Physical trauma occurs in approximately 1 : 12 pregnancies[3,4]. Most emergency rooms will have experienced initial care of the pregnant trauma victim. As the population of urban working mothers continues to increase, so does the incidence of mothers involved in motor vehicle accidents, the major cause of trauma in pregnancy. One in every 12 women in an inner-city population was battered during pregnancy; of these, significant numbers sustained direct assaults to the abdomen[5]. It has been suggested that the pregnant woman is at increased risk for trauma partly because of the 'clumsiness' associated with alterations of body habitus and the center of gravity[6]. In fact, the risk of trauma increases with advancing pregnancy: 8.8%, 40% and 52% in the first, second and third trimesters, respectively[7]. A recent review of the causes of maternal death over a 4-year period in Cook County (Chicago) found that trauma, at 46.3%, was the leading cause of maternal death[8]. The mechanism of injury in these maternal deaths included the following: gunshot wounds (22.7%), motor vehicle accidents (20.5%), stab wounds (13.6%), strangulations (13.6%), blunt head injuries (9.1%), burns (6.8%), falls (4.5%), toxic exposures (4.5%), drownings (2.3%) and iatrogenic injuries (2.3%)[8].

Several retrospective reviews of institutional or multi-institutional experiences of pregnant trauma patients have reported maternal mortality incidences from 3–10% and perinatal mortality incidences from 15–34% (or 3–5 times higher)[9–12]. For the most part, fetal mortality correlates with the severity of the maternal trauma[13]; however, especially with blunt trauma, insignificant trauma history can occasionally be associated with a lethal fetal outcome[14].

PHYSIOLOGICAL ALTERATIONS IN PREGNANCY

The following physiological alterations associated with pregnancy should be recognized during the assessment and treatment of the pregnant trauma victim.

Cardiopulmonary

Cardiac output increases by 20–30% during the first 10 weeks of gestation and reaches a plateau of 50% by mid-pregnancy which is sustained to term. In late pregnancy, the supine position can decrease the cardiac output by as much as 30% due to vena caval compression. This situation could be critical to the fetus in the face of hypovolemia resulting from blood loss. Trauma patients on a stretcher should be bumped or tilted up on the left side to move the pregnant uterus to the right off the vena cava. Patients with spinal or head injuries should be blocked and immobilized before tilting of the stretcher. The placenta is a large arteriovenous low-resistance shunt that adds to the lowered peripheral vascular resistance of pregnancy, which is reflected in a decrease in the mean arterial blood pressure of 10–15 mmHg. The blood flow to the placenta is dependent on cardiac output so that decreases in cardiac output can affect fetal well-being.

The total blood volume is also increased by 50% in pregnancy. Most of this increase (40%) is plasma volume, resulting in a diluting effect. Hemoglobin and albumin concentration are diluted, resulting in a decrease in colloid oncotic pressure and a physiological anemia. Because of this increase in blood volume, acute blood loss of up to 1 l is tolerated without hemodynamic alterations. Hemodynamic instability requiring transfusion may not occur until blood loss approaches 1.5–2 l; however, under such situations blood pressure is maintained at the expense of splanchnic and uteroplacental blood flow[15]. A urine output of 30 ml/h is an excellent parameter to use to gauge the need for aggressive volume expansion therapy. The uterine arteriolar vascular bed is quite sensitive to vasopressor agents. Peripheral vasopressors, such as epinephrine, norepinephrine and dopamine (> 10 ug/min), may restore maternal mean arterial blood pressure but further decrease uterine blood flow. However, centrally active vasopressors, such as ephedrine and mephentermine, may simultaneously restore maternal blood pressure and uterine blood flow[16]. Maternal heart beat increases by 10–15% during pregnancy, but persistent tachycardia (> 100 beats per min) is significant during pregnancy.

Pregnancy is a hyperventilated state. The functional residual capacity is reduced and the tidal volume of the lung is increased. These changes increase the minute ventilation by 50%, which tends to blow off more CO_2; however, the P_{CO_2} is only slightly decreased, as is the plasma bicarbonate level[17]. The pregnant woman is in a state of compensated respiratory alkalosis and is therefore more prone to acidosis. She is also less tolerant of apnea and will become hypoxemic with short periods of apnea or hypoventilation; with an increased functional residual capacity in the non-pregnant state, she would be more tolerant. Thus, in the pregnant trauma victim, oxygenation by whatever means should be instituted immediately and maintained throughout the management period.

Genitourinary/gastrointestinal

From the beginning of the second trimester, both the full bladder and the pregnant uterus are intra-abdominal organs. As the uterus grows, there is compartmentalization of the large and small intestine into the upper abdominal cavity. Furthermore, peristalsis and gastric emptying functions decrease in pregnancy; thus, if a pregnant patient is given general anesthesia, the risk of aspiration is very high if caution is not exercised. This caution should also be used in semi-comatose and comatose patients. The renal collection system, especially the right side, dilates during pregnancy. The distended pregnant abdomen may mask evidence of acute bowel injury in penetrating injuries, owing to difficulty in assessing peritoneal irritation[18].

GENERAL PRINCIPLES IN THE MANAGEMENT OF PREGNANT TRAUMA VICTIMS

For optimal perinatal outcome in the pregnant trauma victim, specific considerations must be given to the physiological demands of the fetus and alterations of physiological response of the pregnant patient[4]. There must be an organized and co-ordinated approach to resuscitation and teamwork among all professionals on the trauma care team[19]. Maternal resuscitation is the only means of fetal resuscitation. Therefore, meticulous attention must be given to the airway, breathing and circulation, the 'ABC' of resuscitation, with minor modifications which include:

(1) Cervical spine immobilization prior to tilting the stretcher;

(2) Liberal use of oxygen;

(3) Rapid expansion of the intravascular volume by intravenous access with a large-bore (16-gauge) catheter (critical);

(4) Mandatory rapid endotracheal intubation and mechanical ventilation in the absence of spontaneous ventilation.

As mentioned above, all pregnant victims must be considered to have a full stomach, and one must be on guard for regurgitation and aspiration. Administration of an antacid, such as sodium citrate, may decrease the aspiration risk. For the massively bleeding patient, rapid replacement of intravascular volume is critical; therefore, while waiting for blood products, crystalloid replacement with an approximate ratio of 3 ml fluid for every 1 ml of blood loss is appropriate. If emergency transfusion is needed before rhesus-antigen status is established, rhesus-negative blood should be used. A baseline coagulation panel can be valuable, especially when blunt abdominal trauma is encountered in combination with abruptio placentae. A rapid assessment can be accomplished by placing venous blood into a red top tube; a prompt clot formation (within 5 min) makes a clinically significant coagulopathy highly unlikely. Placement of a Foley catheter in the urinary bladder is valuable to assess intravascular fluid status as well as the integrity of the bladder. In the unconscious victim, placement of a nasogastric tube should be considered and the gastric aspirate be tested for blood in the blunt abdominal trauma victim. Diagnostic testing, including radiological evaluation, is performed as necessary based on the principle that the mother's life must not be jeopardized to avoid fetal risks. However, consideration should be given to limit radiation exposure to the fetus by shielding the gravid uterus with a lead apron. Adverse fetal effects are unlikely with fetal exposures of 10 rad or less in pregnancy. A single pelvic film is well under 1 rad.

Roentgenography of the chest, head and neck produces negligible fetal exposure. Abdominopelvic computerized tomography (CT) exposure of greater than 5–10 rad has been associated with teratogenic risks; however, there have been no adverse effects on the fetus in small numbers of pregnant women[11,20]. Continuous external fetal heart-rate monitoring should be instituted soon after the maternal condition is stabilized, even with seemingly minor injuries (particularly with blunt abdominal trauma). In large trauma centers, a long line or telephone transmission through a dedicated phone line could be linked to labor and delivery from the emergency room or intensive care unit to help in the co-operative management of the pregnant trauma victim. Of course, if the victim can be moved safely from the emergency room or the intensive care unit, transport to the obstetrics area would be preferable. Finally, when prompt response to cardiopulmonary resuscitation efforts is not evident in a serious trauma victim, consideration should be given to perimortem Cesarean delivery if the fetus is viable[21]. There are many anecdotal experiences where maternal cardiopulmonary resuscitation was greatly aided by prompt Cesarean section of the term or near-term fetus[22]. In recent times, the normal survival of infants following postmortem Cesarean section has been primarily limited to instances when delivery has occurred within 5 min after maternal death[21]. The current consensus is that a viable fetus can be delivered by postmortem Cesarean section even without the consent of a family member.

BLUNT ABDOMINAL TRAUMA

Blunt abdominal trauma usually results from motor vehicle accidents, falls and direct assaults. Impact trauma to the gravid abdomen produces excessive shear forces that can detach the placenta. With maternal survival, the most common cause of fetal death in blunt abdominal traumas is placental abruption. Even minor motor vehicle trauma has precipitated late placental abruption and fetomaternal hemorrhage[23–25]. A recent study of blunt trauma victims revealed a positive Kleihauer–Betke test in 28% of patients, indicating that fetomaternal transfusion is a relatively common event in traumatized pregnant victims[26]. Thus, continuous external fetal monitoring of pregnancies greater than 20–24 weeks' gestation should be instituted as soon as possible, even in minor motor vehicle accident patients. Monitoring periods of 2–6 h are adequate if there are no uterine contractions, the fetal heart-rate patterns are normal, and no uterine tenderness or vaginal bleeding is observed[27]. Increased uterine activity (more than one contraction every 10 min), late deceleration and a sinusoidal pattern may suggest the possibilities of abruptio placentae or fetal anemia due to fetomaternal hemorrhage. Direct fetal injury, although

infrequent, from blunt abdominal trauma most often involves the fetal skull and brain. The most common mechanism of fetal head injury involves simultaneous fracture of the maternal pelvis (usually the pubic rami) in late pregnancy when the fetal head is engaged. Significant fetal intracranial trauma, even in the non-vertex fetus with a history of minor trauma, may occur, presumably by a contra-coup mechanism[28]. Lower abdominal trauma may cause pelvic fractures. Unstable fractures can injure the uterus, urethra and bladder. However, vaginal delivery is still possible with pelvic fractures[29]. Blunt abdominal trauma to the late-pregnant victim can cause uterine rupture by acutely increasing intrauterine pressure[30]. This can result in extrusion of the intrauterine contents into the peritoneal cavity, fetal death and maternal hemorrhagic shock. Diagnosis of intraperitoneal bleeding in the pregnant trauma victim is hampered by the large uterus. When the trauma victim sustains a major blunt abdominal injury with clinical shock, altered mental status and/or neurological deficit, intra-abdominal bleeding and abruptio placentae must be ruled out. Diagnostic peritoneal lavage of intra-abdominal bleeding has proved to be safe and accurate (92% overall) in pregnant trauma victims[31]. Open peritoneal lavage with sharp dissection and opening of the peritoneum under direct vision, usually infraumbilically, is advocated over blind needle insertion to avoid injury to the uterus or other displaced organs[32]. The infusate used is 1 l of warmed Ringer's lactate solution. Retroperitoneal bleeding due to renal fracture or contusion can be ruled out by CT scan.

In summary, the blunt abdominal trauma victim is at risk for intra-abdominal and fetal injury. Following maternal stabilization, consideration should be given to possible unrecognized intraperitoneal injury, abruptio placentae and fetomaternal hemorrhage.

PENETRATING ABDOMINAL TRAUMA

Most penetrating trauma to the pregnant abdomen is caused by gunshot and stab wounds[18]. In late pregnancy, the enlarged uterus is most likely to be injured by penetrating wounds. Penetration of the upper abdomen is likely to injure the intestines, since they are compartmentalized above the uterine fundus. Unlike blunt abdominal trauma, penetrating abdominal trauma has a low maternal mortality, but is associated with a perinatal mortality of 41–71%[33]. The extent and severity of injury due to gunshot wounds depends on numerous factors: size and velocity of the bullet, anatomic region of penetration and angle of entry, deflection of trajectory and fetal age.

Management schemes for penetrating abdominal trauma in pregnancy have changed over the years. In a patient with a gunshot entry wound below the fundus of the uterus, observation is recommended. If maternal vital signs and fetal heart-rate tracings are stable and there is no evidence of maternal compromise or intra-abdominal hemorrhage, radiological location of the bullet is pursued. Continued observation is recommended if the bullet is within the uterus. If any of the above conditions fail, especially if there is evidence of fetal or maternal compromise or if the wound entry is above the level of the uterine fundus, the patient should undergo an exploratory laparotomy. Cesarean delivery is not necessary unless there is evidence of fetal compromise or injury. If the fetus is dead, conservative measures are followed.

Stab wounds to the abdomen in pregnancy are less common and result in a much lower mortality than that from gunshot wounds. Stab wounds to the upper abdomen above the level of the uterine fundus require a laparotomy and complete 'running' of the intestines. Management of the lower abdominal stab wound is less clear. A report of 14 cases of stab wounds to the gravid uterus was reviewed[34]. Even though 50% of the fetuses were injured, either expectant or aggressive (laparotomy) management did not significantly alter outcomes. Expectant management of stab wounds to the lower abdomen may be possible if the maternal condition is stable and fetal assessment by external fetal monitoring is feasible. Peritoneal lavage, laparoscopy or even a fistulogram may reduce the incidence of laparotomy[35,36]. Management is therefore highly individualized, and a conservative approach with vigilant observation of maternal and fetal well-being is often successful.

THERMAL INJURY

Although infrequent, 5–10% of women of reproductive age admitted to burns units with significant burns (greater than 20% of the body surface area with full thickness injury) are pregnant[36]. Perinatal mortality is high (50%) in these patients. Maternal survival is about 97% if the burned area is less than 40% of the body surface area[37]. Premature labor or fetal death generally occurs within the first week in the burns unit. It is often preceded by episodes of maternal hypotension (difficult fluid balance) or hypoxia from shock, sepsis or respiratory failure. Fluid and electrolyte management, sepsis control and respiratory care are key elements leading to a successful outcome. Tocolysis with magnesium sulfate is recommended to treat premature labor. If possible, fetal monitoring in a viable pregnancy should be initiated. The data could be transmitted by telephone line to the obstetric unit. Delivery when fetal viability is reached should be considered in patients sustaining burns greater than 60% of the body surface area for both fetal and maternal indications. In these patients, fetal death usually occurs within the first few days of the burn injury, and maternal outcome may be improved if the pregnancy

is terminated[37–41]. Early wound excision and skin grafting may improve both maternal and fetal outcomes[40]. Smoke inhalation can cause severe maternal respiratory distress; these pregnant victims require close fetal monitoring for fetal well-being because the affected pregnant patients tend to experience desaturation episodes. The timing of delivery of the fetus is individualized and depends on the clinical situation.

SUMMARY

Trauma in pregnancy is a relatively frequent occurrence that all obstetricians should be prepared to manage. Optimal maternal and perinatal outcomes require a clear understanding of the physiological changes associated with pregnancy, as well as all of the ramifications of the type of injury sustained, and a co-ordinated and multidisciplinary approach by the trauma care team. The first priority is treatment and stabilization of the mother. Only then should attention be directed to the fetus, where therapy will require individualization based on as comprehensive a database as one can reasonably gather, including radiological and ultrasound examinations and laboratory studies.

REFERENCES

1. Zerbe M. Clinical management of the pregnant trauma victim. *AACN Clin Issues Crit Care Nurs* 1990;1:479–94
2. National Safety Council. Accident Facts. Chicago: National Safety Council, 1975
3. Peckham CH, King RW. A study of intercurrent conditions observed during pregnancy. *Am J Obstet Gynecol* 1963;87:609–24
4. Pearlman MD, Tintinalli JR, Lorenz RP. Blunt trauma during pregnancy. *N Engl J Med* 1990;323:1609–13
5. Helton AS, McFarlane J, Anderson ET. Battered and pregnant: a prevalence study. *Am J Public Health* 1987;77:1337–9
6. Crosby WM. Trauma during pregnancy: maternal and fetal injury. *Obstet Gynecol Surv* 1963;87:683–99
7. Fort AJ, Harlin RS. Pregnancy outcome after noncatastrophic maternal trauma during pregnancy. *Obstet Gynecol* 1970;35:912–5
8. Fildes J, Reed L, Jones N, *et al.* Trauma: the leading cause of maternal death. *J Trauma* 1992;32:643–5
9. Timberlake GA, McSwain NE Jr. Trauma in pregnancy: a 10-year perspective. *Am Surg* 1989;55:151–3
10. Kissinger DP, Rozycki GS, Morris JA Jr, *et al.* Trauma in pregnancy: predicting pregnancy outcome. *Arch Surg* 1991;126:1079–86
11. Esposito TJ, Gens DR, Smith LG, *et al.* Trauma during pregnancy: a review of 79 cases. *Arch Surg* 1991;126:1073–8
12. Drost TF, Rosemurgy AS, Sherman HF, *et al.* Major trauma in pregnant women: maternal/fetal outcome. *J Trauma* 1990;30:574–8
13. Scorpio RJ, Esposito TJ, Smith LG, Gens DR. Blunt trauma during pregnancy: factors affecting fetal outcome. *J Trauma* 1992;32:213–16

14. Sidky IH, Daikoku NJ, Gopal J. Insignificant blunt maternal trauma with lethal fetal outcome: a case report. *Maryland Med J* 1991;40:1083–5

15. Marx G. Shock in the obstetric patient. *Anesthesiology* 1965;26:151–65

16. Patterson RM. Trauma in pregnancy. *Clin Obstet Gynecol* 198;27:32–8

17. Prowse CM, Gaensler EAL. Respiratory and acid base changes during pregnancy. *Anesthesiology* 1965;26:381–92

18. Lavin JP, Polsky SS. Abdominal trauma during pregnancy. *Clin Perinatol* 1983;10:423–38

19. Manley L, Santanello S. Trauma in pregnancy: uterine rupture. *J Emerg Nurs* 1991;17:279–81

20. Wagner LK, Lester RG, Szldzna LR. *Exposure of the Pregnant Patient to Diagnostic Radiation: A Guide to Medical Management.* New York: Lippincott, 1985

21. Katz VL, Dotters DJ, Droegemueller W. Perimortem Cesarean delivery. *Obstet Gynecol* 1986;68:571–6

22. Marx G. Cardiopulmonary resuscitation of the late pregnant woman. *Anesthesiology* 1982;56:156

23. Higgens, SD, Garite TJ. Late abruptio placentae in trauma patients: implications for monitoring. *Obstet Gynecol* 1984;63:10S–12S

24. Kettel LM, Branch DW, Scott JR. Occult placental abruption after maternal trauma. *Obstet Gynecol* 1988;71:449–53

25. Fries MH, Hankins GDV. Motor vehicle accident associates with minimum maternal trauma but subsequent fetal demise. *Ann Emerg Med* 1989;18:301–4

26. Rose PG, Strohm PG, Zuspan FP. Fetomaternal hemorrhage following trauma. *Am J Obstet Gynecol* 1985;153:844–7

27. American College of Obstetricians and Gynecologists. *Technical Bulletin no. 161*, November 1991. Washington DC: ACOG

28. Stafford PA, Biddinger PW, Zumwalt RE. Lethal intrauterine fetal trauma. *Am J Obstet Gynecol* 1988;159:485–9

29. Smith CV, Phelan JP. Trauma in pregnancy. In Clark SL, Phelan JP, Cotton DB, eds. *Critical Care Obstetrics.* New Jersey: Medical Economics, 1987:382–402

30. Crosby WM, Snyder RG, Snow CC, *et al.* Impact injuries in pregnancy. I. Experimental studies. *Am J Obstet Gynecol* 1965;101:100–10

31. Esposito TJ, Gens DR, Smith LG, Scorpio R. Evaluation of blunt abdominal trauma occurring during pregnancy. *J Trauma* 1989;29:1628–32

32. Rothenberger DA, Quattlebaum FW, Zabel J, *et al.* Diagnostic peritoneal lavage for blunt trauma in pregnant women. *Am J Obstet Gynecol* 1977;129:479–81

33. Franger AL, Buchsbaum JH, Peaceman AM. Abdominal gunshot wounds in pregnancy. *Am J Obstet Gynecol* 1989;160:1124–8

34. Buchsbaum JH. *Trauma in Pregnancy.* Philadelphia: WB Saunders, 1979

35. Haycock CE. Penetrating trauma in pregnancy. In Haycock CE, ed. *Trauma and Pregnancy.* Littleton, NA: PSG Publishing, 1985

36. Cornell WP, Ebert PA, Zuidema GD. X-ray diagnosis of penetrating wounds of the abdomen. *J Surg Res* 1965;5:142–5

37. Matthews RN. Obstetric implications of burns in pregnancy. *Br J Obstet Gynaecol* 1982;89:603–9

38. Smith BK, Rayburn WF, Feller I. Burns and pregnancy. *Clin Perinatol* 1983;10:383–98

39. Akhtar MA, Mulawkar PM, Kulkarni HR. Burns in pregnancy: effect on maternal and fetal outcomes. *Burns* 1994;20:351–5

40. Prasanna M, Singh K. Early burn wound excision in major burns with pregnancy – a preliminary report. *Burns* 1996;22:234–7

41. Unsur V, Oztopcu C, Atalay C, *et al.* A retrospective study of 11 pregnant women with thermal injuries. *Eur J Obstet Gynecol Reprod Biol* 1996;64:55–8

Section VI

Fetal disorders

49

Alloimmune thrombocytopenia

A.B. Levine and R.L. Berkowitz

PATHOGENESIS

Alloimmune thrombocytopenia (AIT) is a syndrome which develops as a result of maternal sensitization to fetal platelet antigens. These women who themselves lack the specific antigen produce immunoglobulin G (IgG) antibodies directed against a platelet antigen that the fetus inherits from its father. The antibodies are then transported across the placenta to the fetal circulation where they result in the destruction of fetal platelets. Thus, the pathogenesis of alloimmune thrombocytopenia is analogous to that of hemolytic (Rh) disease of the newborn. However, unlike Rh disease, prior sensitization to the platelet antigen is not necessary since approximately half of the clinically evident cases of AIT occur in first pregnancies. This suggests that either the fetal platelets gain access to the maternal circulation more easily than red blood cells, and/or the platelet antigens are highly provocative and therefore stimulate production of IgG antibodies during the first pregnancy[1]. In a family with a previously affected infant, the rate of recurrence with an antigen positive fetus is estimated to be at least 90%[2,3]. Additionally, it has been a uniform finding that the severity of thrombocytopenia in subsequent infants is either the same or worse than that of the first affected child.

PLATELET SEROLOGY

Platelets possess specific alloantigens that are expressed on surface membrane glycoproteins. There are five major platelet alloantigen systems, all with biallelic polymorphism and inherited as codominant traits[4]. The difference in alleles results from a single base substitution in the glycoprotein deoxyribonucleic acid (DNA) sequence which ultimately results in a protein recognized as different from its allele[5]. The most common antigen associated with alloimmune thrombocytopenia is HPA-1A, accounting for approximately 80% of reported cases[6]. Other platelet antigen systems involved in alloimmune thrombocytopenia are shown in Table l. The frequency of phenotypes and genotypes for each antigen differs in different ethnic groups.

Table 1 Platelet-specific alloantigen systems involved in alloimmune thrombocytopenia

Nomenclature		Platelet Glycoprotein (GP)	Alleles
New	*Old*		
HPA-1	PL, Zw	GP IIIa	HPA-1a, 1b
HPA-2	Ko	GP Ib	HPA-2a, 2b
HPA-3	Bak	GP IIb	HPA-3a, 3b
HPA-4	Pen, Yuk	GP IIIa	HPA-4a, 4b
HPA-5	Br	GP Ia	HPA-5a, 5b

INCIDENCE/GENETIC ASPECTS OF MATERNAL IMMUNE RESPONSE

Based on prospective analysis, the incidence of alloimmune thrombocytopenia is estimated to be between 1 per 1000 and 1 per 2000 births[6,7]. The expected incidence in Caucasians based on the 98% frequency of the HPA-A1 allele is 1 to 2 per 100 births. This discrepancy between expected and observed incidence suggests that additional factors contribute to the maternal immune response. The risk of sensitization in HPA-A1 negative women is correlated with the presence of specific maternal HLA-associated immune response genes, namely HLA-DR3, and more specifically HLA-DRW52[8]. The immune response markers are contributory, but not sufficient for the development of alloimmunization, as not all HPA-A1 negative women with an HLA-DRW52 haplotype will deliver thrombocytopenic infants[9]. The role of immune responsiveness for other platelet antigens has not yet been established.

CLINICAL PRESENTATION

In typical cases of alloimmune thrombocytopenia, the mother is healthy (without thrombocytopenia) and her pregnancy, labor and delivery are uncomplicated. The neonates who are otherwise normal, present with symptomatic thrombocytopenia within several hours of birth. Affected infants often develop a generalized distribution of petechiae, as well as ecchymoses over the presenting fetal part. Visceral bleeding and bleeding during circumcision or venipuncture may be present. Of greatest consequence is the risk of intracranial hemorrhage, occurring in up to 30% of cases[3] and responsible for the 6.5% mortality rate[10] and the significant long-term neurologic sequelae, including hydrocephaly and porencephaly. Laboratory data are remarkable for an isolated and often severe thrombocytopenia, with normal or increased numbers of megakaryocytes found on bone marrow aspirate. The hematocrit may be decreased if significant bleeding has occurred. A definitive diagnosis can be made by phenotyping parental platelets, and demonstrating antiplatelet antibodies in the serum of the mother which are specific for the antigen incompatibility identified.

Neonatal alloimmune thrombocytopenia is usually a self-limiting disorder, often resolving over the course of several weeks, as maternal antiplatelet antibodies disappear from the neonatal circulation. The most serious and feared complication is intracranial hemorrhage (ICH), and until recently it had been believed that the greatest risk of ICH was at the time of labor and delivery. Hence, obstetric management had focused on the peripartum period, and elective Cesarean section at term was advocated[11,12]. In the neonatal period, the goal was to replenish the neonate's circulating platelets in order to prevent complications secondary to bleeding. These infants should receive compatible antigen negative platelets from either the mother or from compatible donors[13]. If the mother's platelets are used, they must be carefully washed in order to avoid introducing additional antiplatelet antibodies into the neonatal circulation. High dose intravenous immunoglobulin therapy (1–2 g/kg over 1–5 days) may provide an additional or alternative therapy[14,15] especially when matched platelets are unavailable.

EVIDENCE OF ANTENATAL INTRACRANIAL HEMORRHAGE

In 1979, Zalneraitis *et al.* reported two cases of AIT in which there was good evidence that intracranial hemorrhage had occurred *in utero*[16]. Both infants had enlarged heads (> 97%) at birth. The first had bifrontal and left posterior fossa cysts with obstructive hydrocephalus, and the second had a large right parieto-occipital hematoma followed by the development of hydrocephaly and a porencephalic cyst in the same location. Examination of the cyst contents obtained at the time of shunt placement revealed fluid filled with hemosiderin-laden macrophages in the first case and liquified, 'rusty' fluid in the second. The pathologic findings placed the time of bleeding at several months, and 1–2 weeks prior to delivery in these two cases, respectively.

Stronger confirmation that AIT could be responsible for cerebral hemorrhage *in utero* was presented in a series of cases where the diagnosis of porencephaly was made by ultrasound examination in the third trimester in fetuses suspected, and later confirmed, to have this disorder[17].

It is now known that up to 50% of intracranial hemorrhages secondary to alloimmune thrombocytopenia occur *in utero*[3]. Fetal platelet antigens may be expressed as early as 13 weeks' gestation and intracranial hemorrhage may be present by 16 weeks' gestation[18]. Hence, in order to be maximally effective, the treatment of AIT must begin *in utero*.

ANTENATAL MANAGEMENT

Since routine screening for fetomaternal platelet incompatibility is not performed, identifying those fetuses at risk for AIT almost always consists of obtaining the history of a previously affected sibling or other positive family history. The risk to future pregnancies depends on the zygosity of the father. When the father is a heterozygote for the alloantigen, each fetus has a 50% chance of inheriting the antigen. In these cases, DNA-based testing of fetal amniocytes or chorionic villi has enabled typing of fetal platelet antigens[5,8]. Those fetuses who are antigen negative can be managed routinely, while those found to possess the antigen are managed aggressively.

The optimal antenatal management of alloimmune thrombocytopenia is still debated in the literature. One approach consists of serial *in utero* platelet transfusions with antigen negative platelets[19,20]. Evaluation of fetal platelet counts before and after these procedures reveals that platelet transfusions are effective. However, the platelet count remains normal for less than 10 days, and hence platelet transfusions must be administered weekly. This approach subjects the pregnancy to the risk of fetal loss due to repetitive invasive procedures, which is especially significant in that fetuses with AIT are at increased risk for fetal exsanguination associated with cordocentesis[21]. A less invasive alternative involves the use of maternally administered intravenous gamma globulin (IVIG). In the pilot study of 18 patients[22], IVIG with and without steroid therapy was found to significantly increase the fetal platelet count and decrease the risk of intracranial hemorrhage. No cases of intracranial hemorrhage occurred in that series, in contrast to 10/21 (48%) in untreated siblings.

The largest prospective study of the antenatal management of AIT is a randomized trial designed to determine whether the addition of daily low dose steroid therapy (1.5 mg dexamethasone) to IVIG (1 gm/kg/week) was more efficacious than IVIG alone in preventing severe thrombocytopenia and intracranial hemorrhage[3]. Of the 54 women treated, the majority responded to therapy with success rates between 62% and 85%, depending on the definition of response. The addition of low dose dexamethasone was not found to increase the effectiveness of IVIG alone. In this series, there were no cases of intracranial hemorrhage compared with 10 previously affected siblings, and no differences in response when steroids were used concomitantly. Ten initial nonresponders were entered into the 'salvage arm', which consisted of 60 mg of prednisone daily in addition to IVIG. Half of these patients responded with an increased platelet count.

While these findings are quite promising, there have been reports of unsuccessful response (i.e. intracranial hemorrhage *in utero*) to antenatal IVIG therapy[23,24]. The knowledge that (1) not all fetuses will respond to IVIG therapy and (2) salvage therapy (high dose prednisone or platelet transfusions) is available, underscores the need to assess response to therapy by fetal blood sampling to obtain fetal platelet counts. As fetuses with alloimmune thrombocytopenia are at increased risk for fatal bleeding at the time of cordocentesis[21], it seems prudent to have compatible platelets available and to transfuse if the platelet count is found to be < 50 000.

CONCLUSIONS

At present, the prospective diagnosis of a fetus affected with alloimmune thrombocytopenia relies almost exclusively on the history of a previously affected sibling or other positive family history. Since this disorder can potentially result in death or permanent neurologic sequelae as a result of intracranial hemorrhage, the concept of routine screening of pregnant women to detect fetomaternal platelet incompatibility has been proposed. There are limitations to routine antenatal screening. Not all affected pregnancies may not demonstrate detectable anti HPA-A1 antibodies and conversely the presence of anti HPA-A1 antibodies does not invariably predict fetal thrombocytopenia. In addition, not all fetuses with alloimmune thrombocytopenia will develop intracranial hemorrhage. Fetuses at greatest risk include those with severe thrombocytopenia and those with a previously affected sibling with intracranial hemorrhage. Antenatal therapy needs to be directed at this small group of fetuses at risk for intracranial hemorrhage *in utero*.

The optimal antenatal management for alloimmune thrombocytopenia is still unknown. Serial platelet transfusions are efficacious, but necessitate weekly invasive procedures with the additive risks of pregnancy loss. Medical management with maternally administered intravenous gamma globulin appears to be effective in the majority of, but not all, cases. The mechanism(s) of action of IVIG in preventing severe thrombocytopenia is unknown but may reflect (1) decreased maternal antibody production, (2) antibody Fc receptor blockade in the placenta, and/or (3) antibody Fc receptor blockade in the fetal reticuloendothelial system. The mechanism by which IVIG prevents

intracranial hemorrhage in cases where it does not prevent severe thrombocytopenia has also not been elucidated. It is interesting to note that the HPA-A1 antigen is expressed on human endothelial cells as well as platelets. Hence, it has been proposed that HPA-A1 antibodies may damage these cells resulting in vascular injury[21] and predisposition to intracranial bleeding. IVIG may interfere with this endothelial cell–antiplatelet antibody interaction. Lastly, the gestational age at which therapy should be initiated has yet to be established, given the fact that severe thrombocytopenia has been documented as early as 13 weeks' gestation.

REFERENCES

1. Shulman NR, Jordon JV. Platelet immunology. In Coleman RW, Hirsch J, Marder VJ, *et al*. eds. *Hemostasis and Thrombosis*. Philadelphia: JB Lippincott, 1982: 274–342
2. Kaplan C, Daffos F, Forestier F, *et al*. Management of alloimmune thrombocytopenia: antenatal diagnosis and in utero transfusion of maternal platelets. *Blood* 1988;72:340–3
3. Bussel JB, Berkowitz RL, Lynch L, *et al*. Antenatal management of alloimmune thrombocytopenia with intravenous gamma globulin: a randomized trial of the addition of low dose steroid to gamma globulin. *Am J Obstet Gynecol* 1996;174:1414–23
4. Menell JS, Bussel JB. Antenatal management of the thrombocytopenias. *Clin Perinatol* 1994;21:591–614
5. Khouzami A, Kickler TS, Bray PF, *et al*. Molecular genotyping of fetal platelet antigens with uncultured amniocytes. *Am J Obstet Gynecol* 1995;173:1202–6
6. Mueller-Eckhardt C, Kiefel V, Grubert A, *et al*. 348 cases of suspected neonatal alloimmune thrombocytopenia. *Lancet* 1989;1:363–6
7. Blanchette V, Chen L, Defreidberg Z, *et al*. Alloimmunization to the PLA1 platelet antigen: results of a prospective study. *Br J Haematol* 1990;74:209–15
8. Valentin N, Vergracht A, Bignon J, *et al*. HLA-DRW52 a is involved in alloimmunization against PL-A1 antigen. *Hum Immunol* 1990;27:73–9
9. Panzer S, Auerbach L, Cechova E, *et al*. Maternal alloimmunization against fetal platelet antigens: a prospective study. *Br J Haematol* 1995;90:655–60
10. Murphy MF, Metcalfe P, Waters AH. Antenatal management of severe feto-maternal alloimmune thrombocytopenia: HLA incompatibility may affect responses to fetal platelet transfusions. *Blood* 1993;81: 2174–9
11. Mennuti M, Schwarz RH, Gill F. Obstetric management of isoimmune thrombocytopenia. *Am J Obstet Gynecol* 1974;118:565–6
12. Sitarz AL, Driscoll JM, Wolff JA. Management of isoimmune neonatal thrombocytopenia. *Am J Obstet Gynecol* 1976;124:39–42
13. Adner MM, Fisch GR, Starobin SG, *et al*. Use of "compatible" platelet transfusions in treatment of congenital isoimmune thrombocytopenic purpura. *N Engl J Med* 1969;280:244–7

14. Sidiropoulos D, Straume B. The treatment of neonatal isoimmune thrombocytopenia with intravenous immunoglobulin. *Blut* 1984;48:383–6

15. Derycke M, Dreyfus M, Roper JC, *et al*. Intravenous immunoglobulin for neonatal isoimmune thrombocytopenia. *Arch Dis Child* 1985;50:667–9

16. Zalneraitis EL, Young RKS, Krishnamoorthy KS. Intracranial hemorrhage in utero as a complication of isoimmune thrombocytopenia. *J Pediatr* 1979;95:611–4

17. Herman JH, Jumbelic MI, Ancona RJ, *et al*. In utero cerebral hemorrhage in alloimmune thrombocytopenia. *Am J Pediatr Hematol Oncol* 1986;8:312–17

18. Johnson JM, MacFarland JG, Blanchette VS, *et al*. Prenatal diagnosis of neonatal alloimmune thrombocytopenia using an allele specific oligonecleotide probe. *Prenat Diagn* 1993;13:1037–42

19. Nicolini U, Rodeck CH, Kochenour NK, *et al*. In utero platelet transfusions for alloimmune thrombocytopenia. *Lancet* 1988;2:506

20. Murphy MF, Pullon HW, Metcalfe P, *et al*. Management of fetal alloimmune thrombocytopenia by weekly in utero platelet transfusions. *Vox Sang* 1990;58:45–9

21. Paidas MJ, Berkowitz RL, Lynch L, *et al*. Alloimmune thrombocytopenia: fetal and neonatal losses related to cordocentesis. *Am J Obstet Gynecol* 1995;172:475–9

22. Lynch L, Bussel JB, McFarland JG, *et al*. Antenatal treatment of alloimmune thrombocytopenia. *Obstet Gynecol* 1992;80:67–71

23. Kroll H, Kiefel V, Giers G, *et al*. Maternal intravenous immunoglobulin treatment does not prevent intracranial hemorrhage in fetal alloimmune thrombocytopenia. *Transfusion Med* 1994;4:293–6

24. Bussel JB, Zabusky MR, Berkowitz RL, *et al*. Fetal alloimmune thrombocytopenia. *N Engl J Med* 1997;337:22–6

50

Antepartum fetal heart rate monitoring

M.L. Druzin

INTRODUCTION

Continuous intrapartum fetal heart rate monitoring was specifically developed for use in labor, but indirect methods of fetal monitoring may be used in the antepartum patient who is not in labor. The 'natural' stress of uterine contractions was used to determine whether or not the fetus could withstand repetitive decreases in intervillous blood flow[1]. The oxytocin challenge test (OCT) was developed as the original antepartum fetal test. The term 'contraction stress test' (CST) may be more accurate because contractions are not always induced by erogenous oxytocin. Late decelerations, previously described as being indicative of uteroplacental insufficiency in labor, were shown to have the same predictive value in the antepartum period for subsequent labor events and perinatal outcome[2,3]. Accelerations above the baseline of the fetal heart rate, incidentally detected during the performance of stress testing, were associated with a decreased incidence of abnormal CSTs[4,5]. It had also been demonstrated that certain characteristics of the fetal heart rate in response to fetal movement were predictive of fetal condition[6,7]. Subjective assessment of fetal movement by a pregnant patient has long been used as a test of fetal health. This has been quantitatively evaluated and been correlated with abnormal fetal heart rate monitoring and perinatal outcome[8].

In combining maternal perception of fetal movement with recorded fetal heart rate accelerations, the concept of the non-stress test (NST) was proposed. The relationship between fetal heart rate accelerations and subsequent excellent perinatal outcome was demonstrated in numerous studies[4,9–12]. The advantage of the NST was the ease of performance, ease of interpretation, lack of requirement to use oxytocin, and decrease in the time required to perform the test. These important characteristics as well as the predictive reliability of the test made the NST the primary modality of fetal evaluation[10,13,14].

There is still some controversy concerning the ideal sequence of testing. Non-stress testing for primary surveillance is well accepted. In a few centers, the primary surveillance technique is the CST[3,15]. It has been demonstrated that perinatal outcome is improved whichever sequence of testing is used[15,16].

The primary goal of antepartum fetal heart rate testing (AFHRT) is to prevent fetal death, and both NST and CST have low false-negative rates[11,17]. Newer techniques such as the biophysical profile (BPP) were developed in order to decrease the relatively high false-positive rate (false abnormal rate) and to thus lower the incidence of unnecessary delivery[18,19]. By extrapolation, therefore, AFHRT should have predictive reliability for total perinatal outcome.

The well known relationship between fetal movement and fetal heart rate accelerations depends on the integration of peripheral receptors, spinal cord, brain, autonomic nervous system and intact myocardium[20]. The many factors that can influence this well coordinated cascade of events range from physiological to pathological. Lack of accelerations may merely be due to fetal rest–activity cycles or may be secondary to medication, hypoxia, or acidosis[20,21]. The human fetus is known to exhibit highly organized and integrated behavioral states[22,23]. Fetal heart activity may thus be influenced by many stimuli. Chronic hypoxia may modify the parasympathetic response (vagus) prior to sympathetic activation[24]. Acute hypoxemia leads to redistribution of cardiac output, secondary to baroreceptor activation and changes in peripheral vascular resistance[25,26]. The decrease in intervillous blood flow during contractions is well tolerated by the healthy fetus with a normally functioning feto-placental unit. Inadequate placental reserve may manifest clinically as late decelerations[27,28].

INDICATIONS FOR ANTEPARTUM FETAL HEART RATE TESTING (AFHRT)

Indications for the AFHRT include diabetes mellitus, post-term pregnancy, hypertensive disorders of pregnancy, intrauterine growth retardation, history of previous stillbirth, anemia, hemoglobinopathies, decreased fetal movements, premature labor and premature rupture of the membranes and other disorders associated with increased perinatal loss.

In general, the decision of when to initiate AFHRT should be based on the risk of intrauterine death and at a point in gestation when therapy or intervention by delivery gives the infant a reasonable chance of survival. In healthy pregnant patients, whose only obstetric risk factor is a history of stillbirth in previous pregnancies, fetal surveillance could be initiated at about 32 weeks of gestation since the risk of fetal demise before 32 weeks is quite low in this population[29].

THE NON-STRESS TEST

The NST is relatively simple to perform and has the advantage over the contraction stress test with more rapid testing sequence, no contraindications, and no intravenous oxytocin infusion requirement.

The NST is performed using an external system to monitor fetal movement, uterine contractions, and fetal heart rate (FHR). Uterine activity is obtained with a tocodynamometer strapped to the abdomen in conjunction with manual palpation of the uterus by the examiner. This method will register the frequency and relative duration but not the actual strength of the contractions. The patient is given an 'event marker' with which she can register perceived fetal movements on the strip chart. Thus, the patient and the examiner may both record fetal movements.

The FHR can be derived from ultrasonic, phonocardiogram or abdominal wall electrocardiogram signals. Ultrasound will provide an adequate FHR tracing in up to 95% of the cases, while the success rate of the other two methods has been reported as 40–60% of cases.

INTERPRETATION OF THE NST

The NST is usually used as a primary screening test, with BPP and/or CST performed in cases of abnormal NST.

The NST is an observational test in which the FHR response to fetal movement is noted. An NST is considered reactive (normal) if there are two accelerations of the FHR, equal to or greater than 15 beats per minute above the baseline, lasting at least 15 seconds, associated with fetal movement in a 20 minute period. Various other criteria have been used in many centers and a careful evaluation of the data reveals similar perinatal outcomes, irrespective of the criteria used. The number of accelerations required for the NST varies from one acceleration for 10 beats per minute[30] through two accelerations[16,31], three accelerations[4], four accelerations[32] and five accelerations[33,34]. Accelerations without perceived fetal movement are acceptable. After 20 minutes of a non-reactive NST, vibroacoustic stimulation (VAS) is performed over the fetal vertex for three seconds and the patient is monitored until a reactive NST is obtained, or a second 20 minute period passes. If these criteria are not met in two successive 20 minute periods, a BPP and/or CST is performed unless medically contraindicated. Accelerations meeting the criteria for a reactive NST which occur during the performance of the CST qualify the test as reactive.

A reactive NST is usually repeated in seven days, although more frequent testing may be indicated in conditions where sudden deterioration of the fetoplacental unit may occur, such as diabetes mellitus and fetal growth retardation. Initially, both a reactive NST (normal) and a non-reactive NST (abnormal) followed by a negative CST (normal) were repeated in seven days, while a non-reactive NST (abnormal) with positive CST (abnormal) led to consideration for delivery. This protocol was amended in 1979 following re-evaluation of the non-reactive NST with negative CST. It was found that this combination was associated with a higher antepartum death rate than a reactive NST[35]. The non-reactive NST with negative CST is now considered equivocal and is repeated in 24 hours rather than seven days.

An NST is considered abnormal, whether it is reactive or non-reactive, if severe FHR decelerations exist. Severe FHR deceleration is defined as a FHR decrease from the baseline of at least 40 beats per minute, or an absolute heart rate of 90 beats per minute or less, lasting 60 seconds or longer[36,37]. In such cases, delivery is considered unless fetal lung immaturity is documented. If delivery is not attempted, continuous FHR monitoring for 12–24 hours and daily testing for three days is performed. Decreased frequency of testing can be instituted if testing becomes normal for three consecutive days.

The testing interval varies with the clinical situations. If frequent non-periodic variable decelerations occur during the NST, an evaluation of amniotic fluid volume is performed. Variable decelerations may be indicative of umbilical cord compression which is often associated with decreased amniotic fluid volume. Any deterioration in the clinical situation, irrespective of the diagnosis, should be an indication for more frequent testing.

THE CONTRACTION STRESS TEST

The CST is performed while the patient is in the semi-Fowler's position to avoid the supine-hypotensive syndrome. A baseline period of 10–15 minutes is used to assess FHR characteristics and the possibility of periodic changes. Blood pressure should be monitored every 10 minutes to identify supine hypotension that might provoke an abnormal CST. Uterine activity is evaluated for spontaneous contractions. Adequate uterine contractions is defined as having three contractions over a 10-minute interval. If recurrent late decelerations occur with more than 50% of uterine contractions, the test is interpreted as positive. The CST test is negative if there is no late deceleration associated with any contraction. The CST is equivocal if the late decelerations are associated with less than 50% of uterine contractions, or if late decelerations occur in the presence of uterine hyperstimulation. The latter exists if there are more than five uterine contractions over a 10-minute interval. If patients have less than three spontaneous contractions in a 10-minute interval in which no decelerations are noted, stimulation of the nipple by the patient may be performed to produce adequate uterine contractions without using intravenous oxytocin. Nipple stimulation can result in a qualifying CST in over 70% of cases[38–40].

The CST may be contraindicated in the presence of previous vertical uterine incision, placenta previa, premature rupture of the amniotic membranes, polyhydramnios, and third trimester bleeding.

OTHER CONSIDERATIONS OF FHR TESTING

Fetal state

Arbitrary time periods used in AFHRT do not take individual fetal variation into account. The standard 10, 20, and 40 minute rules allow for standardized testing, but may not reflect physiologic reality. Fetal inactivity can last as long as 80–120 minutes[41]. The same investigators showed that observation periods of up to 80 minutes may be necessary to observe fetal accelerations[42]. Sleep–wake cycles may vary from 20 minutes up to three hours[43]. When the total NST time was extended to 90 minutes, a marked reduction in the false-positive rate (false nonreactive rate) was observed[44].

Baseline heart rate and beat to beat variability

The normal fetal heart rate baseline is 110–160 beats per minute. Many factors can influence baseline heart rate. Factors causing an increase in baseline FHR include maternal fever, maternal thyrotoxicosis, and chronic fetal hypoxia. A decrease in heart rate may be due to acute fetal hypoxia, local anesthetics and congenital heart block[24]. In the human fetus, it has been demonstrated that in the second half of gestation, baseline FHR declines, but remains within normal range from 20 to 40 weeks[45]. A deviation from the baseline FHR deserves further investigation.

'Beat to beat variability' is the term used to describe beat to beat variation of the FHR, mediated by the autonomic nervous system. This is the difference between each successive R-R intervals of the fetal electrocardiogram, expressed as a rate. The presence of variability is thought to reflect an intact pathway from cerebral cortex, through the midbrain and to the vagus and conducting system of the heart itself. Thus, cerebral tissue oxygenation is normal with normal FHR variability, and this is important clinically[46]. In external monitoring, using mainly ultrasound derived FHR, the appearance of beat to beat variability is often

artefactual. If beat to beat variability is absent based on indirect methods of monitoring, there is often true decreased beat to beat variability, and a search for the cause of this must be undertaken. Disappearance of beat to beat variability may be ominous[47–49]. However, fetal beat to beat variability may be decreased in response to barbiturates, narcotics, and prematurity. Fetal sleep is probably the most common single cause of decreased beat to beat variability[24].

Since the variability of external FHR monitoring cannot be accurately evaluated by human eyes, assessment of the FHR long-term and short-term variations on the NST could be accomplished by using a computer such as the System 8000 (Oxford Sonicaid, Oxford, United Kingdom). A long-term variation of FHR over a minute of > 30 ms is defined as normal. The short-term variation of FHR is defined as the average pulse intervals between 3.75 s epochs. Low FHR variation by computer analysis is significantly associated with fetal distress during labor and fetal acidemia in the pregnancies complicated by post-term pregnancy or fetal growth retardation[50,51].

Fetal heart rate decelerations during AFHRT

The presence or absence of accelerations of the FHR is the basic information required for the interpretation of the NST. However, other characteristics of the FHR are helpful in further evaluating the fetus. Nonperiodic decelerations of the fetal heart, whether spontaneous or related to fetal movement, are important during AFHRT. The presence of variable type decelerations – 15 beats per minute for 15 seconds – has been correlated with a greater likelihood of poor perinatal outcome[52,53]. This is true irrespective of whether the NST is reactive or not[54].

The occurrence of fetal bradycardia during AFHRT is potentially predictive of perinatal complications. This pattern was originally correlated with an increased incidence of fetal distress in labor when delivery was instituted within 24 hours[36]. Two subsequent studies in which delivery was not instituted based on the appearance of bradycardia confirmed the markedly increased risk of fetal death[55,56]. The importance of this pattern in predicting perinatal morbidity has recently been confirmed in a large series of cases mainly in patients with gestational ages greater than 32 weeks[37]. In the majority of instances in these four series, pregnancies greater than 32 weeks' gestation were evaluated. In a specific group of patients, namely systemic lupus erythematosus with antiphospholipid antibodies, bradycardia may be associated with intrauterine growth retardation, fetal death, or congenital heart block[57]. Elective preterm delivery may be indicated in selected cases.

Gestational age

Gestational age has been shown to be correlated with fetal reactivity[58,59]. The general consensus is that the preterm fetus is more likely to be non-reactive (lack of accelerations) than the fetus at term[60,61]. In these cases, the criteria for reactivity used were identical for term and preterm gestations. Rates of reactivity became similar after 30–32 weeks[62]. Thus, the fetus at gestational ages of 30 weeks or less may be non-reactive based on gestational age alone. The use of identical criteria for reactivity at all gestational ages has recently been questioned[59]. Further large-scale studies with clinical application of different criteria are necessary. Use of the same criteria for all gestational ages may be less confusing and more clinically applicable until further information is available.

In the study of gestational age and the NST[60], those fetuses who were reactive at an early gestational age, even as early as 20–24 weeks, remained so until term with normal outcome. The CST has been shown to be predictive at early gestational ages, less than 34 weeks. Thus, an abnormal screening NST (which may be so because of prematurity) can be followed reliably with a CST[63]. The BPP is being used more frequently in these cases because the CST is often contraindicated in preterm pregnancies. Many preterm fetuses are being monitored in situations such as premature rupture of the membranes, preterm labor, multiple gestation, and placenta previa, which are all relative contraindications to the CST. Thus, management decisions can be made with some degree of confidence in terms of impending fetal compromise.

Application of the NST to gestational ages < 28 weeks awaits further study. Use of the biophysical profile and other parameters of testing may be of use in ascertaining those fetuses who are at risk prior to 28 weeks' gestation[19]. In some conditions, such as collagen-vascular disease and severe hypertensive diseases, there are fetuses who may be compromised prior to 28 weeks (birthweight approximately 1000 g), or prior to 26 weeks (birthweight approximately 800 g). Identification of such a group would lead to optimum use of fetal surveillance techniques at later gestational ages and consideration of elective premature delivery[57].

Extrinsic factors affecting fetal testing

It has been demonstrated that cigarette smoking[64] and phenobarbital[21] are associated with an increased incidence of non-reactive NSTs. It has become common practice to suggest that glucose-containing drinks will shorten time to reactivity, thus increasing the percentage of reactive NSTs. Our experience suggests that glucose ingestion by the mother compared with ingestion of an identical volume of tap water has no effect on time to reactivity, or the incidence of reactive NSTs[65]. Recent data suggest that simple manual manipulation of the fetus neither decreases the time required for performance of a NST, nor changes the reactive NST to non-reactive NST ratio[66]. There is an increased incidence of abnormal AFHRT in the fetus with major congenital anomalies. Repetitive abnormal AFHRT should prompt evaluation for anomalies[9].

The only external stimulus that has proven to be consistently reliable in altering fetal reactivity has been vibroacoustic stimulation (VAS). An earlier study showing improved rates of reactivity[67] was followed by numerous attempts to integrate this into clinical practice[12,68].

A retrospective analysis of the adjunctive use of VAS demonstrated a 50% reduction in the number of non-reactive NSTs[69]. Consequently, a prospective randomized clinical trial was undertaken to compare the standard NST with the fetal VAS test. Those patients randomized to the VAS test underwent transabdominal acoustic stimulation with a Model SC electronic artificial larynx. The incidence of non-reactive tests was 14% in the control group and 9% in the study group ($p = 0.004$). A significant reduction in testing time was also observed[70].

In another study, Smith *et al.*[71] further assessed the usefulness of transabdominal VAS of the fetus and demonstrated an approximately 50% reduction in the number of non-reactive tests and a shorter testing time. No change in the predictive reliability of a reactive test was observed. There was no difference in the incidence of meconium stained amniotic fluid, depressed one or five minute Apgar scores, or operative intervention for fetal distress between the group that was reactive without VAS and the group that required VAS. A reactive test evoked by VAS is as reliable as the traditional NST. Similar data have been reported concerning the use of VAS during BPP[72].

VAS offers distinct advantages to the traditional NST. Fewer non-reactive tests reduce patient anxiety, shorten overall testing time, and allow perinatal resources to be used more efficiently. Although definitive advantages to VAS exist, its routine implementation should await further investigation of its safety and predictive reliability[73].

Amniotic fluid assessment

Amniotic fluid is now recognized as one parameter that is important to assess in an antepartum evaluation scheme. The original BPP proposed by Manning *et al.*[19] gave equal weight to all parameters, irrespective of the mechanism. It is now recognized that fetal movement, fetal breathing, fetal tone, and the NST are likely to be mediated by the central nervous system while amniotic fluid volume (AFV) is an index of fetal renal and/or placental function.

Qualitative AFV assessment was used to predict oligohydramnios and intrauterine growth retardation. A single amniotic fluid pocket of 1 cm or less was highly correlated with intrauterine growth retardation[74]. This measurement was also used as the criterion of AFV in the BPP[19]. Phelan *et al.*[75] found that there were patients with greater than 1 cm pockets of amniotic fluid who gave an overall impression of decreased AFV to the trained observer. In the postdate patients, perinatal morbidity and mortality were high in this specific group.

Chamberlain *et al.*[76] subsequently reported on the 2 cm rule. The next step was the development of the amniotic fluid index (AFI) by Phelan *et al.*[77]. This technique divides the abdomen into four quadrants using the umbilicus as the horizontal line and the linea negra as the vertical line. The vertical diameter of the largest pocket in each quadrant is measured, and the summation of numbers represents the AFI in centimeters. An AFI of 5 cm or less was correlated with increased perinatal morbidity in spite of reactive NST and no fetal heart rate decelerations[59]. The AFI is used as the AFV evaluation in the BPP. A scheme of NST with VAS and AFI has been proposed as the primary form of fetal surveillance[78].

Scoring systems

Some investigators have proposed 'scoring systems' to better quantify changes and predictive reliability in AFHRT schemes[79–81]. While this has been demonstrated to be reliable, it requires a further set of criteria to be memorized. This also leads to reliance on a set of 'numbers' without taking into consideration the clinical implications of that number. It is more clinically applicable to report observations which allow the clinician to form a composite picture of fetal condition.

Multiple gestation

Multiple gestations have increased perinatal morbidity and mortality secondary to increased rates of prematurity and placental insufficiency. The NST has been used reliably in assessing fetal well-being in multiple gestations. Abnormal results were often associated with intrauterine growth retardation[82,83]. With the increased use of techniques to enhance fertility, multiple gestations are presenting more frequently to the practicing obstetrician.

Condition specific antepartum fetal heart rate testing

Frequency of testing will depend on the clinical indication for testing. Once a week testing is suggested as a baseline, but various conditions should prompt more frequent and/or detailed evaluation (e.g. poorly controlled diabetes mellitus, or post-date pregnancies may require two or three times per week testing with evaluation of amniotic fluid). Any change in clinical condition may require modification of a fetal testing scheme.

REFERENCES

1. Pose SV, Castillo JB, Mora-Rojas EO, *et al*. Test of fetal tolerance to induced uterine contractions for the diagnosis of chronic distress. In *Perinatal Factors Affecting Human Development*. Pan Am Health Organization Scientific Publication, 1969:No.185

2. Freeman RK. Clinical value of antepartum fetal heart rate monitoring. In Gluck L, ed. *Modern Perinatal Medicine*. Chicago: Year Book Med Pub Inc, 1974:163

3. Freeman RK, Anderson G, Dorchester W. A prospective multi-institutional study of antepartum fetal heart rate monitoring II. Contraction stress test versus nonstress test for primary surveillance. *Am J Obstet Gynecol* 1982;143:778–81

4. Lee CY, DiLoreto PC, Logrand B. Fetal activity acceleration determination for the evaluation of fetal reserve. *Obstet Gynecol* 1976;48:19–26

5. Trierweiler MW, Freeman RK, James J. Baseline fetal heart rate characteristics as an indicator of fetal status during the antepartum period. *Am J Obstet Gynecol* 1976;125:618–23

6. Hammacher K. The clinical significance of cardiotocography. In Huntington PM, Huter KA, Saline E, eds. *Perinatal Medicine*. Stuttgart: George Shieme Verlagg, 1969:80

7. Kubli FW, Kaeser O, Kinselman M. Diagnostic management of chronic placental insufficiency. In Pecile A, Finzi C, eds. *The FeotoPlacental Unit*. Amsterdam: Excerpta Medica Foundation, 1969:323

8. Sadowsky E, Yaffe H. Daily fetal movement recording and fetal prognosis. *Obstet Gynecol* 1973;41:6

9. Garite TJ, Linzey EM, Freeman RK, *et al*. Fetal heart rate patterns and fetal distress in fetuses with congenital anomalies. *Obstet Gynecol* 1979;53:716–20

10. Phelan JP. The nonstress test: A review of 3000 tests. *Am J Obstet Gynecol* 1981;139:7–10

11. Phelan JP, Cromartie AP, Smith CV. The nonstress test: the false negative test. *Am J Obstet Gynecol* 1982;142:293–6

12. Serafini P, Lindsay MB, Nagey DA, *et al*. Antepartum fetal heart rate response to sound stimulation: the acoustic stimulation test. *Am J Obstet Gynecol* 1984;148:41–5

13. Barrett JM, Salyer SL, Boehm FH. The nonstress test: an evaluation of 1,000 patients. *Am J Obstet Gynecol* 1981;141:153–7

14. Evertson LR, Gauthier RJ, Schifrin BS, *et al*. Antepartum fetal heart rate testing. I. Evolution of the nonstress test. *Am J Obstet Gynecol* 1979;133:29–33

15. Freeman RK, Anderson G, Dorchester W. A prospective multi-institutional study of antepartum fetal heart rate monitoring I. Risk of perinatal mortality and morbidity according to antepartum fetal heart rate test results. *Am J Obstet Gynecol* 1982;143:771–7

16. Schifrin BS, Foye G, Amato J, *et al*. Routine fetal heart rate monitoring in the antepartum period. *Obstet Gynecol* 1979;54:21–5

17. Evertson LR, Paul RH. Antepartum fetal heart rate testing. The nonstress test. *Am J Obstet Gynecol* 1978; 132:895–900

18. Manning FA, Morrison I, Lange IR, *et al*. Fetal assessment based on fetal biophysical profile scoring: experience in 12,620 referred high-risk pregnancies-I. Perinatal mortality by frequency and etiology. *Am J Obstet Gynecol* 1985;151:343–50

19. Manning FA, Platt LD, Sipos L. Antepartum fetal evaluation: development of a fetal biophysical profile. *Am J Obstet Gynecol* 1980;136:787–95

20. Timor-Tritsch IE, Dieker LJ, Hertz RH, *et al*. Studies of antepartum behavioral state in the human fetus at term. *Am J Obstet Gynecol* 1978;132:524–8

21. Keegan KA, Paul RH, Broussar PM, *et al*. Antepartum fetal heart rate testing. III. The effect of phenobarbital on the nonstress test. *Am J Obstet Gynecol* 1979;133: 579–80

22. Martin CB Jr. Behavioural states in the human fetus. *J Reprod Med* 1981;26:425–32

23. Nijhuis JG, Prechtl HFR, Martin CB Jr, *et al*. Are there behavioural states in the human fetus? *Early Hum Dev* 1982;6:177–95

24. Martin CB Jr. Regulation of the fetal heart rate and genesis of FHR patterns. *Semin Perinatol* 1978;2:131–46

25. Cohn HE, Sacks EJ, Heymann MA, *et al*. Cardiovascular responses to hypoxemia and acidemia in fetal lambs. *Am J Obstet Gynecol* 1974;120:817–24

26. Peeters LLH, Sheldon RE, Jones MD Jr, *et al*. Blood flow to fetal organs as a function of arterial oxygen content. *Am J Obstet Gynecol* 1979;135:637–46

27. Caldeyro B, Mendez-Bauer C, Poseior JJ, *et al*. Control of human fetal heart rate during labor. In Cassels EE, ed. *The Heart and Circulation in the Newborn and Infant*. New York: Grune and Stratton, 1966:7

28. Myers RE, Mueller-Heubach E, Adamsons K. Predictability of the state of fetal oxygenation from a quantitative analysis of the components of late deceleration. *Am J Obstet Gynecol* 1973;115:1083–94

29. Weks JW, Asrat T, Morgan MA, *et al*. Antepartum surveillance for a history of stillbirth: when to begin? *Am J Obstet Gynecol* 1995;172:486–92

30. Mendenhall KW, O'Leary JA, Phillips KO. The nonstress test–the value of a single acceleration in evaluating the fetus at risk. *Am J Obstet Gynecol* 1980;136:87–91

31. Keane MWD, Horger EO, Vice L. Comparative study of stressed and non-stressed antepartum fetal heart rate testing. *Obstet Gynecol* 1981;57:320–4

32. Nochimson DJ, Turbeville JS, Terry JE, *et al*. The nonstress test. *Obstet Gynecol* 1978;51:419–21

33. Ingardia CJ, Cetrulo CL, Knuppel RA, *et al*. Prognostic components of the non-reactive non-stress test. *Obstet Gynecol* 1980;56:305–10

34. Weingold AB, Yonekura ML, O'Kieffe J. Non-stress testing. *Am J Obstet Gynecol* 1980;138:195–202

35. Druzin ML, Gratacos J, Paul RH. Antepartum fetal heart rate testing. VI. Predictive reliability of "normal" tests in the prevention of antepartum death. *Am J Obstet Gynecol* 1980;137:746–7

36. Druzin ML, Gratacos J, Keegan KA, *et al*. Antepartum fetal heart rate testing. VII. The significance of fetal bradycardia. *Am J Obstet Gynecol* 1981;139:194–8

37. Druzin ML. Fetal bradycardia during antepartum testing. Further observations. *J Reprod Med* 1989;34:47–51

38. Garite TJ, Freeman RK. Antepartum stress test monitoring. In Quilligan EJ, ed. *Clinics in Obstetrics and Gynecology*. Philadelphia: WB Saunders Co, 1979: 295–307

39. Schifrin BS. Antepartum fetal heart rate monitoring. In Gluck L, ed. *Intrauterine Asphyxia and the Developing Fetal Brain*. Chicago: Year Book Medical Pub Inc, 1977:205

40. Schifrin BS, Lapidus M, Doctor G. Contraction stress test for antepartum fetal evaluation. *Obstet Gynecol* 1975;45:433–8

41. Patrick J, Campbell K, Carmichael L, *et al*. Patterns of gross fetal body movements over 24 hour observation intervals. *Am J Obstet Gynecol* 1982;142:363–71

42. Brown R, Patrick J. The nonstress test: how long is enough. *Am J Obstet Gynecol* 1981;141:646–51

43. Hoppenbrouwers T, Combs D, Ugartechea JC, *et al*. Fetal heart rates during maternal wakefulness and sleep. *Obstet Gynecol* 1981;57:301–9

44. Devoe LD, McKenzie J, Searle NS, *et al*. Clinical sequelae of the extended nonstress test. *Am J Obstet Gynecol* 1985;151:1074–8

45. Druzin ML, Hutson JM, Edersheim T. Relationship of baseline fetal heart rate to gestational age and fetal sex. *Am J Obstet Gynecol* 1986;154:1102–3

46. Schifrin BS. The rationale for antepartum fetal heart rate monitoring. *J Reprod Med* 1979;23:213–21

47. Emmen L, Huisjes HJ, Aarnoudse JG, *et al*. Antepartum diagnosis of the "terminal" fetal state by cardiotocography. *Br J Obstet Gynaecol* 1975;82:353–9

48. Rochard F, Schifrin BS, Goupil F, *et al*. Nonstressed fetal heart rate monitoring in the antepartum period. *Am J Obstet Gynecol* 1976;126:699–706

49. Visser GHA, Huisjes HJ. Diagnostic value of the unstressed antepartum cardiotocogram. *Br J Obstet Gynaecol* 1977;84:321–6

50. Weiner Z, Farmakides G, Schulman H, *et al*. Computerized analysis of fetal heart rate variation in postterm pregnancy: prediction of intrapartum fetal distress and fetal acidosis. *Am J Obstet Gynecol* 1994;171:1132–8

51. Guzman ER, Vintzileos AM, Martins M, *et al*. The efficacy of individual computer heart rate indices in detecting acidemia at birth in growth-restricted fetuses. *Obstet Gynecol* 1996;87:969–74

52. Phelan JP, Lewis PE. Fetal heart rate decelerations during a nonstress test. *Obstet Gynecol* 1981;57:228–32

53. Phelan JP, Platt LD, Yeh SY, *et al*. Continuing role of the nonstress test in the management of the postdates pregnancy. *Obstet Gynecol* 1984;64:624–8

54. Small ML, Phelan JP, Smith CV, *et al*. An active management approach to the postdate fetus with a reactive nonstress test and FHR decelerations. *Obstet Gynecol* 1987;70:636–40

55. Bourgeois FJ, Thiagarajah S, Harbert G Jr. The significance of fetal heart rate decelerations during nonstress testing. *Am J Obstet Gynecol* 1984;150:213–6

56. Dashow EE, Read JA. Significant fetal bradycardia during antepartum heart rate testing. *Am J Obstet Gynecol* 1984;148:187–90

57. Druzin ML, Lockshin M, Edersheim TG, *et al*. Second trimester fetal monitoring and preterm delivery in

pregnancies with systemic lupus erythematosus and/or circulating anticoagulant. *Am J Obstet Gynecol* 1987; 157:1503–10

58. Lavin JP Jr, Miodovnik M, Barden TP. The relationship of nonstress test reactivity and gestational age. *Obstet Gynecol* 1984;63:338–44

59. Sorokin Y, Dierker LJ, Pillay SK, *et al.* The association between fetal heart rate patterns and fetal movements in pregnancies between 20 and 30 weeks' gestation. *Am J Obstet Gynecol* 1982;143:243–9

60. Druzin ML, Fox A, Kogut E, *et al.* The relationship of the nonstress test to gestational age. *Am J Obstet Gynecol* 1985;153:383–9

61. Smith CV, Phelan JP, Paul RH. A prospective analysis of the influence of gestational age on the baseline fetal heart rate and reactivity in a low-risk population. *Am J Obstet Gynecol* 1985;153:780–2

62. Natale R, Nasello C, Turliuk R. The relationship between movements and accelerations in fetal heart rate at twenty-four to thirty-two weeks gestation. *Am J Obstet Gynecol* 1984;148:591–5

63. Gabbe SG, Greeman RK, Goebelsmann U. Evaluation of contraction stress test before 33 weeks gestation. *Obstet Gynecol* 1978;52:649–52

64. Goodman LDS, Visser FGA, Dawes GS. Effects of maternal cigarette smoking on fetal trunk movements, fetal breathing movements and the fetal heart rate. *Br J Obstet Gynaecol* 1984;91:657–61

65. Druzin ML, Foodim J. Effect of maternal glucose ingestion compared with maternal water ingestion on the nonstress test. *Obstet Gynecol* 1986;67:425–6

66. Druzin ML, Gratacos J, Paul RH, *et al.* Antepartum fetal heart rate testing. XII. The effect of manual manipulation of the fetus on the nonstress test. *Am J Obstet Gynecol* 1985;151:61–64

67. Read JA, Miller FC. Fetal heart rate acceleration in response to acoustic stimulation as a measure of fetal well-being. *Am J Obstet Gynecol* 1977;129:512–17

68. Ohel G, Birkenfeld A, Rabinowitz R, *et al.* Fetal response to vibratory acoustic stimulation in periods of low heart rate activity. *Am J Obstet Gynecol* 1986; 154:619–21

69. Smith CV, Phelan JP, Broussard PM, *et al.* Fetal acoustic stimulation testing: a retrospective analysis of the fetal acoustic stimulation test. *Am J Obstet Gynecol* 1985; 153:567–9

70. Smith CV, Phelan JP, Platt LD, *et al.* Fetal acoustic stimulation testing. II. A randomized clinical comparison with the nonstress test. *Am J Obstet Gynecol* 1986; 155:131–4

71. Smith CV, Phelan JP, Broussard P, *et al.* Fetal acoustic stimulation testing. III. Predictive value of a reactive test. *J Reprod Med* 1988;33:217–18

72. Inglis S, Druzin ML, Wagner W, *et al.* Predictive reliability of normal biophysical profile (BPP) following vibro-acoustic stimulation (VAS) is equivalent to normal BPP without VAS. *Am J Obstet Gynecol* 1991;164:363, abstr. 424

73. Romero R, Mazor M, Hobbins JC. A critical appraisal of fetal acoustic stimulation as an antenatal test for fetal well-being. *Obstet Gynecol* 1988;71:781–6

74. Manning FA, Hill LM, Platt LD. Qualitative amniotic fluid volume determination by ultrasound. *Am J Obstet Gynecol* 1981;139:254–8

75. Phelan JP, Platt LD, Yeh SY, *et al.* The role of ultra-sound assessment of amniotic fluid volume in the management of the post date pregnancy. *Am J Obstet Gynecol* 1985;151:304–8

76. Chamberlain PF, Manning FA, Morrison E, *et al.* Ultra-sound evaluation of amniotic fluid volume. I. The relationship of marginal decreased amniotic fluid volume to perinatal outcome. *Am J Obstet Gynecol* 1984;150: 245–9

77. Phelan JP, Smith CV, Broussard P, *et al.* Amniotic fluid volume assessment using the four quadrant technique in the pregnancy between 36 and 42 weeks gestation. *J Reprod Med* 1987;32:540–2

78. Phelan JP. Antepartum fetal assessment - new techniques. *Sem Perinatol* 1988;12:57–65

79. Devoe LD, Yankowitch G, Azor H. The application of multiparameter scoring to antepartum fetal heart rate testing. *J Reprod Med* 1981;26:250–4

80. Krebs HB, Petres RE. Clinical application of a scoring system for evaluation of antenatal fetal heart rate monitoring. *Am J Obstet Gynecol* 1978;130:765–72

81. Lyons ER, Bylsma HM, Shams S, *et al.* A scoring system for nonstressed antepartum fetal heart rate monitoring. *Am J Obstet Gynecol* 1979;133:242–6

82. Knuppel RA, Pawan KR, Scerbo JC, *et al.* Intrauterine fetal death in twins after 32 weeks of gestation. *Obstet Gynecol* 1985;65:172–5

83. Lenstrup C. Predictive value of antepartum nonstress test in multiple pregnancies. *Acta Obstet Gynecol Scand* 1984;63:597–601

51

Doppler velocimetry for fetal surveillance: principles and practice

D. Maulik

INTRODUCTION

Doppler sonography, a technique based upon the physical phenomenon first described by Austrian mathematician and physicist Christian Andreas Doppler in 1841, has made non-invasive assessment of circulation possible, thereby revolutionizing medical diagnostics. Doppler first reported this phenomenon at a meeting of the Natural Sciences Section of the Royal Bohemian Society in Prague, a meeting with only five members of the Society in attendance and a transcriber. His paper, entitled 'On the Colored Light of the Double Stars and Certain Other Stars of the Heavens' was published in 1843 in the society's proceedings[1]. To Doppler's disappointment, however, the paper was not enthusiastically received by the scientific community of his time, although his principle has been extensively used in science and technology since the beginning of the twentieth century.

The premier medical use of Doppler sonography occurred during the late 1950s. The first prototype Doppler ultrasound device for medical application was developed by Satomura, a researcher from the Institute of Scientific and Industrial Research for Osaka University in Japan[2], who also suggested the potential use for percutaneous evaluation of blood flow. Satomura and Kaneko in 1959 were the first to report the construction of an ultrasonic flowmeter[3]. Baker, Watkins and Reid at the University of Washington in Seattle were the first in the United States to develop pulsed Doppler equipment[4]. Other pioneers of pulsed Doppler include Wells in the United Kingdom[5], Peronneau and Leger[6], and Plainol, Pourcelot and co-workers[7] in France.

The use of Doppler sonography for the investigation of human fetal circulation was first reported by FitzGerald and Drumm in 1977[8]. Their work gave rise to a rich period in medicine during which this technique was used by many investigators to characterize most major fetal circulatory systems (Table 1). Many clinical studies, mostly confirming, but occasionally refuting, the diagnostic efficacy of Doppler velocimetry in various pregnancy disorders have since been published. Furthermore, the benefits of Doppler fetal

Table 1 Feasibility of Doppler velocimetry of fetal and uteroplacental circulations

Circulation	Year	Investigators
Umbilical artery	1977	FitzGerald and Drumm[8]
Umbilical vein	1979	Gill[12]
Fetal aorta	1980	Eik-Nes and associates[13]
Uteroplacental	1983	Campbell and associates[20]
Fetal inferior vena cava	1983	Chiba and associates[97]
Fetal cardiac	1984	Maulik and associates[4]
Fetal cerebral	1986	Arbeille and associates[90]
	1986	Wladimiroff and associates[89]
Renal	1988	Vyas and associates[103]

surveillance have been investigated extensively by randomized clinical trials. In subsequent years, most of the relevant issues pertaining to Doppler ultrasound measurement of maternal–fetal hemodynamics which had been raised in the National Institute of Child Health and Development Health Workshop of 1986[9] were addressed. The diagnostic efficacy and clinical effectiveness of the Doppler technique has been extensively investigated. Of the various modalities of fetal surveillance, only the Doppler method shows evidence of improved fetal outcome based on randomized clinical trials and meta-analyses and has now become a standard for fetal surveillance in most parts of the world. This chapter examines the following issues related to the obstetrical use of this technique:

(1) Principles of Doppler velocimetry and the hemodynamic foundation of its use.

(2) Doppler velocimetry of the fetal and uteroplacental circulation.

(3) Clinical efficacy of Doppler velocimetry for fetal surveillance.

(4) Guideline for the clinical application of the Doppler technique.

For a more comprehensive review of the various clinical and basic aspects of Doppler sonography, however, a dedicated text or reference book is recommended[10].

DOPPLER FREQUENCY SHIFT

When relative motion occurs between a source of wave transmission and an observer, the observed changes in the frequency of energy wave transmission is defined as the Doppler effect. The change in the frequency is called the Doppler frequency shift or just the Doppler shift:

$$f_d = f_t - f_r \qquad (1)$$

where f_d is the Doppler shift frequency, f_t is the transmitted frequency and f_r is the received frequency. When the source and the observer move closer, the wavelength decreases and the frequency increases. Conversely, when the source and the observer move apart, the wavelength increases and the frequency decreases. The principle applies to all forms of energy wave propagation including sound. The utility of the Doppler effect originates from the fact that the shift in the frequency is proportional to the speed of movement between the source and the receiver and therefore can be used to assess this speed.

The phenomenon of the Doppler effect is observed when an ultrasound beam encounters a scatterer in motion. The scatterer acts first as a moving receiver and then as a moving source[11]. This forms the basis for restating equation (1) as:

$$f_d = 2f_t v/c \qquad (2)$$

where f_d represents the Doppler frequency shift, f_t the frequency of the incident beam (transducer frequency), v the velocity of the scatterer in a given direction, and c the propagation speed of sound in the medium. Note that the transmitted ultrasound undergoes double Doppler shift before returning to the receiving transducer, the scatterer acting first as a receiver and then as a transmitter. This accounts for the factor of 2 in the above equation. In blood circulation, millions of red cells act as moving scatterers of an incident ultrasound which consequently will undergo frequency shift proportional to the speed of red-cell movement and therefore to blood-flow velocity.

When the incident beam incurs an angle (θ) to the direction of blood flow, the v in the Doppler equation is replaced by the component of the velocity in the direction of the flow obtained by the cosine of the angle (cos θ) (Figure 1):

$$f_d = 2(f_t \cos \theta\, v)/c \qquad (3)$$

To determine the velocity of the scatterer, equation (3) can be rewritten as follows:

$$v = f_d\, c/2f_t \cos \theta \qquad (4)$$

Thus if the angle of beam incidence and the Doppler shift are known, the velocity of blood flow is also known assuming that the transducer frequency and the velocity of sound in tissue remain relatively

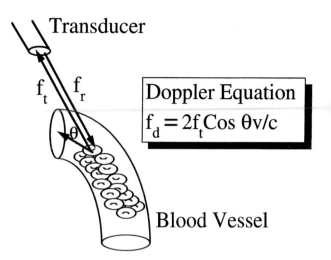

Figure 1 Graphic depiction of the principles of Doppler equation and the proportional relationship between the Doppler shift and the velocity of blood flow. f_t, Doppler frequency shift; f_r, transmitted frequency; f_d, Doppler frequency shift; v, velocity of blood flow; θ, the angle of insonation between the ultrasound beam and the direction of flow; c, velocity of sound in tissue

Table 2 Hemodynamic information from Doppler sonography

- Presence of normal flow in expected location
- Presence of flow in unexpected location
- Absence of flow in expected location
- Speed of blood flow
- Direction of flow
- Circulatory impedance in the arterial circulation
- Volumetric flow
- Disturbed hemodynamics, e.g. turbulent flow

constant. The above equation forms the basis for the clinical application of the Doppler principle.

CIRCULATORY INFORMATION FROM DOPPLER SHIFT

Doppler sonography can yield a variety of clinically useful hemodynamic information. This includes quantification of flow and study of the flow velocity waveform (Table 2). Volumetric flow can be measured by integrating the average velocity across the vascular lumen with the vascular cross-sectional area. In the fetus, the Doppler technique has been used to measure umbilical venous flow[12], descending aortic flow[13] and fetal cardiac output[14]. However, Doppler flow quantification has been of little practical use because of the inherent unreliability of the technique. Consequently, the main perinatal use for Doppler sonography has been indirect assessment of downstream impedance by Doppler waveform analysis.

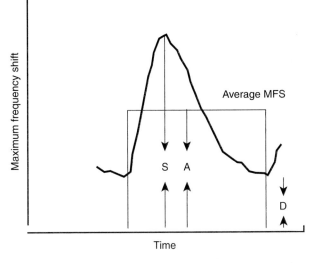

Figure 2 Doppler indices estimated from the maximum frequency shift (MFS) envelope.
S, peak systolic frequency shift value of the envelope; *D*, end-diastolic frequency shift value of the envelope; *A*, average value of the envelope over one cardiac cycle, RI = (S–D)/S[6]; PI = (S–D)/A[5]; S/D Ratio[7]; D/A Ratio[9]
With permission from Maulik D, Yarlagadda P, Youngblood JP, Ciston P. Comparative efficacy of umbilical arterial Doppler indices for predicting adverse perinatal outcome. *Am J Obstet Gynecol* 1991;164:1434

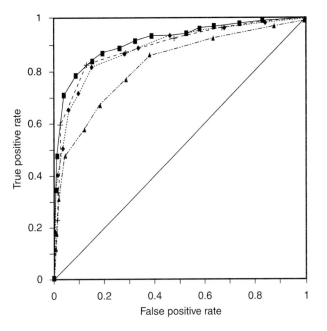

Figure 3 Receiver operating characteristic curves of umbilical arterial Doppler indices. Data points are the measured values of indices. Note that the RI shows the most and the PI the least diagnostic efficacy.
–■–, RI; –+··, S : D; ···◆···, D : A; –▲··, PI.
With permission from Maulik D, Yarlagadda P, Youngblood JP, Ciston P. Comparative efficacy of umbilical arterial Doppler indices for predicting adverse perinatal outcome. *Am J Obstet Gynecol* 1991;164:1434

Doppler waveform analysis

Doppler waveform analysis is usually based on the following characteristics of the maximum frequency shift envelope (Figure 2): the peak systolic value (*S*), end-diastolic value (*D*), and the average value over the cardiac cycle (*A*). These three parameters have been used to develop indices describing the pulsatility of the Doppler waveform. A Doppler index is calculated as a ratio and is, therefore, virtually independent of the angle of insonation. Of the numerous indices, the pulsatility index (PI)1[5], the resistance index (RI)[16], and the *S* : *D* ratio[17] are most commonly used in obstetrical applications. Maulik *et al.*[18] used the receiver operating characteristic (ROC) technique (Figure 3) to investigate the comparative efficacy of the umbilical arterial Doppler indices for predicting adverse perinatal outcome and showed that the RI had the best discriminatory ability when compared with the *S* : *D* ratio ($p < 0.05$), the PI ($p < 0.001$) and the *D* : *A* ratio ($p < 0.05$). Although several workers have described more comprehensive approaches to Doppler waveform analysis[19–22], there is little evidence that these are superior to the traditional Doppler indices. The hemodynamic, angiomorphological and pathophysiological justifications for Doppler waveform analysis are discussed below.

Hemodynamic rationale of Doppler waveform analysis

The rationale is that the Doppler waveform from an arterial source represents the arterial velocity waveform and is configured by both the upstream and downstream circulatory factors. Analysis of the waveform should, therefore, yield information on downstream impedance to flow. Obviously, this requires verification. Although the term 'peripheral vascular resistance' has been traditionally used for describing opposition to flow in an arterial tree, it is applicable only to a steady non-pulsatile flow state. Opposition to flow in a pulsatile circulation is more accurately expressed by the concept of vascular impedance which also includes the resistance. An integral component of this concept is the phenomenon of wave reflection in a vascular tree. Configuration of pressure and flow waves at a specific location results from the interaction of the forward propagating (orthograde) waves with the reflected backward propagating (retrograde) waves[23,24]. The observed pressure waves, which are produced by the summation of orthograde and retrograde waves, show an 'additive' effect; in contrast, the observed flow (or flow velocity) waves demonstrate a 'subtractive' effect (Figure 4). Wave reflections arise whenever there is a significant alteration or mismatching in vascular

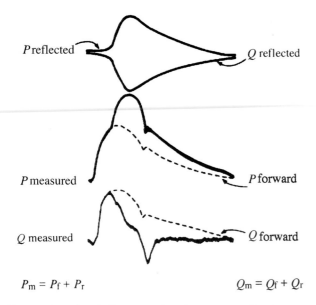

$$P_{\mathrm{m}} = P_{\mathrm{f}} + P_{\mathrm{r}} \qquad\qquad Q_{\mathrm{m}} = Q_{\mathrm{f}} + Q_{\mathrm{r}}$$

Figure 4 The influence of pulse wave reflections on ascending aortic pressure (P) and flow (Q) waveforms. Incident or forward (f) and backward or reflected (r) pressure and flow waves are summed to yield measured (m) pressure and flow waveforms. The forward pressure and flow waves are identical, and so are the reflected waves except that the reflected flow wave is inverted with impact to the reflected pressure wave. With permission from Nichols, *et al*. Age related changes in left ventricular/arterial coupling. In *Ventricular/Vascular Coupling*. Yin FCP, ed. New York: Springer Verlag, 1987:79

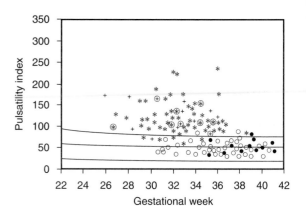

Figure 5 Pulsatility indices of the uteroplacental arteries, measured prior to delivery, plotted on the reference curve. The curve is shown in the format of centiles (3rd, 50th, 97th centiles). The cases with normal placental bed biopsies are marked by open circles, those with pathological classification by stars. The pulsatility index values in the 25 excluded cases are also plotted to show their distribution among the selected suitable cases, which fulfilled the histological criteria of a true placental bed biopsy. The healthy cases are marked by solid circles, the pathological cases by crosses. The pulsatility index values in the group with uteroplacental insufficiency but no hypertension are marked by circled stars and crosses, showing that they are similar to the group with hypertension. Exclusion of the unsuitable cases did not bias the results. With permission from Voigt HJ, Becker V. Uteroplacental insufficiency – comparison of uteroplacental blood flow velocimetry and histomorphology of placental bed. *J Matern Fetal Invest* 1992;2:251

impedance in a circulation. Current evidence suggests that the arterial–arteriolar junctions serve as the main source of wave reflections in an arterial tree. Vasodilation leads to a fall and vasoconstriction to a rise in impedance and wave reflection.

The hemodynamic validation studies may be grouped as those relating to the peripheral resistance and those involving the impedance. Studies in the former group demonstrated a significant relationship between the Doppler indices and the vascular resistance[25–28]. However, as mentioned above vascular impedance is a more appropriate descriptor of opposition to pulsatile flow than resistance. The second group of studies addressed this issue. Maulik and co-workers[29] used an *in vitro* circulatory simulation system for hydrodynamic validation of the Doppler indices. The impedance to flow was progressively increased by sequentially occluding the vessels of the branching model. The Doppler indices correlated significantly ($P < 0.01$) with the parameters of downstream impedance. This was also investigated by Downing and co-workers of the same group[30,31] in a chronic lamb model and it was observed that a significant correlation exists between the PI and the impedance parameters provided the reflex heart rate changes are suppressed. Evidently, the Doppler indices reflect changes in the

downstream impedance. However, the indices may also be affected by heart-rate variations which may obfuscate the former's ability to reflect impedance.

Angiomorphological validation of the Doppler indices

A number of investigators have also addressed the issue of angiomorphological basis for umbilical and uterine arterial velocimetry. Giles and co-workers[32] observed a statistically significant decrease ($p < 0.01$) in the model small arterial count (arteries in the tertiary stem villi measuring < 90 μm in diameter) in abnormal pregnancies with an abnormal umbilical arterial $S : D$ ratio. A similar observation has been reported in relation to the uteroplacental vascular bed and the uteroplacental Doppler waveform. Voigt and Becker[33] performed placental bed biopsies in pregnancies complicated by pre-eclampsia or fetal growth retardation delivered by Cesarean section, and in a control group of healthy pregnancies delivered by Cesarean section for labor dysfunction or malpresentation. Figure 5 summarizes the results. The uteroplacental PI predicted abnormal uteroplacental vascular

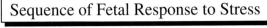

Sequence of Fetal Response to Stress

Sequence may vary according to the etiology and progression

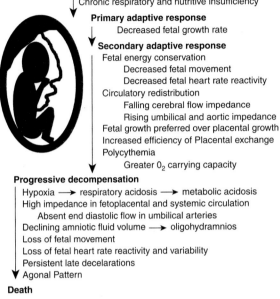

Stress
│ Chronic respiratory and nutritive insufficiency
▼
Primary adaptive response
Decreased fetal growth rate
▼
Secondary adaptive response
Fetal energy conservation
Decreased fetal movement
Decreased fetal heart rate reactivity
Circulatory redistribution
Falling cerebral flow impedance
Rising umbilical and aortic impedance
Fetal growth preferred over placental growth
Increased efficiency of Placental exchange
Polycythemia
Greater O_2 carrying capacity
▼
Progressive decompensation
Hypoxia ⟶ respiratory acidosis ⟶ metabolic acidosis
High impedance in fetoplacental and systemic circulation
Absent end diastolic flow in umbilical arteries
Declining amniotic fluid volume ⟶ oligohydramnios
Loss of fetal movement
Loss of fetal heart rate reactivity and variability
Persistent late decelerations
▼ Agonal Pattern

Death

Figure 6 Summary of fetal sequential response to progressive stress. Note that the depicted sequence is an approximation and the actual course may vary depending on the characteristics of the chronic deprivation and the individual fetal ability to cope. With permission from Maulik D. Doppler velocimetry for fetal surveillance: adverse perinatal outcome and fetal hypoxia. In Maulik D, ed. *Doppler Ultrasound in Obstetrics and Gynecology*. New York: Springer-Verlag, 1997:349

pathology with an accuracy of 90%, a sensitivity of 90%, and a specificity of 95%.

These observations suggest the following vascular and hemodynamic mechanisms for the abnormal Doppler waveforms. Fetoplacental or uteroplacental vaso-obliterative pathology results in an increase in the arterial impedance, which is necessarily associated with enhanced pressure and flow velocity wave reflections. The reflected flow velocity waves propagate retrogradely and change the shape of arterial flow velocity waves. Doppler insonation of the appropriate arterial tree identifies this circulatory phenomenon by demonstrating abnormal Doppler waveforms and indices.

Pathophysiological rationale for Doppler fetal surveillance

Antepartum challenge to fetal well being may arise from chronic nutritive and respiratory deprivation. A spectrum of obstetrical complications, including fetal growth retardation and hypertension, may expose the fetus to such risks. Although an immense amount of information is available on acute and subacute fetal

respiratory deficit, the pathophysiological mechanism of chronic fetal stress has been less clear. However, significant advances have been made recently providing considerable insight into the mechanisms of fetal compensation and decompensation. There is emerging evidence that, encountering sustained stress, the fetus appears to mobilize a spectrum of defensive responses which include preferential preservation of fetal growth over placental growth, changes in fetal movement pattern, and the eventual deceleration of the fetal growth rate (Figure 6).

In the face of continuing deprivation, compensation gives way to decompensation. For example, growth-restricted human fetuses have been shown to develop chronic hypoxia and acidosis. A critical component of fetal homeostatic response involves flow redistribution which favors perfusion of the vital organs (the brain, heart and adrenals) at the expense of flow to muscle, viscera, skin and other less critical tissues and organs[34]. Underlying this phenomenon are the diverse changes in blood-flow impedance in fetal regional circulations. The ability of Doppler indices to reflect changes in flow impedance has been conclusively demonstrated. It also has been shown that fetoplacental or uteroplacental vaso-obliterative pathology results in an increase in the arterial impedance, which is reflected by the abnormal Doppler indices. Doppler velocimetry thus elucidates these circulatory changes associated with fetal compromise and allows perinatal prognostication. This constitutes the rationale for using Doppler ultrasound for fetal surveillance in complicated pregnancies.

DOPPLER VELOCIMETRY OF UMBILICAL ARTERIAL CIRCULATION: NORMATIVE DATA

The umbilical artery was the first fetal vessel to be evaluated by Doppler velocimetry and has since become the most widely investigated fetal circulation. Typically, Doppler interrogation of the umbilical arterial circulation is performed during fetal apnea (see below). In our experience, the inter- and intra-observer variances of the $S:D$ ratio and the RI, as determined by continuous-wave Doppler, were 9.8 and 11.1%, and 4 and 8%, respectively[35]. In normal pregnancy, the umbilical arterial Doppler indices are affected by gestational age, fetal heart rate, fetal breathing and the site of measurement in the cord.

As pregnancy advances, umbilical arterial Doppler waveforms show a progressive rise in the end-diastolic velocity which results in a concomitant fall in the pulsatility (Figure 7). This trend is consistent with a gradual decline in the fetoplacental flow impedance with the advancing gestation[36]. The Doppler indices reflect these changes in the waveform (Figure 8). A statistically significant effect of the heart rate on

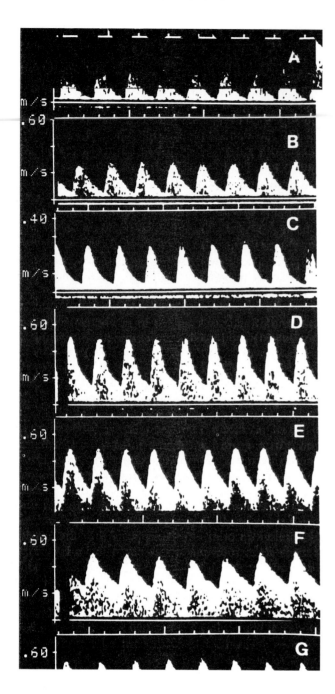

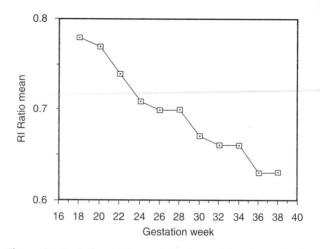

Figure 8   Variation in the umbilical arterial resistance index (RI) at different stages of gestation. With permission from Maulik D. Basic principles of Doppler ultrasound as applied to obstetrics. Clin Obstet Gynecol 1989;32:641

Doppler indices has been reported by a number of investigators[37,38]. It has been shown that changes in the heart rate occur primarily due to alterations in the duration of the diastolic component of the cardiac cycle[39,40], and that the effect of the fetal heart rate may contribute to 15–18% of the variance of the Doppler indices[35]. However, it is not certain that correcting the Doppler indices for fetal heart rate changes would improve the diagnostic efficacy of the indices. Substantial changes in the intrathoracic pressure and central hemodynamics occur during fetal breathing, which produce dynamic variability in the umbilical arterial Doppler waveform and, therefore, in the Doppler indices. This severely compromises the utility of the Doppler indices during fetal breathing and provides the rationale for measuring the indices only during fetal apnea. The location of the Doppler sampling site in the umbilical cord affects the Doppler waveform and therefore the Doppler indices[35,41], which are higher at the fetal than at the placental end of the cord. With the continuous-wave Doppler devices, which are incapable of range resolution, sampling location remains undetermined. There is no evidence, however, that the pulsed-wave Doppler duplex system, which allows range resolution, offers any diagnostic superiority over the continuous-wave Doppler. Finally, the indices do not appear to be affected by fetal behavioral states[42,43].

UMBILICAL ARTERIAL DOPPLER IN FETAL GROWTH RESTRICTION (FGR)

It has been the conventional wisdom that FGR is associated with uteroplacental and fetal circulatory insufficiency. This is supported by the observation that a substantial fall in the umbilical blood flow and subsequent FGR can be produced by microsphere embolization of the uteroplacental circulation in a ewe model[44].

Figure 7   Gestational age effect on the umbilical arterial Doppler frequency shift waveforms. Panels are organized from the top to the bottom according to advancing gestation. A, waveforms at 16 weeks; B, waveforms at 20 weeks; C, waveforms at 24 weeks; D, waveforms at 28 weeks; E, waveforms at 32 weeks; F, waveforms at 36 weeks; G, waveforms at 40 weeks. Note the progressive increase in the end-diastolic velocity and the concomitant fall in the pulsatility as the gestation advances. With permission from Maulik D. Umbilical arterial Doppler velocimetry: normative data and diagnostic efficacy. In Maulik D, ed. *Doppler Ultrasound in Obstetrics and Gynecology.* New York: Springer-Verlag, 1997:129

It has also been demonstrated that when fetal growth is compromised in human pregnancies, the spiral endometrial arterioles often lack appropriate trophoblastic invasion of the media and may display atherosclerotic changes[45]. Although early clinical studies indicated a strong association between abnormal umbilical arterial Doppler indices and suboptimal fetal growth, subsequent experience, however, was mixed (Table 3)[46–53]. This may be partly explained by the considerable amount of ambiguity that surrounds the use of the terms FGR and small for gestational age (SGA). It is well recognized that neither all growth-restricted fetuses are SGA, nor are all SGA infants growth compromised. Furthermore, being SGA does not necessarily mean a compromised outcome. It is apparent that not all FGR or SGA fetuses may suffer from *in utero* compromise in terms of asphyxia, which correlates better with absent end-diastolic velocity in the umbilical artery than with subnormal fetal abdominal circumference (< 5th percentile) as measured by ultrasound[54]. This issue, however, is apparently controversial and is further discussed in the next section. With regard to the various sonographic modalities for recognizing an SGA infant, the majority of studies have demonstrated that conventional fetal ultrasound biometry is more sensitive than umbilical arterial Doppler velocimetry[55–57]. This should not be surprising as fetal size is expected to be better expressed by sonographic measurement of fetal dimensions than by Doppler velocimetry which assesses the hemodynamic state; unless the latter is compromised, the Doppler indices will not change.

UMBILICAL ARTERIAL DOPPLER VELOCIMETRY AND ANTEPARTUM FETAL HYPOXIA–ASPHYXIA

The purpose of fetal surveillance is to detect fetal compromise from *in utero* hypoxia and asphyxia. Fetal homeostatic response to hypoxic and asphyxial challenge has been well described in animals[58]. A central manifestation of this response is the flow redistribution which favors perfusion of the vital organs (the brain, the heart, and the adrenals) at the expense of less critical organs and tissues. This compensatory phenomenon provided the justification for investigating the efficacy of the Doppler velocimetry in identifying fetal hypoxia and asphyxia. Both clinical and animal experimental studies have been reported to address this issue.

Further insight may be obtained from experimental studies conducted in animal models. Many of the relevant findings in this area have been reviewed[59]. In relation to umbilical arterial circulation in the lamb fetus, it appears that the Doppler waveform changes only with severe hypoxia or acidosis[60]. Often, such alterations in the waveform may merely reflect fetal bradycardia induced by acute hypoxia[42]. Similarly, it has been[56] noted that in the aorta of the fetal lamb, significant changes in the Doppler waveform occur only when the oxygen saturation declines to 10–15% or the fetal pH drops to < 7.15. Apparently, in an ovine fetus, hypoxia and acidosis may significantly affect umbilical and aortic velocity waveforms but only as a late phenomenon.

More significantly, a number of clinical studies have been reported in which the association between the Doppler findings and fetal blood gases has been investigated[57,61–68]. These are summarized in Table 4. The studies employed two distinct approaches for the assessment of fetal asphyxia. In four studies, umbilical cord-blood sampling was performed at the time of elective Cesarean section. Obviously, these studies are limited because blood gases measured in this manner may not reflect fetal acid–base status *in utero*. In the remaining five studies, blood gases were determined on fetal blood samples collected by cordocentesis. Most studies used Doppler assessment of the umbilical artery, whereas one used aortic mean velocity, and another added aortic and carotid Doppler assessment. All studies measured pH, most performed PO_2, and some also measured PCO_2 and lactate. Most investigators found a significant association between Doppler assessment of fetal circulation and fetal acid–base

Table 3 Diagnostic efficacy of umbilical arterial Doppler in intrauterine growth retardation

Investigators	Doppler index	Prevalence rate (%)	Sensitivity (%)	Specificity (%)	Positive predictive value (%)
Fleischer *et al.* (1985)	$S:D > 3.0$	16.8	78	83	49
Arduini *et al.* (1987)	PI > 1 SD	30.7	60.8	73	50
Berkowitz *et al.* (1988)	$S:D > 3.0$	25	55	92	73
Divon *et al.* (1988)	$S:D > 3.0$	35.4	49	94	81
Gaziano *et al.* (1988)	$S:D > 4.0$	9.4	79	66	79
Ott (1990)	$S:D > 3.0$	10.4	59	84	29
Maulik *et al.* (1990)	$S:D > 2.9$	12.3	75	71	27
Lowery *et al.* (1990)	$S:D > 4.0$	22.6	65	66	24

$S:D$ ratio, systolic/diastolic ratio; PI, pulsatility index. Modified with permission from Maulik D. Doppler ultrasound in obstetrics. In *Williams Obstetrics*, Cunningham *et al.* eds. 19th edn. Suppl 16

Table 4   Association between fetal Doppler results and fetal blood gases

Author (reference)	Patient population	Patient risk category	Cord blood sampling	Doppler assessment	Acid–Base parameters	Association correlation
Soothill	29	SGA	Cordocentesis	Aortic MV	pH, P_{O_2}, P_{CO_2}	Present
Nicolaides	59	SGA	Cordocentesis	Umbilical arterial AEDV	pH, P_{O_2}	Present
Ferrazzi	14	High risk	Cesarean section	Umbilical arterial PI	pH, P_{CO_2} lactate	Present
Tyrell	112	Unselected	Cesarean section	Umbilical arterial AEDV	pH, P_{O_2}	Present
Bilardo	51	SGA, AGA	Cordocentesis	Umbilical arterial, aortic, carotid PI, RI, MV	pH, P_{O_2}	Present
Vintzileos[*]	62	High risk	Cesarean section	Umbilical arterial $S : D$	pH	Absent
Yoon[*]	105	Unselected	Cesarean section	Umbilical arterial PI	pH, P_{O_2}, P_{CO_2}	Present
Pardi[**]	21	SGA	Cordocentesis	Umbilical arterial PI	pH, P_{O_2}, P_{CO_2}, lactate	Present
Yoon[*]	24	High risk	Cordocentesis	Umbilical arterial PI	pH, P_{O_2}, P_{CO_2}	Present

SGA, small for gestational age; AGA, appropriate for gestational age; AEDV, absent end diastolic velocity; MV, mean velocity; PI, pulsatility index; RI, resistance index; $S : D$, systolic diastolic ratio. [*]Studies compared the Doppler method with the biophysical profile. [**]Study compared fetal-heart rate monitoring with the Doppler method. With permission from Maulik D. *Doppler Ultrasound in Obstetrics and Gynecology*. New York: Springer-Verlag, 1996

compromise. The response of fetal cerebral Doppler waveform presents another perspective on fetal hypoxia and acidosis. This is discussed later in the section dealing with fetal cerebral circulation.

UMBILICAL ARTERIAL DOPPLER VELOCIMETRY AND ADVERSE PERINATAL OUTCOME

The discriminatory efficacy of Doppler velocimetry for predicting perinatal outcome is briefly in this section. A fetal surveillance test may be used either as a diagnostic test for identifying the fetal compromise in high-risk pregnancies, or as a screening test in general obstetrical population at low risk for fetal compromise. Both are presented below. In evaluating this information, we need to recognize the imprecision inherent in the available criteria for defining adverse perinatal outcome.

High-risk pregnancies

Several preliminary studies indicate that the Doppler indices may be powerful predictors of adverse perinatal outcome in complicated pregnancies. The diagnostic efficacy of umbilical arterial $A : B$ (systolic, diastolic) ratio was investigated by Trudinger and co-workers[69] in 170 high-risk patients. The parameters of fetal compromise included birthweight below the 10th percentile or an Apgar score of < 7 at 5 minutes. The fetal heart rate was assessed in terms of reactivity and a modified Fischer score. The Doppler results revealed a sensitivity of 60%, a specificity of 85%, and a positive predictive value of 64%. For the fetal heart-rate reactivity, the corresponding results were 17%, 97%, and 69%, respectively. The values for the Fischer score

results were 36%, 88%, and 58%, respectively. In this study, the umbilical arterial $S : D$ ratio appeared to be more sensitive, but less specific than the electronic fetal heart rate monitoring techniques. Farmakides *et al.*[70] investigated the diagnostic efficacy of the non-stress test (NST) and of the umbilical arterial $S : D$ ratio in 140 pregnancies. The measures of outcome included FGR, fetal distress, Cesarean section for fetal distress, and admission to the neonatal intensive care unit. Fetuses with a normal NST but abnormal $S : D$ ratio had an outcome worse than those with an abnormal NST and a normal $S : D$ ratio; however, those with both tests abnormal experienced the worst outcome. In another study, Brar *et al.*[71] noted that patients with an umbilical arterial $S : D$ ratio > 3 had a significantly greater incidence of SGA infants, fetal distress in labor, presence of meconium at delivery, Cesarean sections, and 5-minute Apgar scores < 7.

Maulik and co-workers[62] studied the diagnostic efficacy of the umbilical arterial $S : D$ ratio for predicting adverse perinatal outcome in 350 high-risk pregnant patients utilizing the ROC technique and other traditional parameters of testing a test. The latter included sensitivity, specificity and the predictive values. The kappa index was used to investigate the degree of agreement between the test and the outcome. The abnormal outcome parameters included SGA (< 10th percentile), Apgar score at 5 minutes > 7, fetal distress (late and severe variable decelerations, absent variability, fetal scalp pH < 7.20), umbilical cord arterial pH < 7.20, presence of thick meconium, and admission to neonatal intensive care unit (> 48 hours). The study indicated that the ratio well predicted the general adverse perinatal outcomes; however, the diagnostic efficacy was better when the SGA infants were excluded (Table 5).

Table 5   Diagnostic efficacy of systolic/diastolic ratio cutoff point of 3.0 to predict the various abnormal outcomes

Category	Sensitivity	Specificity	Positive predictive value	Negative predictive value	Kappa index
General abnormal outcome	0.79	0.93	0.83	0.91	0.73
SGA only	0.75	0.77	0.32	0.95	0.33
Fetal distress, Apgar, pH, NICU	0.86	0.88	0.68	0.96	0.69
Fetal distress, Apgar, pH, NICU, and meconium	0.82	0.92	0.81	0.92	0.74

NICU, neonatal intensive care unit admission; SGA, small for gestational age. With permission from Maulik D, *et al*. The diagnostic efficacy of the umbilical arterial systolic/diastolic ratio as a screening tool: a prospective blinded study. *Am J Obstet Gynecol* 1990;162:1518

Low-risk pregnancies

Although the above findings are very encouraging, there are a few recent reports that demonstrate the inadequate discriminatory efficacy of Doppler velocimetry of the umbilical artery as a screening test in a general obstetrical population at a low risk for adverse perinatal outcome. In a large prospective study involving 2097 singleton pregnancies, Beattie and Dornan[72] evaluated the capability of umbilical arterial Doppler indices (PI, $A:B$ ratio, RI) to detect FGR and perinatal compromise. It was noted that the indices did not adequately predict any of the parameters of adverse perinatal outcome. The suboptimal efficacy of umbilical Doppler insonation in a low-risk population has been corroborated by others[73–75]. Beattie and associates[76] performed Bayesian analysis of the above four studies to determine the post-test probability of an abnormal outcome for an individual patient. The post-test probabilities of an adverse outcome was determined for an individual in terms of positive and negative likelihood ratios and are summarized in Table 6. It is evident that umbilical arterial Doppler velocimetry is of limited utility in a low-risk obstetrical population.

SIGNIFICANCE OF ABSENT END-DIASTOLIC VELOCITY IN THE UMBILICAL ARTERY

It is apparent from cumulative experience that the end-diastolic component of the Doppler waveform is of crucial importance in fetal prognostication[77,78]. Indeed, an absent (Figure 9) or reversed end-diastolic flow velocity is known to be associated with a remarkably adverse perinatal outcome, particularly a very high perinatal mortality rate (Table 7). Most remarkably, this group also demonstrates a high risk of chromosomal abnormalities with a predominance of trisomy 13, 18 and 21. There is also a high association between absent end-diastolic flow and a variety of congenital anomalies

Table 6   Post-test probability of an adverse outcome and umbilical arterial Doppler in low-risk pregnancies: a summary of four studies

Outcome	Positive likelihood ratio	Negative likelihood ratio
Small for gestational age (birth weight < 10th centile)	+ 1.1 to + 4.2	− 0.8 to − 1.0
Adverse perinatal outcome (Apgar < 7 at 1 min, umbilical arterial pH < 7.2, operative delivery for fetal distress, abnormal fetal heart rate)	+ 1.0 to + 3.1	− 0.9 to − 1.0

Modified from Beattie RB, Hannah ME, Dornan JC. Compound analysis of umbilical artery velocimetry in low-risk pregnancy. *J Matern Fetal Invest* 1992;2:269

(Table 8). It has been observed, however, that absent end-diastolic flow may improve, although often only transiently, and that weeks or more may elapse before the fetus may show additional evidence of compromise.

Obviously the presence of absent end-diastolic flow should warn the physician of significantly increased fetal risk and should, therefore, mandate appropriate surveillance measures; however, the benefits of emergency delivery for this phenomenon remain uncertain at present. Furthermore, the homeostatic significance of absent end-diastolic velocity in relation to the alterations in other components of fetal circulation and other parameters of fetal wellbeing needs clarification. Recent reports provide considerable insight in this area. Teyssier and co-workers[79] observed, in an animal model, a hierarchical sequence in the fall in the end-diastolic flow in the fetal circulation when fetoplacental vascular resistance in increased; flow in the aortic isthmus was affected first, followed by flow in the descending aorta and the umbilical artery. Preliminary

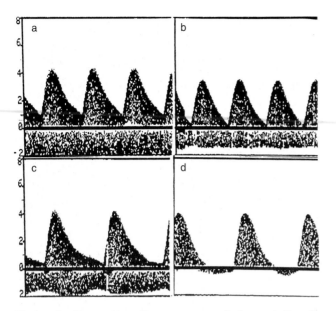

Figure 9 Progressive disappearance of the end-diastolic frequency shift in the umbilical arterial Doppler waveforms from a pregnancy complicated with severe fetal growth restriction at 33 weeks' gestation. (**a**) Presence of the end-diastolic frequency shift, although the Doppler indices were high for the gestational age (*S : D* ratio 5; resistance index 0.8). (**b**) Absence of the end-diastolic frequency shift. (**c**) Spontaneous deceleration with prolongation of the diastolic phase and the appearance of umbilical venous pulsation. (**d**) Progression to the reversal of the end-diastolic frequency shift. With permission from Maulik D. Absent end-diastolic velocity in the umbilical artery and its clinical significance. In Maulik D, ed. *Doppler Ultrasound in Obstetrics and Gynecology.* New York: Springer-Verlag, 1997:363

Table 7 Absent and reverse end-diastolic frequency in the umbilical artery and adverse perinatal outcome

Perinatal outcome	Mean	Range
Perinatal mortality	45%	17–100%
Gestational age	31.6 weeks	29–33 weeks
Birthweight	1056 g	910–1481 g
Small for gestational age	68%	53–100%
Cesarean section for fetal distress	73%	24–100%
Apgar score at 5 min < 7	26%	7–69%
Admission to neonatal intensive care unit	84%	77–97%
Congenital anomalies	10%	0–24%
Aneuploidy	6.4%	0–18%

Modified with permission from Maulik D. Doppler ultrasound in obstetrics. In Cunningham FG, *et al.*, eds. *Williams Obstetrics.* 19th edn. Stamford CT: Appleton & Lange, Suppl 16

clinical observations tended to confirm this[80]. It has also been demonstrated that in fetuses with the absence of end-diastolic velocity in the umbilical artery, ominous patterns develop in the fetal heart-rate tracings when the middle cerebral artery begins to

Table 8 Absent end-diastolic velocity (AEDV) and congenital malformations

Cardiovascular system
  Ventricular septal defect
  Hypoplastic left-heart syndrome
  Double-outlet right ventricle
  Ebstein anomaly
  Arrhythmia – congenital heart block
Central nervous system
  Hydrocephaly
  Holoprosencephaly
  Agenesis of corpus callosum
Urogenital system
  Renal agenesis
  Hydronephrosis
Gastrointestinal system/abdominal wall
  Esophageal atresia
  Omphalocele
  Gastroschisis
Skeletal system
  Polydactyly
  Dysplasia

With permission from Maulik D. *Doppler Ultrasound in Obstetrics and Gynecology.* New York: Springer-Verlag, 1997

lose its compensatory vasodilation[81]. The latter manifests as increases in the PI of the artery and concomitant increases in the cerebral : umbilical arterial PI ratio. These changes are also associated with a significant fall in the left-ventricular output.

Multiple pregnancy

The diagnostic role of Doppler velocimetry in multiple gestation has been evaluated by several investigators. Giles and co-workers[82] studied umbilical arterial *A : B* ratio (same as *S : D* ratio) in 65 twin gestations using a continuous-wave Doppler system. One or both the twins were SGA in 33 cases. In all these, the *A : B* ratio was elevated in at least one twin. Farmakides *et al.*[83] investigated umbilical arterial *S : D* ratio in 43 twin pregnancies and noted that an *S/D* ratio difference of 0.4 or more between the twins predicted a weight difference greater than 349 g with a sensitivity of 73%, and a specificity of 82%. Nimrod and co-workers[84] employed a duplex pulsed Doppler instrument to measure umbilical arterial *S : D* ratio in 30 twin pregnancies. The authors observed that for diagnosing discordant twin growth, the *S : D* ratio had a sensitivity of 50% and a specificity of 82%. In comparison, the sensitivity and specificity of ultrasound measurement of biparietal diameters were 45% and 84%, respectively, whereas abdominal circumferences showed a sensitivity and specificity of 22% and 74%, respectively. More recently, Gaziano and co-workers[85] compared the efficacy of sonographically estimated fetal weight (EFW) with pulsed Doppler umbilical arterial $S:D$ ratio in 101 patients with multiple gestation (94 twin pairs, seven sets of triplets with completed data on 207 fetuses). The authors found that for predicting SGA, the sensitivity of the Doppler measurement was 44%, and that of the EFW (< 10th percentile for gestational age) was 50%. The pulsed-wave Doppler alone did not increase the sensitivity and specificity or positive predictive value for SGA diagnosis when compared to ultrasound estimated weight.

Giles and co-workers[86] have suggested that the incorporation of the Doppler technique in the clinical management of twins may improve the perinatal outcome. A decline in corrected perinatal deaths from 42.1 in 1000 to 8.9 in 1000 was noted in their study. Although this was not a randomized trial, such an impressive decline in the perinatal mortality justifies further rigorous investigation of the role of Doppler velocimetry in managing multiple pregnancies. More recently, Gaziano and associates[87] observed, in 94 twin pairs and seven sets of triplets, that an abnormal pulsed Doppler velocimetry showed high correlation with adverse pregnancy events and that those with abnormal Doppler findings tended to be born 3–4 weeks earlier and to exhibit a greater number of stillbirths, malformations, and greater morbidity. It appears that Doppler velocimetry may assist in identifying the fetus at risk, although no randomized trials have specifically investigated yet the benefits of the Doppler method in multifetal gestations.

DOPPLER ASSESSMENT OF FETAL CEREBRAL CIRCULATION

Pulsed-wave Doppler interrogation of the fetal cerebral circulation has been described by various authors. Marsal and co-workers[88] were the first to describe the interrogation of the common carotid artery in the human fetus. This was followed by reports of flow velocity characterization of the internal carotid[89] and the cerebral vessels[90]. A pulsed-wave Doppler duplex system is essential for identification and interrogation of this circulation. As depicted in Figure 10, cerebral arterial Doppler waveforms typically demonstrate continuing forward flow in diastole. During the second half of pregnancy, fetal cerebral arterial Doppler indices show a progressive decline in the pulsatility consequent to a progressive increase in the end-diastolic flow velocity. These indices are affected by fetal breathing, fetal behavioral state and fetal heart rate[91]. Human and ovine fetal cerebral circulation have been shown to be responsive to fetal hypoxia and hypercapnia[92–94]. When hypoxia progresses to asphyxia, no further fall occurs in the cerebral arterial impedance and, with the eventual diappearance of autoregulation, cerebral vessels may actually demonstrate increased impedance.

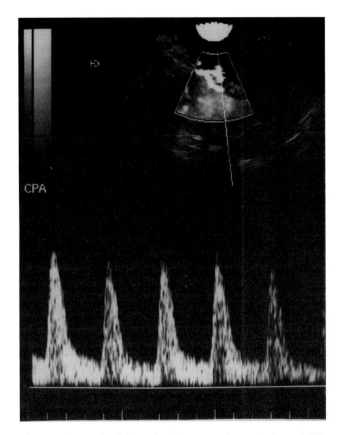

Figure 10 Pulsed Doppler interrogation of the middle cerebral artery in a human fetus at 32 weeks of gestation. The inset in the upper left corner shows two-dimensional image of the fetal head and the location of the Doppler sample volume. The Doppler waves demonstrate continuing forward flow at the end diastolic. Vertical arrows mark the peak systolic and the end-diastolic frequency shifts. With permission from Maulik D. Doppler ultrasound in obstetrics. In Cunningham FG, *et al.*, ed. *Williams Obstetrics.* 19th edn. Stamford CT: Appleton & Lange, Suppl 16

Although cerebral Doppler indices have been studied in high-risk pregnancies such as those with FGR, its main potential appears to rest with its use in conjunction with the umbilical arterial Doppler indices[95,96]. In human fetuses, Arbeille and co-workers[95] investigated the relationship between the Doppler indices from the arteries supplying the brain and those from the umbilical artery to reflect circulatory redistribution that occurs as a compensatory response to hypoxia. This was expressed as cerebroplacental ratio (CPR) in which the cerebral RI is the numerator and the umbilical arterial RI is the denominator. In an ovine model of acute asphyxia, a significant relationship was observed between the CPR and fetal hypoxia in the absence of acidosis[95]. In normal pregnancy, the CPR is > 1 (Figure 11), as the fetoplacental circulatory impedance is lower than the cerebral circulatory impedance. A ratio of < 1 is considered pathological. The utility of CPR in clinical practice remains to be clarified.

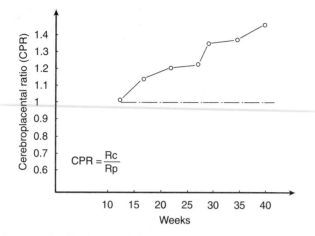

Figure 11 Evolution of the cerebroplacental ratio during a normal pregnancy. Note that the cerebral resistance is superior to the placental resistance at any gestational age and therefore the cerebroplacental ratio is > 1. With permission from Arbeille *et al.* Cerebral Doppler in the assessment of the IUGR and the fetal hypoxia. *J Matern Fetal Invest* 1991; 1:51–56

VENOUS CIRCULATION OF THE FETUS

There has been considerable recent interest in the Doppler evaluation of fetal venous circulation. Doppler characterization of the fetal inferior vena caval (IVC) flow velocity waveform was first reported by Chiba and co-workers[97]. Several reports have appeared since to further elucidate the changes in these waves under normal and pathological conditions. Although Doppler interrogation can be performed at various locations along the IVC, it has been shown that the optimal sampling site is the segment of the IVC between the entrance of the renal vein and the ductus venosus[98]. In a normal fetus with apnea, the IVC flow wave demonstrates a triphasic flow pattern (Figure 12). There are two peaks of forward flow. The first one coincides with the atrial diastole and the ventricular systole; the second forward flow coincides with the ventricular diastole. Finally, there is the third component which is comprised of a variable degree of reverse flow corresponding to the atrial systole. Fetal breathing profoundly affects IVC flow waveform. Aberrations of the waveform are observed in various fetal complications. The latter include fetal cardiac rhythm disturbances[99,100], fetal cardiac failure as manifested by hydrops fetalis[101], and FGR[102]. Although these findings suggest that the Doppler velocimetry of IVC may be useful for fetal surveillance, its practical utility remains to be proven.

OTHER CIRCULATIONS OF THE FETUS

This section deals with Doppler assessment of human fetal aortic and renal circulations, none of which have

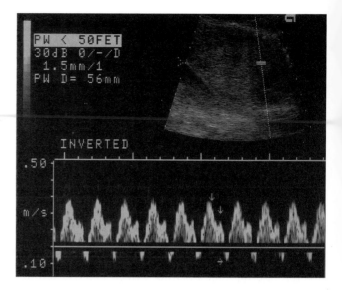

Figure 12 Spectral Doppler waveforms from the inferior vena cava in a human fetus. The upper panel shows the two-dimensional image of the location of the Doppler sample volume. Note the triphasic nature of the Doppler wave. The first forward wave (vertical arrow) coincides with atrial diastole and ventricular systole; the second forward wave (vertical arrow) coincides with ventricular diastole; the retrograde flow wave (horizontal arrow) correspond with the atrial systole

shown any significant potential as a fetal monitor yet. The end-diastolic component of the aortic Doppler waveform progressively increases and the pulsatility decreases as the sample volume is moved sequentially from the aorta to the umbilical arteries. Aortic Doppler waveforms do not demonstrate significant gestational age related changes during the second half of pregnancy. However, they are affected by the behavioral state of the fetus[32]. Vyas and co-workers[103] observed gestational age-dependent decline in the renal arterial PI, and significantly higher renal arterial PI values in a group of SGA fetuses. In a similar study, Veille and Kanaan[104] observed a significantly higher renal arterial PI in the growth-restricted group. However, there were no significant differences in the $S:D$ ratio between the two groups. There is no evidence at present that fetal renal velocimetry has any significant clinical utility.

Doppler assessment of uteroplacental circulation

Doppler waveforms of the uteroplacental vessels have been characterized by several investigators[30,105,106]. Both pulsed-wave and continuous-wave Doppler modes have been used. More recently, transvaginal sonography has also been used. It has often been difficult to ascertain the vascular location in interrogating the uteroplacental vessels. This has seriously limited the ability to repeat the test in the same vessel during a follow-up examination. This may account for the

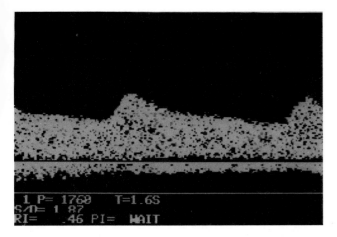

Figure 13 Uterine artery flow velocity waveforms at term pregnancy. The artery was interrogated with a continuous wave Doppler ultrasound device. Note the impressive forward flow at the end diastole

wide range of variability that can be as high as 17% in the same patient tested at different times[107]. During the second half of pregnancy, uteroplacental Doppler waveforms demonstrate a substantial increase in end-diastolic velocities (Figure 13). The diastolic notch that is present in the uterine arterial waveform in early pregnancy disappears between 24 and 26 weeks of gestation. The $S:D$ ratio and other indices of pulsatility progressively decline until week 26 of pregnancy; no further decline is noted following this for the duration of the pregnancy. These changes reflect a marked decrease in the uteroplacental circulatory impedance. An increased pulsatility of the uterine arterial Doppler waveform, persistence of the notch and a significant difference between the right- and the left-uterine arteries have been reported to be associated with FGR, pregnancy-induced hypertension, and adverse perinatal outcome[108–110]. Of the above criteria, a persistent notch is of worst prognostic significance. It has also been suggested that a combination of the uterine and umbilical Doppler indices may offer prognostic insight into the hypertensive complication of pregnancy[112]. With this problem the maternal and fetal prognosis was best when both umbilical and uterine Doppler indices were normal, and worst when both were abnormal. In contrast, others have failed to find any prognostic value in uterine arterial $S:D$ ratio in cases with absent end-diastolic velocity in the umbilical artery[112].

Evidence for clinical efficacy of Doppler velocimetry: randomized trials

The cumulative clinical and experimental evidence strongly affirms the potential of Doppler velocimetry of the fetal circulation as an effective tool for recognizing fetal compromise in high-risk pregnancies. This has prompted many to propose its introduction as a standard for fetal surveillance. However, such enthusiasm must be tempered by a critical appraisal of the efficacy and benefits of the technique. Introduction of a new diagnostic test involves the sequential and often parallel developmental process which transforms the promises of a new technique into an effective diagnostic tool which delivers tangible benefits. The steps include the demonstration of feasibility, association with disease processes and diagnostic efficacy of the technique; but in the end it must be shown without bias that the technique improves the clinical outcome. This can be accomplished only by the randomized clinical trials (RCT). It is encouraging to note that so far twelve such trials[113–126] have been fully reported in the literature. All the RCT studies evaluated umbilical arterial velocimetry; a few also used uterine arterial velocimetry. While most were conducted in high-risk patients, many were used in low-risk mothers. Considerable heterogeneity exists among the trials regarding the selection criteria, the study design, and the measures of pregnancy outcome. Furthermore, most studies do not have any protocol of management based on the test results. These studies are summarized in Table 9 and are further described below.

The twelve peer reviewed studies include a total population of 17 048. These studies can be categorized into two groups according to the population characteristics. In one group, the trials were performed in a selected pregnant population at a higher risk for complications or adverse outcome. However, there was no uniformity among the studies in their selection criteria. The other group includes trials conducted on unselected pregnant mothers. Although presumed to be representative of the general obstetrical population, studies often included patients from university medical centers which tend to attract more complicated cases. This was exemplified by the Utrecht study which was conducted on unselected pregnant mothers but was found to include approximately 50% high-risk patients.

The high-risk group was comprised of seven studies and a total of 5129 patients. Of these, four studies with a population of 1438 showed a beneficial outcome because of Doppler intervention. The remaining three studies with a population of 3691 failed to show any benefit. The unselected group included five trials and a total of 11 919 patients. Beneficial effects were observed in two trials with a population of 4585, but not in the three remaining studies with a population of 7334.

There were differences among the studies regarding the type of patient population, the purpose of the trial, the study design and the method of randomization, the outcome parameters, and the management approach. Furthermore, most studies did not appear to have any defined management protocol to translate fetal surveillance findings into any specific intervention. In the face of such heterogeneity, it is rather difficult to use these findings to develop and recommend a specific management protocol.

Table 9   Summary of all randomized trials of Doppler ultrasound for fetal surveillance fully reported in peer reviewed journals

Author (year)	Reference	Total population	Subject category	Doppler index	Study design	Defined protocol	Benefits
Trudinger *et al.* (1987)	*Lancet* 1:188	300	High risk	UA *S : D*	R/C	No	Yes
Tyrell *et al.* (1990)	*Br J Obstet Gynaecol* 97:909	500	High risk	UA *S : D*	Y/N	No	Yes
				Ut *S : D*			
Hofmeyr *et al.* (1991)	*Obstet Gynecol* 78:359	897	High risk	UA *S : D*	Y/N	No	No
Newnham *et al.* (1991)	*Br J Obstet Gynaecol* 98:956	505	High risk	UA *S : D*	R/C	No	No
				Ut *S : D*			
Davies *et al.* (1992)	*Lancet* 340:1299	2475	Unselected	UA *S : D*	Y/N	No	No
				Ut *S : D*			
Almstrom *et al.* (1992)	*Lancet* 340:936	426	High risk	UA BFC	Y/N	Yes	Yes
Mason *et al.* (1993)	*Br J Obstet Gynaecol* 100:130	2025	Unselected	UA *S : D*	Y/N	No	No
Johnstone *et al.* (1993)	*Br J Obstet Gynaecol* 100:733	2289	High risk	UA RI	Y/N	No	No
Newnham *et al.* (1993)	*Lancet* 342:887	2834	Unselected	UA *S : D*	Y/N	Yes	No
				Ut *S : D*			
Whittle *et al.* (1994)	*Am J Obstet Gynecol* 170:555	2986	Unselected	UA *S : D*	R/C	No	Yes
Omtzigt *et al.* (1994)	*Am J Obstet Gynecol* 170:625	1599	Unselected	UA *S : D*	Y/N	Yes	Yes
Pattinson *et al.* (1994)	*Br J Obstet Gynaecol* 101:104	212	High risk	UA *S : D*	R/C	Yes	Yes

UA, umbilical artery; Ut, uterine artery; S : D, systolic/diastolic ratio; RI, resistance index; BFC, blood flow classes; R/C, Doppler velocimetry results were either revealed or concealed; Y/N = yes, no; Doppler velocimetry was either performed or not performed. Modified with permission from Maulik D. *Doppler Ultrasound in Obstetrics and Gynecology.* New York, Springer-Verlag, 1997

Meta-analysis of Doppler trials

Although the traditional review of clinical trials of Doppler velocimetry as presented above is very informative, it does not assist in arriving at a definitive conclusion regarding its efficacy nor does it provide us with a measure of the magnitude of benefit that may result from its use in clinical practice for fetal surveillance. A better approach is to perform a meta-analysis which involves aggregating and statistically analyzing data from the various trials to derive a valid quantitative conclusion. The technique has been used widely for systematic review of scientific research in social sciences, and has been extensively applied later to clinical research in medicine. Traditionally, the method for deriving the average estimate of the effect size has been to use one of the fixed effects models which takes into account intrastudy but not interstudy variance. This model was developed by Mantel and Haentzel[127] and was subsequently modified by Yusuf *et al.*[128]. When the fixed effects model is used, a separate statistical test (such as the χ^2 distribution) is usually performed to determine whether the variations in the results can be explained by chance. However, this is a relatively insensitive tool to test for homogeneity[129]. Although the fixed-effects model is the most widely used method in meta-analysis in the medical field, there has been significant criticism of its exclusive use. The alternative method, the random effects model, originally suggested by Cochran[130] and subsequently developed by DerSimonian and Laird[131], deals with study to study variations in the analytic process. There has been a substantial support for this approach, particularly when one is aiming to apply the meta-analytic inference to the future application of the treatment rather than to the past trials under investigation[132,133].

Alfirevic and Neilson[134] recently reported a meta-analysis of published and unpublished randomized Doppler trials in high-risk pregnancies. Of the twelve studies included, six were peer reviewed original publications, two were unpublished (personal communication), two appeared to be abstracts published in conference proceedings, and two were review articles. The trials were subjected to a quality-assessment program proposed by Chalmers and associates[135] and were found to be eligible for inclusion in the systematic review process. This report suggested a significant reduction in the perinatal deaths of normally formed fetuses consequent to the use of umbilical arterial Doppler surveillance (Figure 14). The decline in the odds of perinatal mortality was by 38%. A significant decrease was also noted in the number of antepartum admissions to the hospital (44%), induction of labor (20%) and Cesarean section for fetal distress (52%). Moreover, a significant decline was observed in elective delivery, intrapartum fetal distress and hypoxic encephalopathy on *post hoc* analyses (Figure 15). Obviously, this last group of benefits require further investigation. Noting that the statistical method utilized in this meta-analysis was based on the fixed model, we undertook a random effects model approach as described by DerSimonian and Laird to reanalyze the data pertaining to perinatal deaths as collated by Alfirevic and Neilson[134]. The data are presented in Figure 16 which confirms the results from the fixed-model analysis. The random-effect model

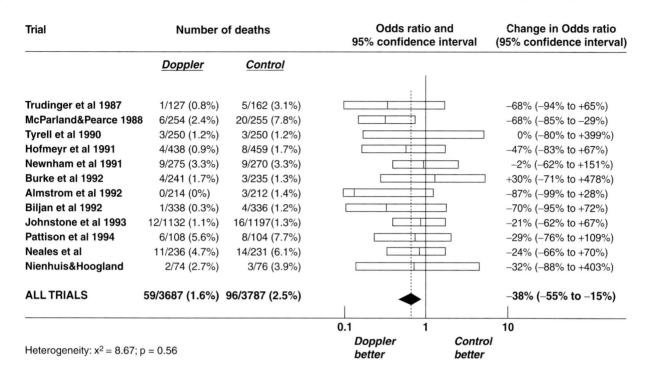

Trial	Number of deaths		Odds ratio and 95% confidence interval	Change in Odds ratio (95% confidence interval)
	Doppler	*Control*		
Trudinger et al 1987	1/127 (0.8%)	5/162 (3.1%)		−68% (−94% to +65%)
McParland&Pearce 1988	6/254 (2.4%)	20/255 (7.8%)		−68% (−85% to −29%)
Tyrell et al 1990	3/250 (1.2%)	3/250 (1.2%)		0% (−80% to +399%)
Hofmeyr et al 1991	4/438 (0.9%)	8/459 (1.7%)		−47% (−83% to +67%)
Newnham et al 1991	9/275 (3.3%)	9/270 (3.3%)		−2% (−62% to +151%)
Burke et al 1992	4/241 (1.7%)	3/235 (1.3%)		+30% (−71% to +478%)
Almstrom et al 1992	0/214 (0%)	3/212 (1.4%)		−87% (−99% to +28%)
Biljan et al 1992	1/338 (0.3%)	4/336 (1.2%)		−70% (−95% to +72%)
Johnstone et al 1993	12/1132 (1.1%)	16/1197(1.3%)		−21% (−62% to +67%)
Pattison et al 1994	6/108 (5.6%)	8/104 (7.7%)		−29% (−76% to +109%)
Neales et al	11/236 (4.7%)	14/231 (6.1%)		−24% (−66% to +70%)
Nienhuis&Hoogland	2/74 (2.7%)	3/76 (3.9%)		−32% (−88% to +403%)
ALL TRIALS	**59/3687 (1.6%)**	**96/3787 (2.5%)**		**−38% (−55% to −15%)**

Heterogeneity: $x^2 = 8.67$; $p = 0.56$

Figure 14 Proportional effect of Doppler ultrasonography on number of dead babies (stillbirths and neonates) when used in high risk pregnancy. With permission from Alfirevic Z, Nielson JP. Doppler ultrasonography in high risk pregnancies: systematic review with meta-analysis. *Am J Obstet Gynecol* 1995;172:1379

Outcome (Number of trials)	Number of deaths		Odds ratio and 95% confidence interval	Change in Odds ratio (95% confidence interval)	Heterogeneity
	Doppler	*Control*			
Delivery					
Elective delivery (g)	1190/2902(41.3%)	1338/2971(45.0%)		−16% (−24% to −6%)	p = 0.02
Fetal distress antepartum (1)	19/254 (7.5%)	24/251 (9.6%)		−33% (−59% to +43%)	
Fetal distress after induction (2)	37/381 (9.7%)	29/413 (7%)		+32% (−21% to +121%)	p = 0.61
Fetal distress after spont. labour (2)	16/381 (4.2%)	21/413 (5.1%)		−21% (−59% to +54%)	p = 0.05
Fetal distress in labour (4)	95/648 (14.7)	130/681 (19.1%)		−31% (−48% to −7%)	p = 0.01
Caesarean section in labour (5)	214/1837 (11.6%)	240/1926 (12.5%)		−7% (−23% to +14%)	p = 0.01
Neonatal outcome					
Birthweight < 10 centile (1)	93/275 (33.85)	89/270 (32.9%)		+4% (−27% to +48%)	
Low Apgar at 1 min (5)	193/1202 (16.1%)	185/1223 (15.1%)		+6% (−16% to +32%)	p = 0.04
Treatment with oxygen (2)	58/402 (14.4%)	74/432 (17.1%)		−18% (−43% to +19%)	p = 0.40
Hypoxic encephalopathy (1)	0/247 (0%)	5/249 (2%)		−87% (−98% to −22%)	

Figure 15 Effects of Doppler ultrasonography on perinatal outcome in high risk pregnancies. *Post hoc* analysis. With permission from Alfirevic Z, Nielson JP. Doppler ultrasonography in high risk pregnancies: systematic review with meta-analysis. *Am J Obstet Gynecol* 1995;172:1379

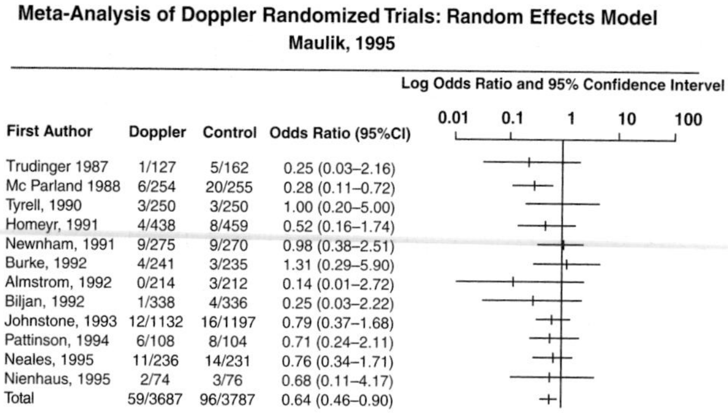

Meta-Analysis of Doppler Randomized Trials: Random Effects Model
Maulik, 1995

First Author	Doppler	Control	Odds Ratio (95%CI)
Trudinger 1987	1/127	5/162	0.25 (0.03–2.16)
Mc Parland 1988	6/254	20/255	0.28 (0.11–0.72)
Tyrell, 1990	3/250	3/250	1.00 (0.20–5.00)
Homeyr, 1991	4/438	8/459	0.52 (0.16–1.74)
Newnham, 1991	9/275	9/270	0.98 (0.38–2.51)
Burke, 1992	4/241	3/235	1.31 (0.29–5.90)
Almstrom, 1992	0/214	3/212	0.14 (0.01–2.72)
Biljan, 1992	1/338	4/336	0.25 (0.03–2.22)
Johnstone, 1993	12/1132	16/1197	0.79 (0.37–1.68)
Pattinson, 1994	6/108	8/104	0.71 (0.24–2.11)
Neales, 1995	11/236	14/231	0.76 (0.34–1.71)
Nienhaus, 1995	2/74	3/76	0.68 (0.11–4.17)
Total	59/3687	96/3787	0.64 (0.46–0.90)

Figure 16 Meta-analysis of Doppler randomized clinical trials performed on high-risk pregnancies utilizing the random effects model of DerSimonian and Laird. The analysis shows effect on perinatal mortality. With permission from Maulik D. Doppler velocimetry for fetal surveillance: randomized clinical trials and implications for practice. In Maulik D, ed. *Doppler Ultrasound in Obstetrics and Gynecology.* New York: Springer-Verlag, 1997:376

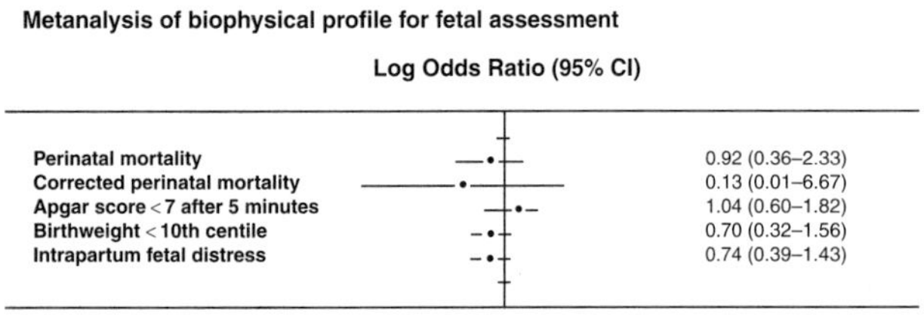

Metanalysis of biophysical profile for fetal assessment

Log Odds Ratio (95% CI)

Perinatal mortality	0.92 (0.36–2.33)
Corrected perinatal mortality	0.13 (0.01–6.67)
Apgar score < 7 after 5 minutes	1.04 (0.60–1.82)
Birthweight < 10th centile	0.70 (0.32–1.56)
Intrapartum fetal distress	0.74 (0.39–1.43)

Figure 17 Meta-analysis of randomized trials of antepartum non-stress cardiotocography for fetal surveillance. With permission from Nielson JP. Biophysical profile for antepartum fetal assessment. The Cochrane Pregnancy and Childbirth Database, 1995

analysis suggests that the use of umbilical arterial Doppler velocimetry for fetal surveillance in complicated pregnancies may lead to a 36% decline in the perinatal deaths (confidence interval, CI −54% to −10%).

It should also be noted that a meta-analysis does not replace the value of a randomized clinical trial based on a sufficient sample size. Depending on the choice of the outcome parameter and the effect size, it will probably require thousands of patients involving multiple centers to conduct such a study. It would be a tremendous challenge to organize and obtain sufficient resources for a trial of this magnitude.

It is of interest to note that the other biophysical modes of fetal surveillance are not based on any demonstration of benefits by RCT. None of the four RCTs performed on the non-stress test showed any benefits and their meta-analysis corroborates this (Figure 17)[136], whereas contraction stress test and fetal biophysical profile have not been subjected to any reported RCT investigations.

GUIDELINES FOR UMBILICAL ARTERIAL DOPPLER FETAL SURVEILLANCE

Based upon the above evidence of clinical efficacy of umbilical arterial Doppler indices, the following practical recommendations for its usage in managing high-risk pregnancy is recommended. These guidelines incorporate the existing modalities of fetal surveillance although some investigators advise the use of Doppler as the exclusive primary tool for fetal surveillance. Such a recommendation may not be pragmatic and pathophysiologic evidence suggests a more comprehensive approach for fetal surveillance.

Indications for Doppler velocimetric fetal surveillance

Doppler velocimetry is indicated in pregnancies where the fetus is at risk for chronic nutritive and respiratory stress. A variety of pregnancy complications such as FGR and hypertensive disease can cause such stress. Common indications for performing Doppler surveillance of the fetus are listed in Table 10 and are discussed below. Umbilical arterial Doppler velocimetry is predictive of adverse perinatal outcome in well-defined high-risk pregnancies including FGR, pre-eclampsia and the concurrence of both. Although umbilical arterial Doppler has been recommended in the past for identifying an SGA infant, sonographic measurement is the better predictor of fetal size. Unless the fetal hemodynamic state is compromised from stress, the Doppler indices will not change. Consistent with this, it has been shown that, in high-risk pregnancies, abnormal umbilical arterial Doppler indices correlate with antepartum fetal asphyxia. The indices, therefore, may be helpful in distinguishing a growth-restricted and compromised SGA fetus from a constitutionally SGA fetus. Finally, and most importantly, randomized trials have shown significant

Table 10 Indications for umbilical arterial Doppler velocimetry

- Small-for-gestational-age fetus (< 10th centile)
- Pre-eclampsia (primary and superimposed)
- Secondary hypertension
- Maternal renal disease
- Autoimmune vascular disease
    Systemic lupus erythematosus
    Antiphospholipid antibody syndrome
    Other
- Pregestational diabetes mellitus
- Sickle cell disease
- Multiple gestation

With permission from Maulik D. Doppler velocimetry in fetal surveillance. In *Current Therapy in Obstetrics and Gynecology.* Zuspan FP, Quilligan EJ eds. Philadelphia: WB Saunders improvement in the rate of perinatal mortality from the use of umbilical arterial Doppler in managing pregnancies complicated with clearly defined FGR and hypertension.

Doppler velocimetry is also useful in managing pregnancies affected by autoimmune disorders including systemic lupus erythematosus and antiphospholipid syndrome. Similarly, umbilical arterial Doppler is helpful in recognizing fetal compromise in multiple pregnancies, particularly in those with discordant growth and twin transfusion syndrome. Doppler methodology is also recommended for fetal surveillance in pregnancies with pregestational diabetes, especially when vasculopathy is present; however, it should not be used to assess the quality of glucose control. Finally, the utility of umbilical arterial Doppler in managing postdated pregnancies remains to be defined.

Technique of umbilical arterial Doppler interrogation

Before Doppler examination, the mother is appropriately counseled regarding the reason for the test, the nature of the information generated by the device, its reliability and safety, and other relevant issues. Similar to the procedure in fetal heart-rate (FHR) monitoring, the mother lies in a semirecumbent position with a slight lateral tilt to minimize the risk of significant caval compression. Examination should be conducted only during fetal apnea and in the absence of fetal hiccup or excessive movement. Doppler insonation of the umbilical arterial circulation can be performed by either a continuous-wave Doppler device or a pulsed Doppler duplex system.

Continuous-wave Doppler sonography of the uterine artery is a relatively simple procedure and can be performed in the office using a free-standing Doppler instrument. The transducer is usually a pencil-shaped probe with an operating frequency of 2–4 MHz. The transducer is placed on the mother's abdomen overlying the fetus with an acoustic coupling jelly intervening between the transducer face and the maternal abdominal skin. The method is essentially a blind technique, similar to that used for listening to fetal heart tones with the simpler Doppler devices. The transducer is systematically manipulated to obtain the characteristic Doppler frequency shift waveforms which are visualized in the display screen. The process of identification is facilitated by listening to the typical audible sound of the uterine arterial Doppler shift. Complete Doppler insonation of the artery is ensured by obtaining the umbilical venous Doppler signals simultaneously with the arterial signals.

With a pulsed-wave duplex Doppler system, an obstetrical scan is initially performed to identify the loops of the cord (Figure 18). Unlike the continuous-wave mode, the pulsed-wave Doppler insonation

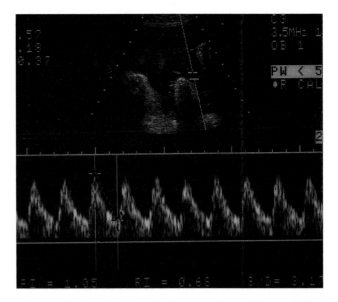

Figure 18   Duplex Doppler interrogation of the umbilical artery. The upper panel demonstrates the placement of the Doppler sample volume in a loop of the umbilical cord. The lower panel shows the Doppler frequency shift waveforms from the interrogated artery

permits selection of the location in the umbilical cord for interrogation. Usually a free-floating loop of the cord is insonated. The cursor line representing the beam path is aligned to intersect the umbilical vessels at the selected location and the Doppler sample volume is placed in that location. The Doppler mode is then activated and the Doppler waveforms are recorded and analyzed.

Management of high-risk pregnancy using Doppler sonography

Principles of managing a high-risk pregnancy utilizing uterine arterial Doppler velocimetry in conjunction with other fetal surveillance test findings will be described in this section. Abnormal elevation of the umbilical arterial Doppler indices usually precedes ominous changes in other tests including poor FHR variability, cessation of fetal movement and a poor fetal biophysical profile (BPP) score. Thus a high or increasing $S:D$ ratio warrants more intense fetal surveillance which consists of weekly or biweekly umbilical Doppler, the non-stress test (NST) and the BPP. If these tests are assuring, fetal surveillance should continue unless intervention is indicated because of other complications. On the other hand, if these tests indicate fetal compromise, delivery should be planned. The latter may be accomplished either by induction of labor or by Cesarean section depending on other obstetric factors and according to the current standards of practice.

In contrast to an elevated $S:D$ ratio, the development of absent end diastolic velocity (AEDV) indicates more urgent action as it is associated with an unusually adverse perinatal outcome. Management of this condition depends on several factors (including gestational age and the probability of fetal pulmonic maturity, additional indicators of fetal jeopardy, the presence of fetal aneuploidy and malformations), and is discussed below and outlined in the algorithm in Figure 19.

AEDV and near-term pregnancy

The development of AEDV should prompt consideration of delivery when fetal lung maturity is anticipated or proven. Although the prudence of emergency delivery for this complication has been questioned, randomized clinical trials and their meta-analyses have shown improved outcome from obstetric interventions based on uterine arterial Doppler velocimetry. It is recommended therefore that the mother should be delivered when this complication develops in a pregnancy at or near term (> 36 weeks) when continuation of the pregnancy presents a greater threat to fetal safety and wellbeing.

The mode of delivery is determined by assessing relevant obstetric factors including cervical status, fetal presentation and the severity of fetal compromise. If reversed end-diastolic velocity develops in the uterine artery, the probability of impending fetal death is very high; therefore, it may be more prudent to deliver the infant promptly by Cesarean section rather than to test its tolerance to the rigors of labor induction. The above management approach, however, is not applicable if lethal aneuploidy or malformation is present (see below).

AEDV and preterm pregnancy

In preterm pregnancy (6 36 weeks) when significant risk of fetal pulmonic immaturity is present, the management is conservative and further assurance of fetal wellbeing should be sought from daily surveillance by uterine arterial Doppler, NST and BPP. Delivery is indicated when a single test or a combination of these tests indicates imminent fetal danger. The ominous signs include the reversal of end-diastolic component of the uterine arterial Doppler waveform non-reactive NST, poor FHR baseline variability, persistent late decelerations, oligohydramnios, and BPP score < 4. The optimal mode of delivery should be decided by assessing relevant obstetric factors as stated above in relation to the term pregnancy.

An alternative, more aggressive, approach proposes obstetric intervention at 34 completed weeks of gestation when many consider the fetal risk from a hostile intrauterine environment to be greater than that from pulmonic immaturity. A further modification of this approach involves confirmation of fetal pulmonic maturity in preterm pregnancies between 34 and 36 weeks by lecithin/sphingomyelin and phosphatidylglycerol determination; delivery is recommended if the test results are assuring.

AEDV with fetal malformation or aneuploidy

When absent or reversed end-diastolic velocity develops early in the third trimester, especially in the absence of any pregnancy complications associated with AEDV, the fetus should be assessed to rule out any malformations or aneuploidy. Fetal anatomic integrity is evaluated using carefully performed tertiary-level ultrasound scanning. Fetal karyotype should be determined if an increased risk of aneuploidy is suggested by clinical or ultrasound information. The latter includes the presence of multiple anomalies, other sonographic markers of chromosomal aberrations and normal amniotic fluid volume (suggesting the absence of chronic fetal deprivation and stress). However, it should be noted that, contrary to the conventional wisdom, fetuses with chromosomal aberrations are not more prone to symmetrical growth restriction. If these fetal investigations identify lethal aneuploidy (trisomy 13 or 18) or malformations, an appropriate management plan should be instituted.

It should be noted that these recommendations do not provide a solution for every contingency that may develop in the course of a high-risk pregnancy. The physician must individualize the care in light of the myriad of variations in the clinical situation. The information presented in this chapter should be used

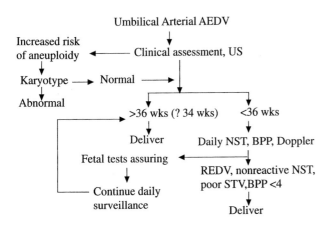

Figure 19 Algorithm for managing absent end-diastolic velocity in the umbilical artery. AEDV, absent and diastolic velocity; US, ultrasound; BPP, biophysical profile; NST, non-stress test; UA, umbilical artery. With permission from Maulik D. Doppler velocimetry in fetal surveillance. In *Current Therapy in Obstetrics and Gynecology*. Zuspan, Quilligan, eds. Philadelphia: WB Saunders, 199

as a pragmatic guideline which integrates the new modality with the existing standards of fetal surveillance. As new evidence accumulates and experience grows, evidence-based integration of the various modalities of fetal monitoring in appropriate sequence and frequency will add further refinement to this plan of management.

CONCLUSION

Introduction of Doppler velocimetry has allowed noninvasive assessment of the fetal and uteroplacental circulations. Hemodynamic, angiomorphological and pathophysiological evidence affirms the rationale of using the method for fetal surveillance. Numerous studies, as reviewed in this chapter, have established a noteworthy correlation between abnormal Doppler indices and various pregnancy disorders and adverse perinatal outcome. Furthermore, the majority of clinical investigations suggest that, in high-risk pregnancies, umbilical arterial Doppler indices may be a reliable predictor of perinatal problems including fetal death. However, before the technique can be accepted as a standard method of fetal surveillance, perinatal benefits from its use in clinical management must be clearly established. It is noteworthy that most randomized trials on Doppler velocimetry to date have yielded very positive results, the most promising benefit seeming to be a significant reduction in the number of preventable fetal deaths. Current evidence clearly indicates that Doppler velocimetry should be an essential component of antepartum fetal surveillance in high-risk pregnancies. Clearly, no single testing modality should be regarded as the exclusive method for fetal monitoring as these tests reveal different aspects of fetal pathophysiology, often in a complementary manner. Further investigation is necessary to determine the effectiveness of Doppler velocimetry of other fetal circulations such as the middle cerebral artery for improving the perinatal outcome.

REFERENCES

1. Doppler C. Uber das farbige Licht der DoppIesterne und einiger anderer Gestirne des Himmels. *Abhandl Konigl Bohm Ges Ser* 1843;2:465–82
2. Satomura S. Ultrasonic Doppler method for the inspection of cardiac functions. *J Acout Soc Am* 1957; 29:1181–3
3. Satomura S, Kaneko Z. Ultrasonic blood rheograph. In *Proceedings of the 3rd International Conference on Medical Elect* 1960:254
4. Baker DW. Pulsed ultrasonic Doppler blood flow sensing. *IEEE Trans Sonic Ultrasonics SU-17* 1970;3: 170–85
5. Wells PNT. A range gated ultrasonic Doppler system. *Med Biol Eng* 1969;7:641–52
6. Peronneau PA, Leger F. Doppler ultrasonic pulsed blood flowmeter. In *Proceedings of the 8th Conference on Medical and Biological Engineering* 1969:10–11
7. Plainol T, Pourcelot L, Pottier JM, Degiovanni E. Study of carotid circulation by means of ultrasonic methods and thermography. *Revue Neurologique* 1972;126:127–41
8. FitzGerald DE, Drumm JE. Noninvasive measurement of the fetal circulation using ultrasound: a new method. *BMJ* 1977;2:1450–1
9. Maulik D, McNellis D, eds. *Doppler Ultrasound Measurement of Maternal-Fetal Hemodynamics*. Ithaca, NY: Perinatology Press, 1987
10. Maulik D, ed. *Doppler Ultrasound in Obstetrics and Gynecology*. New York: Springer-Verlag New York Inc., 1997
11. Atkinson P, Woodcock JP. *Doppler Ultrasound*. London: Academic Press, 1982
12. Gill RW. Pulsed Doppler with B-mode imaging for quantitative blood flow measurements. *Ultrasound Med Biol* 1979;5:223–7
13. Eik Nes SH, Brubakk AO, Ulstein MK. Measurement of human fetal blood flow. *Br Med J* 1980;28:283–4
14. Maulik D, Nanda NC, Saini VD. Fetal Doppler echocardiography: methods and characterization of normal and abnormal hemodynamics. *Am J Cardiol* 1984;53:572–8
15. Gosling RG, King DH. Ultrasound angiology. In Marcus AW and Adamson J, eds. *Arteries and Veins*. Edinburgh: Churchill Livingstone, 1975:61
16. Pourcelot L. Applications cliniques de l'examen Dopple transcutane: velocimetric ultrasone Doppler. In Pourcelot L, ed. *Velocimetric Ultrasonore Doppler*. Seminaire INSERM 1974;34:213–40
17. Stuart B, Drumm J, FitzGerald DE, Duigan NM. Fetal blood velocity waveform in normal and complicated pregnancy. *Br J Obstet Gynaecol* 1980;87:780–5
18. Maulik D, Yarlagadda P, Youngblood JP, Ciston P. Comparative efficacy of the umbilical arterial Doppler indices for predicting adverse perinatal outcome. *Am J Obstet Gynecol* 1991;164:1434–40
19. Maulik D, Saini VD, Nanda NC, Rosenzweig MS. Doppler evaluation of fetal hemodynamics. *Ultrasound Med Biol* 1982;8:705–10
20. Campbell S, Diaz-Recasens J, Griffin DR, *et al*. New Doppler technique for assessing uteroplacental blood flow. *Lancet* 1983;1:675–7
21. Thompson RS, Trudinger JB, Cook CM. Doppler ultrasound waveforms in the fetal umbilical artery: quantitative analysis technique. *Ultrasound Med Biol* 1985;11:707–14
22. Marsal K. Ultrasound assessment of fetal circulation as a diagnostic test: a review. In Lipshitz J, Maloney J, Nimrod C, Carson G, eds. *Perinatal Development of the Heart and Lung*. Ithaca, NY: Perinatology Press, 1987:127
23. Westerhof N, Sipkema P, Van den Bos GC, Elzinga G. Forward and backward waves in the arterial system. *Cardiovasc Res* 1972;6:648–56
24. Murgo JP, Westerhof N, Giolma JP, Altobelli SA. Manipulation of ascending aortic pressure and flow wave reflections with Valsalva maneuver: relationship to input impedance. *Circulation* 1981;63:122–32

25. Spencer JAD, Giussani DA, Moore PJ, Hanson MA. *In vitro* validation of Doppler indices using blood and water. *J Ultrasound Med* 1991;10:305–8

26. Maulik D, Yarlagadda P, Nathanielsz PW, Figueroa JP. Hemodynamic validation of Doppler assessment of fetoplacental circulation in a sheep model system: *J Ultrasound Med* 1989;8:177–81

27. Trudinger BJ, Stevens D, Connelly A, *et al.* Umbilical artery velocity waveform and placental resistance: the effects of embolization of the umbilical circulation. *Am J Obstet Gynecol* 1987;157:1443–8

28. Morrow RJ, Adamson SL, Bull SB, Knox Ritchie JW. Effect of placental embolization on the umbilical arterial velocity waveform in fetal sheep. *Am J Obstet Gynecol* 1989;161:1055–60

29. Maulik D, Yarlagadda P. Hemodynamic validation of the Doppler indices: an *in vitro* study. *3rd Congress of the International Doppler Society, Malibu, USA.* Abstract, 1990

30. Downing GJ, Yarlagadda AP, Maulik D. Comparison of the pulsatility index and input impedance parameters in a model of altered hemodynamics. *J Ultrasound Med* 1991;10:317–21

31. Downing GJ, Maulik D. Correlation of the pulsatility index (PI) with input impedance parameters during altered hemodynamics (Abstract). *J Matern Fetal Invest* 1991;2:114

32. Giles WB, Trudinger JB, Baird PJ. Fetal umbilical artery flow velocity waveforms and placental resistance: pathologic correlation. *Br J Obstet Gynaecol* 1985;92:31–8

33. Voigt HJ, Becker V. Uteroplacental insufficiency – comparison of uteroplacental blood flow velocimetry and histomorphology of placental bed. *J Matern Fetal Invest* 1992;2:251–5

34. Peeters LLH, Sheldon RE, Jones MD, *et al.* Blood flow to fetal organs as a function of arterial oxygen content. *Am J Obstet Gynecol* 1979;135:637–46

35. Maulik D, Yarlagdda AP, Youngblood JP, Willoughby L. Components of variability of umbilical arterial Doppler velocimetry – a prospective analysis. *Am J Obstet Gynecol* 1989;160:1406–12

36. Dawes GS. *Fetal and Neonatal Physiology*, Chicago, IL: Yearbook Medical Publishers, 1968:66

37. Mires G, Dempster J, Patel NB, *et al.* The effect of fetal heart rate on umbilical artery flow velocity waveform. *Br J Obstet Gynaecol* 1987;94:665–9

38. Yarlagadda AP, Willoughby L, Maulik D. Effect of fetal heart rate on umbilical arterial Doppler indices. *J Ultrasound Med* 1989;8:215–18

39. Maulik D, Downing GJ, Yarlagadda AP. Umbilical arterial Doppler indices in acute uteroplacental flow occlusion. *Echocardiography* 1990;7:619–27

40. Downing G, Yarlagadda P, Maulik D. Effects of acute hypoxemia on umbilical arterial Doppler indices in a fetal ovine model. *Early Human Dev* 1991;25:1–10

41. Abramowicz JS, Warsof SL, Arrington J, Levy DL. Doppler analysis of the umbilical artery: the importance of choosing the placental end of the cord. *J Ultrasound Med* 1989;8:219–21

42. van Eyck J, Wladimiroff JW, v.d. Wijngaard JA, *et al.* The blood flow velocity waveform in the fetal internal carotid and umbilical artery; its relationship to fetal

43. van Eyck J, Wladimiroff JW, v.d. Wijngaard JA, *et al.* The blood flow velocity waveform in the fetal descending aorta; its relationship to fetal behavioral states in growth retarded fetuses at 37–38 weeks of gestation. *Early Hum Dev* 1986;14:99–107

44. Clapp JF, Szeto JF, Larrow R, *et al.* Umbilical blood flow response to embolization of the uterine circulation. *Am J Obstet Gynecol* 1980;138:60–6

45. Brosens I, Dixon AG, Robertson WB. Fetal growth retardation in the arteries of the placental bed. *Br J Obstet Gynaecol* 1977;84:656–63

46. Fleischer A, Schulman H, Farmakides G, *et al.* Umbilical artery velocity waveforms and intrauterine growth retardation. *Am J Obstet Gynecol* 1985;152:502–5

47. Arduini D, Rizzo G, Romannini C, Mancuso S. Fetal blood flow velocity waveforms as predictors of growth retardation. *Obstet Gynecol* 1987;70:7–10

48. Berkowitz GS, Chitkara U, Rosenberg J, *et al.* Sonographic estimation of fetal weight and Doppler analysis of umbilical artery velocimetry in the prediction of intrauterine growth retardation: a prospective study. *Am J Obstet Gynecol* 1988;158:1149–53

49. Divon MY, Guidetti DA, Braverman JJ, *et al.* Intrauterine growth retardation – a prospective study of the diagnostic value of real-time sonography combined with umbilical artery flow velocimetry. *Obstet Gynecol* 1988;72:611–14

50. Gaziano E, Knox GE, Wager GP, *et al.* The predictability of the small-for-gestational-age infant by real-time ultrasound-derived measurements combined with pulsed Doppler umbilical artery velocimetry. *Am J Obstet Gynecol* 1988;158:1431–9

51. Ott WJ. Comparison of dynamic image and pulsed Doppler ultrasonography for the diagnosis of intra-uterine growth retardation. *J Clin Ultrasound* 1990;18:3–11

52. Maulik D, Yarlagadda P, Youngblood JP, Ciston P. The diagnostic efficacy of the umbilical arterial systolic/diastolic ratio as a screening tool: a prospective blinded study. *Am J Obstet Gynecol* 1990;162(6):1518–25

53. Lowery CL, Henson BV, Wan J, Brumfield CG. A comparison between umbilical artery velocimetry and standard antepartum surveillance in hospitalized high-risk patients. *Am J Obstet Gynecol* 1990;162:710–14

54. Nicolaides KH, Bilardo CM, Soothill PW, *et al.* Absence of end diastolic frequencies in umbilical artery: a sign of fetal hypoxia and acidosis. *Br Med J* 1988;297:1026–7

55. Chambers SE, Hoskins PR, Haddad NG, *et al.* A comparison of fetal abdominal circumference measurements and Doppler ultrasound in the prediction of small-for-dates babies and fetal compromise. *Br J Obstet Gynaecol* 1989;96:803–8

56. Malcus P, Hokegard KH, Kjellmer I, *et al.* The relationship between arterial blood velocity waveforms and acid–base status in fetal lamb during acute experimental asphyxia. *J Matern Fetal Invest* 1991;1:29–34

57. Soothill PW, Nicolaides KH, Bilardo K, *et al*. Uteroplacental blood velocity resistance index and umbilical venous P_{O_2}, P_{CO_2}, pH, lactate and erythroblast count in growth retarded fetuses. *Fetal Ther* 1986;1:176–9

58. Cohn H, Sachs E, Heymann M, Rudolph A. Cardiovascular responses to hypoxemia and acidemia in fetal lambs. *Am J Obstet Gynecol* 1974;120:817–24

59. Hasaart THM, Maulik D, Morrow RJ. Validation of fetal flow velocimetry: a review of *in vitro* and *in vivo* modeling. *J Matern Fetal Invest* 1993;3:95–104

60. Copel JA, Woudstra BR, Wentworth R, *et al*. Hypoxia cannot be detected by the umbilical *S* : *D* ratio in fetal lambs. *J Matern Fetal Invest* 1991;1:219–21

61. Nicolaides KH, Bilardo CM, Soothill PW, Campbell S. Absence of end diastolic frequencies in umbilical artery: a sign of fetal hypoxia and acidosis. *Br Med J* 1988;297:1026–7

62. Ferrazzi E, Pardi G, Bauscaglia M. The correlation of biochemical monitoring versus umbilical flow velocity measurements of the human fetus. *Am J Obstet Gynecol* 1988;159:1081–7

63. Tyrrell S, Obaid AH, Lilford RJ. Umbilical artery Doppler velocimetry as a predictor of fetal hypoxia and acidosis at birth. *Obstet Gynecol* 1989;74:332–7

64. Bilardo CM, Nicolaides KH, Campbell S. Doppler measurements of fetal and uteroplacental circulations: relationship with umbilical venous blood gases measured at cordocentesis. *Am J Obstet Gynecol* 1990;162:115–20

65. Vintzileos AM, Campbell W, Rodis J, *et al*. The relationship between fetal biophysical assessment, umbilical artery velocimetry, and fetal acidosis. *Obstet Gynecol* 1991;77:622–6

66. Yoon BH, Syn HC, Kim SW. The efficacy of Doppler umbilical velocimetry in identifying fetal acidosis. A comparison with fetal biophysical profile. *J Ultrasound Med* 1992;11:1–6

67. Pardi G, Cetin I, Marconi AM, *et al*. Diagnostic value of blood sampling in fetuses with growth retardation. *New Engl J Med* 1993;328:692–6

68. Yoon BH, Romero R, Roh CR, *et al*. Relationship between the fetal biophysical profile score, umbilical artery Doppler velocimetry, and fetal blood acid–base status determined by cordocentesis. *Am J Obstet Gynecol* 1993;169:1586

69. Trudinger BJ, Cook CM, Jones L, Giles WB. A comparison of fetal heart rate monitoring and umbilical artery waveforms in the recognition of fetal compromise. *Br J Obstet Gynaecol* 1986;93:171

70. Farmakides G, Schulman H, Winter D, *et al*. Prenatal surveillance using non-stress testing and Doppler velocimetry. *Obstet Gynecol* 1988;71:184

71. Brar HS, Medearis AL, DeVore GR, Platt LD. A comparative study of fetal umbilical velocimetry with continuous and pulsed wave Doppler ultrasonography in high risk pregnancies: relationship to outcome. *Am J Obstet Gynecol* 1989;160:375

72. Beattie RB, Dornan JC. Antenatal screening for intrauterine growth retardation with umbilical artery Doppler ultrasonography. *Br Med J* 1989;298:631

73. Hanretty KP, Primrose MH, Neilson JP, Whittle MJ. Pregnancy screening by Doppler uteroplacental and umbilical waveforms. *Br J Obstet Gynaecol* 1989;96:1163–7

74. Newnham JP, Patterson LL, James IR, *et al*. An evaluation of the efficacy of Doppler flow velocity waveform analysis as a screening test in pregnancy. *Am J Obstet Gynecol* 1990;162:403–10

75. Sijmons EA, Reuwer PJ, van Beek E, Bruinse HW. The validity of screening for small-for-gestational-age and low-weight-for-length infants by Doppler ultrasound. *Br J Obstet Gynaecol* 1989;96:557–61

76. Beattie RB, Hannah ME, Dornan JC. Compound analysis of umbilical artery velocimetry in low-risk pregnancy. *J Matern Fetal Invest* 1992;2:269

77. Woo JSK, Liang ST, Lo RLS. Significance of an absent or reversed end-diastolic flow in Doppler umbilical artery waveforms. *J Ultrasound Med* 1987;6:291

78. Rochelson B, Schulman H, Farmakides G, *et al*. The significance of absent end-diastolic velocity in umbilical artery velocity waveforms. *Am J Obstet Gynecol* 1987;156:1213

79. Teyssier G, Fouron JC, Maroto D, *et al*. Blood flow velocity in the fetal aortic isthmus: a sensitive indicator of changes in systemic peripheral resistances. I. Experimental studies. *J Matern Fetal Invest* 1993;3:213

80. Fouron JC, Teyssier G, Bonnin P, *et al*. Blood flow velocity in the fetal aortic isthmus: a sensitive indicator of changes in systemic peripheral resistances. II. Preliminary observations. *J Matern Fetal Invest* 1993;3:219

81. Weiner Z, Farmakides G, Schulman H, Penny B. Central and peripheral hemodynamic changes in fetuses with absent end-diastolic velocity in umbilical artery; correlation with computerized fetal heart rate pattern. *Am J Obstet Gynecol* 1994;170:509

82. Giles WB, Trudinger BJ, Cook CM. Fetal umbilical artery flow velocity–time waveforms in twin pregnancies. *Br J Obstet Gynaecol* 1985;92:490

83. Farmakides G, Schulman H, Saldana LR, *et al*. Surveillance of twin pregnancy with umbilical artery velocity. *Am J Obstet Gynecol* 1985;153:789

84. Nimrod C, Davies D, Harder J, *et al*. Doppler ultrasound prediction of fetal outcome in twin pregnancy. *Am J Obstet Gynecol* 1987;156:402–6

85. Gaziano EP, Calvin S, Bendel RP, *et al*. Pulsed Doppler umbilical artery waveforms in multiple gestation: comparison with ultrasound estimated fetal weight for the diagnosis of small for gestational age infant. *J Matern Fetal Invest* 1992;1:277–80

86. Giles WB, Trudinger BJ, Cook CM, *et al*. Umbilical artery flow velocity waveforms and twin pregnancy outcome. *Obstet Gynecol* 1988;72:894–7

87. Gaziano EP, Knox H, Ferrera B, *et al*. Is it time to reassess the risk for the growth-retarded fetus with normal Doppler velocimetry of the umbilical artery? *Am J Obstet Gynecol* 1994;170:1734–41

88. Marsal K, Lingman G, Giles W. Evaluation of the carotid, aortic and umbilical blood velocity (Abstract). *Proceedings from Society for the Study of Fetal Physiology, 11th Annual Conference, Oxford*, 1984

89. Wladimiroff JW, Tonge HN, Stewart PA. Doppler ultrasound assessment of cerebral blood flow in the human fetus. *Br J Obstet Gynaecol* 1986;93:471–5

90. Arbeille P, Tranquart F, Body G, *et al*. Evolution de la circulation arterielle ombilicale et cérébrale du foetus au cours de la grossesse. *Progr Neonatologie* 1986; 6:30–7

91. van Eyck J, Wladimiroff JW, van den Wijngaard JAGW, *et al*. The blood flow velocity waveform in the fetal internal carotid and umbilical artery; its relationship to fetal behavioural states in normal pregnancy at 37–38 weeks of gestation. *Br J Obstet Gynaecol* 1987; 94:736–41

92. Vyas S, Nicolaides KH, Bower S, Campbell S. Middle cerebral artery flow velocity waveforms in fetal hypoxaemia. *Br J Obstet Gynaecol* 1990;97:797–803

93. Arbeille P, Maulik D, Fignon A, *et al*. Assessment of the fetal P_{O_2} changes by cerebral and umbilical Doppler on lamb fetuses (Abstract). *J Matern Fetal Invest* 1992;2:34

94. Arbeille P, Maulik D, Fignon A, *et al*. Assessment of the fetal P_{O_2} changes by cerebral and umbilical Doppler on lamb fetuses during acute hypoxia. *Ultrasound Med Biol* 1995;21:861–70

95. Arbeille P, Roncin A, Berson M, *et al*. Exploration of the fetal cerebral blood flow by duplex Doppler – linear array system in normal and pathological pregnancies. *Ultrasound Med Biol* 1987;13:329–37

96. Wladimiroff JW, van den Wijngaard JAGW, Degani S, *et al*. Cerebral and umbilical blood flow velocity waveforms in normal and growth retarded pregnancies; a comparative study. *Obstet Gynaecol* 1987;69:705–9

97. Chiba Y, Utsu M, Kanzaki T, Hasegawa T. Changes in venous flow and intratracheal flow in fetal breathing movements. *Ultrasound Med Biol* 1983;11:43–9

98. Rizzo G, Arduini D, Caforio L, Romanini C. Effects of sampling sites on inferior vena cava flow velocity waveform. *J Matern Fetal Invest* 1992;2:153–6

99. Reed KL, Appleton CP, Anderson CF, *et al*. Doppler studies of vena cava flows in human fetuses – insights into normal and abnormal cardiac physiology. *Circulation* 1990;81:498–505

100. Kanzaki T, Murakami M, Kobayashi H, Chiba Y. Characteristic abnormal blood flow pattern of the inferior vena cava in fetal arrhythmia. *J Matern Fetal Invest* 1991;1:35–9

101. Gudmundsson S, Huhta JC, Wood DC, *et al*. Venous Doppler ultrasonography in the fetus with nonimmune hydrops. *Am J Obstet Gynecol* 1991;164:33–7

102. Rizzo G, Arduini D, Romanini C. Inferior vena cava flow velocity waveforms in appropriate for gestational age fetuses. *Am J Obstet Gynecol* 1992;166:1271–80

103. Vyas S, Nicolaides KH, Campbell S. Renal artery flow–velocity waveforms in normal and hypoxemic fetuses. *Am J Obstet Gynecol* 1988;161:168–72

104. Veille JC, Kanaan C. Duplex Doppler ultrasonographic evaluation of the fetal renal artery in normal and abnormal fetuses. *Am J Obstet Gynecol* 1989;161:1502–7

105. Trudinger BJ, Giles WB, Cook CM. Flow waveforms in the maternal uteroplacental and fetal umbilical placental circulation. *Am J Obstet Gynecol* 1985;152:155–63

106. Stabile I, Bilardo C, Panella M, *et al*. Doppler measurement of uterine blood flow in the first trimester of normal and complicated pregnancies. *Trophoblast Res* 1988;3:301–7

107. Rightmire DA, Campbell S. Fetal and maternal Doppler blood flow parameters in posterm pregnancies. *Obstet Gynecol* 1987;69:891–4

108. Campbell S, Pearce JMF, Hackett G, *et al*. Qualitative assessment of utero-placental blood flow: early screening test for high risk pregnancies. *Obstet Gynecol* 1986; 68:649–53

109. Trudinger BJ, Giles WB, Cook CM. Uteroplacental blood flow velocity–time waveforms in normal and complicated pregnancy. *Br J Obstet Gynaecol* 1985;92:39

110. Schulman H, Ducey J, Farmakides G, *et al*. Uterine artery Doppler velocimetry: the significance of divergent systolic/diastolic ratios. *Am J Obstet Gynecol* 1987; 157:1539–42

111. Ducey J, Schulman H, Farmakides G, *et al*. A classification of hypertension in pregnancy based on Doppler velocimetry. *Am J Obstet Gynecol* 1987;157:660

112. Thaler I, Wiener Z, Itskovitz J, Brandes JM. Uterine blood flow patterns in patients with absent of reverse end diastolic flow velocity in umbilical artery waveforms. *J Matern Fetal Invest* 1991;1:83–6

113. Trudinger BJ, Cook CM, Giles WB, *et al*. Umbilical artery flow velocity waveforms in high risk pregnancy: randomised controlled trial: *Lancet* 1987;1:188

114. Tyrrell SN, Lilford RJ, Macdonald HN, *et al*. Randomized controlled trial (RCT) clinical trial. *Br J Obstet Gynaecol* 1990;97(10):909–12

115. Hofmeyr GJ, Pattinson R, Buckley D, *et al*. Umbilical artery resistance index as a screening test for fetal well-being. II. Randomized feasibility study. *Obstet Gynecol* 1991;78:359–62

116. Newnham JP, O'Dea MA, Reid KP, Diepeveen DA. Doppler flow velocity waveform analysis in high risk pregnancies: a randomized controlled trial. *Br J Obstet Gynaecol* 1991;98:956–60

117. Davies JA, Gallivan S, Spencer JAD. Randomised controlled trial of Doppler ultrasound screening of placental perfusion during pregnancy. *Lancet* 1992; 340:1299–303

118. Almstrom H, Axelsson O, Cnattingius S, *et al*. Comparison of umbilical artery velocimetry and cardiotocography for surveillance of small for gestational age fetuses: a multi-center randomized controlled trial. *J Matern Fetal Invest* 1991;1:127 (Abstract)

119. Almstrom H, Axelsson O, Cnattingius S, *et al*. Comparison of umbilical artery velocimetry and cardiotocography for surveillance of small for gestational age fetuses: a multi-center randomized controlled trial. *Lancet* 1992;340:936–40

120. Mason GC, Lilford RJ, Porter J, Nelson E. Randomised comparison of routine versus highly selective use of Doppler ultrasound in low risk pregnancies. *Br J Obstet Gynaecol* 1993;100:130–3

121. Johnstone FD, Prescott R, Hoskins P, *et al*. The effect of introduction of umbilical Doppler recordings to obstetric practice. *Br J Obstet Gynaecol* 1993;100: 733–41

122. Newnham JP, Evans SF, Michael CA, *et al*. Effects of frequent ultrasound during pregnancy: a randomised controlled trial. *Lancet* 1993;342:887–91

123. Whittle MJ, Hanretty KP, Primrose MH, Neilson JP. Screening for the compromised fetus: a randomized

trial of umbilical artery velocimetry in unselected pregnancies. *Am J Obstet Gynecol* 1994;170:555–9

124. Omtzigt AWJ. Clinical Value of Umbilical Doppler Velocimetry. Doctoral thesis. University of Utrecht, The Netherlands, 1990

125. Omtzigt AMWJ, Reuwer PJHM, Bruinse HW. A randomized controlled trial on the clinical value of umbilical Doppler velocimetry in antenatal care. *Am J Obstet Gynecol* 1994;170:625–34

126. Pattinson RC, Norman K, Odendal HJ. The role of Doppler velocimetry in the management of high risk pregnancies. *Br J Obstet Gynaecol* 1994;101:114–20

127. Mantel N, Haentzel W. Statistical aspects of the analysis of data from retrospective studies of disease. *J Natl Cancer Inst* 1959;22:719

128. Yusuf S, Peto R, Lewis J, *et al*. Beta blockade during and after myocardial infarction: an overview of the randomized trials. *Prog Cardiovasc Dis* 1985;27:335

129. Chalmers TC, Buyse MEB. Meta-analysis. In Chalmers TC, ed. *Data Analysis for Clinical Medicine: The Qualitative Approach to Patient Care in Gastroenterology*. Rome: International University Press, 1988

130. Cochran WG. The combination of estimates from different experiments. *Biometrics* 1954;10:101

131. DerSimonian R, Laird N. Meta-analysis in clinical trials. *Controlled Clin Trials* 1986;8:177

132. Demets DL. Methods for combining randomized clinical trials: strengths and limitations. *Stat Med* 1987;6:341

133. Bailey KR. Inter-study differences: how should they influence the interpretation and analysis of results? *Stat Med* 1987;6:351

134. Alfirevic Z, Nielson JP. Doppler ultrasonography in high risk pregnancies: systematic reviews with meta-analysis. *Am J Obstet Gynecol* 1995;172:1379–87

135. Chalmers TC, Smith H Jr, Blackburn M, *et al*. A method for assessing the quality of a randomized control trial. *Clin Trials* 1981;2:31

136. Neilson JP. Doppler ultrasound (all trials). In *Pregnancy and Childbirth Module*. Enkin MW, Kierse MJNC, Renfrew MJ, Neilson JP, eds. *Cochrane Database of Systematic Reviews*. Disk Issue 2, Review No. 07337. Oxford: Update Software

52

Erythroblastosis fetalis

P.N. Rauk and A. Daftary

INTRODUCTION

Hydrops fetalis was observed centuries before the cause was identified. Not until the early 1940s was isoimmunization to the rhesus blood group antigen, Rh(D), proposed as the cause of erythroblastosis fetalis[1]. Between 1940 and 1970, a further understanding of the pathophysiology of isoimmunization led to the routine use of Rh immune globulin for the prevention of Rh disease. Liley[2] further discovered that the severity of Rh disease could be predicted by amniotic fluid bilirubin level and pioneered intrauterine transfusion for the treatment of severe anemia. Few areas of obstetrics have benefited more from the introduction of ultrasound and cordocentesis than in the treatment of isoimmunization. The morbidity and mortality due to hemolytic disease of the newborn has been dramatically reduced only through these technologies.

This chapter discusses the incidence, pathogenesis, diagnosis, management and treatment of isoimmunization with an emphasis on anti-Rh(D) disease. The pathophysiology of fetal hydrops and the role of amniocentesis, ultrasound, Doppler and intrauterine transfusion in the management of rhesus isoimmunization is emphasized.

INCIDENCE AND SOURCES OF RHESUS ISOIMMUNIZATION

The incidence of anti-D isoimmunization relates to the number of Rh(D)-positive fetuses born to Rh-negative mothers, the rate of transplacental passage of fetal blood cells, and the immunological response of the mother. The frequency of Rh-negative genotype varies considerably by race. Fifteen percent of whites are Rh-negative compared with 6% of blacks and 1% of Orientals[3]. Given random mating of Rh-negative white females with Rh-positive males, the expected frequency of a Rh-positive conceptus is 9.2%. The actual rates of isoimmunization in white gravidas six months post-delivery are 6.9% and 12.6% after delivery of a first and second Rh-positive infant, respectively[4]. The antepartum rate of isoimmunization is between 1 and 2%[5].

Rh isoimmunization results when Rh-positive cells enter the maternal circulation and stimulate an immune response. Pollack[6] in 1971, using Rh-negative volunteers, showed that 65% of individuals are immunized after a single injection of 37.5 ml of packed Rh-positive red blood cells. Even following as much as 500 ml of Rh-positive blood, only 80% of volunteers become sensitized. Thus one in four Rh-negative individuals will not become sensitized when exposed to Rh-positive blood.

The rate of isoimmunization is also modified by the ABO status of the mother and fetus. Stern and Goodman[7], in 1961, demonstrated the protective effect of ABO incompatibility on Rh immunization in Rh-negative volunteers. Rh antibodies developed in only 16% of individuals given Rh-positive, ABO-incompatible blood compared with 70% given ABO-compatible blood. Ascari observed that following delivery of an ABO-compatible Rh-positive fetus the incidence of isoimmunizations was 17%[8]. The observed incidence of Rh isoimmunization in group O mothers with maternal–fetal ABO incompatibility was 9–13%. Rh isoimmunization during pregnancy or within three days of delivery occurs in 0.6% of ABO incompatible pregnancies versus 2.0% in ABO compatible pregnancies[5].

Fetal–maternal hemorrhage (FMH) is the major source of Rh isoimmunization. As early as 1941, Levine proposed the passage of fetal cells into the maternal circulation caused isoimmunization[9]. The actual volume of red blood cells necessary for Rh sensitization is unknown. Sensitization in Rh-negative volunteers has been produced with as little as 0.1 ml of red blood cells[10].

Spontaneous FMH is the most common cause of sensitization during pregnancy, labor and delivery. Fetal red blood cells have been detected in the maternal circulation at six weeks of gestation. Generally, fetal cells are detected in the maternal circulation using acid elution techniques or the Kleihauer– Betke smear. Although as few as 1 : 1 000 000 or 0.004 ml of fetal cells can be detected, considerable variation in sensitivity is observed among various laboratories. Among ABO-compatible pregnancies, FMH occurs in the first trimester in 6.7%, the second trimester in 15.9% and the third trimester in 28.9%[11]. FMH occurs in 50% of women at delivery and is > 24 ml of fetal red cells in 0.7%[11].

FMH occurs after both induced and spontaneous abortion. Among first-trimester abortions, rates of

FMH are 9.9% at 5–6 weeks, 16.7% at 6–7 weeks and 18.6% at 7–8 weeks[12]. Rates of iso-immunization, however, correlate poorly with the demonstration of FMH. The average rate of sensitization following spontaneous and induced abortion without Rh immune globulin is 8.4% (range 0–13%)[13].

Rh isoimmunization can also occur following ectopic pregnancy. FMH occurs in 24% of ruptured ectopic pregnancies[14]. This rate is higher than for unruptured ectopics and may represent the transperitoneal passage of fetal red blood cells[14].

Amniocentesis leads to FMH even when the placenta is localized with ultrasound. FMH was demonstrated in 5.4% of patients when the placenta was partially anterior compared with 15.8% with an anterior placenta[15]. Despite avoidance of an anterior placenta, the rate of FMH is 4.7%, with 2.6% > 0.1 ml of blood[16]. Chorionic villous sampling also increases the risk for FMH. Blakemore[17] noted a rise in maternal serum alpha-fetoprotein in 50% of women following first trimester chorionic villous sampling.

RHESUS BLOOD GROUP SYSTEM

The rhesus antigen was discovered when rabbits were administered rhesus monkey blood and the rabbit derived antibody agglutinated human red blood cells. The rhesus factor, now Rh(D) antigen, is found on 85% of human red blood cells. The Rh system is, however, more accurately identified by many red cell antigens. Three systems of nomenclature, the Fischer–Race, Weiner, and Rosenfield models, are currently used to describe an individual's Rh genotype.

(1) The Fischer–Race model assumes three closely linked genes each coding for a pair of alleles. These alleles code for antigens identified by antisera and have been denoted as D, C, c, E, and e antigens[18]. No d antigen has yet been discovered. The presence of the antigen D denotes Rh positivity. Each individual carries two sets of the three antigens. The population frequency of each genotype is known, and the most probable genotype for any individual can be assumed based on the phenotype identified by blood typing. Some sets of antigens are more common than others (Table 1).

Table 1 Rhesus system nomenclature

Rosenfield	Weiner	Fisher–Race
1	Rho	D
2	rh′	C
3	rh″	E
4	hr′	c
5	hr″	e

Modified from Rote, NS. Pathophysiology of Rh isoimmunization. *Clin Obstet Gynecol* 1982;25:243

(2) Weiner[19], in describing the Rh system, identifies each set of the three antigenic determinates D, C(c), and E(e), as a single product of a gene locus with multiple alleles. The system also uses an abbreviated nomenclature for each genotype (Table 1). Thus the genotype CDe/cde is represented by R1,r and contains the alleles Rho, rh′, hr″, and hr′. The gene R1 codes for CDe and r for cde.

(3) Rosenfield and co-workers[20], in 1962, proposed a system which assigned a number to the gene product or allele. Utilizing this system the complexity inherent in the Rh system can be adequately characterized (Table 2).

The Rh system includes many more antigens than D, C, c, E, and e. The antigen D^μ deserves further discussion. D^μ is a weakened form of D and is found in 0.6% of the Caucasian population. D^μ is identified when direct agglutination is equivocal or negative but antiglobulin tests detect D positivity. D^μ cells are also less immunogenic than D cells. D^μ cells from a fetus can be destroyed by anti-D in the mother. D^μ fetal cells may also stimulate an anti-D response in the mother. Generally D^μ positive individuals are considered Rh- positive. The identification of D^μ the first time in a woman following delivery may be due to a large FMH of D-positive fetal cells. All women identified as D^μ at delivery require a Kleihauer–Betke smear to rule out large FMH.

Regardless of the nomenclature used, the gene(s) in the Rh system code for proteins which are essential structural elements of the red cell membrane. The Rh antigens are unique to red cell membranes and are not found in other cell types.

Table 2 Genotype frequencies in Rh(D)-positive individuals

Phenotype	Frequency*	Genotypes (%)
cDe/ce	2.1	cDe/cde(96.8), cDe/cDe(3.2)
CDe/ce	35.0	CDe/cde(93.7), CDe/cde(6.2), cDe/Cde(0.1)
CDe/Ce	18.5	CDe/CDe(95.6), cDe/Cde(4.4)
cDE/cE	11.8	cDE/cde(92.4), cDE/cDe(6.1), cDe/cdE(0.5)
cDE/cE	2.3	cDE/cDE(85.6), cDE/cdE(14.4)
CDe/cE	13.1	CDe/cDE(90.3), CDe/cdE(7.6), cDE/Cde(2.1)
CDE/ce	0.2	CDE/cde(93.7), CDE/cDe(6.2), cDe/CdE(0.1)
CDE/Ce	0.2	CDE/CDe(95.8), CDE/Cde(2.2), cDe/CdE(2.0)
CDE/cE	0.1	CDE/cDE(90.5), CDE/cdE(7.6), CDe/CdE(1.8)
CDE/CE	rare	CDE/CDE(98.3), CDE/CdE(1.7)

*Total 83.2% in white population

METHODS OF ANTIBODY DETECTION

The Rh status and antibody status of all women should be identified at the first prenatal visit. In Rh-negative women, an antibody screen should be repeated at 28 weeks. An antibody screen not only identifies antibodies to D but to the other rhesus antigens and atypical antigens. Antibodies are identified by the agglutination of specific red cell preparations by the test serum. The agglutination reaction is performed in both saline and colloid media. In saline, IgM antibodies are able to crosslink red cells and produce agglutination due to the multiple antigen-binding sites on the IgM molecule. IgG antibodies are identified by agglutination in colloid media such as albumin. The albumin reduces the electrostatic repulsion between red cells and allows IgM molecules to crosslink the red cells. Therefore, the antibody titer in saline reflects the IgM component only, while the titer in albumin media reflects both IgG and IgM. The distinction between IgM and IgG antibodies is important as IgM antibodies do not cross the placental barrier and thus do not affect the fetus.

Several methods are available to enhance the agglutination reaction to identify IgG, or incomplete, antibodies at lower titers. An indirect antiglobulin titer utilizes Coombs serum or antihuman immnunoglobulin to accentuate agglutination. With this method, the test serum is incubated with red blood cells, washed, and Coombs serum is added. The Coombs serum crosslinks the antibody-coated cells and produces agglutination. Generally, the indirect antiglobulin assay is more sensitive than agglutination in saline or colloid and titers are higher. The use of enzymatically altered red cells is the most sensitive manual technique for identifying antibody titers. Automated techniques for identifying anti-D antibodies are also available. However, antibodies identified by automated methods alone and not by manual methods may not be used to establish a case of Rh isoimmunization. Automated methods detect antibody at low concentration, 1–8 ng/ml, compared with direct agglutination, 10–200 ng/ml[21]. Thus very weak antibodies at low concentration may be detected. These antibodies rarely cause hemolytic disease.

PATHOGENESIS AND SCOPE OF HEMOLYTIC DISEASE OF THE FETUS AND NEWBORN

Pathogenesis

D antigen is present on the surface of fetal red blood cells, and is demonstrable by anti-D agglutination, as early as 38 days postconception[22]. (Trophoblast may express the D antigen[23], but this has not been consistently verified.) At the end of the first trimester, erythropoiesis is evident in the spleen and liver. By the end of the second trimester, the responsibility for blood production has shifted to the bone marrow. At term, erythropoiesis is exclusively a marrow function.

Fetomaternal hemorrhage is presently the most common pathway for maternal exposure to 'foreign' red cell antigens. (There are no known 'naturally occurring' Rh antigens.) Sensitization then takes place: the Rh-negative mother is exposed to Rh(D) antigen on fetal red blood cells and, after recognizing this as foreign, generates a competent primary immune response. This immune response has been well studied in Rh-negative volunteers exposed to Rh-positive red cells. Generally, several injections are needed to produce an antibody response in the majority of individuals. Antibody evidence appears slowly (2–6 months after initial exposure), is weak, and is mostly IgM. IgM has a molecular weight of 900 000 and cannot traverse the placenta. IgM titers then rapidly fall and IgG titers gradually rise. IgG has a molecular weight of 160 000 and can cross the placenta. Without sensitization, the secondary response that causes fetal red blood cell hemolysis cannot take place. As has previously been noted, one-quarter of Rh-negative women are 'non-responders' to Rh(D) antigen. With subsequent exposures to Rh(D) antigen, there is a prompt (in days) anamnestic secondary response in the form of IgG (mostly IgG_1 and IgG_3). The dose of antigen required is very small. The secondary response is heightened by repetitive exposure and it is more pronounced (increased titers and avidity) with longer intervals between exposures. This secondary response may account for the appearance of anti-Rh antibodies during pregnancy in individuals with prior negative screens.

IgG anti-D is actively transported across the placental barrier in endocytic vacuoles and released intact, by exocytosis, into the fetal circulation. It then binds fetal red blood cells and initiates the process of red cell destruction, the basic pathogenesis of hemolytic disease of the fetus and newborn (HDFN). The strength of antibody binding will vary with antigen density on the fetal red blood cells, antibody titers, and avidity.

Anti-D IgG is not known to activate complement, but rather initiates immune identification (via its Fc portion) by macrophages and polymorphonuclear white blood cells. By virtue of multiple Fc receptors, these cells become surrounded by 'rosettes' of antibody-coated red cells. This occurs in the reticuloendothelial system (RES), primarily the spleen. The slower circulation here allows for more intimate contact. These white cells then initiate extravascular hemolysis by pseudopods which fragment the red cell membrane. Loss of membrane substance causes sphering of the red cells, decreased deformability, and increased osmotic fragility. This leads to phagocytosis and lysis of the red cells. Antibody-dependent cellular cytotoxicity (ADCC), where lymphoid K cells and monocytes bind antibody coated red cells and initiate lysis, remains an *in vitro* phenomenon and has not yet been demonstrated with respect to HDFN *in vivo*.

Fetal response to anemia

The extravascular hemolysis causes formation of red cell degradation products (hemoglobin, stromal elements) and anemia. The degradation products undergo placental clearance and do not impact on HDFN until after birth. The severity of anemia determines the compensatory response and thus the extent of intrauterine disease. There is much variability in fetal response and the factors determining individual capacity for compensation are not well understood. Extent of manifestation may range from hydrops with intrauterine demise to mild neonatal anemia.

In normal fetuses, hemoglobin concentration increases linearly with gestational age, from a mean of 11 g/dl at 17 weeks to a mean of 15 g/dl at 40 weeks[24] (Figure 1). This is consistent with a response to a linear decrease in umbilical venous P_{O_2}. This allows the umbilical venous oxygen content to be maintained[25].

Between gestational weeks 10–24, hemopoiesis primarily takes place in the liver and spleen. However, from week 16 onward, there is a rapid decrease in extramedullary hemopoiesis (EMH) and a concomitant increase in medullary contribution. In the liver, as in other sites of EMH, there is no mechanism for preventing the release of nucleated red blood cell precursors into the circulation. In contrast, in the bone marrow, only the reticulocyte has the deformability and motility necessary to be released into the circulation. The liver, however, releases proportionately more reticulocytes. Thus, along with the increase in hemoglobin concentration, there is a linear decrease in reticulocyte count and an exponential decrease in erythroblast count with advancing gestation[26]. Since erythroblasts are released only by extramedullary sites, the erythroblast count may be considered an indirect measure of EMH.

Hemolysis is reflected in a decreased oxygen-carrying capacity. The fetus initially compensates by increasing cardiac output. This is probably accomplished by decreasing peripheral vascular resistance. Doppler studies show increased velocity of flow in the descending thoracic aorta and the common carotid artery[27–29]. Erythropoietin concentration increases with mild-to-moderate levels of anemia (hemoglobin deficit of 2–7 g/dl from the mean for gestational age). The bone marrow is very responsive to this, and intramedullary hemopoiesis increases. This is reflected in a linear increase in reticulocyte count with progressive anemia (Figure 2)[25]. With progressive anemia and hemoglobin deficits > 7 g/dl, there is a significant increase in plasma and amniotic fluid erythropoietin concentration[30]. This causes recruitment of EMH sites including the liver, spleen, kidneys, adrenals, intestinal

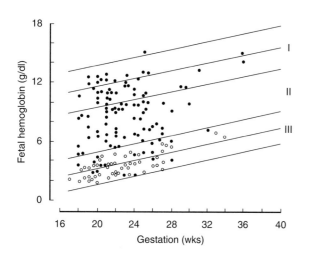

Figure 1 Initial hemoglobin concentration in isoimmunized fetuses at first blood sampling. O, Hydropic fetuses; ●, non-hydropic fetuses. Zone I = the 85% confidence intervals of the named hemoglobin for estimated gestational age and zone III does the same for hydropic fetuses. Zone II = moderate anemia. Reprinted with permission from reference 24

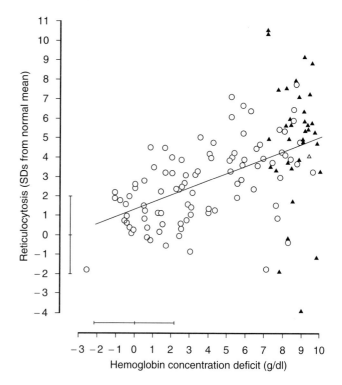

Figure 2 Hemoglobin deficit from mean for estimated gestational age (EGA) vs. reticulocytosis (in number of standard deviations from mean for EGA) in isoimmunized fetuses (O); ▲, hydropic fetuses. Reprinted with permission from reference 25

mucosa, lymph nodes and placenta. This is reflected in an exponential rise in the erythroblast count (Figure 3)[25]. Thus, the term 'erythroblastosis fetalis'. As can be seen in Figure 1[24], hydropoic fetuses also demonstrate a linear relationship between hemoglobin concentration and gestational age. They have hemoglobin deficits that range from > 7 g/dl to < 10 g/dl below the mean. Presumably, a hemoglobin deficit of 10 g/dl is the minimum hemoglobin concentration necessary to ensure intrauterine survival. The variability in fetal response to anemia can be seen in figure 3. There are several fetuses with hemoglobin deficits > 7 g/dl that do not show stigmata diagnostic of hydrops. Previous reports have shown hydrops to be associated with hemoglobin < 4 g/dl[31], < 5 g/dl[32], and hematocrit < 15%[33].

In some fetuses, destruction of red cells exceeds increase in production and anemia progresses. As oxygen content decreases, blood flow to all tissues increases until some 'critical level' is reached where hypoxia ensues. At this point, a redistribution in blood flow takes place in favor of the most vital organs, leaving an even greater inadequacy of blood flow/oxygen to the remaining organs[34]. When hemoglobin deficit is > 3 standard deviations (SD) below the mean, umbilical artery lactate concentration increases. When the hemoglobin deficit reaches > 7 SD below the mean for gestational age (roughly equivalent to oxygen content < 2 m mol/l), umbilical vein lactate concentration increases. The P_{O_2} and P_{CO_2} do not change in either umbilical vessel with any degree of anemia and the pH in the umbilical artery only decreases once hemoglobin deficit is > 7–8 g/dl[35]. Thus, at mild-to-moderate degrees of hemoglobin deficit, the placenta clears lactate that has accumulated in umbilical arterial blood. Once placental capacity for lactate clearance is exceeded, systemic metabolic acidosis ensues.

As EMH increases, important structural changes occur in the liver. Islands of hemopoiesis enlarge and compress on vasculature and normal parenchyma, thus compromising function. Venous compression may cause venous stasis and decreased blood supply, thus altering substrate uptake as well as liberation of synthetic products. With parenchymal damage, protein production may be diminished, resulting in hypoalbuminemia and hypoproteinemia[36,37]. In one study, total protein was > 2 SD below the mean for gestational age in all hydropic and in six of ten non-hydropic fetuses while albumin was > 2 SD below the mean in six of seven hydropic and two of ten non-hydropic fetuses[36]. Coupled with this decrease in systemic oncotic pressure is hypoxic endothelial damage that may contribute to extravascular fluid/protein loss and the development of ascites, anasarca, and serous cavity effusions. Venous stasis in the hepatic bed may also increase hydrostatic pressure in the placental vasculature, thus altering fluid dynamics and nutrient exchange. Placental size will increase with placental edema and the altered fluid dynamics may contribute to hydramnios formation[38].

In some fetuses, a downward spiraling course ensues. Worsening anemia, acidosis, liver failure and cardiovascular compromise culminate in hydrops and fetal demise[32]. The concept that the fetus is in congestive heart failure at the time of death has not been substantiated: normal fetal–placental blood volume (FPBV) has been seen even in hydropic fetuses[39–41]. Doppler studies, however, have shown a decrease in mean velocity of aortic blood flow in some hydropic fetuses with hemoglobin deficits > 7 g/dl. This could suggest some form of myocardial decompensation secondary to hypoxia/acidosis and decreased venous return secondary to hepatic infiltration[28]. Cordocentesis data in cases of irreversible fetal compromise leading to demise indicate that the terminal events are severe mixed acidosis and hypoxia[32].

Scope of HDFN

Bowman[42] describes three basic categories regarding severity of fetal/neonatal disease. Approximately one-half of affected fetuses are mildly affected and will not require treatment after delivery. They have a positive direct Coombs test of cord blood (diagnostic of HDFN) and are mildly anemic (cord hemoglobin concentration > 12–13 g/dl) and mildly hyperbilirubinemic with cord bilirubin concentration < 3.0–3.5 mg/dl. These neonates develop normally without significant neonatal anemia or hyperbilirubinemia.

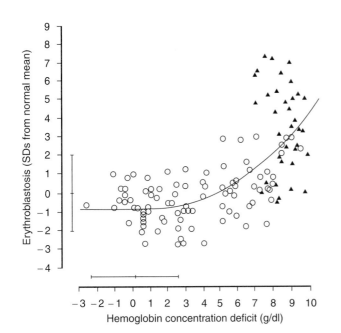

Figure 3 Hemoglobin deficit vs. erythroblastosis in isoimmunized fetuses (O); ▲, hydropic fetuses. Reprinted with permission from reference 25

Twenty-five percent of affected fetuses and neonates have moderate disease. These fetuses can compensate for hemolysis sufficiently to maintain adequate hemoglobin concentration without developing hydrops. Following delivery, the neonate must now metabolize the products of hemolysis (heme and unconjugated bilirubin – previously metabolized by the mother via placental transfer) on its own. Newborns, especially if premature, have delayed production of albumin and their livers are deficient in both the bilirubin-conjugating enzyme glucuronyl transferase and transport protein Y. They cannot adequately metabolize indirect bilirubin to the direct form nor is there an adequate concentration of albumin to transport indirect bilirubin in plasma. Thus, the concentration of the lipid-soluble indirect bilirubin increases. Diffusion into tissues with high membrane lipid content occurs, predominantly the neurons of the basal ganglia, hippocampal cortex, and subthalamic nuclei in the brain. Unconjugated bilirubin interferes with mitochondrial function and is therefore cytotoxic. Hypoxia and acidosis may potentiate this effect. The dead neurons are yellow-stained secondary to the accumulation of bilirubin, thus the term 'kernicterus'. Kernicterus (bilirubin encephalopathy) is associated with 80–90% mortality. Those neonates that survive may have severe morbidity, including hypertonicity, profound sensorineural hearing loss, choreoathetoid cerebral palsy, and mental retardation.

The remaining 25% of affected fetuses will develop severe disease. Without *in utero* therapy, these fetuses will develop hydrops fetalis secondary to progressive anemia. Fifty percent of these fetuses will do so prior to 34 weeks' gestation.

MONITORING THE PREGNANCY AT RISK

Detecting sensitization

All women registering for prenatal care should have their blood typed and an indirect Coombs antibody screen performed at their first prenatal visit. This should be done with all pregnancies regardless of prior screening tests. Rh-negative women may show new evidence of anti-D sensitization and all pregnant women regardless of Rh status may show sensitization to 'atypical' antigens. If the indirect Coombs test is positive, antigen specificity and antibody titer or concentration are determined.

Management of the Rh-negative woman with a negative antibody screen

The patient's ABO grouping and the ABO/Rh status of the baby's father should be determined. If he is Rh-negative, the fetus should also be. Repeating the antibody screen at 28 weeks is advocated to look for new evidence of sensitization. The baby's Rh status is confirmed from cord blood studies at birth. Antenatal Rh immune globulin (RHIG) is not necessary if the father of the baby is Rh-negative. If the father is Rh-positive, his ABO group and Rh phenotype should be established. From this, his likely Rh genotype (and therefore zygosity for D) can be determined, and thus the risk of sensitization can be estimated. A maternal antibody screen is repeated at 28 weeks and RHIG is given if the screen is still negative[43]. Some advocate serial screening of this group of women starting at 18–20 weeks[42,44]. At the time of delivery, neonatal ABO grouping and Rh status is determined from cord blood. Maternal antibody screen is repeated. If the neonate is Rh-positive and the maternal antibody screen is negative, RHIG 300 µg intramuscularly is given. If significant FMH is suspected, the Kleihauer–Betke screen for fetal red cells in maternal serum is done to estimate the volume of exchange. The RHIG dose can then be adjusted accordingly. The cost effectiveness of universally using the Kleihauer–Betke test has not been established. If at any point in pregnancy the antibody screen becomes positive, the mother is managed accordingly (see below).

The Rh-positive woman with a negative antibody screen does not need further evaluation as she is not likely to develop significant atypical antigen sensitization during her pregnancy[43].

Management of the Rh-negative woman with a positive antibody screen

Antibody testing

Once it is established that the antibody specificity is for a red cell antigen associated with HDFN, the antigen status and zygosity of the fetus's father is determined. This is done in order to ascertain if the fetus is at risk. (If it cannot be determined, he is assumed to be antigen positive.) If he is homozygous negative for the antigen, the fetus is not at risk and the mother undergoes routine prenatal care. If the father is homozygous positive or heterozygous for the antigen, maternal antibody titer is assessed. If antibody titrations are performed in the same laboratory by experienced technologists, they can be of value in determining only if the fetus is at risk for HDFN. They cannot, however, predict severity of disease accurately enough to undertake therapy based on them alone. The concept of the 'critical' antibody titer at which the fetus is at risk for severe HDFN must be established for each laboratory and is based on the experience at that particular medical center. Some advocate following antibody titer serially starting at 16–18 weeks and then each 2–4 weeks[42,43] until a critical titer is reached. In general, it is felt that in an initial immunized pregnancy, the fetus is not at significant risk if the titer remains < 1 : 16[43].

The accuracy and value in following titers in subsequent pregnancies or once the critical titer is reached is likely to be low. The target of investigation at that point should be the fetus.

In some centers, if paternity is in doubt, paternal blood cannot be obtained, or testing indicates paternal heterozygosity with a < 90% probability that the fetus has the particular antigen, direct fetal blood sampling by cordocentesis is done at 18–20 weeks' gestational age[45]. The fetal ABO/Rh status is determined, along with a direct Coombs test and a hemoglobin and hematocrit. If the fetus is antigen negative, further maternal and fetal testing is obviated. If the fetus is antigen positive, severity of fetal disease can be determined from the hemoglobin and hematocrit and intrauterine transfusion therapy can be initiated. If the fetus is not anemic, serial evaluations with ultrasound and amniocentesis can be done.

Predicting severity

Obstetric history is of some value in determining if the fetus is at risk for severe disease. In general, disease severity tends to worsen with subsequent pregnancies. (Occasionally, severity may remain the same or lessen.) Past history of hydrops fetalis, *in utero* therapy, stillbirth, or neonatal exchange transfusions is considered significant. With a positive past obstetrical history, surveillance in subsequent pregnancies is begun at the same gestational age or earlier. Obstetrical history is of little benefit if the father is heterozygous. Coupled with the antibody titers, it can be decided if the fetus is at risk. Once this is done, assessment of severity of disease is undertaken.

Amniocentesis and amniotic fluid ΔOD_{450} evalutaion

With hemolysis, heme is liberated and metabolized to indirect or unconjugated bilirubin by the fetus. This bilirubin can be excreted into the amniotic fluid, primarily via the tracheopulmonary secretions, but also some via fetal urine. Bilirubin has a characteristic absorption pattern on spectrophotometry with a peak at 450 nm. The relative concentration of bilirubin in amniotic fluid can be assessed by drawing a tangent between the absorbances at 365 and 550 nm and determining the change (Δ) in optical density at 450 nm (ΔOD_{450}) due to bilirubin[2]. This is measured vertically and plotted on semilog paper with wavelength as the linear horizontal coordinate and optical density as the logarithmic vertical coordinate (Figure 4). The ΔOD_{450} is then plotted on a graph using gestational age as the horizontal coordinate (Figure 5)[43]. This is necessary because unaffected fetuses produce bilirubin early in gestation: there is a statistically significant rise between 14 and 20 weeks, a

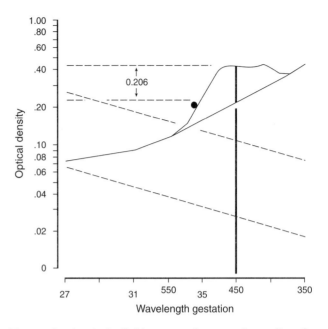

Figure 4 Amniotic fluid spectrophotometric reading for ΔOD_{450} determination. The value in this example is 0.206 and falls within Liley zone 3. Reprinted with permission reference 42

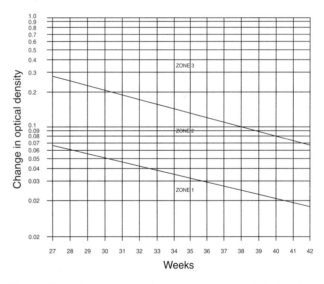

Figure 5 Liley graph with zones demarcated indicating degrees of severity of HDFN. Reprinted with permission from reference 43

peak between 22 and 26 weeks, and then a downward trend after 26 weeks[46]. This third-trimester downward trend is the basis for the Liley determinations[2]. Liley examined amniotic fluid within a week of birth in 101 pregnancies from 27 weeks estimated gestational age to term. He correlated this with the cord blood hemoglobin and the degree of HDFN and was able to divide the spectrophotometric graph into three zones. He found that the severity of HDFN could be predicted from the size and trend to the ΔOD_{450} peak in relation to gestational age. Zone 1 (lower zone) indicates unaffected or mildly affected fetuses. Zone 3 (upper zone) contains severely affected fetuses including those with hydrops, severe anemia, or those destined for imminent fetal death within several days. Zone 2 (midzone) contained fetus with intermediate disease. Severity increases as values approach zone 3.

Indications for and timing of the procedure Determination of ΔOD_{450} is a valuable indirect means of determining severity of fetal involvement. Indications include significant past obstetrical history or obtainment of a 'critical' antibody titer. If past history is significant or if 'critical' antibody titer is present before 20 weeks, initial amniocentesis can be carried out as early as 17–18 weeks. Nicolaides and co-workers[47] evaluated Rh-isoimmunized pregnancies between 18 and 25 weeks' estimated gestational age by fetoscopy for fetal blood sampling and by amniotic fluid sampling for ΔOD_{450} determination. They found little, if any, correlation between the ΔOD_{450} and concurrent fetal hemoglobin concentration. There was no ΔOD_{450} value or Liley zone (extrapolated back to 18 weeks) that clearly separated severely anemic (hemoglobin concentration < 6 g/dl) from non-anemic (hemoglobin concentration > 9.7 g/dl) fetuses. Trends in ΔOD_{450} values also were not predictive. It was their conclusion that the only reliable method to determine severity of HDFN in the third trimester is the determination of fetal hemoglobin concentration by fetal blood sampling. Other authors dispute this[44,48,49] and claim that single ΔOD_{450} values if high enough (range 0.15–0.40) or with a trend rising toward or above this value, can also predict severe disease. If there is any question as to extent of disease, fetal blood sampling is indicated.

In patients without significant obstetrical history and in whom a 'critical' antibody titer is reached after 26 weeks, amniocentesis for ΔOD_{450} determination should be done and plotted on a Liley graph. A correlation between Liley graph values/zones and fetal hematocrit within one week are excellent with around 95% predictivity of severe disease[50]. Subsequent amniocenteses are timed according to the prior ΔOD_{450} value and the trend of values. If values remain in or fall into zone 1, repeat tests can be done every 3–4 weeks. If the values are in zone 2, repeat evaluations should be done every 1–2 weeks, increasing in frequency as values rise in zone 2. If values reach high zone 2 or into zone 3, fetal blood sampling is indicated to assess the hemoglobin concentration[3].

Technique To decrease the risk of FHM and possibly worsening sensitization[51], amniocentesis is done aseptically under ultrasound guidance to avoid placental trauma. If transplacental access is necessary, going

through the thinnest available area and with a smaller gauge needle may minimize the possible exchange. A Kleihauer–Betke assay may be helpful here to determine the volume of fetal blood exchanged. The fluid is protected from light and centrifuged as soon as possible. Spectrophotometric measurements are done along with pulmonary maturity assays if the fetus is > 32 weeks' estimated gestational age. There is no consistent evidence that lung maturation is either delayed or accelerated in the isoimmunized pregnancy[52].

Sources of error If amniotic fluid is not protected from light (which degrades bilirubin), the resultant ΔOD_{450} will be artifactually low. With ultrasound guidance, it is unlikely that maternal or fetal urine or fetal ascites would be obtained. Urine has no 450-nm peak and ascitic fluid has a very high peak frequently requiring dilution. Fetal or maternal blood (oxyhemoglobin) contamination of the sample produces sharp peaks at 415, 540, and 575 nm thus obscuring the bilirubin peak. Small amounts of fetal plasma (containing bilirubin) intermixed with amniotic fluid will falsely elevate the 450-nm peak with subsequent misinterpretation of disease severity. Meconium has strong peaks at 405–410 and 450 nm and thus will obscure the 450-nm peak[53]. Contamination by meconium or red cells and their breakdown products can be overcome in large part with chloroform-extraction methods[54].

Certain congenital anomalies are associated with falsely elevated ΔOD_{450} values (i.e. anencephaly, proximal gastrointestinal obstructive anomalies, fetal nephrosis, etc.)[53]. Also, sickle cell disease with hemolysis and increased maternal bilirubin may be associated with elevated amniotic fluid ΔOD_{450} values (i.e. maternal to fetal transfer of bilirubin) and thus give incorrect predictions of fetal severity[55].

Of paramount importance is early establishment or verification of gestational age as this not only impacts significantly on the correct evaluation of ΔOD_{450} values, but also determines the timing of interventions and/or delivery.

Other avenues for fetal assessment

An important goal in the management of fetuses at risk for HDFN is to identify fetuses whose condition is deteriorating but who have not become hydropic. Intervention at an earlier, less severe, stage of disease may improve survival.

Ultrasound Various fetal anatomic changes noted by ultrasound, though not specific, suggest moderate-to-severe HDFN with imminent development of hydrops. Unfortunately, absence of these signs does not mean the fetus is only mildly affected. If these signs do develop, there is no consistent sequence to their development.

Enlargement of the right atrium or heart[56], 'bowel halo' sign within the peritoneal cavity[57] and/or pericardial effusion[58] have all been touted as the earliest ultrasound findings in severe hemolytic disease. Hydramnios is common and thought to be the most consistent sign of significant disease[31,33]. Nicolaides and co-workers[31] carried out serial ultrasound measurements of placental thickness, umbilical vein diameter, abdominal circumference, intraperitoneal volume and head circumference to abdominal circumference ratio in 50 affected pregnancies at 18–26 weeks. They showed that, in the absence of hydrops, these signs were unreliable predictors of severe disease. Hydropic changes include ascites (> 5 mm), skin edema (> 5–7 mm skin thickness), hydramnios, and serous cavity (pleural, pericardial) effusions[32], though criteria vary from author to author. Occasionally, with serious fetal compromise, oligohydramnios may develop.

Serial ultrasound examinations are done weekly or every 2 weeks starting at 16–18 weeks to assess the fetus for the above-mentioned signs. Since many are subjective, it is important they be assessed serially by the same individual or individuals. Ultrasound also allows demonstration of fetal growth, which is usually normal in HDFN, and in defining fetal and placental location for invasive procedures.

Doppler assessment   Reasonable relationships have been found between increased systolic velocities (in the descending thoracic aorta and common carotid artery) and the degree of fetal anemia[27,28,59,60]. This may be consistent with a hyperdynamic circulation in anemic fetuses. Cardiac output has also been noted to be increased in anemic fetuses[61]. The highest correlations are seen in previously untransfused fetuses. Several authors have proposed formulas for deriving fetal hemoglobin concentration estimations in untransfused fetuses[27,60]. These have not withstood prospective evaluation at this juncture (in the non-hydropic fetus)[62]. In this series, Copel and co-workers concluded that Doppler flow–velocity waveform indices were of limited usefulness in the prediction of fetuses requiring transfusion or in the timing of a series of transfusions.

Fetal behavioral assessment   Currently, fetal behavior is best assessed using the biophysical profile (BPP) as the framework. Fetal movement has long been used as an indicator of fetal wellbeing but may be present until the time of death. Decreased fetal movement associated with decreased or absent fetal breathing movements in a hydropic fetus indicates a moribund fetus, impending demise, and the need for immediate intervention[63]. Amniotic fluid volume may be normal even at this stage.

The accuracy of fetal heart-rate monitoring for evaluation of fetal wellbeing and predicting anemia in Rh disease is debated. Some authors[44] have noted a decrease in fetal heart-rate variability with fetal hemoglobin concentrations between 4 and 8 g/dl. Others[64] have claimed that spontaneous late decelerations and the presence of sinusoidal fluctuations indicate fetal hypoxia, thus permitting conservative management in pregnancies with normal heart rate tracings. Nicolaides and co-workers[65] found abnormal fetal heart rate patterns to be more common in anemic (hemoglobin deficit >2 g/dl) than non-anemic fetuses, but there was a large overlap. Therefore, reliance on FHR monitoring can be of poor predictive value in assessing the degree of fetal disease. They did, however, note that abnormal fetal heart-rate patterns were more closely related to fetal oxygenation than to hemoglobin concentration.

Polymerase chain reaction testing   With the discovery of the Rh(D) gene and its sequencing, it has now become possible to identify the Rh genotype of a fetus in a Rh-negative woman by polymerase chain reaction (PCR) of DNA extracted from amniocytes obtained by amniocentesis. This method was first published by Bennett and co-workers[66]. By using an internal control to test the adequacy of DNA obtained from amniocytes, all Rh-positive and Rh-negative fetuses can be identified. The sensitivity and specificity of this testing is reported as 99.7% and 94% respectively[67]. Fisk and co-workers have suggested that this method has two advantages[68]. Testing for fetal Rh genotype can be made earlier in gestation than can be done with fetal blood sampling. The test is available for both amniocentesis and chorionic villous sampling (CVS) material. It is therefore recommended that PCR be performed to test fetal genotype when the father is heterozygous and severe disease has occurred early in a previous pregnancy, at the time of initial amniocentesis for standard OD_{450} measurements, and whenever either CVS or amniocentesis is indicated for other reasons. As the gene sequences of more blood group antigens are identified, PCR may also be offered for the genotyping of fetuses at risk for hemolytic disease from antibodies to non-Rh antigens.

MANAGEMENT
Mild-to-moderately affected fetuses

These fetuses typically are not at risk for hydrops fetalis. Either amniocentesis has not been required or all ΔOD_{450} values have remained below the middle of zone 2. Serial ultrasounds have shown no signs of hydrops or 'prehydrops'. Serial biophysical profiles have been reassuring. These mothers should be allowed to deliver spontaneously and at term. Induction may be carried out once pulmonary maturity is assured and the cervix is favorable. The fetus will not be hydropic but may be hyperbilirubinemic and anemic at birth thus requiring prompt transfusion therapy. For this reason, delivery should take place in an institution capable of rendering appropriate care.

Severely affected fetuses

This is the fetus at risk for hydrops fetalis; half will manifest before 34 weeks. In this group, serial amniocentesis and ultrasounds will have been done starting in the mid-second trimester. If the obstetrical history and antibody titer in the second trimester were suggestive of increased likelihood of severe disease, fetal blood sampling may also have been undertaken. Weekly or twice weekly non-stress tests and biophysical profiles will also have been done. Indications for intervention (delivery vs. *in utero* transfusion) include ΔOD_{450} values in high zone 2 or in zone 3, ultrasound evidence of 'prehydrops' or hydrops, fetal anemia (hemoglobin < 10 g/dl or hematocrit < 30%[44]) at fetal blood sampling, or abnormal fetal behavioral evaluation. The particular mode of therapy undertaken will depend on estimated gestational age, fetal condition, and the approach favored by the perinatal/neonatal team (Table 3).

In most centers, early delivery and neonatal therapy are the rule after pulmonary maturity is confirmed. If fetal lungs are immature, steroids can be administered to the mother followed in 24–48 hours by fetal (*in utero*) blood transfusion (IUT). As mentioned previously, assessment of fetal lung profiles in the face of isoimmunization is unaltered. Caritis and co-workers[69] noticed a sudden and dramatic decrease in ΔOD_{450} values following maternal administration of betamethasone. The significance and etiology of this is unclear, but this should be taken into account if further fetal amniotic fluid evaluations, and not immediate delivery, are entertained. (Modes of delivery will be addressed at the end of this section.)

Liley[70] was the first to describe intraperitoneal blood transfusion (IPT) to improve survival. Several authors utilized this mode of therapy with varying degrees of success[50,71–73]. In 1981, direct intravascular transfusion (IVT) through a needle introduced via fetoscope into an umbilical vessel was described[74]. This was followed rapidly by ultrasound guided IVTs via a needle directed into the hepatic portion of the umbilical vein[75,76], the heart[77], and the umbilical cord[37,78–81]. Both IPT and IVT will be described and compared.

Table 3 The severely-affected fetus

< 32 weeks EGA	32–34 weeks EGA	> 34 weeks EGA
In utero transfusions, deliver when pulmonary maturity at > 32–34 weeks	Deliver if pulmonary maturity or single *in utero* transfusion	Deliver

EGA, estimated gestational age

Intraperitoneal transfusion (IPT)

Erythrocytes injected into the peritoneal cavity are absorbed intact via the mesenteric and subdiaphragmatic lymphatics. They then enter the central jugular venous system via the thoracic duct. In non-hydropic fetuses, absorption takes place at the rate of 10–15% (of the injected volume) per 24 hours. Other authors noted complete absorption in 3–4 days[82]. In the face of ascites, absorption is slow and very erratic[42]. Since plasma is absorbed preferentially to cells, packing the cells tightly (i.e. to hematocrit > 85%) will aid absorption. The volume of blood injected is limited by the size of the peritoneal cavity. If intraperitoneal pressure exceeds umbilical venous pressure, it is thought placental circulation and fetal venous return will decrease and intrauterine demise may occur. The following formula was developed to prevent this[83]:

IPT volume (ml) = [weeks' gestation – 20] × 10

Typically, IPTs are spaced in the following manner: 7–10 days until the second transfusion, then every 3–4 weeks between subsequent transfusions. This can be altered or accelerated by evidence of more rapid fetal deterioration on serial ultrasounds or behavioral assessment or by calculating residual donor hemoglobin concentration and transfusing when this decreases to approximately 10–11 g/dl[42]. The formula used is:

$$\text{Hb}_{\text{residual}} = \frac{(0.55) \times \text{Hb}_{\text{donor}}}{85 \times \text{EFW (g)}} \times \frac{120 - \text{interval (days)}}{120}$$

where EFW = estimated fetal weight. This formula assumes: (1) following IPT, 55% of infused red cells will be in circulation within the fetus; (2) 85 ml/kg is the estimated fetal blood volume; and (3) 120 days is the lifespan of the donor cells.

Fetal disease is rarely treated by a single IPT. The goal is to halt progression of hemolysis. The second IPT generally accomplishes inhibition of fetal hemopoiesis and complete replacement with non-antigenic donor blood. Subsequent IPTs are designed to keep pace with the increasing blood volume requirements of the growing fetus.

The technique of IPT has undergone many modifications since Liley first described it. The most significant modification is the use of realtime ultrasound to guide the proper placement of the needle and catheterization of the fetal peritoneal cavity[71,73]. Ultrasound is performed before the procedure to assess fetal lie, placental location, and presence or absence of ascites. It is preferable to have the fetus in a lateral or abdominal anterior position. Abdomen posterior positions contraindicate the procedure. A posterior or lateral placenta is also preferred. Under maternal sedation, aseptic conditions, and local anesthesia, the 15–16-gauge Tuohy needle is guided via ultrasound into the fetal abdomen. Premedications may also include tocolytics and prophylactic antibiotics[73]. Blood is then transfused either through the needle or an 18-gauge epidural catheter which has been threaded into the peritoneal cavity. Fresh, type O negative, leukocyte-poor, irradiated, cytomegalovirus (CMV) negative, HIV negative, high hematocrit, maternally cross-matched blood is then transfused at rates up to 5–10 ml/min. Volume is calculated by the formula given previously. If ascites is present, typically a volume 20–30 ml in excess of the planned transfusion volume is removed, if possible. If the fetus is hydropic, intraperitoneal digoxin may also be given[73]. Fetal heart rate is monitored, by ultrasound, intermittently during the procedure. If the fetus is in good condition, a tachycardia will be noted; bradycardia at any point is ominous. After the procedure, fetal heart rate is again monitored. This may be done intermittently if the fetus is < 26 weeks' estimated gestational age and the mother may be discharged soon if all is satisfactory. If gestational age is > 26 weeks, the fetus is monitored continuously in labor and delivery. If the fetus does well, the mother may be discharged at the physician's discretion. If fetal distress is identified, emergent delivery can be accomplished. Subsequent follow-up by ultrasound and fetal behavioral tests may be done as frequently as once per week in non-hydropic fetuses and twice weekly for hydropic fetuses[73].

Intravascular transfusion (IVT)

As mentioned previously, investigators have utilized several portions of the umbilical vein for fetal blood sampling and IVT. Most prefer the segment just proximal to the cord insertion site into the placenta. Free loops of cord or the cord insertion site into the abdomen may also be used if fetal or placental position precludes the use of the placental insertion site[81]. One contraindication to using the placental insertion site would be velamentous insertion of the cord. The risk of vascular trauma and excessive bleeding is high without the mechanical and coagulative properties of Wharton's jelly. (The intrahepatic portion of the umbilical vein and fetal cardiac puncture are used rarely secondary to increased risks of morbidity and mortality.) The use of premedications (i.e. prophylactic antibiotics or tocolytics, use of digoxin/diuretics, use of paralytics, etc.) vary between authors as does the needle gauge used, hemoglobin/hematocrit of donor blood and the hemoglobin/hematocrit goal of transfusion (Table 4). The common threads seem to be the use of ultrasound guidance, maternal sedation, and donor blood that is relatively fresh, tightly packed, leukocyte-poor, irradiated, CMV and HIV negative and cross-matched/compatible with maternal serum[37,80,81,84–87].

First, ultrasound assessment of fetal/placental position is completed. Feasibility of IVT is determined by careful identification of the target. The mother is premedicated, the abdomen aseptically prepared and draped, and local anesthetic given at the abdominal needle insertion site. Figure 6 shows a typical sampling and transfusion apparatus. The needle is guided by ultrasound into the target vessel and fetal blood is aspirated. The sample is tested at the bedside for fetal origin. This can be done several ways. The Singer alkaline-denaturation test gives rapid evaluation: alkaline solution denatures maternal hemoglobin to produce a brown/green color while samples containing only fetal hemoglobin remain pink (this test obviously is effective only in the untransfused fetus). Bedside automated cell sorters are also available and effective (fetal

Table 4 Intravascular transfusion

First author	Premedication	Fetal medication	Needle (g)	Donor hematocrit (%)	Hematocrit goal (%)	Transfusion rate (ml/min)	Notes
Rodeck[84]	Sedatives	Furosemide, if hydrops	26	60–80%	35–45%	1–3	Fetoscopy
Berkowitz[81,87]	Meperidine, prochlorperazine, diazepam, cefazolin	Atracurium	20,22	NA	35–50%	1–2	
Grannum[37]	Meperidine, diazepam, terbutaline	Pancuronium	22	85–95%	30–40%	1–3	Exchange and simple
Socol[77]	Meperidine, diazepam	NA	22	85%	35–45%	1–3	
Weiner[89]	NA	Pancuronium, furosemide	22	70%	45–50%	NA	Needle-Guide
Laifer[96]	Narcotic, benzodiazepine	Atracurium, pancuronium	22	70%	13–16 Hb (g/dl)	5	

NA, not available

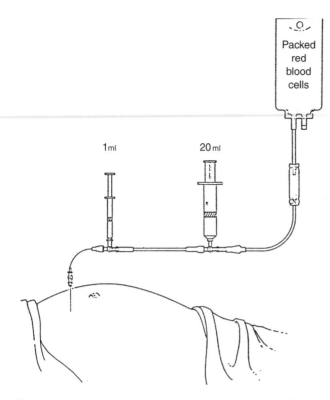

Figure 6 Intravascular transfusion apparatus with two three-way stopcocks permitting minimization of needle movement during sampling and transfusion. Reprinted with permission from reference 87

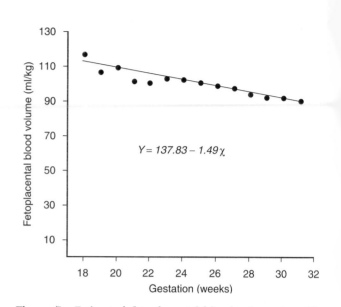

$$Y = 137.83 - 1.49\chi$$

Figure 7 Estimated fetoplacental blood volume in ml/kg estimated fetal weight. Reprinted with permission from reference 40

red blood cells have larger mean corpuscular volume than adult red cells[32]. The hemoglobin value can also be determined rapidly and accurately at the bedside with an automated instrument[88], thus allowing rapid determination of the need for transfusion. Time does not allow for Kleihauer–Betke testing for fetal blood determination to be used at the bedside but this can be sent to the lab along with the other fetal evaluative studies: complete blood count with platelet count/differential, blood grouping/direct Coombs, albumin/total protein, bilirubin, alanine aminotransferase/aspartate aminotransferase, and blood gases (which umbilical vessel is accessed must be known for proper interpretation). All these tests can be done on a few milliliters of fetal blood[32].

Action now is based on the results. Fetuses with hemoglobin concentrations within 2 g/dl of the mean for gestational age are not transfused[24]. Others use cut-offs such as hematocrit < 30% or hemoglobin < 10 g/dl[44,89]. Infusion is also carried out under ultrasound visualization with notation of turbulence from blood streaming within the umbilical vessels. If no streaming is seen, the transfusion is halted as the needle may have become dislodged and embedded in the Wharton's jelly. Injection of blood could therefore compress the umbilical vessels. The volume of infusion needed (V_d) can be calculated from the estimated

FPBV for gestational age (V_i), the initial fetal hematocrit (H_i), the hematocrit of donor blood (H_d), and the desired final hematocrit (H_f), according to the formula[40,41]:

$$V_d = V_i(H_f - H_i) / (H_d - H_f)$$

Estimated FPVB has been calculated by these authors to be (mean) 94.0 ml/kg[41] to 101 ± 14 ml/kg[40] with a significant decrease with advancing gestation (Figure 7). Fetal–placental blood volume ranges from 117 ml/kg at 18 weeks to approximately 93 ml/kg at 31 weeks[40]. These values replace the value of 160 ml/kg[90] determined by using radiolabeled proteins which gives overestimations of blood volumes due to rapid loss from the circulation[40,41]. One group[91] formulated tables (Tables 5 and 6) based on estimated fetal weight or gestational age while another[24] developed nomograms (Figure 8) based on H_i, H_d, and gestational age. Transfusion is carried out diligently (at rates 6 15 ml/min[79]) while intermittently observing the fetal heart rate. The same caveats apply as for IPT. Once the transfusion is completed, the needle is flushed and a postransfusion sample is drawn for determination of hematocrit. If the H_f goal has not been reached, a new V_d can be estimated using the current hematocrit as H_i. Calculations of the mean attrition rate of donor red cell hematocrit range from 1.1 ± 0.6% per day (range 0.4–3.8) in non-hydropic fetuses to 1.7 ± 1.1% per day (range 0.6–3.5) in hydropic fetuses[91]. The combined mean decline is 1.3 ± 1.1% per day[91,92]. Plans for repeat transfusion should be made once the hemoglobin or hematocrit is estimated to have decreased to the transfusion cut-offs

Table 5 Predicted volume of packed red cells (hematocrit) required for desired level of hematocrit increase according to estimated fetal weight

EFW (g)	Level of desired increase in hematocrit*				
	10%	15%	20%	25%	30%
500	12.5	16.1	19.7	23.2	26.8
600	14.8	19.1	23.4	27.7	32.0
700	17.2	22.2	27.2	32.2	37.2
800	19.5	25.2	31.0	36.7	42.4
900	21.8	28.3	34.7	41.2	47.6
1000	24.2	31.3	38.5	45.7	52.8
1100	26.5	34.4	42.3	50.1	58.0
1200	28.8	37.4	46.0	54.6	63.2
1300	31.2	40.5	49.8	59.1	68.4
1400	33.5	43.5	53.5	63.6	73.6
1500	35.8	46.6	57.3	68.1	78.8
1600	38.1	49.6	61.1	72.5	84.0
1700	40.5	52.7	64.8	77.0	89.2
1800	42.8	55.7	68.6	81.5	94.4
1900†	45.1	58.7	72.4	86.0	99.6
2000†	47.5	61.8	76.1	90.5	104.8
2100†	49.8	64.8	79.9	94.9	110.0
2200†	52.1	67.9	83.7	99.4	115.2
2300†	54.5	70.9	87.4	103.9	120.4
2400†	56.7	73.9	91.0	108.2	125.4
2500†	59.0	76.9	94.8	112.7	129.6

EFW, estimated fetal weight; *Volume of packed red cells in ml
†Extrapolated from the following equation:
Volume (ml) = 0.888 + 0.00895 (EFW) − 0.00177[hematocrit increase] + 0.00143[EFW × hematocrit increase]

Table 6 Predicted volume of packed red cells (hematocrit) required for desired level of hematocrit increase according to gestational age

GA (weeks)	Level of desired increase in hematocrit*				
	10%	15%	20%	25%	30%
21	13.1	14.2	15.2	16.3	17.3
22	13.7	15.8	17.9	19.9	22.0
23	14.8	17.9	21.1	24.2	27.3
24	16.5	20.6	24.8	30.0	33.1
25	18.7	23.9	29.1	34.3	39.5
26	21.4	27.7	33.9	40.2	46.4
27	24.7	32.0	39.3	46.6	53.9
28	28.6	36.9	45.3	53.6	61.9
29	33.0	42.4	51.7	61.1	70.5
30	37.9	48.4	58.8	69.2	79.6
31	43.4	54.9	66.4	77.8	89.3
32†	49.5	62.0	74.5	87.0	99.5
33†	56.0	69.6	83.2	96.7	110.3
34†	63.2	77.8	92.4	107.0	121.6

GA, gestational age; *Volume of packed red cells in ml
†Extrapolated from the following equation:
Volume (ml) = 169.43 − 13.29 [GA] + 0.274 [GA²] − 4.17[hematocrit increase] + 0.209[GA × hematocrit increase]

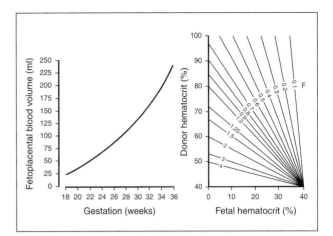

Figure 8 To estimate volume of blood transfusion necessary to achieve a post-transfusion hematocrit of 40%, multiply the estimated fetoplacental blood volume for gestational age by the factor *F* (determined by initial fetal hematocrit and the hematocrit of donor blood). Reprinted with permission from reference 24

Table 7 Intrauterine transfusion complications

Fetal	Maternal	Fetomaternal
Overtransfusion	PROM	Fetomaternal exchange
Exsanguination	Chorioamnionitis	
Cord hematoma	Preterm labor	
Fetal distress	Abruptio placenta	
In utero demise	Emergent Cesarean section	

PROM, preterm rupture of membranes

mentioned previously. When H_i is measured at the subsequent transfusion, the attrition rate for that particular fetus can be calculated by subtracting the current hematocrit from the previous post-transfusion hematocrit and dividing by the interval in number of days between transfusions. This now can be used to determine further transfusion intervals. Surveillance following IVT is similar to that used with IPT consisting of daily fetal-kick counts and frequent use of ultrasound, non-stress tests, and biophysical profiles.

Complications following transfusions

Intraperitoneal vs. intravascular transfusions Table 7 summarizes the general complications of both IPT and IVT. For IPT, procedure-related death rates range from 0%[73] up to 5–10%[48,71,84] depending on technique and patient population. For IVT, mortality rates per procedure range from 1.5 to 2%[84] up to 4%[86]. Daffos and co-workers[78] performed 606 cordocenteses in the second and third trimesters under ultrasound guidance and had a procedure-related death rate of < 1%. Their procedures were done predominantly to rule out congenital infection and therefore, higher traumatic death rates would be expected in severe Rh-affected fetuses and with the use of *in utero* transfusions. Daffos and co-workers[78] also noted no bleeding following the procedure in approximately 60% of cases, < 1 min of bleeding in another 30% of cases and only > 2 min of bleeding in 2% of cases. The risks of elevating antibody concentration with invasive procedures can be significant: upwards of 40–75% with fetoscopy and ultrasound-guided procedures[51]. This could have the impact of worsening fetal disease, if not in the current pregnancy then in future pregnancies.

The effects of replacing fetal hemoglobin with adult hemoglobin on blood gases and acid–base balance were evaluated[93]. Some authors found that fetuses with adult hemoglobin had lower umbilical artery blood pH and higher base excess while the Po_2, Pco_2 and bicarbonate concentrations remained the same. In the umbilical vein, blood with adult hemoglobin had a significantly higher Po_2 while the other parameters remained unchanged. This indicates that oxygen delivery to fetal tissues is worse with adult hemoglobin (i.e. decreased pH, increased base excess in the umbilical artery). However, acidosis (through the Bohr effect) would shift the hemoglobin dissociation curve to the right, thus promoting oxygen release. Umbilical venous Po_2 was increased suggesting that a healthy uteroplacental circulation can increase oxygen transfer if needed.

Survival following in utero transfusion (IUT)   See Table 8 for a compilation of various studies, time of study, form of IUT used, and success rates in terms of live births. In the ultrasound era, survival with IPT has ranged from as low as 49%[71] up to rates as high as 80–90%[42,73,84]. For hydropic fetuses alone, IPT survival rates are between 51 and 75%[48,73].

For IVT, the experience is more recent and consequently involves a smaller number of patients. Survival rates range from 75–85%[37,43,84–86] up to

100%[80]. Considering only hydropic fetuses, survival rates average 75–80%[37,43,84,85].

Reversal of hydrops with IVT has also been accomplished by several authors, some starting with IUTs at < 20 weeks' gestational age[3,37,80,84]. In one study[3], two-thirds of the hydropic fetuses had reversal with all showing resolution of hypoalbuminemia, hypoproteinemia, and elevated liver transaminase values concomitant with sustained hematocrit > 15%.

Intraperitoneal vs. intravascular transfusion: a comparison

Intravascular transfusion is now clearly favored over intraperitoneal transfusion in most, if not all, circumstances. It allows direct access to the fetal compartment and determination of fetal status with regard to anemia, acid–base balance, liver function, etc. By being able to determine pre- and post-transfusion hematocrits, the transfusion can be tailored to that particular fetus. This consequently allows for rational planning of future transfusions. The formulas used for IPT are empiric and rely only on gestational age. As some non-hydropic fetuses can be severely anemic (hemoglobin < 4 g/dl or > 7 g/dl below the mean for gestational age), it is obvious that formulas based solely on gestational age can be erroneous.

Intravascular transfusion seems to be more effective in hydropic fetuses. These fetuses absorb intraperitoneal blood more slowly and erratically in the face of ascites. It is also easier to accomplish in cases of anterior placenta (risks of IPT triple in this situation[42]) and if the fetal lie is with the back anterior. Although it is possible to do both IPT and IVT prior to 20 weeks, the risk of traumatic morbidity with IPT is increased at earlier gestations due to the smaller fetal size and the large gauge Tuohy needle used. Also, overall, the traumatic mortality rate per procedure with IVT is significantly lower than with IPT at any gestational age.

Table 8   Survival after *in utero* transfusion (IUT)

First author	Dates of study	Form of IUT	Fetuses (n)	Transfusions (n)	EGA range (weeks)	Survival		
						Non-hydropic (%)	Hydropic (%)	Overall (%)
Frigoletto[71]	1978–9	IPT	35	87	21–31	61%	28%	49%
Harman[73]	1980–2	IPT	24	62	NA	100%	75%	92%
Bowman[48]	1970–8	IPT	113	293	NA	78%	50%	70%
Rodeck[84]	1982–4	IVT, fetoscopy	25	77	19–28	70%	73%	72%
Berkowitz[86]	1984–7	IVT	17	45	21–31	NA	NA	76%
Grannum[85]	pre-1986	IVT, exchange	4	9	22–31	–	75%	75%
Grannum[3]	1984–8	IVT, exchange, and simple	50	162	NA	71%	89%	79%
Socol[80]	pre-1987	IVT	3	12	< 26	–	100%	100%

EGA, estimated gestational age; IPT, intraperitoneal transfusion; IVT, intravascular transfusion; NA, not available

Table 9 Intraperitoreal transfusion (IPT) vs. intravascular transfusion (IVT)

Parameter assessed	IPT	IVT	Comment
Mean EGA at first transfusion (weeks)	26.5	26.5	44 patients, each group
Procedures per fetus (*n*)	2.4	3.9	
Attempts per successful transfusion (*n*)	1.8	1.2	
Percentage maternal complications per procedure	12.5%	3.0%	Infection, ROM, emergent
Traumatic deaths (*n*)	8	1	Cesarean section, etc.
Mean treatment duration (days)	34.4	53.2	
Mean EGA, delivery (weeks)	30.7	34.1	
Neonatal exchange transfusions per child (*n*)	1.8	0.8	
Survivals			
Percentage overall	66%	91%	
Percentage hydropic fetuses	48%	86%	
Percentage non-hydropic fetuses	83%	96%	

EGA, estimated gestational age; ROM, rupture of membranes

Harman and co-workers[94] performed a matched case-comparison for IPT and IVT. Results are summarized in Table 9. Several points can be emphasized.

(1) Although IVT required more attempts per fetus, it was associated with fewer complications and fewer consequences of failure with a sharp increase in traumatic death.

(2) There was a significant prolongation of gestation with not only improved survival rates in both hydropic and non-hydropic fetuses, but also improved 'quality' of survival. The authors concluded IVT was the procedure of choice for all levels of fetal disease.

Intraperitoneal transfusion may yet still have a role in modern management of the severely affected fetus. It is easy to do, and by using it in combination with IVT, the volume of transfusion given can be increased and thus it is possible to increase the interval between transfusions, decrease the total number of procedures per pregnancy, and decrease the risk of morbidity to the fetus.

(One group advocated using exchange transfusions via the intravascular route[92] based on the theory that the tenuous cardiovascular system in a severely anemic fetus could be compromised or overburdened by a bolus simple transfusion. Subsequent experience in their laboratory and by others has shown that even a hydropic fetus tolerates simple transfusions quite well[3,79]. Also, exchange transfusions have the drawback of increased operative time thus increasing the risk of morbidity and complications.)

Timing and mode of delivery

This group of infants should be delivered in a tertiary referral center where the nursery is capable of caring for a potentially very sick and/or hydropic premature neonate. Delivery should be accomplished as soon as pulmonary maturity is reached.

Trial of labor induction and vaginal delivery is appropriate and successful in the majority of cases. The use of cervical-ripening agents may increase the rate of successful inductions. Fetal heart rate should be monitored continuously and by fetal scalp electrode as indicated. Fetal scalp blood for determination of pH and blood gases should be obtained for suspicious heart rate tracings (interpretation may be difficult in the fetus with scalp edema). The ability to intervene rapidly is a must. Threshold for a Cesarean section is often low, especially in the hydropic fetus. Fetal malpresentation is also an indication for Cesarean section.

Development in survivors of in utero transfusions

Physical and intellectual development in the short term seems to be normal in the vast majority of children who received IUT; 83–87% are completely normal[42,95]. Approximately 4% of these children have major CNS sequelae (sensorineural deafness, athetosis, aphasia) of which approximately 75% can be attributed to sequelae of HDFN and 25% can be attributed to sequelae of prematurity. The remaining have minor CNS sequelae, the majority of which are secondary to prematurity[95].

ALTERNATIVE STRATEGIES FOR THE MODULATION OF SENSITIZATION

Potential methods for the *in utero* treatment of Rh isoimmunization aside from intrauterine transfusion have been proposed. These methods which include the use of corticosteroids, promethazine, immune globulin, and plasmapheresis show little promise in suppressing antibody production or preventing severe hemolytic disease. Corticosteroids are thought to reduce hemolysis in patients with autoimmune anemias by interfering with antibody production and antibody-coated red cell destruction. No reports have demonstrated a benefit in Rh isoimmunization[97]. Corticosteroids also reduce levels of bilirubin in amniotic fluid and may mask ongoing severe hemolysis. Promethazine reduces the coating of red cells by antibody but has failed to reduce hemolytic disease in several studies[97]. Immune globulin has been used in an attempt to block ongoing antibody production. The benefit for Rh disease has not been substantiated. Though plasmapheresis reduces antibody concentration temporarily a rebound in antibody production occurs following cessation of therapy[97]. Bowman has recommended plasmapheresis only in women with a partner homozygous for the antigen which has produced hydrops in previous pregnancies in the early mid-trimester[97].

ANTI-D IMMUNOGLOBULIN (RHIG)

The efficacy of anti-D immunoglobulin (RHIG) in preventing Rh isoimmunization has been clearly established. The ability of passively administered immunoglobulin to prevent antigen-stimulated immune response was established many years before the method was applied to rhesus isoimmunization. Freda and co-workers[98] in the 1960s successfully prevented immunization in 14 of 14 Rh-negative volunteers given RHIG 72 hours after being given Rh-positive blood. Six of 13 controls became sensitized. At the same time, Clarke and co-workers[99] in Great Britain using a similar antibody preparation demonstrated the protection of RHIG. Pollack[6] in 1971 further established that each 20 µg of RHIG prevented sensitization to 1 ml of Rh-positive red blood cells.

The first clinical trials of RHIG were initiated in the late 1960s. RHIG was given within 72 hours of delivery in Rh-negative mothers delivered of an ABO-compatible Rh-positive baby. Of 3389 women treated in several multicenter trials, only 0.18% became sensitized in the first six months after delivery versus 6.9% of controls[4]. In a subsequent pregnancy delivering a Rh-positive infant the rate of isoimmunization was reduced ten-fold (12.9% controls vs. 1.3% treated). At the McMaster Conference in 1977 on the prevention of Rh isoimmunization, a review of all clinical trials demonstrated a reduction in sensitization within six months after receiving 300 µg RHIG at delivery from 5.2% to between 0 and 0.6%. This reduction was observed over a five-year period[100].

Rh isoimmunization occurs in 1.8% of Rh-incompatible ABO compatible pregnancies prior to delivery. These women would not be protected by RHIG given after delivery. Bowman therefore initiated a clinical trial of antepartum RHIG in Canada in 1968[5]. Of 62 women immunized during pregnancy, 92% were detected after 28 weeks' gestation. RHIG (300 µg) was given at 28–34 weeks' gestation. None of the treated patients showed immunization at the time of delivery. Tovey[101] in Yorkshire, UK demonstrated a reduction of isoimmunization by eight-fold with antepartum RHIG. At the McMaster Conference a review of all trials demonstrated a reduction in sensitization from 1.2% to 0.16% at delivery and for up to six months postpartum[100]. Thus despite the increased cost of antepartum RHIG and the fact that women carrying Rh-negative fetuses will receive unnecessary RHIG, a significant reduction in new cases of sensitization is achieved.

The mechanism of action of RHIG is not entirely understood. The RHIG may bind to Rh-positive fetal cells and accelerate their clearance from the circulation. The suppression of immunization, however, has been successful despite normal clearance of red blood cells[102]. RHIG may block antigen sites on red cell membranes preventing their exposure to macrophages. With the dose of RHIG given, only a small fraction of the antigenic sites on each red cell are blocked. The most likely explanation involves the inhibition or modulation of the mechanism of immune response involving macrophages and T-helper and T-suppressor cells.

RHIG is licensed in the USA at an intramuscular dose of 300 µg. As little as 100 µg is used after a full-term delivery in other countries. A controlled trial of doses ranging from 20 to 200 µg showed equal efficacy of 100 and 200 µg[103]. Doses of 20 and 50 µg were less effective. No prospective trial has compared 200 µg and 300 µg directly. RHIG at 50 µg is completely effective in preventing sensitization following first-trimester abortion[104]. Currently, RHIG is administered within 72 hours of delivery. The 72-hour rule is arbitrary. It was established solely on the availability of prisoner volunteers at Sing Sing prison in the work done by Freda and co-workers[98]. No clinical trials have established the rate of sensitization after a delay of > 72 hours. A single study evaluating administration of RHIG to Rh-negative volunteers 13 days after being given injections of Rh-positive blood showed prevention of sensitization[105]. RHIG should therefore be given after 72 hours even if a failure of administration within the 72-hour time period is discovered.

Current recommendations for the use of RHIG are included in Table 10. D[µ]-positive individuals identified prior to delivery do not require RHIG. D[µ] positivity identified after delivery requires a quantitation of the extent of FMH to rule out a large FMH which may incorrectly be identified as D[µ] positivity. Rh(D)-negative, D[µ]-negative women who deliver a D[µ]-positive fetus require RHIG. Whether RHIG prevents sensitization to D[µ] fetal cells is controversial.

Table 10 Recommendations for the use of anti-D immuno-globulin (RHIG)

Indication	Dose
First-trimester abortion	50 µg
Second-trimester abortion	300 µg
Ectopic pregnancy	300 µg
Chorionic villus sampling	50 µg
Amniocentesis	300 µg
28-week prophylaxis	300 µg
Abdominal trauma or external version	300 µg
Postpartum Rh-positive fetus	
6 15-ml fetal–maternal hemorrhage	300 µg
> 15-ml fetal–maternal hemorrhage	20 µg/ml

Sources of RHIG failures

Despite the routine use of RHIG, Rh isoimmunization has not been eliminated. Several sources of RHIG failure are identified: isoimmunization prior to the use of RHIG, failure to identify the patient who needs RHIG, and failure to administer adequate doses of RHIG. Sensitization occurs prior to 28 weeks' gestation in 8% of women who show sensitization by delivery[5]. Sensitization, theoretically, may occur secondary to exposure of Rh-negative infants to the transplacental passage of maternal Rh-positive red cells at birth. Bowen and Renfield[106] demonstrated anti-D by automated methods in 11% of Rh-negative infants born to Rh-positive mothers. Other reports have failed to show this high rate of newborn anti-D[107]. Thus sensitization prior to pregnancy in nulliparas or prior to 28 weeks' gestation may account for cases of sensitization not preventable with RHIG.

Tovey analyzed all new cases of Rh isoimmunization between 1980 and 1984 in Yorkshire, UK to identify sources of prophylaxis failure[108]. Of 163 new cases, 22% failed to receive RHIG after abortion and full-term delivery. Other sources of failure included primigravidas sensitized prior to delivery (16%), prior sensitizing pregnancy before the use of RHIG (16%), and failures of protection (46%). In the 1970s, various programs were instituted to increase RHIG utilization. By increasing utilization from 93% to 99.5%, new cases of sensitization were reduced from 4.5% to 1.2%[109].

Despite the administration of 300 µg of RHIG at delivery, failures do occur. Maternal–fetal hemorrhages > 15 ml of fetal red cells account for a majority of failures. Approximately 0.7% of pregnancies will have a maternal–fetal hemorrhage > 15 ml of red cells. Identification of the percentage of fetal cells in the maternal circulation by the Kleihauer–Betke acid-elution technique would prevent isoimmunization in this small fraction of patients. An assessment of the volume of fetal–maternal transfusion should be made following all deliveries. When routine quantitation of FMH is not practical, those cases known to be associated with large FMH should be screened. These include placenta previa, abruptio placenta, maternal abdominal trauma, manual removal of the placenta and multifetal gestation. Procedures including external cephalic version, percutaneous umbilical blood sampling, and intrauterine transfusion for antibodies other than anti-D in Rh-negative women may be associated with large FMH and require an assessment of the degree of FMH using a Kleihauer–Betke smear. Despite the transfusion of whole units of Rh-positive cells into Rh-negative individuals, correct calculation and administration of the RHIG dose prevent sensitization[110]. With large MFH or transfusion of Rh-positive blood, the calculated dose of RHIG should be divided into six doses given at 12-hour intervals[111]. As much as 1200 µg of RHIG may be given at a single time intramuscularly.

IRREGULAR ANTIBODIES

Since the 1970s the routine use of RHIG has dramatically reduced the number of cases of isoimmunization to the D antigen. Today hemolytic disease secondary to other Rh and irregular blood group antigens is increasing in frequency. This increase is also due to a more liberal use of transfusion in the last two decades in women of child-bearing age. Of the antigens in the Rh system, c and E are more often associated with severe hemolytic disease[112]. Of 733 Rh-positive women identified with blood group antibodies over a thirty-year period in Wales, 78% were of the Rh system with 53% E and 24% c[113]. Of the other antibodies, anti-Kell was the most common, comprising 13%. The sources of sensitization in the rhesus system were primarily maternal and fetal incompatibility, while a history of prior blood transfusion comprised the major source of sensitization to antibodies in other systems.

Sensitized pregnancies involving non-D rhesus antibodies and other blood group antibodies are managed in the same manner as anti-D. Table 11 shows the severity of hemolytic disease associated with each antigen. The pathogenesis of hemolytic disease due to atypical antibodies is similar to that with Rh(D). The standard management of Kell-sensitized pregnancies is controversial. Caine and Mueller-Heubach[114] in 1986 suggested that the ΔOD_{450} results were less predictive of the severity of disease with anti-Kell. Most authors manage ΔOD_{450} results with anti-Kell the same as with anti-D. However, close surveillance of fetal well-being and fetal hydrops is advisable even in the presence of normal ΔOD_{450}. As with anti-D, a critical titer must be established at each institution for irregular blood-group antibodies.

Whenever an atypical antibody is identified in the pregnant patient, an assessment of paternal genotype is necessary. The genotype of the father establishes the

Table 11   Irregular blood-group antibodies

Blood group system	Antigen	Severity of HDN
Rhesus	C	Mild to moderate
	c	Mild to severe
	E	Mild to severe
	e	Mild to moderate
Kell	K	Mild to severe
	k	Mild
Duffy	Fya	Mild to severe
	Fyb	Not a cause of HDN
Kidd	Jka	Mild to severe
	Jkb	Mild to severe
MNSs	M	Mild to severe
	N	Mild
	S	Mild to severe
	s	Mild to severe
	U	Mild to severe
Lutheran	Lua	Mild
	Lub	Mild
Diego	Dia	Mild to severe
	Dib	Mild to severe
Lewis	Lea	Not a cause of HDN
	Leb	Not a cause of HDN

HDN, Hemolytic disease of the newborn
Modified from reference 115

probability of the antigen being present on fetal cells. As with anti-Kell, 0.2% of the population are homozygous for Kell (KK), 8.7% are heterozygous for Kell (Kk), and the majority, 91%, are homozygous for k (kk)[115]. The majority of couples will therefore be at low risk for conceiving a Kell-positive fetus.

REFERENCES

1. Levine P, Burnham L, Katzin GM, *et al*. The role of isoimmunization in the pathogenesis of erythoblastosis fetalis. *Am J Obstet Gynecol* 1941;42:925–37
2. Liley AW. Liquor amnii analysis in the management of pregnancy complicated by rhesus sensitization. *Am J Obstet Gynecol* 1961;82:1359–70
3. Grannum PAT, Copel JA. Prevention of Rh isoimmunization and treatment of the compromised fetus. *Semin Perinatol* 1988;12:324–35
4. Freda VJ. Rh immunization – experience with full term pregnancies. *Clin Obstet Gynecol* 1971;14:594–610
5. Bowman JM, Chown B, Lewis M, Pollack JM. Rh isoimmunization during pregnancy: antenatal prophylaxis. *Can Med Assoc J* 1978;118:623–7
6. Pollack W, Ascari WQ, Kochesky RJ, *et al*. Studies on Rh prophylaxis. 1. Relationship between doses of anti-Rh and size of antigenic stimulus. *Transfusion* 1971;11:333–9
7. Stern K, Goodman HS, Berger M. Experimental isoimmunization to hemoantigens in man. *J Immunol* 1961;67:189–98
8. Ascari WQ, Levine P, Pollack W. Incidence of maternal Rh isoimmunization by ABO compatible and incompatible pregnancies. *Br Med J* 1969;1:399–401
9. Levine P, Katzin EM, Bunham L. Isoimmunization in pregnancy: its possible bearing on the etiology of erythroblastosis fetalis. *J Am Med Assoc* 1941;116:825–7
10. Zipursky A, Israels LG. The pathogenesis and prevention of Rh immunization. *Can Med Assoc J* 1967;97:1245–57
11. Cohen F, Zueler WW, Gustafson DC, Evans MM. Mechanism of isoimmunization. I. The transplacental passage of fetal erythrocytes in homospecific pregnancies. *Blood* 1964;23:621–46
12. Leong M, Duby S, Kinch RAH. Fetal–maternal transfusion following early abortion. *Obstet Gynecol* 1979;54:424–6
13. Ascari WQ. Abortion and maternal Rh immunization. *Clin Obstet Gynecol* 1971;14:625–34
14. Katz J, Marcus RG. The risk of Rh isoimmunization in ruptured tubal pregnancy. *Br Med J* 1972;3:667–9
15. Menutti MT, Brummond W, Crombleholme WR, *et al*. Fetal–maternal bleeding associated with genetic amniocentesis. *Obstet Gynecol* 1980;55:48–54
16. Bowman JM, Pollack JM. Transplacental fetal hemorrhage after amniocentesis. *Obstet Gynecol* 1985;66:749–54
17. Blakemore KJ, Baumgarten A, Schoenfeld-Dimaio M, *et al*. Rise in maternal serum alpha fetoprotein concentration after chorionic villus sampling and possibility of isoimmunization. *Am J Obstet Gynecol* 1986;155:988–93
18. Race RR. The Rh genotype and Fisher's theory. *Blood* 1948;3:27–42
19. Weiner AS. The RH series of allelic genes. *Science* 1944;100:595–7
20. Rosenfield R, Allen FH, Rubenstein P. Genetic model for the Rh blood-group system. *Proc Natl Acad Sci USA* 1973;70:1303–7
21. Mollison PL. Techniques for detecting red cell antigens and antibodies. In Mollison PL, ed. *Blood Transfusion in Medicine*, 7th edn. Cambridge, MA: Blackwell Scientific Publications, 1983
22. Keith L, Davis RP, Berger GS. Clinical experience with the prevention of Rh-isoimmunization: a historical comparative analysis. *Am J Reprod Immunol* 1984;5:84–9
23. Goto S, Nishi H, Tomoda Y. Blood group Rh-D factor in human trophoblast determined by the immunofluorescent method. *Am J Obstet Gynecol* 1980;137:707–12
24. Nicolaides KH, Soothill PW, Clewell WH, *et al*. Fetal hemoglobin measurement in the assessment of red cell isoimmunization. *Lancet* 1988;1:1073–5
25. Nicolaides KH, Thilaganatha NB, Mibasha NRS, Rodeck CH. Erythroblastosis and reticulocytosis in anemic fetuses. *Am J Obstet Gynecol* 1988;159:1063–5
26. Nicolaides KH. Studies on fetal physiology and pathophysiology in rhesus disease. *Semin Perinatol* 1989;13:328–37
27. Rightmire DA, Nicolaides KH, Rodeck CH, Campbell S. Fetal blood velocities in Rh isoimmunization: relationship to gestational age and fetal hematocrit. *Obstet Gynecol* 1986;68:233–6
28. Bilardo CM, Nicolaides KH, Campbell S. Doppler studies in red cell isoimmunization. *Clin Obstet Gynecol* 1989;32:719–27

29. Warren PS, Gill RW, Fisher CC. Doppler flow studies in rhesus isoimmunization. *Semin Perinatol* 1987;11:375–8

30. Finne PH. Erythropoietin production in fetal hypoxia and in anaemic uraemic patients. *Ann NY Acad Sci* 1968;149:497–503

31. Nicolaides KH, Fontanarosa M, Gabbe S, Rodeck CH. Failure of ultrasonographic parameters to predict the severity of fetal anemia in rhesus isoimmunization. *Am J Obstet Gynecol* 1988;158:920–6

32. Harman CR. Fetal monitoring in the alloimmunized pregnancy. *Clin Perinatol* 1989;16:691–733

33. Chitkara U, Wilkins I, Lynch L, *et al.* The role of sonography in assessing severity of fetal anemia in Rh- and Kell-isoimmunized pregnancies. *Obstet Gynecol* 1988;71:393–8

34. Soothill PW, Nicolaides KH, Rodeck CH. Effect of anemia on fetal acid–base status. *Br J Obstet Gynaecol* 1987;94:880–3

35. Soothill PW, Nicolaides KH, Rodeck CH, *et al.* Relationship of fetal hemoglobin and oxygen content to lactate concentration in Rh isoimmunized pregnancies. *Obstet Gynecol* 1987;69:268–71

36. Nicolaides KH, Warenski JC, Rodeck CH. The relationship of fetal plasma protein concentration and hemoglobin level to the development of hydrops in rhesus isoimmunization. *Am J Obstet Gynecol* 1985;152:341–4

37. Grannum PAT, Copel JA, Moya FR, *et al.* The reversal of hydrops fetalis by intravascular intrauterine transfusion in severe isoimmune fetal anemia. *Am J Obstet Gynecol* 1988;158:914–19

38. Hansen TN, Gest AL. Hydrops fetalis. In Brace RA, Ross MG, Robillard JE, eds. *Reproductive and Perinatal Medicine*, Vol. XI. *Fetal and Neonatal Body Fluids*. Ithaca, NY: Perinatology Press, 1989

39. Phibbs RH, Johnson P, Tooley WH. Cardio-respiratory status of erythroblastotic newborn infants. II. Blood volume, hematocrit, and serum albumin concentration in relation to hydrops fetalis. *Pediatrics* 1974;53:13–23

40. Nicolaides KH, Clewell WH, Rodeck CH. Measurement of human fetal–placental blood volume in erythroblastosis fetalis. *Am J Obstet Gynecol* 1987;157:50–13

41. MacGregor SN, Socol ML, Pielet BW, *et al.* Prediction of fetoplacental blood volume in isoimmunized pregnancy. *Am J Obstet Gynecol* 1988;159:1493–7

42. Bowman JM. Hemolytic disease. In Creasy RK, Resnik R, eds. *Maternal-Fetal Medicine: Principles and Practice*, 2nd edn. Philadelphia, PA: WB Saunders, 1989

43. American College of Obstetrics and Gynecology, Technical Bulletin number 148. Management of Isoimmunization in Pregnancy. Washington, DC: ACOG, 1990

44. Parer JT. Severe Rh isoimmunization: current methods of *in utero* diagnosis and treatment. *Am J Obstet Gynecol* 1988;158:1323–9

45. Reece EA, Copel JA, Scioscia AL, *et al.* Diagnostic fetal umbilical blood sampling in the management of isoimmunization. *Am J Obstet Gynecol* 1988;159:1057–62

46. Ananth U, Warsof SL, Coulehan JM, *et al.* Mid-trimester amniotic fluid delta optical density at

450 nm in normal pregnancies. *Am J Obstet Gynecol* 1986;155:664–6

47. Nicolaides KH, Rodeck CH, Mibashan RS, Kemp JR. Have Liley charts outlived their usefulness? *Am J Obstet Gynecol* 1986;155:90–4

48. Bowman JM. The management of Rh-isoimmunization. *Am J Obstet Gynecol* 1978;52:1–16

49. Ananth U, Queenan JT. Does midtrimester ΔOD_{450} of amniotic fluid reflect severity of Rh disease? *Am J Obstet Gynecol* 1989;161:47–9

50. Bowman JM, Pollock JM. Amnionic fluid spectrophotometry and early delivery in the management of erythroblastosis fetalis. *Pediatrics* 1965;35:815–35

51. Bowell PJ, Sellinger M, Ferguson J. Antenatal fetal blood sampling for the management of autoimmunized pregnancies: effect upon maternal anti-D potency levels. *Br J Obstet Gynaecol* 1988;95:759–64

52. Horenstein J, Golde SH, Platt LD. Lung profiles in the isoimmunized pregnancy. *Am J Obstet Gynecol* 1985;153:443–7

53. Liley AW. Errors in the assessment of hemolytic disease from amniotic fluid. *Am J Obstet Gynecol* 1963;86:485–94

54. Brazie JV, Bowes Jr WA, Ibbott FA. An improved, rapid procedure for the determination of amniotic fluid bilirubin and its use in the prediction of the course of Rh-sensitized pregnancies. *Am J Obstet Gynecol* 1969;104:80–6

55. Lindsay MK, Lypo VR. Nonpredictive value of measurements of ΔOD_{450} in SS disease. *Am J Obstet Gynecol* 1985;153:75–6

56. Birnholz JC. Fetal behavior and condition. In Callen PW, ed. *Ultrasonography in Obstetrics and Gynecology.* Philadelphia, PA: WB Saunders, 1983

57. Benacerraf BR, Frigoletto FD. Sonographic sign for the detection of early fetal ascites in the management of severe isoimmune disease without intrauterine transfusion. *Am J Obstet Gynecol* 1985;152:1039–41

58. DeVore GR, Ackerman RJ, Cabal L, *et al.* Hypoalbuminemia: the etiology of antenatally diagnosed pericardial effusion in rhesus-hemolytic anemia. *Am J Obstet Gynecol* 1982;142:1056–7

59. Kirkinen P, Jouppila P, Eik-Nes S. Umbilical vein blood flow in rhesus-isoimmunization. *Br J Obstet Gynaecol* 1983;90:640–3

60. Copel JA, Grannum PAT, Belanger K. Pulsed Doppler flow–velocity waveforms before and after intrauterine intravascular transfusions for severe erythroblastosis fetalis. *Am J Obstet Gynecol* 1988;158:768–74

61. Copel JA, Grannum PAT, Green JJ, *et al.* Fetal cardiac output in the isoimmunized pregnancy: a pulsed Doppler echocardiographic study of patients undergoing intravascular intrauterine transfusion. *Am J Obstet Gynecol* 1989;161:361–5

62. Copel JA, Grannum PAT, Green JJ, *et al.* Pulsed Doppler flow–velocity waveforms in the prediction of fetal hematocrit of the severely isoimmunized pregnancy. *Am J Obstet Gynecol* 1989;161:341–4

63. Harman CR, Manning FA, Bowman JM, *et al.* Use of intravascular transfusion to treat hydrops fetalis in a moribund fetus. *Can Med Assoc J* 1988;138:827–30

64. Visser GH. Antepartum sinusoidal and decelerative fetal heart rate patterns in Rh disease. *Am J Obstet Gynecol* 1982;143:538–44

65. Nicolaides KH, Sadovsky G, Cetin E. Fetal heart rate patterns in red blood cell isoimmunized pregnancies. *Am J Obstet Gynecol* 1989;161:351–6

66. Bennett PR, Kim CLV, Colin Y, *et al.* Prenatal determination of fetal RhD type by DNA amplification. *New Engl J Med* 1993;329:607–10

67. Yankowitz J, Li S, Murray JC. Polymerase chain reaction determination of RhD blood type: an evaluation of accuracy. *Obstet Gynecol* 1995;86:214–17

68. Fisk NM, Bennett P, Warwick RM, *et al.* Clinical utility of fetal RhD typing in alloimmunized pregnancies by means of polymerase chain reaction on amniocytes or chorionic villi. *Am J Obstet Gynecol* 1994:171:50–4

69. Caritis SN, Mueller-Heubach E, Edelstone DI. Effect of betamethasone on analysis of amniotic fluid in the rhesus-sensitized pregnancy. *Am J Obstet Gynecol* 1977;127:529–32

70. Liley AW. The technique of foetal transfusion in the treatment of severe hemolytic disease. *Aust NZ J Obstet Gynaecol* 1964;4:145–8

71. Frigoletto FD, Umansky I, Birnholz J, *et al.* Intrauterine fetal transfusion in 365 fetuses during 15 years. *Am J Obstet Gynecol* 1981;139:781–90

72. Watts DH, Luthy DA, Benedetti TJ, *et al.* Intraperitoneal fetal transfusion under direct ultrasound guidance. *Obstet Gynecol* 1988;71:84–8

73. Harman CR, Manning FA, Bowman JM, Lange IR. Severe Rh disease – poor outcome is not inevitable. *Am J Obstet Gynecol* 1983;145:823–9

74. Rodeck CH, Holman CA, Karnicki J, *et al.* Direct intravascular fetal transfusion by fetoscopy in severe rhesus isoimmunization. *Lancet* 1981;1:652–7

75. Ch de Crespigny LC, Robinson HP, Quinn M, *et al.* Ultrasound-guided fetal blood transfusions for severe rhesus isoimmunization. *Obstet Gynecol* 1985;66:529–32

76. Bang J, Bock TE, Trolle D. Ultrasound-guided fetal intravenous transfusion for severe rhesus hemolytic disease. *Br Med J* 1982;284:373–4

77. Westgren M, Selbing A, Stangenberg M. Fetal intracardiac transfusions in patients with severe rhesus isoimmunization. *Br Med J* 1988;296:885–6

78. Daffos F, Capella-Paulovsky M, Forestier F. Fetal blood sampling during pregnancy with the use of a needle guided by ultrasound: a study of 606 consecutive cases. *Am J Obstet Gynecol* 1985;153:655–60

79. Nicolaides KH, Soothill PW, Rodeck CH, Clewell W. Rh disease: intravascular fetal blood transfusion by cordocentesis. *Fetal Ther* 1986;1:185–92

80. Socol ML, MacGregor SN, Pielet BW, *et al.* Percutaneous umbilical transfusion in severe rhesus isoimmunization. *Am J Obstet Gynecol* 1987;159:1369–75

81. Berkowitz RL, Chitkara U, Goldberg JD, *et al.* Intrauterine intravascular transfusions for severe red blood cell isoimmunization: ultrasound-guided percutaneous approach. *Am J Obstet Gynecol* 1986;155:574–81

82. Harman CR, Biehl DR, Pollock DJ, *et al.* Intrauterine transfusion: kinetics of absorption of donor cells in fetal lambs. *Am J Obstet Gynecol* 1983;145:803–6

83. Halitsky V, Krumholz BA. Estimation of red cell volume requirements for intrauterine transfusion. *Obstet Gynecol* 1968;31:543–50

84. Rodeck CH, Nicolaides KH, Warsof SL, *et al.* The management of severe rhesus isoimmunization by fetoscopic intravascular transfusions. *Am J Obstet Gynecol* 1984;150:769–77

85. Grannum PAT, Copel JA, Plaxe SC, *et al. In utero* exchange transfusion by direct intravascular injection in severe erythroblastosis fetalis. *New Engl J Med* 1986;314:1431–4

86. Berkowitz RL, Chitkara U, Wilkens IA, *et al.* Intravascular monitoring and management of erythroblastosis fetalis. *Am J Obstet Gynecol* 1988;158:783–95

87. Berkowitz RL, Chitkara U, Wilkens IA, *et al.* Technical aspects of intravascular transfusions: lessons learned from 33 procedures. *Am J Obstet Gynecol* 1987;157:4–9

88. Laifer SA, Kuller JA, Hill LM. Rapid assessment of fetal hemoglobin concentration using the Hemocue system. *Obstet Gynecol* 1990;76:723–4

89. Weiner CP, Pelzer GD, Heilskov J, *et al.* The effect of intravascular transfusion on umbilical venous pressure in anemic fetuses with and without hydrops. *Am J Obstet Gynecol* 1989;161:1498–1501

90. Morris JA, Hustead RF, Robinson RG, *et al.* Measurement of fetoplacental blood volume in human previable fetus. *Am J Obstet Gynecol* 1974;118:927–34

91. Plecas DV, Chitkara U, Berkowitz G, *et al.* Intrauterine intravascular transfusion for severe erythroblastosis fetalis: how much to transfuse? *Obstet Gynecol* 1990;75:965–9

92. MacGregor SN, Socol ML, Pielet BW, *et al.* Prediction of hematocrit decline after intravascular fetal transfusion. *Am J Obstet Gynecol* 1989;161:1491–3

93. Soothill PW, Nicolaides KH, Rodeck CH, Bellingham AJ. The effect of replacing fetal hemoglobin with adult hemoglobin on blood gas and acid–base parameters in human fetuses. *Am J Obstet Gynecol* 1988;158:66–9

94. Harman CR, Bowman JM, Manning FA, Menticoglou SM. IUT–intraperitoneal vs. intravascular approach: a case–control comparison. *Am J Obstet Gynecol* 1990;162:1053–9

95. Halitsky V. Sequelae in children who survived *in utero* fetal transfusion: a comparison with those who underwent postpartum exchange transfusion only. In Tejani N, ed. *Obstetrical Events and Developmental Sequelae.* Boca Raton, FL: CRC Press, 1990

96. Laifer SA, Kuller JA, Hill LM. *In utero* intravascular transfusion for treating fetal hemolytic disease. *Surg Gynecol Obstet* 1991;172:319

97. Bowman JM. Antenatal suppression of Rh alloimmunization. *Clin Obstet Gynecol* 1991;34:296–303

98. Freda VJ, Gorman JG, Pollack W. Successful prevention of experimental Rh sensitization in man with an anti-Rh gamma-2-globulin antibody preparation: a preliminary report. *Transfusion* 1964;4:26–32

99. Clarke CA, Donohoe WTA, Finn R, *et al.* Further experimental studies on the prevention of Rh haemolytic disease. *Br Med J* 1963;1:979–84

100. Davey MG, Zipursky A. McMaster Conference on prevention of Rh immunization: first report of the western Canadian trial. *Can Med Assoc J* 1969;100:1021–4

101. Grannum PAT, Copel JA. Prevention of Rh isoimmunization and treatment of the compromised fetus. *Semin Perinatol* 1988;12:324–35

102. Pollack W. Recent understanding for the mechanism by which passive administered Rh antibody suppresses the immune response to Rh antigen in unimmunized Rh-negative women. *Clin Obstet Gynecol* 1982;25:255–65

103. Mollison PL, Barron SL, Bowley C, *et al*. Controlled trial of various anti-D dosages in suppression of Rh sensitization following pregnancy. *Br Med J* 1974;2:75–80

104. Stewart FH, Bernhill MS, Bozorgi N. Reduced dose of Rh immunoglobulin following first trimester pregnancy termination. *Obstet Gynecol* 1978;51:318–22

105. Samson D, Mollison PL. Effect of primary Rh immunization of delayed administration of anti-Rh. *Immunology* 1975;28:349–57

106. Bowen FW, Renfield M. The detection of anti-D in Rho(D)-negative infants born to Rho(D)-positive mothers. *Pediatr Res* 1976;10:213–15

107. Scott JR, Beer AE, Guy LR, *et al*. Pathogenesis of Rh immunization in primigravidas: fetomaternal versus maternofetal bleeding. *Obstet Gynecol* 1977;49:9–14

108. Tovey LAD. Haemolytic disease of the newborn – the changing scene. *Br J Obstet Gynaecol* 1986;93:960–6

109. Berger GS, Keith L. Utilization of Rh prophylaxis. *Clin Obstet Gynecol* 1982;25:267–75

110. Pollack W, Ascari WQ, Crispen JF. Studies on Rh prophylaxis. 2. Rh immune prophylaxis after transfusion with Rh-positive blood. *Transfusion* 1971;11:340–4

111. Bowman HS, Mohn JF, Lambert RM. Prevention of maternal Rh immunization after accidental transfusion of D(Rho)-positive blood. *Vox Sang* 1972;22:385–96

112. Kornstad L. New cases of irregular blood group antibodies other than anti-D in pregnancy: frequency and clinical significance. *Acta Obstet Gynecol Scand* 1983;62:431–6

113. Hardy J, Napier JAF. Red cell antibodies detected in antenatal tests on rhesus positive women in south and mid Wales, 1948–1978. *Br J Obstet Gynaecol* 1981;88:91–100

114. Caine ME, Mueller-Heubach E. Kell sensitization in pregnancy. *Am J Obstet Gynecol* 1986;154:85–90

115. Weinstein L. Irregular antibodies causing hemolytic disease of the newborn: a continuing problem. *Clin Obstet Gynecol* 1982;25:321–32

53
Fetal age assessment

C.M. Martin

Fetal age and fetal growth assessment are undoubtedly the most common issues dealt with in the modern field of obstetric ultrasound. Correct gestational age assignment is critical when problems such as fetal macrosomia, intrauterine growth retardation, or other conditions which may mandate delivery at a time other than the anticipated due date confront the clinician later in gestation. In this day of readily available high-resolution sonography, iatrogenic prematurity related to elective operative delivery or induction of labor should never occur.

Prior to the advent of sonography, clinical history, last menstrual period and uterine size on initial pelvic examination were the hallmarks of gestational dating. Even under the best of circumstances, these parameters are fraught with inaccuracies. Menstrual irregularities, ovulation disorders and patient error while using oral contraceptives can all lead to erroneous assignment of gestational age based upon menstrual history. The variations in patient body habitus and ease of examination coupled with anatomic alterations such as uterine myomata may lead to further compounded errors in assignment of gestational age which may have dire consequences for the patient and her baby later in pregnancy when critical issues surrounding the appropriate timing of delivery are encountered.

Direct evaluation of the developing fetus with ultrasound has enabled us to recognize discrepancies in fetal size vs. menstrual and clinical dating at a time when it is still feasible to estimate accurately and to reassign an estimated date of confinement. The key to reassignment of due date, however, lies in early fetal assessment before that time in gestation when growth disorders such as macrosomia, symmetrical large-for-gestational-age fetal growth, intrauterine growth retardation and symmetrical small-for-gestational-age fetal growth patterns become apparent. Detailed discussion of growth disorders will be undertaken in subsequent chapters, but these disorders must be considered in the differential diagnosis of size vs. dates discrepancies whenever a patient presents for initial assessment in the late second or third trimester of pregnancy. The first trimester is considered to extend to the end of 12 weeks' menstrual age.

THE FIRST TRIMESTER OF PREGNANCY

The advent of transvaginal sonography has greatly increased the ability to observe the earliest sonographic events in both normal and pathological early gestation. This technology, coupled with very sensitive quantitative measurements of serum β-human chorionic gonadotropin (β-hCG) by radioimmunoassay or enzyme-linked immunosorbent assay (ELISA) of the intact hCG molecule, has led us to the point where it is possible to identify serological evidence of pregnancy at the time of the anticipated menstrual period, and serially to follow the sonographic development of these early gestations in a variety of common situations. These include early first-trimester bleeding, progesterone deficiency, recurrent pregnancy wastage and previous history of ectopic pregnancy. Early recognition of pathological trends in either the serum hCG level or the sonographic findings (Table 1) may trigger intervention that could salvage the gestation or minimize the morbidity to the patient resulting from delay in diagnosis[1–3].

The first structure to be observed in early gestation is the gestational sac. Using high-resolution transvaginal ultrasound, the gestational sac can be imaged by the

Table 1 β-Human chorionic gonadotropin (β-hCG) measurements (U/l) and sonographic markers

| Marker | Gestational age (weeks) | Radioimmunoassay | | ELISA intact hCG |
		2nd International Reference Standard	1st International Reference Preparation	
Gestational sac	4.3	500	1000	1000
Yolk sac	4.9	1400	3000	2800
Embryo	5.4	5000	10 000	10 000
Heartmotion	5.8	10 000	20 000	20 000

5th week of amenorrhea. The gestational sac can be identified as a hypoechoic circular or oval structure within the uterus, immediately adjacent to the endometrial echo, and surrounded by a well developed echodense ring of decidual reaction (Figure 1). In early studies utilizing transabdominal imaging, measurements of gestational sac size and mean sac diameter were utilized to assign gestational age. Convention dictates that the gestational sac size is obtained by measuring the length and anteroposterior dimensions of the sac from sagittal images of the uterus, and the transverse uterine image is used to measure the width of the sac at its maximal transverse dimension. The average of these three measurements is the mean sac diameter. When the gestational sac is measured, measurements include the anechoic area only, and the decidual reaction surrounding the sac is not included (Figure 2). Hellman and associates[4] were able to predict gestational age from mean gestational sac size, utilizing the following formula:

$$\text{Gestational age (weeks)} = \frac{\text{mean gestational sac diameter (cm)} + 2.543}{0.702}$$

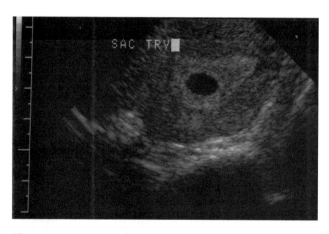

Figure 1 Very early gestational sac surrounded by echogenic ring of decidual tissue

Joupilla[5] evaluated the accuracy of dating derived from the size of the early gestational sac and found it to be ± 7 days.

The yolk sac is the next structure to appear. The yolk sac can be identified within the gestational sac within days of its appearance. The yolk sac is a smooth, round structure with fine margins (Figure 3). The yolk sac slowly enlarges to a maximum of roughly 4–5 mm in diameter and slowly regresses in the later weeks of the first trimester. Its persistent presence in the first trimester and its extra-amniotic location must be kept in mind, so that it is not confused with an anomalous fetal structure. Abnormalities of the yolk sac such as the calcified yolk sac and the hydropic yolk sac have been linked to first-trimester loss[6–8].

The fetal pole is first seen as an area of increased echoes at one margin of the yolk sac. The duplex of fetal pole and yolk sac has a 'signet ring' appearance initially (Figure 4). Gradually the fetal pole enlarges to the point that it dwarfs the yolk sac. By the time that the fetal pole has reached a crown–rump length of 3–5 mm, the first fetal heart motion can be identified with high-resolution transvaginal sonography. The crown–rump length is the first fetal measurement used to assign gestational age. The measurement is made along the long axis of the embryo. Transvaginal sonography can resolve the early fetal neural tube adequately to begin to recognize cranial and caudal poles of the embryo as early as the 7th week of amenorrhea. This polarity enables accurate recognition of the true long axis of the embryo.

The measurement of crown–rump length (Figure 5) is used throughout the first trimester from first visualization of the fetal pole to approximately the 11th week of amenorrhea. Late in the first trimester, curling of the fetus can lead to underestimation of the crown–rump length, and inaccurate gestational age assignment. Multiple images with the fetus in a position of maximal extention will help to avoid this pitfall. By 11–12 weeks of gestation, the head is easily

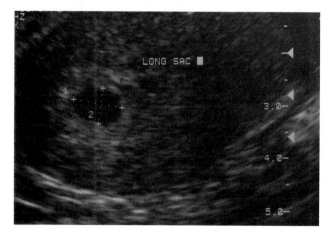

Figure 2 Electronic calipers mark the borders of the gestational sac

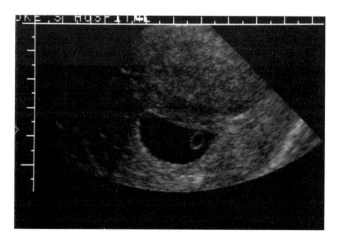

Figure 3 The yolk sac is seen as a distinct circular structure within the gestational sac

identified and has sufficient intracranial anatomy visible for accurate biparietal diameter measurements to be used to assign fetal age. Crown–rump length has been shown to be accurate to within ± 5–7 days of the predicted date of confinement[9] and is as accurate as a second-trimester biparietal diameter in the prediction of the date of confinement[10].

THE SECOND AND THIRD TRIMESTERS OF PREGNANCY

The accuracy of gestational age assignment increases with decreasing gestational age. The earlier we study the fetus, the more accurately we can assign gestational age. In the second trimester, ultrasound may be used to assess gestational age as well as fetal growth and evaluation of fetal anatomy. Because it is very rare to find growth retardation in the early to mid-second trimester in the absence of chromosomal or gross anatomical abnormalities, we can still focus on assigning a due date in this time frame if this is the first opportunity we are afforded for fetal assessment. The second trimester is a period in which there is linear fetal growth, which exhibits fairly large incremental increases. In the second trimester, evaluation of the overall status of the fetus requires multiple fetal biometric assessments. In the second trimester, gestational age assignment can be made with accuracy up to the 24th week of gestation. After this time, variations in fetal growth due to hereditary, metabolic or uteroplacental factors may begin to become manifest, and these factors render later attempts at dating quite inaccurate. Prior to 25 weeks of gestation, sonographically determined due dates are accurate to ± 10 days.

Measurements that are routinely useful in the assessment of gestational age in the second trimester include the biparietal diameter (Figure 6) and the femur length (Figure 7). The biparietal diameter was the first fetal parameter to be measured and formed the earliest 'gold standard' for assessing gestational age and fetal growth[11]. An entire body of literature exists dealing with the sonographic measurement of the fetal head. In situations in which abnormalities of the fetal head render the biparietal diameter useless as a measurement of gestational age, the femur length may be used in its place. The femur length, as well as the lengths of the other long bones of the fetal limbs, bear a direct relationship to fetal age[12,13]. The femur is the most widely used long bone for age assessment. The accuracy of femur length measurement is equivalent to the accuracy of gestational age assignment based on the fetal biparietal diameter at any given gestational age. Estimation based on the femur length, like the biparietal diameter, is most accurate at early gestational ages. Below 20 weeks of gestation, an estimated date of confinement based upon femur length alone is accurate to ± 7 days[14].

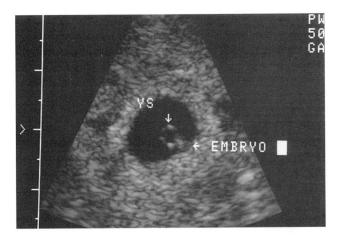

Figure 4 The early embryo is first visualized as a thickening along one border of the yolk sac (YS)

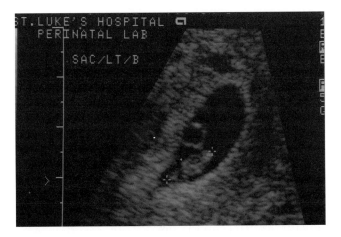

Figure 5 Electronic calipers mark the crown–rump length of the embryo. The yolk sac lies to the left of the embryo

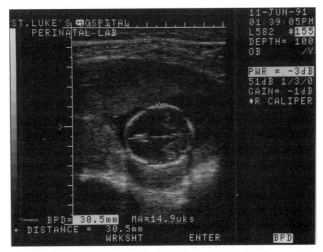

Figure 6 Electronic calipers positioned correctly for measurement of the biparietal diameter. Measurements are taken from the outer margin of the anterior parietal bone to the inner table of the posterior parietal bone

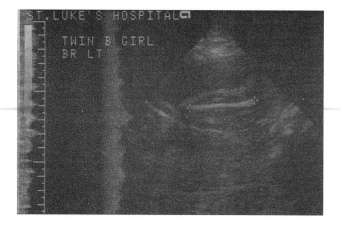

Figure 7 Femur length is measured along the shaft of the long bone. Electronic calipers show the appropriate plane of measurement

The head and abdominal circumferences are actually measurements of fetal growth rather than fetal age, but these parameters are also measured when overall gestational age assignment is made in the second trimester. Multiparametric evaluation allows one to measure linear (femur length), concentric (biparietal diameter and head circumference) fetal growth. A number of nomograms for each of the above fetal measurements have been developed. These are based upon local population and demographic patterns which are peculiar to the area in which the research was conducted, so that there are minor variations from author to author among the nomograms.

Measurement of the fetal head by both biparietal diameter and head circumference will allow for internal quality control of these measurements. The head circumference will remain unaffected by situations in which the fetal head is molded by compression due to malpresentation or oligohydramnios. When the fetal head is molded, the biparietal diameter may be artifactually smaller (dolichocephalic) or larger (brachycephalic) than expected when compared to the other fetal measurements or compared to the clinical estimation of gestational age. The head circumference should not be altered by molding, so that variations in shape will not be reflected in inaccuracies in head circumference measurement. The degree of molding of the fetal head may be determined by using the cephalic index[15]. The cephalic index is independent of gestational age and is determined by the ratio of the outer to outer edge measurements of the biparietal diameter and the occipitofrontal diameter[16]:

$$\text{Cephalic index} = \frac{\text{outer to outer edge biparietal diameter}}{\text{outer to outer edge occipitofrontal diameter}} \times 100$$

The mean cephalic index is 78.3, with a 2SD range of 70–86. When the cephalic index is low, the head is dolichocephalic or compressed along the biparietal diameter. When the cephalic index is high, the head is brachycephalic or compressed along the occipitofrontal diameter. The finding of an abnormal cephalic index will allow the observer either to correct the biparietal diameter to take into account the effect of molding, or to use other parameters as a substitute for the biparietal diameter in assigning gestational age and estimating fetal weight. Visually apparent variations in shape of the fetal head can be appreciated at ± 1SD (i.e. cephalic index ≤ 74 or ≥ 83). For this reason, we apply the formula for cephalic index to all head measurements made in our laboratory and apply a correction[17] for the biparietal diameter in all instances in which cephalic index is within ± 1SD.

$$\text{Corrected biparietal diameter} = \frac{\text{biparietal diameter} + \text{occipitofrontal diameter}}{2.265}$$

When fetal measurements are made in the second trimester, the multiple biometric parameters should lie within ± 10 days of each other to be judged internally consistent and confirmatory of the clinical gestational age based upon the last menstrual period. If the parameters are more than ± 10 days discrepant from each other, one of several situations may be operative. Either the measurements are erroneous or there is some reason for fetal dyssymmetry which requires further investigation. In the first case, diligent reassessment of representative images of the fetal measurements should be undertaken and remeasurement of the fetus in the case of poor image quality should be performed. If the image quality is optimal, then careful reassessment of the fetus for the presence of stigmata of genetic or anatomic abnormalities should be performed. In the absence of any recognizable congenital anomalies, consideration of some abnormality of fetal growth remains to be addressed. This situation can be best assessed by remeasurement of the fetus after an appropriate interval to allow for sufficient growth. An optimal interval of 2–3 weeks is desirable, unless there is a maternal or fetal condition which would contraindicate waiting this long for reassessment. Too frequent measurement of the fetus can result in confusing results due to the additive effects of very small growth increments and interobserver variations in measurement.

Use of the head and abdominal circumferences (Figures 8 and 9) in the second trimester serves to confirm the other fetal measurements and also helps to assess the nutritional status of the fetus. In the situation of asymmetric intrauterine growth retardation, the fetal head is preserved at the expense of the fetal abdomen, with the net result of a markedly smaller than expected abdominal circumference when compared to the fetal head circumference. In the opposite situation of fetal macrosomic growth, the abdominal circumference is inordinately larger than expected for

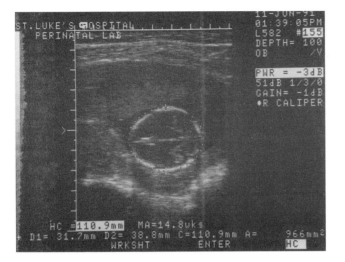

Figure 8   Head circumference as measured by perimeter tracing

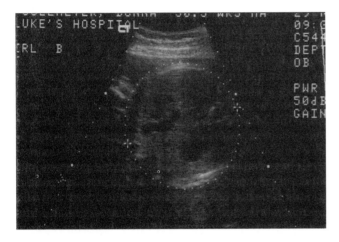

Figure 9   Abdominal circumference as determined at the level of the 'V-shaped' junction of umbilical vein and portal sinus

gestational age, due to the excessive deposition of subcutaneous fat in the abdominal wall and the larger amount of glycogen stored in the fetal liver. These growth disorders will be discussed in greater detail in later chapters.

In the situation in which a first-trimester crown–rump length has already been used to assign gestational age, the fetal measurements obtained in the second trimester should be looked at as a reflection of appropriateness of interval fetal growth since the previous evaluation and confirmation of the gestational age. Inappropriate interval growth or failure to corroborate previous sonographic gestational age assignment should be looked at in the light of a newly uncovered disturbance of fetal growth. Once a gestational age has been sonographically established early in gestation, there is no reason to modify the estimated

date of confinement which has been given. Interval fetal assessment that reflects deficient or excessive interval change in fetal size or the development of internal fetal asymmetry should reinforce the need for a careful surveillance for fetal growth disorders.

THE THIRD TRIMESTER OF PREGNANCY

In the third trimester, the widening of variation in normal fetal growth makes accurate assessment of gestational age subject to great error. Gestational ages assigned late in gestation may carry an error of ± 3–4 weeks because of the great variations in normal infants at term as well as the impact of fetal growth disorders in this period of gestation. In the case in which an initial sonographic assessment is carried out in the third trimester in a patient who has no clinically reliable information for gestational age assignment, a reliable estimated date of confinement cannot be assigned. In this scenario, the fetal biometry, if internally consistent, may be compared to average fetuses at a given gestational age to obtain a rough estimate of where this individual fetus may fall on standard nomograms. Interval assessment of fetal measurements may then be carried out to determine whether the interval fetal growth is appropriate. If the interval growth is appropriate, the fetus can be managed until it reaches a theoretical 40 weeks of gestation based upon the first evaluation. From this point on, it can be treated as a post-dates fetus and managed with standard post-dates evaluation until labor ensues or it is deemed appropriate to induce labor because of cervical changes or fetal indications of the post-maturity syndrome.

If inappropriate interval growth is encountered on serial assessment, the growth disorder should be categorized and the management should be individualized on the basis of the particular disorder suspected. If elective delivery is desired, assessment of fetal lung maturity may be necessary.

Other markers of gestational age

Because the variation in fetal growth is so wide in the third trimester, investigators have looked for other fetal parameters such as ossification centers to assess gestational age.

The distal femoral epiphysis, proximal tibial epiphysis and proximal humeral epiphysis have all been shown to be useful markers to assign gestational age in late pregnancy. The distal femoral epiphysis is not visualized before 28 weeks of gestation and is reliably visualized after 32 weeks of gestation. The proximal tibial epiphysis is absent before 34 weeks of gestation and is reliably present after 36 weeks. The proximal humeral epiphysis is reliably present at 40 weeks[18,19].

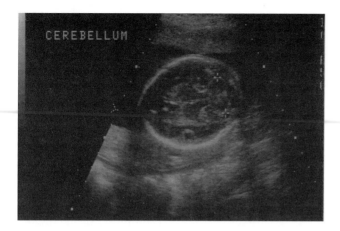

Figure 10   When the posterior fossa is imaged, the transverse diameter of the cerebellum can readily be measured

The clavicle is another bone that has been used to estimate gestational age when the fetus is in either the occipitoanterior or occipitoposterior position. In such a position the biparietal diameter cannot be easily measured, but the clavicle is readily apparent. The clavicular length measurement in millimeters is roughly equivalent to the mean gestational age in weeks. However, for a given gestation, the range of normal from the 5th to the 95th centiles may encompass 10 weeks (mean gestational age ± 5 weeks)[20].

The transverse cerebellar diameter (Figure 10) is another parameter that may be used to assess gestational age during the second trimester, because it has been shown to be well preserved even in cases of severe intrauterine growth retardation. For this reason it may serve both as a parameter for gestational age assignment and for an internal quality control standard to which other measurement results may be compared[21].

CONCLUSIONS

Gestational age assessment is the cornerstone of standard obstetric care today. Conscientious early confirmation or reassignment of clinical dates is vital to the appropriate management of a variety of obstetric complications which may result in early delivery. In many cases, accurate gestational age assignment may obviate the need for invasive tests of pulmonary maturity. Once it is appropriately established by early ultrasonography, the gestational age or estimated date of confinement should never be changed. Variations from the originally determined estimated date of confinement which appear in later gestation should always be considered to be due to growth abnormalities, and the fetus should be managed in that light. Early gestational age assessment also provides a baseline fetal evaluation to which all subsequent evaluations may be compared in the event of an abnormality of fetal growth. The use of multiple parameters provides a thorough base for fetal evaluation which takes into account the complexities of fetal growth and development.

REFERENCES

1. Nyberg DA, Filly RA, Mahoney BS, *et al*. Early gestation: correlation of hCG levels and sonographic identification. *Am J Roentgenol* 1985;144:951
2. Gast MJ, Pineda J, Martin CM, *et al*. Serum intact hCG assay for the evaluation of early pregnancy and its disorders. *Am J Gynecol Health* 1990;4:120
3. Kivikoski AI, Martin CM, Smeltzer JS. Transabdominal and transvaginal ultrasonography in the diagnosis of ectopic pregnancy: a comparative study. *Am J Obstet Gynecol* 1990;163:123
4. Hellman LF, Kobayashi M, Fillisti L, Lavenhar M. Growth and development to the human fetus prior to the twentieth week of gestation. *Am J Obstet Gynecol* 1969;103:789
5. Joupilla PC. Length and depth of the uterus and the diameter of the gestation sac in normal gravidas during early pregnancy. *Acta Obstet Gynecol Scand* 1971; 50(15 suppl):29
6. Reece EA, Scioscia AL, Pinter E, *et al*. Prognostic significance of the human yolk sac assessed by ultrasonography. *Obstet Gynecol* 1988;159:1191
7. Ferrazzi E, Brambati A, Oldrini A, *et al*. The yolk sac in early pregnancy failure. *Am J Obstet Gynecol* 1988; 158:137
8. Harris R, Vincent L, Askin F. Yolk sac calcification: a sonographic finding associated with intrauterine embryonic demise in the first trimester. *Radiology* 1988;166:109
9. Robinson HP, Fleming JEE. A critical evaluation of sonar 'crown–rump length' measurements. *Br J Obstet Gynaecol* 1975;82:702
10. Kopta MM, May RR, Crane JP. A comparison of the reliability of the estimated date of confinement predicted by crown–rump length and biparietal diameter. *Am J Obstet Gynecol* 1983;145:562
11. Hadlock FP, Deter RL, Harrist RB, Park SK. Fetal biparietal diameter: a critical re-evaluation of the relation to menstrual age by means of realtime ultrasound. *J Ultrasound Med* 1982;1:97
12. Jeanty P, Kirkpatrick C, Dramaix-Wilmet M, *et al*. Ultrasound evaluation of fetal limb growth. *Radiology* 1981;140:165
13. O'Brien GD, Queenan JT. Growth of the ultrasound fetal femur during normal pregnancy. *Am J Obstet Gynecol* 1981;141:833
14. Hadlock FP. Determination of fetal age. In Athey PA, Hadlock FP, eds. *Ultrasound in Obstetrics and Gynecology*. St Louis: CV Mosby, 1985
15. Hadlock FP, Deter RL, Carpenter RJ, Park SK. Estimating fetal age: effect of head shape on BPD. *Am J Roentgenol* 1984;142:797
16. Hohler CW. Cross-checking pregnancy landmarks by ultrasound. *Contemp Obstet Gynecol* 1982;20:169
17. Doubilet PM, Greenes RA. Improved prediction of gestational age from fetal head measurements: *Am J Roentgenol* 1984;142:797

18. Goldstein I, Lockwood C, Belanger K, Hobbins J. Ultrasonographic assessment of gestational age with the distal femoral and proximal tibial ossification centers in the third trimester. *Am J Obstet Gynecol* 1988;158:127

19. Chan WF, Ang AH, Soo YS. The value of lower limb ossification centers in the radiological estimation of fetal maturity. *Aust NZ J Obstet Gynaecol* 1972;12:55

20. Yarkoni S, Schmidt W, Jeanty P. Clavicular measurement: a new biometric parameter for fetal evaluation. *J Ultrasound Med* 1985;4:467

21. Reece EA, Goldstein I, Geanluigi P, *et al*. Fetal cerebellar growth unaffected by intrauterine growth retardation: a new parameter for prenatal diagnosis. *Am J Obstet Gynecol* 1987;157:632

54
Fetal anomalies

H.N. Winn

INTRODUCTION

About 27 per 1000 births in the USA are associated with major fetal malformations of which the majority can be diagnosed by ultrasonography *in utero*. Prenatal detection of a fetal anomaly could alter the obstetric management to reduce the fetal morbidity. Antenatal diagnosis of conditions such as omphalocele, gastroschisis, and diaphragmatic hernia allows prompt evaluation and management during the perinatal period. In addition, patients may elect to terminate pregnancies having fetuses with devastating conditions detected during the first and early second trimester. In addition, a prior knowledge of anatomically or genetically lethal anomalies, such as anencephaly, bilateral renal agenesis, and trisomy 13, could avert a Cesarean delivery for fetal distress or malpresentation.

The question of whether each obstetric patient should have an ultrasound examination to screen for fetal anomalies remains unanswered. If ultrasound screening ever becomes a reality, one scan at 18 to 20 weeks' gestation should be sufficient for both gestational dating and assessment of fetal anatomy. This timing is subject to change, however, in view of the constantly improving resolution of new ultrasound equipment, which makes the detailed evaluation of fetal anatomy during the first trimester feasible. The following section deals with the sonographic features of the more common fetal anomalies.

CENTRAL NERVOUS SYSTEM

The anatomy of the fetal brain can be well delineated by current high-resolution ultrasound equipment. To assess the fetal brain and spine thoroughly, multiple scans are required. At the level of the BPD, the following structures can be visualized: the thalami, the cavum septa pellucid, the frontal horns, and the pulsating middle cerebral arteries in the sylvanian fissures (Figure 1). The slit-like third ventricle is occasionally visible between the thalami (Figure 2). The bodies of the lateral ventricles can be seen on the axial plan rostrad to the BPD plane. At this level, the ratio of lateral ventricular width to cerebral hemisphere width (LVW : HW) is determined to aid in the diagnosis of hydrocephaly (Figure 3). Nomograms for this ratio have been developed[1,2]. It should be noted that the

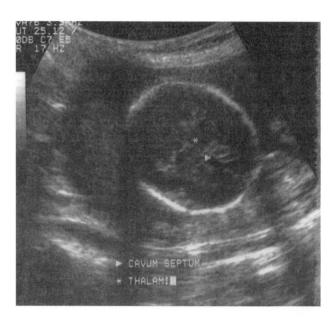

Figure 1 Axial view of a normal fetal brain at the level of the thalami. The cavum septum can be seen anterior to the thalami

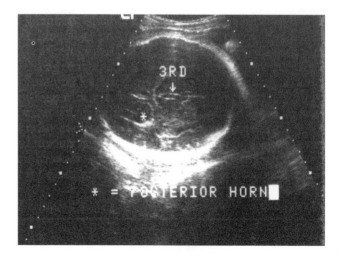

Figure 2 Axial view of a normal fetal brain shows the third ventricle as a slit between the thalami

LVW : HW ratio decreases from a mean of 55% at 15 weeks to a mean of about 30% throughout the third

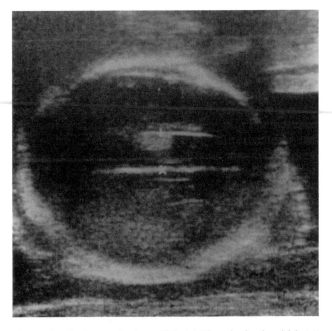

Figure 3   Left ventricular width (+) / hemispheric width (×) ratio of the lateral ventricles. The hemispheric width is measured from the midline to the inner table of the skull

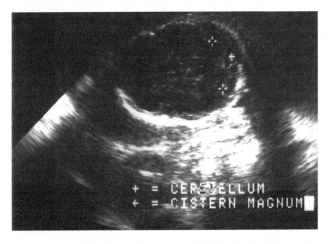

Figure 4   Axial view of a normal fetal brain shows the posterior fossa containing the cerebellum and the cistern magnum

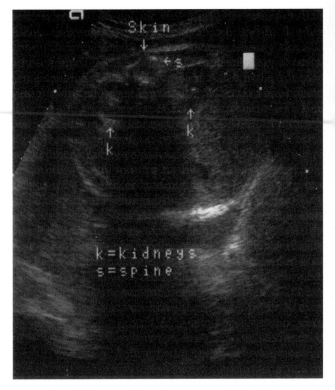

Figure 5   Axial view of a normal fetal spine shows the three ossification centers forming a triangle and the overlying skin

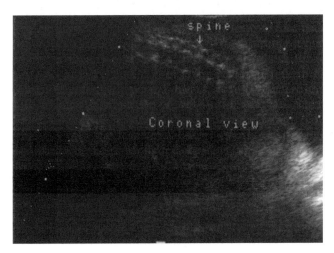

Figure 6   Coronal view of a normal fetal spine shows the three parallel lines corresponding to the bodies and lateral pedicles of the spines. A spine curvature can be appreciated from this view

trimester. The posterior fossa, which houses the cerebellum, the fourth ventricle, and the cistern magna, can be viewed by obtaining an axial plane caudad to the BPD plane with a slightly posterior inclination (Figure 4).

Each fetal vertebra has three ossification centers corresponding to the two lateral pedicles and the body. These ossification centers are responsible for the triangular configuration and the three parallel lines seen on the cross section (Figure 5) and coronal section (Figure 6) of the spine, respectively. The spinal curvature is best evaluated by sagittal section. It is important to demonstrate the presence of the overlying soft tissue and skin.

Hydrocephalus

Hydrocephalus is the condition that has both ventriculomegaly and increased intracranial pressure. Congenital hydrocephalus usually arises from obstruction of the normal flow of cerebrospinal fluid. It is subdivided into communicating and non-communicating

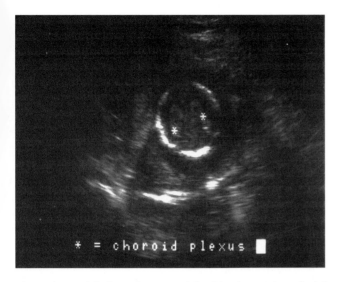

Figure 7 Axial view of a normal fetal brain at 16 weeks of gestation shows the lateral ventricles filled with choroid plexus

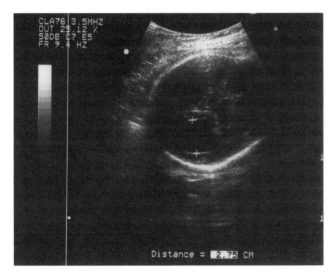

Figure 8 Ventriculomegaly. Axial view of the fetal brain reveals dilated posterior horns of the lateral ventricles as evidenced by the increased ventricular width

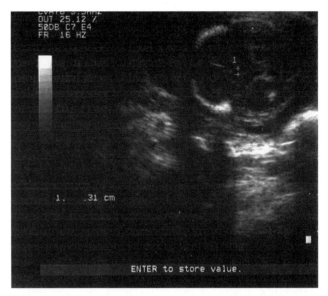

Figure 9 Aqueductal stenosis. Axial view of the fetal brain at 21 weeks of gestation reveals the dilated third ventricle (+ +)

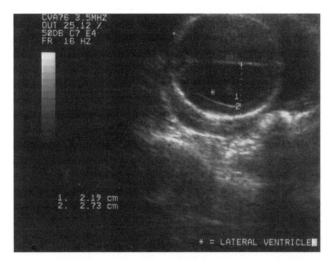

Figure 10 Aqueductal stenosis. Axial view of the fetal brain at 21 weeks of gestation (the same fetus as in Figure 9) at a more rostrad position reveals dilated lateral ventricles. The LVW/HW ratio is about 80%

hydrocephalus. The latter includes Dandy–Walker malformation and aqueductal stenosis. The incidence of congenital hydrocephalus is usually quoted as 1 per 2000 births, but it ranges from 0.12 to 2.5 per 1000 births[3]. Since the intracranial pressure (ICP) cannot be readily measured *in utero*, the diagnosis of fetal hydrocephalus rests on the morphologic changes presumably resulting from increased ICP or ventriculomegaly. During the early second trimester, the bodies and the atria of the lateral ventricles are filled with the choroid plexus (Figure 7). Anterior displacement or relative reduction in the choroid plexus size appear to be more sensitive indicators of mild hydrocephalus than is the LVW : HW ratio during this early stage of pregnancy[4].

The gross distortion of the choroid plexus as an early sign of hydrocephalus may be detected by transvaginal ultrasonography as early as 15 weeks of gestation[5]. Advanced hydrocephalus can be readily diagnosed by the apparent ventriculomegaly with elevated LVW : HW ratio and/or macrocrania (Figure 8).

Aqueductal stenosis is the most common type of hydrocephalus and accounts for 43% of cases[6]. It can be diagnosed by the presence of dilated third and lateral ventricles and normal posterior fossa (Figures 9 and 10). Aqueductal stenosis may be transmitted as an

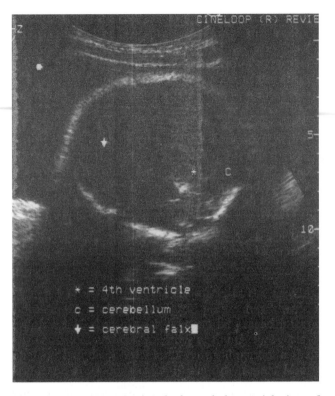

Figure 11 Communicating hydrocephalus. Axial view of the fetal brain reveals dilatation of the fourth ventricle and the cistern magnum in the posterior fossa. This fetus also has dilated lateral ventricles

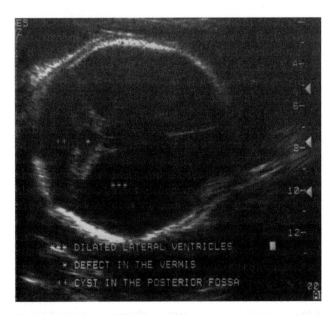

Figure 12 Dandy–Walker malformation. Axial view of the fetal brain reveals dilated lateral ventricles, a cyst in the posterior fossa and a defect in the cerebellar vermis

X-linked recessive disorder[7–10]. In this situation, an adducted thumb may be an additional feature[8]. Communicating hydrocephalus occurs in 38% of the

cases[6] and is characterized by dilatation of all the ventricles, i.e. the lateral, third, and fourth ventricles. The differentiation between aqueductal stenosis and communicating hydrocephalus is not always possible if the fourth ventricle is only minimally dilated. Demonstration of a dilated subarachnoid cistern is diagnostic of communicating hydrocephalus[11] (Figure 11). The classic Dandy–Walker malformation consists of hydrocephalus, a cyst in the posterior fossa, and defective cerebellar vermis (Figure 12). It accounts for 2–4% of hydrocephalus[12]. Dandy–Walker malformation variants which occur from either cerebellar dysgenesis or hypoplasia possess a cyst in the posterior fossa and a defective vermis, but usually lack ventriculomegaly[12,13]. Both Dandy–Walker malformation and its variants have an associated risk of chromosomal abnormalities of about 30%[13,14]. Unilateral hydrocephalus may arise from agenesis or stenosis of the foramen of Monro, or transient obstruction of the foramen of Monro due to either intraventricular hematoma or brain dysplasia[15]. The foramen of Monro provides the communication between the third and lateral ventricles.

For patients with a family history of hydrocephalus, a normal ultrasound examination before 20 weeks of gestation is reassuring, but a repeat scan later in the gestation is recommended because of the possibility of either false-negative findings or delayed manifestation[7,16,17]. Once the diagnosis of fetal hydrocephalus is made, a detailed sonographic examination of the fetus, including fetal echocardiography, is essential because of the high incidence of associated intracranial and extracranial anomalies such as agenesis of the corpus callosum, neural tube defects, and cardiac anomalies, which ranges from 20% to 85%[11,17]. In addition, genetic amniocentesis is recommended because chromosomal abnormalities such as trisomy 21, trisomy 18, and mosaicism have been observed in about 10% of cases[11,16]. The incidence of chromosomal abnormalities increases with the presence of associated anomalies. The prognosis of congenital hydrocephalus depends mainly on the underlying pathology, the severity and progression of ventriculomegaly, and the presence of associated anomalies[18]. The cortical mantle thickness is not an accurate predictor of subsequent mental and neurologic development[19]. Normal intelligence and physical development have been reported in cases of severe hydrocephalus, especially those without severe associated anomalies[19,20]. Fetuses with mild ventriculomegaly (maximum LVW : HW ratio of 0.55) who do not require postnatal surgical intervention have an excellent chance of normal mental development[18]. Fetuses with unilateral hydrocephalus or aqueductal stenosis requiring postnatal ventri-culoperitoneal shunting have about 60% chance of normal mental development[15,18]. Ventriculomegaly by itself does not appear to predispose a fetus to intrauterine demise.

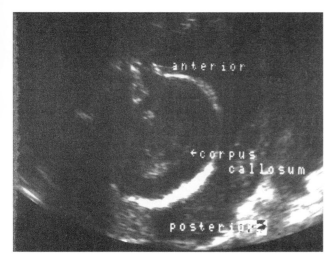

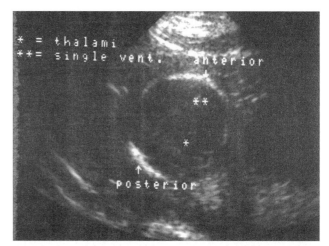

Figure 13 Sagittal view of a normal fetal brain at the midplane shows the corpus callosum as a curved echogenic band above the thalami

Figure 14 Holoprosencephaly. Coronal view of a fetal brain reveals a single ventricle and fused thalami

Severe associated anomalies account for the high perinatal mortality of up to 50% among continuing pregnancies. Intrapartum cephalocentesis is associated with perinatal mortality of more than 90%[20,21].

Pregnancy may continue to term if the ventriculomegaly is stable without macrocrania, otherwise delivery may be attempted at 34–36 weeks after fetal lung maturity is documented. Cesarean section is performed in the absence of lethal anomalies for obstetrical indications such as fetal distress, malpresentation or cephalopelvic disproportion from macrocrania. *In utero* ventriculoamniotic shunt is no longer performed because of the high procedure-related perinatal mortality of up to 10.25% and the uncertain benefit[22].

Agenesis of the corpus callosum

The corpus callosum connects the two cerebral hemispheres and can be visualized in either a sagittal or a coronal plane (Figure 13). Prenatal diagnosis of agenesis of the corpus callosum is possible after 4.0 months of gestation when it is usually completely developed[23,24]. Common ultrasonographic findings include: (1) ventriculomegaly of the lateral ventricles or third ventricle; (2) marked separation of the lateral ventricles; and (3) interposition of the dilated third ventricle between the lateral ventricles from upward displacement[23–25]. The complete fetal anatomy should be carefully assessed because of the commonly associated fetal anomalies[23–25]. The risk of chromosomal abnormalities with only agenesis of the corpus callosum is probably low. However, determination of fetal chromosomes is advisable especially if there are other associated anomalies. In a recent study, karyotyping was done on 12 fetuses who had agenesis of the corpus callosum; only one fetus with polydactyly had an abnormal

chromosome, trisomy 13[24]. Family history is important because it may be transmitted as X-linked recessive and autosomal recessive as a part of more complex syndromes[24,26]. Fetal prognosis depends on the associated chromosomal and structural abnormalities. Patients who have only complete agenesis of the corpus callosum are likely to develop normally[24,26]. Mental retardation and epilepsy are possible postnatal complications[26].

Holoprosencephaly

Holoprosencephaly arises from a failed cleavage of the primitive prosencephalon. The condition occurs in 1 : 16 000 liveborn infants and 1 : 250 induced abortions[27]. It is associated with chromosomal abnormalities (trisomy 13, trisomy 18, or triploidy), mendelian inheritance (autosomal dominant, autosomal recessive, or X-linked recessive) and diabetes[28,29]. The defective genes on which the defects, such as a deletion, may result in holoprosencephaly have been identified on chromosomes 2, 7, 18, and 21[29–31]. The phenotypic expression is quite variable. Three types of holoprosencephaly have been recognized: alobar, semilobar or lobar depending on the degree of cleavage of the prosencephalon[32]. In alobar holoprosencephaly there is a prominent single ventricle without the interhemispheric fissure, and fused thalami without the third ventricle[33] (Figures 14 and 15). Semilobar holoprosencephaly has a variable length of the posterior interhemispheric fissure[34]. In lobar holoprosencephaly, there may be only a mild lateral ventriculomegaly[35]. Detailed examination of the fetal anatomy, especially the face, is important because of the frequent association of other anomalies. Median facial defects such as cleft palate, cleft lip, cyclopia, anophthalmia, or proboscis nose are commonly present[36] (Figure 16). The severity of the mental retardation associated with holoprosencephaly varies, with the alobar type of

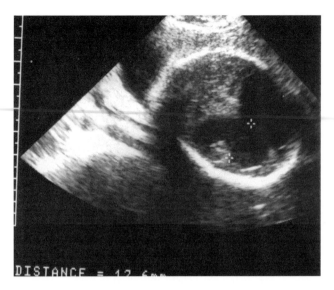

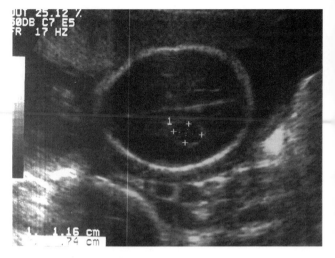

Figure 17   Unilateral choroid plexus cyst. Axial view of the fetal brain reveals a unilateral choroid plexus cyst

Figure 15   Holoprosencephaly. Axial view of the brain (the same fetus as in Figure 14) reveals a single ventricle (*)

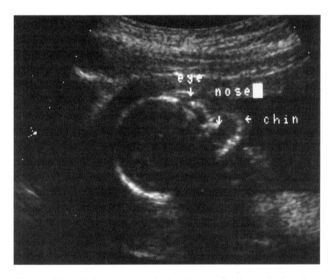

Figure 16   Holoprosencephaly. Coronal view of the face (the same fetus as in Figure 14) reveals many features associated with holoprosencephaly: hypotelorism, a peaked nose and a small chin

holoprosencephaly being the most severe, followed by semilobar then lobar ones. In fact, alobar holoprosencephaly is usually considered lethal. Genetic amniocentesis is recommended because of the increased risk of chromosomal abnormalities.

Choroid plexus cyst

A choroid plexus cyst is a well defined margin cyst in the choroid plexus of the lateral ventricles (Figure 17). The cysts can occur unilaterally or bilaterally in about 1% of fetuses who have ultrasound examinations during the second trimester[37,38]. The presence of a choroid

plexus cyst necessitates a detailed assessment of fetal structural anatomy because of the associated anomalies. Hydrocephalus, agenesis of the corpus callosum, cardiac defects (ventricular septal defect, single outflow tracts, complex heart defects, atrioventricular canal defect, and overriding aorta), esophageal atresia, and multicystic kidneys have been reported[37,38]. The incidence of chromosomal abnormalities in isolated choroid plexus cysts is up to 4% and does not appear to be affected by the size or bilaterality of the cysts[37,39]. Abnormal karyotypes associated with isolated choroid plexus cysts include trisomy 18, trisomy 21, and balanced translocation[25,37]. The presence of other associated anomalies increases the incidence of abnormal chromosomes in fetuses with choroid plexus up to 75% depending on the nature of associated anomalies[37,38]. About 94% of isolated choroid plexus cysts regress in 4–6 weeks[37,38]. Normal neonatal outcomes occur in all fetuses having isolated choroid plexus with normal chromosomes[37–40]. Chromosomal analysis could be offered to patients whose fetuses have isolated choroid plexus cysts. Some patients may prefer to have chromosomal analysis only if the choroid plexus cysts persist on a repeat ultrasound examination in 4–6 weeks since normal chromosomes are likely in this setting[40].

Neural tube defects

The neural tube is temporarily open during early normal embryogenesis. Failure of the neural tube to close gives rise to a variety of neural tube defects (NTDs), including anencephaly, encephalocele, and spina bifida. The incidence of NTDs is affected by ethnic background, gender and geography[41]. In the USA, the incidence of NTDs among caucasians is 1 to 3 per 1000 births. Females are more likely to be affected with female : male ratios up to 3 : 1 and 2 : 1 for anencephaly and spina bifida respectively. The gradual decline in the birth prevalence of NTDs has been attributed to widespread prenatal diagnosis, recent maternal intake of folate supplementation and other not yet identified environmental factors[41]. Neural tube defects is a multifactorial disorder with an overall recurrence risk of 2%. If one parent is affected, the risk of having a child with a NTD is about 1%[42–44]. Currently, screening for NTDs by maternal serum alpha-fetoprotein (MSAFP) is being routinely offered to pregnant women as part of prenatal care. Ultrasonography plays a very crucial role in the mass screening program by dating the pregnancy, ruling out multiple gestation or fetal demise, and ultimately detecting fetal anomalies[45]. It should be emphasized that the targeted (level II) ultrasound examination in order to confirm or rule out an NTD lesion or other anomalies should be performed by an experienced ultrasonographer, since diagnostic accuracy depends on experience[46]. At present, amniocentesis for amniotic AFP and acetylcholinesterase is often recommended to patients in whom no etiology can be found to account for the elevated MSAFP. Ultrasound examination alone could miss about 10% of open NTDs in patients with elevated MSAFP[47,48]. It remains to be determined if a detailed ultrasonographic examination of the fetus by an experienced ultrasonographer with improved equipment is sufficient for diagnostic purposes without resorting to the invasive amniocentesis procedure.

The risk of NTDs could be reduced with folate supplementation. A multi-center randomized double-blind study demonstrated that maternal intake of 4 mg of folic acid daily during the periconception period had a 72% protective effect of reducing the risk of NTDs in patients having had a previous pregnancy with a NTD. No apparent adverse maternal–fetal effects were noted[49]. Other non-randomized studies showed that maternal intake of 0.4–1.0 mg daily also reduced the risk of NTDs in patients without a prior NTD-affected pregnancy[50–52]. The United States Public Health Service recommends: (1) women who have had a previous NTD-affected pregnancy should take 4 mg of folic acid daily during the periconception period; and (2) all women of child-bearing age who are capable of becoming pregnant should consume 0.4 mg of folic acid daily[53]. It should be cautioned that taking 4 mg of folic acid daily may mask pernicious anemia, the latter caused by vitamin B12 deficiency.

Anencephaly

Anencephaly is a lethal condition characterized by the absence of the cranium and cerebral hemispheres (Figure 18). It occurs in 0.6 to 0.8 per 1000 live births[42]. The diagnosis can be made by 12 weeks and,

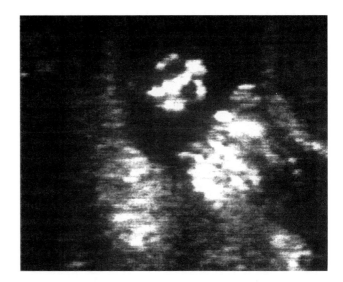

Figure 18 Anencephaly. Coronal view of the fetal head reveals absence of the cranium and cerebral hemispheres above the eyes

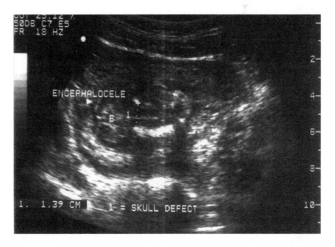

Figure 19 Encephalocele. Axial view of the fetal brain with occipital encephalocele reveals a skull defect through which the brain tissue (B) herniates

in some cases, even earlier by transvaginal ultrasonography. A normal crown–rump length measured during the first trimester may not exclude this condition[54]. Polyhydramnios is an almost constant finding.

Encephalocele

An encephalocele simply connotes the presence of brain tissue within a meningeal sac. The condition can be diagnosed by demonstrating a defect in the skull through which the meningeal sac containing intracranial tissue protrudes (Figure 19). When there is no brain tissue in the sac, the condition is called a meningocele. The occipital site is most commonly involved. The incidence of encephalocele is about 1 in

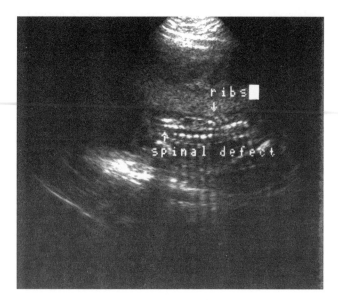

Figure 20 Spinal defect. Coronal view of the fetal spine reveals a defect involving the second and third sacral spines

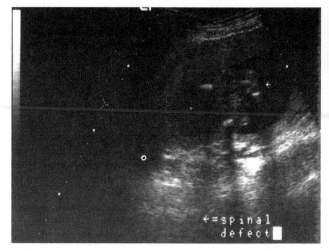

Figure 21 Open spinal defect. Axial view of the spine (the same fetus as in Figure 20) reveals splaying of the lateral processes without the covering skin

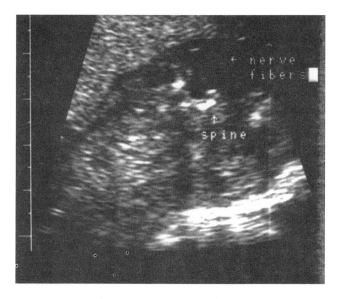

Figure 22 Myelomeningocele. This view demonstrates the presence of neural tissues extending from the open spinal defect into the sac of the myelomeningocele

2000 live births[55]. Encephalocele may be an isolated finding or part of a syndrome, such as Meckel's syndrome, an autosomal recessive condition with a recurrence risk of 25%[56]. Meckel's syndrome consists of encephalocele, polycystic kidneys, polydactyly, and a variety of other anomalies. Hydrocephalus is frequently associated with encephalocele. The prognosis is poor and depends on the degree of brain herniation. Lorber reported a mortality of 44% and 0% for encephalocele and occipital meningocele, respectively, in a 5 year study from 1959 to 1963[57]. Death was mainly attributed to affected vital medullar centers, meningitis, or other concomitant lethal anomalies. The incidence of mental or physical handicaps was higher among the survivors of encephalocele (80%) compared with the survivors of meningocele (40%)[57].

Spina bifida

Spina bifida is a condition in which there is an incomplete fusion of the vertebrae along the midline. The lesion can be further subdivided into closed (occult) or open (aperta) defects depending on whether or not there is intact soft tissue and skin over the lesion. The incidence of spina bifida aperta detected by MSAFP screening is about 1.5 per 1000 pregnancies[58,59]. Ultrasonographically, spina bifida is characterized by splaying of the lateral processes, which is apparent on coronal as well as cross-sectional planes (Figures 20 and 21). In myelomeningocele, the open defect is covered by the meningeal sac, which contains the neural tissue (Figure 22). Meningocele is simply a meningeal sac devoid of neural tissue. Hydrocephalus is commonly seen in spina bifida aperta, presumably due to

the obstruction of the cerebrospinal fluid circulation as a result of the downward displacement of the brain stem and cerebellar herniation into the cervical spinal column (a type II Arnold–Chiari malformation)[60,61]. The cistern magnum is thus affected. A normal cistern magnum is 4–9 mm in depth and is usually reduced in size, or obliterated in the presence of an open NTD[62]. Other cranial changes secondary to open spina bifida, such as scalloping of the frontal bones 'lemon sign' (Figure 23) at the BPD level and cerebellar abnormalities, have been described. The cerebellum is either absent or is reduced in size with increased anterior curvature 'banana sign'[63] (Figure 24). At a gestation age of

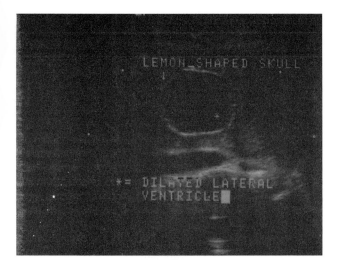

Figure 23 Open spina bifida. Axial view of the brain (the same fetus as in Figure 20) reveals the lemon-shaped skull and dilated lateral ventricles

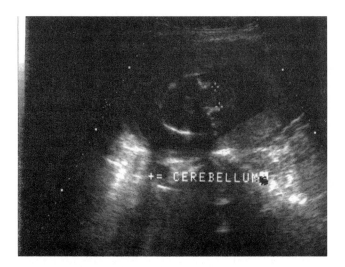

Figure 24 Open spina bifida. Axial view of the posterior fossa of the fetal brain reveals the 'banana sign' of the reduced-sized cerebellum

24 weeks or less, the positive predictive values of lemon sign and cerebellar changes in detecting an open NTD by ultrasonography are 92% and 100% respectively. Beyond 24 weeks of gestation, the positive predictive value of a lemon sign (Figure 23) or cerebellar changes in detecting an open NTD is 100%. While greater than 95% of fetuses with an open NTD demonstrate both the lemon sign and cerebellar changes at 24.0 weeks of gestation or less, only 13% and 91% of fetuses with open NTD show the lemon sign or cerebellar changes, respectively, at a later gestation. In addition, the banana sign is the main cerebellar abnormality seen at 24 weeks or less and absent cerebellum is usually seen at a later gestation[63].

The prognosis for infants with spina bifida depends on the type (open versus closed), the level, and the extent of the lesion, the presence of associated hydrocephalus or myelomeningocele, and the treatment utilized. The survival rates at 2 years of age for infants with spina bifida vary from 90% to 50%, depending on whether or not a concomitant hydrocephalus exists. The increased mortality associated with hydrocephalus is probably due to compression of the brain stem as a part of the Arnold–Chiari malformation. The best prognosis is associated with a low sacral lesion without coexisting hydrocephalus[64]. A retrospective study suggests that fetuses with meningocele without concomitant chromosomal abnormalities or other lethal structural anomalies have a better postnatal motor function if delivered by Cesarean section before the onset of labor. Severe hydrocephalus is defined as head circumferences of at least 4 standard deviations above the mean and cerebral mantle thickness of less than 1 cm[65,66]. However, the optimal mode of delivery for fetuses with open NTDs remains to be determined by a prospective randomized study.

CHEST

Diaphragmatic hernia

Diaphragmatic hernia occurs in a range of 1 per 2200 births to 1 per 5000 births[67]. There is a defect, usually 2–3 cm in diameter, in the diaphragm through which the abdominal viscera such as intestines, stomach, liver, spleen, pancreas, or kidneys herniate into the chest cavity. The defect occurs at one of the four locations on the diaphragm: posterolateral (80–90% of the cases), parasternal, central tendon, and esophageal orifice. The posterolateral defect (Bochdalek) involves the left, right or both sides in 80%, 15% and 5% of the cases, respectively[67–70]. The heart may be shifted within the chest. Congenital diaphragmatic hernia (CDH) occurs sporadically and is transmitted as a multifactorial inheritance with a recurrence risk of about 2%[71]. Familial cases have been reported[72,73]. Associated structural anomalies may occur up to 95% of stillborn and 20% of liveborn infants with CDH and may involve many systems such as the nervous system, gastrointestinal system, skeletal system, cardiovascular system and genitourinary system[68,69,74]. In addition, there are also associated chromosomal abnormalities such as trisomy 21, trisomy 18, or trisomy 13 which occur in about 16% of cases[70,74,75]. The condition can be prenatally diagnosed by an ultrasound examination demonstrating the presence of an abdominal organ and usually the shifting of the heart within the chest (Figures 25, 26 and 27). Peristalsis of the intestines may be visualized. In right-sided CDH, the only ultrasound finding may be the presence of the gallbladder in the chest[76]. Herniation of the liver into the chest makes the primary closure of the defect more difficult with

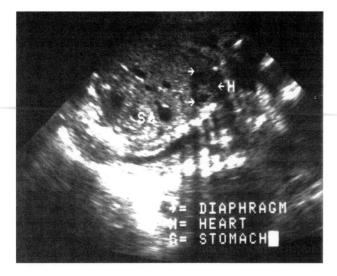

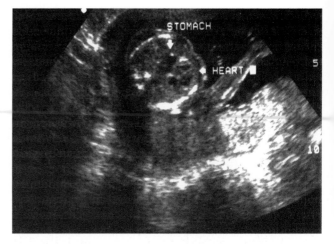

Figure 25 Coronal view of the fetal body shows the diaphragm separating the chest from the abdomen. The stomach is located in the left side of the abdomen below the heart

Figure 27 Congenital diaphragmatic hernia. Axial view of the chest (the same fetus as in Figure 26) reveals the presence of the stomach next to the heart inside the chest

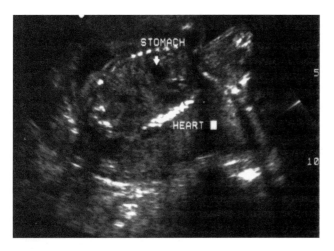

Figure 26 Congenital diaphragmatic hernia. Coronal view of the fetal body reveals the stomach is inside the chest above the diaphragm

potential kinking of the umbilical vessels causing fetal bradycardia and fetal demise[77]. The presence of the stomach in posterior or midthoracic regions of the chest or coursing of the portal vein toward the diaphragm predicts the presence of liver herniation with 100% accuracy[77]. Polyhydramnios, probably arising from the obstruction of the gastrointestinal tract, is often present. Fetal prognosis depends on the presence of associated anomalies, the timing of herniation and the volume of the abdominal viscera in the chest. Pulmonary hypertension and pulmonary hypoplasia are the major cause of neonatal death[78]. Dismal prognosis is associated with a herniation of a large volume of abdominal organs into the chest at an early

gestational age[67]. The prognostic value of polyhydramnios remains to be determined. While some investigators found polyhydramnios associated with much higher perinatal mortality, others have not found it to be a useful predictor of perinatal outcomes[75,79,80]. The overall perinatal mortality is about 75%[75,79]. Once the diagnosis of CDH is made, a detailed assessment of fetal anatomy and determination of fetal chromosomes are recommended. Although open fetal surgery has been successfully attempted[67,81], the role of fetal surgery in the treatment of CDH requires much further investigation. CHD *per se* is not an indication for Cesarean section. Delivery at a tertiary care center is strongly recommended so that surgical and medical intervention can be promptly initiated.

Chylothorax

Isolated pleural effusion can result from erythroblastosis fetalis or from nonimmune causes such as infection, or chylothorax. Pleural effusion can be demonstrated by ultrasound examination as a sonolucent area within the chest (Figure 28). Chylothorax exists if more than 80% of cells in the pleural fluid are lymphocytes. The pleural fluid can be obtained by fetal thoracentesis. The overall perinatal mortality is 53%[82]. Mild isolated chylothorax may resolve spontaneously. Severe chylothorax may necessitate decompression by intermittent thoracentesis or thoracoamniotic shunt to minimize the potential pulmonary hypoplasia[82,83]. The latter may be considered when pleural effusion rapidly reaccumulates after thoracentesis. We have seen cases of unilateral pleural effusion resolved after only one or two fetal thoracenteses with excellent neonatal outcomes. Serial ultrasound examinations to assess the progression of the pleural effusion are recommended. Thoracentesis before delivery may facilitate the postnatal

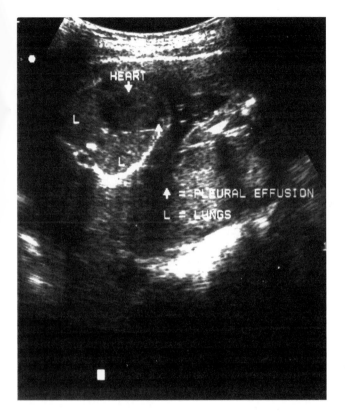

Figure 28 Axial view of the fetal chest shows unilateral pleural effusion appearing as a sonolucent area at the costophrenic angle

resuscitation. Chylothorax is not an indication for Cesarean section delivery.

Abdominal wall defects

The two common anterior ventral wall defects are omphalocele and gastroschisis. Both are associated with elevation of MSAFP and amniotic fluid AFP. The sensitivity for detecting omphalocele and gastroschisis by MSAFP are 42% and 77%, respectively. The sensitivity of detecting either of the conditions by amniotic fluid AFP is 93%[84]. Since other associated anomalies, such as NTDs and cardiac and gastrointestinal abnormalities can exist, detailed ultrasonographic examination of the fetus is indicated. The risk of abdominal wall defects from elevated MSAFP is much reduced after a normal detailed ultrasound examination by an experienced ultrasonographer[85]. This information may be useful to the patients in deciding whether to undergo a genetic amniocentesis for elevated MSAFP. The optimal route of delivery remains controversial. A recent retrospective study demonstrated that there was no significant difference in neonatal outcomes such as necrotizing enterocolitis, meconium aspiration, sepsis, respiratory distress syndrome, staged abdominal closure, Apgar scores at five minutes and mortality

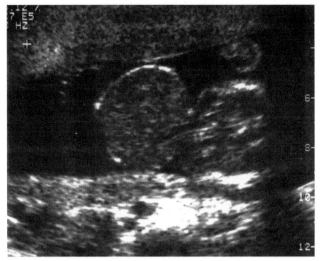

Figure 29 Omphalocele. Axial view of the fetal abdomen reveals the abdominal wall defect through which the liver and intestines herniate. The herniated organs are contained within the amnioperitoneal sac

between infants delivered by the vaginal route and those delivered by Cesarean section. Fetuses with extracorporeal liver were excluded from the study[86]. We perform Cesarean section when a large abdominal wall defect with herniation of many major abdominal organs such as the liver is present. Accurate prenatal diagnosis, prompt surgical intervention, and the availability of total parenteral nutrition all have a beneficial impact on the perinatal mortality and morbidity associated with these two ventral wall defects.

Omphalocele

Omphalocele is defined as an amnioperitoneal sac that contains herniated intra-abdominal organs. The condition results from a defective embryonic body folding. The incidence of omphalocele varies from 0.2 to 0.4 per 1000 live births[87,88]. The diagnosis of omphalocele can be made by demonstrating the herniated abdominal organs being covered by the amnioperitoneal membranes into which the umbilical cord is inserted (Figure 29). An incidence of associated congenital structural anomalies, such as cardiac, genitourinary, and NTD and chromosomal abnormalities, of up to 64% and 37% of cases, respectively, has been reported[84,88]. Amniocentesis for karyotyping is indicated when omphalocele is prenatally diagnosed. The prognosis for infants with omphalocele depends primarily on the severity of the coexisting anomalies. A mortality of 12% for isolated omphalocele has been noted. The causes of death include respiratory distress syndrome, subarachnoid hemorrhage, volvulus and peritonitis, meconium aspiration, and unknown cardiorespiratory arrest[89].

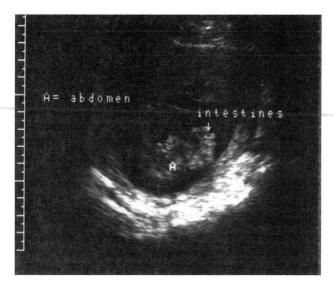

Figure 30   Gastroschisis. Axial view of the fetal abdomen reveals the free loops of intestines extruding from the abdomen. The free loops of intestines appear like 'cauliflower'

Gastroschisis

Gastroschisis implies a ventral abdominal wall defect through when the abdominal organs prolapse. The defect involves the whole thickness of the abdominal wall and is usually situated to the right of the normally inserted umbilical cord. *In utero* interruption to the omphalomesenteric artery has been proposed to explain the constellation of findings associated with gastroschisis[90]. The incidence of gastroschisis is about 0.1 per 1000 live births[87,88]. Diagnosis of gastroschisis should be considered on visualizing the free loops of intestines floating in the amniotic sac (Figure 30). Differentiation between a ruptured omphalocele and gastroschisis is not always possible. Involvement of the liver usually occurs with the former condition. In contrast to omphalocele, gastroschisis is associated with a lower incidence of concomitant anomalies (5 to 38%), increased incidence of chromosomal abnormality, and lower mortality rate (7.7 to 27%)[84,88,89]. Gastroschisis is not associated with an increased incidence of chromosomal abnormalities. Intestinal complications, such as perforation, multiple bowel atresia, and infection, are the major causes of perinatal mortality and morbidity. Serial ultrasound examinations are recommended to monitor the fetal growth because of the high incidence of intrauterine growth restriction and the status of the bowels[88].

OBSTRUCTION

Ultrasonography provides a new dimension in the dynamic evaluation of the gastrointestinal tract. Fetal swallowing and intestinal motility can be readily assessed. Polyhydramnios usually occurs when there is a mechanical or functional obstruction to the flow of the amniotic fluid through the upper gastrointestinal tract. Severe polyhydramnios can cause preterm labor and significant maternal discomfort. Therapeutic amniocentesis may be necessary. The prognosis of a variety of obstructive lesions of the digestive tract depends on the presence of associated structural and chromosomal anomalies and prematurity. Surgical correction of these lesions is feasible during the neonatal period. At present, ultrasonography is the only non-invasive and safe means for the prenatal diagnosis of digestive tract obstruction.

Esophageal atresia

Esophageal atresia occurs as result of maldevelopment of the rostral portion of the foregut, which gives rise to both the trachea and the esophagus. As a consequence, esophageal atresia is almost always associated with one of the forms of tracheoesophageal fistula. The incidence of esophageal atresia with tracheoesophageal fistula is about 1 per 2500 births[91]. Esophageal atresia should be suspected when polyhydramnios coexists with a non-visualized stomach. If there is a tracheoesophageal fistula, a stomach can be usually seen. Since there is an increased incidence of associated structural and chromosomal abnormalities, a thorough examination of the fetus and genetic amniocentesis are indicated.

Duodenal atresia

Duodenal atresia can arise from failure of the lumen to recanalize, compression from the annular pancreas, or occlusion of the vascular supply to the duodenum[92]. The incidence of duodenal atresia is 1 per 10 000 live births[93]. The diagnosis of duodenal atresia is supported by the presence of a connecting double-bubble sign on cross section image of the abdomen, representing the distended stomach and the proximal duodenum (Figure 31)[94]. Increased peristalsis can usually be observed in the distended organs. There is a high incidence of associated anomalies in this condition with the more commonly affected organs being the heart, vertebral column, intestine, and kidneys. Down syndrome is present in 30% of the cases[95]. The prognosis is excellent if other anomalies are not present.

Intestinal atresia or stenosis

Intestinal atresia or stenosis is another common cause of bowel obstruction that can be prenatally diagnosed. Atresia of the intestine is about 20 times as common as stenotic lesions. The colon is rarely involved[96]. Ischemia has been proposed as the cause of congenital intestinal atresia[97]. Similar lesions have been produced by interrupting the blood supply to the intestine of fetal dogs. Further evidence to support this theory includes failure to observe the solid stage in the intestine beyond the duodenum during embryogenesis and

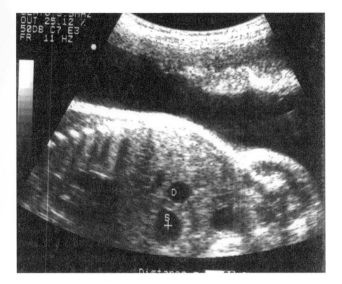

Figure 31 Duodenal atresia. Coronal view of the fetal abdomen reveals the 'double-bubble' sign representing the dilated stomach (S) and duodenum (D)

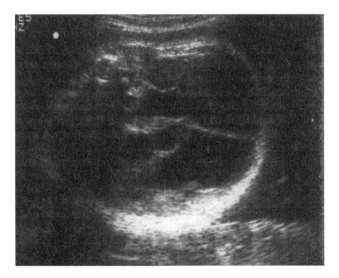

Figure 32 Intestinal atresia. Axial view of the fetal abdomen with obstruction of the small intestines reveals multiple loops of dilated, thick-walled small intestines

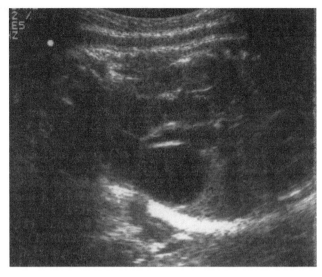

Figure 33 Intestinal atresia. Coronal view of the abdomen with obstruction of the small intestines (same fetus as in Figure 32) reveals multiple loops of dilated, thick-walled small intestines

observation of bile in the meconium in some cases of intestinal atresia[97,98]. This theory cannot account for all the cases of intestinal atresia because patent vessels feeding the atretic segment of the intestine have been demonstrated[99]. The incidence of small intestine atresia or stenosis varies from 1/1000 to 1/5000 live births while that of colon atresia or stenosis is 1/20 000 live births[100]. The diagnosis of intestinal atresia or stenosis should be considered when multiple dilated loops of bowel are present (Figures 32 and 33). Associated polyhydramnios may contribute to preterm labor and delivery. Genetic amniocentesis is not indicated for simple intestinal atresia or stenosis because concomitant chromosomal abnormalities are not generally seen. Serial ultrasound examinations are indicated to evaluate the status of the intestine. The prognosis depends on the type and extent of intestinal atresia, gestational age, and associated anomalies. The advent of hyperalimentation has significantly contributed to the reduced mortality and morbidity associated with this condition. A 100% survival rate for intestinal atresia without concomitant cystic fibrosis has been reported[101].

URINARY TRACT

Ultrasonography provides an invaluable tool to evaluate the fetal urinary tract. The fetal kidneys can be visualized by the 10th week of gestation[102]. Early in pregnancy, they appear as two oval hypoechogenic structures on either side of the spine. As pregnancy advances, the cortex, the renal echogenic parenchyma, and the sonolucent pelvis can be readily differentiated (Figure 5). The kidneys enlarge with advancing gestational age, and the renal circumference to abdominal circumference ratio remains somewhat constant at about 0.30 throughout gestation[103]. The ureters are normally not visible, and the bladder appears as a sonolucent structure in the fetal pelvis and can be recognized consistently by 12 weeks[102]. Serial examinations 30 minutes apart may be necessary to identify the bladder, since the fetus voids about every 60 minutes. Furthermore, since complete emptying of the bladder occurs infrequently, the bladder should be visualized during the period of examination most of the time[104]. The amniotic fluid is a dialysate of fetal blood until about 17 weeks of gestation when keratinization of the fetal skin begins. During early gestation, the fetal skin is readily permeable to water, and concentrations of sodium and urea are similar to those of fetal serum[105]. Keratinization of the fetal skin is complete by 25 weeks gestation[106]. The fetal kidneys start to produce urine and demonstrate the ability to reabsorb sodium from urine as early as 12 weeks of gestation[105]. After 17 weeks, urine production significantly contributes to the volume of amniotic fluid. Near term, the urine output increases linearly from 12.2 ml/h at 32 weeks to 28.2 ml/h at 40 weeks' gestation[104].

Detailed examination of the fetal urinary tract should be carried out whenever oligohydramnios is present. Pulmonary hypoplasia may result from oligohydramnios and is the major cause of perinatal mortality and morbidity associated with urinary tract abnormality[107]. Other factors may play a role in the pathogenesis of pulmonary hypoplasia, at least in the case of bilateral renal agenesis, where a reduction in airway development has been reported[108]. This observation suggests an insult to lung development between 12 and 16 weeks of gestation, when oligohydramnios is not a major factor. A brief review of different urinary tract abnormalities, such as bilateral renal agenesis, multicystic kidney disease, infantile polycystic kidney disease, and obstructive uropathy is discussed in the following sections.

Bilateral renal agenesis

Bilateral renal agenesis (BRA) is a lethal condition resulting from defective development of the kidneys during embryogenesis. It can occur as an isolated anomaly or as part of a multiple anomaly syndrome. The classic Potter's syndrome consists of BRA, pulmonary hypoplasia, unusual facial features, and abnormal positioning of the hands and feet. The severe oligohydramnios in BRA has been implicated as the cause of Potter's syndrome[109].

The incidence of bilateral renal agenesis ranges from 0.1 to 0.3 per 1000 births, with a male to female ratio of 2.5 : 1[110,111]. The recurrence risk for isolated BRA is 3.5%[110]. The diagnosis can be made by demonstrating the absence of fetal kidneys, a non-visualized bladder, and oligohydramnios[112]. Visualization of the kidneys in the presence of severe oligohydramnios can be very difficult and may be facilitated by instillation of warm saline. A potential pitfall in diagnosis of BRA is the tendency to mistake adrenals for kidneys (Figure 34). Administration of furosemide to the mother to induce fetal diuresis has been suggested to assess fetal renal function. However, false-negative results have been reported with this test, and there is some suggestion that the diuretic crosses the placenta poorly[113].

Infantile polycystic kidney disease

Infantile polycystic kidney disease (IPKD), or Potter's type I cystic dysplasia, is another form of renal tubular

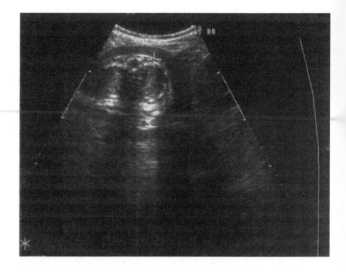

Figure 34   Renal agenesis. Axial view of the fetal abdomen reveals absent kidneys and prominent adrenal glands. This fetus also has oligohydramnios

maldevelopment during embryogenesis. The incidence of IPKD is 2 per 100 000 births[114]. It is an autosomal recessive disease with a recurrence risk of 25%. Infantile polycystic kidney disease may be a part of Meckel's syndrome, which, in addition, mainly consists of occipital encephalocele and postaxial polydactyly. Prenatal diagnosis of IPKD by ultrasonography before the 24th week of gestation has been reported, and the typical ultrasound features may not emerge until after the 20th week of gestation[115,116]. The ultrasonographic features include hyperechogenic, enlarged kidneys, oligohydramnios, and non-visualized bladder[116] (Figure 35). The hyperechogenicity reflects the presence of multiple microcysts as a result of proliferation and dilatation of renal proximal tubules. Progressive enlargement of these kidneys has been observed. The prognosis of IPKD is generally lethal.

Multicystic kidneys

Multicystic kidney disease (MKD), or Potter's type II cystic dysplasia, arises from a developmental abnormality of the renal tubules and is manifested as cystic changes throughout the kidneys. The incidence of bilateral MKD is about 1 per 10 000 births, with a very low recurrence rate. The diagnosis of MKD should be considered when cysts of variable shapes and sizes are present throughout the renal parenchyma, with the largest usually located in the periphery (Figure 36)[117–119]. Since the affected kidney is non-functional, bilateral MKD is a lethal condition associated with oligohydramnios and non-visualized bladder. About two thirds of the patients with unilateral MKD have either a pathologic contralateral kidney or other associated anomalies. Hypertension may develop in patients who have unilateral MKD[120].

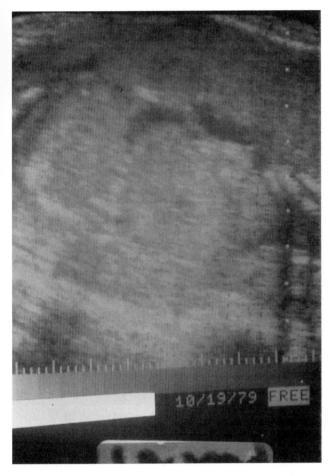

Figure 35 Infantile polycystic kidney. Axial view of the fetal abdomen reveals bilateral enlarged, echogenic kidneys

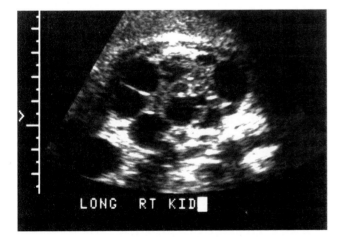

Figure 36 Multicystic kidney. Longitudinal view of the fetal abdomen reveals multiple cysts of variable shapes and sizes scattered throughout the right kidney's parenchyma

Obstructive uropathy

Obstructive uropathy usually occurs at three levels, the uteropelvic junction (UPJ), the uterovesical junction

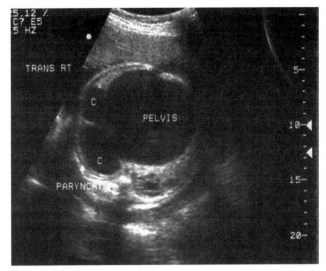

Figure 37 Grade 4 hydronephrosis with cystic dysplasia. Axial view of the fetal abdomen reveals cysts extending from the dilated renal pelvis as result of ureteropelvic junction obstruction. The parenchyma is thin

(UVJ), and the urethra. Dilatation of the urinary tract proximal to the obstructive site will ensue, and type IV cystic dysplasia may develop. Ultrasonographically, type IV cystic dysplasia is characterized by the presence of multiple cysts radiating from the dilated pelvis (Figure 37). Differentiation between type II and severe type IV cystic dysplasia is not always possible, however. The concomitant distended bladder and/or dilated ureter would support the diagnosis of the latter. The ureter and urethra are not usually visible unless they become dilated because of obstruction. It should be noted that the ureters can be dilated to an enormous size, resulting in abdominal distention. A possible mechanism of obstructive uropathy is a defective recanalization of the ureters resulting partial UPJ or UVJ obstruction[121].

The prognosis of infants with obstructive uropathy depends on the degree of hydronephrosis and cystic dysplasia of the kidneys, which are in turn affected by the timing, the duration, and the severity of the obstruction. The Society for Fetal Urology has proposed a system of grading hydronephrosis for postnatal evaluation of fetal hydronephrosis, based on the degree of the dilatation of the renal pelvis and calyces on the longitudinal view of the kidney[122]. This system may be used to grade fetal hydronephrosis prenatally. Grade 0 has no splitting of the normally echogenic central renal complex (CRC). Grade 1 has minimal splitting of CRC (Figure 38), right kidney. Grade 0 and 1 are considered to be normal. Grade 2 has splitting of CRC confined to the renal pelvis, and a few calyces (Figure 39). Grade 3 has thick renal parenchyma (more than 1/2 of the parenchyma of the normal kidney) and dilatation of the renal pelvis and all calyces (Figure 40). Grade 4 has thin renal parenchyma (< 1/2 of the parenchyma

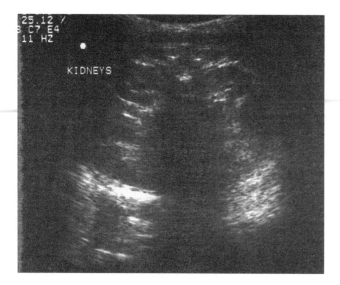

Figure 38 Hydronephrosis. Axial view of the fetal abdomen reveals mild dilatation of the renal pelvis with intact calyces of the right kidney

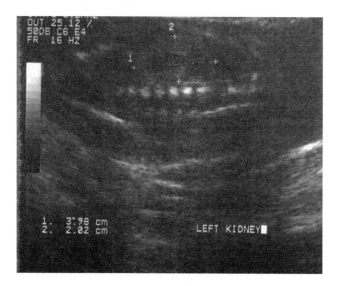

Figure 39 Grade 2 hydronephrosis. Longitudinal view of the fetal abdomen reveals dilatation of the renal pelvis, not renal calyces, from partial ureteropelvic junction obstruction

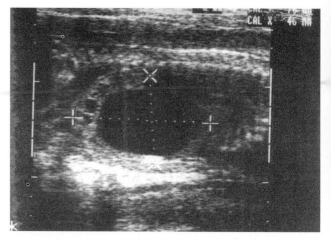

Figure 40 Grade 3 hydronephrosis. Longitudinal view of the fetal abdomen reveals severe dilated renal pelvis and development of multiple cysts in the renal cortex as a result of ureteropelvic junction obstruction

of the normal kidney) and dilatation of the renal pelvis and calyces (Figure 37).

The overall renal prognosis for either UPJ or UVJ obstruction is good. In most cases, conservative management is appropriate and immediate postnatal surgery is seldom indicated[123,124]. Irreversible renal damage may occur if there is complete obstruction before 20 weeks of gestation[125,126]. The presence of oligohydramnios and severe cystic dysplasia denotes a very poor prognosis, whereas a normal amount of amniotic fluid and mild hydronephrosis are associated with good outcomes[125,127]. The appearance of renal

cortical cysts (Figure 40) implies dismal renal function with a sensitivity and specificity of 44% and 100%, respectively[128]. Analysis of urine obtained from the fetal bladder by percutaneous cystocentesis can provide valuable prognostic information. Poor renal function is associated with fetal urine sodium, chloride concentrations, and osmolarity of > 100 mEq/ml, > 90 mEq/ml, and > 210 mOsm, respectively. These values probably reflect the kidney's inability to reabsorb sodium, chloride, and other electrolytes. Lower levels of these parameters indicate better outcomes[126]. Interestingly, proton nuclear magnetic resonance spectroscopy of the fetal urine amino acids valine, alanine, and threonine appears to better differentiate fetuses with normal renal function from those with abnormal renal function[129]. The prognosis also depends on the presence of associated extraurinary anomalies and chromosomal abnormality, with the incidence ranging from 28 to 50% and from 8 to 23%, respectively[114,125,130]. Trisomy 13 and trisomy 18 are the two most common chromosomal abnormalities observed. Genetic amniocentesis and a detailed ultrasonographic examination of the fetus are indicated when severe obstructive uropathy is detected. Serial ultrasound examinations are necessary to evaluate the progression of hydronephrosis and renal status.

The obstetric management of patients whose fetuses have stable obstructive uropathy accompanied by a good prognosis should not be altered. In other situations, perinatal care should be individualized. *In utero* treatment of obstructive uropathy has been attempted with percutaneous placement of a chronic vesicoamniotic shunt. This procedure would not benefit fetuses with vesicourethral reflux. The procedure-related perinatal mortality is 4%. Improved survival rates are noted for the prune-belly syndrome and posterior

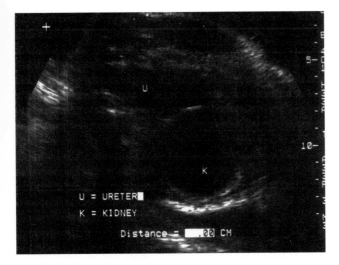

Figure 41 Ureterovesical junction obstruction. Longitudinal view of the fetal abdomen reveals dilated ureter (U) and grade 4 hydronephrosis with severely dilated renal pelvis (K)

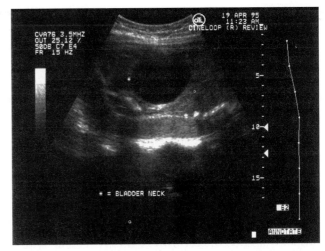

Figure 43 Posterior urethral valve. Coronal section of the fetal abdomen reveals dilated bladder (cystic structure in the center) and dilated urethra at the bladder neck (*)

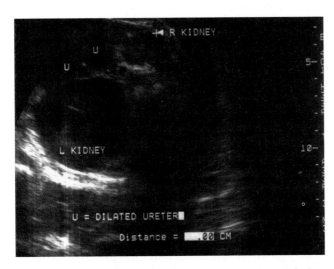

Figure 42 Ureterovesical junction obstruction. Axial view of the fetal abdomen (same fetus as in Figure 41) reveals severely dilated renal pelvis and dilated ureter (U)

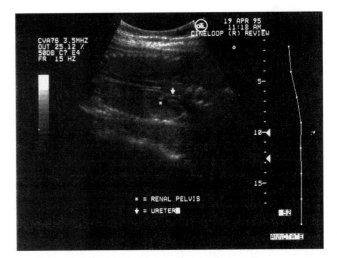

Figure 44 Posterior urethral valve. Longitudinal view of the fetal abdomen (same fetus as in Figure 43) reveals dilated renal pelvis (*) and ureter

urethral valve syndrome[22]. Vesicoamniotic shunts may reduce the perinatal mortality and morbidity in selected cases of obstructive uropathy.

Ureteropelvic junction obstruction

UPJ obstruction is characterized by pelvic dilatation and/or type IV cystic dysplasia of the kidneys. It occurs unilaterally in about 90% of the cases, with the left kidney being involved twice as frequently as the right one. The male to female sex ratio is about 2.0 : 1[131]. The risk of recurrence is low because it is a sporadic

event in most cases. The etiology of UPJ obstruction remains unclear. Functional rather than mechanical abnormality accounts for most cases of UPJ obstruction. At the UPJ area, excessive collagen fibers between constantly contracted smooth muscle cells have been observed with electron microscopy[132]. The natural history of unilateral UPJ obstruction is generally benign[133]. About 85% of fetuses with unilateral UPJ have a good renal function without postnatal surgical intervention[133]. Furthermore, renal function improves after elective pyeloplasty in the remaining cases[133]. The renal prognosis of bilateral UPJ obstruction depends on other factors as mentioned above.

Ureterovesical junction obstruction

Obstruction at the UVJ is characterized by dilatation of the ureters and/or renal pelvis (Figures 41 and 42). A type IV cystic dysplasia of the kidneys may occur in a long-standing obstruction. The obstruction at this level is most likely due to a developmental rather than an extrinsic problem[134,135]. The prognosis, the recurrence risk, and perinatal management of this condition are similar to those of UPJ obstruction.

Posterior urethral valve

Posterior urethral valve denotes the presence of a membranous structure in the posterior wall of the urethra. It accounts for 36% of the cases of obstructive uropathy and occurs exclusively in male fetuses[125]. Any of the following ultrasonographic features – dilated bladder, hydroureter, hydronephrosis, and type IV cystic dysplasia – may occur singly or in combination, depending on the timing, duration, and severity of the obstruction (Figures 43 and 44).

Vesicoureteral reflux

Vesicoureteral reflux can occur either unilaterally or bilaterally and account for about 25% of cases of fetal hydronephrosis[123]. Prenatal ultrasonographic findings of vesicoureteral reflux include dilated ureters, and/or dilated renal pelves and type IV cystic dysplasia of the kidneys similar to those of UVJ obstruction. The diagnosis can only be made postnatally with a voiding cystourethrogram. Postnatal management consists of prophylactic antibiotics to prevent urinary tract infection, expectant management with possible spontaneous resolution of the hydronephrosis, reimplantation of the ureters, or nephrectomy for non-functional kidneys[123].

CONCLUSION

Ultrasonography has made a significant contribution to our much greater understanding of the complex, intricate life *in utero*. There remain many questions and challenges ahead of us that require further investigation. These include prenatal diagnosis of congenital anomalies at the earlier stage of pregnancy, *in utero* therapeutic intervention for congenital hydrocephalus and twin-to-twin transfusion, and a deeper understanding of human fetal physiology in healthy and disease states; undoubtedly, ultrasonography continues to play an essential role in this human endeavor.

REFERENCES

1. Denkhaus H, Winsberg F. Ultrasonic measurement of the fetal ventricular system. *Radiology* 1979;131:781–7
2. Jeanty P, Dramaix-Wilmet M, Delbeke D, *et al.* Ultrasonic evaluation of fetal ventricular growth. *Neuroradiology* 1981;21:127–31
3. Shapiro K. Hydrocephaly. In Buyse ML, ed. *Birth Defects Encyclopedia*. 1st ed. Cambridge, MA: Blackwell Scientific Publications, Inc., 1990:887–8
4. Chinn DH, Callen PW, Filly RA. The lateral cerebral ventricle in early second trimester. *Radiology* 1983;148:529–31
5. Bronshtein M, Ben-Shlomo I. Choroid plexus dysmorphism detected by transvaginal sonography: the earliest sign of fetal hydrocephalus. *J Clin Ultrasound* 1991;19:547–53
6. Burton BK. Recurrence risks for congenital hydrocephalus. *Clin Genet* 1979;16:47–53
7. Benke P, Strassbel LR. Prenatal study of X-linked aqueductal stenosis. *J Med Genet* 1980;17:158
8. Brocard O, Ragage C, Vilbert M, *et al.* Prenatal diagnosis of X-linked hydrocephalus. *J Clin Ultrasound* 1993;21:211–4
9. Bickers DS, Adams RD. Hereditary stenosis of the aqueduct of Sylvius as a cause of congenital. *Brain* 1949;72:246
10. Holmes LB, Nash A, Zurhein GM, *et al.* X-linked aqueductal stenosis: clinical and neuropathological findings in two families. *Pediatrics* 1973;51:697–704
11. Pilu G, Rizzo N, Orsini LF, *et al.* Antenatal recognition of cerebral anomalies. *Ultrasound Med Biol* 1986;12:319–26
12. Hirsch JF, Pierre-Kahn A, Renier D, *et al.* The Dandy-Walker malformation: a review of 40 cases. *J Neurosurg* 1984;61:515–22
13. Russ PD, Pretorius DH, Johnson MD. Dandy-Walker syndrome. A review of fifteen cases evaluated by prenatal sonography. *Am J Obstet Gynecol* 1989;161:401–6
14. Estroff JA, Scott MR, Benacerraf BR. Dandy-Walker variant: prenatal sonographic features and clinical outcome. *Radiology* 1992;185:755–8
15. Patten RM, Mack LA, Finberg HJ. Unilateral hydrocephalus: prenatal sonographic diagnosis. *AJR Am J Roentgenol* 1991;156:359–63
16. Chervenak FA, Berkowitz RL, Romero R, *et al.* The diagnosis of fetal hydrocephalus. *Am J Obstet Gynecol* 1983;147:703–16
17. Chervenak FA, Berkowitz RL, Tortora M, *et al.* Diagnosis of ventriculomegaly before fetal viability. *Obstet Gynecol* 1984;64:652
18. Drugan A, Krause B, Zador IE, *et al.* The natural history of prenatally diagnosed cerebral ventriculomegaly. *J Am Med Assoc* 1989;261:1785–8
19. Lorber J. The results of early treatment of extreme hydrocephalus. *Dev Med Child Neurol* 1968;16(suppl):21–9
20. Chervenak FA, Duncan C, Ment LR, *et al.* Outcome of fetal ventriculomegaly. *Lancet* 1984;2:179–81
21. Chervenak FA, Berkowitz RL, Tortora M, *et al.* The management of fetal hydrocephalus. *Am J Obstet Gynecol* 1985;151:933–42
22. Manning FA. International fetal surgery registry: 1985 update. *Clin Obstet Gynecol* 1986;29:551–7
23. Loeser JD, Alvord EC Jr. Agenesis of the corpus callosum. *Brain* 1968;91:553–70
24. Patrizia V, Alessandro G, Strobelt N, *et al.* Prognostic indicators in the prenatal diagnosis of agenesis of the corpus callosum. *Am J Obstet Gynecol* 1994;170:753–8

25. Gebarski SS, Gebarski KS, Bowerman RA, *et al*. Agenesis of the corpus callosum: sonographic Features. *Radiology* 1984;151:443–8

26. Loeser JD, Alvord EC Jr. Clinicopathological correlations in agenesis of the corpus callosum. *Neurology* 1968;18:745–56

27. Cohen MM Jr. Perspectives on holoprosencephaly: Part 1. Epidemiology, genetics, and syndromology. *Teratology* 1989;40:211–35

28. Munke M. Clinical, cytogenetic, and molecular approaches to the genetic heterogeneity of holoprosencephaly. *Am J Med Genet* 1989;34:237–45

29. Munke M, Emanuel BS, Zakai EH. Holoprosencephaly: association with intestitial deletion of 2p and review of the cytogenetic literature. *Am J Med Genet* 1988; 30:929–38

30. Frezal J, Schinzel A. Report of the committee on clinical disorders, chromosomes aberrations, and uniparental disomy. *Cytogenet Cell Genet* 1991;58:986–1052

31. Gurrieri F, Trask BJ, van den Engh G, *et al*. Physical mapping of the holoprosencephaly critical region on chromosome 7q36. *Nature Genet* 1993;3:247–51

32. DeMyer W. Classification of cerebral malformations. *Birth Defects* 1971;7:78–93

33. Filly RA, Chinn DH, Callen PW. Alobar holoprosencephaly: ultrasonographic prenatal diagnosis. *Radiology* 1984;151:455–9

34. Cayea PD, Balcar I, Alberti O, *et al*. Prenatal diagnosis of semilobar holoprosencephaly. *AJR Am J Roentgenol* 1984;142:401–2

35. Hoffman-Tretin JC, Horoupian DS, Koenigsberg M, *et al*. Lobar holoprosencephaly with hydrocephalus: antenatal demonstration and differential diagnosis. *J Ultrasound Med* 1986;5:691–7

36. DeMyer W, Zeman W, Palmer CG. The face predicts the brain: diagnostic significance of median facial anomalies for holoprosencephaly (arhinencephaly). *Pediatrics* 1964;34:256

37. Kupferminc MJ, Tamura RK, Sabbagha RE, *et al*. Isolated choroid plexus cyst(s): an indication for amniocentesis. *Am J Obstet Gynecol* 1994;171:1068–71

38. Platt LD, Carlson DE, Medearis AL, *et al*. Fetal choroid plexus cysts in the second trimester of pregnancy: a cause for concern. *Am J Obstet Gynecol* 1991;164:1652–6

39. Nadel AS, Bromley BS, Frigoletto FD Jr, *et al*. Isolated choroid plexus cysts in the second-trimester fetus: is amniocentesis really indicated? *Radiology* 1992; 185:545–8

40. Clark SL, DeVore GR, Sabey PL. Prenatal diagnosis of cysts of the fetal choroid plexus. *Obstet Gynecol* 1988; 72:585–7

41. Yen IH, Khoury MJ, Erickson D, *et al*. The changing epidemiology of neural tube defects: United States, 1968–1989. *Am J Dis Child* 1992;146:857–61

42. Alter M. Anencephalus, hydrocephalus and spina bifida. Epidemiology with special reference to a survey in Charleston, S.C., *Arch Neurol* 1962;7:411

43. Cohn HE, Sacks EJ. Cardiovascular response to hypoxemia and acidemia in fetal lambs. *Am J Obstet Gynecol* 1974;120:817–24

44. Milunsky A. Prenatal detection of neural tube defects. VI. Experience with 20 000 pregnancies. *J Am Med Assoc* 1980;244:2731–5

45. Hobbins JC, Venus I, Tortora M, *et al*. Stage II ultrasound examination for the diagnosis of fetal abnormalities with an elevated amniotic fluid alpha fetoprotein concentration. *Am J Obstet Gynecol* 1982; 142:1026–9

46. Roberts CJ, Evans KT, Hibbard BM, *et al*. Diagnostic effectiveness of ultrasound in detection of neural tube defect. The South Wales experience of 2509 scans (1977–1982) in high-risk mothers. *Lancet* 1983;2:1068

47. Platt LD, Feuchtbaum L, Filly R, *et al*. The California maternal serum-fetoprotein screening program: the role of ultrasonography in the detection of spina bifida. *Am J Obstet Gynecol* 1992;166:1328–9

48. Tabor A, Philip J, Madsen M, *et al*. Randomized controlled trial of genetic amniocentesis in 4606 low-risk women. *Lancet* 1986;1:1287–93

49. MRC Vitamin Study Research Group 1991. Prevention of neural tube defects: results of the Medical Research Council vitamin study. *Lancet* 1991;338:131–7

50. Mulinare J, Cordero JF, Erickson JD, *et al*. Periconceptional use of multivitamins and the occurrence of neural tube defects. *J Am Med Assoc* 1988;260: 3141–5

51. Bower C, Stanley FJ. Dietary folate as a risk factor study in Western Australia. *Med J Aust* 1989;150:613–9

52. Milunsky A, Jick H, Jick SS, *et al*. Multivitamin/folic acid supplementation in early pregnancy reduces the prevalence of neural tube defects. *J Am Med Assoc* 1989;262:2847–52

53. Centers for Disease Control 1993. Recommendations for the use of folic acid to reduce the number of cases of spina bifida and other neural tube defects. *MMWR Morb Mortal Wkly Rep* 1992;41(RR-14):1–7

54. Goldstein RB, Filly RA, Callen PW. Sonography of anencephaly: pitfalls in early diagnosis. *J Clin Ultrasound* 1989;17:397–402

55. Shapiro K. Encephalocele. In Buyse ML, ed. *Birth Defects Encyclopedia*. 1st ed. Cambridge, MA: Blackwell Scientific Publications, Inc., 1990:614–5

56. Mecke S, Passarge E. Encephalocele, polycystic kidneys and polydactyly as an autosomal recessive trait simulating certain other disorders. The Meckel syndrome. *Ann Genet* 1971;14:97–103

57. Lorber J. The prognosis of occipital encephalocele. *Dev Med Child Neurol* (Suppl)1967;13:75–86

58. Burton BK, Sowers SG, Nelson LH. Maternal serum alpha-fetoprotein screening in North Carolina: experience with more than twelve thousand pregnancies. *Am J Obstet Gynecol* 1983;146:439–44

59. Milunsky A, Alpert E. Results and benefits of a maternal serum alpha-fetoprotein screening program. *J Am Med Assoc* 1984;252:1438–42

60. Lorber J. Systemic ventriculographic studies in infants born with meningomyelocele and encephalocele. The incidence and development of hydrocephalus. *Arch Dis Child* 1961;36:381

61. Russell DS, Donald C. The mechanism of internal hydrocephalus in spina bifida. *Brain* 1935;58:203

62. Goldstein R, Podrasky AE, Filly RA, *et al*. Effacement of the fetal cistern magna in association with myelomeningocele. *Radiology* 1989;172:409–13

63. Van den Hof MC, Nicolaides KH, Campbell J, *et al*. Evaluation of the lemon and banana signs in one

hundred thirty fetuses with open spina bifida. *Am J Obstet Gynecol* 1990;162:322–7

64. Ames MD, Schut L. Results of treatment of 171 consecutive myelomeningoceles – 1963–1968. *Pediatrics* 1972;50:466–70

65. Luthy DA, Wardinsky T, Shurtleff D, *et al.* Cesarean section before the onset of labor and subsequent motor function in infants with meningomyelocele diagnosed antenatally. *New Engl J Med* 1991;324:662–6

66. Friedrichs PE. Cesarean section before labor for infants with meningomyelocele. *New Engl J Med* 1991;325:359

67. Adzick NS, Harrison MR. The Unborn surgical patient. *Curr Probl Surg* 1994;31:9–67

68. Butler NR, Claireaux AE. Congenital diaphragmatic hernia as a cause of perinatal mortality. *Lancet* 1962; 1:659

69. David TJ, Illingworth CA. Diaphragmatic hernia in the south-west of England. *J Med Genet* 1976;13:253–62

70. Hansen J, James S, Burrington J, *et al.* The decreasing incidence of pneumothorax and improving survival of infants with congenital diaphragmatic hernia. *J Pediatr Surg* 1984;19:385–8

71. Lipson AK, Williams G. Congenital diaphragmatic hernia in half sibs. *J Med Genet* 1985;22:145–7

72. Mishalany H, Grodo J. Congenital diaphragmatic hernia in monozygotic twins. *J Pediatr Surg* 1976;21:372–4

73. Frey P, Glanzmann R, Nars P, *et al.* Familial congenital diaphragmatic defect: transmission from father to daughter. *J Pediatr Surg* 1991;26:1396–8

74. Greenwood RD, Rosenthal A, Nadas AS. Cardiovascular abnormalities associated with congenital diaphragmatic hernia. *Pediatrics* 1976;57:92–7

75. Adzick NS, Vacanti JP, Lillehei CW, *et al.* Fetal diaphragmatic hernia: ultrasound diagnosis and clinical outcome in 38 cases. *J Pediatr Surg* 1989;24:654–8

76. Nicolaides KH, Blott M. Prenatal diagnosis of congenital diaphragmatic hernia. In Puri P, ed. *Congenital Diaphragmatic Hernia*. Basel: Karger, 1989:62–8

77. Bootstaylor BS, Filly RA, Harrison MR, *et al.* Prenatal sonographic predictors of liver herniation in congenital diaphragmatic hernia. *J Ultrasound Med* 1995; 14:515–20

78. Adzick NS, Harrison MR, Glick PL, *et al.* Diaphragmatic hernia in the fetus: prenatal diagnosis and outcome in 94 cases. *J Pediatr Surg* 1985;20:357–61

79. Sharland GK, Lockhart SM, Heward AJ, *et al.* Prognosis in fetal diaphragmatic hernia. *Am J Obstet Gynecol* 1992;166:9–13

80. Crawford DC, Wright VM, Drake DP, *et al.* Fetal diaphragmatic hernia: the value of fetal echocardiography in the prediction of postnatal outcome. *Br J Obstet Gynaecol* 1989;96:705–10

81. Harrison MR, Adzick NS, Longaker MT, *et al.* Successful repair *in utero* of a fetal diaphragmatic hernia after removal of herniated viscera from the left thorax. *New Engl J Med* 1990;32:1582–4

82. Longaker MT, Lagerge JM, Dansereau J, *et al.* Primary fetal hydrothorax: natural history and management. *J Pediatr Surg* 1989;24:573–6

83. Rodeck CH, Fisk NM, Fraser DI, *et al.* Long-term *in utero* drainage of fetal hydrothorax. *N Engl J Med* 1988;319:1135–8

84. Mann L, Ferguson-Smith MA, Desai M, *et al.* Prenatal assessment of anterior abdominal wall defects and their prognosis. *Prenat Diagn* 1984;4:427–35

85. Thornton JG, Lilford RJ, Newcombe RG. Tables for estimation of individual risks of fetal neural tube and ventral wall defects, incorporating prior probability, maternal serum fetoprotein levels, and ultrasonographic examination results. *Am J Obstet Gynecol* 1990;163:773–5

86. Lewin DF, Towers CV, Garite TJ, *et al.* Fetal gastroschisis and omphalocele: is Cesarean section the best mode of delivery? *Am J Obstet Gynecol* 1990;196:773–5

87. Baird PA, MacDonald ED. An epidemiologic study of congenital malformations of the anterior abdominal wall in more than half a million consecutive live births. *Am J Hum Genet* 1981;33:470–8

88. Carpenter MW, Curci MR, Dibbins AW, *et al.* Perinatal management of ventral wall defects. *Obstet Gynecol* 1984;64:646–51

89. Stringel G, Filler RM. Prognostic factors in omphalocele and gastroschisis. *J Pediatr Surg* 1979;14:515–19

90. Hoyme HE, Higginbottom MC, Jones KL. The vascular pathogenesis of gastroschisis: intrauterine interruption of the omphalomesenteric artery. *J Pediatr* 1981; 98:228–9

91. Roberts CC, Ashcraft KW. Esophageal atresia. In Buyse ML, ed. *Birth Defects Encyclopedia*. 1st ed. Cambridge, MA: Blackwell Scientific Publications, Inc.; 1990: 641–2

92. Fonkalsrud EW, deLorimier AA, Hays DM. Congenital atresia and stenosis of the duodenum. A review compiled from the members of the Surgical Section of the American Academy of Pediatrics. *Pediatrics* 1969; 43:79–83

93. Besser AS. Duodenal atresia or stenosis. In Buyse ML, ed. *Birth Defects Encyclopedia*. 1st ed. Cambridge, MA: Blackwell Scientific Publications, Inc.; 1990:549–50

94. Duenhoelter JH, Santos-Ramos R, Rosenfeld CR, *et al.* Prenatal diagnosis of gastrointestinal tract obstruction. *Obstet Gynecol* 1976;47:618–20

95. Atwell JD, Klidjian AM. Vertebral anomalies and duodenal atresia. *J Pediatr Surg* 1982;17:237–40

96. Freeman NV. Congenital atresia and stenosis of the colon. *Br J Surg* 1966;53:595

97. Louw JH, Barnard CN. Congenital intestinal atresia. Observations on its origin. *Lancet* 1955;2:1065

98. Lynn HB, Espino S. Intestinal atresia: an attempt to relate location to embryologic process. *Arch Surg* 1959;79:357

99. Nixon HH, Tawes R. Etiology and treatment of small intestinal atresia: analysis of a series of 127 jejunoileal atresias and comparison with 62 duodenal atresias. *Surgery* 1971;69:41–51

100. Besser AS. Intestinal atresia or stenosis. In Buyse ML, ed. *Birth Defects Encyclopedia*. 1st ed. Cambridge, MA: Blackwell Scientific Publications, Inc.; 1990:975–6

101. Martin LW, Zerella JT. Jejunoileal atresia: a proposed classification. *J Pediatr Surg* 1976;11:399–403

102. Green JJ, Hobbins JC. Abdominal ultrasound examination of the first trimester fetus. *Am J Obstet Gynecol* 1988;159:165–75

103. Grannum PAT, Bracken M, Silverman R, *et al.* Fetal kidney size in normal gestation by comparison of ratio

of kidney circumference to abdominal circumference. *Am J Obstet Gynecol* 1980;136:249–54

104. Cambell S, Wladimiroff JW, Dewhurst CJ. The antenatal measurement of fetal urine production. *J Obstet Gynaecol Br Commonw* 1973;80:680–6

105. Lind T, Kendall A, Hytten FE. The role of the fetus in the formation of amniotic fluids. *J Obstet Gynaecol Br Commonw* 1972;79:289–98

106. Hashimoto K, Gross BG, DiBella RJ, *et al*. The ultrastructure of the skin of human embryos. IV. The epidermis. *J Invest Derm* 1966;47:317–35

107. Perlman M, Levin M. Fetal pulmonary hypoplasia, anuria, and oligohydramnios: clinicopathologic observations and review of the literature. *Am J Obstet Gynecol* 1974;118:1119–21

108. Hislop A, Hey E, Reid L. The lungs in congenital bilateral renal agenesis and dysplasia. *Arch Dis Child* 1979;54:32–8

109. Potter EL. Bilateral absence of ureters and kidneys: a report of 50 cases. *Obstet Gynecol* 1965;25:3

110. Carter CO, Evans K, Pescia G. A family study of renal agenesis. *J Med Genet* 1979;16:176–88

111. Carter CO, Evans K. Birth frequency of bilateral renal agenesis, (Letter). *J Med Genet* 1981;18:158

112. Romero R, Cullen M, Grannum PAT, *et al*. Antenatal diagnosis of renal anomalies with ultrasound. III. Bilateral renal agenesis. *Am J Obstet Gynecol* 1985;151:38–43

113. Harman CR. Maternal furosemide may not provoke urine production in the compromised fetus. *Am J Obstet Gynecol* 1984;150:322–3

114. Potter EL. Type I cystic kidney: tubular gigantism. In *Normal and Abnormal Development of the Kidney*. Chicago: Yearbook Medical Publishers, 1972:141–53

115. Habif DV Jr, Berdon WE, Yeh MN. Infantile polycystic kidney disease: *in utero* sonographic diagnosis. *Radiology* 1982;142:475–7

116. Romero R, Cullen M, Jeanty P, *et al*. The diagnosis of congenital renal anomalies with ultrasound. II. infantile polycystic kidney disease. *Am J Obstet Gynecol* 1984;150:259–62

117. Beretsky I, Lankin DH, Russell JH. Sonographic differentiation between the multicystic dysplastic kidney and the ureteropelvic junction obstruction *in utero* using high resolution real-time scanners employing digital detection. *J Clin Ultrasound* 1984;12:429–33

118. D'Alton M, Romero R, Grannum PAT, *et al*. Antenatal diagnosis of renal anomalies with ultrasound. IV. Bilateral multicystic kidney disease. *Am J Obstet Gynecol* 1986;54:532–7

119. Sanders RC, Hartman DS. The sonographic distinction between neonatal multi-cystic kidney and hydronephrosis. *Radiology* 1984;151:621–5

120. Greene LF, Feinzaig W, Dahlin DC. Multicystic dysplasia of the kidney with special reference to the contralateral kidney. *J Urol* 1971;105:482–7

121. Ruano-gil D, Coca-Payeras A, Tejedo-Mateu A. Obstruction and normal recanalization of the ureter in the human embryo. Its relation to congenital ureteric obstruction. *Eur Urol* 1975;1:287–93

122. Fernbach SK, Maizels M, Conway JJ. Ultrasound grading of hydronephrosis: introduction to the system used by the Society of Fetal Urology. *Pediatr Radiol* 1993;23:478–80

123. Steinhardt GF, Luisiri A, Goodgold H. The long-term outcome of fetally diagnosed uropathies. *J Mat Fetal Med* 1992;1:277–85

124. Blachar A, Blachar Y, Pinchas LD, *et al*. Clinical outcome and follow-up of prenatal hydronephrosis. *Pediatr Nephrol* 1994;8:30–5

125. Hobbins JC, Romero R, Grannum PAT, *et al*. Antenatal diagnosis of renal agenesis with ultrasound. I. Obstructive uropathy. *Am J Obstet Gynecol* 1984;148:868–77

126. McFayden JR, Wigglesworth JS, Dillon MJ. Fetal urinary tract obstruction: is active intervention before delivery indicated? *Br J Obstet Gynaecol* 1983;90:342–9

127. Glick PL, Harrison MR, Golbus MS, *et al*. Management of the fetus with congenital hydronephrosis II. Prognostic criteria and selection for treatment. *J Pediatr Drug* 1985;20:376

128. Mahoney BS, Filly RA, Callen PW, *et al*. Fetal renal dysplasia: sonographic evaluation. *Radiology* 1984;152:143–6

129. Eugene M, Muller F, Dommergues M, *et al*. Evaluation of postnatal renal function in fetuses with bilateral obstructive uropathies by proton nuclear magnetic resonance spectroscopy. *Am J Obstet Gynecol* 1994;170:595–602

130. Nicolaides KH, Rodeck CH, Gosden CM. Rapid karyotyping in non-lethal fetal malformations. *Lancet* 1986;1:283

131. Johnston JH, Evans JP, Glassbert KI, *et al*. Pelvic hydronephrosis in children: a review of 219 personal cases. *J Urol* 1977;117:97–101

132. Hanna MK, Jeffs RD, Sturgess JM, *et al*. Ureteral structure and ultrastructure. Part II. Congenital ureteropelvic junction obstruction and primary obstructive megaureter. *J Urol* 1976;116:725–30

133. Freedman ER, Rickwood AMK. Prenatally diagnosed pelviureteric junction obstruction: a benign condition. *J Pediatr Surg* 1994;29:769–72

134. Tokunaka S, Tomohiko K, Tsuji I. Two infantile cases of primary megaloureter with uncommon pathological findings: ultrastructural study and its clinical implication. *J Urol* 1980;123:214–17

135. Wood BP, Ben-ami T, Teele RL, *et al*. Ureterovesical obstruction and megaloureter: diagnosis by real-time ultrasound. *Radiology* 1985;156:79–81

55
Fetal biophysical profile

A.M. Vintzileos, W.A. Campbell and J.F. Rodis

INTRODUCTION

The antepartum detection of fetal asphyxia has been a major challenge in perinatal medicine. The purpose of antepartum surveillance in terms of biophysical monitoring is the detection of fetal hypoxia and acidosis for timely intervention, thereby avoiding fetal death *in utero*. After the introduction of electronic fetal heart rate monitoring, the non-stress stress test (NST) and the contraction stress test (CST) became widely used in antepartum fetal surveillance. Both tests have relatively low false-negative rates (< 1–2.7%) but high false-positive rates (50% to > 75%)[1–5]. Moreover, the CST is theoretically contraindicated in patients with premature rupture of the membranes, multiple gestations, incompetent cervix, preterm labor or vaginal bleeding. The combination of low false-negative and high false-positive rates of the NST and CST is a testimony to the fact that these tests predict fetal health reasonably well. However, they are much less accurate in the prediction of fetal compromise. The inability of these two tests to differentiate between fetal compromise and sleep is due to the fact that both tests utilize only one biophysical variable, the fetal heart rate. If heart rate alone is the only information available, it is impossible to differentiate between coma and sleep in the adult patient. With the introduction of realtime ultrasound, a direct examination of the fetus became a reality. Acute fetal markers such as fetal movements, fetal breathing movements and tone, as well as assessment of the intrauterine environment, i.e. estimation of amniotic fluid volume and placental grading, could be objectively evaluated. The combination of biophysical variables as means of antepartum fetal surveillance was first introduced by Manning *et al.* in 1980[6]. The fetal biophysical profile was developed to decrease the false-positive results. The most important element of this testing method is the combination of acute and chronic markers of the fetal condition.

Acute markers

The acute markers of the fetal condition are fetal heart rate reactivity, fetal movements, fetal breathing movements and fetal tone. These activities are initiated and regulated by the fetal central nervous system (CNS). The presence or absence of these markers may reflect fetal acid–base status at the time of testing. The presence of a normal biophysical activity implies that the CNS center that controls the activity is intact and functioning and therefore non-hypoxic. However, the absence of a single fetal biophysical activity is not always due to hypoxia and acidosis; in fact, it is most frequently due to normal periodicity or CNS depressants. Normal periodicity of fetal biophysical activities such as fetal breathing movements and fetal body movements have been documented in normal and high-risk pregnancies. The periodicity of these biophysical activities is short term (20–40 minutes) or long term similar to those diurnal rhythms of extrauterine life. Periodicity has also been documented in fetal heart-rate variability. Presence or absence of periodicity in fetal tone and/or fetal heart rate accelerations has not been reported. Maternal administration of CNS depressants and sedatives (e.g. morphine, meperidine, barbiturates, Valium) and drugs such as heroin and methadone may inhibit fetal biophysical activities. Central nervous system stimulants such as hyperglycemia and catecholamines may increase biophysical activities. The effect of hypoxia and acidosis on the fetal biophysical profile depends on the severity, duration, chronicity, and frequency of the insult(s). Fetal hypoxia may be transient without acidosis, or prolonged with associated metabolic or mixed acidosis, thus affecting multiple organs. Acute fetal hypoxia produces a definite decrease of fetal heart rate reactivity (non-reactive NST) and fetal breathing movements, and when severe will abolish fetal movements and fetal tone[7,8].

The fetal CNS centers which control the fetal biophysical activities are shown in Table 1. Published data indicate that there are variations in the sensitivity of these centers to hypoxia and acidosis[7,8]. The biophysical activities which become active first in fetal neurodevelopment are the last to become compromised during intrauterine asphyxia. The fetal tone center begins functioning at 7½–8½ weeks' gestation and the fetal movement center begins functioning at approximately 9 weeks' gestation. These two centers are the last to become compromised during asphyxia. The fetal breathing movement center, which starts operating after 20–21 weeks' gestation, and the fetal heart-rate reactivity center, which starts operating by the end

Table 1   Fetal central nervous system centers

FT	Cortex (subcortical area?)	Embryogenesis	↑
FM	Cortex nuclei		
FBM	Ventral surface of fourth ventricle		
NST	Posterior hypothalamus, medulla	Hypoxia	↓

FT, fetal tone; FM, fetal movements; FBM, fetal breathing movements; NST, non-stress test. Reprinted with permission from reference 7

of the second trimester or early third trimester, are the most sensitive to asphyxia. Data from our institution indicate that fetal heart rate reactivity and fetal breathing are abolished when the fetal pH is < 7.20, whereas fetal movement and tone are abolished at pH values < 7.10. The clinical meaning of this 'gradual hypoxia concept' is that the first manifestations of fetal asphyxial compromise are non-reactive NST and absent fetal breathing, whereas in advanced stages, fetal movements and tone are also absent. In our experience, poor fetal tone is associated with the highest perinatal death rate (42.8%)[7]. The concept of a different level of sensitivity to hypoxia of the fetal CNS centers is a prerequisite for the correct clinical application of the information derived from the biophysical assessment. In addition, it allows for assessment of the degree of fetal compromise.

Chronic markers

The amniotic fluid volume is not influenced by acute changes in fetal CNS function. Chronic fetal hypoxia is frequently associated with redistribution of cardiac output away from non-vital to vital fetal organs. The result may be decreased lung and kidney perfusion with decreased urine production and, therefore, oligohydramnios. Fetuses with oligohydramnios are not only chronically stressed but also at high risk for cord compression and *in utero* death. Several studies have demonstrated a strong correlation between oligohydramnios and increased incidence of adverse perinatal outcome. In structurally normal fetuses, a perinatal mortality rate of 1.97 in 1000 has been reported in the presence of normal qualitative amniotic fluid volume (largest pocket > 2 cm and < 8 cm), whereas the perinatal mortality rates in fetuses with marginal (largest pocket 1–2 cm) and decreased amniotic fluid (largest pocket < 1 cm) have been 37.7 in 1000 and 109.4 in 1000, respectively[9]. Most fetal biophysical assessment schemes consider oligohydramnios as an abnormal assessment even if all the remaining parameters are normal. The presence of oligohydramnios has been considered by us and others as an indication for delivery[6,8,10,11]. In structurally normal viable fetuses, the simultaneous presence of oligohydramnios and spontaneous fetal heart-rate variable decelerations constitutes an indication for delivery regardless of gestational age. Placental grading has also been included by us in the fetal biophysical profile. The reason for including placental grading is our previous finding that patients with grade 3 placentas have an increased incidence of abnormal intrapartum fetal heart rate patterns (44.4%) and abruptio placenta (14.8%) during labor[7]. In our view, the inclusion of grade 3 placentas makes sense because it alerts the obstetrician during the intrapartum period of these patients.

Since the early 1980s, attempts have been made to give a score to each biophysical variable to produce a 'fetal biophysical profile score'. There are currently two types of scoring systems: one proposed by Manning and co-workers (Table 2) and the other by Vintzileos and co-workers (Table 3). In both scoring systems, a score of > 8 is reassuring of fetal wellbeing. A score of < 8 is non-reassuring and repeat testing or delivery is suggested. In both systems, the presence of oligohydramnios constitutes an abnormal biophysical assessment even if all the remaining biophysical variables are normal.

FETAL BIOPHYSICAL PROFILE AND FETAL ACID–BASE STATUS

In most studies, the last biophysical assessment within a week of delivery has been used for correlation with fetal condition at birth. The disadvantages of such studies, however, are the long interval between performing the biophysical assessment and the birth of the infant, as well as the effects of labor and drugs on the fetus, i.e. factors that can alter fetal condition. To correlate the fetal biophysical profile with fetal acid–base studies at the time of testing and to further explore the issue of variations in sensitivity to acidemia at which the fetal biophysical activities become compromised, Vintzileos and co-workers[8] studied 124 consecutive patients with singleton pregnancies and gestational ages between 26 and 43 weeks undergoing Cesarean section prior to the onset of labor. All patients had a biophysical profile performed within six hours of the Cesarean section. This biophysical profile was correlated with fetal acid–base status as determined by umbilical cord blood pH measurements. Figure 1 illustrates the relationship between the fetal biophysical score and cord arterial pH. One hundred and two fetuses had a score of > 8; in this group of fetuses, the cord arterial pH was 7.28 ± 0.04 (mean ± SD); two fetuses (2%) were acidotic among these 102 fetuses. Thirteen fetuses with scores of 5–7 had a cord arterial pH of 7.19 ± 0.06 (mean ± SD); 9 fetuses (69%) were acidotic among these 13 fetuses. Nine fetuses with scores of 6 4 had a cord arterial pH of 6.99 ± 0.10 (mean ± SD), and all were acidotic. The three groups

Table 2 Fetal biophysical profile scoring according to Manning and co-workers[6]

Variable	Score 2	Score 0
Fetal breathing movements (FBM)	The presence of at least 30 s of sustained FBM in 30 min of observation.	Less than 30 s of FBM in 30 min.
Fetal movements	Three or more gross body movements in 30 min of observation. Simultaneous limb and trunk movements are counted as a single movement.	Two or less gross body movements in 30 min of observation.
Fetal tone	At least one episode of motion of a limb from a position of flexion to extension and a rapid return to flexion.	Fetus in a position of semi- or full-limb extension with no return to flexion with movement. Absence of fetal movement is counted as absent tone.
Fetal reactivity	The presence of two or more fetal heart rate accelerations of at least 15 bpm and lasting at least 15 s and associated with fetal movement in 40 min.	No acceleration or less than two accelerations of the fetal heart rate in 40 min of observation.
Qualitative amniotic fluid volume	A pocket of amniotic fluid that measures at least 1 cm in two perpendicular planes.	Largest pocket of amniotic fluid measures < 1 cm in two perpendicular planes.
Maximal score	10	–
Minimal score	–	0

Reprinted with permission from reference 6

Table 3 Criteria for scoring biophysical variables according to Vintzileos and co-workers[7]

Non-stress test
  Score 2 (NST 2): five or more FHR accelerations of at least 15 bpm in amplitude and at least 15 s duration associated with fetal movements in a 20-min period.
  Score 1 (NST 1): two to four accelerations of at least 15 bpm in amplitude and at least 15 s duration associated with fetal movements in a 20-min period.
  Score 0 (NST 0): one or fewer accelerations in a 20-min period.
Fetal movements
  Score 2 (FM 2): at least three gross (trunk and limbs) episodes of fetal movements within 30 min. Simultaneous limb and trunk movements were counted as a single movement.
  Score 1 (FM 1): one or two fetal movements within 30 min.
  Score 0 (FM 0): absence of fetal movements within 30 min.
Fetal breathing movements
  Score 2 (FBM 2): at least one episode of fetal breathing of at least 60 s duration within a 30-min observation period.
  Score 1 (FBM 1): at least one episode of fetal breathing lasting 30–60 s within 30 min.
  Score 0 (FBM 0): absence of fetal breathing or breathing lasting < 30 s within 30 min.
Fetal tone
  Score 2 (FT 2): at least one episode of extension of extremities with return to position of flexion, and also one episode of extension of spine with return to position of flexion.
  Score 1 (FT 1): at least one episode of extension of extremities with return to position of flexion, or one episode of extension of spine with return to position of flexion.
  Score 0 (FT 0): extremities in extension. Fetal movements not followed by return to flexion. Open hand.
Amniotic fluid volume
  Score 2 (AF 2): fluid evident throughout the uterine cavity. A pocket that measures > 2 cm in vertical diameter.
  Score 1 (AF 1): a pocket that measures < 2 cm but more than vertical diameter.
  Score 0 (AF 0): crowding of fetal small parts. Largest pocket < 1 cm in vertical diameter.
Placental grading
  Score 2 (PL 2): placental grading 0, 1, or 2.
  Score 1 (PL 1): placenta posterior difficult to evaluate.
  Score 0 (PL 0): placental grading 3.

NST, non-stress test; FHR, fetal heart rate; bpm, beats per minute; FM, fetal movements; FBM, fetal breathing movements; FT, fetal tone; AF, amniotic fluid; PL, placental grading. Maximal score 12; minimal score 0. Reprinted with permission from reference 7

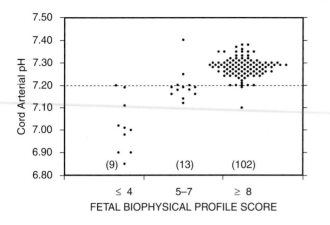

Figure 1 Relationship between the fetal biophysical profile score and cord arterial pH. (Number of fetuses in parentheses.) Reprinted with permission from reference 8

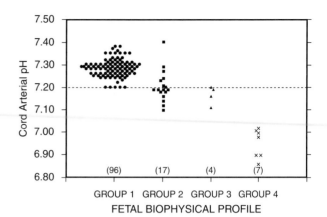

Figure 3 Relationship between the fetal biophysical activities (acute markers) and cord arterial pH. (Number of fetuses in parentheses.) ●, R-NST and/or FBM +; ▲, NR-NST, FBM −; FM, FT ±; ■, NR-NST, FBM −; FM, FT +; ✕, NR-NST, FBM −; FM, FT −. Reprinted with permission from reference 8

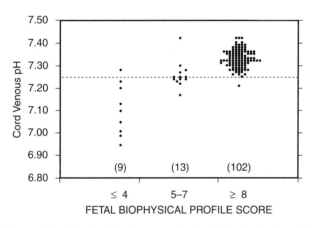

Figure 2 Relationship between the fetal biophysical profile score and cord venous pH. (Number of fetuses in parentheses.) Reprinted with permission from reference 8

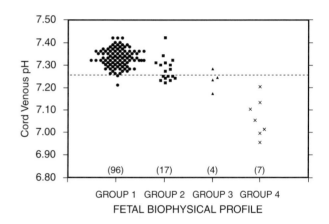

Figure 4 Relationship between the fetal biophysical activities (acute markers) and cord venous pH. (Number of fetuses in parentheses.) ●, R-NST and/or FBM +; ▲, NR-NST, FBM −; FM, FT ±; ■, NR-NST, FBM −; FM, FT +; ✕, NR-NST, FBM −; FM, FT −. Reprinted with permission from reference 8

had statistically different cord arterial pH values. The relationship between the biophysical score and cord venous pH was similar and is illustrated in Figure 2. Figure 3 illustrates the relationship between the individual biophysical activities and the cord arterial pH values. Group 1 consisted of 96 fetuses with reactive NST and/or fetal breathing present (lasting > 30 s); none of these fetuses were acidotic. The common characteristic of groups 2, 3, and 4 was that all fetuses had non-reactive NST and no breathing present. However, group 2 (17 fetuses) had normal movements (three or more body movements) and tone; the mean pH of this group was 7.20, and 10 (59%) fetuses were acidotic in this group. Group 3 (four fetuses) had compromised movements (one or two body movements) or tone; the mean cord arterial pH was 7.16, and three (75%) were acidotic. Group 4 (seven fetuses) had all biophysical activities absent. The mean cord arterial pH of this

group was 6.95, and all seven (100%) fetuses were acidotic at birth (cord arterial pH < 7.20). The relationship between the individual biophysical activities and cord venous pH measurements was similar (Figure 4). Careful observation of the results illustrated in Figure 3 suggests that there are different levels of sensitivity to hypoxia and acidosis at which the fetal biophysical activities become compromised. The fetal heart rate reactivity and fetal breathing seem to be compromised when the pH is lower than 7.20. At pH values of 7.10–7.20, fetal movements and tone are still present but not normal and at pH values < 7.10, movements and tone are totally absent. The ability of the individual biophysical components alone and in combination to predict fetal acidemia are shown in Table 4. Of the individual biophysical components, fetal heart-rate reactivity and fetal breathing had 100% sensitivities and negative predictive values, an observation that suggests that either test is a reasonable choice for primary fetal surveillance. The combination of non-reactive NST and no fetal breathing (as the 'abnormal test') improved the specificity and positive predictive values to 92 and 71%, respectively. Fetal tone has the highest positive predictive value (100%) but low sensitivity (45%), an observation that suggests that fetal tone alone should not be used for primary fetal surveillance.

The relationship of fetal biophysical profile and cord blood gas values at cordocentesis has recently been studied by Ribbert and co-workers[12]. In that study, 14 severely growth-retarded fetuses had a bio-physical profile assessment prior to fetal blood sampling by cordocentesis. The fetal biophysical profile was correlated with blood pO_2, pH, oxygen saturation, and oxygen content. It was found that the fetal biophysical profile was a good indicator of the degree of fetal acidemia. Of the individual fetal biophysical activities, fetal heart rate reactivity was compromised for Δ pH (observed pH subtracted from the appropriate mean for gestation) below – 2 SDs; the fetal breathing movements were compromised at Δ pH values below – 3 SDs; fetal body movements and fetal tone were compromised for Δ pH values below – 4 SDs. These preliminary data using fetal blood-gas values obtained at cordocentesis confirmed the observations of Vintzileos and co-workers in that the fetal biophysical profile can predict the degree of fetal acidemia and that the fetal heart-rate reactivity and fetal breathing movements are the first, whereas fetal gross body movements and tone are the last, biophysical activities to be compromised during acidemia.

In another study of 62 patients undergoing Cesarean section prior to the onset of labor, the relationship between fetal biophysical assessment performed within three hours of delivery and cord blood gases was investigated[13]. Our observations were extended to include not only cord blood pH values, but also pO_2, pCO_2, bicarbonate and base excess. It was found that non-reactive non-stress testing was associated with lower pH, pO_2, bicarbonate and base excess, but not significantly different pCO_2 as compared to reactive non-stress testing. Similar differences were observed between the presence versus absence of fetal breathing. The absence of fetal movements and/or tone was associated with lower pH, pO_2, bicarbonate and base excess, and a higher pCO_2 as compared to the presence of body movements and tone. These blood-gas differences were noted in both cord arterial and venous blood. Comparison of the different levels of cord blood gases at which the biophysical activities are compromised revealed that not only acidemia but also progressive hypoxemia and hypercapnea are initially associated with loss of fetal heart-rate reactivity and breathing and in advanced stages with loss of movements and tone. These most recent observations suggest that the first manifestations of fetal hypoxemia and acidemia are non-reactive NST and absence of fetal breathing. In advanced hypoxemia, hypercapnea and acidemia, fetal movements and tone are absent.

Table 4 Efficacy of the fetal biophysical variables to predict fetal acidemia

Biophysical variable(s)	Definition of the abnormal test	Sensitivity (%) (n)	Specificity (%) (n)	Positive predictive value (%) (n)	Negative predictive value (%) (n)
Biophysical score	6 7	90% (18/20)	96% (100/104)	82% (18/22)	98% (100/102)
Non-stress test, fetal breathing movements	Non-reactive NST and no breathing	100% (20/20)	92% (96/104)	71% (20/28)	100% (96/96)
Non-stress test	Less than one acceleration in 20 min	100% (20/20)	76% (79/104)	44% (20/45)	100% (79/79)
Fetal breathing movements	< 30 s	100% (20/20)	64% (67/104)	35% (20/57)	100% (67/67)
Fetal movements	Less than three	50% (10/20)	96% (100/104)	71% (10/14)	91% (100/110)
Fetal tone	Compromised or absent	45% (9/20)	100% (104/104)	100% (9/9)	90% (104/115)
Amniotic fluid	< 1 cm	35% (7/20)	93% (97/104)	50% (7/14)	88% (97/100)
Amniotic fluid	< 2 cm	45% (9/20)	86% (89/104)	38% (9/24)	89% (89/100)
Placental grading	Grade 3	5% (1/20)	94% (98/104)	14% (1/7)	84% (98/117)

n, number of fetuses
Reprinted with permission from reference 12

CLINICAL EXPERIENCE WITH THE FETAL BIOPHYSICAL PROFILE

The quantitative and qualitative variations of the individual biophysical components are gestational age dependent. To determine whether or not these variations could normally change the biophysical profile and scoring of the healthy fetus throughout gestation, Vintzileos and co-workers[14] studied 210 patients with intact membranes and normal pregnancy outcome. These patients had a total of 951 serial examinations from 25 to 44 weeks' gestation. The frequency of the individual biophysical components from 25 to 44 weeks are shown in Table 5. As shown, there is a significant increase in reactive NSTs after 32 weeks while fetal breathing and amniotic fluid volume are decreased after 40 weeks. The incidence of grade 3 placentas increases significantly after 32 weeks. The fetal movements and fetal tone remain stable from 25 to 44 weeks. These variations in the frequencies of the fetal biophysical components from 25 to 44 weeks' gestation agree with the findings of several other investigators[15–18]. It should be noted, however, that the frequency of reassuring biophysical scores (> 8) did not change significantly from 25 to 44 weeks' gestation.

At this point, it should be emphasized that the changes in the biophysical components as shown in Table 5 pertain to the biophysical profile scoring as defined by our criteria (Table 3) for the purpose of antepartum fetal surveillance. Using the scoring criteria of Manning and co-workers, Baskett and co-workers[19] had similar findings regarding the changes of the biophysical components throughout gestation. Their study involved pregnancies with normal perinatal outcome (5582 fetuses/11 012 biophysical profiles). There was an increased number of reactive NSTs and fetal breathing movements at 34 to 41 weeks as compared to earlier gestations. The NST, fetal breathing movements, fetal tone and amniotic fluid volume were more likely to be abnormal in prolonged gestations (42–44 weeks) as compared to term gestations (37–41 weeks). Although changes in the individual biophysical components were noted, the frequency of normal biophysical scores (> 8) did not change significantly throughout gestation. The understanding of the gestational age-dependent changes of the biophysical components is mandatory for the proper clinical application of the biophysical profile, especially when one manages very preterm gestations.

Table 5 Frequency of individual biophysical variables and biophysical scoring of > 8 in pregnancies with intact membranes (scoring according to the criteria by Vintzileos and co-workers)[*]

	Gestation (weeks)								
	25–28 n = 61 (6.4%)	*p value*	29–32 n = 192 (20.1%)	*p value*	33–36 n = 347 (36.4%)	*p value*	37–40 n = 257 (27.0%)	*p value*	41–44 n = 94 (9.8%)
NST-2	22 (36.0%)	NS	82 (42.7%)	<0.01	223 (64.2%)	NS	188 (73.1%)	NS	77 (81.9%)
NST-1	19 (31.1%)	NS	68 (35.4%)	<0.01	86 (24.7%)	NS	44 (17.1%)	NS	9 (9.5%)
NST-0	20 (32.7%)	NS	42 (21.8%)	<0.01	38 (10.9%)	NS	25 (9.7%)	NS	8 (8.5%)
FBM-2	36 (59.0%)	NS	143 (74.4%)	NS	264 (76.0%)	NS	181 (70.4%)	<0.05	52 (55.3%)
FBM-1	4 (6.5%)	NS	15 (7.8%)	NS	31 (8.9%)	NS	20 (7.7%)	NS	6 (6.3%)
FBM-0	21 (34.4%)	NS	34 (17.7%)	NS	52 (14.9%)	NS	56 (21.7%)	<0.05	36 (38.3%)
FM-2	61 (100%)	NS	188 (97.9%)	NS	331 (95.3%)	NS	242 (94.1%)	NS	86 (91.4%)
FM-1	0 (0.0%)	NS	4 (2.0%)	NS	14 (4.0%)	NS	12 (4.6%)	NS	5 (5.3%)
FM-0	0 (0.0%)	NS	0 (0.0%)	NS	2 (0.5%)	NS	3 (1.1%)	NS	3 (3.1%)
FT-2	61 (100.0%)	NS	182 (94.7%)	NS	324 (93.3%)	NS	232 (90.2%)	NS	79 (84.0%)
FT-1	0 (0.0%)	NS	9 (4.6%)	NS	21 (6.0%)	NS	24 (9.3%)	NS	12 (12.7%)
FT-0	0 (0.0%)	NS	1 (0.5%)	NS	2 (0.5%)	NS	1 (0.4%)	NS	3 (3.1%)
AF-2	58 (95.0%)	NS	189 (98.4%)	NS	331 (95.3%)	NS	231 (89.8%)	<0.01	70 (74.4%)
AF-1	1 (1.6%)	NS	3 (1.5%)	NS	11 (3.1%)	NS	22 (8.5%)	<0.01	16 (17.0%)
AF-0	2 (3.2%)	NS	0 (0.0%)	NS	5 (1.4%)	NS	4 (1.5%)	<0.01	8 (8.5%)
PL-2	61 (100.0%)	NS	189 (98.4%)	NS	321 (92.5%)	NS	212 (82.4%)	<0.01	64 (68.0%)
PL-1	0 (0.0%)	NS	3 (1.5%)	NS	12 (3.4%)	NS	10 (3.8%)	<0.01	13 (13.8%)
PL-0	0 (0.0%)	NS	0 (0.0%)	<0.05	14 (4.0%)	<0.01	35 (13.6%)	<0.01	17 (18.0%)
Total score of > 8	61 (100%)	NS	186 (96.8%)	NS	341 (98.2%)	NS	249 (96.8%)	NS	83 (88.2%)

[*]See Table 3

NST, non-stress test; FBM, fetal breathing movements; FM, fetal movements; FT, fetal tone; AF, amniotic fluid volume
PL, placental grading; NS, not significant. Reprinted with permission from reference 14

Table 6 Management scheme based on biophysical profile scoring

Score	Recommended management
8–10	Repeat in 1 week. In diabetic (insulin-dependent) and postdate patients, repeat twice weekly. No indication for active intervention.
4–6	If fetal pulmonary maturity assured and cervix favorable, delivery, otherwise repeat in 24 hours. If persistent score of 4–6, deliver if fetal pulmonary maturity certain. Otherwise treat with steroid and deliver in 48 hours.
0–2	Evaluate for immediate delivery. In cases of certain pulmonary immaturity, give steroids and deliver in 48 hours.

Reprinted with permission from reference 20

In their initial study of the fetal biophysical profile score, Manning and co-workers[6] reported on 216 patients who were solely managed by the NST results. The results of the other biophysical components were not taken into consideration and, therefore, the biophysical score did not influence patient management. There was a significant correlation between abnormal biophysical profile score and low 5-minute Apgar scores, fetal distress in labor and perinatal death rate. The most accurate differentiation of the sleeping normal fetus from the compromised fetus was obtained when all biophysical variables were used. When all biophysical components were normal (score 10) the perinatal death rate was zero. When all biophysical components were abnormal (score 0) the perinatal death rate was 600 per 1000 and the fetal death rate was 400 per 1000. Based on the results of this study, Manning and colleagues suggested a management protocol according to the biophysical profile scoring as outlined in Table 6. This protocol was put forward for patient management in a subsequent study by the same investigators, involving 1184 consecutive referred high-risk patients who had 2238 fetal biophysical scores performed[20]. The purpose of the study was to assess the impact of using the biophysical score on perinatal death rate among referred high-risk patients. There were six perinatal deaths in the study group for a perinatal mortality of 5.06 per 1000 which was significantly less than the predicted rate for a similar high-risk population (65 per 1000) and also the general population (14.3 per 1000) in Manitoba. Only one fetus died after a reassuring biophysical score, thus giving a true false-negative rate of 0.8 per 1000. Moreover, 13 of 19 (68.4%) fetuses with major congenital anomalies were prenatally diagnosed as a result of realtime scanning. Of the 13 major congenital anomalies detected, 8 were lethal. In two cases the antepartum detection of the anomaly helped neonatal survival. Platt and co-workers[21] studied 283 patients who had a total of 1112 biophysical profiles. Patients were managed according to the NST results and not the results of the biophysical profile. The perinatal mortality rate for all patients delivered in their institution during the study period was 22.6 per 1000 as opposed to 14 per 1000 (corrected 7 per 1000) for the study population and 7.4 per 1000 for fetuses with a biophysical score of > 8. The authors questioned the predictive accuracy of the biophysical score as compared to the NST alone.

A comparison between fetal biophysical profile scoring (375 patients) and NST testing (360 patients) showed that the fetal biophysical profile scoring scheme had a significantly higher predictive value in regard to low Apgar scores[22]. Also, the sensitivity and specificity were higher with fetal biophysical profile scoring, but these did not reach statistical significance. The negative predictive powers of the two testing schemes were similar. All fetal anomalies were detected during realtime ultrasound scanning. However, none of the fetal anomalies were detected by NST testing. In another study, Platt and co-workers[23] randomized patients into two groups: one managed with NST (373 patients) and the other managed with fetal biophysical profile score (279 patients) as a primary test for fetal surveillance. The correlated perinatal mortality in the NST group was 7 per 1000 and the biophysical profile group was 5 per 1000. The perinatal mortality rate in their hospital during the study period was 19 per 1000. The study suggested that, except for the negative predictive value of low 5-minute Apgar scores, the diagnostic values for all other outcome parameters (perinatal mortality, fetal distress in labor and intrauterine growth retardation) were consistently higher in the fetal biophysical profile as compared to the NST group. However, only the positive predictive value of overall abnormal outcome and the negative predictive value of small for gestational age infants were significantly better with the biophysical profile.

Baskett *et al.*[24] reported on the management of 2400 high-risk pregnancies which had a total of 5618 biophysical profile scores performed. During the study period, the overall perinatal mortality in their hospital was 14.5 per 1000. The perinatal mortality in the study population was only 9.2 per 1000. Structurally normal fetuses with a normal biophysical score had a perinatal mortality of 1 per 1000. Fetuses with very abnormal scores (0–4) had a perinatal mortality rate of 292 per 1000. In this study, abnormal perinatal outcome was defined as intrapartum fetal distress, low 5-minute Apgar score (< 7), intrauterine growth retardation, and perinatal death. The positive predictive value of an abnormal biophysical score for an abnormal perinatal outcome was 79.2%. This predictive power was significantly better as compared to the NST, fetal breathing movements, and fetal tone; however, it did not reach statistical significance when compared to fetal movement and amniotic fluid volume. In another study, Manning and co-workers[11] reported on 12 620 high-risk patients who had 26 257 biophysical profile scores. There were 93 perinatal deaths of which 24 occurred in structurally normal, non-isoimmunized fetuses (corrected perinatal mortality rate 1.9 per 1000). Eight of these structurally normal fetuses died within one week after a normal biophysical profile (corrected false-negative rate of 0.634 per 1000). The uncorrected stillbirth rate was 3.64 per 1000 and the uncorrected neonatal death rate was 3.72 per 1000. When the perinatal mortality was correlated to the biophysical score results, it was found that the overall mortality ranged from as low as 0.652 per 1000 tests (with a normal score of > 8) to as high as 187 per 1000 tests (with a score of 0). The overwhelming majority of the biophysical profiles (97.5%) were normal and only 0.76% had a score of 6 4. The same authors subsequently reported their experience with 19 221 high-risk pregnancies which were managed by 44 828 biophysical profiles[25]. The frequency of intrauterine death among structurally normal fetuses after a reassuring biophysical profile was 0.726 per 1000 (14 deaths). Because four of these deaths occurred owing to cord prolapse, the false-negative rate of a normal test, under the most ideal circumstances, could have been as low as 0.518 per 1000 (10 deaths). Eight of the antepartum fetal deaths occurred 3–7 days after a normal biophysical profile. Therefore, it is possible that increased frequency of testing (i.e. twice a week) could have prevented some or all of these fetal deaths. The usefulness of the fetal biophysical profile in predicting perinatal death has also been investigated by Baskett and co-workers[26] in 4184 fetuses. The overall perinatal mortality in the study population was 7.6 per 1000. Fetuses with a normal biophysical score (score 8–10), had a perinatal mortality rate of 1, fetuses with an equivocal score (score 6) 31.3, and fetuses with an abnormal score (score 0–4) had a perinatal mortality of 200 per 1000. The false-negative rate was 0.7 per 1000, very similar to the false-negative rate reported by Manning and co-workers (0.726 per 1000).

The selective use of the NST was reported by Manning and co-workers[27], who omitted the NST from the initial biophysical evaluation and included only the other four biophysical components (fetal breathing movements, fetal movements, fetal tone, and amniotic fluid volume). The authors studied 2712 patients who had a total number of 7851 tests and showed that the test accuracy was not compromised[27]. In addition, the need for NST was reduced to only 2.7% of the cases.

The selective use of the NST improved the efficacy of the authors' testing unit, shortened the duration of the test, and increased the number of patients that could be tested daily. A recent study, however, by Eden and co-workers[28], questioned the wisdom of omitting the NST from the initial biophysical evaluation, as fetuses with all normal biophysical components but variable decelerations during NST testing had increased frequency of abnormal perinatal outcome. More recently, Mills and co-workers[29] proposed a two-tier approach to biophysical assessment of the fetus by a retrospective review of 2038 biophysical assessments in 500 high-risk pregnancies. The authors compared the efficacy of the NST vs. biophysical profile in predicting fetal asphyxia in fetuses with normal and abnormal growth. The sensitivity, specificity, positive predictive value and negative predictive value of the NST to predict lethal fetal asphyxia were 100%, 77.5%, 0.4% and 100%, whereas of the fetal biophysical profile were 100%, 99.7%, 33.3% and 100%, respectively. The authors suggested that the biophysical evaluation of the fetus should be rationalized on the basis of the clinical problem and fetal growth. According to the authors, if the fetal growth is normal, as judged by ultrasound evaluations every four weeks, no biophysical assessment is necessary. If the growth is abnormal, biweekly NSTs and fetal growth checks by ultrasound every two weeks are indicated. The authors concluded that the fetal biophysical profile should be reserved for those cases where the NST is abnormal or equivocal. By using this testing method, the authors speculated that they could theoretically reduce their work load of NSTs by > 60% and biophysical profiles by > 75%.

The use of the biophysical profile in postdates has been reported by Johnson and co-workers[30], who managed 307 consecutive post-term pregnancies with twice-weekly biophysical profiles. The study suggested that if the biophysical score is reassuring, waiting for spontaneous onset of labor is advisable as it results in good outcome with a much lower Cesarean section rate (15% vs. 42% for induction patients)[30]. The same authors also reported on the use of the fetal biophysical profile in managing 238 diabetic pregnancies who had a total number of 1028 profiles performed[31]. In patients with an abnormal score, there was a high rate of intensive- care nursery admissions and Cesarean section rate (50%). Of the fetuses with normal biophysical profile scores, 57.4% entered spontaneous labor, 31.3% were induced, and the remaining 11.3% were delivered by elective repeat or primary Cesarean section. Stillbirths were prevented and 87% of the patients delivered at or near term with minimal maternal or neonatal morbidity. Abnormal biophysical profile scoring was associated with a significantly higher rate of operative intervention and neonatal morbidity. According to the authors, the fetal biophysical profile allows for a safe expectant management in the diabetic pregnancy.

More recently, Manning and co-workers[32] reported on the positive predictive accuracy of the very abnormal biophysical profile score (score 0). Twenty-nine of 28 655 fetuses (0.092%) had a last biophysical profile score of 0 prior to delivery. A score of 0 was defined as the absence of fetal movements, fetal tone, fewer than three gross body movements and a vertical diameter of the maximal pocket of amniotic fluid < 2 cm. The perinatal death rate in this group of 29 fetuses was 48.3% (14 of 29) and the majority (11 of 14) were stillborn. Death occurred as early as 30 minutes and as long as 11 days after the last test. Three asphyxia-related neonatal deaths occurred despite immediate and aggressive intervention. Perinatal morbid outcomes in this study were: fetal distress in labor, 5-minute Apgar score < 7, umbilical vein pH < 7.20 or admission to a neonatal intensive care unit for over 24 hours for reasons unrelated to prematurity. Morbid perinatal outcome was defined as the presence of at least one of these four outcomes. The positive predictive value of a biophysical profile score of 0, with mortality and morbidity used as endpoints, was 100%. The authors emphasized that the very abnormal fetal biophysical profile (score = 0) is a perinatal emergency. Since there were some fetuses who survived after delivery, procrastination based upon the belief that the outcome would be dismal should be discouraged in the presence of a score of 0. In another study of 26 780 fetuses, Manning and co-workers[33] studied the relationship between the last biophysical profile score and various perinatal morbid outcomes and mortality. A highly significant inverse linear correlation was observed between biophysical profile score and fetal distress, admission to neonatal intensive care unit, intrauterine growth retardation, low 5-minute Apgar score (< 7), and umbilical cord pH < 7.20. No correlation was found between fetal biophysical profile score and the incidence of meconium or major anomaly. A highly significant inverse exponential (log 10) relationship was observed between biophysical score and perinatal mortality. The authors interpreted the data as suggesting that the biophysical profile scoring provides insight into the extent and degree of fetal compromise.

The usefulness of the fetal biophysical profile in twin gestations has been studied by Lodeiro and co-workers[34]. Forty-nine twin gestations with additional high-risk factors such as suspected growth retardation of one or both twins, maternal chronic hypertension, or pregnancy-induced hypertension were followed with weekly biophysical profiles. The sensitivity, specificity, positive predictive value, and negative predictive value of the biophysical assessment in predicting fetal distress were 83.3, 100, 100 and 97.7%, respectively. The false-negative rate was 2.2%. This was due to one twin pair delivered at 26 weeks' gestation, where both neonates died because of extreme prematurity. Four twin gestations had fetal distress in only one of the twins and all eight fetuses (four pairs) had non-reactive NSTs. The biophysical profile accurately predicted the distressed twin of each of the four pairs, and it also correctly identified wellbeing for its counterpart twin. The authors concluded that the biophysical profile is a safe and effective tool in the antepartum fetal surveillance of twin gestations.

Vintzileos and co-workers[7] reported on their initial experience with 150 high-risk pregnancies, which had a total of 342 biophysical profiles. The patients were managed according to the NST–CST results. There was a good correlation between biophysical score and adverse perinatal outcomes such as abnormal intrapartum fetal heart-rate patterns, meconium during labor, fetal distress and perinatal mortality rate. Fetal biophysical scores of > 8 were associated with good pregnancy outcome in all cases and very abnormal scores (6 4) were almost always associated with fetal distress. The absence of fetal movements was the best predictor of abnormal intrapartum heart-rate patterns (80%), non-reactive NST was the best predictor of meconium stained fluid (33.3%), oligohydramnios was the best predictor of fetal distress (37.5%) and absent fetal tone was the best predictor of fetal death rate (42.8%). Eleven fetuses were born acidemic (cord arterial pH < 7.20). Prior to delivery, all had non-reactive NSTs and none had fetal breathing. There were two fetuses with normal fetal movement and both survived. Of five fetuses with movement present but compromised (one or two body movements in 30 minutes) only one died. Of four fetuses who had absent fetal movement, three died, all three also having absent fetal tone. These observations suggested that the biophysical components do not contribute to the predictive accuracy in an equally proportionate manner. The wisdom of arbitary assignment of equal score weights for the biophysical components has also been recently questioned by Manning and co-workers[35]. In a recent study of 525 fetuses, they studied the relationship between the last abnormal biophysical profile score, in total and by variable composition, and a variety of abnormal perinatal outcomes such as fetal distress in labor, low 5-minute Apgar score (< 7), intrauterine growth retardation and admission to the neonatal intensive care unit for > 24 hours. It was found that all variable combinations for the same score subsets (score 6, 4 and 2) are not equal in predictive accuracy. For a biophysical score of 6, the probability of fetal distress or death was significantly higher when the NST and fetal tone were abnormal, whereas the probability of fetal distress was significantly lower when fetal tone and fetal breathing movements were absent. Significant variations in positive predictive accuracy also occurred within subsets of variable combinations yielding a biophysical profile score of 4; these variations, however, disappeared with a biophysical profile score of 2. Overall, the NST, amniotic fluid volume, and fetal breathing movements emerged as the most powerful variables for all perinatal outcome measures. Fetal tone seemed to play a lesser role, and fetal movement was found to be important only for predicting fetal distress.

Protocol of antepartum fetal biophysical assessment

Considering the 'gradual hypoxia concept', and also the 100% sensitivity for predicting the acidemic fetus by using the combination of 'non-reactive NST and absent fetal breathing' as the abnormal test, Vintzileos and co-workers have recommended a modified fetal evaluation scheme for patients with intact membranes. This scheme is based on the individual biophysical components rather than the score (Figure 5)[8,10]. It should be noted that this scheme is also supported by the recent data of Manning and co-workers[35] which suggest that the NST, amniotic fluid volume and breathing movements are the most powerful predictors.

This protocol includes assessment of an acute (NST or fetal breathing) and a chronic (amniotic fluid volume) marker. A reactive NST or fetal breathing lasting > 30 s (even in the presence of a non-reactive NST) excludes the possibility of fetal asphyxia at the time of testing. In the presence of a non-reactive NST, the differentiation should be made between fetal sleep and asphyxia. To do so, realtime scanning is performed. If fetal breathing is detected (lasting > 30 s), the examination is terminated and further management is based on the amniotic fluid volume assessment. If all biophysical activities (non-reactive NST, fetal breathing, fetal movements, and fetal tone) are absent after 30 minutes of continuous observation, prompt delivery is undertaken. If the fetus has a non-reactive NST and breathing is absent, while movements and tone are normal, extended testing is undertaken to differentiate fetal sleep from asphyxia. The NST is continued until a reactive pattern is observed or until 120 minutes have elapsed. If the NST is still non-reactive, the realtime examination is repeated. If no fetal breathing is observed, then delivery is considered, if the gestational age is > 32 weeks. In very preterm gestations (< 32 weeks) in the absence of fetal heart rate cyclicity, in addition to non-reactive NST and absent fetal breathing, delivery is also considered[36]. If fetal heart rate cyclicity and body movements are both present and normal, then expectant management is indicated.

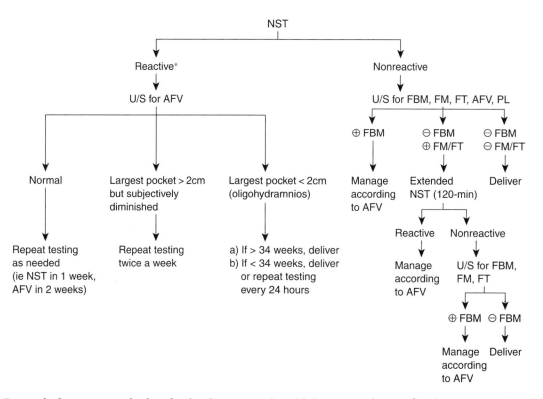

Figure 5   Protocol of antepartum fetal evaluation in pregnancies with intact membranes. *In the presence of variable decelerations and oligohydramnios, consider delivery; in the presence of variable decelerations and normal AFV, consider extended (120 minutes) or repeat NST within 24 hours. NST, non-stress test; U/S, ultrasound; AFV, amniotic fluid volume; FBM, fetal breathing; FM, fetal movement; FT, fetal tone; PL, placental grading, +, present/normal; –, absent/abnormal. Reprinted with permission from *Am J Obstet Gynecol* 1987;157:627–631.)

Another question to be addressed is whether or not the fetus is chronically stressed and therefore a candidate for a cord accident. This determination is made by assessing the presence or absence of oligohydramnios and/or variable decelerations during non-stress testing. When there is a normal amount of amniotic fluid and no variable decelerations, expectant management is indicated. The presence of oligohydramnios in a term or a near-term gestation with intact membranes is an indication for delivery regardless of how normal or abnormal the other biophysical components are. In our view, a < 2-cm largest pocket is qualified for the definition of oligohydramnios. The combination of oligohydramnios and variable decelerations during the NST constitutes an indication for delivery in viable, structurally normal fetuses, regardless of gestational age. In very preterm gestations (< 32 weeks) in the presence of oligohydramnios and no identifiable fetal anomalies, individualization should be the rule. If delivery is not undertaken, frequent testing (every 24 hours) is an alternative logical plan of management. In this group of fetuses, we have recently used continuous or pulsed Doppler studies to decide proper management. We have applied this scheme of antepartum fetal evaluation to 12 684 fetuses over an eight-year period, and we have encountered only two deaths of structurally normal fetuses within a week after a reassuring biophysical assessment. This alternative protocol of antepartum fetal evaluation, without including the scoring of the biophysical variables, not only increases the sensitivity of the method but also shortens the testing time. The understanding of the different degrees of fetal acidemia at which the fetal biophysical activities become compromised, as well as the significance of oligohydramnios, is mandatory to avoid errors that may result in unnecessary interventions or adverse perinatal outcome. The most common errors in the interpretation and application of the fetal biophysical profile have been when management decisions are based on the score alone without considering the individual biophysical components or the overall clinical context of each case, inappropriate interval between testing, and hesitancy to act promptly on the abnormal test results. The use and misuse of the fetal biophysical profile has been described in detail by Vintzileos and co-workers[10].

Computer-assisted biophysical profile

The biophysical methods currently used in clinical practice are arbitrary since they do not provide exact quantification of the biophysical activities over a long period, nor do they account for the occasionally long intervals of fetal inactivity which are frequently observed in normal fetuses. To circumvent these drawbacks, an extended period of concurrent observation of the biophysical activities has been attempted by using computer-assisted systems[37] or phonographic transducers[38]. Devoe and co-workers[39] have reported their experience by using a computerized system which allowed analysis of the simultaneously acquired biophysical activities in 200 term high-risk fetuses. The biophysical activities obtained for each high-risk fetus were compared with previously established nomograms. The results correlated with the presence or absence of perinatal mortality, fetal distress, a low 5-minute Apgar score (< 7), and intrauterine growth retardation. A test was considered abnormal if two or more biophysical activities quantitatively fell > 2 SD below the population mean. A decreased frequency of fetal body movements, decreased amniotic fluid volume, and decreased frequency of fetal heart rate accelerations were the most common abnormalities. When fetuses with normal or abnormal perinatal outcomes were classified by the last computerized biophysical test, the sensitivity was 86%, specificity 89%, positive predictive value 75%, negative predictive value 93%, and overall diagnostic accuracy 86.2%. This diagnostic accuracy was significantly better as compared to the arbitrary scoring system of Manning and co-workers. However, this comparison was not based on a randomized trial; in addition, it was not clear whether or not the computer-assisted biophysical profile results influenced patient management.

USE OF THE FETAL BIOPHYSICAL PROFILE IN PATIENTS WITH PREMATURE RUPTURE OF THE MEMBRANES (PROM)

The effect of PROM on the fetal biophysical profile and scoring throughout gestation has been investigated by Vintzileos and co-workers[14] in a retrospective analysis of 1151 fetal biophysical profiles associated with good pregnancy outcome. In that study normal fetal biophysical profiles and scores were determined from 25 to 44 weeks in patients with intact membranes (Table 5) and compared with profiles and scores of a group of patients with PROM and good pregnancy outcome (Table 7). Good pregnancy outcome was defined as the absence of congenital anomalies, infection, fetal distress, perinatal mortality, and morbidity. As shown in Table 7, in PROM patients there was more amniotic fluid volume after 32 weeks and more grade 3 placentas after 40 weeks. The frequency of reactive NSTs, fetal breathing, fetal movements, and fetal tone did not change from 25 to 44 weeks in patients with PROM. In most gestational ages the presence of PROM, as compared to intact membranes, was associated with higher frequency of reactive NSTs, absence of fetal breathing, and reduced amniotic fluid volume. The frequency of non-reactive non-stress testing at less than 32 weeks' gestation was only 13.5% in the presence of ruptured membranes. The overall biophysical

Table 7 Frequency of individual biophysical variables and biophysical scoring of > 8 in pregnancies with ruptured membranes (scoring according to the criteria by Vintzileos and co-workers)[*]

	Gestation (weeks) $n = 200$ (%)								
	25–28 $n = 30$ (15%)	*p* value	29–32 $n = 72$ (36%)	*p* value	33–36 $n = 76$ (38%)	*p* value	37–40 $n = 20$ (10%)	*p* value	41–44 $n = 2$ (1%)
NST-2	17 (56.6%)	NS	52 (72.2%)	NS	56 (73.6%)	NS	20 (100.0%)	NS	2 (100.0%)
NST-1	9 (30.0%)	NS	10 (13.8%)	NS	16 (21.0%)	NS	0 (0.0%)	NS	0 (0.0%)
NST-0	4 (13.3%)	NS	10 (13.8%)	NS	4 (5.2%)	NS	0 (0.0%)	NS	0 (0.0%)
FBM-2	10 (33.3%)	NS	38 (52.7%)	NS	49 (64.4%)	NS	13 (65.0%)	NS	2 (100.0%)
FBM-1	1 (3.3%)	NS	5 (6.9%)	NS	8 (10.5%)	NS	4 (20.0%)	NS	0 (0.0%)
FBM-0	19 (63.3%)	NS	29 (40.2%)	NS	19 (25.0%)	NS	3 (15.0%)	NS	0 (0.0%)
FM-2	30 (100%)	NS	69 (95.8%)	NS	73 (96.0%)	NS	20 (100.0%)	NS	2 (100.0%)
FM-1	0 (0.0%)	NS	3 (4.1%)	NS	3 (3.9%)	NS	0 (0.0%)	NS	0 (0.0%)
FM-0	0 (0.0%)	NS	0 (0.0%)	NS	0 (0.0%)	NS	0 (0.0%)	NS	0 (0.0%)
FT-2	30 (100.0%)	NS	69 (95.8%)	NS	74 (97.3%)	NS	20 (100.0%)	NS	2 (100.0%)
FT-1	0 (0.0%)	NS	3 (4.2%)	NS	2 (2.6%)	NS	0 (0.0%)	NS	0 (0.0%)
FT-0	0 (0.0%)	NS	0 (0.0%)	NS	0 (0.0%)	NS	0 (0.0%)	NS	0 (0.0%)
AF-2	19 (63.3%)	NS	46 (63.8%)	<0.05	66 (86.8%)	NS	16 (80.0%)	NS	0 (0.0%)
AF-1	5 (16.6%)	NS	17 (23.6%)	<0.05	7 (9.2%)	NS	1 (5.0%)	NS	0 (0.0%)
AF-0	6 (20.0%)	NS	9 (12.5%)	<0.05	3 (3.9%)	NS	3 (15.0%)	NS	2 (100.0%)
PL-2	29 (96.6%)	NS	72 (100.0%)	NS	71 (93.4%)	NS	17 (85.0%)	<0.05	0 (0.0%)
PL-1	0 (0.0%)	NS	0 (0.0%)	NS	2 (2.6%)	NS	0 (0.0%)	NS	0 (0.0%)
PL-0	1 (3.3%)	NS	0 (0.0%)	NS	3 (3.9%)	NS	3 (15.0%)	<0.05	2 (100.0%)
Total score of > 8	26 (86.6%)	NS	70 (97.2%)		75 (98.6%)	NS	18 (90.0%)	NS	2 (100.0%)

[*]See Table 3

NST, non-stress test; FBM, fetal breathing movements; FM, fetal movements; FT, fetal tone; AF, amniotic fluid volume

PL, placental grading; NS, not significant. Reprinted with permission from reference 14

Table 8 Changes in fetal biophysical profile caused by PROM

- Increase in fetal heart-rate reactivity
- Decrease in fetal breathing movements
- No change in fetal movements
- No change in fetal tone
- No change in the overall biophysical score

scoring was not altered by the presence of PROM. The changes in the fetal biophysical profile caused by PROM are summarized in Table 8.

A prospective study by Vintzileos *et al.*[40] using frequent fetal biophysical assessments in patients with PROM showed that an abnormal biophysical profile was an early indicator of intra-amniotic infection. Seventy-three patients with no clinical signs of labor or infection were included in the study. A fetal biophysical profile was performed on admission and was repeated every 24–48 hours. The last biophysical assessment before delivery was correlated with the development of clinical amnionitis, possible neonatal sepsis and neonatal sepsis. The diagnosis of possible neonatal sepsis was made when there was strong clinical and laboratory evidence of neonatal infection but the cultures were

negative. The diagnosis of neonatal sepsis was made in the presence of positive cultures of blood, urine, or cerebrospinal fluid. There was no correlation between the fetal biophysical assessment and intra-amniotic infection in the 20 of the 73 patients who delivered > 24 hours from the last biophysical assessment. There were 53 patients who delivered in < 24 hours of the last examination; in these patients, a biophysical score of > 8 was associated with an infection rate of 2.7%, and an abnormal biophysical score (6 7) was associated with an overall infection rate of 93.7%. The first manifestations of fetal intra-amniotic infection were non-reactive non-stress testing and absence of fetal breathing. Loss of fetal movement and absent fetal tone were late findings in the process of infection. The best predictor of infection was the overall biophysical score. Of the individual biophysical components, the NST, fetal breathing movements, fetal movement, and fetal tone were found to be important in the above order. The fetal biophysical score was 6 7 in all 14 cases with possible neonatal sepsis or neonatal sepsis. No difference in the mean cord pH between the infected and non-infected cases was found, an observation that suggests that the low scores of the infected group were not due to hypoxia, but rather to infection.

In patients with PROM, the degree of oligohydramnios, as one of the components of the biophysical profile, is strongly correlated to pregnancy prolongation, intrapartum fetal heart rate patterns consistent with umbilical cord compression, Cesarean section rate, fetal distress, infection, and perinatal mortality rate. The correlation between the degree of oligohydramnios and pregnancy outcome in 90 patients with PROM and no signs of infection or labor has been reported by Vintzileos and co-workers[41]. Patients with severe oligohydramnios (largest amniotic fluid pocket < 1 cm) had the highest frequency of amnionitis (47.3%), possible neonatal sepsis (26.3%), and neonatal sepsis (31.5%); the frequency of amnionitis, possible neonatal sepsis, and neonatal sepsis in patients with largest amniotic fluid pocket > 2 cm was 9.2, 3.7, and 1.8%, respectively. The authors concluded that patients with PROM and severe oligohydramnios should be followed with daily fetal biophysical profiles.

The usefulness of the NST in following patients with PROM was determined by a retrospective analysis of 127 consecutive patients with PROM[42]. These patients had NSTs every 24–48 hours as part of the fetal biophysical profile. Based on the last NST result prior to delivery the sensitivity, specificity, positive predictive value, and negative predictive value to predict infection outcome were calculated to be 78.1, 86.3, 67.7, and 92.1%, respectively. Analysis of the longitudinal trend of the NST results showed that patients who initially had a reactive NST and subsequently converted to a non-reactive NST developed clinical intra-amniotic infection in almost 90% of the cases.

The usefulness of fetal breathing, lasting > 30 s, to predict intra-amniotic infection has also been investigated in 130 patients with PROM who were followed with assessments every 24–48 hours[43]. The sensitivity, specificity, positive predictive value, and negative predictive value of fetal breathing to predict intra-amniotic infection were 91.6, 64.8, 50, and 95.3%, respectively. Of the individual biophysical components, the presence of fetal breathing has been the most reliable in ruling out fetal infection, if observed within 24 hours prior to delivery.

Vintzileos and co-workers[44] have presented a comparison between daily fetal biophysical profile determinations and amniocentesis (for Gram stain and culture) in 58 patients who presented with preterm PROM and no apparent infection or labor. In addition to the usual indications for delivery, a positive Gram stain or culture of the transabdominally obtained amniotic fluid, or a persistently abnormal biophysical score (6 7 on two examinations, 2 hours apart, in the presence of a non-reactive NST and absence of fetal breathing) were also considered as indications for delivery. The last biophysical profile prior to delivery and amniocentesis results on admission were correlated with infection outcome. All but one of the 13 cases with

neonatal infection were associated with an abnormal biophysical assessment. There were two cases with amnionitis without neonatal infection; both cases had normal biophysical profiles. The sensitivity, specificity, positive predictive value, and negative predictive value of the biophysical profile were 80, 97.6, 92.3 and 93.3%, respectively. The sensitivity, specificity, positive predictive value, and negative predictive value of the Gram stain were 60, 81.3, 52.9, and 85.3%, respectively, whereas the amniotic fluid cultures were 60, 86, 60, and 86%, respectively. The authors concluded that in preterm PROM daily biophysical profiles are more efficacious than amniocentesis on admission in selecting those patients who are having or are candidates for intra-amniotic infection and therefore in need of prompt delivery. Moreover, the fetal biophysical profile is simple, non-invasive, it can be repeated daily, or even more frequently, and it is applicable to all patients.

The question of whether or not the pregnancy outcome is improved by using daily biophysical profiles has been investigated by Vintzileos and co-workers[45]. In that study, the study group (73 consecutive patients with PROM) were managed with daily biophysical profiles according to the protocol illustrated in Figure 6. The pregnancy outcome of this group was compared with the outcomes of two other historic groups: one control group managed conservatively (73 consecutive patients with PROM) and the other managed with amniocentesis on admission (73 consecutive patients with PROM). Maternal and neonatal infection rates, as well as low 5-minute Apgar scores were significantly less in the study than in the control group. The percentage of mother–infant pairs who developed infection in the study group (10.9%) was significantly less than in the control group (30.1%). Clinical amnionitis was reduced from 20.5 to 5.4%. The frequencies of possible neonatal sepsis and neonatal sepsis were also lower in the study group as compared to the control group (5.4 vs. 13.6% and 1.3 vs. 9.5%, respectively). As compared with the amniocentesis group, the study group had significantly less neonatal sepsis (1.3 vs. 12.3%). The authors concluded that the use of amniocentesis may decrease the incidence of clinical amnionitis, but it does not improve the neonatal infection outcome. The neonatal infection outcome was, however, reduced by using daily biophysical assessment.

Mechanism by which fetal biophysical activities are compromised in the presence of intra-amniotic infection

In order to investigate the role of fetal acidemia in causing diminished biophysical activities in the setting of subclinical infection and PROM, Vintzileos and co-workers[46] have undertaken a prospective evaluation of 53 consecutive patients with preterm PROM who

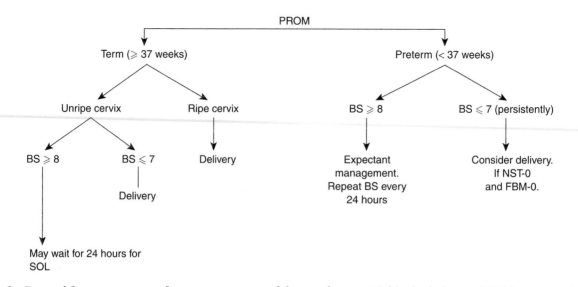

Figure 6 Protocol for management of premature rupture of the membranes. BS, biophysical score, NST-0, non-reactive non-stress test, FBM-0, fetal breathing absent; SOL, spontaneous onset of labor. Reprinted with permission from reference 40

were delivered because of an abnormal fetal biophysical assessment as the only indication. Fetal acidemia at birth was defined as cord artery pH < 7.20. Of the 53 fetuses, 19 developed no maternal or neonatal infection and none was acidemic at birth. Seventeen fetuses developed possible neonatal sepsis and none was acidemic at birth. Fifteen fetuses developed neonatal sepsis and only five were acidemic at birth. Two fetuses developed clinical amnionitis and only one was acidemic at birth. While fetal acidosis could explain the diminished fetal biophysical activities in five of the 15 fetuses who developed neonatal sepsis and in one with clinical amnionitis, this mechanism could not explain the compromised biophysical activities in the remaining 10 fetuses with neonatal sepsis and all 17 fetuses who developed possible neonatal sepsis. A possible explanation for the diminished biophysical activities of the infected non-acidemic fetus may be an increased production of prostaglandins, perhaps through interleukin-1 release. Interleukin-1, which is the main fever mediator, induces changes in the electroencephalogram that may be responsible for the decreased motor activity during fever in both animals and humans[47]. Since interleukin-1 is capable of stimulating prostaglandin production from macrophages and other cell types, it has been suggested that this effect may be responsible for the decrease in fetal breathing observed not only prior to labor but also in the setting of subclinical infection. This increased prostaglandin secretion may be responsible for the direct inhibitory effect on the fetal CNS centers or indirectly may lead to increased peripheral vascular resistance through vasoconstriction of the umbilical and chorionic vessels[48,49]. Since there are experimental data to suggest

that prostaglandins increase placental vascular resistance through vasoconstriction of umbilical and chorionic vessels, it seems reasonable to investigate the role of Doppler umbilical artery velocimetry in this group of patients. In our institution the relationships among umbilical artery velocimetry, fetal biophysical profile and placental inflammation in patients with PROM have recently been examined[50]. Our preliminary results involved 28 consecutive patients with preterm PROM who were followed with daily fetal biophysical profiles and systolic : diastolic (S : D) ratios as determined by a continuous wave Doppler. After delivery, placental pathologic examination for evidence of inflammation was performed in all cases. When only the last examination, within 24 hours of delivery, was considered, patients with placental inflammation (choriodeciduitis, umbilical and/or chorionic vasculitis) had higher mean S : D ratio (2.92 ± 0.62 versus 2.29 ± 0.25) and lower biophysical score (6.2 ± 2.3 versus 9.1 ± 2.1) as compared to those without evidence of placental inflammation. It should be noted that the mean S : D ratio value 24 hours prior to delivery in cases with placental inflammation was 2.92, which is not necessarily higher than the normal range. Fetuses with placental infection increased their S : D ratio during the last 24 hours prior to delivery approximately 30% (which was statistically significant) over the mean value of the preceding days. Our preliminary data suggest that larger studies are needed to more accurately determine the value of the longitudinal trend in S : D ratios in regard to being an additional non-invasive means of identifying subclinical intra-amniotic infection. The increase in umbilical vascular resistance supports a role for vasoactive substances, i.e. prostaglandins, as mediators of infection causing vasoconstriction of umbilical and chorionic vessels. This increase in vascular resistance may compromise uteroplacental circulation and diminish biophysical activities prior to the development of fetal acidemia.

REFERENCES

1. Evertson LR, Gauthier RJ, Schifrin BS, *et al*. Antepartum fetal heart rate testing. I. Evolution of the nonstress test. *Am J Obstet Gynecol* 1979;133:29–33

2. Schifrin BS. The rationale of antepartum fetal heart rate monitoring. *J Reprod Med* 1979;23:213–21

3. Christie GB, Cudmore W. The oxytocin challenge test. *Am J Obstet Gynecol* 1979;118:327–30

4. Gauthier RJ, Evertson LR, Paul RH. Antepartum fetal heart rate testing. II. Intrapartum fetal heart rate testing and neonatal outcome following a positive contraction stress test. *Am J Obstet Gynecol* 1979;133:34–9

5. Ray M, Freeman R, Pine S, *et al*. Clinical experience with the oxytocin challenge test. *Am J Obstet Gynecol* 1972;114:1–9

6. Manning FA, Platt LD, Sipos L. Antepartum fetal evaluation. Development of a fetal biophysical profile score. *Am J Obstet Gynecol* 1980;136:787–95

7. Vintzileos AM, Campbell WA, Ingardia CJ, *et al*. The fetal biophysical profile and its predictive value. *Obstet Gynecol* 1983;62:271–8

8. Vintzileos AM, Gaffney SE, Salinger LM, *et al*. The relationship between fetal biophysical profile and cord pH in patients undergoing Cesarean section before the onset of labor. *Obstet Gynecol* 1987;70:196–201

9. Chamberlain PFC, Manning FA, Morrison I, *et al*. Ultrasound evaluation of amniotic fluid volumes. I. The relationship of marginal and decreased amniotic fluid volumes to perinatal outcome. *Am J Obstet Gynecol* 1984;150:245–9

10. Vintzileos AM, Campbell WA, Nochimson DJ, *et al*. The use and misuse of the fetal biophysical profile. *Am J Obstet Gynecol* 1987;156:527–33

11. Manning FA, Morrison I, Lange IR, *et al*. Fetal assessment based on fetal biophysical profile scoring: experience in 12 620 referred high risk pregnancies. I. Perinatal morbidity by frequency and etiology. *Am J Obstet Gynecol* 1985;151:343

12. Ribbert LSM, Snijders RJM, Nicolaides KH, *et al*. Relationship of fetal biophysical profile and blood gas values at cordocentesis in severely growth-retarded fetuses. *Am J Obstet Gynecol* 1990;163:569–71

13. Vintzileos AM, Fleming AD, Scorza WE, *et al*. Relationship between fetal biophysical activities and umbilical cord blood gases. *Am J Obstet Gynecol* 1991;165:707–13

14. Vintzileos AM, Feinstein SJ, Lodeiro JG, *et al*. Fetal biophysical profile and the effect of premature rupture of the membranes. *Obstet Gynecol* 1986;67:818–23

15. Hopper KD, Komppa GH, Bice P, *et al*. A reevaluation of placental grading and its clinical significance. *J Ultrasound Med* 1984;3:261–6

16. Lavin JP, Miodovnik M, Barden TP. Relationship of nonstress test reactivity and gestational age. *Obstet Gynecol* 1984;63:338–44

17. Queenan JT, Thompson W, Whitfield CR, *et al*. Amniotic fluid volume in normal pregnancies. *Am J Obstet Gynecol* 1972;114:34–8

18. Sadovsky E, Laufer N, Allen JW. The incidence of different types of fetal movement during pregnancy. *Br J Obstet Gynaecol* 1979;86:10–14

19. Baskett TF. Gestational age and fetal biophysical assessment. *Am J Obstet Gynecol* 1988;158:332–4

20. Manning FA, Morrison I, Lange IR. Fetal biophysical profile scoring: a prospective study of 1184 high-risk patients. *Am J Obstet Gynecol* 1981;140:289–94

21. Platt LD, Eglington GS, Sipos L, *et al*. Further experience with the fetal biophysical profile score. *Obstet Gynecol* 1983;61:480–5

22. Manning FA, Lange IR, Morrison I, *et al*. Fetal biophysical profile score and the nonstress test: a comparative trial. *Obstet Gynecol* 1984;64:326–31

23. Platt LD, Walla CA, Paul RH, *et al*. A prospective trial of fetal biophysical profile versus the nonstress test in the management of high risk pregnancies. *Am J Obstet Gynecol* 1985;153:624–33

24. Baskett TF, Gray JH, Prewett SJ, *et al*. Antepartum fetal assessment using a fetal biophysical profile score. *Am J Obstet Gynecol* 1984;148:630–3

25. Manning FA, Morrison I, Harman CR, *et al*. Fetal assessment based on fetal biophysical profile scoring: experience in 19 221 referred high risk pregnancies. II. An analysis of false-negative fetal deaths. *Am J Obstet Gynecol* 1987;157:880–4

26. Baskett TF, Allen AC, Gray JH, *et al*. Fetal biophysical profile and perinatal death. *Obstet Gynecol* 1987;70:357–60

27. Manning FA, Morrison I, Lange IR, *et al*. Fetal biophysical profile scoring: selective use of the nonstress test. *Am J Obstet Gynecol* 1987;156:709–12

28. Eden RD, Seifert LS, Kodack LD, *et al*. A modified biophysical profile for antenatal fetal surveillance. *Obstet Gynecol* 1988;71:365–9

29. Mills MS, James DK, Slade S. Two-tier approach to biophysical assessment of the fetus. *Am J Obstet Gynecol* 1990;163:12–17

30. Johnson JM, Harman CR, Lange IR, *et al*. Biophysical profile scoring in the management of postterm pregnancy: an analysis of 307 patients. *Am J Obstet Gynecol* 1986;154:269–73

31. Johnson JM, Lange IR, Harman CR, *et al*. Biophysical profile scoring in the management of the diabetic pregnancy. *Obstet Gynecol* 1988;72:841–6

32. Manning FA, Harman CR, Morrison I, *et al*. Fetal assessment based on fetal biophysical profile scoring. III. Positive predictive accuracy of the very abnormal test (biophysical profile score = 0). *Am J Obstet Gynecol* 1990;162:398–402

33. Manning FA, Harman CR, Morrison I, *et al*. Fetal assessment based on fetal biophysical profile scoring. IV. An analysis of perinatal morbidity and mortality. *Am J Obstet Gynecol* 1990;162:703–9

34. Lodeiro JG, Vintzileos AM, Feinstein SJ, *et al.* Fetal biophysical profile in twin gestations. *Obstet Gynecol* 1986;67:824–7

35. Manning FA, Morrison I, Harman CR, *et al.* The abnormal fetal biophysical profile score. V. Predictive accuracy according to score composition. *Am J Obstet Gynecol* 1990;162:918–24

36. Vintzileos AM, Campbell WA, Bors-Koefoed R, *et al.* The relationship between cyclic variation of fetal heart rate patterns and cord pH in preterm gestations. *Am J Perinatol* 1989;6:310–13

37. Devoe LD, Searle N, Phillips M, *et al.* Computer-assisted assessment of the fetal biophysical profile. *Am J Obstet Gynecol* 1985;153:317–21

38. Colley N, Southall DP. Biophysical profile in the fetus from a phonographic sensor. *Eur J Obstet Gynecol Reprod Biol* 1986;23:261–6

39. Devoe LD, Castillo RA, Searle N, *et al.* Prognostic components of computerized fetal biophysical testing. *Am J Obstet Gynecol* 1988;158:1144–8

40. Vintzileos AM, Campbell WA, Nochimson DJ, *et al.* The fetal biophysical profile in patients with premature rupture of the membranes – an early predictor of fetal infection. *Am J Obstet Gynecol* 1985;152:510–16

41. Vintzileos AM, Campbell WA, Nochimson DJ, *et al.* Degree of oligohydramnios and pregnancy outcome in patients with premature rupture of the membranes. *Obstet Gynecol* 1985;66:162–7

42. Vintzileos AM, Campbell WA, Nochimson DJ, *et al.* The use of the nonstress test in patients with premature rupture of the membranes. *Am J Obstet Gynecol* 1986;155:149–53

43. Vintzileos AM, Campbell WA, Nochimson DJ, *et al.* Fetal breathing as a predictor of infection in premature rupture of the membranes. *Obstet Gynecol* 1986;67:813–17

44. Vintzileos AM, Campbell WA, Nochimson DJ, *et al.* Fetal biophysical profile versus amniocentesis in predicting infection in preterm premature rupture of the membranes. *Obstet Gynecol* 1986;68:488–94

45. Vintzileos AM, Bors-Koefoed R, Pelegano JF, *et al.* The use of fetal biophysical profile improves pregnancy outcome in premature rupture of the membranes. *Am J Obstet Gynecol* 1987;157:236–40

46. Vintzileos AM, Petrikovsky BM, Campbell WA, *et al.* Cord blood gases and abnormal fetal biophysical assessment in preterm premature rupture of the membranes. *Am J Perinatol* 1991;8:155–60

47. Baracos V, Rodemann P, Dinarello CA, *et al.* Stimulation of muscle protein degradation and prostaglandin E_2 release by leukocytic pyrogen interleukin-1. *New Engl J Med* 1983;308:553–8

48. Howard RB, Hosokawa T, Maquire MH. Pressor and depressor actions of prostanoids in the intact human fetoplacental vascular bed. *Prostaglandins, Leukotrienes Med* 1986;21:323–30

49. Mak KK-W, Gude NM, Walters WAW, *et al.* Effects of vasoactive autacoids on the human umbilical–fetal placental vasculature. *Br J Obstet Gynaecol* 1984;91:99–106

50. Fleming DA, Salafia C, Vintzileos AM, *et al.* The relationships among umbilical arterial velocimetry, fetal biophysical profile and placental inflammation in preterm premature rupture of the membranes. *Am J Obstet Gynecol* 1991;164:38–41

56
Fetal blood sampling

F. Daffos

INTRODUCTION

Modern technology has enhanced the study of fetal physiology, a unique state characterized by maternal dependence via the placenta and gestational age changes. A valued technique, fetal blood sampling facilitates biophysical intrauterine evaluation of the fetus and is vital to the growing clinical discipline of fetal medicine.

TECHNIQUE
Procedure

Fetoscopic blood sampling has been replaced by an ultrasound-guided puncture of the umbilical cord[1]. A high-resolution, realtime ultrasonographic machine is used to locate the placental insertion of the umbilical cord. Under an aseptic condition and direct ultrasonographic guidance, a long 20- or 22-guage needle is introduced near the ultrasound transducer, in the plane of the ultrasound image, and passed through the maternal abdominal wall. The needle is guided toward the vessels of the cord, which subsequently are punctured at about 1 cm from insertion into the placenta. The cord insertion is used as opposed to free loops of the cord because the cord insertion is fixed (Figure 1). The punctured vessel is usually the vein, due to its larger diameter, rather than the artery. Depending on gestational age, 1–3 ml of fetal blood are taken, which is usually < 5% of the feto-placental blood volume.

Fetal blood sampling can be accomplished as early as week 18 of gestation. The procedure can be performed using local anesthesia with xylocaine without premedications. Repeated samplings allow the physician to follow progression of a fetal disease and response to therapy. Our experience has revealed that the procedure takes < 10 min in 92% of cases and has a success rate of 97%, with one single puncture of the mother's abdominal wall.

Special considerations

Fetal blood sampling technique may be difficult in the following situations:

(1) Maternal obesity impairs image quality and necessitates a longer needle which is more difficult to guide into the vessels.

(2) Oligohydramnios, polyhydramnios or the large size of a term fetus may visually hamper the funicular insertion. Puncturing the cord near the insertion to the fetal abdomen or a free loop of umbilical cord near the cord insertion may be necessary. When encountering oligohydramnios, filling the amniotic cavity with warm, normal saline may improve visualization. In the case of polyhydramnios, removal of a substantial amount of amniotic fluid to reduce the distance between the abdominal wall and the point of the cord insertion may improve visualization and facilitate needle guidance.

(3) Fetal movements may dislodge the needle from the cord prematurely and cause severe fetal bleeding, especially in the case of velamentous insertion of the cord.

(4) In twin pregnancies, it is essential to ascertain the fetus to whom the punctured cord belongs.

When encountering difficulty during a fetal blood sampling, do not persist for > 15 min. Instead, schedule another sampling a few days later.

Complications

According to Hohlfeld and co-workers[2]: 'The risk of complications and fetal death after fetal blood

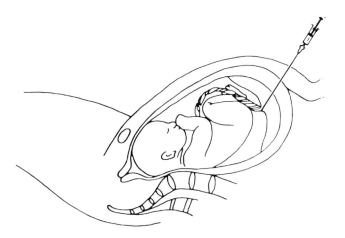

Figure 1 Fetal blood sampling from the umbilical vein with the use of a needle guided by ultrasound

sampling (FBS) varies according to the underlying fetal disorder, the gestational age and the operator's experience. In low-risk situations, such as prenatal diagnosis of congenital toxoplasmosis, the risk of early fetal loss (within 3 weeks of the sampling) was 0.60%, and the total spontaneous fetal loss was 1.29% in our series of 2731 consecutive cases. Furthermore, in our experience, no fetal or neonatal death was observed in the case of FBS performed past the 36th week of gestation (*n* = 365). Sampling should only be considered when the maternal bleeding time is normal and platelet count > 50 × 10^9^/l. At risk pregnant women should be specifically instructed to avoid acetylsalicylic acid and other drugs interfering with platelet function. In this series, thrombocytopenia, however severe, never led to serious funicular hemorrhage after FBS.'

The most frequently encountered complications are as follows.

- *Chorioamnionitis* correlates with the number of punctures through the maternal abdominal wall. Our experience suggests that this complication rises when more than two punctures occur for each sampling attempt. Chorioamnionitis may be associated with peritonitis, which occurs when the needle passes through the bowel.

- *Premature ruptured membranes* and *uterine contractions* occur more frequently as the gestational age advances, especially in the presence of preexisting spontaneous contractions and/or polyhydramnios.

- *Bleeding* from the point of puncture is observed in 60% of the cases. The bleeding stops spontaneously within two minutes in 93% of the cases. Seldom does it cause fetal anemia, but it can occasionally bring about fatal exsanguination when the fetus has a hemorrhagic disorder (e.g. Glanzmann's thrombasthenia or thrombocytopenia).

- *Fetal bradycardia* during or immediately following the procedure is observed in 10% of the cases. It is most often transient. In the early gestational age (18–20 weeks of amenorrhea), however, fetal bradycardia may fail to subside and may bring about fetal death within a few hours (0.25% of cases).

- *Spasm of the punctured artery* may account for the abnormalities of the fetal cardiac rhythm which may necessitate delivery once fetal viability is reached[3]. Spasm also may induce cord hematoma and thrombosis of the punctured vessel.

- *Fetomaternal hemorrhage* may occur in > 50% of the cases (< 5 ml in two-thirds of cases) particularly when funicentesis is transplacental, which may result in erythroblastosis fetalis. The rhesus blood group of the fetus should therefore be assessed. If the mother is rhesus negative and the fetus is rhesus positive, the mother should receive Rhogam ®(Johnson and Johnson; anti-D gamma-globulins). The amount of Rhogam to be given can be determined from the Kleihauer–Betke test done within 24 h of the procedure. A positive maternal indirect Coombs test indicates that a sufficient quantity of Rhogam is administered.

Assessment of fetal blood purity

The blood sampling may be contaminated by maternal blood or diluted by amniotic fluid. Its purity should be ensured prior to interpretation of biological results[4]. Maternal blood contamination may be associated with the presence of IgM in fetal blood; this could lead to a misdiagnosis of fetal congenital infection.

Similarly, a substantial contamination by amniotic fluid can falsely suggest fetal anemia. A minute dilution with amniotic fluid can cause thrombocytopenia and activate the coagulation cascade which could lead to the misdiagnosis of fetal coagulopathy.

CLINICAL APPLICATIONS OF FETAL BLOOD SAMPLING

Initially, fetal blood sampling was limited to determination of fetal karyotype during the third trimester of gestation, and existence of a protein or an enzyme in fetal blood when hereditary diseases were concerned. Currently, it is possible to diagnose illnesses acquired in the course of pregnancy such as infection, hypoxemia and maternofetal immunological conflicts (Table 1).

The fetal karyotype

Karyotyping from fetal lymphocytes can be obtained within 48–72 h. Indications for fetal karyotyping are:

(1) Presence of fetal structural anomalies, detected by ultrasonography, frequently associated with chromosomal anomaly.

(2) Existence of a mosaicism on chorionic villi or amniotic fluid analysis.

(3) Failure of amniocyte culture after amniocentesis.

(4) Diagnosis of Fragile X after a negative study on amniocytes in a male fetus.

(5) Severe intrauterine growth restriction (IUGR) which carries a high risk for chromosomal abnormality. The associated severe oligohydramnios precludes access to the amniotic cavity.

Hereditary hematological diseases

These are as follows.

(1) Coagulation factor deficiencies.

(2) Hemophilia. The prenatal diagnosis of hemophilia can be facilitated by fetal blood sampling in the following situations:

Table 1   Indications for fetal blood sampling

Prenatal diagnosis	*Assessment of fetal welfare*	*Fetal therapy*	*Fetal pharmacology*

Karyotyping
  Fetal malformation
  Intrauterine growth
    restriction
  Mosaicism on amniotic
    fluid
  Fragile X syndrome
Hereditary diseases
  Coagulopathies
  Hemoglobinopathies
  Immune deficiency
Congenital infections
  Toxoplasmosis
  Rubella, varicella,
    cytomegalovirus
  Parvovirus
	Intrauterine growth
	  restriction
	    Fetal anoxia
	    Nutrition status
	Maternofetal
	  immunological
	  conflict
	    Blood groups
	    Platelet groups
		In utero transfusions
		  Red blood cells, platelets
		Drugs
		  Thyroxine, digitoxin
			Transplacental passage of drugs
			  Pyrimethamine, aspirin,
			    vitamin K_1, low-molecular-
			    weight heparins

no study of the index case is available;

the family is not aware of known DNA polymorphisms;

the patient's first referral is in the second half of pregnancy;

the diagnosis of non-hemophiliac male fetus has been established on DNA by means of extragenic markers carrying a risk of recombinations.

The diagnosis rests on determination of factor VIII or IX activity. The normal values for the fetus during the second trimester are:

factor VIIIc: 40% ± 12% of the adult;

factor IXc: 9.8% ± 1.2% of the adult.

(3) Von Willebrand's disease. This occurs when both parents have Type I or one of the parents has Type IIa.

(4) Hereditary thrombocytopathies and thrombocytopenias:

Glanzmann's thrombasthenia, Jean Bernard and Soulier's thrombocytic dystrophy;

thrombocytopenia with radial aplasia (TAR syndrome).

(5) Hemoglobinopathies (sickle cell disease, beta-thalassemia). The diagnosis is based on:

the study of *in vitro* synthesis of the globin chains by fetal reticulocytes;

the direct study of hemoglobin in fetal erythrocytes by electrofocusing or by chromatography on ion-exchange resin.

Fetal blood sampling may be useful when diagnosis cannot be made from the DNA analysis of

chorionic villi, when the gestational age is too advanced, or a large number of mutations is present (beta-thalassemia).

(6) Hereditary immunodeficiencies. A thorough study of the index case is a prerequisite.

(7) Red blood cell enzymatic deficiencies. Funicentesis is indicated in couples who already have had a homozygous child.

Fetal infection

Generally, the earlier in pregnancy the infection occurs, the more severe fetal sequelae are. At about the 18th–20th week of amenorrhea, the fetus is able to synthesize a sufficient quantity of its own specific antibodies. These antibodies can ameliorate fetal infection.

It is possible to diagnose a large number of congenital infections *in utero* (toxoplasmosis, rubella, cytomegalovirus, varicella, parvovirus, chlamydia). As in adult medicine, the diagnosis of fetal infection is based on biological signs such as the presence of a pathogenic element or antibodies in fetal blood or amniotic fluid.

Detection of a parasite or a virus in the fetus can be accomplished with cell culture in continuous lineages or by inoculating the sediment of amniotic fluid centrifugation or fetal blood into animals such as mice.

The rubella virus usually can be cultured from fetal blood. Cytomegalovirus is more often found in the amniotic fluid. *Toxoplasma gondii* may be detected in fetal blood or amniotic fluid (Table 2). It is found in fetal blood when infection occurs shortly before fetal blood sampling[5]. Following a parasitemia of a variable duration, the parasite is eliminated through fetal urines and thus can be assessed by polymerase chain reaction (PCR) techniques from amniotic fluid samples in amniotic fluid[6].

Table 2   Presence of *Toxoplasma gondii* in cases of congenital toxoplasmosis

Time of maternal infection (in weeks of amenorrhea)	Time of fetal blood sampling (in weeks of amenorrhea ± SD)	Inoculation into mice (percentage of positive results)		
		Fetal blood	Amniotic fluid	Both
Between 6 and 16 weeks	23.03 ± 2.5	16%	16%	50%
Between 17 and 25 weeks	26.54 ± 2.4	45%	20%	25%

Fetal synthesis of specific IgM antibodies

The fetus's capacity to synthesize IgM antibodies against fetal infection gradually matures as gestational age advances. Non-specific total IgM is rarely found in fetal blood before 17 weeks of gestation. The rate of IgM synthesis increases rapidly between 17 and 22 weeks of gestation. Beyond 22 weeks of gestation, the fetal production of IgM antibodies in response to infection is universally observed.

The slightest trace of contamination by maternal blood containing specific IgM would misdiagnose fetal infection. Moreover, fetal synthesis of IgM is very low and may be undetected if the assays are not sensitive enough. A reliable result cannot be reasonably expected until week 22 of gestation.

The fetal synthesis of specific IgM antibodies varies with the pathogenic agents and is affected by the blocking effect of maternal IgM antibodies and maternal treatment. For example, whereas specific IgM antibodies are found in nearly all cases of congenital rubella, they are found in only 20% of congenital toxoplasmosis.

Fetal responses to congenital infection may have other manifestations such as leukocytosis, thrombocytopenia and abnormal liver enzymes. These findings may be helpful in the prenatal diagnosis of congenital infection.

Fetal hypoxemia

Intrauterine growth restriction in the non-malformed fetus is a significant cause of perinatal mortality and morbidity. The common denominator is placental dysfunction with a decrease in maternofetal oxygenation. Fetal blood sampling allows the physician to objectively evaluate the degree of fetal hypoxemia. Although the pathophysiology of fetal hypoxemia requires further study, the clinical application of fetal oxygenation and acid–base status is currently in progress. The signs of chronic progressive fetal hypoxia are more stable and reliable than those of acute decompensation, which may vary rapidly in response to maternal oxygenation, uterine contractions and maternal stress caused by the sampling itself[7].

The need to assess the degree and duration of hypoxia must be tempered by the risk of fetal blood sampling in the setting of fetal growth restriction. Fetal growth restriction is a clinical condition for which use of this technique is contentious. Fetuses with IUGR tolerate cord puncture less well than other third-trimester fetuses and thus often exhibit severe bradycardia during, or shortly after, the procedure. Since Doppler investigation provides an indirect, non-invasive, means to assess fetal hypoxia and acidemia, blood sampling should be reserved for those fetuses with severe IUGR in early gestation whereby more information is required for management.

The maternofetal immunological conflict

Red blood cell fetomaternal incompatibilities

While Rhogam has reduced the incidence of anti-D alloimmunization, severe rhesus hemolytic disease still exists. Failure or insufficient administration of Rhogam accounts for 75% of the cases of rhesus isoimmunization. Management of rhesus isoimmunization includes:

(1) Patient history. The disease intensifies with subsequent pregnancy.

(2) Evaluation of maternal specific IgG titer, the critical value being 1 μg/ml with the indirect Coombs titer being at least 1:16.

(3) The ultrasonographic findings of fetal hydrops which are associated with significant fetal anemia.

(4) Determination of the bilirubin index of the amniotic fluid from amniocentesis, starting at 26–28 weeks of gestation. This is an indirect reflection of fetal hemolysis.

Funicentesis can be utilized for both diagnosis and treatment of this condition[8]. Fetomaternal incompatibilities of c, C, E and Kell antigens may also be as early and severe as rhesus D incompatibilities. When the father is known to be c positive or Kell positive, the antenatal management is similar to that of rhesus D incompatibility.

Fetal thrombocytopenia

The three major causes of severe fetal thrombocytopenia are alloimmunization in the platelet PlA$_1$ (or ZWA) system, idiopathic thrombocytopenic purpuras (ITP), and asymptomatic thrombocytopenias (AST) near the end of pregnancy.

The use of fetal blood sampling in ITP has become controversial. The data in Table 3 deal with fetal platelet counts < 150 000/μl (3–150 000/μl), found during blood sampling for a variety of maternal/fetal conditions. Fetal platelet counts < 50 000/μl emanated mostly from patients with alloimmune thrombocytopenia, ITP, or infection. In ITP, maternal platelet count and the level of platelet-associated IgG do not correlate with fetal platelet count[2].

There is no doubt that alloimmune thrombocytopenia represents a significant threat to the fetus and fetal blood sampling plays an extremely important role in the diagnosis and treatment of this disease. Fetal blood sampling reveals the early appearance (week 20 of amenorrhea) of severe fetal thrombocytopenias (< 10 000/μ) in cases of anti-PLA$_1$ alloimmunization. This may explain the 10% incidence of fetal intracerebral hemorrhages occurring *in utero* before delivery.

Normal fetal biology

A large number of fetal blood samplings have been performed in order to diagnose congenital toxoplasmosis in a population where only 5% of the fetuses were infected. These samplings have helped establish the normal fetal biological parameters in 95% of fetuses born without any infection[9]. Two major basic principles must be considered in understanding and interpreting the fetal biological parameters:

(1) The progressive maturation of different systems in the fetus, including hematology, biochemistry, acid–base balance and oxygenation. For example, hematopoiesis is first achieved in the thymus, proceeding to the liver, and then bone marrow. The normal values of the various fetal hematological parameters vary with gestational age.

(2) Transplacental passage depends on molecular size and net charge. For example, IgG antibodies cross the placenta readily while IgM antibodies do not because of larger molecular size. Fetal

Table 3 Etiologies of fetal thrombocytopenias. Mean platelet count: $85 \pm 51 \times 10^3/\mu$ (range 3–150)

Etiology	Percentage of cases
Infections (toxoplasmosis, rubella)	46.5%
Antiplatelet (PLA$_1$, Bak system) alloimmunizations	16.6%
Fetal malformations	11.8%
Intrauterine growth restriction	11.1%
Idiopathic thrombocytopenic purpura	7.7%
Rhesus alloimmunization	3.5%
Miscellaneous	2.8%

creatininemia levels have no diagnostic value since fetal serum values are similar to maternal values. There is no correlation between maternal and fetal lactate dehydrogenase (LDH) activities. Consequently, fetal LDH value can be used to assess fetal status.

Fetal therapy and prenatal pharmacology

The fetus can be treated either through the mother, or directly by fetal intravascular injection. In either case, fetal blood sampling is essential. When fetal treatment is administered maternally, repeated fetal blood samplings allow for evaluation of fetal response to therapy (steroids or immunoglobulins in the case of fetal immunological thrombocytopenia).

Drugs such as digitoxin and levothyroxin can also be injected directly into fetal circulation. Common fetal therapies by intravenous access include transfusions of red blood cells in cases of rhesus alloimmunizations, and of platelets in cases of alloimmune thrombocytopenia.

Simultaneous access to blood from either side of the placental barrier, maternal or fetal blood, has offered exceptional opportunities to address such issues as whether a drug passes through the placental barrier or whether a drug affects fetal physiology. The answers to both questions are not necessarily correlated. For instance, Tables 4 and 5[10] show that while vitamin K$_1$ easily passes through the placental barrier, it has no effect on the fetal synthesis of vitamin K$_1$-dependent

Table 4 Transplacental passage of vitamin K$_1$ (in pg/ml) during second and third trimesters of pregnancy after maternal ingestion of 20 mg of vitamin K$_1$/day over 3–7 days before sampling

Gestation stage (pg/ml)	Non-supplemented (pg/ml)	Supplemented (pg/ml)
Second trimester		
Mother	565	81 130
Fetus	30	765
Birth		
Mother	395	45 190
Fetus	21	783

Table 5 Prothrombin activity in fetal plasma during second and third trimesters of pregnancy as related to maternal vitamin K$_1$ supplementation

Gestation stage	Non-supplemented	Supplemented
Second trimester	16.5%	16.9%
Birth	49.5%	47.8%

Prothrombin activity expressed as a percentage of normal adult plasma

coagulation factors. These remain very low in the fetus, most likely due to the immaturity of hepatic synthesis rather than to hypovitaminosis K_1.

REFERENCES

1. Daffos F, Capella-Pavlovsky M, Forestier F. Fetal blood sampling during pregnancy with use of a needle guided by ultrasound: a study of 606 consecutive cases. *Am J Obstet Gynecol* 1985;153:655–60
2. Hohlfeld P, Forestier F, Kaplan C, *et al*. Fetal thrombocytopenia: a retrospective survey of 5194 fetal blood samplings. *Blood* 1994;84:1851–6
3. Muller J, Giovangrandi Y, Parnet-Mathieu F, *et al*. Acute fetal distress after fetal blood sampling (case report). *Eur J Obstet Gynecol Reprod Biol* 1988;28:269–72
4. Forestier F, Daffos F, Rainaut M, Cox WL. The assessment of fetal blood samples. *Am J Obstet Gynecol* 1989; 158:1184–8
5. Daffos F, Forestier F, Capella-Pavlovsky M, *et al*. Prenatal management of 746 pregnancies at risk for congenital toxoplasmosis. *N Engl J Med* 1988; 318:271–5
6. Hohlfeld P, Daffos F, Costa JM, *et al*. Prenatal diagnosis of congenital toxoplasmosis with a polymerase chain reaction test on amniotic fluid. *N Engl J Med* 1994;331:695–9
7. Cox WL, Daffos F, Forestier F, *et al*. Physiology and management of intrauterine growth restriction: a biologic approach with fetal blood sampling. *Am J Obstet Gynecol* 1988;159:36–41
8. Grannum PAT, Copel JA, Moya F, *et al*. The reversal of hydrops fetalis by intravascular intrauterine transfusion in severe isoimmune fetal anemia. *Am J Obstet Gynecol* 1988;159:1135–6
9. Daffos F, Forestier F. *Medicine et Biologie du Foetus Humain*. Paris: Maloine Editeur, 1988
10. Forestier F. Some aspects of fetal biology. *Fetal Ther* 1987;2:181–7

57

Fetal demise

J.M. Shyken

INTRODUCTION

One of the greatest tragedies encountered by obstetricians is that of intrauterine fetal demise. Prior to 20 weeks, fetal death is generally discussed in the context of missed or spontaneous abortion, and after 20 weeks, as intrauterine fetal demise (IUFD)[1]. Fortunately, this complication occurs rarely. In pregnancies known to be viable at 8 weeks, 90–97% survive to viability.

The etiologic factors contributing to an IUFD are diverse and numerous. About 50% of antepartum fetal demise is thought to be preventable with risk screening and selective application of antepartum surveillance techniques. As such, the diagnosis of fetal demise, determination of etiology, and obstetric management require a systematic approach. Maternal grief, guilt, and overwhelming social stress should be anticipated and handled in a rational, compassionate manner.

EPIDEMIOLOGY

A fetal death is defined as one that occurs prior to the complete expulsion of the products of conception, regardless of gestational age. Death is defined by the lack of heartbeat, umbilical cord pulsation, respirations, or voluntary muscle movement. The stillbirth, or fetal mortality, rate is a summation of both intrapartum and antepartum fetal losses and is most accurately expressed per total births. The fetal death or fetal mortality ratio, on the other hand, is the summation of all antepartum and intrapartum deaths expressed per 1000 live births. The National Center for Health Statistics compiles data for fetal deaths; however, interstate differences in reporting requirements make comparability of data somewhat difficult. About 48% of reported fetal deaths occur prior to 20 weeks' gestation, but it is clear that fetal deaths are under-reported in the earliest stages of gestation, as reports are not required in all states. To enhance comparability, demises reported, or presumed to be at greater than or equal to 20 weeks are generally used for epidemiologic comparisons and for the calculation of fetal mortality rates[2,3].

Antepartum death of a fetus after 20 weeks of gestation occurs in about 1% of pregnancies[4] or approximately 7.5/1000 live births in the USA[2]. This represents about 50% of perinatal mortality[1]. Since the widespread use of intrapartum fetal monitoring and improvements in neonatal, obstetrical, and anesthesiologic care, intrapartum and neonatal mortality have improved. Therefore, since the 1970s, antepartum fetal demise represents a greater proportion of total perinatal mortality.

The risk of fetal death is a function of gestational age. The fraction of pregnancies lost per unit time is significantly higher in the weeks preceding clinical detection of pregnancy than later. Studies of early pregnancy that examine the risk of pregnancy loss prior to clinical recognition of pregnancy, derived from pregnancies diagnosed by elevation of human chorionic gonadotropin (hCG), were reviewed by Boklage[5]. These data compiled from naturally occurring singleton pregnancies indicate 27% survival from fertilization to clinical pregnancy. After clinical pregnancy is recognized, the chance of survival to live birth is 85%–90% and to live birth at term is 76%–90%. Of fertilizations resulting in twins, 32% survive from clinical recognition to term[5]. The prospective risk of stillbirth at 26 weeks is 1/150, and decreases steadily to 1/350 at 37 weeks, 1/475 at 40 weeks, and increases steadily thereafter to 1/375 at 43 weeks[6].

The rate of fetal death has declined steadily since 1942, but has not been symmetric with respect to race. Despite advances in perinatal care, in 1988 the fetal death ratio for African-American women was over double the ratio for Caucasian women, 12.9 and 6.4 per 1000 live births, respectively. It is likely that socioeconomic factors and demographic characteristics that represent barriers to prenatal care are at least partially responsible for this discrepancy. Causes for the decline in fetal death rate since 1969 are felt by some to be related to an increase in state- and federally-funded social and health programs targeted to the maternal–child population. These resulted in expanded use of family planning, Medicaid coverage of prenatal care, and availability of abortion[3]. Also intrapartum electronic fetal monitoring, antepartum fetal surveillance technology, and the increased use of Cesarean section are felt to be partially responsible.

Other epidemiologic indicators, besides race, compiled by the National Center for Health Statistics and reported with respect to fetal deaths are maternal age, marital status, geographic location, fetal gender, birth weight, and plurality of birth. Risk factors associated with fetal death include maternal age less than 15 or greater than 35, single motherhood, male fetal gender, and multifetal gestation[2]. Comparisons of fetal death by geographic location in the USA are somewhat hampered by the inconsistencies of reporting between states. Other risk factors include inadequate prenatal care, maternal smoking, low maternal weight, history of pregnancy loss[7], and low socio-economic status.

ETIOLOGY

No universal classification system for the etiology of antepartum fetal demise exists. The causes of fetal death have changed since the 1960s, with a large decline in deaths due to intrapartum asphyxia and Rh isoimmunization. Smaller declines in unexplained deaths, and deaths due to intrauterine fetal growth retardation (IUGR) have been realized, but no change in the fetal death rate due to intrauterine infection or abruptio placentae are seen[7]. In depth discussion of these etiologic agents are discussed elsewhere in the text and therefore are mentioned here only briefly. The cause of IUFD is inapparent in at least 25 to 50% of cases[4,7]. It should be remembered that etiologies of fetal death are rarely single or independent, rather, they overlap significantly. Further 'causes of death' listed on the birth certificate may not correlate with the 'cause of death' indicated by necropsy.

Chromosomal causes

The frequency of chromosomal aberrations seen in fetal deaths is about 5% to 8%[8,9]. This frequency, while considerably less than the frequency of chromosomal abnormalities seen with spontaneous abortions in the first trimester, is clearly higher than the frequency among liveborn infants (0.6% per year). Aneuploidies account for 95% of the chromosome abnormalities that are seen in fetal deaths, and structural chromosomal abnormalities account for the remainder. Fetuses born who are phenotypically normal have an abnormal karyotype in about 2% of cases[8].

Non-chromosomal anomalies

Dysmorphic features or congenital anomalies occur in about 12–20% of stillbirths[9–11]. In the USA, CNS malformations are most common among stillbirths (74.5%), followed by musculoskeletal (11.1%), genitourinary (7.9%), cardiovascular (5.6%), and gastrointestinal (0.9%) malformations[10]. Included among these are the amniotic band disruption sequence, congenital malformations due to teratogens, multiple congenital anomalies of unknown cause, and other genetic, nonchromosomal syndromes. Disruption of developmental sequences that may occur as a result of early

Table 1 Infectious causes of fetal death

Bacterial
  Listeria monocytogenes
  Enteric organisms
  Ureaplasma species
  Mycoplasma species
  Chlamydia trachomatis
  Group B beta-hemolytic streptococci
  Fusobacterium
  Brucella abortus
  Clostridium species
  Salmonella

Spirochetal infections
  Leptospira species
  Treponema pallidum

Mycotic (rare)
  Candida species
  Coccidiomycosis

Protozoan
  Plasmodium species
  Trypanosoma cruzi (Chagas disease)
  Toxoplasma gondii

Viral
  Parvovirus B19
  Rubella
  Varicella
  Cytomegalovirus
  Coxsackie B
  ECHO viruses

amnion disruption, vascular interruption in development, or twin-to-twin vascular complications account for 2.4% of stillbirths[12].

Infectious causes

Infectious causes of fetal death are either ascending, from colonization of the lower genital tract, or transplacental transmission. Infection of the intrauterine fetus is either primary, occurring in a live fetus, or secondary, occurring after an intrauterine demise. The recognition of infectious diseases as a cause of fetal demise is important prognostic information for counseling in subsequent pregnancies. The more common agents associated with fetal death are listed in Table 1. Bacterial infections causing chorioamnionitis, from ascending intrauterine infection, may rarely cause intrauterine fetal demise through decidual necrosis with abruptio placenta; however, they are more likely to be a cause of preterm delivery. Primary ascending infection may occur in the absence of rupture of the amniochorion and in association with conditions such as cervical incompetence or retained intrauterine device. Agents often isolated in such cases of stillbirths include enteric organisms, *Mycoplasma*, *Chlamydia*, *Ureaplasma*, group B streptococci, and anaerobes[13].

Listeria monocytogenes, on the other hand, tends to be asymptomatic in the mother, yet fatal for the fetus *in utero*. The mode of infection is transplacental following maternal septicemia. As a result, fetal sepsis and abscesses in the placenta and fetal lung, liver, adrenal, and brain occur. Perinatal mortality is said to be 60[14]. Other rarer causes that have been reported to be associated with fetal death include leptospirosis with fever, *Brucella*, *Clostridia*, *Salmonella*, and fungal infections[14].

Parasitic infections have been demonstrated to cause fetal death. Fetal death due to malaria may be associated with high maternal fever rather than the infectious particle. Even in endemic areas, there is the very low frequency of congenital infection of 0.3%. Chagas disease, caused by the agent *Trypanosoma cruzi* is an important cause of hydrops and fetal death in South America and Brazil, but of little significance in the USA. These parasitic infections, however, should be considered among pregnant patients who travel to endemic areas. Toxoplasmosis, on the other hand, is a more important cause of fetal disease in the USA, as the cat is the reservoir for the organism. It appears to be a relatively uncommon, yet recognized, cause of IUFD[14].

Viral infections, such as rubella, are known to cause fetal death through endothelial damage and thromboses in placental and fetal vessels. Fetal infection with Coxsackie virus B3, seen relatively frequently in neonates, may also cause fetal myocarditis with hydrops and IUFD[14]. Varicella viral infection in pregnancy may be particularly severe for the gravida, with pneumonia or encephalitis. Transplacental infections may result in fetal embryopathy, but the rare fetal wastage described is likely due to maternal hypoxia and febrile disease.

Cytomegalovirus (CMV) infection is the most common congenital viral infection, seen in 1% of newborns, though the majority are asymptomatic. The embryopathy caused by this organism is well-described, with widespread organ involvement and intrauterine growth retardation. Prenatal CMV disease is also characterized by chronic placental villitis. Major fetal or placental vessel thrombosis, fetal hydrops, and fetal death are also described[14].

Human Parvovirus B19 infection in pregnancy is associated with fetal death and hydrops. The risk of fetal death after known Parvovirus B19 infection in pregnancy is under investigation, but appears to be less than 10%[15].

The incidence of syphilis is increasing in many areas of the USA with an attendant increase in the number of cases of congenital syphilis. The spirochete *Treponema pallidum* causes transplacental infection which may result in preterm delivery, congenital infection, stillbirth, or intrauterine fetal demise.

Isoimmunization

Isoimmunization by Rh or other blood group antigens is a decreasing cause of fetal death, according to a recent Canadian study. Fretts and her co-workers[7] found the fetal death rate due to isoimmunization decreasing from 4.3/10 000 in the 1960s, to 0.7/10 000 at present, representing a fall of 95%. This important cause of fetal death has diminished due to the widespread use of Rh immune globulin and improved techniques in the care of isoimmunized pregnancies. When isoimmunization occurs, the cause of fetal death is due to fetal hydrops arising from severe fetal anemia, caused by intravascular hemolysis and fetal extramedullary hematopoiesis, resulting in compression and destruction of normal hepatocytes. The resultant impairment of hepatic function leads to hypoproteinemia which contributes to fetal hydrops.

Fetal growth restriction

The presence of intrauterine growth restriction (IUGR) indicates a degree of uteroplacental insufficiency that compromises provision of nutrients to the fetus and in its most severe degree can result in fetal death. Intrauterine growth restriction may result from medical, toxicologic, immunologic, infectious, chromosomal, or obstetric conditions. However, almost 50% of IUGR is idiopathic. The relative risk of fetal death due to SGA vs. AGA is 11.8 (95% confidence interval 8.09–17.1)[7].

Abruptio placenta

Since the 1980s, abruptio placenta, defined as the premature separation of a normally implanted placenta, is the leading known cause of fetal death. Hemorrhage which occurs at the periphery of the placenta (marginal abruption) and basal decidual hemorrhage (concealed or basal abruption) causes disruptions of maternal–fetal exchange at those sites. These can be associated with basal decidual necrosis, overlying placental infarction, and acute or chronic decidual inflammation[13]. Abruptio placentae occur in about 1% of pregnancies and in association with a large number of maternal and obstetrics conditions, including a prior history of abruption, tobacco smoking, low socio-economic status, unmarried status, undernutrition, increased parity or gravidity, age less than 20 or greater than 30, and use of cocaine. Saftlas *et al.*[16] identified the association of twin gestation, preterm premature rupture of membranes, chorioamnionitis, chronic hypertension, and pre-eclampsia/eclampsia with abruption. In addition, women with placental abruption are 11 times more likely to have a stillbirth than those without[16].

Medical diseases complicating pregnancy

Intrauterine asphyxia may result from conditions that cause maternal hypoxia or profound metabolic derangement, including maternal sepsis, shock, poisoning, or metabolic or respiratory acidosis. Chronic vascular or metabolic disease may manifest as uteroplacental insufficiency leading to IUGR.

Maternal diabetes, formerly an important cause of fetal death, is now associated with a fetal death rate of 1–6/10 000[7]. Fetal death *in utero* occurs most commonly after 36 weeks in patients with poor glycemic control which may manifest as polyhydramnios or fetal macrosomia. The cause of demise in fetuses of diabetic mothers is not known precisely. IUFD may be due to metabolic derangement including hyperglycemia, hyperinsulinemia, and ketoacidosis. These in turn may cause chronic intrauterine hypoxia from alterations in fetal red blood cell oxygen release and decreased placental and uterine blood flow[17]. The most common cause of death in these fetuses, however, is congenital malformations. Vascular disease and pre-eclampsia also contribute to fetal death among diabetic women.

Autoimmune causes

Autoimmune phenomena leading to fetal death indicate damage by maternal autoantibodies directed against maternal–fetal antigens. Systemic lupus erythematosus (SLE), the most common autoimmune disease in pregnancy, is associated with fetal death in 19% when antiphospholipid antibodies are not present, and 73% when present[18]. Even in patients without SLE, the presence of the lupus anticoagulant factors is associated with an increased risk of fetal losses beyond the first trimester[19,20]. Controversy still exists regarding the role of antiphospholipid antibodies and fetal death[18,21], considering that some women who have antiphospholipid antibodies have normal pregnancies[21]. It is postulated that the cause of fetal death in these cases is related to placental thrombosis because the lupus anticoagulant and anticardiolipin antibodies are associated with thrombosis and/or thrombocytopenia. Abnormalities in the fetoplacental barrier probably play a role in the antiphospholipid antibody-mediated fetal losses because unexplained elevated maternal serum α-fetoprotein (MSAFP) in the presence of elevated IgG anticardiolipin antibodies or lupus anticoagulants is associated with a high risk (62%) of fetal losses[22].

Hypertensive diseases

The causes of fetal deaths *in utero* associated with hypertension, whether chronic or pre-eclampsia, result from chronic uteroplacental insufficiency and abruption. By the time the diagnosis of pre-eclampsia is made, significant reduction in uteroplacental blood flow has already occurred. The risk of IUFD appears to increase dramatically when pre-eclampsia is superimposed upon chronic hypertension, or when severe pre-eclampsia is seen[23].

Other causes

The rate of unexplained antepartum, asphyxial, fetal deaths declined in the 1980s to 13.6/10 000 births, but accounts for 27% of fetal deaths. Postmaturity, historically a major contributor to the fetal death rate, contributes to a negligible degree at present[7], presumably due to intensive antepartum surveillance. Types of cord accidents reported include prolapse, true knots, torsion, thrombosis, and strangulation by amniotic bands. Taken together, these account for between 2.5 and 11.9% of fetal deaths in the series reviewed by Kochenour[24]. Unfortunately, these complications are largely unpreventable.

Cocaine abuse is an increasingly recognized cause of fetal death. This occurs as a result of dose-dependent maternal hypertension, catecholamine-induced reduction of uterine arterial blood flow with fetal hypoxemia, abruptio placenta, and prematurity[25]. Other drugs of abuse, including heroin, have been known to cause fetal death, presumably due to fetal withdrawal and hypoxia[26].

Caffeine intake of more than 321 mg per day during the month before conception, or of more than 163 mg per day during pregnancy, have been significantly associated with an increased risk of fetal losses. It should be noted that a cup of coffee, a cup of tea, or a can of soda contains an average of 107 mg, 34 mg and 47 mg of caffeine respectively[27].

Catastrophic and non-catastrophic trauma to the pregnant woman complicates 6% to 7% of all pregnancies, but fetal death due to this cause occurs much less commonly. Motor vehicle accidents represent the greatest proportion of trauma to pregnant women, but assaults, penetrating trauma, falls, and burns occur in reportable numbers. Clearly, maternal death, maternal shock, and abruptio placenta are important factors contributing to fetal loss. In general, greater degrees of maternal injury and hypoxia predict fetal death[28]. Fetomaternal hemorrhage can occur in association with abruption, trauma, or obstetric manipulation, and has been associated with IUFD.

Abnormally deep placental implantation, as in the circumvallate or circummarginate placenta or placenta percreta may be associated with fetal death due to marginal, basal, or intraplacental hemorrhage[13].

Other causes of fetal death include placental tumors including gestational trophoblastic neoplasia and chorioangioma. Non-immune hydrops may also result in IUFD, which is discussed elsewhere in this textbook.

Multifetal gestation

Twins and higher order multifetal gestations represent a special situation with respect to the epidemiology and etiology of IUFD. They are over-represented in the group of fetuses with congenital malformations and fetal death at any gestational age. The rate of fetal death among twins also represents an excess of concordant deaths. Twins represent 8% of all stillbirths, versus 2% of all births[5].

Single fetal demise complicates 0.5 to 6.8% of multiple gestations[29]. Specific causes of fetal death in twins include abruptio placenta, twin–twin transfusion, congenital malformations, IUGR, cord complications, umbilical cord prolapse, and complications associated with gestational hypertension.

Risk of recurrence

The risk of recurrence of antepartum fetal demise or stillbirth is largely predicated upon the cause, when discernible. Fretts *et al.*[7] found that in the 1960s, the risk of recurrent stillbirth was fourfold greater than the risk of stillbirth in the general population, but in the 1980s, a history of stillbirth was no longer associated with a significantly increased risk of fetal death. In 1985, Freeman *et al.*[30] demonstrated a higher risk of abnormal antepartum fetal heart rate tracing, induction of labor, or Cesarean section for fetal/maternal complications in patients having experienced a stillbirth in a previous gestation. Nonetheless, perinatal mortality was not increased over controls. These findings are presumably due to intensive antepartum surveillance directly preventing IUFD. Abruption carries a 5.5 to 16.6% chance of recurrence in a subsequent pregnancy, but in the face of abruptio placenta complicating two pregnancies, the risk of a third rises to 25%[31]. Whenever a non-recurring cause for fetal death is identified, the parents should be counseled and reassured.

PATHOPHYSIOLOGY AND COMPLICATIONS

Since fetal demise may occur as a result of a number of maternal and fetal conditions, pathophysiologic principles are discussed in the context of those disorders elsewhere in this text. It is, however, appropriate to discuss the complication of acquired coagulopathy as a result of a retained dead fetus, or the 'dead fetus syndrome'. Fetal death incites the clotting cascade through the very slow release of tissue thromboplastin into the amniotic fluid which slowly crosses into the maternal circulation. Disseminated intravascular coagulation results with consumption of clotting factors, thrombocytopenia, intravascular fibrin formation with resultant fibrinolysis, and fibrin degradation product formation. The net result is a cycle of vascular occlusion, inhibition of coagulation, and coagulopathy. The 'dead fetus syndrome' is rare because of the availability of methods for pregnancy termination. When seen, it is very unusual with retention of a dead fetus for less than four weeks[32].

Maternal death associated with IUFD occurs rarely. Causes of these deaths include coagulopathy and hemorrhage, amniotic fluid embolism, or underlying maternal disease[1].

DIAGNOSIS

Clinical findings associated with IUFD, while not diagnostic, provide the impetus for further investigation to confirm fetal viability. These clinical findings include loss of previously perceived fetal activity, failure of growth in uterine size, regression of the symptoms of pregnancy (including breast changes), and weight loss. Loss of maternal perception of fetal activity may be due to changes in fetal state, environmental influences, or relative insensitivity of the mother to small fetal movements. It is nonetheless prudent to investigate reports of loss of fetal activity without delay.

A finding of elevation of maternal serum alpha-fetoprotein (MSAFP) may first initiate the cascade of events that lead to the diagnosis of IUFD. After exclusion for incorrect dates and twins with MSAFP < 4.5 multiples of the median, the incidence of fetal death is 14% in women with elevations in MSAFP[33]. When MSAFP levels are unusually high (greater than 4 to 5 multiples of the median), intrauterine fetal demise is more likely.

The diagnosis of intrauterine fetal demise can be made readily using real-time ultrasound. In the absence of auscultatory evidence of fetal viability, real-time ultrasonography should be employed to establish the diagnosis of fetal viability or of intrauterine fetal demise. From 5.5 to 8 weeks' gestation, vaginal probe sonography may be necessary to detect fetal cardiac activity, but is generally not necessary after this time. The diagnosis of IUFD is confirmed by the absence of fetal cardiac activity. Associated findings may be fetal anomalies, abnormal posturing, excessive curvature of the spine, overlapping of the fetal cranial bones, or oligohydramnios. In addition, fetal scalp edema, apparent as a hypoechoic zone surrounding the fetal cranium (also known as the 'halo' sign), may be appreciated[34].

Radiologic signs, pathognomonic of IUFD, are rarely sought since the availability of real-time ultrasonography. With the exception of the use of serial hCG and progesterone measurements in the first trimester as an adjunct to ultrasound for the diagnosis of missed abortion or ectopic pregnancy, biochemical monitoring has little or no place in the diagnosis of IUFD.

MANAGEMENT OF FETAL DEMISE

Once the diagnosis of fetal death is confirmed, a management plan is devised. Expectant management is safe in view of the very slow development of hypofibrinogenemia, beginning about 4 weeks after IUFD[32]. Conversely, injudicious attempts at immediate delivery may be hazardous for the mother. Spontaneous delivery should be expected to occur within 14 days in 90%, and within 21 days in 93%[35]. While awaiting spontaneous delivery, fibrinogen, platelet count, and fibrin split product levels should be monitored weekly. Consider induction of labor if spontaneous labor has not occurred 2–3 weeks after fetal demise; induction of labor should be begun if spontaneous delivery has not occurred by 4 weeks after IUFD, or if there is chemical or clinical evidence of maternal coagulopathy. Some women, emotionally devastated, may consider continued retention of their dead fetus abhorrent. Counseling regarding expectant management versus induction of labor should include weighing the potential psychic complications versus medical and surgical risks. At times, in consideration of the mother's psychological well-being, judicious termination of pregnancy should be attempted. In all cases, management is individualized.

Cervical dilation followed by mechanical evacuation or suction of the uterus is best undertaken if the uterus is less than or equal to 14 weeks' size. Few are sufficiently skilled or experienced at dilation and evacuation of larger uteri.

Up to 28 weeks' gestation, delivery can be accomplished in over 90% of cases[36], using prostaglandin (PG) preparations. The most widely used form is the PGE_2 20 mg, intravaginal suppository, placed every 4 hours until delivery. Frequently, uterine curettage is necessary to remove retained placental fragments after expulsion of the fetus[36]. Systemic side effects, including pyrexia, tachycardia, diarrhea, and vomiting, are frequent. Use of prostaglandin suppositories after 28 weeks may increase the risk of uterine rupture via hyperstimulation. Prostaglandin E_2 is contraindicated in the presence of prior sensitivity to prostaglandins, active cardiac, pulmonary, renal, or hepatic disease. Recently, intravaginal misoprostol (PGE_1) has been recognized as a safe and effective alternative for pregnancy termination for fetal death when used in doses of 100–200 mg every 6–12 h[37,38].

When the cervix is favorable for induction, the intravenous administration of oxytocin can be used to effect labor. Prior to 28 weeks the uterus may be insufficiently sensitive to the effects of oxytocin. Whenever oxytocin is administered, water intoxication is prevented by avoiding administration of large volumes of electrolyte-free solutions during a long induction of labor. Care is taken to avoid uterine overstimulation. After rupture of the membranes, an intrauterine pressure catheter should be placed.

When the cervix is not favorable, cervical ripening with prostaglandin E_2 gel (0–5 mg in 2.5 ml methylcellulose gel) can precede induction of labor. Sequential intracervical applications of PGE_2 gel at 6-hour intervals may be necessary to achieve significant cervical readiness[39]. Oxytocin should be withheld for 4 to 6 hours after the gel is placed. Cervidil (Forest Pharmaceuticals Inc., St Louis, MO), a 10-mg dinoprostone insert, can be used to deliver PGE_2 at 0.3 mg/h vaginally. Alternately, laminaria tents or synthetic cervical dilators, such as Lamicel (Cabot Medical Corp., Langhorne, PA) or Dilapan (Gynotech, Inc., Lebanon, NJ), can be used to ripen the unfavorable cervix.

INVESTIGATION INTO THE CAUSE OF FETAL DEATH

Careful maternal history and physical examination may provide an explanation for IUFD and obviate the need for expensive laboratory investigations. Queries should include genetic, obstetric, and medical information, as well as exposure to medications and recreational drugs.

The karyotype of the delivered fetus should be obtained when the fetus is macerated, has ambiguous genitalia, non-immune hydrops, oligohydramnios sequence, or multiple anatomic defects. Fetal tissue for cytogenetic analysis should be collected in a clean, closed container, without addition of extra fluid for transport. The likelihood of successful cell culture and karyotype obtained from the stillborn infant is inversely related to the time between fetal death and delivery. When the fetus is macerated, placental tissue may prove a better source for cell culture. Other sources for chromosome studies include cord or cardiac blood, skin, or fascia lata.

Amniotic fluid cytogenetic analysis has also been described in order to successfully identify chromosomal abnormalities in the fetus. Amniotic fluid obtained by amniocentesis shortly after the diagnosis of IUFD has been demonstrated superior in achieving a successful karyotype to fascia lata obtained from the infant at delivery[40]. When managing a woman with an IUFD expectantly, if delivery is anticipated to occur more than a few days after the time of fetal death, amniocentesis at the time of diagnosis of IUFD should be considered.

Selected cases with suspicion of infectious etiologies should have microbiologic studies. Membrane sections may be cultured, as well as various fetal specimens, including cerebrospinal fluid, blood, lung, or liver tissue. Aside from standard organisms, cultures should include *Listeria monocytogenes*. Fetuses affected by intrauterine growth restriction, non-immune hydrops, or a clinical history of infection, in particular, should have microbiologic evaluation. Maternal and fetal cord blood for TORCH (toxoplasmosis, rubella, cytomegalovirus, herpes), Parvovirus, and VDRL titers should be obtained in selected cases[13].

When fetal hydrops is evident, additional studies recommended are hemoglobin and hematocrit, albumin, and hemoglobin electrophoresis. Maternal blood type, Rh, and antibody status should be rechecked to rule out erythroblastosis fetalis.

Recurrent fetal loss suggests immunologic causes which may be manifestations of the antiphospholipid antibody syndrome. A search for anticardiolipin antibodies and lupus anticoagulant should be undertaken in women with systemic lupus erythematosus or related autoimmune disease, recurrent pregnancy loss, and unexplained fetal deaths. The utility of routinely obtaining antiphospholipid antibody studies in women with fetal demise is not certain at this time.

Recently, Gregory[41] reviewed laboratory studies performed routinely to characterize stillbirths. The studies that were positive most often were TORCH titers (16.6%), urine drug screens (15.4%), anti-nuclear antibody (9.7%), and VDRL (8.3%). Kleihauer–Betke stain was positive in 4.9% and prothrombin time, fibrinogen, and hemoglobin A1C were abnormal less frequently. In our experience, urine drug toxicology screening is helpful in identifying fetal deaths associated with abruption and cocaine use.

Pitkin[4] recommends obtaining four tests when searching for the cause of IUFD: karyotype, listeria culture, Kleihauer–Betke stain of peripheral blood, and PTT screen for the lupus anticoagulant. Routine use of a large number of laboratory tests to characterize fetal demise is not indicated; rather, limited studies should be obtained, based on clinical risks.

Pathologic examination of the fetus

After consent, gross autopsy is indicated. A gross description of the fetus, including appropriate anthropomorphic and radiologic studies, and photographs should be performed. Detection of congenital or genetic abnormalities is facilitated by a systematic approach by a geneticist or pathologist experienced in such evaluations. The value of routine microscopic examination of the fetal organs is not clear, but most pathologists choose to submit representative sections. Histologic examination is indicated for certain cardiac and renal anomalies, obstructive uropathy, congenital infections, fetal tumors, growth failure, skeletal abnormalities, and ambiguous genitalia[42].

Pathologic examination of the placenta

Placental lesions, generally inflammatory or vascular, are seen in at least 43–50% of cases of fetal death[43]. The pathologist should investigate the placenta grossly to determine if there are gross areas of hemorrhage, and look for areas of deciduitis and arterial and venous lesions. Examination of the placenta, membranes, and umbilical cord may identify abnormalities of cord insertion, umbilical vessel number, thrombosis of vessels, placental tumors, and other findings. Fetal death is associated with extensive placental infarcts, relatively low placental weight for gestational age, and excessive intervillous fibrin deposition[13]. Fetal death by infectious or inflammatory causes may best be diagnosed through placental histologic examination.

Emotional aspects of fetal demise

Attention to the psychosocial needs of the patient should be foremost from the first mention of fetal demise, through labor, delivery, postpartum and recovery period. Respect for her feelings of vulnerability and those of her family are central to the disclosure and explanation of her pregnancy loss. Few other situations test the patient–doctor relationship, or underscore the necessity for compassionate and open communication, so acutely. At the time of diagnosis of fetal demise, due to overwhelming grief and perhaps guilt, the gravida might be unwilling to submit herself or her fetus to examinations that might explain the IUFD. Symptoms of maternal grief include sleep disturbance, depression, anorexia and weight loss, nervousness, social withdrawal, guilt, anger, hostility, and morbid preoccupation with the baby[44].

Because the process of maternal–fetal psychologic attachment begins prenatally, it is ill-advised to protect the mother from the grief of her stillbirth by isolating her from the deceased infant. Rather, parents should be encouraged to hold their baby, name their child and plan a memorial service or funeral consistent with their religious practices. Parents should be given photographs and other keepsakes of the baby. They should be encouraged to explore and verbalize their feelings about their baby's death as a normal part of the grieving process. Literature regarding perinatal bereavement should be provided. Planned supportive counseling following hospital discharge has been demonstrated to shorten the bereavement process[44].

SUMMARY

The predicament of intrauterine fetal demise is emotionally challenging for the both the patient and the obstetrician. Diagnosis is greatly simplified by the use of real-time ultrasonography. Likewise, management, which is gestational age-dependent, is facilitated via availability of laminaria and prostaglandin E_2 gel or suppositories. Decisions regarding timing of delivery should be made with the emotional, social, and medical needs of the parturient in mind. Of utmost importance is the thorough, systematic investigation into the cause of the IUFD. Only if the etiology is known can the patient be adequately counseled about the chance of recurrence and the potential for prevention in future gestations.

REFERENCES

1. Diagnosis and management of fetal death. ACOG Technical Bulletin # 176, January 1993, American College of Obstetricians and Gynecologists, Washington, DC, 176:1–8
2. Vital statistics of the United States. 1988; Mortality, vol II, part A. National Center for Health Statistics, DHHS Publication No. (PHS) 911101, Hyattsville, MD, 1991
3. Pettiti DB. The epidemiology of fetal death. *Clin Obstet Gynecol* 1987;30:253–8
4. Pitkin RM. Fetal death: diagnosis and management. *Am J Obstet Gynecol* 1987;157:583
5. Boklage CE. Survival probability of human conceptions from fertilization to term. *Int J Fertil* 1990;35:75–94
6. Feldman GB. Prospective risk of stillbirth. *Obstet Gynecol* 1992;79:547–53

7. Fretts RC, Boyd ME, Usher RH, *et al*. The changing pattern of fetal death, 1961–1988. *Obstet Gynecol* 1992;79:35–9

8. Warburton D. Chromosomal causes of fetal death. *Clin Obstet Gynecol* 1987;30:268–77

9. Pauli RM, Reiser CA. Wisconsin Stillbirth Service Program: II. Analysis of diagnoses and diagnostic categories in the first 1000 referrals. *Am J Med Genet* 1994;50:135–53

10. Kalter H. Five-decade international trends in the relation of perinatal mortality and congenital malformations: stillbirth and neonatal death compared. *Int J Epidemiol* 1991;20:173–9

11. Pauli RM, Reiser CA, Lebovitz M, *et al*. Wisconsin Stillbirth Service Program:I. Establishment and assessment of a community-based program for etiologic investigation of intrauterine deaths. *Am J Med Genet* 1994;50:116–34

12. Luebke HJ, Reiser CA, Pauli RM. Fetal disruptions: assessment of frequency, heterogeneity, and embryologic mechanisms in a population referred to a community-based stillbirth assessment program. *Am J Med Genet* 1990;36:56–72

13. Curry CJR, Honore LH. A protocol for the investigation of pregnancy loss. *Clin Perinatol* 1990;17:723–42

14. Benirschke K, Robb JA. Infectious causes of fetal death. *Clin Obstet Gynecol* 1987;30:284–94

15. Center for Disease Control. Risks associated with human Parvovirus B19 infection. *Morbid Mortal Weekly Rep* 1989;38:81–8

16. Saftlas AF, Olson DR, Atrash HK, *et al*. National trends in the incidence of abruptio placentae, 1979–1987. *Obstet Gynecol* 1991;78:1081–6

17. Landon MB, Gabbe SG. Fetal surveillance in the pregnancy complicated by diabetes mellitus. *Clin Obstet Gynecol* 1991;34:535–43

18. Derksen RHWM, Bouma BN, Kater L. The striking association between lupus anticoagulant and fetal loss in systemic lupus erythematosus patients. *Arthritis Rheum* 1986;29:695–6

19. Out HJ, Bruinse HW, Christiaens GC, *et al*. A prospective, controlled multicenter study on the obstetric risk of pregnant women with antiphospholipid antibodies. *Am J Obstet Gynecol* 1992;167:26–32

20. Oshiro RT, Silver RM, Scott JR, *et al*. Antiphospholipid antibodies and fetal death. *Obstet Gynecol* 1996;87:489–93

21. Infante-Rivard C, David M, Gauthier R, *et al*. Lupus anticoagulants, anticardiolipin antibodies, and fetal loss: a case-control study. *N Engl J Med* 1991;325:1063–6

22. Silver RM, Draper ML, Byrne JL, *et al*. Unexplained elevations of maternal serum alpha-fetoprotein in women with antiphospholipid antibodies: a harbinger of fetal death. *Obstet Gynecol* 1994;83:150–5

23. Sibai BM, Spinnato JA, Watson DL, *et al*. Pregnancy outcome in 303 cases with severe preeclampsia. *Obstet Gynecol* 1984;64:319–25

24. Kochenour NK. Other causes of fetal death. *Clin Obstet Gynecol* 1987;30:312–21

25. Woods JR, Plessinger MA, Clark KE. Effect of cocaine on uterine blood flow and fetal oxygenation. *J Am Med Assoc* 1987;257:957–61

26. Rementeria JL, Nunag NN. Narcotic withdrawal in pregnancy: stillbirth incidence with a case report. *Am J Obstet Gynecol* 1973;116:1152–6

27. Infante-Rivard C, Fernandez A, Gauthier R, *et al*. Fetal loss associated with caffeine intake before and during pregnancy. *J Am Med Assoc* 1993;270:2940–43

28. Hoff WS, D'Amelio LF, Tinkoff GH, *et al*. *Surg Gynecol Obstet* 1991;172:175–80

29. Dudley DKL, D'Alton ME. Single fetal death in twin gestation. *Semin Perinatol* 1986;10:65–72

30. Freeman RK, Dorchester W, Anderson G, *et al*. The significance of a previous stillbirth. *Am J Obstet Gynecol* 1985;151:7–13

31. Hibbart BM, Jeffcoate TNA. Abruptio placentae. *Obstet Gynecol* 1966;27:155–67

32. Pritchard JA. Fetal death *in utero*. *Obstet Gynecol* 1959;14:573–80

33. Robinson L, Grau P, Crandall BF. Pregnancy outcomes after increasing maternal serum alpha-fetoprotein levels. *Am J Obstet Gynecol* 1989;74:17–20

34. Cubberly DA. Diagnosis of fetal death. *Clin Obstet Gynecol* 1987;30:259–67

35. Tricomi V, Kohl SG. Fetal death *in utero*. *Am J Obstet Gynecol* 1957;74:1092–7

36. Kochenour NK. Management of fetal demise. *Clin Obstet Gynecol* 1987;30:322–30

37. Bugalho A, Bigue C, Machungo F, *et al*. Induction of labor with intravaginal misoprostol in intrauterine fetal death. *Am J Obstet Gynecol* 1994;171:538–41

38. Jain JK, Mishell DR. A comparison of intravaginal misoprostol with prostaglandin E_2 for termination of second-trimester pregnancy. *N Engl J Med* 1994;331:290–3

39. Mainprize T, Nimrod C, Dodd G, *et al*. Clinical utility of multiple dose administration of prostaglandin E2 gel. *Am J Obstet Gynecol* 1987;156:341–3

40. Brady K, Duff P, Harlass FE, *et al*. Role of amniotic fluid cytogenetic analysis in the evaluation of recent fetal death. *Am J Perinatol* 1991;8:68–70

41. Gregory K, Settledge R, Paul R. Stillbirths: what laboratory studies are helpful? *Am J Obstet Gynecol* 1992;166:310

42. Tyson W, Manchester D. Pathologic aspects of fetal death. *Clin Obstet Gynecol* 1987;30:331–41

43. Ornoy A, Salamon-Arnon J, Ben-Zur Z, *et al*. Placental findings in spontaneous abortions and stillbirths. *Teratology* 1981;24:243–52

44. Zeanah CH. Adaptation following perinatal loss: a critical review. *J Am Acad Child Adolesc Psychiatry* 1989;28:467–80

58

Fetal echocardiography: prenatal diagnosis of congenital heart disease

G. Pilu, S. Gabrielli, A. Perolo and D. Prandstraller

ULTRASOUND EVALUATION OF ANATOMY AND FUNCTION OF THE FETAL HEART

Pioneer studies on the ultrasound investigation of the fetal heart were reported in the early 1970s[1-3]. Since high-resolution real-time ultrasound was introduced in the late 1970s, reports on ultrasound assessment of fetal cardiac anatomy and function have been appearing with increasing frequency in both the obstetric and the cardiological literature. Currently, fetal echocardiography is a well established technique for prenatal diagnosis of cardiac defects[4-7]. However, the diffusion of this technique is still limited, as it requires both a very experienced operator and an extremely meticulous scanning. Screening the entire obstetric population, therefore, does not seem possible, and fetal echocardiography should be directed towards selected pregnancies carrying a higher than normal risk for fetal cardiac anomalies. The commonly accepted indications are reported in Table 1. Despite the fact that echocardiography should not be recommended in all pregnancies, several authors have suggested that during routine ultrasound examinations some views of the fetal heart should be obtained by any obstetric sonographer even without specific training. The use of such views, the four-chamber view being the most representative example[6], would seem to be a reasonable compromise between screening the entire obstetric population and completely ignoring the fetal heart during obstetric ultrasound examination.

By using a high-frequency transducer (5–7 MHz) the main cardiac connections can be consistently imaged starting from 14 weeks' gestation. From a technical point of view, however, the optimal period for fetal echocardiography is probably between 20 and 26 weeks. In later gestation, increasing calcification of fetal ribs and a relative decrease in amniotic fluid volume hinder the examination and it is rare that this can be satisfyingly accomplished at term. The sequential approach to the evaluation of cardiac anatomy, originally suggested for pathological and angiographic studies[8], is very suitable for fetal echocardiography.

The left and right sides of the fetus are assessed by determining the relative position of the head and spine. The visceral situs is then assessed by demonstrating the relative position of the stomach, hepatic vessels, abdominal aorta and inferior vena cava (Figure 1). A transverse section of the fetal chest allows demonstration of the four-chamber view (Figure 2). This view is easily obtained, even by sonographers who are not specifically trained, allowing identification of many cardiac anomalies[6]. The elements that are relevant in the analysis of the four-chamber view are the following: position of the heart inside the thorax (the heart is normally positioned in the left side of the chest, with the apex pointing to the left); integrity of the ventricular and atrial septum; equal size of the left and right ventricles and atria. The patency of the atrioventricular valves can be demonstrated by real-time imaging of the movements of the leaflets. Additional elements include the more apical insertion of the tricuspid valve compared to the mitral valve and the presence of the moderator band of the trabecula septomarginalis at the apex of the right ventricle. These elements are both of value in distinguishing the morphological left from the right ventricle.

Table 1 Indications for fetal echocardiography

Maternal and familial indications
Familial history of congenital heart disease
Maternal diabetes
Maternal drug exposure during pregnancy
Maternal infections during pregnancy
Maternal alcoholism[*]
Maternal connective tissue disease
Maternal phenylketonuria

Fetal indications
Polyhydramnios
Non-immune hydrops
Dysrhythmias
Extracardiac anomalies
Chromosomal aberrations
Symmetrical intrauterine growth retardation

[*] The interested reader is referred to a review paper: Copel JA, Pilu G, Kleinman CS. Congenital heart disease and extracardiac malformations. Associations and indications for fetal echocardiography. *Am J Obstet Gynecol* 1986;154:1121

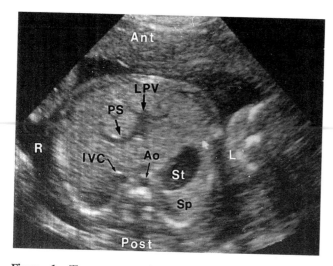

Figure 1 Transverse section of the upper abdomen in a mid-trimester fetus demonstrating the visceral situs. The portal sinus (PS) corresponds to the hilum of the liver and it, as well as the inferior vena cava (IVC), are normally seen to the right (R). The stomach (St), spleen (Sp) and descending aorta (Ao) are normally seen to the left (L). Ant, anterior; Post, posterior; LPV, left portal vein

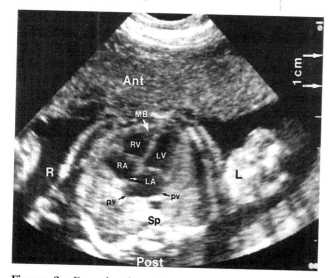

Figure 2 Four-chamber view of the heart in a mid-trimester fetus. Left and right ventricular and atrial chambers (LV, RV, LA, RA) are easily identified. The widely patent foramen ovalis centrally interrupts the atrial septum. Note the pulmonary veins (pv) entering the right atrium and the moderator band (MB) at the apex of the right ventricle. Sp, fetal spine; Ant, anterior; Post, posterior; R, right; L, left

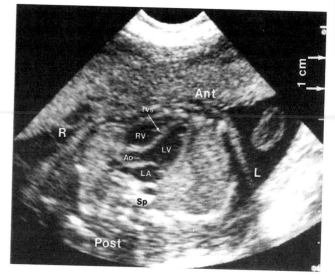

Figure 3 Long-axis view of the left ventricle (LV) demonstrating the left ventriculoarterial connection. There is a normal continuity between the anterior wall of the ascending aorta (Ao) and the ventricular septum (ivs) and between the posterior wall of the aorta and the anterior leaflet of the mitral valve. Ant, anterior; Post, posterior; R, right; L, left; RV, right ventricle; LA, left atrium

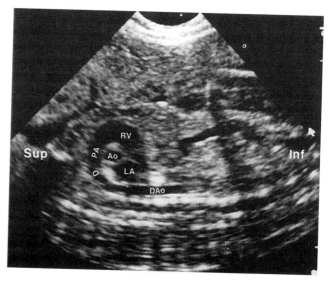

Figure 4 The right ventriculoarterial connection. In this scanning plane the outflow tract of the right ventricle (RV) encircles the ascending aorta (Ao) and gives rise to the pulmonary artery (PA), which is in turn connected to the ductus arteriosus (D). DAo, descending aorta; Sup, superior; Inf, inferior; LA, left atrium

Tilting the transducer cephalad, the left ventriculoarterial connection is identified (Figure 3). Slight angulations allow the visualization of the right outflow tract and main pulmonary artery, ductus arteriosus (Figure 4) and aortic arch (Figure 5).

M-mode ultrasound evaluation of the fetal heart is easily performed by using the currently available real-time directed M-mode apparatuses[9,10]. Movements of the cardiac valves and walls can be studied with this technique (Figure 6). The tracings are remarkably similar to those that have been described after birth. M-mode has also been used to derive nomograms of the normal size of the ventricular chambers and great vessels[9,11,12]. Measurement of ventricular chambers and determination of contractility have been suggested as a means of assessment of cardiac function[11], although the clinical value of such evaluation is still undetermined.

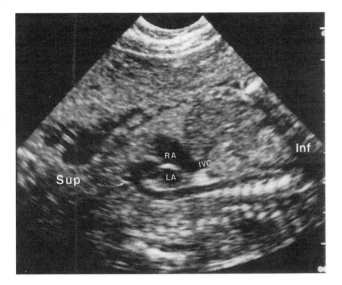

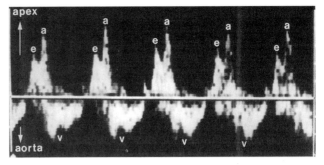

Figure 5 The aortic arch. Branching of the brachiocephalic vessels is evident (small arrow). IVC, inferior vena cava; RA, right atrium; LA, left atrium; Sup, superior; Inf, inferior

Figure 7 Pulsed Doppler sonogram of the left ventricle. A large sampling gate is used, including both the inlet and the outlet tract. Blood moves towards the apex of the heart during passive ventricular filling (e point), and an acceleration is noted corresponding to atrial systole (a). Note that the a wave is dominant over the e wave. Opposite movement of blood, directed towards the outflow tract and aorta, is identified during ventricular systole (v)

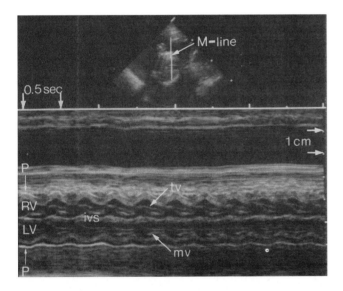

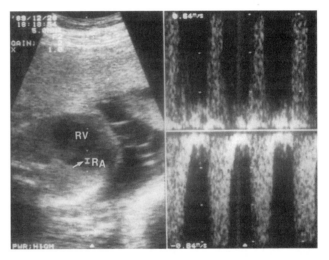

Figure 6 Real-time directed M-mode sonogram of ventricular chambers in a mid-trimester fetus. The M-line is directed across the right ventricle (RV), tricuspid valve (tv), interventricular septum (ivs), left ventricle (LV) and mitral valve (mv). Dense echoes arise from the pericardium (P). The undulations of ventricular walls and septum reflect ventricular contractions

Figure 8 Severe tricuspid insufficiency. The sampling gate is positioned in the right atrium (RA) above the tricuspid valve, and pulsed Doppler registers a regurgitant jet of blood. Signal aliasing suggests very high velocities

M-mode ultrasound is currently particularly valuable in the identification and differential diagnosis of fetal dysrhythmias[13–16].

Pulsed Doppler ultrasound evaluation has been applied to the study of the heart function in the live human fetus[17–25]. Adequate recordings of velocity waveforms of the blood flow through the atrioventricular valves, great vessels and inferior vena cava can be obtained in almost all cases, starting from 18–20 weeks

(Figure 7). Several authors have pointed out remarkable differences between *in utero* and postnatal Doppler studies. The higher velocity in the flow at the ventricular inlet that is dependent upon atrial contraction when compared to passive venous filling has been interpreted as a sign of the physiological 'stiffness' of the fetal myocardium[19]. Pulsed Doppler ultrasound, in combination with two-dimensional and M-mode sonography, has proved useful in the evaluation of both fetal dysrhythmias and structural anomalies. In this light, Doppler is of value for documenting atrioventricular valve insufficiency (Figure 8). It has recently been demonstrated that the association of structural heart disease, hydrops and atrioventricular valve insufficiency carries a very poor prognosis[18]. It has also been found that in normal fetuses the peak velocity in both ascending aorta and pulmonary artery is less than 1 m/s[21]. This observation is relevant for the prenatal diagnosis of pulmonary and aortic stenosis, associated with post-stenotic turbulence.

The use of Doppler in the fetus, however, is still an area of ongoing research. Sophisticated analyses of cardiac function are appearing with increasing frequency. Color Doppler ultrasound is a remarkable example in this regard, allowing rapid identification of blood flow and blood flow direction in the different chambers of the fetal heart (Figures 9–12).

INCIDENCE AND ETIOLOGY OF CONGENITAL HEART DISEASE

The incidence of congenital heart diseases (CHD) is currently estimated to be 8–9 out of 1000 live births[26,27]. Ventricular septal defects, pulmonary stenosis and atrial septal defects are most commonly encountered.

The very high frequency of CHD among spontaneous abortions is well established[28]. The discrepancy between prenatal and postnatal series is thought to be the consequence of spontaneous selection of fetuses with chromosomal aberrations and/or multiple anomalies.

CHD is thought to be a multifactorial disorder in over 90% of cases[29]. The recurrence risk after the birth of one affected child is about 2–5%. An unusually high frequency of cardiac anomalies has been reported in children of mothers with CHD[30]. These observations have prompted the hypothesis that cytoplasmic inheritance or teratogens may play a role in the etiology of CHD. Table 2 reports the recurrence risks that are suggested by Nora and Nora[30].

Monogenic inheritance is thought to account for 1–2% of cases[29]. This figure includes both cases of

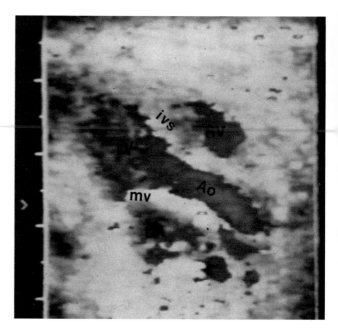

Figure 10   Color Doppler investigation of left heart shown in gray scale. Movement of blood across the mitral valve (mv) towards the left ventricle (LV) is reflected in a red stream of color. Opposite flow towards the outflow tract and ascending aorta (Ao) is coded blue. RV, right ventricle; ivs, interventricular septum

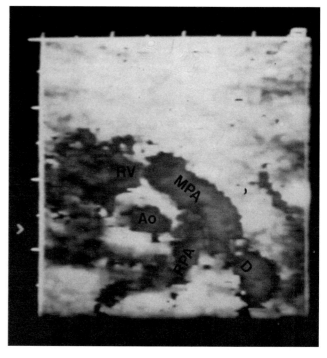

Figure 11   Color Doppler investigation of right heart hemodynamics. Blood flow along the main pulmonary artery (MPA), right pulmonary artery (RPA) and ductus arteriosus (D) is moving away from the transducer. RV, right ventricle

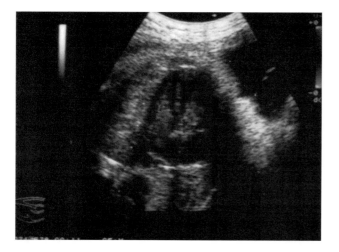

Figure 9   Color Doppler investigation of ventricular filling shown in gray scale. The parallel color streams indicate movement of blood across the atrioventricular valves during diastole

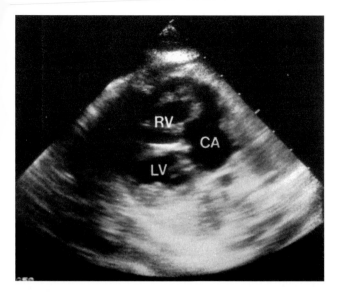

Figure 12   Partial atrioventricular canal with a common atrium (CA). The entire atrial septum is defective in this fetus with left isomerism and complex congenital heart disease. Note the insertion of the atrioventricular valves at the same level on the interventricular septum. RV, right ventricle; LV, left ventricle

isolated cardiac anomalies transmitted as single gene disorders and cases of CHD occurring with a variable degree of penetrance in syndromes with monogenic inheritance. Chromosomal aberrations are found in 4–5% of infants with CHD. Environmental factors, mostly rubella infection, are probably implicated in no more than 1–2% of cases.

In this chapter prenatal diagnosis of CHD is reviewed. The categorization and nomenclature of cardiac anomalies that we have adopted follows the approach suggested by Becker and Anderson[8].

ATRIAL AND VENTRICULAR SEPTAL DEFECTS

The atrial septal defects (ASDs) are commonly divided into *primum* and *secundum* types. Primum ASD is the simplest form of the atrioventricular defects that cover a wide spectrum of severity, the most severe being the complete atrioventricular canal. Atrioventricular canal is found in more than 50% of infants with trisomy 21[31]. Secundum ASD may be a part of the Holt–Oram syndrome, with autosomal dominant transmission.

Owing to the presence of the foramen ovalis valve, it is usually difficult to achieve proper assessment of the integrity of the septum secundum in the fetus, and it is questionable whether isolated, small defects in this area can be recognized *in utero*. We have never detected a secundum ASD prior to birth. Conversely, primum ASDs are easily seen. The complete atrioventricular canal is featured by the association of an ASD with a ventricular septal defect and a common atrioventricular valve. The insertion of the two atrioventricular valves at the same level of the ventricular septum is a useful echocardiographic sign of this anomaly (Figures 12 and 13).

ASDs are not a cause of impairment of cardiac function *in utero*, as a large right-to-left shunt at the level of the atria is a physiological condition in the fetus. Most affected infants are asymptomatic even in the neonatal period. In the complete form of atrioventricular canal, the common atrioventricular valve may be incompetent, and systolic blood regurgitation from the ventricles to the atria may give rise to congestive heart failure[32]. Doppler ultrasound allows identification of the regurgitant jet[23].

Ventricular septal defects (VSDs) are probably the most common congenital cardiac defect. The echocardiographic diagnosis depends upon the demonstration of a dropout of echoes in the ventricular septum (Figure 14). Obviously, VSDs smaller than 1–2 mm will fall beyond the resolution power of current ultrasound equipment and will escape detection. There is no evidence that VSDs are responsible for hemodynamic compromise *in utero*. Even a large interventricular communication probably gives rise to only small, bidirectional shunts in the fetus, as during intrauterine life the right and left ventricular pressures are believed to be equal[33]. The vast majority of infants are not symptomatic in the neonatal period[34].

Table 2   Recurrence risks (%) of congenital heart disease

| | Recurrence Risks | | |
Defect	One sibling affected*	Father affected†	Mother affected†
Aortic stenosis	2	3	13–18
Atrial septal defect	2.5	1.5	4–4.5
Atrioventricular canal	2	1	14
Coarctation	2	2	4
Patent ductus arteriosus	3	2.5	3.5–4
Pulmonary stenosis	2	2	4–6.5
Tetralogy of Fallot	2.5	1.5	2.5
Ventricular septal defect	3	2	6–10

*Data derived from reference 29; †data derived from reference 30

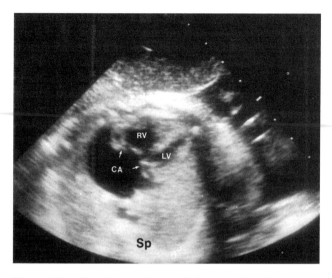

Figure 13 Complete atrioventricular canal. A single atrioventricular valve with leaflets opening centrally (arrows) is seen. A common atrium (CA) is present. RV, right ventricle; LV, left ventricle; Sp, spine

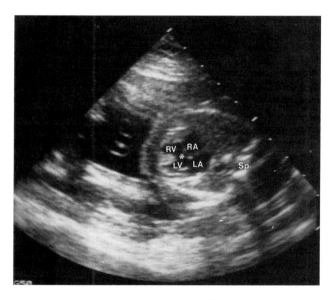

Figure 14 Ventricular septal defect (*) in a mid-trimester fetus. RV, right ventricle; LV, left ventricle; RA, right atrium; LA, left atrium; Sp, spine

PULMONARY STENOSIS

The most common form of pulmonary stenosis is the valvular type, owing to the fusion of the pulmonary leaflets. The hemodynamics is altered proportionally to the degree of stenosis. The work of the right ventricle is increased, as well as the pressure, leading to hypertrophy of the ventricular walls. In the most severe cases, right ventricular overload results in congestive heart failure.

Postnatal diagnosis of pulmonary stenosis depends upon cross-sectional demonstration of doming of the

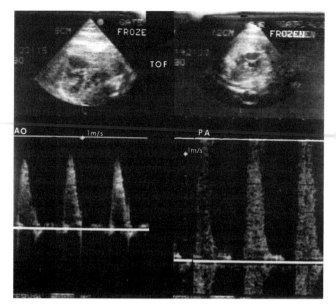

Figure 15 Pulmonary stenosis in a fetus with tetralogy of Fallot demonstrated by pulsed Doppler echocardiography. Peak velocity in the pulmonary artery (PA) exceeds 1 m/s and results in aliasing. Peak velocity in the ascending aorta (AO) is within normal limits

pulmonary cusps and post-stenotic turbulence detected by Doppler ultrasound[35]. M-mode examination is unreliable. Prenatal diagnosis is probably difficult, as only a few, very severe, cases have been described in the literature, particularly cases with enlargement of the right ventricle and/or post-stenotic enlargement or hypoplasia of the pulmonary artery. Demonstration with pulsed Doppler of increased blood velocities in the pulmonary artery may assist the diagnosis (Figure 15).

AORTIC STENOSIS

Aortic stenosis is commonly divided into supravalvular, valvular and subaortic forms. The subaortic forms include a fixed type, representing the consequence of a fibrous or fibromuscular obstruction, and a dynamic type, which is due to a thickened ventricular septum obstructing the outflow tract of the left ventricle. The latter is also known as asymmetric septal hypertrophy or idiopathic hypertrophic subaortic stenosis. In the most severe cases, the association of left ventricular pressure overload and subendocardial ischemia, owing to a decrease in coronary perfusion, may lead to early intrauterine impairment of cardiac function[36]. Insufficiency of the mitral valve and systolic regurgitation may ensue. Intrauterine hemodynamic perturbation following aortic stenosis is indirectly attested to by the very high incidence of intrauterine growth retardation in infants affected by this anomaly[37]. Neither supravalvular nor subaortic stenosis are usually manifested clinically in newborns.

The same considerations previously reported for the prenatal diagnosis of pulmonary stenosis apply to aortic stenosis. Severe cases of this condition have been described frequently in the current literature[36,38]. Pulsed Doppler ultrasound is valuable in assessing both increased velocities in the ascending aorta and the occasional presence of mitral valve insufficiency[23].

Asymmetric septal hypertrophy has been identified in a fetus[39]. The only reported case, however, is likely to be an exception, as there is evidence indicating that this anomaly usually has a progressive course, and is not apparent in the neonatal period[40]. We are not aware of any case of supravalvular aortic stenosis detected *in utero*.

TETRALOGY OF FALLOT

Tetralogy of Fallot is characterized by the following conditions: a ventricular septal defect, usually located in the perimembranous area; an infundibular pulmonary stenosis; aortic valve over-riding the ventricular septum; and hypertrophy of the right ventricle. Both pathological studies in infants and echocardiographic studies in live fetuses seem to agree in documenting a late onset of right ventricular hypertrophy[11,41].

In the most severe cases, the infundibulum of the right ventricle and the pulmonary artery may be atretic, and the anomaly is commonly referred to as pulmonary atresia with VSD. Associated defects, including atrial septal defects and bicuspid or absent pulmonary valve, are frequently seen. The main factor affecting hemodynamics is the degree of hypoplasia of the right ventricular outflow tract, as this causes both a decrease in pulmonary blood flow and a right-to-left shunt at the level of the ascending aorta, with decreased oxygen saturation. Tetralogy of Fallot, however, does not seem to cause hemodynamic compromise *in utero*. Even in case of very tight infundibular stenosis or pulmonary atresia, the combined output of both ventricles is directed towards the aorta, and the pulmonary vascular bed is supplied by reverse flow through the ductus arteriosus. This concept is supported by the observation of normal intrauterine fetal growth in affected fetuses[37]. Congestive heart failure is very rarely seen in neonates, and it usually occurs only in those with an absent pulmonary valve.

Echocardiographic diagnosis can be made by demonstrating the aorta over-riding the ventricular septum[11,32] (Figure 16). Caution is recommended, as artifacts are frequently seen. In our experience, all fetuses with tetralogy of Fallot had a strikingly enlarged ascending aorta on real-time examination, which should raise the index of suspicion. Study of the right ventricular outflow tract and pulmonary artery provides important clinical information, by allowing assessment of the degree of infundibular stenosis. Doppler ultrasound is valuable in assessing

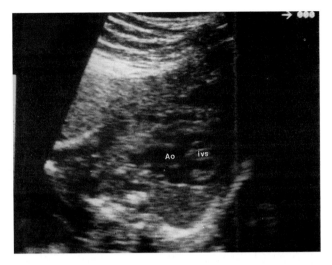

Figure 16 In this mid-trimester fetus with tetralogy of Fallot, the long-axis view of the left ventricle reveals a large ascending aorta (Ao) over-riding the interventricular septum (ivs)

the presence of blood flow in the pulmonary artery. Enlargement of the right ventricle, main pulmonary trunk and pulmonary artery suggests absence of the pulmonary valve[32].

TRANSPOSITION OF THE GREAT ARTERIES

Transposition of the great arteries (TGA) is commonly subdivided into two types: complete TGA and corrected TGA. In complete TGA, the aorta arises from the morphological right ventricle and the pulmonary artery from the left ventricle in the presence of a normal atrioventricular connection. Associated cardiac anomalies are frequently found. According to Becker and Anderson[8] three main varieties can be distinguished: transposition with intact ventricular septum, with or without pulmonary stenosis; transposition with ventricular septal defect; and transposition with ventricular septal defect and pulmonary stenosis. Other anomalies commonly found include abnormalities of the atrioventricular valves, underdevelopment of either the right or the left ventricle and coarctation of the aorta.

Corrected TGA is featured by the association of an atrioventricular and a ventriculoarterial discordance. The right atrium is connected to the left ventricle, which is connected to the pulmonary artery; the left atrium is connected to the right ventricle, which is connected to the ascending aorta.

Fetal echocardiography allows identification of abnormalities of the ventriculoarterial connections. In both complete and corrected transposition, the two great vessels arise parallel from the base of the heart. By careful scanning, the aorta and the pulmonary artery can be identified and their relationship with each ventricle can be assessed (Figures 17 and 18). The differential diagnosis between complete and corrected TGA depends upon identification of the morphological right and left ventricle by visualization of the moderator band, papillary muscles and insertion of atrioventricular valves. The atrioventricular connection can be further recognized by demonstration of

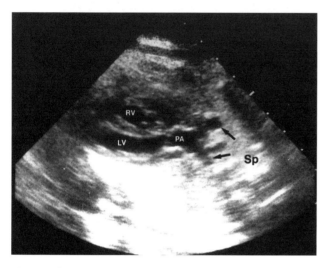

Figure 17 Complete transposition of the great arteries. The vessel arising from the left ventricle (LV) can be identified as the pulmonary artery (PA) by the fact that it has a posterior course and bifurcates (arrows). RV, right ventricle; Sp, spine

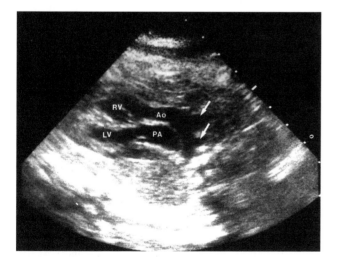

Figure 18 Same case as Figure 17. The vessel arising from the right ventricle (RV) can be identified as the ascending aorta (Ao) by the fact that it has a long upward course and gives rise to the brachiocephalic vessels (arrows). In this scanning plane, the parallel relationship of aorta and pulmonary artery (PA) typical of transpositions is demonstrated. LV, left ventricle

systemic and pulmonary venous return. Fetuses with uncomplicated complete TGA usually do not undergo hemodynamic compromise *in utero*. Survival after birth depends upon the persistence of the fetal circulation. In corrected TGA, the discordance between the atrioventricular and ventriculoarterial connections cancel each other and ideally there should not be any hemodynamic imbalance. Corrected TGA may be an occasional finding at autopsy. Important associated cardiac anomalies, however, are found in the vast majority of cases (ventricular septal defects, pulmonary stenosis, abnormalities of the atrioventricular valves, atrioventricular block).

DOUBLE-OUTLET RIGHT VENTRICLE

In double-outlet right ventricle (DORV) most of the aorta and the pulmonary artery arise from the right ventricle (Figure 19). The relationship between the two great vessels may vary. A defect of the ventricular septum is almost always associated, as well as other anomalies, such as atrial septal defects, pulmonary stenosis, or abnormalities of the atrioventricular valves. By definition, the term DORV includes those cases of tetralogy of Fallot in which the aorta predominantly arises from the right ventricle. Prenatal diagnosis of DORV has been reported[42]. Differentiation from other conotruncal anomalies, however, such as TGA and tetralogy of Fallot, is notoriously difficult[43].

HYPOPLASTIC LEFT HEART SYNDROME

Hypoplastic left heart syndrome (HLHS) is characterized by a very small left ventricle, with mitral and/or aortic atresia. Blood flow to the head and neck vessels and coronary artery is supplied in a retrograde manner via the ductus arteriosus. HLHS is frequently associated with intrauterine heart failure. The prognosis is always extremely poor. Untreated infants die usually in the very first days of life. Palliative procedures have been proposed and long-term survivors have been reported. Recently, cardiac transplantation in the neonatal period has also been attempted.

Echocardiographic diagnosis of HLHS in the fetus depends upon the demonstration of a diminutive left ventricle[44,45]. The ascending aorta is severely hypoplastic. The right ventricle, right atrium and pulmonary artery are usually enlarged (Figure 20). Color and pulsed Doppler ultrasound may assist the diagnosis by demonstrating retrograde blood flow in the ascending aorta and a regurgitant jet in those cases with associated tricuspid valve insufficiency. In most cases, the ultrasound appearance is self-explanatory, and the diagnosis an easy one.

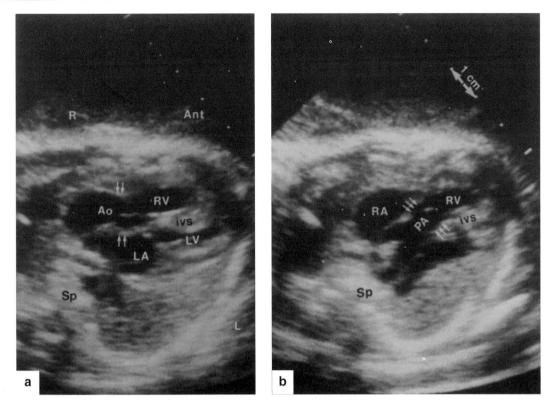

Figure 19 Double-outlet left ventricle. The pulmonary artery (PA) and most of the ascending aorta (Ao) are seen arising from the right ventricle (RV). The aorta over-rides a defect of the interventricular septum (ivs)

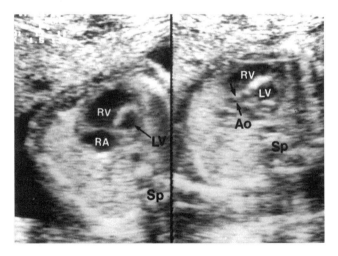

Figure 20 Hypoplastic left heart in a mid-trimester fetus. The diminutive left ventricle (LV) is connected to a severely hypoplastic ascending aorta (Ao). RV, right ventricle; RA, right atrium; Sp, spine

PULMONARY ATRESIA WITH INTACT VENTRICULAR SEPTUM

Pulmonary atresia with intact ventricular septum (PA:IVS) in infants is usually associated with a hypoplastic right ventricle. In fetuses, cases with enlarged right ventricle and atrium have been described with unusual frequency[46]. Although prenatal series are small, it is possible that the discrepancy with the pediatric literature is due to the very high perinatal loss rate that is found in 'dilated' cases. Enlargement of the ventricle and atrium is probably the consequence of tricuspid insufficiency. Prenatal diagnosis of PA:IVS relies upon the demonstration of a small pulmonary artery with an atretic pulmonary valve. Real-time two-dimensional ultrasound diagnosis can be assisted by demonstrating with Doppler ultrasound the absence of anterograde blood flow within the main pulmonary trunk and the presence of reverse flow through the ductus arteriosus.

UNIVENTRICULAR HEART

According to Becker and Anderson[8], the term 'univentricular heart' defines a group of anomalies characterized by the presence of an atrioventricular junction that is entirely connected to only one chamber in the ventricular mass. By adhering to this approach, the univentricular heart includes both those cases in which two atrial chambers are connected, by either two distinct atrioventricular valves or by a common one, to a main ventricular chamber (classic 'double-inlet single ventricle') as well as those cases in which, because of the absence of one atrioventricular connection

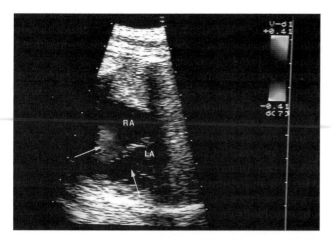

Figure 21 Double-inlet single ventricle. Color Doppler in this diastolic frame depicts blood entering from the right and left atria (RA, LA) into a single ventricular chamber, crossing two separate atrioventricular valves

(tricuspid or mitral atresia), one of the ventricular chambers is either rudimentary or absent. The main ventricular chamber may be of either the left or right type, and in some cases may be of indeterminate type. A rudimentary ventricular chamber lacking an atrioventricular connection is a frequent but not constant finding. Antenatal echocardiographic diagnosis is usually easy. An example of double-inlet univentricular heart is shown in Figure 21. Figure 22 displays a case of mitral atresia. The hemodynamics may vary greatly from case to case, depending upon the type of ventriculoarterial connection and the sum of the associated cardiac anomalies that are very frequently seen.

CARDIOMYOPATHIES

Congenital cardiomyopathies include a heterogeneous group of myocardial disorders, commonly subdivided into non-obstructive and obstructive forms. The etiology of the former type includes inborn errors of metabolism, muscular dystrophies and infections. Obstructive forms include hypertrophic cardiomyopathy of infants of diabetic mothers and asymmetric septal hypertrophy, which has been previously considered. Hypertrophic cardiomyopathy is found in 30–50% of infants of diabetic mothers, although it is clinically evident in a much smaller proportion[47]. The etiology of this condition is controversial, but it is commonly accepted that it represents the final consequence of fetal hyperglycemia and hyperinsulinemia.

Cardiomyopathies of both obstructive and non-obstructive types share in common – either as a consequence of pump failure and/or valvular regurgitation, or of obstruction to ventricular outflow – a more or less marked tendency to congestive heart failure. The onset and extent of symptoms is extremely variable from case to case. Most newborns are asymptomatic, but cases associated with intrauterine heart failure have been described[11,48].

Echocardiographic diagnosis of non-obstructive forms relies upon demonstration of cardiomegaly and poor contractility of ventricular chambers[48]. In obstructive forms, thickening of the interventricular septum has been reported[39,49] (Figure 23).

COARCTATION OF THE AORTA

The pathogenesis of coarctation of the aorta is controversial. Three hypotheses were suggested. Coarctation may be a true malformation, due to an embryogenetic abnormality; or the consequence of aberrant ductal tissue in the aortic wall, resulting in narrowing of the isthmus at the time of closure of the ductus (the so-called Skodaic theory); or, finally, the anatomic result of an intrauterine hemodynamic perturbation due to an intracardiac anomaly diverting blood flow from the aorta into the pulmonary artery and the ductus arteriosus. There is clinical as well as pathological evidence supporting at least the last two hypotheses.

A discrete shelf between the isthmus and the descending aorta is the most common finding at anatomic dissection. Tubular hypoplasia of a segment of the aortic arch is seen less frequently. Coarctation may be a postnatal event, and this limits prenatal diagnosis in many cases. This anomaly, however, has been described in the fetus, although only in late pregnancy[50]. In one case seen in our laboratory, echocardiography was negative at 20 weeks. At 30 weeks, enlargement of the right ventricle was found and the aortic isthmus appeared to be severely narrowed (Figure 24). As the blood flow through the isthmus is minimal during intrauterine life, the descending aorta being mainly supplied via the ductus arteriosus, isolated coarctation is not expected to alter the hemodynamics significantly. However, cases with tubular hypoplasia of the aortic arch may result in a greater hemodynamic burden, and this could explain the dilatation of the right heart that has been documented with echocardiography prior to birth.

FETAL DYSRHYTHMIAS

Irregular patterns of fetal heart rhythms are a frequent finding. Short periods of tachycardia, bradycardia and ectopic beats as well are very commonly seen, and in the vast majority of cases have no clinical significance. The electrical instability of the fetal heart has not yet received a clear explanation. Catecholamine release or accessory pathways have been suggested to play a role. Even with the realization that a clear differentiation between physiological variations and pathological alterations is not possible in many cases, a distinction

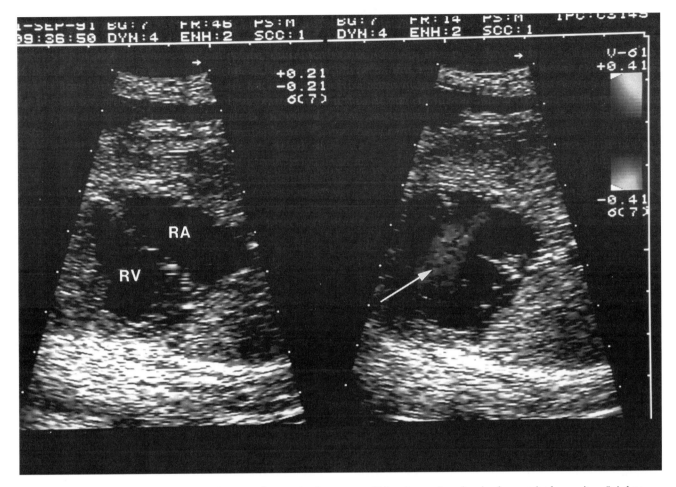

Figure 22 Mitral atresia. Color Doppler reveals one single stream of blood entering the single ventricular cavity of right type (RV) from the right atrium (RA)

should be attempted for practical clinical purposes. According to Allan and colleagues[13], a sustained bradycardia of less than 100 beats/min, a sustained tachycardia of more than 200 beats/min and irregular beats occurring more than one in ten should be considered abnormal and require further investigation.

The fetal electrocardiogram is of little value in the prenatal diagnosis of dysrhythmias, as a satisfactory transbdominal recording can be obtained in a minority of cases. At present, M-mode and pulsed Doppler ultrasound are the best available techniques for the assessment of irregular fetal heart rhythm.

The study of the mechanical events of the sequence of contraction may be accomplished in different ways[18–20]. Simultaneous visualization of atrioventricular valves and ventricular wall motion, aortic valve opening and atrial wall movement with M-mode and sampling of the ventricular inlet or inferior vena cava with M-mode can be used from time to time. The sequence of excitations can be reasonably inferred by the sequence of contractions (Figures 25 and 26).

Premature atrial and ventricular contractions

Premature atrial and ventricular contractions are the most frequent fetal dysrhythmias[19] (Figure 27). Repeated premature contractions can give rise to complex rhythm patterns. Premature atrial contractions may be either conducted to the ventricles or blocked, depending upon the time of the cardiac cycle in which they occur, thus resulting in either an increased or a decreased ventricular rate. Blocked premature atrial contractions should be differentiated from atrioventricular block. Premature atrial and ventricular contractions are considered to be a benign condition[19]. They probably do not induce any hemodynamic perturbation, do not appear to be associated with an increased risk of structural abnormalities and usually disappear *in utero* or soon after birth. However, as there is at least a theoretical possibility that in a few cases an ectopic beat triggers a re-entrant tachyarrhythmia, serial monitoring of the fetal heart during pregnancy is suggested.

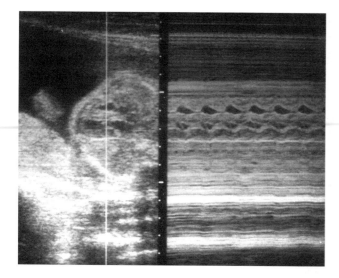

Figure 23   In this mid-trimester fetus echocardiography was motivated by a previous sibling who died in infancy with severe hypertrophic cardiomyopathy. At 22 weeks, an unusual thickness of the interventricular septum was noted. At 24 weeks, these findings were confirmed. Termination of pregnancy was performed upon request of the couple and necropsy revealed severe hypertrophic cardiomyopathy associated with a small ventricular septal defect that had not been detected by antenatal sonography

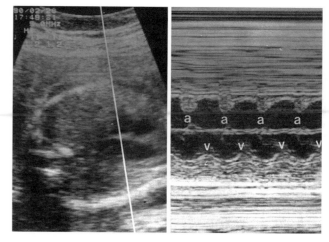

Figure 25   M-mode echocardiogram in the mid-trimester demonstrating the atrioventricular sequence of contraction. The M-line is directed across the anterior wall of the right atrium and posterior wall of the left ventricle and demonstrates fluctuations reflecting atrial (a) and ventricular (v) systole

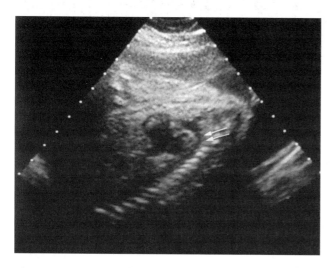

Figure 24   In this 30-week fetus with enlarged right heart, a seemingly narrow aortic arch is noted (arrows). Severe coarctation was confirmed at birth

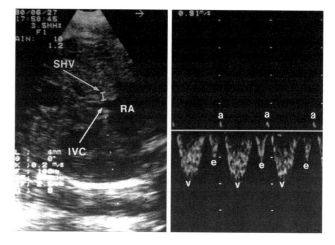

Figure 26   Pulsed Doppler sonography of the sagittal suprahepatic vein (SHV). The sampling gate is positioned close to the connection with the inferior vena cava (IVC). Pulsatile blood flow is commonly recorded in this vessel during fetal life. Three separate peaks can be recognized: blood moves fast towards the heart in two separate waves reflecting ventricular systole (v) and passive venous filling (e). During atrial systole (a), retrograde flow is recorded. Analysis of these waveforms allows inferance of the atrioventricular sequence of contraction similar to the M-mode tracings of cardiac chambers

Supraventricular tachyarrhythmias

Supraventricular tachyarrhythmias include supraventricular paroxysmal tachycardia (SVT), atrial flutter and atrial fibrillation. SVT is characterized by an atrial frequency between 200 and 300 beats/min and a 1 : 1 atrioventricular conduction rate. It can occur by one of two mechanisms: automaticity and re-entry. In the former case, an irritable ectopic focus discharges at high

frequency. In the latter case, an electrical impulse re-enters the atria, giving rise to repeated electrical activity. Re-entry may occur at the level of the sinoatrial node, inside the atrium, the atrioventricular node and the His Purkinje system. Re-entry may also occur along an anomalous atrioventricular connection such

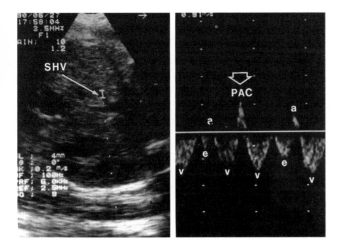

Figure 27 In this fetus with premature atrial contractions, an abnormal waveform was recorded in the suprahepatic vein (SHV) by pulse Doppler sonography. The normal sequence is interrupted by premature atrial contractions (PAC). Note that peak velocity is higher with this abnormal beat than with regular atrial systole. The following sequence of waves suggest that the premature atrial beat is conducted to the ventricle

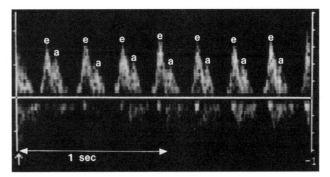

Figure 28 Pulsed Doppler evaluation of ventricular inlet in a fetus with supraventricular tachycardia (240 beats/min). Compare this image with Figure 7. With fetal tachycardia the e wave appears dominant over the a wave, the opposite of normal. This is thought to represent failure of diastolic filling

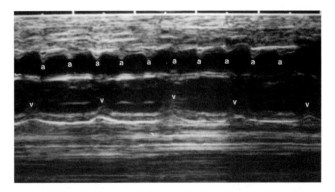

Figure 29 Complete atrioventricular block in a third-trimester fetus. Fluctuations of the atrial wall (a) suggest a regular atrial rate of about 120 beats/min. Ventricular systole (v) occurs at a much lower rate (60 beats/min) and is totally dissociated from atrial systole

as the Kent bundle in the Wolff–Parkinson–White (WPW) syndrome. In atrial flutter the atrial rate ranges from 300 to 400 beats/min. Owing to variable degrees of atrioventricular block, the ventricular rate ranges between 60 and 200 beats/min. In atrial fibrillation, the atrial rate is more than 400 beats/min and the ventricular rate ranges between 120 and 200 beats/min. Atrial flutter and fibrillation often alternate, and are thought to arise from similar mechanisms, which include circus movement of the electrical impulse, ectopic formation, multiple re-entry and multifocal impulse formation. SVT is by far the most common tachyarrhythmia in children. The most frequent form is that caused by atrioventricular nodal re-entry.

Diagnosis of fetal tachyarrhythmia can be easily accomplished by direct auscultation or continuous Doppler examination. M-mode and/or pulsed Doppler ultrasound allow identification of the precise heart rate and recognition of the atrioventricular sequence of contraction.

The association between fetal tachyarrhythmia and non-immune hydrops is well established[32,51]. It has been postulated that a fast ventricular rate results in suboptimal filling of the ventricle. This would lead to decreased cardiac output, right atrial overload and congestive heart failure[51]. Pulsed Doppler analysis of ventricular filling in tachyarrhythmic fetuses would seem to support such a view[51] (Figure 28).

Intrauterine pharmacological cardioversion of fetal tachyarrhythmia by maternal administration of drugs has been attempted with success in many cases. The optimal approach to the treatment of this condition is still uncertain and is a matter of controversy. Digoxin, verapamil, propranolol, quinidine, procainamide, flecainide and amiodarone have all been used. Cardioversion in the setting of fetal hydrops is felt to be difficult to obtain with maternal drug administration, and direct injection into the umbilical vein by funipuncture has been proposed in these cases. The interested reader is referred to specific works on this subject[51–53].

Atrioventricular block

Atrioventricular block can result from immaturity of the conduction system, absence of connection to the atrioventricular node or abnormal anatomic position of the atrioventricular node. Atrioventricular block is commonly classified into three types. First degree-atrioventricular block corresponds to a simple conduction delay, which is associated with a prolongation of the PR interval on the EKG. Second-degree atrioventricular block is subdivided into Mobitz types I and II. Mobitz type I consists of a progressive prolongation of the PR interval that finally leads to the blocking of one atrial impulse (Luciani–Wenckebach phenomenon). In Mobitz type II the ventricular rate is a submultiple of the atrial rate (e.g. 2 : 1, 3 : 1). In third-degree or complete atrioventricular block, there is a complete dissociation of atria and ventricles, usually with independent and slow activation of the ventricles (Figure 29). Third-degree atrioventricular block is widely reported to be associated in over half of the cases with cardiac structural anomalies[54], including corrected transposition, univentricular heart, cardiac tumors and cardiomyopathies. Although in the cases without structural cardiac diseases the etiology is unknown, there is growing evidence suggesting an association with the presence of maternal antibodies against antigens associated with Sjögren syndrome, such as SSA/Ro and SSB/la antigens. Transplacental passage of these antibodies would lead to inflammation and damage of the conduction system. Anti-SSA antibodies have been reported in over 80% of mothers who delivered infants with atrioventricular block, although only 30% had clinical evidence of connective tissue disease, mostly lupus erythematosus[55–58].

First- and second-degree atrioventricular block are not usually associated with any significant hemodynamic perturbtion. Third-degree atrioventricular block may lead to important bradycardia, resulting in a decreased cardiac output and congestive heart failure *in utero*[19,32]. The obstetric management of this condition is uncertain. A multicenter study including 55 cases diagnosed *in utero* suggested that the presence of structural cardiac defects, hydrops and a ventricular rate of less than 55 beats/min are poor prognostic factors[59].

Maternal plasmapheresis and administration of steroids have been proposed for the antenatal treatment of third-degree atrioventricular block associated with maternal autoantibodies[60]. The available experience, however, is scanty[60]. Both in our experience and in that of others[59], the maternal administration of β-mimetics had little effect on fetal ventricular rate.

Intrauterine ventricular pacing has been attempted in one case. A lead was inserted through the maternal abdominal and uterine walls and the fetal thorax and placed inside the right ventricle. Although a regular ventricular frequency was obtained, fetal death ensued a few hours later[61].

REFERENCES

1. Winsberg F. Echocardiography of the fetal and newborn heart. *Invest Radiol* 1972;7:152
2. Ianniruberto A, Iaccarino M, De Luca I, *et al.* Analisi delle strutture cardiache fetali mediante ecografia. Nota tecnica. *Proceedings of the 3rd National Congress of the SISUM*, Terlizzi, 24–25 September 1977:285–90
3. De Luca I, Ianniruberto A, Colonna L. Aspetti ecografici del cuore fetale. *G Ital Cardiol* 1978;8:776
4. Kleinman CS, Hobbins JC, Jaffe CC, *et al.* Echocardiographic studies of the human fetus: prenatal diagnosis of congenital heart disease and cardiac dysrhythmias. *Pediatrics* 1980;65:1059
5. Allan LD, Crawford DC, Anderson RH, *et al.* Echocardiographic and anatomical correlates in fetal congenital heart disease. *Br Heart J* 1984;52:542
6. Copel JA, Pilu G, Green JJ, *et al.* Fetal echocardiographic screening for congenital heart disease: the importance of the four-chamber view. *Am J Obstet Gynecol* 1987;157:648
7. Pilu G, Baccarani G. Prenatal diagnosis of cardiac structural abnormalities. *Fetal Ther* 1986;1:73
8. Becker AE, Anderson RH. *Pathology of Congenital Heart Disease*. London: Butterworths, 1981
9. Allan LD, Joseph MC, Boyd EGCA, *et al.* M-mode echocardiography in the developing human fetus. *Br Heart J* 1982;47:573
10. DeVore GR, Donnerstein RL, Kleinman CS, *et al.* Fetal echocardiography 1. Normal anatomy as determined by real-time directed M-mode ultrasound. *Am J Obstet Gynecol* 1982;144:249
11. DeVore GR, Siassi B, Platt LD. Fetal echocardiography. IV. M-mode assessment of ventricular size and contractility during the second and third trimester of pregnancy in the normal fetus. *Am J Obstet Gynecol* 1984;150:981
12. St John Sutton MG, Gewitz MH, Shah B, *et al.* Quantitative assessment of growth and function of the cardiac chambers in the normal human fetus. A prospective longitudinal echocardiographic study. *Circulation* 1984;69:645
13. Allan LD, Anderson RH, Sullivan ID, *et al.* Evaluation of fetal arrhythmias by echocardiography. *Br Heart J* 1983;50:240
14. Kleinman CS, Donnerstein RL, Jaffe CC, *et al.* Fetal echocardiography. A tool for evaluation of *in utero* cardiac arrhythmias and monitoring of *in utero* therapy: analysis of 71 patients. *Am J Cardiol* 1983;51:237
15. DeVore GR, Siassi B, Platt LD. Fetal echocardiography. 111. The diagnosis of cardiac arrhythmias using real-time directed M-mode ultrasound. *Am J Obstet Gynecol* 1983;146:792
16. Stewart PA, Tonge HM, Wladimiroff JW. Arrhythmias and structural abnormalities of the fetal heart. *Br Heart J* 1983;50:550
17. Huhta JC, Strasburger JF, Carpenter RJ, *et al.* Pulsed Doppler fetal echocardiography. *J Clin Ultrasound* 1985;13:247
18. Silverman NH, Kleinman CS, Rudolph AM, *et al.* Fetal atrioventricular valve insufficiency associated with nonimmune hydrops. A two dimensional echocardiographic and pulsed Doppler ultrasound study. *Circulation* 1985;72:825
19. Reed KL, Shan DJ, Scagnelli S, *et al.* Doppler echocardiographic studies of diastolic function in the human fetal heart. Changes during gestation. *J Am Coll Cardiol* 1986;8:391
20. Kenny JF, Plappert T, Doubilet P, *et al.* Changes in intracardiac blood flow velocities and right and left ventricular stroke volumes with gestational age in the normal human fetus: a prospective Doppler echocardiographic study. *Circulation* 1986;74:1208
21. Reed KL, Meijboom EJ, Sahn DJ, *et al.* Cardiac Doppler flow velocities in human fetus. *Circulation* 1986;73:41

22. Lingman G, Marsal K. Circulatory effects of fetal cardiac arrhythmias. *Pediatr Cardiol* 1986;7:67

23. Kenny JF, Plappert T, Doubilet P, *et al*. Effects of heart rate on ventricular size, stroke volume, and output in the normal human fetus: a prospective Doppler echocardiographic study. *Circulation* 1987;76:52

24. Machado MVL, Chita SC, Allan LD. Acceleration time in the aorta and pulmonary artery measured by Doppler echocardiography in the midtrimester normal human fetus. *Br Heart J* 1987;58:15

25. De Smedt M, Visser GHA, Meijboom EJ. Fetal cardiac output estimated by Doppler echocardiography during mid- and late gestation. *Am J Cardiol* 1987;60:338

26. Mitchell SC, Korones SB, Berendes HW. Congenital heart disease in 56,109 births. Incidence and natural history. *Circulation* 1971;43:323

27. Hoffman JI, Christianson R. Congenital heart disease in a cohort of 19,502 births with long-term follow-up. *Am J Cardiol* 1978;42:641

28. Gerlis LM. Cardiac malformations in spontaneous abortions. *Int J Cardiol* 1985;7:29

29. Nora JJ, Nora AH. *Genetics and Counselling in Cardiovascular Disease*. Springfield, IL: Charles C Thomas, 1978

30. Nora JJ, Nora AH. Maternal transmission of congenital heart disease: new recurrence risk figures and the questions of cytoplasmic inheritance and vulnerability to teratogens. *Am J Cardiol* 1987;59:459

31. Rowe RD, Uchida IA. Cardiac malformation in mongolism. A prospective study of 184 mongoloid children. *Am J Med* 1961;31:726

32. Kleinman CS, Donnerstein RL, DeVore GR, *et al*. Fetal echocardiography for evaluation of *in utero* congestive heart failure: a technique for study of nonimmune fetal hydrops. *N Engl J Med* 1982;306:568

33. Rudolph AM. *Congenital Disease of the Heart*. Chicago: Year Book Medical Publisher, 1974

34. Hoffman JIE, Rudolph AM. The natural history of ventricular septal defects in infancy. *Am J Cardiol* 1965; 16:634

35. Feigenbaum H. *Echocardiography*, 3rd edn. Philadelphia: Lea & Febiger, 1981

36. Allan LD, Little D, Campbell S, *et al*. Fetal ascites associated with congenital heart disease. Case report. *Br J Obstet Gynaecol* 1981;88:453

37. Reynolds JL. *Intrauterine Growth Retardation in Children with Congenital Heart Disease. Its Relation to Aortic Stenosis*. Birth Defects Original Articles Series 1972; 8:143

38. Huhta JC, Carpenter RJ, Moise KJ, *et al*. Prenatal diagnosis and postnatal management of critical aortic stenosis. *Circulation* 1987;75:573

39. Stewart PA, Buis-Liem T, Verwey RA, *et al*. Prenatal ultrasonic diagnosis of familial asymmetric septal hypertrophy. *Prenat Diagn* 1986;6:249

40. Wright GB, Keane JF, Nadas AS, *et al*. Fixed subaortic stenosis in the young. Medical and surgical course in 83 patients. *Am J Cardiol* 1983;52:830

41. Lev M, Rimoldi HJA, Rowlatt UF. The quantitative anatomy of cyanotic tetralogy of Fallot. *Circulation* 1964;30:531

42. Stewart PA, Wladimiroff JW, Becker AE. Early prenatal detection of double outlet right ventricle by echocardiography. *Br Heart J* 1985;54:340

43. Sanders SP, Bierman FZ, Williams RG. Conotruncal malformations. Diagnosis in infancy using subxyphoid 2-dimensional echocardiography. *Am J Cardiol* 1982; 50:1361

44. Sahn DJ, Shenker L, Reed KL, *et al*. Prenatal ultrasound diagnosis of hypoplastic left heart syndrome *in utero* associated with hydrops fetalis. *Am Heart J* 1982; 104:1368

45. Silverman NH, Enderlein MA, Goibus MS. Ultrasonic recognition of aortic valve atresia *in utero*. *Am J Cardiol* 1984;53:391

46. Allan LD, Crawford DC, Tynan MJ. Pulmonary atresia in prenatal life. *J Am Coll Cardiol* 1986;8:1131

47. Walther FJ, Siassi B, King J, *et al*. Cardiac output in infants of insulin-dependent diabetic mothers. *J Pediatr* 1985;107:109

48. Bovicelli L, Picchio FM, Pilu G, *et al*. Prenatal diagnosis of endocardial fibroelastosis. *Prenat Diagn* 1984;4:67

49. Romero R, Pilu G, Jeanty P, *et al*. Cardiomyopathies. In *Prenatal Diagnosis of Congenital Anomalies*. Norwalk: Appleton & Lange, 1987:178–80

50. Allan LD, Crawford DC, Tynan MJ. Evolution of coarctation of the aorta in intrauterine life. *Br Heart J* 1984;52:471

51. Kleinman CS, Copel JA, Weinstein EM, *et al. In utero* diagnosis and treatment of fetal supraventricular tachycardia. *Semin Perinatol* 1985;9:113

52. Hansmann M, Gembruch U, Manz M, *et al*. Fetal tachyarrhythmias – transplacental and direct treatment of the fetus – a report of 60 cases. *Ultrasound Obstet Gynecol* 1991;1:162

53. Kleinman CS, Copel JA. Electrophysiological principles and fetal antiarrhythmic therapy. *Ultrasound Obstet Gynecol* 1991;1:286

54. Griffiths SP. Congenital complete heart block. *Circulation* 1971;43:615

55. Chameides L, Truex RC, Vetter V, *et al*. Association of maternal systemic lupus erythematosus with congenital complete heart block. *N Engl J Med* 1977;297:1204

56. Mc Cue CM, Mantakas ME, Tingelstad JB, *et al*. Congenital heart block in newborns of mothers with connective tissue disease. *Circulation* 1977;56:82

57. Scott JS, Maddison PJ, Taylor, PV, *et al*. Connective tissue disease, antibodies to ribonucleoprotein and congenital heart block. *N Engl J Med* 1983;309:209

58. Singsen BH, Akthar JE, Weinstein MM, *et al*. Congenital complete heart block and SSA antibodies. Obstetric implications. *Am J Obstet Gynecol* 1985; 152:655

59. Schmidt KG, Ulmer HE, Silverman NH, *et al*. Perinatal outcome of fetal complete atrioventricular block: a multicenter experience. *J Am Coll Cardiol* 1991;91:1360

60. Olah KS, Gee H. Fetal heart block associated with maternal anti-Ro (SS-A) antibody. Current management. A review. *Br J Obstet Gynaecol* 1991;98:751

61. Carpenter RJ, Strasburger JF, Garson A, *et al*. Fetal ventricular pacing for hydrops secondary to complete atrioventricular block. *J Am Coll Cardiol* 1986;8:1434

59

Fetal growth restriction

M.Y. Divon

INTRODUCTION

Low birthweight is an important predictor of neonatal morbidity and mortality. This condition can be the result of either preterm delivery or fetal growth restriction. Fetuses whose growth has been restricted by a process of intrauterine growth restriction (IUGR) have an increased incidence of perinatal morbidity and mortality[1]. Heinonen *et al.*[2] have recently studied the fetal to first-year survival of preterm infants born at 26–32 weeks' gestation and concluded that IUGR was associated with a three-fold increase in neonatal mortality. Relative to infants with normal growth, IUGR is associated with a higher incidence of low Apgar scores, perinatal asphyxia, hypothermia, polycythemia, hypocalcemia, pulmonary hemorrhage, and impaired immune function[3].

DEFINITION AND CLASSIFICATION OF IUGR

Intrauterine growth rates are measured by relating the size of the infant at birth to an expected norm for gestational age. Birthweight is the most accessible and reliable measure of the newborn and is, therefore, widely used for this purpose.

Fetal size and fetal growth are often confused in clinical practice. Intrauterine growth restriction denotes a pathological process stemming from growth restriction. In contrast, small-for-gestational age (SGA) identifies the infant whose birthweight is below an arbitrary percentile for gestational age. The 10th percentile is often used for this purpose; however, birthweights below the 25th, 15th, and 5th percentile or 2 standard deviations (SD) below the mean have also been used in the past. Using birthweight criteria as the gold standard for intrauterine growth presents a few problems. First, the diagnosis of growth restriction is based on a single observation (birthweight) made at an endpoint (gestational age at delivery). Fetal growth, however, cannot be estimated from less than two measurements separated by a 'reasonable' interval.

Second, not every infant whose birthweight is below the 10th percentile for gestational age is small because of a pathological growth-restrictive process. The constitutionally small infant is indeed small but shows appropriate growth and has no other complications.

The converse is also a problem. A dysmature, postdate infant may be subjected to severe growth restriction, yet, its birthweight is often above the 10th percentile for gestational age. Thus, a tall and very thin infant may be misclassified as appropriately grown. Third, estimation of gestational age presents recurrent problems. An infant may be assigned different gestational ages depending on the specific method used to establish this age (i.e. last menstrual period, early clinical examination, early ultrasound examination or neonatal assessment).

Several 'commonly used' norms for birthweight as a function of gestational age have been described[4]. Differences between these norms are due to different geographical origin (differences in altitude are of primary importance), race, ethnicity, parity and neonatal sex. The mean birthweight at 40 weeks' gestation reported by Lubchenco and co-workers[5] at Denver (high altitude) was 120 g smaller than that reported by Brenner and co-workers[6] who studied an east coast (sea-level), racially mixed population (Table 1).

Despite all of these concerns, and probably due to a lack of a more dynamic definition, IUGR is often defined as birthweight below the 10th percentile for

Table 1 10th percentile birthweight values as a function of gestational age

	Birthweight (g)	
Gestational age (weeks)	Lubchenco et al.[5]	Brenner et al.[6]
28	860	770
29	970	900
30	1075	1030
31	1180	1170
32	1290	1310
33	1480	1490
34	1670	1670
35	1860	1930
36	2050	2190
37	2240	2350
38	2430	2510
39	2530	2630
40	2630	2750
41	2675	2790
42	2720	2830

gestational age. By definition, the incidence of this condition is 10%. Variations of this proportion are caused by using the wrong norm for the population under study.

Growth and symmetry are affected by the nature and severity of the underlying growth-restrictive process as well as its timing and duration. In 1963, Gruenwald[7] identified two distinct patterns of decreased growth – symmetric and asymmetric. Early-phase growth disturbance (typically first trimester and early second trimester) often culminates in symmetric growth retardation. Since growth in this phase is primarily due to cell hyperplasia, restriction of growth results in a lower cell number. Thus, the newborn is symmetrically small (i.e. concomitant decrease in the size of the head, trunk, length, and all other body organs). This pattern is often seen in growth disturbance associated with chromosomal anomalies, congenital malformations and transplacental infections. In the asymmetric type, the growth rate of the trunk is smaller than that of other organs. This is caused by relative depletion of the actively growing liver combined with decreased subcutaneous fat deposition. Third-trimester growth abnormalities, such as those seen with maternal vascular disease, restrict fetal growth during the hypertrophic growth phase. Due to preferential perfusion of the brain and adequate linear growth, the asymmetrically growth-restricted newborn is identified by either an abnormally increased head circumference to abdominal circumference ratio or by an abnormal ponderal index. The neonatal ponderal index has been suggested as a measure of the proportion between neonatal body mass and length[8]. This index is defined as a percentage of birthweight (in grams) divided by body length (in centimeters) cubed. Theoretically, an abnormal ponderal index should differentiate the normal from the wasted and malnourished infant. Miller[9] suggested that a low ponderal index indicates asymmetric growth restriction and that it is a more accurate predictor of fetal morbidity than birthweight alone. Defining IUGR by an abnormal ponderal index does, however, suffer from several limitations. First, severe early-onset growth restriction often results in a normal ponderal index due to restriction of both weight and linear growth. Second, accurate measurements of neonatal length are not easy to obtain. A small error in this measurement is cubed when calculating the ponderal index and may lead to erroneous conclusions. Because of these limitations, the ponderal index has not received widespread clinical acceptance in obstetrics. It is necessary to be aware that these symmetric and asymmetric patterns of fetal growth may merge and become indistinguishable. A maternal vascular disease beginning early enough may cause symmetrical growth restriction. Likewise, an asymmetrically growth-restricted fetus can become symmetric once brain sparing or linear growth are no longer

maintained (this phenomenon has been identified as 'late flattening of the biparietal diameter' and is associated with increased neonatal morbidity). It is commonly believed that 'placental insufficiency' results in asymmetrical growth restriction whereas chromosomal abnormalities are associated with symmetrical IUGR. Data presented by Nicolaides and co-workers[10] indicate, however, that fetal genetic disease may be associated with severe asymmetrical growth.

In a study of 752 consecutively born, single, white, term infants, Miller[11] has noted that the ratio of asymmetric to symmetric to 'mixed' types of IUGR is 4.7 : 2.7 : 1.0, respectively. Basel and co-workers[12] reported on longitudinal sonographic biometry performed on fetuses with decreased growth rates and concluded that the type of IUGR is determined to a large extent by the timing and duration of the insult rather than the specific etiology.

ETIOLOGY OF IUGR

Various disease processes may result in IUGR. The final fetal size is determined by the severity, gestational age at onset and duration of the underlying pathology.

Abrams and Newman[13] have examined the relationship between maternal characteristics and the risk of delivering a growth-restricted neonate (birthweight < 10th percentile for gestational age) in 2228 women. These authors used multivariate analysis to show that the following variables are significant risk factors for IUGR: cigarette smoking (odds ratio = 3.18), low maternal weight gain (odds ratio = 2.96), black ethnicity (odds ratio = 2.60), prepregnancy underweight (odds ratio = 2.36), Asian ethnicity (odds ratio = 1.88), primiparity (odds ratio = 1.85) and low maternal height (odds ratio = 1.63). It should be noted that Asian ethnicity and low maternal height may represent predisposing factors for normal, constitutionally small infants. Maternal history of low birthweight and a previous delivery of a low birthweight infant have been added to the above list by Kramer[14,15].

The etiological factors that result in restriction of fetal growth potential can be grouped into intrinsic and extrinsic categories (Table 2). Intrinsic fetal abnormalities, such as genetic and congenital anomalies

Table 2 Etiological factors in IUGR

Intrinsic factors	*Extrinsic factors*
Chromosomal aberrations	Maternal–placental–fetal
Congenital structural defects	infections
Constitutional (genetic	Uteroplacental perfusion
heritage)	Chronic maternal
	disease
	Substrate availability
	Toxins

(Tables 3 and 4) often result in a symmetrical IUGR. The incidence of chromosomal aberrations in growth-retarded, live fetuses varies from 30% in severe, early onset cases to approximately 2.2% for term deliveries[16,17]. IUGR and polyhydramnios were the most common associated finding in 386 structurally anomalous fetuses (52% and 54.5%, respectively) reported by Wladimiroff *et al.*[18] Symmetric growth restriction is also seen commonly with fetal infections (Table 5) and teratogenic agents (Table 6). Other extrinsic conditions, such as maternal vascular and placental causes of IUGR (Table 5), often result in an asymmetrical growth restriction pattern. Structural anomalies of the placenta and the umbilical cord (Table 7) have not been associated with a particular form of growth restriction.

Antenatal identification of the cause of IUGR is probably possible in as many as 50% of cases. Various etiological factors require management decisions and have important neonatal implications. An intensive survey of maternal history (Table 8), physical examination, blood tests and genetic studies is recommended.

Table 3   Chromosomal anomalies associated with IUGR

Common	Rare
Trisomy 13	Trisomy 22
Trisomy 18	Turner's Syndrome
Trisomy 21	4p and 4q syndromes
	5p and 5q syndromes
	13q syndrome
	18p and 18q syndromes
	Trisomy 9 mosaic syndrome
	Triploidy syndrome
	Partial trisomy 10q syndrome
	Ring 1
	Ring 22

Table 4   Fetal structural anomalies associated with IUGR

Neural tube defects
Renal anomalies (Potter's syndrome)
Anencephaly
Pancreatic agenesis
Congenital heart defects
Dwarfism syndromes
Chondrodystrophies
Osteogenesis imperfecta
Primordial short stature

Table 5   Maternal causes of IUGR

Chronic disease
  Hypertension
  Collagen vascular disease
  Renal disease
  Cyanotic cardiopulmonary disease
  Thyrotoxicosis
  Advanced diabetes mellitus
  Hemoglobinopathies
  SS hemoglobin

Pre-eclampsia

Malnutrition

Infection
  Toxoplasmosis
  Malaria
  Rubella
  Cytomegalovirus
  Herpes
  Syphilis
  Listeriosis

Table 6   Drugs and medications associated with IUGR

Marijuana
Heroin, methadone
Cocaine
Cigarette smoking
Alcohol
Aminopterin
Coumarin derivatives
Cytotoxic drugs
Isotretinoin
Lithium
Paramethadione
Phenytoin

Table 7   Placental factors in IUGR

Placenta previa
Chronic placental abruption
Decreased uteroplacental perfusion
Chorioangioma
Partial molar pregnancy
Twin-to-twin transfusion
Single umbilical artery

Table 8   Screening for IUGR by history

Smoking
Altitude
Malnutrition (poor weight gain)
Previous IUGR
Medications
Recreational drugs
Alcohol
Chronic maternal disease

Genetic anomalies
  Maternal age
  Family history
  Habitual abortion
  Alpha-fetoprotein
  Environmental: lead, mercury, copper

First-trimester vaginal bleeding
Parent's size

The astute clinician should also realize that the fetus of constitutionally small parents will most likely express its genetic heritage in its pattern of intrauterine growth.

DIAGNOSIS OF IUGR

When growth restriction is recognized, intensive monitoring of the affected pregnancy is required, and early intervention on behalf of the compromised fetus may be advisable. Screening for IUGR by serial fundal height and maternal weight-gain assessments should be routinely performed during prenatal care. Decreased fundal height may be associated with IUGR (oligohydramnios, wrong dates and fetal malposition should also be considered). The sensitivity of this test may be as high as 50%[19]. The false-positive rate is, however, quite high at approximately 56%[20]. Beazly and Kurjak[21] reported that 25% of such assessments performed beyond 36 weeks' gestation were inaccurate by > 500 g and that the error increased at the extremes of the birthweight range (when this information is most useful). Similar results were reported by Loeffler[22].

Pregnant women whose weight gain is inadequate or fundal height is decreased stand an increased risk of having an infant who will develop fetal growth restriction. Clinical risk assessment does not, however, appear to adequately and consistently predict IUGR. Further evaluation by sonographic assessment should be offered to patients with risk factors and a high index of suspicion.

Intrauterine growth restriction can be manifest by a variety of combinations of decreased fetal weight, body length, head circumference, abdominal circumference and soft tissue mass. Ultrasound is the only direct method available for assessing fetal size. It also provides for an assessment of factors associated with IUGR such as fetal anomalies, oligohydramnios, and increased placental impedance. A thorough evaluation should include a detailed study of fetal, umbilical and placental structural anomalies as well as measurements of the biparietal diameter (BPD), head circumference (HC), abdominal circumference (AC), femur length (FL), and a semiquantitative assessment of amniotic fluid volume in the form of the amniotic fluid index (AFI). Morphometric ratios such as the HC : AC and FL : AC as well as a sonographic estimate of fetal weight (EFW) can then be derived from these measurements. Umbilical artery Doppler velocity studies provide data regarding placental impedance to blood flow and may be constructive in patients who are at increased risk for IUGR.

Several studies have evaluated the ability of both single and serial BPD measurements to identify IUGR. The results vary widely, with sensitivities ranging from 44% to 90%[23]. These measurements may not identify the symmetrically small fetus.

A strong correlation between fetal femur length and neonatal crown to heel length can been demonstrated[24].

The experience with this measurement as an independent predictor of IUGR is limited. O'Brien and Queenan[25] have shown that the femur length helps differentiate between symmetrical and asymmetrical patterns of growth restriction. Overall, both the size of the fetal head and length of the femur are affected late in most cases of IUGR and, therefore, these measurements are too insensitive to be used as independent predictors of IUGR.

Measurements of the fetal abdominal circumference are commonly used as a means for identification of the growth-restricted fetus. This measurement reflects the size of the liver (which correlates with the degree of fetal malnutrition) as well as the volume of subcutaneous fat. In addition, the abdominal circumference is decreased in both symmetric and asymmetric growth restriction. Therefore, it is not surprising that sonographic measurements of the abdominal circumference predict growth restriction more accurately than either the biparietal diameter or the femur length. In a large study of 3616 sonographically dated pregnancies, Warsof and co-workers[26] have shown that abdominal circumference measurements predicted IUGR with a sensitivity of 61%, specificity of 95%, true-positive rate of 86% and true-negative rate of 83%. Their results also indicate that the optimal gestational age to screen for IUGR is approximately 34 weeks. Similarly, other investigators[27–29] have reported relatively high positive predictive values for this measurement (ranging from 84% to 100%). Fernazzi and co-workers[30] noted that the positive predictive value of the abdominal circumference for detection of the growth-restricted fetus increases with gestational age (from 51% at 29–30 weeks' gestation to 71% at term).

Accurate pregnancy dating is essential for the interpretation of abdominal circumference measurements. However, uncertainty about gestational age occurs frequently and makes the differentiation between the appropriate-for-gestational age and the growth-restricted fetus difficult. Because growth of the fetal abdomen is linear from 15 weeks of gestation onward, determination of the rate of growth offers a gestational age-independent parameter to identify the IUGR fetus. Divon and co-workers[31] found a significant difference in the rate of growth of the fetal abdominal circumference between IUGR fetuses and fetuses that were appropriate for gestational age (6.0 ± 4.9 mm/14 days and 14.7 ± 7.1 mm/14 days, respectively). An increase in fetal abdominal circumference of < 10 mm/14 days had a sensitivity of 85% in identifying the IUGR fetus. Thus, the use of serial measurements of abdominal circumference offers an attractive method of identifying the IUGR fetus, especially when gestational age is uncertain.

The comparison of growth in some body organs relative to others has led to the development of a number of morphometric ratios. These ratios are useful in the diagnosis of asymmetrical IUGR where the abdominal circumference is smaller than expected when compared to the size of the head or the length of the body. Consequently, abnormally elevated FL/AC or HC/AC ratios aid in the identification of the asymmetrically growth-restricted fetus. The average value of HC/AC decreases in a linear fashion from 16 to 40 weeks of gestation. A HC/AC > 2 standard deviations above the mean has been suggested as an abnormal value[32]. Kurjak and co-workers[28] correctly identified 80% of growth-restricted fetuses with the use of this ratio. In contrast, Divon and co-workers[33] applied this ratio to a population of IUGR fetuses of mixed etiologies and reported a relatively low sensitivity of 36%, with specificity of 90%, positive predictive value of 67% and negative predictive value of 72%. These authors concluded that the HC/AC tends to be a better predictor of IUGR in situations related to third trimester 'placental insufficiency' resulting in asymmetric fetal growth.

Hadlock and co-workers[34] reported on the use of the FL/AC ratio as a gestational age-independent index of fetal growth. From 21 weeks' gestation to term, the normally grown fetus has an FL/AC of 22% ± 2% (± SD). An FL/AC > 23.5% was associated with a sensitivity of 60% and a specificity of 90% for identification of the growth-restricted fetus. Similarly, Divon and co-workers[31] reported a sensitivity of 55% for the same cut-off value and concluded that this parameter is fairly useful in differentiating between the fetus demonstrating appropriate growth and the growth-restricted fetus when gestational age is uncertain.

The most commonly used definition of IUGR is a birthweight < 10th percentile for gestational age. Therefore, it seems reasonable to use sonographic estimation of fetal weight to diagnose IUGR in the antenatal period. This parameter would also allow the clinician to evaluate changes in interval growth as compared to normative standards available throughout the latter part of pregnancy. Various equations which incorporate different variables (i.e. BPD, HC, AC and FL) have been proposed in an attempt to accurately estimate the fetal weight[35]. In general, these estimates are associated with a mean percentage absolute error of approximately 7–10%[36]. Several investigators have evaluated the ability of fetal weight estimates to identify the fetus with growth restriction. Divon and co-workers[33] estimated fetal weight using Hadlock's formula based on BPD, abdominal circumference, and femur length in a population of 127 high-risk patients, 45 of whom delivered IUGR neonates. They reported a sensitivity and specificity of 87%, positive predictive value of 78%, and negative predictive value of 92% for estimated fetal weight < 10th percentile for gestational age. Compared with other indices used to detect IUGR, such as HC : AC ratio, FL : AC ratio, amniotic fluid volume, and Doppler velocimetry, the best predictor appeared to be an estimated fetal weight of

< 10th percentile. Ott and Doyle[37] evaluated 595 pregnancies in which ultrasound examinations were performed within 72 h of delivery. Fetal weight was estimated using measurements of the BPD and abdominal circumference. They reported a sensitivity of 90% and a specificity of 80%. All infants with severe growth restriction (birthweight < 3rd percentile) were correctly identified, for a sensitivity of 100%.

Not surprisingly, equations that incorporate head and body proportions as well as body length seem to provide more accurate sonographic estimates of fetal weight. This has been shown to be especially true for the IUGR fetus. Guidetti and co-workers[38] showed that estimates of fetal weight that include abdominal circumference and femur length correlated best with birthweight. Overall, 75% of the estimates using the BPD–AC–FL equation were within 10% of the actual birthweight. Clearly, as long as the definition of IUGR is based on birthweight and gestational age criteria, the ability to diagnose fetal growth restriction is significantly dependent on the accuracy of the estimated fetal weight.

Oligohydramnios has long been recognized as a complication of fetal growth restriction. This is probably caused by decreased urination secondary to decreased renal perfusion reflecting redistribution of blood flow from non-vital to vital organs.

Manning and co-workers[39] used realtime sonography to qualitatively assess amniotic fluid volume in 120 pregnancies in which fetal growth restriction was suspected. Defining oligohydramnios as the largest vertical pocket of fluid measuring < 1 cm, they reported a sensitivity of 84%, specificity of 97%, positive predictive value of 90%, and negative predictive value of 95%. Other investigators, however, have not confirmed these results. Divon and co-workers[33] evaluated 127 patients referred with a clinical suspicion of IUGR. Oligohydramnios was defined by the vertical dimension of the largest pocket of fluid measuring < 2 cm. They reported a sensitivity of only 16% and a specificity of 98%. The low sensitivity and high specificity of amniotic fluid volume as an indicator of IUGR have also been shown by others[40–42].

An amniotic fluid index of 6 5 cm has been suggested as a sonographic marker of oligohydramnios[43]. However, the reported experience with this cut-off value and its relationship with either diagnosis or outcome in pregnancy complicated by IUGR is limited. The presence of oligohydramnios assumes increased importance when gestational age is questionable. If oligohydramnios is present in the absence of ruptured membranes, congenital anomalies or postdatism, IUGR is the most likely explanation. Thus, the presence of oligohydramnios can be considered a gestational age-independent predictor of IUGR. Its presence is considered an ominous sign with respect to fetal distress and is generally accepted as an indication for delivery[39,41–43].

A variety of new concepts for diagnosing IUGR have been reported in recent years. These include placental grading, thigh–calf circumference, transverse cerebellar diameter, thoracic to abdominal circumference ratio and magnetic resonance imaging. Although some of these concepts appear promising, they must be confirmed by additional studies.

In conclusion, despite the recent advances in ultrasound and Doppler technologies, reliable growth assessment of the fetus continues to present a clinical challenge. As the neonatal diagnosis of IUGR is commonly based on birthweight for gestational age criteria, it could be assumed that fetal growth could be accurately assessed whenever gestational age is known and estimated fetal weight is calculated with a reasonable accuracy. In addition, the finding of abnormally elevated morphometric ratios indicates asymmetric fetal growth. Indicators of fetal growth that are independent of gestational age (such as FL : AC, oligohydramnios and serial sonographic measurements of fetal abdominal circumference) should be applied whenever gestational age is unknown.

ANTEPARTUM FETAL TESTING

Intensive fetal surveillance should be instituted once growth restriction is detected or suspected. The nonstress test (NST) is most commonly used for this purpose. A reactive NST indicates that the fetal central nervous system is well oxygenated and has the ability to integrate autonomic nervous system reflexes that are initiated with body movements and result in an acceleration of the fetal heart rate. A growth-restricted fetus may be moving less frequently in order to conserve energy as well as being asphyxiated as a result of decreased supply of nutrients or failure of placental respiratory function. Under these circumstances the NST is likely to be non-reactive. A review[44] of NSTs has suggested that fetuses with normal growth have a lower incidence of non-reactive tests when compared to growth-restricted fetuses.

A reactive NST is highly indicative of a well-oxygenated fetus. The false-negative rate of a reactive NST performed twice weekly is approximately 2–3 in 1000. The converse, however, is not true. The association between a non-reactive NST and fetal hypoxia is rather low. The false-positive rate of a 40-minute non-reactive NST is approximately 80% and, therefore, in addition to fetal hypoxia other causes of non-reactivity should be considered (i.e. fetal sleep–wake cycles, prematurity, congenital anomalies, maternal use of medications and drugs). A non-reactive fetal heart rate (FHR) pattern with or without spontaneous decelerations may be the first sign of fetal structural anomalies associated with IUGR[45]. Therefore, a detailed sonographic evaluation, combined with analysis of fetal karyotype if significant fetal anomalies are found,

should be considered under these conditions. In addition, the growth-restricted fetus is at an increased risk of spontaneous variable FHR decelerations due to cord decompression resultant from oligohydramnios and/or decreased Wharton's jelly. Therefore, an ultrasound assessment of the amount of amniotic fluid should be performed whenever variable decelerations are detected during non-stress testing.

Several authors have suggested that the presence of severe oligohydramnios in a growth-restricted fetus should be used as an indication for delivery. Recent Doppler studies have shown that oligohydramnios in IUGR fetuses is associated with increased resistance to blood flow in the fetal renal artery[46,47]. Decreased renal perfusion in these fetuses is probably part of a compensatory mechanism resulting in redistribution of blood flow from non-vital to vital organs. As long as the central nervous system is adequately perfused, other tests of fetal well being (such as the NST, contraction stress test (CST) or fetal breathing movements) will be normal. Under theses conditions, most clinicians would intervene before the fetus decompensates (decompensation would be indicated by the presence of oligohydramnios combined with an abnormal NST, CST or biophysical profile score).

Chamberlain and co-workers[41] applied a 2-cm vertical 'depth' rule to define oligohydramnios and concluded that its presence is an ominous sign with respect to fetal health. The corrected perinatal mortalities for fetuses with marginal and decreased amniotic fluid volume were 37.7 in 1000 and 109.4 in 1000, respectively. These authors concluded that the presence of oligohydramnios should prompt a discussion regarding the need for a timely delivery.

Additional causes of oligohydramnios should be considered prior to intervention. It is relatively easy to exclude premature rupture of the membranes or an obstructive uropathy. Differentiating renal agenesis from a structurally normal but growth-restricted fetus may be more difficult. Fetuses with renal agenesis are often growth-restricted. In addition, visualization of the fetal kidneys may be impossible in the presence of oligohydramnios. Instillation of normal saline into the amniotic cavity may improve the quality of the sonographic image.

When FHR late decelerations occur persistently with spontaneous uterine contractions, fetal hypoxia should be suspected. If the pattern is inconsistent (i.e. an occasional FHR deceleration) a CST may be considered. Approximately 50% of positive CSTs are associated with fetal hypoxia. This positive predictive value increases dramatically when, in addition to the presence of late decelerations, the baseline FHR is non-reactive. Similarly, the prognosis of a positive CST with a reactive baseline FHR is much better than that of a positive CST with a non-reactive FHR baseline. Growth-restricted fetuses account for approximately one-third of positive tests in all patients undergoing CSTs and the incidence of a positive CST is higher in growth-restricted fetuses than in fetuses with normal growth (30–40% vs. 7–12%, respectively)[44].

The high false-positive rate of abnormal NST requires additional testing prior to intervention on a presumed diagnosis of fetal distress. In the face of a non-reactive NST, fetal wellbeing is commonly established by biophysical profile scoring. As stated earlier, the presence of oligohydramnios should raise the issue of delivery. Otherwise, a biophysical profile score of 8–10/10 is associated with a low risk for either fetal asphyxia or imminent fetal death. In general, as the biophysical profile score decreases, the likelihood of fetal asphyxia increases. As with non-stress testing and contraction stress testing, biophysical profile scores are, in general, lower in IUGR fetuses when compared to other 'high-risk' fetuses. Devoe and co-workers[48] noted that their IUGR patients accounted for 33% of all abnormal biophysical profile scores, although they constituted only 20% of the tested population.

Gradual deterioration of fetal health is reflected by decreased or absent fetal activity. Therefore, biophysical profile testing represents a rational approach for fetal surveillance. Baskett and co-workers[49] reported that growth-restricted fetuses were more likely to have perinatal complication with oligohydramnios (30%), decreased fetal body movements (23%) and decreased fetal tone (21%).

Pollack and co-workers[50] have recently reported on 4727 patients undergoing non-stress testing followed by biophysical profile testing when indicated. IUGR was the primary indication for fetal testing in 478 (10%) patients. No fetal deaths were reported in the tested IUGR population. In a large study of 19 221 patients, Manning and co-workers[51] noted that 4 of 14 fetal deaths, following normal tests, occurred in IUGR pregnancies. These results underscore the fact that intensive fetal testing is associated with an extremely low false-negative rate.

DOPPLER VELOCIMETRY

Normal fetal growth is determined by multiple maternal–fetal variables. Continuous blood flow on either side of the placenta and adequate fetal perfusion are obviously an absolute necessity. Indeed, fetal growth restriction is associated with various abnormalities of the uteroplacental, umbilical and fetal circulations[52,53]. Doppler devices allow for a non-invasive evaluation of blood flow by displaying Doppler-shifted frequencies which are proportional to the velocity of red blood cells. Qualitative assessment of these waveforms is provided by angle-independent indices which are based on various ratios between the systolic and diastolic components of the waveform. Most studies concur that the simplest index (i.e. the systolic:diastolic ratio,

S:D) is clinically as useful as any of the more complicated indices (such as the resistance index or the pulsatility index).

Maternal and fetal blood-flow velocity waveforms are influenced by the stroke volume, pressure gradient, heart rate, vessel wall elasticity and blood viscosity. Fast heart rates result in a relatively high end-diastolic component, while increased downstream impedance causes low end-diastolic flows. Since blood flow during diastole is mostly passive, as placental impedance increases, the umbilical arterial end-diastolic flow decreases. Therefore, severe placental impedance is associated with low, absent or reversed end-diastolic umbilical blood flow.

On the maternal side, some evidence[54] suggests that changes in uterine artery velocity waveforms (arcuate arteries) may be detected as early as the second trimester in some pregnancies which eventually develop pre-eclampsia or IUGR. Other investigators[55–57] have also reported that in some cases of IUGR, abnormal uterine perfusion may be the first sign of a developing disease process. In contrast, Newnham and co-workers[58], who evaluated uteroplacental blood flow at 14, 18, 24, 28 and 34 weeks of gestation, reported that abnormal waveforms were significantly correlated with the future development of fetal hypoxia; however, they were not predictive of subsequent development of IUGR. Both Chambers and co-workers[27] and Jacobson and co-workers[59] concluded that Doppler studies of the uteroplacental perfusion are of a limited clinical value due to their poor sensitivity and high false-positive rate.

On the fetal side, many studies have reported a significant decrease in end-diastolic flow of the umbilical artery and the descending aorta of the growth-retarded fetus[53]. These studies indicate that some forms of IUGR may result from 'placental insufficiency' defined by increased placental impedance reflecting a decrease in the number of intraplacental arterial channels[60–62]. A decreased pulsatility index in the internal carotid arteries[63] reported in some of these fetuses reflects enhanced perfusion of the brain and is probably indicative of redistribution of blood flow resulting in the 'brain sparing effect'.

Trudinger and co-workers[64] have recently reported on 2178 high-risk pregnancies on whom umbilical artery velocity waveforms were evaluated. The incidence of IUGR (birthweight < 10th percentile) in this population was 27%; 50% of their IUGR fetuses had an abnormal (> 95th percentile) umbilical arterial S:D ratio. The odds ratio of a fetus with an abnormal arterial velocity waveform for being diagnosed as growth-restricted by birthweight criteria was 5.9 (95% confidence interval of 4.7–7.3). Moreover, preterm infants with abnormal S:D ratios spent twice as long in the neonatal intensive care unit than those with normal velocity waveforms. Based on their large

Table 9   Umbilical artery velocimetry for prediction for IUGR in high-risk pregnancies

First author	Study patients, n (prevalence of IUGR)	Definition of IUGR	Definition of abnormal waveform	Odds ratio (95% confidence interval)
Divon (1988)[33]	127 (35%)	BW 6 10th percentile	S : D > 3.0	14.7 (4.6–50.5)
Berkowitz (1988)[84]	168 (25%)	BW 6 10th percentile	S : D > 3.0	6.6 (2.7–16.4)
Schulman (1989)[85]	255 (9%)	BW < 15th percentile	S : D > 3.0	19.9 (6.9–59.0)
Dempster (1989)[86]	205 (40%)	BW < 10th percentile	S : D > 95th percentile	3.3 (1.6–6.5)
Sijmons (1989)[87]	400 (22%)	BW < 10th percentile	PI > 95th percentile	4.4 (2.0–9.4)
Lowery (1990)[88]	146 (14%)	BW < 10th percentile	S : D > 4.0	10.9 (3.8–32.5)
Gudmundsson (1991)[89]	139 (51%)	BW < 15th percentile	PI > 2 SD above mean	7.1 (3.0–17.2)
Kay (1991)[68]	48 (37.5%)	BW < 10th percentile	S : D > 2 SD above mean	11.3 (2.1–52.0)
Trudinger (1991)[64]	2178 (27%)	BW < 10th percentile	S : D > 95th percentile	5.9 (4.7–7.3)

BW, birthweight; S : D, systolic : diastolic ratio; PI, pulsatility index

study population, these authors concluded that 'in high risk pregnancy Doppler umbilical artery flow velocity waveforms predict the most compromised fetuses in terms of growth retardation and requirement for neonatal intensive care'.

The ability to detect IUGR with Doppler velocimetry varies considerably (Table 9). Overall, the odds ratios presented demonstrate a significantly increased likelihood of delivering an IUGR newborn once the Doppler study is abnormal. These studies are hampered by the absence of standard definitions for both IUGR and abnormal velocity waveforms. In addition, most studies have preferentially evaluated high-risk populations with an abnormally high incidence of IUGR.

A few studies have evaluated the usefulness of screening the general population for IUGR with the use of umbilical artery velocimetry. Beattie and Dornan[65] evaluated a total of 2097 singleton pregnancies at 28, 34 and 38 weeks of gestation. Less than 20% of this population was defined as 'high-risk' pregnancies. The sensitivity of an abnormal S : D ratio for prediction of IUGR was rather low (from 31% to 40% depending on the gestational age at the time of the study). Bruinse and co-workers[66] studied an unselected population of 405 pregnant women at 28 and 34 weeks of gestation. Doppler screening for IUGR had a low sensitivity of 17% and 22%, respectively. Hanretty and co-workers[67] screened uteroplacental and umbilical arteries in 543 unselected patients at 20–30 and 34–36 weeks' gestation. They found no difference in outcome

of pregnancies with normal or abnormal uteroplacental waveforms. However, birthweights were significantly lower in patients with an abnormal umbilical artery waveform at either gestational age. Based on these studies, it is possible to conclude that Doppler screening of the general population is associated with a low yield. The cost : benefit ratio of such screening programs is yet to be studied.

The combined use of Doppler velocimetry with real-time ultrasound for the diagnosis of IUGR was reported by Divon and co-workers[33]. The study population consisted of 127 patients referred with a clinical suspicion of IUGR. Forty-five infants (35%) were identified as IUGR by birthweight 6 10th percentile for gestational age. These authors concluded that neither sonographic nor Doppler tests were uniformly successful in identifying the growth-restricted infant. Overall, the best prediction was offered by sonographic estimates of fetal weight which correctly identified 39 of the 45 IUGR infants. An S : D ratio > 3 was seen in 49% of the IUGR fetuses. All indices performed similarly in predicting the non-IUGR infant (range of specificities: 87–98%). Similar results were reported by Kay and co-workers[68] on 48 patients who underwent sonographic measurements and Doppler evaluations of the uterine and umbilical vasculatures. A comparison of fetal abdominal circumference measurements and Doppler velocimetry for the prediction of IUGR was carried out by Chambers and co-workers[27]. These authors studied 145 pregnancies suspected of being small for dates and found that sonographic measurements of the fetal abdominal circumference were superior to umbilical artery velocimetry for prediction of IUGR with sensitivities of 73% and 47%, respectively. It should, however, be emphasized that Doppler can be used as a gestational age independent index of IUGR (i.e. S : D > 3.0 is abnormal after 30 weeks' gestation) while evaluation of the abdominal circumference requires accurate gestational dating.

The utility of Doppler velocimetry in the prediction of adverse outcome in pregnancies at risk for IUGR was investigated by Berkowitz and co-workers[69]. These authors reported that approximately 50% of their IUGR infants had abnormal umbilical artery velocity waveforms and that these waveforms were valuable in identifying the growth-restricted infant who was at increased risk for one or more of the following outcome criteria: early delivery, reduced birthweight, oligohydramnios, neonate intensive-care unit admission and prolonged hospital stay. Similar results, indicating that Doppler velocimetry allows accurate and early recognition of those growth-restricted fetuses who will become distressed antenatally were reported by Reuwer and co-workers[70]. Several investigators have noted that all their IUGR-related neonatal deaths and a majority of their intensive-care admissions were confined to those fetuses with abnormal Doppler velocimetry results[71,72]. Reviewing these studies, it becomes obvious that a normal umbilical artery velocity waveform does not always guarantee ideal fetal outcome. Drogtrop and co-workers[73] reviewed cases of documented fetal distress with a normal umbilical artery Doppler study and have reached the same conclusion.

Extreme forms of increased placental impedance are sometimes coupled with absent or reversed diastolic velocities. This situation is clearly abnormal and is often associated with maternal hypertension and severe fetal growth restriction[74]. Several studies have described the ominous outcome found in fetuses with extremely abnormal umbilical artery velocity waveforms[75–77]. Due to high mortality rates of 50–90%, some authors have suggested that an 'aggressive' management protocol is justified[78–81]. Wenstrom and co-workers[82] studied 450 high-risk pregnancies who underwent level II sonograms after 20 weeks' gestation. Twenty-two of these patients had absent or reversed diastolic flow in the umbilical artery. Ten had IUGR, 10 had either congenital malformations or were aneuploid, and in two cases, the etiology was not identified. Among the four cases with fetal aneuploidy, one had multiple severe anomalies including holoprosencephaly, renal agenesis and polydactyly, and the other three had IUGR. Therefore, a thorough evaluation of fetal anatomy and search for the underlying etiology which causes absent or reversed diastolic blood flow should be attempted when managing a patient with IUGR. Whether a karyotype should also be obtained in patients with absent diastolic or reversed

diastolic flow without major congenital anomalies or severe symmetrical IUGR, needs further evaluation. Guidelines for the clinical management of the fetus with markedly diminished umbilical artery end-diastolic flow have been suggested by Divon and co-workers[83]. Fifty-one fetuses with an S : D > 2 SD above the mean for gestational age were managed conservatively with intensive daily fetal monitoring. Their results suggest that immediate delivery of the fetus with diminished end-diastolic flow may not be mandatory. These authors concluded that the combined use of fetal biophysical testing with commonly used maternal and fetal indications for delivery results in acceptable fetal outcome and prolongation of gestational age.

It would be impossible to conclude from these studies that umbilical artery velocimetry is a rational test to perform when IUGR is suspected. It is useful in both establishing the diagnosis and determining the intensity of subsequent fetal surveillance. However, its utility in screening the general population for IUGR or otherwise adverse outcome seems limited.

MANAGEMENT

Once the diagnosis of IUGR is suspected, several management issues should be considered. These include parental counseling regarding a search for the etiology of growth restriction, fetal surveillance, timing of delivery, and neonatal outcome. In addition, the need for bedrest and adequate maternal nutrition should be discussed with the patient. The use of alcohol, tobacco or any other unnecessary toxins should be discouraged.

The increased incidence of perinatal morbidity and mortality among IUGR pregnancies often necessitates early delivery (as soon as lung maturity can be demonstrated). Preterm delivery should be considered in the growth-restricted fetus when fetal surveillance indicates a high probability of fetal asphyxia. Management of the IUGR pregnancy with a known fetal anomaly or an abnormal karyotype should be tailored to the specific abnormality.

Various opinions have been voiced with respect to early delivery of the fetus with poor or absent growth. While some have questioned the accuracy of the diagnosis, others have argued that a slow rate of growth is a compensatory mechanism enhancing fetal survival. In addition, it has been pointed out that this condition indicates that the intrauterine environment is inadequate and that the fetus may benefit from an early delivery. Current evidence is insufficient to resolve this debate. The risks of iatrogenic prematurity should always be weighed against the potential benefits of early delivery. Amniocentesis for documentation of lung maturity should be considered when poor fetal growth is clearly demonstrated. The benefits of conservative management in the presence of documented lung

Table 10   Indications for delivery in IUGR

Fetal compromise
Deteriorating maternal condition
Term pregnancy with a favorable cervix
Term pregnancy with markedly abnormal umbilical
    artery velocity waveform
Absence of fetal growth with documented lung maturity
Oligohydramnios

maturity are probably limited. Additional indications for delivery are shown in Table 10.

CONCLUSION

Intrauterine growth is an important sign of fetal well-being. The clinical significance of fetal growth restriction stems from it being a significant predictor of perinatal morbidity and mortality. Intrauterine growth restriction is an entity whose definition is controversial and whose etiology and natural history are poorly understood. Its antenatal diagnosis is less then optimal and many management issues remain unresolved. Nonetheless, it is a condition of paramount importance to the obstetrician who can optimize perinatal outcome by timely and accurate diagnosis coupled with appropriate intervention. Further research is needed to improve our understanding, diagnosis and management of fetal growth restriction.

REFERENCES

1. Starfield B, Shapiro S, McCormick M, *et al.* Mortality and morbidity in infants with intrauterine growth retardation. *Pediatrics* 1982;101:978
2. Heinonen K, Hakulinen A, Jokela V. Survival of the smallest; time trends and determinants of mortality in a very preterm population during the 1980s. *Lancet* 1988;2:204
3. Kazzi NJ, Poland RL. Neonatal risks associated with intrauterine growth retardation. In *Intrauterine Growth Retardation – A Practical Approach.* Gross TL, Sokol RJ, eds. Chicago: Year Book Medical Publishers, 1989
4. Goldberg RL, Cutter GR, Hoffman HJ, *et al.* Intrauterine growth retardation: standards for diagnosis. *Am J Obstet Gynecol* 1989;161:271
5. Lubchenco LO, Hansman C, Dressler, *et al.* Intrauterine growth as estimated from liveborn birthweight data at 24 to 42 weeks of gestation. *Pediatrics* 1963;32:793
6. Brenner WE, Edelman DA, Hendricks CH. A standard of fetal growth for the United States of America. *Am J Obstet Gynecol* 1976;126:555
7. Gruenwald P. Chronic fetal distress and placental insufficiency. *Biol Neonate* 1963;5:215
8. Rohrer F. Der Index der Körperfulle als Mars des Ernährungszustandes. *Münch Med Wochenschr* 1921; 68:580
9. Miller HC. Intrauterine growth retardation: an unmet challenge. *Am J Dis Child* 1981;135:944
10. Nicolaides KH, Snijders RJM, Noble P. Cordocentesis in the study of growth retarded fetuses. In *Abnormal Fetal Growth*, Divon MY, ed. New York: Elsevier Science, 1991
11. Miller HC. Prenatal factors affecting intrauterine growth retardation. *Clin Perinatol* 1985;12:307
12. Basel D, Lederer R, Diamant YZ. Longitudinal ultrasonic biometry of various parameters in fetuses with abnormal growth rate. *Acta Obstet Gynecol Scand* 1987; 66:143
13. Abrams B, Newman V. Small for gestational age birth: maternal predictors and comparison with risk factors of spontaneous preterm delivery in the same cohort. *Am J Obstet Gynecol* 1991;164:785
14. Kramer MS. Intrauterine growth and gestational duration determinants. *Pediatrics* 1987;80:502
15. Kramer MS. Determinants of low birth weight, methodological assessment and meta-analysis. *Bull WHO* 1987;65:663
16. Weiner CP, Williamson RA. Evaluation of severe growth retardation using cordocentesis – hematologic and metabolic alterations by etiology. *Obstet Gynecol* 1989; 73:225
17. Chen AT, Falek A, Lester W. Chromosome aberrations in full-term low birthweight neonates. *Hum Genet* 1974; 21:13
18. Wladimiroff JW, Sachs ES, Reuss A, *et al.* Prenatal diagnosis of chromosome abnormalities in the presence of fetal structural defects. *Am J Med Genet* 1988;29:289
19. Rosenberg K, Grant JM, Aitchison T. Measurement of fundal height as screening test for fetal growth retardation. *Br J Obstet Gynaecol* 1981;88:115
20. Welch RA, Wolfe HM, Sokol RJ. The role of clinical determinants in predicting intrauterine growth retardation. In *Intrauterine Growth Retardation*. Gross TL, Sokol RJ, eds. Chicago: Year Book Medical Publishers, 1989
21. Beazly JM, Kurjak A. Prediction of foetal maturity and birthweight by abdominal palpation. *Nursing Times* 1973;June 14:763
22. Loeffler FE. Clinical foetal weight prediction. *J Obstet Gynaecol Br Commonw* 1967;74:675
23. Guidetti DA, Divon MY. Sonographic detection of the IUGR fetus. In *Abnormal Fetal Growth*, Divon MY, ed. New York: Elsevier Science, 1991
24. Ott WJ. Fetal femur length, neonatal crown–heel length and screening for intrauterine growth retardation. *Obstet Gynecol* 1985;65:460
25. O'Brien GP, Queenan JT. Ultrasound fetal femur length in relation to intrauterine growth retardation. *Am J Obstet Gynecol* 1982;144:35
26. Warsof SL, Cooper DJ, Little D, Campbell S. Routine ultrasound screening for antenatal detection of intrauterine growth retardation. *Obstet Gynecol* 1986; 67:33
27. Chambers SE, Haskins PR, Haddad NG, *et al.* A comparison of fetal abdominal circumference measurements and Doppler ultrasound in the prediction of small for dates babies and fetal compromise. *Br J Obstet Gynaecol* 1989;96:803
28. Kurjak A, Kirkinen P, Latin V. Biometric and dynamic ultrasound assessment of small for dates infants: report of 260 cases. *Obstet Gynecol* 1980;56:281

29. Hadlock FP, Deter RL, Harrist RB, *et al.* A date independent predictor of intrauterine growth retardation: femur length/abdominal circumference ratio. *Am J Roentgenol* 1983;141:979

30. Fernazzi E, Nicolini V, Kustermann A, Pardi G. Routine obstetric ultrasound: effectiveness of cross-sectional screening for fetal growth retardation. *J Clin Ultrasound* 1986;14:17

31. Divon MY, Chamberlain PF, Sipos L, *et al.* Identification of the small for gestational age fetus with the use of gestational age independent indices of fetal growth. *Am J Obstet Gynecol* 1986;155:1197

32. Campbell S, Thoms A. Ultrasound measurement of the fetal head to abdominal circumference ratio in the assessment of growth retardation. *Br J Obstet Gynaecol* 1977;84:165

33. Divon MY, Guidetti DA, Braverman JJ, *et al.* Intrauterine growth retardation – a prospective study of the diagnostic value of real time sonography combined with umbilical artery flow velocimetry. *Obstet Gynecol* 1988; 72:611

34. Hadlock FP, Deter FL, Harris RB, *et al.* A date-independent predictor of intrauterine growth retardation: femur length : abdominal circumference ratio. *Am J Roentgenol* 1983;141:979

35. Woolf J, Divon MY. Microcomputer program for fetal growth assessment. In *Abnormal Fetal Growth*, Divon MY, ed. New York: Elsevier Science, 1991

36. Pollack RN, Divon MY. Problems in detecting fetal macrosomia. *Contemporary Obstet Gynecol* 1991:9–13

37. Ott WJ, Doyle S. Ultrasonic diagnosis of altered fetal growth by use of a normal ultrasonic fetal weight curve. *Obstet Gynecol* 1984;63:201

38. Guidetti DA, Divon MY, Braverman JJ, *et al.* Sonographic estimates of fetal weight in the IUGR population. *Am J Perinatol* 1990;7:5

39. Manning FA, Hill LM, Platt LD. Qualitative amniotic fluid volume determination by ultrasound: antepartum detection of intrauterine growth retardation. *Am J Obstet Gynecol* 1981;129:255

40. Patterson RM, Prihoda TJ, Pouliot MR. Sonographic amniotic fluid measurement and fetal growth retardation: an appraisal. *Am J Obstet Gynecol* 1987; 157:1406

41. Chamberlain PF, Manning FA, Morrison I, *et al.* Ultrasound evaluation of amniotic fluid volume. I. The relationship of marginal and decreased amniotic fluid volumes to perinatal outcomes. *Am J Obstet Gynecol* 1984;150:245

42. Philipson EN, Sokol RJ, Williams T. Oligohydramnios: clinical association and predictive values for intrauterine growth retardation. *Am J Obstet Gynecol* 1983;146:271

43. Rutherford SE, Phelan JP, Smith CV, *et al.* The four quadrant assessment of amniotic fluid volume: an adjunct to antepartum fetal heart rate testing. *Obstet Gynecol* 1987;70:353

44. Devoe LD: Antenatal evaluation of the growth retarded fetus. In *Abnormal Fetal Growth*, Divon MY, ed. New York: Elsevier Science, 1991

45. Nayot P, Moryosef S, Granat M, *et al.* Antepartum fetal heart rate patterns associated with major congenital anomalies. *Obstet Gynecol* 1984;63:414

46. Veille JC, Kanaan C. Duplex Doppler ultrasongraphic evaluation of the fetal renal artery in normal and abnormal fetuses. *Am J Obstet Gynecol* 1989;161:1502–7

47. Arduini D, Rizzo G. Fetal renal artery velocity waveforms and amniotic fluid volume in growth retarded and post-term fetuses. *Obstet Gynecol* 1991;77:370

48. Devoe LD, Castillo RA, Searle N, Searle J. Prognostic components of computerized fetal biophysical testing. *Am J Obstet Gynecol* 1988;158:1144

49. Baskett TF, Grady JH, Prevett SS, *et al.* Antepartum fetal assessment using a fetal biophysical profile score. *Am J Obstet Gynecol* 1984;148:630

50. Pollack RN, Divon MY, Henderson CE, *et al.* Is 'acute placental abruption' a chronic process? *J Matern Fetal Invest* 1994;4:5

51. Manning FA, Morrisson I, Harman CR, *et al.* Fetal assessment based on fetal biophysical profile scoring: experience in 19 221 referred high risk pregnancies. II. An analysis of false negative fetal deaths. *Am J Obstet Gynecol* 1987;157:880

52. Fleischer A, Guidetti D, Sublemuller P. Umbilical artery velocity waveforms in the intrauterine growth retarded fetus. *Clin Obstet Gynecol* 1989;32:660

53. Divon MY, Hsu HW. Maternal and fetal velocity waveforms in IUGR. *Clin Obstet Gynecol* 1992;35:156

54. Campbell S, Pearce JM, Hackett G, *et al.* Qualitative assessment of uteroplacental blood flow: early screening test for high-risk pregnancies. *Obstet Gynecol* 1986; 68:649

55. Cohen-Overbeek, Pearce JM, Campbell S. The antenatal assessment of uteroplacental and fetoplacental blood flow using Doppler ultrasound. *Ultrasound Med Biol* 1985;11:329

56. Trudinger BJ, Giles WB, Cook C. Uteroplacental blood flow velocity time waveforms in normal and complicated pregnancy. *Br J Obstet Gynaecol* 1985;92:39

57. Trudinger BJ, Giles WB, Cook C. Flow velocity waveforms in the maternal uteroplacental and fetal umbilical placental circulations. *Am J Obstet Gynecol* 1985; 152:155

58. Newnham JP, Patterson LL, James IR, *et al.* An evaluation of the efficacy of Doppler flow velocity waveform analysis as a screening test in pregnancy. *Am J Obstet Gynecol* 1990;162:403

59. Jacobson SL, Imhof R, Manning N, *et al.* The value of Doppler assessment of the uteroplacental circulation in predicting preeclampsia or intrauterine growth retardation. *Am J Obstet Gynecol* 1990;162:110

60. Giles WB, Trudinger BJ, Baird P. Fetal umbilical artery flow velocity waveforms and placental resistance: pathological correlation. *Br J Obstet Gynaecol* 1985;92:31

61. McCowan LM, Mullen BM, Ritchie K. Umbilical artery flow velocity waveforms and the placental vascular bed. *Am J Obstet Gynecol* 1987;157:900

62. Fox RY, Pavlova Z, Benirschke K, *et al.* The correlation of arterial lesions with umbilical artery Doppler velocimetry in the placentas of small-for-dates pregnancies. *Obstet Gynecol* 1990;75:578

63. Wladimiroff JW, Wijngaard JAGW, Degani S, *et al.* Cerebral and umbilical arterial blood flow velocity waveforms in normal and growth retarded pregnancies. *Obstet Gynecol* 1987;69:705

64. Trudinger BJ, Cook CM, Giles WB, *et al.* Fetal umbilical artery velocity waveforms and subsequent neonatal outcome. *Br J Obstet Gynaecol* 1991;98:378

65. Beattie RB, Dornan JC. Antenatal screening for intrauterine growth retardation with umbilical artery Doppler ultrasonography. *Br Med J* 1989;298:631

66. Bruinse HW, Sijmons EA, Reuwer PJHM. Clinical value of screening for fetal growth retardation by Doppler ultrasound. *J Ultrasound Med* 1989;8:207

67. Hanretty KP, Primrose MH, Neilson JP, Whittle MJ. Pregnancy screening by Doppler uteroplacental and umbilical artery waveforms. *Br J Obstet Gynaecol* 1989;96:1163

68. Kay HH, Carrol BB, Dahmus M, Killam AP. Sonographic measurements with umbilical artery Doppler analysis in suspected intrauterine growth retardation. *J Reprod Med* 1991;36:65

69. Berkowitz GS, Mehalek KE, Chitkara U, *et al.* Doppler umbilical velocimetry in the prediction of adverse outcome in pregnancies at risk for intrauterine growth retardation. *Obstet Gynecol* 1988;71:742

70. Reuwer PJHM, Sijmons EA, Rietman GW, *et al.* Intrauterine growth retardation: prediction of perinatal distress by Doppler ultrasound. *Lancet* 1987;2:415

71. Rochelson BL, Schulman H, Fleischer A, *et al.* The clinical significance of Doppler umbilical artery velocimetry in the small-for-gestational age fetus. *Am J Obstet Gynecol* 1987;156:1223

72. McCowan LM, Erskine LA, Ritchie K. Umbilical artery Doppler blood flow studies in the preterm, small-for-gestational age fetus. *Am J Obstet Gynecol* 1987;156:655

73. Drogtrop AP, Bruinse HW, Reuwer PJH. Normal umbilical artery Doppler sonography does not exclude fetal distress. *Acta Obstet Gynecol Scand* 1990;69:351

74. Rochelson B. The clinical significance of absent end diastolic velocity in the umbilical artery waveforms. *Clin Obstet Gynecol* 1989;32:692

75. Arabin B, Siebert M, Jimenez E, Saling E. Obstetrical characteristics of a loss of end diastolic velocities in the fetal aorta and/or umbilical artery using Doppler ultrasound. *Gynecol Obstet Invest* 1988;25:173

76. Brar HS, Platt LD. Antepartum improvement of abnormal umbilical velocimetry: does it occur? *Am J Obstet Gynecol* 1989;160:36

77. Reed KL, Anderson CF, Shenker L. Changes in intracardiac Doppler blood flow velocities in fetuses with absent umbilical artery diastolic flow. *Am J Obstet Gynecol* 1987;157:774

78. Brar HS, Platt LD. Reverse end diastolic flow velocity on umbilical artery velocimetry in high risk pregnancies: an ominous finding with adverse pregnancy outcome. *Am J Obstet Gynecol* 1988;159:559

79. Hsieh FJ, Chang FM, Ko TM, *et al.* Umbilical artery flow velocimetry waveforms in fetuses dying with congenital anomalies. *Br J Obstet Gynaecol* 1988;95:478

80. Woo JSK, Liang ST, Lo RLS. Significance of an absent or reversed end diastolic flow in Doppler umbilical artery waveforms. *J Ultrasound Med* 1987;6:291

81. Schulman H. The clinical implications of Doppler ultrasound analysis of the uterine and umbilical arteries. *Am J Obstet Gynecol* 1987;156:889

82. Wenstrom K, Weiner CP, Williamson R. Diverse maternal and fetal pathology associated with absent end diastolic flow in the umbilical artery of the high-risk fetuses. *Obstet Gynecol* 1991;77:375

83. Divon MY, Girz BA, Lieblich L, Langer O. Clinical management of the fetus with markedly diminished umbilical artery end-diastolic flow. *Am J Obstet Gynecol* 1989;161:1523

84. Berkowitz G, Chitkara U, Rosenberg J, *et al.* Sonographic estimation of fetal weight and Doppler analysis of umbilical artery velocimetry in the prediction of intrauterine growth retardation: a prospective study. *Am J Obstet Gynecol* 1988;158:1149

85. Schulman H, Winter D, Farmakides G, *et al.* Pregnancy surveillance with Doppler velocimetry of uterine and umbilical arteries. *Am J Obstet Gynecol* 1989;160:192

86. Dempster J, Mires GJ, Patel N, Taylor DJ. Umbilical artery velocity waveforms: poor association with small-for-gestational age babies. *Br J Obstet Gynaecol* 1989;96:692

87. Sijmons EA, Reuwer PJHM, Beek EV, Bruinse HW. The validity of screening for small-for-gestational age and low-weight-for-length infants by Doppler ultrasound. *Br J Obstet Gynaecol* 1989;96:557

88. Lowery CL, Henson BV, Wan J, Brumfield CG. A comparison between umbilical artery velocimetry and standard antepartum surveillance in hospitalized high-risk patients. *Am J Obstet Gynecol* 1990;162:710

89. Gudmundsson S, Maruisal K. Blood velocity waveforms in the fetal aorta and umbilical artery as predictors of fetal outcome: a comparison. *Am J Perinatol* 1991;8:1–6

60

Fetal lung maturity

J.A. Bartelsmeyer

INTRODUCTION

Assessment of fetal pulmonary maturity is one of the most critical issues confronting obstetricians. Prematurity with fetal lung immaturity is far and away the leading cause of neonatal morbidity and mortality. Obstetricians are constantly challenged by clinical situations where the status of fetal pulmonary maturity has direct bearing on the decision making process. As recently as fifteen years ago, iatrogenic prematurity was a major etiology of neonatal respiratory distress syndrome (RDS)[1]. Iatrogenic prematurity with RDS has been associated, for the most part, with elective repeat Cesarean sections, a procedure that continues in modern obstetrics. For these reasons a large amount of research over the last thirty years has dealt specifically with developing tests that accurately predict which fetuses are at risk for RDS. The development of tests, coupled with widespread dissemination of knowledge and almost universal availability of testing, has considerably decreased the incidence of iatrogenic prematurity and RDS. These tests enable the clinician to make clinical decisions more confidently when an elective delivery is contemplated during a complicated pregnancy.

Unfortunately, too often a newborn is admitted to the neonatal intensive care unit with a diagnosis of RDS following an elective delivery in an uncomplicated pregnancy. In a different situation, a mother and a fetus may be placed in unnecessary jeopardy by continued intrauterine treatment of an obstetrical problem because methods available to document fetal lung maturity are not utilized. To avoid these types of dilemmas, the clinician needs to know in which circumstances a determination of fetal maturity is indicated, what studies are available and which particular test is best suited to the clinical situation. Unfortunately, the available technology cannot meet the demands of all possible situations and quite often physicians must rely upon their clinical experience.

The American College of Obstetricians and Gynecologists (ACOG) published a committee opinion in September 1991 that addressed the issue of assessing fetal pulmonary maturity[2] (Table 1). It is important to note that the ACOG committee opinion does not consider a known last menstrual period and an early examination reliable indicators of fetal maturity.

Table 1 Fetal maturity assessment prior to elective repeat Cesarean delivery (ACOG, 1991)

The assessment of fetal maturity is important in determining the timing of a repeat Cesarean delivery. For patients being considered for elective repeat Cesarean deliveries, if one of the following criteria is met, fetal maturity may be assumed and amniocentesis need not be performed:

1. Fetal heart tones have been documented for 20 weeks by nonelectronic fetoscope or for 30 weeks by Doppler.
2. It has been 36 weeks since a positive serum or urine human chorionic gonadotropin pregnancy test was performed by a reliable laboratory.
3. An ultrasound measurement of the crown-rump length, obtained at 6–11 weeks, supports a gestational age of > 39 weeks.
4. An ultrasound, obtained at 12–20 weeks, confirms the gestational age of > 39 weeks determined by clinical history and physical examination.

These criteria are not intended to preclude the use of menstrual dating. If any one of the above criteria confirms gestational age assessment on the basis of menstrual dates in a patient with normal menstrual cycles and no immediately antecedent use of oral contraceptives, it is appropriate to schedule delivery at > 39 weeks by the menstrual dates. Ultrasound may be considered confirmatory of menstrual dates if there is gestational age agreement within 1 week by crown–rump measurement obtained at 6–11 weeks or within 10 days by the average of multiple measurements obtained at 12–20 weeks.

Awaiting the onset of spontaneous labor is another option.

Reprinted with permission from reference 2

These guidelines are intended to be used when an elective delivery in a relatively normal pregnancy is contemplated. In instances where maternal disease or other obstetrical problems are present, these rules may not apply. Using a similar set of guidelines, Frigoletto and co-workers[3] reported an incidence of 0.13% iatrogenic prematurity with RDS over a three-year span covering more than 1500 repeat Cesarean sections.

The committee opinion of the ACOG suggests that a biochemical test of amniotic fluid be performed to determine pulmonary maturity when the criteria outlined are not met or when there is reason to suspect that delayed maturation could be present. The lecithin : sphingomyelin (L : S) ratio has been the standard test of fetal lung maturity against which all other tests are compared since 1971 when Gluck and associates[4] first published their data. Numerous other tests using biochemical assays, ultrasound findings and other markers of lung maturity have been introduced since that time. While some of these are clinically useful and others have promise for the future, many of them are only of historical interest. This chapter includes a review of the presently useful assays and those that may be useful in the future. Each method will be judged by its correlation to the L : S ratio, its accuracy in indicating fetuses at risk for RDS (Table 2), its ease of performance, the time it takes to obtain results and the cost of the test. A brief review of fetal pulmonary development will be presented in the first part of the chapter.

FETAL LUNG DEVELOPMENT

Anatomical development

Functional neonatal gas exchange is dependent upon normal structural lung development, including alveoli, and the production of sufficient amounts of surfactant, a complex mixture containing phospholipids that facilitate expansion and prevent collapse of the alveoli.

The initial sign of lung development occurs during the early embryonic period when the lung buds appear[5]. Sequential branching during the next 16–20 weeks results in development of the bronchial tree. By 20–24 weeks, the terminal bronchioles are present; distal to these are the alveoli, the respiratory units of the lung. For the remainder of the pregnancy, there is a progressive maturation of the alveoli preparing for extrauterine gas exchange. The alveolar epithelium, which initially is composed of a cuboidal epithelium, begins to flatten. Eventually a thin layer of

epithelium, the Type I alveolar cells, covers most of the surface of the alveoli with occasional interspersed Type II alveolar cells. Mature alveoli capable of functional gas exchange are not usually present until approximately 26 weeks' gestation. The lungs continue to develop and at term approximately 50% of the adult alveoli are present.

Progressive vascularization occurs during lung maturation and follows a branching pattern similar to the bronchioles. Eventually a capillary meshwork is adjacent to each alveolus at which time blood is separated from the lung space by two endothelial surfaces, the respiratory and vascular endothelium, and a thin layer of connective tissue.

Surfactant production

Surfactant is a phospholipid rich substance that decreases the surface tension of the air–water interface in the alveolus preventing atelectasis or collapse of the terminal respiratory unit during respiration. It is a complex mixture containing 70–80% phospholipids, 10% protein and 10% neutral lipids, primarily cholesterol[6]. The principal phospholipids found in human surfactant include phosphatidylcholine (lecithin), phosphatidylinositol, phosphatidylglycerol and sphingomyelin. This combination of phospholipids is unique when compared to lipid or membrane fractions from other organs. In fact, phosphatidylglycerol is entirely unique to surfactant. Most of the phosphatidylcholine found in surfactant is saturated with two fatty acids, predominately palmitic acid, esterified to the phospholipid backbone. This disaturated phospholipid, dipalmitoylphosphatidylcholine, is the principal surface-active component of surfactant. Almost all of the saturated phosphatidylcholine found in lung effluent is associated with surfactant. In contrast, large amounts of the unsaturated lecithin measured in amniotic fluid is not an integral part of surfactant. Normal surfactant action necessary for neonatal respiratory function is dependent upon predictable changes in the relative contributions of each phospholipid[7] (Figure 1). Sphingomyelin is found in low amounts from early in the second trimester and is present in relatively low concentrations throughout gestation. Lecithin is first detectable around 24–26 weeks' gestation and increases in concentration for the remainder of pregnancy. The concentrations of lecithin and sphingomyelin are equal around 32 weeks' gestation and at approximately 35 weeks, lecithin is found in amounts two times that of sphingomyelin. Phosphatidylinositol can be detected in amniotic fluid during the second trimester and subsequently peaks at 5–10% of total phospholipids between 35 and 37 weeks, then falls off afterwards. Phosphatidylglycerol is not normally present until 35–37 weeks, after which time levels continue to rise until the end of gestation[8] (Figure 2). A

Table 2   Accuracy of tests to determine fetal lung maturity

Sensitivity	*Specificity*
Ability of test to correctly identify all fetuses at risk for RDS (if the test is able to identify all fetuses at risk for RDS, it is 100% sensitive).	Ability of test to correctly identify all fetuses not at risk for RDS. (If only one-half of all fetuses who will not develop RDS are identified as not being at risk, then the test is only 50% specific.)
False-positive rate	*False-negative rate*
Percentage of fetuses identified as being at risk for RDS but do not develop RDS.	Percentage of fetuses identified as not being at risk for RDS but do develop RDS.

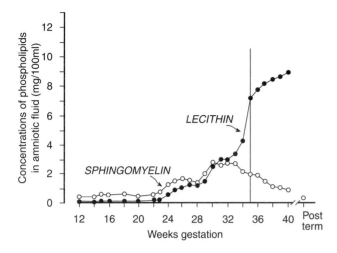

Figure 1 Changes in the mean concentrations of lecithin and sphingomyelin in the amniotic fluid during normal pregnancy. Reprinted with permission from reference 7

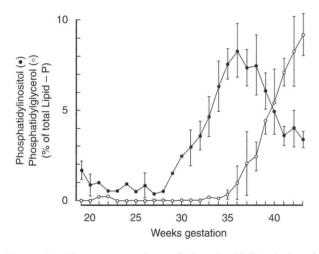

Figure 2 The concentrations of phosphatidylinositol and phosphatidylglycerol in the amniotic fluid during normal pregnancy. Reprinted with permission from reference 8

less-stable and less-active lecithin, palmitoylmyristoyl-lecithin is produced beginning at 20 to 22 weeks. It is felt that the presence of this phospholipid may explain why some very premature infants do not suffer RDS.

In addition to lipids, approximately 10% of surfactant are proteins. Optimal activity of surfactant is dependent upon the presence of specific proteins. Most of the protein associated with surfactant is albumin; many of the other proteins have not been characterized. The major human surfactant associated protein, other than albumin, is an oligo-mer with a molecular weight of 35 kDa. This protein appears in amniotic fluid in increasing concentrations as gestation advances. The exact role of this protein is not known but proposed functions include a role in control of surfactant storage, secretion and reuptaken by Type II alveolar cells[9].

The Type II alveolar cells are cuboidal cells interspersed among respiratory epithelium lining the alveoli. They can be recognized histologically by their characteristic lamellar bodies, the storage granules for surfactant. Soon after their appearance at around 20 weeks, surfactant is released. The mechanism whereby this release takes place, and the agents stimulating it, are poorly understood but probably involves both chemical and mechanical mediators. The composition of surfactant and the timing of surfactant release can be affected by numerous pregnancy related events and pharmacological agents.

DETERMINING FETAL LUNG MATURITY

Many of the original methods developed to assess fetal pulmonary maturity, such as amniotic fluid creatinine, osmolality and percentage of cells staining with Nile Blue sulfate, were extremely unreliable and are mentioned only for historical purposes. For twenty years, the L : S ratio has been the standard test employed because of its high sensitivity to predict RDS in the uncomplicated pregnancy. Significant disadvantages of the L : S ratio are the high rate of false-immature results and the unreliability of the test in many clinical situations, such as diabetes and meconium-stained amniotic fluid. The test is expensive and takes 2–4 hours to complete. The multitude of alternative tests of fetal maturity developed over the last two decades have sought to address these shortcomings. Some caution should be exercised when evaluating the newer methods as claims of reliability are often based upon a small number of patients.

The tests for fetal lung maturity are broken down into the following three categories:

(1) Direct measurements of surfactant or its components.

(2) Indirect measurements of surfactant based upon physiologic properties of amniotic fluid.

(3) Correlation of fetal lung maturity with ultrasound findings.

Measurements of surfactant components

Amniotic fluid phospholipids

Gluck and co-workers[4] reported in 1971 that the L : S ratio was correlated with the ability of neonatal lungs to adapt to an extrauterine existence. The authors noted that a dramatic rise in lecithin levels occurred near the end of pregnancy. An L : S ratio of 2.0 was achieved around 35 weeks and correlated with fetal lung maturity. Subsequent articles reporting over 2000 patients confirmed that the L : S ratio of 2.0 was able to predict the occurrence of RDS with a sensitivity of 97–98%[10,11].

The validity of an L : S ratio of 2.0 to predict fetal pulmonary maturity is dependent upon the methodology used to determine the ratio. Alterations in methodology can change results significantly. The most common method uses an acetone precipitation step to separate the phospholipids, particularly the lecithin, into non-acetone precipitable and acetone precipitable components. The acetone precipitable lecithin represents the disaturated phosphatidylcholine, the major surface active component of surfactant. If the acetone precipitation step is eliminated, measurements will reflect total lecithin which may falsely elevate the L : S ratio.

The phospholipids are separated by thin-layer chromatography. The corresponding spots can then be measured with reflectance densitometry or planimetric techniques. Either method of determining the L : S ratio will yield equivalent results up to a ratio of 3.0[12].

Although the L : S ratio is a sensitive measurement of RDS it does so with low specificity. Harvey et al.[10] found that an L : S ratio < 2.0 predicts RDS only 53% of the time. Herbert[13] evaluated the frequency and severity of RDS in infants with L : S ratios < 2.0 and found that: at extremely low L : S ratios, < 0.5, 100% of infants developed RDS and over 70% died; when the L : S ratio was between 0.5 and 0.99, almost 50% of the neonates developed RDS but only 15% required ventilatory support; when the L : S ratio exceeded 1.0, < 5% of infants developed RDS; no infant with an L : S ratio > 0.8 died from RDS and; infants with L : S ratios as low as 0.6 did not acquire RDS. Donald[14] found a 63% morbidity and 23% mortality when the L : S ratio was < 2.0. The risk of neonatal morbidity or mortality associated with a low L : S ratio is dependent upon several factors including gestational age, concomitant maternal or fetal disease and intrapartum acidemia and hypoxemia. But an L : S ratio of < 2.0 in most near term fetuses is not a very good indicator of neonatal RDS.

In 1976 Hallman[8] reported on the levels of minor phospholipids, phosphatidylinositol and phosphatidylglycerol, in amniotic fluid during pregnancy. Three years later, the concept of the 'lung profile' was introduced[11]. The lung profile consists of the L : S ratio and the percentages of disaturated (acetone-precipitable) lecithin, phosphatidylinositol and phosphatidylglycerol in amniotic fluid. The information provided by the lung profile enhances the accuracy of diagnosing fetal lung maturity and provides further information on lung development. In a small group of patients, the specificity was increased from 69% to 93% by substituting the lung profile for the L : S ratio[10]. The addition of a test to detect phosphatidylglycerol decreased the rate of false-positives significantly. Other authors have subsequently confirmed that the presence

of phosphatidylglycerol can improve the specificity of the L : S ratio[15]. In general, phosphatidylglycerol is reported as being absent, trace or present, corresponding to phosphatidylglycerol concentrations of 0%, < 5% and > 5% of total phospholipids, respectively. When phosphatidylglycerol is present, RDS does not occur except possibly in cases of intrapartum acidemia and hypoxemia or other fetal disease. With trace amounts of phosphatidylglycerol in amniotic fluid, an incidence of RDS < 1% has been reported[15].

Many factors can affect the L : S ratio. Lecithin is found in many body fluids including blood, vaginal secretions and gastrointestinal fluid. Hence the addition of blood to amniotic fluid will alter the L : S ratio. Buhi and Spellacy[16] found that the L : S ratio of serum was approximately 1.4 which would tend to lower the L : S ratio of amniotic fluid from mature fetuses. Other authors have shown variable results with upward and downward shifts in the L : S ratio of amniotic fluid mixed with blood[17]. The changes are probably dependent upon the initial L : S ratio and the amount of contaminating blood.

The addition of meconium to amniotic fluid has also been associated with inconsistent changes in the L : S ratio[16,18]. Amniotic fluid obtained from a vaginal pool can be used to assess pulmonary maturity. However, in one study 22% of amniotic fluid samples obtained from vaginal pools had higher L : S ratios than paired samples of amniotic fluid obtained from the amniotic sac by amniocentesis[19].

If the analysis of amniotic fluid contaminated with blood, meconium or vaginal secretions does not give reliable L : S ratios, other methods of assessing fetal lung maturity should be used. Phosphatidylglycerol is an appropriate marker of maturity in these situations because it is virtually absent from body fluids other than lung surfactant. This has been confirmed by numerous clinical studies[15,20]. A recent report suggests that vaginal bacterial infections may falsely elevate phosphatidylglycerol levels[21]. The authors describe a case where phosphatidylglycerol was detected in the vaginal pool but not in an amniocentesis specimen and the neonate subsequently developed RDS. The site of sampling during an amniocentesis may also effect the L : S ratio. Dual samples performed on 26 patients at the time of elective Cesarean section found that fluid obtained from close to the fetal mouth has an L : S ratio higher than samples obtained from the caudal pole 81% of the time[22]. The maximum difference between samples was 0.7 and two infants developed RDS, both of whom had L : S ratios obtained from near the fetal mouth of > 2.0 while samples obtained from the alternate site were immature.

Maternal and fetal disease states and other obstetrical problems can affect the timing of fetal lung maturity. It has been widely reported that diabetes may delay pulmonary maturity. Advanced states of diabetes

(White's Classes D, F, R) cause accelerated fetal maturity[23]. Less advanced stages of diabetes have more variable effects on lung development. It appears that pulmonary maturity is delayed and that the L : S ratio may not be a reliable indicator of pulmonary maturity[24]. Other authors noted no difference between diabetic patients and controls[23,25]. When maternal diabetes is well controlled during the pregnancy, there is not a significant delay in pulmonary maturity and the L : S ratio can be used to establish the risk of neonatal RDS[24,26,27]. Although the appearance of phosphatidylglycerol has been reported to be delayed in pregnancies of diabetic women (Classes A, B, C), it remains a reliable predictor of pulmonary maturity[28]. The L : S ratio can be used to assess fetal lung maturity when glucose levels have been well controlled in a diabetic pregnancy. But when control has been erratic or is difficult to assess, positive phosphatidylglycerol or higher L : S ratios (> 2.5) should be used to predict fetal lung maturity. Some obstetrical complications and maternal disease states are thought to 'stress' the pregnancy and accelerate fetal lung development. Chronic hypertension, maternal cardiovascular disease, chronic placental insufficiency and prolonged rupture of membranes appear to accelerate fetal maturity; the impact of pre-eclampsia on fetal lung maturation is uncertain[23,29,30]. If fetal lung maturity is accelerated, phosphatidylglycerol may be present before the mature L : S ratio develops. The effects of maternal isoimmunization on fetal lung maturity and amniotic fluid phospholipid composition is not clear; both delayed maturation and no significant impact are reported[23,31].

Twin gestation by itself may not necessarily accelerate fetal lung maturity. Fetal lung maturation is comparable between singleton and twin pregnancies when preterm labor is the only complication affecting both groups[32]. The fetal lung maturation may occur earlier in twin gestations when accompanied by such complications as pregnancy-induced hypertension, pre-eclampsia, discordance, or premature rupture of membranes[33]. The L : S ratios of twin fetuses tend to be synchronous when the weights are concordant. However, 11% of concordant twins had discordant L : S ratios including one set that was discordant for maturity[33,34]. Fetal lung maturity may differ significantly in the presence of a significant fetal growth discordance. While the smaller twin tends to develop lung maturity earlier than its counterpart, it is not always the case[33,34]. Thus, it would seem prudent to obtain amniotic fluid for lung maturity studies from all fetuses in a multiple gestation, particularly if an elective delivery is contemplated.

The AmnioStat-FLM (Hana Biologics, Beheley, CA, USA) is an easily performed assay of phosphatidylglycerol that provides rapid results with minimal equipment necessary[35-37]. Levels of phosphatidylglycerol as low as 0.5 ng/ml can be detected by this method. This level of detection is equivalent to the lower limit of detection with thin-layer chromatography. When compared to thin-layer chromatography, the Amniostat-FLM has a concordance rate of approximately 90%[35-37]. The level of agreement is greatest at a gestational age of > 34 weeks. As is true with phosphatidylglycerol detection by thin-layer chromatography, the Amniostat-FLM has a false-positive rate > 50%. The specificity is highest if used when the gestational age is > 36 weeks[35-37]. The Amniostat-FLM appears to be accurate in predicting fetal lung maturity from the vaginal pool samples[38]. There are other bedside tests that are quicker, cheaper and have a high sensitivity at this gestational age. For these reasons some authors have questioned if this method of determining fetal lung maturity is cost effective at any gestational age[39].

Amniotic fluid proteins

Approximately 10% of surfactant is composed of proteins, the major one being albumin. The predominant protein involved in surfactant metabolism is a 35-kDa protein, surfactant associated protein 35 (SAP-35). This protein is unique to surfactant and originates from the Type II alveolar cells. A significant increase in amniotic fluid concentrations of SAP-35 occurs near term and a significant correlation with pulmonary maturity has been noted[40,41]. The recent development of a method utilizing enzyme-linked immunosorbent assay (ELISA) and monoclonal antibodies has simplified measurements of this protein and allows routine testing[41]. The test can predict RDS with an accuracy similar to that of the L : S ratio[41]. In high-risk pregnancies such as diabetes or hypertension, the levels of SAP-35 have less correlation with fetal pulmonary maturity and are probably not reliable in these situations[40].

Amniotic fluid neutral lipids

In addition to polar lipids, amniotic fluid contains large amounts of neutral or non-polar lipids. Forty percent of the total non-polar lipid fraction of amniotic fluid at term is cholesterol palmitate. The exact role of cholesterol palmitate is not known but it could serve as a transport mode for palmitic acid which is used in the synthesis of saturated phosphatidylcholine. Ludmir and co-workers[42] reported a simple and rapid method of determining cholesterol palmitate levels in amniotic fluid using thin-layer chromatography and densitometry. In a small number of patients, levels of cholesterol palmitate were correlated with fetal lung maturity. A similar correlation was not demonstrated in diabetic pregnancies[43].

Information about amniotic fluid protein and neutral lipids provide valuable information on surfactant production and lung development. Preliminary results suggest that both assays could be used as a test to determine fetal pulmonary maturity. However, at this time, neither assay offers significant improvement over more widely available tests such as phospholipid assays.

Indirect measurements of surfactant

The 'shake test' and related assays

In 1972 Clements and co-workers introduced the 'shake test' which indirectly measures the concentration of surfactant by measuring the stability of bubbles in a mixture of amniotic fluid and ethanol[44]. The accuracy of the test is comparable to that of the L : S ratio[44,45]. A commercially available kit, Lumadex-Foam Stability Index (Beckman Instruments, Brea, CA, USA) gives similar results[46]. Because this test is rapid and fairly inexpensive, it can be employed as an initial bedside screening test. The shake test and its modifications indirectly measure the concentrations of saturated lecithin in the amniotic fluid. In the presence of maternal diabetes or contamination of amniotic fluid with blood, meconium or vaginal secretions, the test is not a dependable indicator of lung maturity[45,46]. The 'tap test', a modification of the shake test, measures the stability of bubbles in a solution of amniotic fluid, hydrochloric acid and dimethylether. Results from a series of over 300 patients demonstrate that the tap test is as accurate as the L : S ratio or shake test in predicting fetal lung maturity[47].

The obvious values of these tests are the simplicity in performance and the short time required to obtain results. They do not appear to have predictive values that are significantly different from those of the L : S ratio. It is not clear how the results of the assays are affected by maternal diabetes or contamination of amniotic fluid. In normal near-term gestations, a shake test or a related assay performed with uncontaminated amniotic fluid can predict RDS with a high degree of sensitivity but low specificity.

Amniotic fluid optical density

In 1976, Sbarra and co-workers[48] reported that the absorbence of light by amniotic fluid at 400 nm was correlated with the L : S ratio. However, pigmented substances such as bilirubin, blood and meconium also absorb significantly at 400 nm and may falsely elevate results. In a subsequent report, the authors measured the absorption of amniotic fluid at 650 nm and found that an optical density (OD) of > 0.15 was correlated with an L : S ratio 2.0[49]. The correlation between the amniotic fluid OD at 650 nm and the L : S ratio has been confirmed in other studies[50,51]. In more than 500 patients, an OD_{650} reading of > 0.15 resulted in a false-negative rate of < 3%. Amniotic fluid absorbence was also compared with neonatal outcomes[52]. An OD_{650}

of > 0.15 was associated with a rate of neonatal RDS < 5%, which is comparable to those of the L : S ratio. Spectrophotometric analysis of amniotic fluid is not a very specific method of identifying patients at risk for RDS. A low OD_{650} was associated with RDS < 50% of the time.

Particulate matter suspended in the amniotic fluid absorbs light and is responsible for the changes in optical density. Fetal squames, lamellar bodies or other structures may be responsible. Amniotic fluid cell counts[53] and amniotic fluid lamellar body concentrations[54] have been strongly correlated with advancing gestational age and rising L : S ratios. Plauche and co-workers[55] found that OD_{650} readings were most directly associated with amniotic fluid cell counts. In this study, negligible optical absorbence was generated by solutions containing variable concentrations of phospholipids. Based upon these results, optical density at 650 nm may indirectly correlate with pulmonary maturity via a direct measurement of cutaneous maturation.

Spectrophotometric analysis of amniotic fluid is as reliable a predictor of pulmonary maturity as the L : S ratio. The OD_{650} can be performed rapidly, cheaply and with minimal training. Spectrophotometers can be found in most clinical laboratories. As is true with the L : S ratio and shake test, OD_{650} has a low diagnostic specificity for neonatal RDS; thus positive tests should be followed up with additional testing if delivery is indicated. The reliability of the test is unknown in pregnancies complicated by maternal diabetes or contamination of amniotic fluid with bilirubin, meconium or blood; other methods should be employed in these situations.

Fluorescence polarization of amniotic fluid

In 1976, Shinitzky and co-workers[56] employed an alternative method of assessing fetal lung maturity by measuring the fluorescence polarization of amniotic fluid. A fluorescent probe is added to amniotic fluid, the fluid is exposed to a polarizing light and the level of fluorescent polarization is determined. There are at present two systems used to measure fluorescent polarization: the FELMA microviscometer (Elscind, Hackensack, NJ, USA) and the TDx system (Abbott, Irving, TX, USA). The FELMA is a system specifically designed to measure the fluorescent polarization of amniotic fluid. The TDx is an automated fluorescence polarimeter used for the analysis of many types of chemicals in a variety of fluids. Both systems are fairly expensive but the TDx system is available in many clinical laboratories.

The fluorescent probe of the FELMA system is the hydrocarbon DPH, a relatively unstable compound that needs to be prepared daily and is sensitive to light and oxygen. Two fluorescent phosphatidylcholine molecules are used with the TDx system, NDB-PL[57] and PC16[58].

While both probes have similar properties, the structure of PC16 has been modified to enhance its stability.

After the fluorescent probe is added to amniotic fluid, it is incorporated into phospholipid structures, protein and other macromolecules. Incorporation of a particular probe into a macromolecule depends upon the chemical properties of the probe, its interactions with the macromolecules and the concentration of the macromolecules. The solution is exposed to polarized light and components of the emitted fluorescence are measured. The amount and intensity of fluorescence detected is related to ability of the dye to rotate. If the dye is bound to a larger or less fluid structure, there will be less motion between the time of absorption and emission of the protein. This results in higher levels of fluorescence polarization.

The fluorescent polarization of amniotic fluid is in large part determined by the binding of the probe to phospholipid structures and to the predominant protein, albumin[57]. Binding of the dye to endogenous protein will increase the fluorescent polarization because the large size and non-fluid nature of proteins decreases the motion of the probe. Conversely, incorporation of the probe into phospholipid structures will relatively decrease the fluorescent polarization because these are more fluid structures. If the phospholipid membranes contain a large percentage of saturated lecithin, the fluorescent polarization will be even lower.

Fluorescence polarization of amniotic fluid is inversely related to the L : S ratio[58,59]. The ability of fluorescence polarization to predict RDS is similar to the lung profile, very few false-mature results occur while the specificity ranges from 50 to 70%[60,61]. The technique is not reliable when amniotic fluid is contaminated by blood or meconium since both fluids contain lipids and proteins that affect the fluorescent polarization value in an unpredictable manner[57,59].

The fluorescent polarization values are not significantly affected by high-risk pregnancy complications except diabetes[61,62]. Maternal diabetes has variable effects on values, and the test is an unreliable indicator of fetal maturity in this clinical situation.

The TDx system using the PC16 fluorescent probe developed by Russell[58] may have some advantages. The TDx system is widely available in clinical laboratories and the PC16 probe is more stable than NDB-PL. This method utilizes a software package developed by the manufacturer that allows interinstitutional comparisons. In addition, the albumin is measured in each sample and the result is provided as a surfactant: albumin ratio, taking into account the variable concentrations of albumin in amniotic fluid. All three methods have the advantage of providing results rapidly, in 30–45 min, and requiring only 0.5–1.0 ml of fluid.

In a prospective clinical evaluation of the TDx system using the NBD-PL probe, a fluorescent polarization of < 0.260 was 100% sensitive at identifying fetuses who subsequently developed RDS with a specificity of > 70%[63]. In a multicenter evaluation of the TDx system utilizing PC16, sensitivity of 96% and a specificity of 88% were obtained with a cutoff value for maturity set at 50 mg/g (surfactant : albumin value). In this study the corresponding sensitivity and specificity for the L : S ratio was 96 and 83% respectively[64]. In insulin-dependent diabetic patients, a TDx-FLM value of at least 70 mg/g is not associated with RDS requiring intubation[65,66]. These findings suggest that fluorescence polarization may be a reliable alternative to the L : S ratio.

Ultrasonography

Determination of fetal lung maturity by ultrasonography offers many advantages: safety, non-invasiveness and immediate results. The biparietal diameters (BPD), placental grading and fetal ossification centers are the most commonly used parameters for this purpose. Studies indicate that a maximum of 5% of patients, diabetes mellitus excluded, with a BPD > 9.2 cm will develop RDS[67–69]. The predictive values of the BPD increase with known gestational age of > 38 weeks. Similarly, in normal term gestations, grade 3 placentas are highly correlated with fetal pulmonary maturity, as determined by a mature L : S ratio and the absence of neonatal RDS. However, if grade 3 changes do not permeate the entire placenta, there is a small risk of neonatal RDS[70–74]. Fetal pulmonary maturity appears to be correlated with the presence and size of ossification centers[75–80]. In one instance when the distal femoral epiphysis was at least 3 mm and a proximal tibial epiphysis was present, the L : S ratio was > 2.0 in all cases[80]. Although the BPD, placenta grading, and fetal ossification centers may have good predictive values of RDS among term, uncomplicated pregnancies, their values in preterm and complicated pregnancies remain to be evaluated. Further study also is needed in the ultrasonographic assessment of fetal lung maturity pertaining to amniotic fluid turbidity, fetal bowel pattern, relative echogenicity of the fetal liver and lung and fetal lung compressibility[81–84].

CONCLUSION

The level of sensitivity and specificity obtained with a particular test will vary with the threshold chosen to indicate fetal lung maturity. In addition, the sensitivity and specificity achieved with a particular threshold will depend upon the gestational age of the fetus. For example, at a gestational age of 38 weeks, a threshold level may be lowered to increase specificity with only minimal loss in sensitivity because most fetuses will be mature at that gestational age. If the lower threshold is employed at 32 weeks' gestation, a significant rise in the rate of false-negative results may occur because a substantial portion of the fetuses will be immature.

The threshold level that is used to indicate fetal pulmonary maturity should be based upon the gestational age of the fetus and the urgency of the clinical situation. If the mother or her fetus would be placed in substantial jeopardy by continuation of the pregnancy, delivery may be appropriate at a lower cutoff. If possible, the threshold should be set at a level where RDS may occur but mortality is extremely rare. When entirely elective deliveries are being considered or where the clinical urgency is minimal, cutoff points at which there is very little or no risk of RDS should be chosen.

By using a combination of tests in an orderly fashion, results can be achieved more efficiently and with greater levels of specificity. Garite and co-workers[85] used a 'fetal maturity cascade' consisting of the shake test, fluorescent polarization (FELMA) and L : S ratio in 175 patients from 31 to 40 weeks' gestation. The shake test is performed first and if mature, no further test is done. If the shake test is immature, fluorescent polarization was measured, and so on. A sensitivity of 99% was achieved with a specificity of 59%. Only 10% of patients with test results indicating lung maturity needed an L : S ratio performed, representing a substantial reduction in cost. The use of complementary tests is reasonable and justifiable as long as the clinician understands the limitations of such a protocol and will adjust cutoffs depending upon the gestational age and urgency of the situation.

Each obstetrician must be familiar with the assay and methodology employed by the laboratory. It is necessary to know the limitations of the test and of the laboratory performing the test. For a given assay and methodology employed, every laboratory should establish cutoff values that equate with lung maturity and evaluate a new assay or technique prior to clinical application.

REFERENCES

1. Hack M, Fanaroff AA, Klaus MH, *et al*. Neonatal respiratory distress following elective delivery. *Am J Obstet Gynecol* 1976;126:43–7
2. Fetal maturity assessment prior to elective repeat Cesarean delivery. *ACOG Committee Opinion* 98; September 1991
3. Frigoletto FD, Phillippe M, Davies IJ, Ryan KJ. Avoiding iatrogenic prematurity with elective repeat cesarean section without the routine use of amniocentesis. *Am J Obstet Gynecol* 1980;137:521–4
4. Gluck L, Kulovich MV, Borer RC, *et al*. Diagnosis of the respiratory distress syndrome by amniocentesis. *Am J Obstet Gynecol* 1971;109:440–5
5. Assessment of fetal lung maturity. *ACOG Educational Bull* 230; November 1996
6. Ohno K, Akino T, Fujiwara T. Phospholipid metabolism in perinatal lung. In Scarpelli EM and Cosmi EV, eds. *Review in Perinatal Medicine*. New York: Raven Press, 1978
7. Gluck L, Kulovich MV. Lecithin/sphingomyelin ratio in amniotic fluid in normal and abnormal pregnancy. *Am J Obstet Gynecol* 1973;115:539–46
8. Hallman M, Kulovich M, Kirkpatrick E, *et al*. Phosphatidylinositol and phosphatidylglycerol in amniotic fluid. *Am J Obstet Gynecol* 1976;125:613–17
9. King RJ. Composition and metabolism of apolipoprotein of pulmonary surfactant. *Am Rev Physiol* 1985;47:775
10. Harvey D, Parkinson C, Campbell S. Risk of respiratory distress syndrome. *Lancet* 1975;1:42
11. Kulovich MV, Hallman MB, Gluck L. The lung profile. I. Normal pregnancy. *Am J Obstet Gynecol* 1975;135:57
12. Gluck L, Kulovich MV, Borer RC, Keidel WN. The interpretation and significance of the lecithin/sphingomyelin ratio in amniotic fluid. *Am J Obstet Gynecol* 1974;120:142–55
13. Herbert WNP, Tyson J, Jimenez JH. Severity of respiratory distress syndrome with low lecithin/sphingomyelin ratio. *Obstet Gynecol* 1981;57:426–36
14. Donald IR, Freeman RK, Goebelsmann U, *et al*. Clinical experience with the amniotic fluid lecithin/ sphingomyelin ratio. *Am J Obstet Gynecol* 1973;115:547–52
15. Plauche WC, Faro S, Letellier R. Phosphatidylglycerol and fetal lung maturity. *Am J Obstet Gynecol* 1982;144:167
16. Buhi WC, Spellacy WN. Effects of blood or meconium on the determination of the amniotic fluid lecithin/ sphingomyelin ratio. *Am J Obstet Gynecol* 1975;121:321–33
17. Gibbons JM, Huntley TE, Joachim E, *et al*. Effects of maternal blood contamination on amniotic fluid analysis. *Obstet Gynecol* 1974;44:657–61
18. Kulkarni BD, Bieniarz J, Burd L, Scommegna A. Determination of lecithin/sphingomyelin ratio in amniotic fluid. *Obstet Gynecol* 1972;40:173–9
19. Dombroski RA, Mackenna J, Brame RG. Comparison of amniotic fluid lung maturity profiles in paired vaginal and amniocentesis specimens. *Am J Obstet Gynecol* 1981;140:461–4
20. Stedman CH, Crawford S, Staten E, Cherny WB. Management of preterm premature rupture of membranes: assessing amniotic fluid in the vagina for phosphatidylglycerol. *Am J Obstet Gynecol* 1981;140:34–8
21. Schumacher RE, Parisi VM, Steady HM, Jsao FHC. Bacteria causing false positive test for phosphatidylglycerol in amniotic fluid. *Am J Obstet Gynecol* 1985;151:1067–8
22. Worthington D, Smith B. The site of amniocentesis and the lecithin/sphingomyelin ratio. *Obstet Gynecol* 1978;52:552–4
23. Gluck L, Kulovich MV. Lecithin/sphingomyelin ratios in amniotic fluid in normal and abnormal pregnancy. *Am J Obstet Gynecol* 1973;115:539–46
24. Piper JM, Lander O. Does maternal diabetes delay fetal pulmonary maturity? *Am J Obstet Gynecol* 1993;1968:783–6
25. Singh EJ, Mejia A, Zuspan FP. Studies of human amniotic fluid phospholipids in normal, diabetic and drug abuse pregnancy. *Am J Obstet Gynecol* 1974;119:623–9
26. Tabsh KMA, Brinkman CR, Bashore RA. Lecithin/ sphingomyelin ratio in pregnancies complicated by

insulin-dependent diabetes mellitus. *Obstet Gynecol* 1982;59:353–8

27. Farrell PM, Engle MJ, Curet LB, *et al.* Saturated phospholipids in amniotic fluid of normal and diabetic pregnancies. *Obstet Gynecol* 1984;64:77–85

28. Curet LB, Olson RV, Schneider JM, Zachman RD. Effects of diabetes mellitus on amniotic fluid lecithin/sphingomyelin ratio and respiratory distress syndrome. *Am J Obstet Gynecol* 1979;135:10–13

29. Yambao TJ, Clark D, Smith C, Aubry RH. Amniotic fluid phosphatidylglycerol in stressed pregnancies. *Am J Obstet Gynecol* 1981;14:191–4

30. Schiff E, Friedman SA, Mercer BM, Sibai BM. Fetal lung maturity is not accelerated in preeclamptic pregnancies. *Am J Obstet Gynecol* 1993;169:1096–101

31. Quinlan RTJ, Buhi WC, Cruz AC. Fetal pulmonary maturity in isoimmunized pregnancies. *Am J Obstet Gynecol* 1984;148:787–9

32. Winn HN, Romero R, Roberts A, *et al.* Comparison of fetal lung maturation in preterm singleton and twin pregnancies. *Am J Perinatol* 1992;9:326–29

33. Leveno KJ, Quirk JG, Whalley PJ, *et al.* Fetal lung maturation in twin gestation. *Am J Obstet Gynecol* 1984;148:405–11

34. Spellacy WN, Cruz AC, Buhi WC, Birk SA. Amniotic fluid L : S ratio in twin gestation. *Obstet Gynecol* 1977;50:68–70

35. Garite TJ, Yabusaki KK, Moberg LJ, *et al.* A new rapid slide agglutination test for amniotic fluid phosphatidylglycerol. *Am J Obstet Gynecol* 1983;147:681–6

36. Lockitch G, Wittmann BK, Mura SM, Hawkley LC. Evaluation of Amniostat-FLM assay for assessment of fetal lung maturity. *Clin Chem* 1984;3017:1233–7

37. Benoit J, Merrill S, Rundell C, *et al.* An initial clinical trial with both vaginal pool amniocentesis samples. *Am J Obstet Gynecol* 1986;159:65–8

38. Lewis DF, Towers CV, Major CA, *et al.* Use of Amniostat-FLM in detecting the presence of phosphatidylglycerol in vaginal pool samples in preterm premature rupture of membranes. *Am J Obstet Gynecol* 1993;169:573–6

39. Egberts J, Wijnards JBG. Uselessness of the phosphatidylglycerol assay for prediction of lung maturity. *Am J Obstet Gynecol* 1989;161:1417

40. McMahon MJ, Mimouni F, Miodovnik M, *et al.* Surfactant associated protein (SAP-35) in amniotic fluid from diabetic and nondiabetic pregnancies. *Obstet Gynecol* 1987;70:94–8

41. Hallman M, Arjomaa P, Mizumoto M, Akino T. Surfactant proteins in the diagnosis of fetal lung maturity. *Am J Obstet Gynecol* 1988;158:531–5

42. Ludmir J, Alvarez JG, Mennuti MT, *et al.* Cholesterol palmitate as a predictor of fetal lung maturity. *Am J Obstet Gynecol* 1987;157:84–8

43. Ludmir J, Alvarez JG, Landon MB, *et al.* Amniotic fluid cholesterol palmitate in pregnancies complicated by diabetes mellitus. *Obstet Gynecol* 1988;72:360–2

44. Clements JA, Platzker ACG, Tierney OF, *et al.* Assessment of the risk of respiratory-distress syndrome by a rapid test for surfactant in amniotic fluid. *New Engl J Med* 1972;286:1077–81

45. Morrison JC, Whybrew WD, Bucovaz ET. The L : S ratio and shake test in normal and abnormal pregnancies. *Obstet Gynecol* 1978;52:410–4

46. Sher G, Statland BE. Assessment of fetal pulmonary maturity by the Lumadex Foam Stability Index test. *Obstet Gynecol* 1983;61:444–9

47. Sokol ML. The tap test: confirmation of a simple, rapid, inexpensive, and reliable indicator of fetal pulmonary maturity. *Am J Obstet Gynecol* 1990;162:218

48. Sbarra AJ, Michlewitz H, Selvaraj RJ, *et al.* Correlation between amniotic fluid optical density and L : S ratio. *Obstet Gynecol* 1976;48:613–5

49. Sbarra AJ, Selvaraj RJ, Cetrulo CL, *et al.* Positive correlation of optical density at 650 nm with L : S ratios in amniotic fluid. *Am J Obstet Gynecol* 1978;130:788–90

50. Copeland W, Stempel L, Lott JA, *et al.* Assessment of a rapid test on amniotic fluid for estimating fetal lung maturity. *Am J Obstet Gynecol* 1978;130:225–6

51. Arias F, Andrinopoulos G, Pineda J. Correlation between amniotic fluid optical density, L : S ratio and fetal pulmonary maturity. *Obstet Gynecol* 1978;51:152–5

52. Cetrulo CL, Sbarra AJ, Selvaraj RJ, *et al.* Amniotic fluid optical density and neonatal respiratory outcome. *Obstet Gynecol* 1980;55:262–5

53. Hudson EA, Gauntlett J. Amniotic fluid cells and the L : S ratio. *Obstet Gynecol* 1977;49:280–6

54. Lee W, Bell M, Novy MJ. Pulmonary lamellar bodies in human amniotic fluid: their relationship to fetal age and the L : S ratio. *Am J Obstet Gynecol* 1980;136:60–6

55. Plauche WC, Faro S, Vychech J. Amniotic fluid optical density: relationship to L : S ratio, phospholipid content and desquamation of fetal cells. *Obstet Gynecol* 1981;58:309–13

56. Shinitzky M, Goldfisher A, Bruck A, Goldman B, *et al.* A new method for assessment of fetal lung maturity. *Br J Obstet Gynaecol* 1976;83:838–44

57. Tait JF, Franklin RW, Simpson JB, Ashwood ER. Improved fluorescence polarization assay for use in evaluating fetal lung maturity. I. Development of the assay procedure. *Clin Chem* 1986;32:248–54

58. Russell JC. A calibrated fluorescence polarization assay for assessment of fetal lung maturity. *Clin Chem* 1987;33:1177–84

59. Blumenfeld TA, Stark RI, James LS, George JD, *et al.* Determination of fetal lung maturity by fluorescence polarization of amniotic fluid. *Am J Obstet Gynecol* 1978;130:782–7

60. Golde SH, Vogt JF, Gabbe SG, Cabal LA. Evaluation of the FELMA microviscometer in predicting fetal lung maturity. *Obstet Gynecol* 1979;54:639–42

61. Ashwood ER, Tait JF, Foerder CA, *et al.* Improved fluorescence polarization assay for use in evaluating fetal lung maturity. III. *Clin Chem* 1986;32:260

62. Barkai G, Hashiach S, Lanzer D, *et al.* Determination of fetal lung maturity from amniotic fluid microviscosity in high risk pregnancy. *Obstet Gynecol* 1982;59:615–23

63. Tait JF, Foerder CA, Ashwood ER, Benedetti TJ. Prospective clinical evaluation of an improved fluorescence polarization assay for predicting fetal lung maturity. *Clin Chem* 1987;33:554–8

64. Russell JC, Cooper CM, Ketchum CH, *et al.* Multicenter evaluation of TDx test for assessing fetal lung maturity. *Clin Chem* 1980;35:1005

65. Livingston EG, Herbert WN, Hage ML, *et al.* For the Diabetes and Fetal Maturity Study Group: use of the TDx-FLM assay in evaluating fetal lung maturity in an insulin-dependent diabetic population. *Obstet Gynecol* 1995;86:826–9

66. Tanasijevic MJ, Winkelman JW, Wybenga DR, *et al.* Prediction of fetal lung maturity in infants of diabetic mothers using the FLM S/A and disaturated phosphatidylcholine tests. *Am J Clin Pathol* 1996;105:17–22

67. Goldstein P, Gershenson D, Hobbins JC. Fetal biparietal diameter as a predictor of a mature L : S ratio. *Obstet Gynecol* 1976;48:667–9

68. Spellacy WN, Gelman SR, Wood SD, *et al.* Comparison of fetal maturity evaluation with ultrasonic biparietal diameter and amniotic fluid L : S ratio. *Obstet Gynecol* 1978;51:109–11

69. Strassner HT, Platt LD, Whittle M, *et al.* Amniotic fluid phosphatidylglycerol and realtime ultrasonic cephalometry. *Am J Obstet Gynecol* 1979;134:804–8

70. Grannum PAT, Berkowitz RL, Hobbins JC. The ultrasonic changes in the maturing placenta and their relationship to fetal pulmonic maturity. *Am J Obstet Gynecol* 1979;133:915–9

71. Petrucha RA, Golde SH, Platt LD. Real-time ultrasound of the placenta in assessment of fetal pulmonic maturity. *Am J Obstet Gynecol* 1982;142:463–7

72. Harman CR, Manning FA, Stearns E, Morrison I. The correlation of ultrasonic placental grading and fetal pulmonary maturation in five hundred sixty-three pregnancies. *Am J Obstet Gynecol* 1982;143:941–3

73. Tabsh KRA. Correlation of real-time ultrasonic placental grading with amniotic fluid L : S ratio. *Am J Obstet Gynecol* 1983;145:504–8

74. Kazzi GM, Gross TL, Sokol RJ, Kazzi SNJ. Noninvasive prediction of hyaline membrane disease: an optimized classification of sonographic placental maturation. *Am J Obstet Gynecol* 1985;152:213–9

75. Gentilli P, Trasimeni A, Giorlandino C. Fetal ossification centers as predictors of gestational age in normal and abnormal pregnancies. *J Ultrasound Med* 1984;3:193–7

76. Mahoney BS, Callen PW, Filly RA. The distal femoral epiphyseal ossification center in the assessment of third trimester menstrual age. *Radiology* 1985;155:201–4

77. Goldstein I, Lockwood C, Belanger K, Hobbins J. Ultrasonic assessment of gestational age with the distal femoral and proximal tibial ossification centers in the third trimester. *Am J Obstet Gynecol* 1988;158:127–30

78. Mahoney BS, Bowie JD, Killam AP, *et al.* Epiphyseal ossification centers in the assessment of fetal maturity. *Radiology* 1986;159:521–4

79. Tabsh KMA. Correlation of ultrasonic epiphyseal centers and the L : S ratio. *Obstet Gynecol* 1984;64:92–6

80. Goldstein I, Lockwood CJ, Reece A, Hobbins JC. Sonographic assessment of the distal femoral and proximal tibial ossification centers in the prediction of pulmonic maturity in normal women and women with diabetes. *Am J Obstet Gynecol* 1988;159:72–6

81. Gross TL, Wulfson RN, Kuhnert PM, *et al.* Sonographically detected free floating particles in amniotic fluid predict a mature L : S ratio. *J Clin Ultrasound* 1985;13:405–9

82. Helewa M, Manning F, Harman C. Amniotic fluid particles: are they related to a mature amniotic fluid phospholipid profile? *Obstet Gynecol* 1989;74:893–96

83. Zilianti M, Fernandez S. Correlation of ultrasonic images of fetal intestine with gestational age and fetal maturity. *Obstet Gynecol* 1983;62:569–75

84. Birnhulz JC, Farrel EE. Fetal lung development: compressibility as a measure of maturity. *Radiology* 1985;157:495–9

85. Garite TJ, Freema RK, Nageotte MP. Fetal maturity cascade: a rapid and cost-effective method for fetal lung maturity testing. *Obstet Gynecol* 1986;67:619–22

61
Fetal macrosomia

H.N. Winn

INTRODUCTION

Macrosomia, arbitrarily defined as a birthweight of > 4000 g at term, complicates about 10% and 25% of term and post-term pregnancies, respectively[1–4]. It remains an important cause of perinatal morbidity and mortality and maternal morbidity, which arise mainly from birth injury and asphyxia and increased rate of Cesarean section, respectively[5,6]. In addition to the significant immediate complications, the long-term impact of less severe perinatal asphyxia on the mental development of the affected children is unknown. The major obstacle in reducing the perinatal morbidity and mortality associated with fetal macrosomia has been the inability to predict with certainty which fetuses will sustain birth injury prior to delivery. To minimize the adverse perinatal and maternal outcomes associated with this problem, it is important to have a well-planned management scheme for patients with fetal macrosomia, recognizing that there is currently no perfect solution. In the following discussion, the current understanding of fetal macrosomia with regard to risk factors, diagnosis, and intrapartum management will be presented.

RISK FACTORS

The first step in the management of fetal macrosomia is the identification of patients at risk for this condition. It has been shown that patients with such characteristics as diabetes, obesity, advanced age, multiparity, post-term pregnancy, idiopathic polyhydramnios and prior maternal and sibling birthweights of > 4000 g are at risk of having fetal macrosomia[2,5,7–9].

In general, maternal diabetes mellitus doubles the risk of having neonatal macrosomia compared to that of the non-diabetic population. The poorer the glycemic control, the greater the potential of having fetal macrosomia[10–14]. Interestingly, it has been demonstrated that the risk of fetal macrosomia also rises in untreated patients with one abnormal value on a glucose tolerance test (GTT)[15,16], even though these patients may be classified as normal if the criterion of having two abnormal values is used for diagnosing gestational diabetes mellitus. The mechanism of fetal macrosomia in the case of maternal diabetes mellitus as originally proposed by Pederson and co-workers[17] is the acceleration of fetal growth due to fetal hyperinsulinemia in response to fetal hyperglycemia, which is in turn affected by maternal hyperglycemia. This hypothesis is supported by a high degree of correlation between cord serum levels of C-peptide and fetal macrosomia in diabetic patients[18]. Fetal macrosomia and organomegaly of the placenta, liver, and heart have been observed in the chronically maintained euglycemic and hyperinsulinemic rhesus monkey[19]. The direct impact of maternal and fetal hyperglycemia *per se* on fetal macrosomia remains unclear[18,20,21]. It is possible that macrosomic fetuses maintain euglycemia by increased production of insulin. This could explain the similar levels of maternal glycosylated hemoglobin but higher levels of total insulin, free insulin, and C-peptide in cord serum of macrosomic fetuses compared with non-macrosomic ones in diabetic patients[22]. Metabolic factors other than maternal hyperglycemia may play a role in causing fetal macrosomia in the clinical setting.

Since the fetus may continue to grow beyond 37 weeks of gestation, the incidence of fetal macrosomia increases with advancing gestational age with an overall rate of about 25–30% at ⩾ 41 weeks' gestation[1,4]. Maternal obesity (prepregnancy weight of ⩾ 90 kg) is a strong indicator of fetal macrosomia and associated with at least 1.5-fold increased risk[23–26]. The increased incidence of fetal macrosomia in obese patients could be due to multiple factors, such as altered metabolic homeostasis with an inherent risk of abnormal glucose metabolism and heredity. Advanced maternal age (> 35 years old) is also a risk factor for fetal macrosomia even after correction for parity and gestational diabetes[27]. Genetic influence may also account for the high correlation between maternal and sibling birthweights and the current neonate's birthweight. Infants with birthweights of ⩾ 4500 g have a seven-fold increased chance or 22% prevalence of having a subsequent sibling with birthweight of ⩾ 4500 g[28].

DIAGNOSING FETAL MACROSOMIA

The next step in the management of patients at risk for fetal macrosomia at term is estimating fetal weight. This can be done by clinical assessment and/or ultrasound examination. Estimation of fetal weight by clinical examination of fundal height is usually inaccurate, especially at the extremes of fetal sizes. A larger-than-expected fundal height may point to the potential for fetal macrosomia. Ultrasonography provides a more accurate means of obtaining an estimated fetal weight (EFW). In general, by using the fetal abdominal circumference (AC) and the biparietal diameter (BPD) or femur length (FL), fetal weights can be estimated based on the published formulas to within 10% and 5% of the actual weight in 80% and 50% of normal fetuses, respectively[29]. It appears that the Hadlock's[30] formula utilizing the AC and FL

$$\log_{10} [\text{weight}] = 1.304 + 0.05281\,\text{AC} + 0.1938\,\text{FL} - 0.004\,\text{AC} \times \text{FL}$$

provides the best estimation of birthweight of macrosomic fetuses[31]. At present, accuracy in predicting birthweight in macrosomic fetuses remains limited. In fact, one study demonstrated a positive predictive value for fetal macrosomia of only 67% when the birthweight is > 4100 g[32]. Another approach utilized the macrosomic index, which is the difference between the fetal chest circumference and the BPD, to identify macrosomic fetuses in pregnancies complicated by diabetes mellitus. In one study, 87% of macrosomic infants had a macrosomic index of ⩾ 1.4 cm. The utility of this index for the prediction of fetal macrosomia remains to be determined[33]. When the gestational age is known, ultrasound examination during the third trimester can be used to identify large-for-gestational-age (LGA) fetuses who are at risk for being macrosomic at delivery. When the EFW or the AC, the latter reflecting insulin-sensitive tissue, or both are above the 90th percentile, macrosomia can be correctly diagnosed in 74% and 88.8% of infants of diabetic mothers, respectively[34]. In pregnancies complicated by diabetes mellitus, accelerated growth of abdominal circumference (above the 90th percentile), which may become apparent as early as 24 weeks of gestation, is associated with increased risk of fetal macrosomia at term[35]. A growth of abdominal circumference of ⩾ 1.2 cm per week during the gestational interval of 32–39 weeks is noted in about 80% of macrosomic infants of diabetic pregnancies[36]. In pregnancies at risk for fetal macrosomia, serial ultrasound examinations (every 3–4 weeks) for EFW and AC starting at about 32.0 weeks of gestation may be helpful in detecting fetal macrosomia.

INTRAPARTUM MANAGEMENT

Once fetal macrosomia is suspected, termination of pregnancy after fetal lung maturity is documented may be considered. In most situations, a trial of labor can be attempted unless there are contraindications such as absolute cephalopelvic disproportion (CPD), placenta previa, vasa previa, malpresentation of the fetus, previous classical Cesarean section, or an EFW > 5000 g. Fetal lung maturity should be documented prior to induction of labor. Amniocentesis for lecithin : sphingomyelin (L : S) ratio and phosphatidylglycerol is generally utilized to document fetal lung maturity in the following situations: (1) uncertain gestational age; (2) gestational age < 39 weeks in non-diabetic pregnancies; and (3) gestational age of < 40 weeks in diabetic pregnancies.

Induction of labor

One of the major concerns about induction of labor in the presence of an unfavorable cervix, i.e. a Bishop score of ⩽ 5, is failed induction resulting in an increased Cesarean section rate[37]. It has been suggested that the prenatal diagnosis of fetal macrosomia by ultrasound makes the obstetricians more likely to perform Cesarean section delivery[38]. To facilitate the induction, cervical ripening can be accomplished by the use of intracervical artificial laminaria (Lumicil) and low-dose continuous oxytocin infusion overnight. The oxytocin infusion is started at 0.5 mU/min and doubled hourly to a maximum dose of 4 mU/min. Usually, mild uterine contractions are obtained at this low dose. This combination of laminaria and low-dose oxytocin infusion is usually sufficient to make the cervix favorable for a full induction of labor the next morning.

Cervidil, a prostaglandin vaginal insert containing 10 mg of dinoprostone, has been shown to shorten the interval from induction to delivery when it is used for cervical ripening. This vaginal insert releases the medication at a rate of about 0.3 mg/h[39]. Alternatively, misoprostol (Cytotec), a PGE_1 given intravaginally at a dosage of 25 µg every 6 hours for a total of four doses, is also effective for cervical ripening and induction of labor. Hyperstimulation and hypertonus of uterine contractions are potential uncommon complications for both Cervidil and Cytotec[40]. The cost of Cytotec is, however, only a fraction of that of Cervidil. Intravenous oxytocin may be given about 4 h after the last dose of misoprostol or 6–12 h after insertion of Cervidil.

Intravenous oxytocin is the drug of choice for induction of labor in the USA. Recently there has been a shift to a lower total dose by starting at a lower concentration and increasing at longer intervals and lesser increments. This change in the usage of oxytocin for induction of labor has been made for the following reasons.

(1) The steady-state oxytocin concentration is not reached until approximately 40 min from the last dose[41,42].

(2) Effective uterine contractions can occur with an oxytocin infusion rate between 4.0 and 8.0 mU/min in the majority of patients (in fact, 95% of patients will develop progressive cervical dilatation with an oxytocin infusion rate of ⩽ 8.0 mU/min)[42–44].

(3) The incidence of uterine hypercontractility and the resulting abnormal heart rate are reduced.

A protocol for the continuous infusion of oxytocin for induction of labor is the following:

- Oxytocin infusion is started at 0.5 mU/min and then doubled every hour up to the rate of 8 mU/min.
- Thereafter, the dose is increased 4 mU/min every hour until the maximum dose of 20 mU/min is reached.

The dose of oxytocin should not be raised further when adequate uterine contractions (i.e. a frequency of 2–3 min, durations of 40–90 s, and intensities of 40–90 mmHg) or progressive cervical dilatation and descent are obtained regardless of how low the oxytocin dose may be. A lower starting dose of oxytocin is preferable because uterine hyperstimulation may occur at very low doses.

Accurate assessment of uterine contractions and optimal fetal heart-rate monitoring are important whenever induction of labor is attempted. This becomes even more important when induction of labor is carried out for impending fetal macrosomia in view of the increased risk of CPD and birth injury. Labor course should be closely monitored for arrest or protraction disorders[21,45,46]. Thus, intrauterine pressure and direct fetal electronic monitoring should be initiated as soon as it is feasible and safe to do so.

Birth injury and shoulder dystocia

The major complication associated with delivery of a macrosomic fetus is birth trauma such as clavicle fracture and subsequent brachial plexus injury from a difficult vaginal delivery[6,45,47–50]. The overall risk of shoulder dystocia rises sharply from 3% for birthweights < 4000 g to 10.3% and 23.9% for the ranges of birthweights between 4000 and 4500 g and > 4500 g, respectively. When birthweights are > 3500 g, the incidence of shoulder dystocia generally doubles in diabetic patients compared to non-diabetic ones for similar birthweights. Thus, the combination of macrosomia and diabetes places the patient at a high risk for neonatal shoulder dystocia[47]. Similarly, diabetes mellitus increases the risk of neonatal brachial plexus injury from vaginal delivery about three-fold compared to the non-diabetic condition[6]. Although there is a strong correlation between birthweight and brachial plexus injury, the latter occurs as a consequence of shoulder dystocia in a majority of patients[51]. Asphyxia and brachial palsy occur in up to 42% of infants with true shoulder dystocia[52].

Shoulder dystocia is associated with significant perinatal morbidity and mortality and usually occurs unexpectedly. It would be ideal if shoulder dystocia could be anticipated and thus could be avoided in pregnancies at risk for this condition. In general, fetal weight or pelvimetry is a poor indicator of CPD or birth trauma. The fetal–pelvic index (FPI) has been introduced to address this issue[7]. First, the anteroposterior (APD) and transverse (TD) diameters of the fetal head and abdomen and the maternal inlet and midpelvis are determined. Fetal and maternal measurements are obtained by ultrasonography and X-ray pelvimetry, respectively. The corresponding circumferences (C) are calculated from the two perpendicular diameters using the formula:

$$C = \frac{[TD + APD] \times 3.14}{2}$$

The FPI is the sum of the two circumference differences (cephalopelvic differences) as the following:

$$FPI = [HC - IC] + [AC - MC]$$

where HC, IC, AC and MC are head circumference, index circumference, abdominal circumference and midpelvis circumference, respectively. A positive FPI indicates the presence of CPD/shoulder dystocia; a negative FPI indicates their absence. The sensitivity and specificity of the FPI in the diagnosis of CPD/shoulder dystocia are both 94%. Further study is needed to determine the predictive value of the FPI in detecting CPD/shoulder dystocia in pregnancies complicated by fetal macrosomia.

Another approach to the detection of shoulder dystocia utilized fetal biometric evaluation. Studies of neonates have demonstrated significant differences in many neonatal anthropometric measurements between newborn infants with and without dystocia. The mean shoulder circumference was significantly larger when shoulder dystocia had complicated delivery[53]. The neonatal bisacromial diameter is well correlated with the ultrasonographically measured circumferences of the fetal chest and arm[54]. Thus, the relationship between fetal chest circumference and other fetal parameters such as head circumference or abdominal circumference may be potentially useful in predicting shoulder dystocia in pregnancies at risk for this condition.

Once a trial of labor is under way, the course of labor should be closely followed by a cervicographic analysis. Protraction and arrest disorders of labor may be associated with an increased risk for shoulder dystocia. Operative vaginal delivery by itself or in combination with an abnormal course of labor may predispose to shoulder dystocia in the case of fetal macrosomia[47,52,55,56]. Thus, it is necessary to be very cautious when selecting an operative vaginal delivery to correct the arrest or protract disorders of descent or cervical dilatation in the presence of fetal macrosomia, especially in a diabetic mother, even though the sensitivity of these clinical parameters in predicting shoulder dystocia is low.

To minimize the perinatal morbidity and mortality associated with shoulder dystocia once it occurs, it is necessary to be ready to initiate the appropriate steps and maneuvers to effect a timely delivery. Time is a critical factor with regard to perinatal mortality and morbidity. The cardinal diagnostic sign of shoulder dystocia is retraction of the delivered head against the maternal perineum due to the obstruction to the passage of both shoulders at the pelvic inlet. This situation more likely arises when both shoulders present to the pelvic inlet from the anteroposterior position instead of an oblique one, and when the shoulder circumferences are large[53,56,57]. Direct traction on the fetal head may be ineffective unless therapeutic fracture of the clavicles is associated. Because the fetus naturally passes through the birth canal with a screw motion, rotation of the shoulder to reduce the shoulder circumference, or rotation to an oblique position, are the underlying mechanisms of most effective maneuvers, as described below[56,58].

McRobert's maneuver

This easily performed maneuver involves a sharp flexion of the patient's thighs onto the abdomen. It accomplishes a straightening of the maternal sacrum relative to the lumbar spine, thus eliminating the sacral promontory as an obstruction, and effects anterior rotation of the pubic symphysis, thus assisting in bringing the fetal posterior shoulder through the pelvic inlet by simultaneously displacing the fetal anterior shoulder cephalad[59].

Woods' maneuver

Woods first described the principle of rotation of the shoulders rather than direct traction on the fetal head to resolve shoulder dystocia. In this classical approach, delivery of the posterior shoulder is accomplished by pressing on the anterior aspect of the posterior shoulder toward the fetal back, while a gentle pressure is placed on the uterus fundus. The posterior shoulder can usually be delivered under the pubic symphysis after a rotation of 180°. The remaining shoulder is similarly delivered by rotating an arc of 180°, but in the opposite direction with pressure on its anterior aspect[58].

Rubin's maneuver

This maneuver applies the same principle of rotation but differs from Woods' maneuver in that adduction instead of abduction of the shoulders is carried out. Adduction is accomplished by pushing the shoulder toward the fetal chest. It should be reemphasized that the adduction is performed with direct pressure on the fetal shoulder, not by rotating the fetal head. This maneuver results in reduction of the shoulder transverse diameter and circumference as well as rotation of the shoulder to the more oblique position[50].

Delivery of the posterior arm

Performance of this maneuver requires locating the fetal elbow with the operator's hand in the vagina. The fetal forearm is then flexed, drawn across the fetal chest, and delivered through the vaginal opening. It would be easier for the operator to use his or her left or right hand depending on whether the fetal back is facing the maternal left or right side, respectively.

Zavanelli maneuver

This maneuver should be used as the last resort when all other maneuvers to effect a vaginal delivery have failed. The maneuver involves returning the fetal head to the vagina by reversing the sequence of the normal birthing process. The fetus is subsequently delivered by Cesarean section from the cephalic presentation. Excellent neonatal outcomes have been reported with this maneuver[60].

Elective Cesarean section

Although macrosomia is associated with an increased incidence of Cesarean section delivery as a result of abnormal labor, such as arrest of descent or cervical dilatation, an estimated fetal weight in the range 4000–4900 g may not be an absolute indication for elective Cesarean section. A trial of labor in patients with ultrasonographic diagnosis of fetal macrosomia resulted in vaginal delivery in about 72% of cases[61]. Furthermore, vaginal birth after previous Cesarean section was shown to occur in 58% and 43% of patients with infant birthweight ranges 4000–4499 g and ≥ 4500 g, respectively, with no higher risk of uterine rupture[62]. However, elective Cesarean delivery may have a role in the management of pregnancies with fetal macrosomia in certain situations. For example, when EFW is > 4500 g or > 5000 g, the birthweight is likely to be ≥ 4000 g or ≥ 4500 g, respectively, assuming 10% error in the estimation. In this range of birthweights (> 4000 g or > 4500 g for diabetic or non-diabetic patients, respectively), the risk for shoulder dystocia is ≥ 20%[47]. Thus, it would not be unreasonable to offer an elective Cesarean section to patients with a macrosomic fetus having an EFW of ≥ 4500 g or ≥ 5000 g in diabetic or non-diabetic patients, respectively. Of course, vaginal delivery should be attempted even in this weight range if the patient has a history of previous vaginal delivery of other infants of similar size or larger. Interestingly, a decision analytic model reveals that elective Cesarean section to prevent permanent brachial plexus injury appears to be cost-effective for estimated fetal weight of $\geqslant 4000$ g in diabetic patients but not cost-effective for estimated weight of $\geqslant 4500$ g in non-diabetic patients[63]. The best approach in managing patients with fetal macrosomia awaits randomized clinical trials.

Another situation involves breech presentation of a macrosomic fetus for which elective Cesarean section delivery after failed external version may be indicated. The American College of Obstetricians and Gynecologists places the upper limit for fetal size of 4000 g when vaginal delivery of a breech fetus is attempted[64]. The patient's prior obstetric history and the obstetrician's experience with breech delivery certainly play a significant role in the decision.

It should be emphasized that, because good data are lacking, individualization is key to the management of macrosomic fetuses in these clinical settings. Regardless of the method of delivery, patients should be well informed of the risks for shoulder dystocia and its sequelae as well as the available options when macrosomia is suspected.

SUGGESTED MANAGEMENT PROTOCOL

An ultrasound examination for estimating fetal weight and determining fetal presentation should be made as early as 37 weeks of gestation in patients at risk for fetal macrosomia. If there has been a question of gestational age, an ultrasound examination should be made prior to 20 weeks of gestation to confirm the date of confinement. Once fetal macrosomia is suspected, fetal lung maturity must be documented before delivery is attempted. Elective Cesarean section may be considered in cases in which the estimated fetal weight is > 5000 g in non-diabetic pregnancies, > 4500 g in diabetic patients, or > 4000 g in breech presentation, recognizing that the exact cutoff level is influenced by the perceived accuracy of sonographic estimates of fetal weight. External version of the breech fetus may be attempted unless there are contraindications such as bleeding, placenta previa or abruption, certain fetal anomalies, oligohydramnios, or premature rupture of membranes[65,66]. The alternative approach would be to obtain the FPI and select the mode of delivery depending on whether the FPI is positive or negative. It should be noted that the FPI has not been tested in a large population of patients to determine its predictive value. If the fetus has an estimated weight between 4000 and 4900 g and presents as vertex, a trial of labor may be conducted provided there are no contraindications. Internal monitoring of fetal heart rate and uterine pressure should be initiated as soon as it is feasible. The course of labor should be closely followed, keeping in mind that an abnormal course of labor may herald a potential CPD and/or shoulder dystocia. Operative vaginal delivery is not recommended because it may be associated with

an unusually high risk of shoulder dystocia and subsequent birth injury.

If shoulder dystocia occurs in spite of the above precautions, timely application of a preplanned sequence of steps and effective maneuvers should be carried out. Time is critical because the risk of fetal brain injury and death increases as the duration of shoulder dystocia advances. Arbitrarily, we recommend trying the McRobert's maneuver first because of its simplicity and effectiveness, followed by the Rubin's maneuver, Woods' maneuver, suprapubic pressure, fundal pressure, and delivery of the posterior arm in decreasing order of preference. The Zavanelli maneuver should be attempted if the above procedures to effect vaginal delivery have failed and sufficient time has elapsed since the occurrence of shoulder dystocia to raise concern about neonatal asphyxia and/or death.

CONCLUSION

The management of fetal macrosomia with an increased risk of shoulder dystocia and its attendant morbidity and mortality remains a challenge for the modern clinician. In spite of many attempts to identify the patient at risk for fetal macrosomia, the perfect predictor has not yet emerged. The physician must therefore rely on clinical skills in raising his or her index of suspicion for fetal macrosomia, and once it is considered, ancillary diagnostic testing should help to confirm the diagnosis. The summation of this information should then be weighed carefully as the plan for delivery is constructed. A well-orchestrated attempt at vaginal delivery or a timely operative delivery can be carried out with a high probability of excellent maternal and fetal outcomes. In cases in which macrosomia with shoulder dystocia is encountered without antecedent warning, foreknowledge of the serial maneuvers that will enable the delivery of the impacted shoulders can minimize fetal injury.

REFERENCES

1. Arias F. Predictability of complications associated with prolongation of pregnancy. *Obstet Gynecol* 1987;70:101–6
2. Boyd ME, Usher RH, McLean FH. Fetal macrosomia: prediction, risks, proposed management. *Obstet Gynecol* 1983;61:715–22
3. Golditch IM, Kirkman K. The large fetus. Management and outcome. *Obstet Gynecol* 1978;52:26–30
4. Chervenak JL, Divon MY, Hirsch J, *et al*. Macrosomia in the postdate pregnancy: is routine ultrasonographic screening indicated? *Am J Obstet Gynecol* 1989;161:753–6
5. Spellacy WN, Miller S, Winegar A, *et al*. Macrosomia – maternal characteristics and infant complications. *Obstet Gynecol* 1985;66:158–61
6. Ecker JL, Greenberg JA, Norwitz ER, *et al*. Birth weight as a predictor of brachial plexus injury. *Obstet Gynecol* 1997;89:643–7

7. Klebanoff MA, Mills JL, Berendes HW. Mother's birth weight as a predictor of macrosomia. *Am J Obstet Gynecol* 1985;153:253–7

8. Morgan MA, Thurnau GR. Efficacy of the fetal–pelvic index for delivery of neonates weighing 4000 grams or greater: a preliminary report. *Am J Obstet Gynecol* 1988;158:1133–7

9. Sohaey R, Nyberg DA, Sickler GK, *et al.* Idiopathic polyhydramnios: association with fetal macrosomia. *Radiology* 1994;190:393–6

10. Coustan DR, Imarah J. Prophylactic insulin treatment of gestational diabetes reduces the incidence of macrosomia, operative delivery, and birth trauma. *Am J Obstet Gynecol* 1984;150:836–42

11. Goldberg JD, Franklin B, Lasser D, *et al.* Gestational diabetes: impact of home glucose monitoring on neonatal birth weight. *Am J Obstet Gynecol* 1986;154:546

12. Lin CC, River J, River P, *et al.* Good diabetic control early in pregnancy and favorable fetal outcome. *Obstet Gynecol* 1986;67:51–6

13. Morris MA, Grandis AS, Litton JC. Glycosylated hemoglobin concentration in early gestation associated with neonatal outcome. *Am J Obstet Gynecol* 1985;153:651–4

14. Willman SP, Leveno KJ, Guzick DS, *et al.* Glucose threshold for macrosomia in pregnancy complicated by diabetes. *Am J Obstet Gynecol* 1986;154:470–5

15. Langer O, Brustman L, Anyaegbunam A, *et al.* The significance of one abnormal glucose tolerance test value on adverse outcome in pregnancy. *Am J Obstet Gynecol* 1987;157:758–63

16. Lindsay MK, Graves W, Klein L. The relationship of one abnormal glucose tolerance test value and pregnancy complications. *Obstet Gynecol* 1989;73:103–6

17. Pedersen J, Bojsen-Moller B, Paulsen H. Blood sugar in newborn infants of diabetic mothers. *Acta Endocrinol* 1954;15:33–52

18. Sosenko IR, Kitzmiller JL, Loo SW, *et al.* The infant of the diabetic mother. *New Engl J Med* 1979;301:859

19. Susa JB, McCormick KL, Widness JA, *et al.* Chronic hyperinsulinemia in the fetal rhesus monkey: effects on fetal growth and composition. *Diabetes* 1979;28:1058–63

20. Widness JA, Schwartz HC, Thompson D, *et al.* Glyco-hemoglobin (HbA_{1c}): a predictor of birth weight in infants of diabetic mothers. *J Pediatr* 1978;92:8–12

21. Yatscoff RW, Mehta A, Dean H. Cord blood glycosylated (glycated) hemoglobin: correlation with maternal glycosylated (glycated) hemoglobin and birth weight. *Am J Obstet Gynecol* 1985;152:861–6

22. Schwartz R, Gruppuso PA, Petzold K, *et al.* Hyperinsulinemia and macrosomia in the fetus of the diabetic mother. *Diabetes Care* 1994;17:640–8

23. Edwards LE, Dickes WF, Alton IR, *et al.* Pregancy in the massively obese. Course, outcome, and obesity prognosis of the infant. *Am J Obstet Gynecol* 1978;131:479–83

24. Gross T, Sokol RJ, King K. Obesity in pregnancy. Risks and outcome. *Obstet Gynecol* 1980;56:446–50

25. Philipson EH, Kalhan SC, Edelbert SC, *et al.* Maternal obesity as a risk factor in gestational diabetes. *Am J Perinatol* 1985;2:268–70

26. Wolfe HM, Zador IE, Gross TL, *et al.* The clinical utility of maternal body mass index in pregnancy. *Am J Obstet Gynecol* 1991;164:1306–10

27. Kirz DS, Dorchester W, Freeman RK. Advanced maternal age. The mature gravida. *Am J Obstet Gynecol* 1985;152:7–12

28. Davis R, Woelk G, Mueller BA, *et al.* The role of previous birthweight on risk for macrosomia in a subsequent birth. *Epidemiology* 1995;6:607–11

29. Shepard MJ, Richards VA, Berkowitz RL, *et al.* An evaluation of two equations for predicting fetal weight by ultrasound. *Am J Obstet Gynecol* 1982;142:47–54

30. Hadlock FB, Harrist RB, Sharman RS, *et al.* Estimation of fetal weight with the use of head, body, and femur measurements: a prospective study. *Am J Obstet Gynecol* 1985;151:333–7

31. Hirata GI, Medearis AL, Horenstein J, *et al.* Ultrasonographic estimation of fetal weight in the clinically macrosomic fetus. *Am J Obstet Gynecol* 1990;162:238–42

32. Miller JM Jr, Haywood LB, Oscar FK, *et al.* Ultrasonographic identification of the macrosomic fetus. *Am J Obstet Gynecol* 1988;159:1110–4

33. Elliott JP, Garite TJ, Freeman RK, *et al.* Ultrasonic prediction of fetal macrosomia in diabetic patients. *Obstet Gynecol* 1982;60:159–62

34. Tamura RK, Sabbagha RE, Depp R, *et al.* Diabetic macrosomia – accuracy of third trimester ultrasound. *Obstet Gynecol* 1986;67:828–32

35. Keller JD, Metzger BE, Dooley SL, *et al.* Infants of diabetic mothers with accelerated fetal growth by ultrasonography: are they all alike? *Am J Obstet Gynecol* 1990;163:893–7

36. Landon MB, Mintz MC, Gabbe SG. Sonographic evaluation of fetal abdominal growth: predictor of large-for-gestational age infant in pregnancies complicated by diabetes mellitus. *Am J Obstet Gynecol* 1989;160:115–21

37. Combs CA, Singh NB, Khoury JC. Elective induction versus spontaneous labor after sonographic diagnosis of fetal macrosomia. *Obstet Gynecol* 1993;81:492–6

38. Weeks JW, Pitman T, Spinnato JA II. Fetal macrosomia: does antenatal prediction affect delivery route and birth outcome? *Am J Obstet Gynecol* 1995;173:1215–19

39. Rayburn WF. Prostaglandin E_2 gel for cervical ripening and induction of labor: a critical analysis. *Am J Obstet Gynecol* 1989;160:529–34

40. Wing DA, Paul RH. A comparison of differing dosing regimens of misoprostol for cervical ripening and labor induction: interim analysis. *Am J Obstet Gynecol* 1996;175:158–64

41. Amico JA, Seitch J, Robinson AG. Studies of oxytocin in plasma of women during hypocontractile labor. *J Clin Endocrinol Metab* 1984;58:274–9

42. Seitchik J, Castillo M. Oxytocin augmentation of dysfunctional labor. I. Clinical data. *Am J Obstet Gynecol* 1982;144:899–905

43. Baxi LV, Petrie RH, Caritis SN. Induction of labor with low-dose prostaglandin $F_{2\alpha}$ and oxytocin. *Am J Obstet Gynecol* 1980;136:28–31

44. Seitchik J, Castillo M. Oxytocin augmentation of dysfunctional labor. III. Multiparous patients. *Am J Obstet Gynecol* 1983;145:777–80

45. Oppenheim WL, Davis A, Growdon WA, *et al.* Clavicle fractures in the newborn. *Clin Orthop* 1990;250:176–80

46. Turner MJ, Rasmussen MJ, Turner JE, *et al.* The influence of birth weight on labor in nulliparas. *Obstet Gynecol* 1990;76:159–63

47. Acker DB, Sachs BP, Friedman EA. Risk factors for shoulder dystocia. *Obstet Gynecol* 1985;66:762–8

48. Acker DB, Gregory KD, Sachs BP, *et al.* Risk factors for Erb–Duchenne palsy. *Obstet Gynecol* 1988;71:389

49. Gordon M, Rich H, Deutschberger J, *et al.* The immediate and long-term outcome of obstetric birth trauma. I. Brachial plexus paralysis. *Am J Obstet Gynecol* 1973; 117:51–6

50. Rubin A. Management of shoulder dystocia. *J Am Med Assoc* 1964;189:835–7

51. McFarland LV, Raskin M, Daling JR, *et al.* Erb/ Duchenne's palsy: a consequence of fetal macrosomia and method of delivery. *Obstet Gynecol* 1986;68:784–8

52. Gross SJ, Shime J, Farine D. Shoulder dystocia: predictors and outcome. A five-year review. *Am J Obstet Gynecol* 1987;156:334–6

53. Modanlou HD, Komatsu G, Dorchester W, *et al.* Large-for-gestational-age neonates: anthropometric reasons for shoulder dystocia. *Obstet Gynecol* 1982;60:417–23

54. Winn HN, Grasso J, Holcomb W, *et al.* The potential of fetal chest circumference in the prenatal diagnosis of shoulder dystocia. In *Proceedings of the 9th Annual Society of Perinatal Obstetricians Meeting*, New Orleans: Society of Perinatal Obstetricians, 1989:274

55. Benedetti TJ, Gabbe SG. Shoulder dystocia: a complication of fetal macrosomia and prolonged second stage of labor with mid-pelvic delivery. *Obstet Gynecol* 1978; 52:526–9

56. Hopwood HG. Shoulder dystocia: fifteen years' experience in a community hospital. *Am J Obstet Gynecol* 1982; 144:162–6

57. Smeltzer JS. Prevention and management of shoulder dystocia. *Clin Obstet Gynecol* 1986;29:2

58. Woods CE, Westbery A. Principle of physics as applicable to shoulder delivery. *Am J Obstet Gynecol* 1943; 45:796–804

59. Gonik B, Stringer CA, Held B. An alternate maneuver for management of shoulder dystocia. *Am J Obstet Gynecol* 1983;145:882–4

60. Sandberg ED. The Zavanelli maneuver: a potentially revolutionary method for the resolution of shoulder dystocia. *Am J Obstet Gynecol* 1985;152:479–84

61. Delpapa EH, Mueller-Heubach E. Pregnancy outcome following ultrasound diagnosis of macrosomia. *Obstet Gynecol* 1991;78:340–3

62. Flamm BL, Goings JR. Vaginal birth after Cesarean section: is suspected fetal macrosomia a contraindication? *Obstet Gynecol* 1989;74:694–7

63. Rouse DJ, Owen J, Goldenberg RL, *et al.* The effectiveness and cost of elective Cesarean delivery for fetal macrosomia diagnosis by ultrasound. *J Am Med Assoc* 1996;276:1480–6

64. The American College of Obstetricians and Gynecologists. *Management of the breech presentation*. Technical Bulletin number 95. Washington, DC: ACOG, 1986

65. Marchick R. Antepartum external cephalic version with tocolysis: a study of term singleton breech presentations. *Am J Obstet Gynecol* 1988;158:1339–46

66. Morrison JC, Myatt RE, Martin JN, *et al.* External cephalic version of the breech presentation under tocolysis. *Am J Obstet Gynecol* 1986;154:900–3

62

Fetal oxygenation and acidosis

H.N. Winn and R.H. Petrie

INTRODUCTION

All living things, including the human fetus, require energy to carry out the various life functions and processes. The energy form under consideration here is adenosine triphosphate (ATP). The fetus requires ATP to function and carry out appropriate metabolic functions. Normally, ATP is produced by Krebs' cycle, where ATP, water, and carbon dioxide are produced. To function optimally, an adequate supply of oxygen is required in Krebs' cycle. When fetal oxygen deprivation occurs and Krebs' cycle does not produce sufficient ATP, then a non-oxidative process is employed to produce ATP. The Embden–Meyerhof pathway produces smaller amounts of ATP, and the byproducts are pyruvic and lactic acids. Pyruvic acid is rapidly converted into lactic acid. Lactic acid in sufficiently great concentration may cause brain cell damage. The brain cell wall becomes permeable to water, causing the cytoplasm to swell to a point at which cell wall integrity can no longer be maintained, and the brain cell undergoes lysis. Obviously, with sufficient concentrations of lactic acid and the corresponding loss of sufficient numbers of brain cells, fetal neurological damage or even death may ensue.

As it is currently understood, fetal oxygen deprivation is a function of an inadequate supply of oxygen delivered to the fetus as a result of reduced blood flow from the maternal circulation to the placenta and the intervillous space. This form of fetal oxygen deprivation, uteroplacental insufficiency, may have its clinical cause in problems such as maternal hypotension, maternal hypertension, uterine hyperactivity, and severe forms of anemia. In the placental intervillous space, oxygen from the maternal red cell is exchanged for carbon dioxide coming from the fetal circulation as the fetal red cell then takes up oxygen from the mother. Oxygen is then transported to the fetus via the fetal–placental circulation through the umbilical cord. Because the umbilical cord has no rigid protective support, it is possible to interrupt blood flow and the delivery of oxygen to the fetus by umbilical cord compression. Varying degrees of umbilical cord compression, ranging from minor repetitive compression with contractions to the somewhat devastating potential of an umbilical cord prolapse through the cervix with major or total compression, are noted in the majority of all labor processes. Usually, these are minor and do not require major interventions; however, on occasion, cord compression may produce sufficient oxygen deprivation to necessitate an early delivery by the use of early, instrument-assisted delivery or by Cesarean section.

Alteration in blood flow resulting in oxygen deprivation to the fetus may vary in the degree of reduction and duration. Although a fetus may be exposed to reduced oxygenation that is sufficient to cause intrauterine growth restriction over many months, it may cause minimal or no obvious effect on or damage to brain cells. The obstetrician may recognize that chronic fetal oxygen deprivation can be expected in certain disorders, such as the hypertensive diseases in pregnancy, intrauterine growth restriction, diabetes, and prolonged gestation, and that there are few techniques available to detect the degree or severity of chronic fetal oxygen deprivation. In some instances, there may be sufficient oxygen deprivation prior to the onset of labor to cause brain damage. Blood flow and fetal oxygen supply may subsequently be ameliorated, with normal surveillance parameters of fetal oxygenation during labor, and a resultantly impaired neonate may be noted some time following delivery.

The form of intrapartum fetal oxygen deprivation which the obstetrician is currently equipped to recognize and manage is acute fetal oxygen deprivation due to alterations in uteroplacental or fetal–placental blood flow delivery of oxygen to the fetus. Although it is well recognized that severe forms of anemia, abnormal hemoglobin structure, and various anatomical abnormalities may result in fetal oxygen deprivation, by far the most common cause is uteroplacental insufficiency. It is recognized that labor itself provides the potential for primary fetal oxygen deprivation, as well as an additive amount of deprivation that may cause a prelabor borderline supply of oxygen to the fetus to become an overt fetal oxygen deprivation sufficient to cause morbidity or mortality. The manner in which this occurs is relatively simple. The intramyometrial pressure rises during a uterine contraction, as a function of that contraction. If this elevation in pressure becomes greater than the pressure responsible for providing blood flow to the placenta, then a decrease in flow occurs. Normally, the fetus is able to tolerate this; however, if uterine activity is too great in either duration or intensity, there may be sufficient oxygen deprivation to cause a problem. Likewise, fetal–placental blood flow may be interrupted, causing fetal oxygen deprivation by umbilical cord compression, as previously described.

An infant that is markedly depressed at birth, as evidenced by very low Apgar scores, marked fetal metabolic acidosis, seizure activity shortly after birth, and evidence of other neonatal organ system insult or damage, may point to intrapartum fetal oxygen deprivation of the acute type, which is sufficiently severe to bring about permanent neurological impairment[1].

METHODS OF SURVEILLANCE FOR FETAL OXYGEN DEPRIVATION

In the early 1960s, intermittent intrapartum fetal surveillance by the collection of fetal capillary blood for determination of pH was introduced. Subsequently, with the use of fetal pH and P_{CO_2}, levels, bicarbonate and base excess have been available to evaluate fetal oxygenation. This advance occurred at a time when intermittent stethoscopic evaluation of fetal heart rate was the only reliable method of intrapartum fetal surveillance. Normal intermittent intrapartum fetal heart-rate data were very reliable indicators to allow the labor to continue without worry of fetal oxygen deprivation. A number of fetuses demonstrated abnormal fetal heart-rate data during labor, which caused the obstetrician to think about methods that would enhance the diagnosis of significant fetal oxygen deprivation. The use of intermittent pH determinations from fetal scalp capillary blood collection in instances of normal values enabled the obstetrician to extend the time that a fetus could be comfortably left *in utero* when abnormal fetal heart-rate data were obtained. With abnormal pH values, there is an increased probability of fetal oxygen deprivation when both fetal heart rate and acid–base surveillance indicate that the fetus may be experiencing fetal oxygen deprivation.

For almost two centuries, fetal heart rate has been used as a way to determine whether the fetus was alive or dead. More recently, when it became important to evaluate fetal oxygenation, a number of investigators have found that normal intrapartum fetal heart-rate data are highly predictive of a healthy fetus. Abnormal fetal heart-rate data are considerably less predictive of a fetus with significant oxygen deprivation. Accordingly, the principal value of fetal heart-rate surveillance is that normal data, being the most predictive value for a healthy fetus, allow the labor to continue toward its completion without significant concern for fetal damage or death secondary to oxygen deprivation.

Surveillance of the amniotic fluid as a potential marker for fetal oxygen deprivation involves an evaluation for volume as well as for the presence of meconium in the amniotic fluid. The presence of a normal amount of amniotic fluid without the presence of meconium is more significantly associated with a normal fetal oxygenation state than the presence of oligohydramnios is associated with fetal oxygen deprivation. Nevertheless, the presence of oligohydramnios, particularly in conditions such as prolonged gestation, may be associated with an increased likelihood for problems during the intrapartum period, including the potential for fetal oxygen deprivation. Developmental abnormalities, including abnormal chromosomes, and various metabolic and infectious problems, may be associated with abnormal amniotic fluid volumes.

The principal screening surveillance technique for the intrapartum evaluation of the fetal oxygenation state is fetal heart-rate monitoring[2]. The presence of normal fetal heart-rate data during the intrapartum period usually indicates that there is no fetal oxygen deprivation. With normal fetal heart-rate data, most investigators consider that it is safe to allow labor to continue toward completion and delivery. Fetal heart-rate monitoring is accomplished by two methods: intermittent determinations of the fetal heart rate and continuous electronic calculation and recording of the fetal heart rate.

Intermittent fetal heart-rate monitoring

This is currently performed by three different methods. The first is the use of a Doppler/ultrasound device that is handheld with a transducer placed over the gravid abdomen. The fetal heart tones are detected and manual counting is carried out. Each time that the fetal heart rate is determined, it should be recorded in the patient's chart. In a similar technique, a stethoscope is placed over the gravid abdomen and the actual heart tones are obtained, counted, and manually recorded in the patient's chart. The third technique involves the intermittent use of a continuous electronic fetal heart-rate monitor (either external or internal) to detect, instantaneously calculate, and automatically record the fetal heart rate on graphic tracing.

Intermittent fetal heart-rate monitoring is generally performed according to guidelines provided by the American College of Obstetricians and Gynecologists[2]. This technique for the evaluation of fetal oxygenation can be used in almost all low-risk pregnancy labors, as well as most appropriately selected high-risk pregnancy labors. A stethoscope (fetoscope) or a handheld Doppler device is used to listen to the fetal heart tones for evaluation. The interval used for counting fetal heart rate varies from several brief intervals (5–15 s) to longer intervals (30–60 s). Occasionally, listening for several minutes continuously in order to ensure a rate is recommended.

The frequency of fetal heart-rate determinations depends on the probability of fetal oxygen deprivation. It is recommended that for low-risk patients, the fetal heart rate should be determined at least every hour in the latent phase of labor, every 30 min in the active phase of labor, and every 15 min during the second stage of labor. When monitoring high-risk patients, it is recommended that the fetal heart rate be determined every 30 min during the first stage of labor and in latent phase labor, every 15 min in active phase labor, and every 5 min during the second stage of labor. It is important that, when intermittent fetal heart-rate surveillance is used, the frequency of fetal heart-rate determination not only be adhered to by patient risk category, but the rate must be also recorded in the patient's chart on each and every occasion that the fetal heart rate is determined. In addition to these intervals, it is further recommended that the fetal heart rate be taken during labor in the following situations:

(1) initiation of labor-enhancing procedures (e.g. artificial amniotomy);

(2) periods of ambulation;

(3) administration of medication and administration or initiation of anesthesia/analgesia, including recognition of abnormal uterine activity patterns such as increased basal tones or tachysystole;

(4) evaluation of oxytocin (maintenance, increase, or decrease of doses);

(5) administration of medicine (at a time of peak action);

(6) expulsion of an enema; urinary catheterization; vaginal examination; and

(7) evaluation of anesthesia or analgesia (maintenance, increase, or decrease of doses).

When using intermittent Doppler/stethoscopic fetal heart-rate monitoring, traditionally reassuring rates have varied from 110 to 120 beats per minute at the lower range and 150 to 160 beats per minute at the upper range. It is normal to note the presence of fetal heart rate accelerations in the absence of decelerations following contractions. The fetal rate of 100 to 119 beats per minute in the absence of other non-reassuring fetal heart-rate data is generally not associated with fetal compromise. Non-reassuring fetal heart-rate data include baseline fetal heart rate of < 100 beats per minute (it should be noted that a moderate bradycardia of 80–100 beats per minute may be associated with fetal head compression and not necessarily associated with non-reassuring patterns), a fetal heart rate of < 100 beats per minute 30 s after a contraction, an unexplained fetal baseline tachycardia > 160 beats per minute, especially if tachycardia persist through three or more contractions in spite of corrective measures.

Using the intermittent stethoscopic/Doppler form of fetal heart-rate monitoring during labor, when it is ascertained that an abnormality may exist, the use of additional methods of evaluation for potential fetal oxygenation are employed and include external continuous fetal cardiotocography, internal continuous fetal cardiotocography, fetal scalp blood sampling for acid–base determinations, or fetal stimulatory data that correlate fetal heart-rate accelerations to acid–base data to gain commentary regarding fetal acid–base status. This often includes umbilical cord arterial and venous respiratory blood gas determinations at delivery.

Continuous electronic fetal heart-rate monitoring

This is performed by two methods[3,4]. External continuous fetal heart-rate monitoring is carried out extra-amniotically from transducers that are placed on the gravid abdomen overlying the fetal heart. Currently, the most commonly used technique is that of a Doppler/ultrasound device that detects one of four cardiac events (aortic opening, aortic closing, mitral opening, or mitral closing); with each beat of the fetal heart, the cardiotachometer instantaneously calculates and causes the rate to be recorded on a graph. Other signals used for external or extraamniotic fetal heart-rate monitoring include use of an abdominal microphone to detect the 'lub dub' of the fetal heart and instantaneously calculate and record rate. This can also be accomplished by the use of multiple electro-cardiographic electrodes placed on the maternal abdomen to obtain the fetal electrocardiogram (EKG) and thus calculate rate from the 'R' wave of the fetal EKG. Phonocardiographic and electrocardiographic techniques, while they can be used for some patients during labor, are not generally applicable for technical reasons, and the most commonly used external technique for continuous fetal heart-rate monitoring is that of Doppler ultrasound. A tocodynamometer is positioned over the gravid uterus to detect uterine activity from the changing uterus curvature during a contraction.

Once the cervix dilates to 1–2 cm and the chorioamnion is or has been ruptured, an electrode may be applied to the fetal presenting part for the collection of fetal electrocardiographic signals as well as the placement of an intrauterine pressure catheter for measuring intraamniotic pressures. The transducers from the intraamniotic or internal fetal heart-rate monitoring are attached to an electronic monitor, where continuous instantaneously calculated and recorded fetal heart rate is displayed on a continuous graphic tracing. The value of internal continuous electronic monitoring over external continuous fetal heart-rate monitoring and intermittent fetal heart-rate monitoring is that, with an electrode attached to the fetal presenting part and with an intrauterine pressure catheter positioned, precise information regarding fetal heart rate and uterine activity is available on a continuous basis. With external monitoring, some degree of variation in rate may occur due to non-predictability in the selection of one of the four cardiac events (aortic opening, aortic closing, mitral opening, and mitral closing). At the same time, when a tocody-namometer is used to detect uterine activity, precision relating to quantitation of uterine activity in terms of frequency, duration, and amplitude of a contraction is lost, whereas the use of intrauterine pressure to represent uterine contractions is a continuous and quantita-tively precise database for evaluation.

Some critics of continuous fetal heart-rate monitor-ing believe that monitoring requires the patient to stay in bed once monitoring begins, not allowing her to be up walking and moving about. Both internal and external monitoring by radiotelemetry is now possible. Telemetry will allow the entire labor to be accom-plished away from a labor bed while still providing continuous information regarding fetal heart rate and uterine activity.

Using internal monitoring, the 'R' wave from the fetal EKG is obtained and the temporal interval between each 'R–R' interval is measured in milli-seconds. A calculation for rate is made based on the assumption that the 'R–R' interval would be uniform for a whole minute. Each 'R–R' interval's rate is indi-vidually recorded. For a rate of 120 beats per minute, the 'R–R' interval is 500 ms. Instantaneously calcu-lated fetal heart rate and intrauterine pressure are recorded on graph paper that moves uniformly at a given speed. Usually the graph paper speed is 3 cm/min, although 1 cm/min may be used to save paper. Vertical scaling is from 30 to 240 beats per minute and covers a 7-cm vertical distance and from 0 to 100 mmHg over a 4-cm vertical distance. Generally, wider vertical lines occur once every minute (Figure 1). Although graph paper or tracing can be used to write notes upon and record vital signs and time markers for the labor, some manufacturers provide spontaneous documentation of time and the ability to record other clinical information that may be important. After deli-very, the fetal heart rate tracing is generally micro-filmed or electronically stored and becomes available as a permanent part of the patient's medical record.

Intermittent vs. continuous monitoring

A recent meta-analysis comparing intermittent fetal heart rate (FHR) monitoring and continuous electronic fetal monitoring (EFM) reveals that the latter signifi-cantly reduces the incidence of perinatal mortality due to fetal hypoxia by approximately 60%, from 1.8 per 1000 births in the auscultation group to 0.7 per 1000 births in the EFM group[5]. In addition, compared to intermittent fetal heart rate monitoring, EFM also has significantly higher positive and negative predictive val-ues for fetal acidosis, either metabolic, respiratory, or mixed. Fetal acidosis is defined as umbilical artery pH < 7.15 or umbilical vein pH < 7.20[6]. On the other hand, EFM significantly increases the rates of Cesarean sections and operative vaginal deliveries[5]. It is impor-tant to evaluate FHR frequently during the continuous monitoring of FHR so that prompt and proper inter-vention can be done to alleviate fetal hypoxia and/or acidosis. The American College of Obstetricians and Gynecologists recommends that FHR be evaluated at least every 15 min during the active phase of labor and at least every 5 min during the second stage of labor[2].

INTERPRETATION OF ELECTRONIC FETAL HEART-RATE MONITORING
Baseline fetal heart rate

When using continuous FHR monitoring, the baseline FHR is the approximate mean rate rounded to nearest increments of 5 beats per minute during an interval of 10 min or greater, excluding periodic or episodic changes or marked FHR variability. Bradycardia or tachycardia exists if the baseline FHR is < 110 or > 160 beats per minute, respectively[7]. Although the base-line FHR of 110–160 beats per minute is considered the normal range, baseline FHR in the ranges of 90–110 and 160–180 beats per minute is not uncom-mon nor necessarily abnormal in the absence of other abnormal FHR markers. Persistent fetal bradycardia or tachycardia, without other markers, while representing a relatively low potential fetal oxygen deprivation or acidosis, is slightly more likely to be associated with some degree of fetal oxygen deprivation than a normal rate. Other conditions may cause a fetal tachycardia or a fetal bradycardia. Maternal fever, fetal infection, maternal thyrotoxicosis, fetal anemia, fetal infection and fetal tachyarrhythmias may cause fetal tachycardia. Fetal tachycardia may develop after maternal adminis-tration of certain drugs such as beta-sympathomimetic tocolytic agents or vagolytic agents such as scopo-lamine or atropine. Fetal bradycardia may be observed in patients who receive pharmacological agents such as beta-blockers (e.g. propranolol), in fetal posterior cephalic position, and in fetal congenital heart block. At the gestational age of 24–26 weeks, the presence of unexplained fetal bradycardia (< 100 beats per minute) or tachycardia (> 160 beats per minute) within an hour of delivery has been associated with an increased incidence of neonatal death[8].

Sinusoidal fetal heart-rate

A sinusoidal fetal heart rate occurs infrequently, but may be of considerable clinical importance. The baseline rate is usually within the normal range of 110 to 160 beats per minute. The pattern is relatively smooth and has a somewhat undulating pattern of uniform variability with an aptitude of 5–20 beats per minute that resembles a sine wave (Figure 1). The sinusoidal FHR pattern can be seen in fetal anemia, fetal intracranial hemorrhage[9], maternal hypothermia[10], and maternal administration of narcotics such as meperidine, alphaprodine, and butorphanol.

A physiological mechanism for this FHR pattern is unknown. A number of investigators believe that this may represent an abnormal neurological control of the heart rate, which may result from varying degrees of fetal oxygen deprivation. The presence of a persistent non-pharmacologically induced fetal sinusoidal heart rate is generally thought to represent potential fetal oxygen deprivation. To allow labor to continue, it is necessary to obtain information regarding fetal anemia and fetal acid–base status. This may be obtained either by direct capillary blood collection for acid–base status and hematocrit or by stimulation of the fetus to evoke a fetal heart-rate acceleration.

Fetal heart-rate variability

Fetal heart rate variability is defined as fluctuations in the baseline FHR of at least 2 cycles per minute. The distinction between short-term (beat-to-beat) variability and long-term variability is unnecessary because the fluctuations of FHR are visually determined as a unit. The amplitude of FHR variability is measured in beats per minute from the peak to the trough of the baseline FHR fluctuating cycle. The baseline FHR variability is the average of the amplitudes within the 10-min interval and is classified as the following: (1) absent FHR variability: undetectable amplitude; (2) minimal FHR variability: undetectable < amplitude ⩽ 5 beats per minute (Figure 2); (3) moderate FHR variability: 6 beats per minute ⩽ amplitude ⩽ 25 beats per minute (Figure 3); and (4) marked FHR variability: amplitude > 25 beats per minute[7]. Fetal heart-rate variability is perhaps the most reliable indicator of fetal well-being that is available to the obstetrician. Fetal heart-rate variability represents an interplay between the cardio-accelerator and cardio-inhibitor centers in the fetal brain stem. Physiologically under normal nervous system control, it is unusual for the fetal heart rate to be steady at one constant number. Normal fetal heart rate variability recorded on a graph represents one of the best indicators of intact integration between the nervous system of the fetus and the fetal cardiovascular system. Although the loss of fetal heart-rate variability potentially may suggest fetal hypoxia, other factors may be

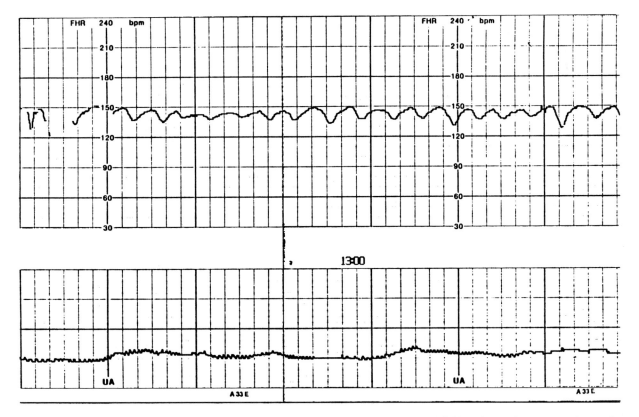

Figure 1 Fetal heart-rate tracing reveals a sinusoidal pattern with a long-term variability of 5–10 beats per minute (bpm). The fetus has severe anemia from erythroblastosis

responsible, including fetal sleep state, pharmacological agents that depress the central nervous system, a fetal tachycardia > 180 beats per minute, and anomalies of the heart and central nervous system. Maternal intake of magnesium sulfate may decrease the FHR beat-to-beat variability but not FHR long-term variability within 1 hour of intravenous administration[11]. It is possible for a fetus of a gestational age of $\geqslant$ 26 weeks to demonstrate normal fetal heart-rate variability.

Marked fetal heart-rate variability may indicate a shift in the P_{O_2}–P_{CO_2} relationship, which the barochemoreceptors mediate without the presence of significant or repetitive fetal heart-rate decelerations. There generally is no significant clinical alteration in fetal oxygenation. The presence of increased fetal heart-rate variability that is followed by loss of FHR variability may indicate potential fetal oxygen deprivation. Without other significant markers of potential fetal oxygen deprivation, a reduction or loss of fetal heart-rate variability represents a potential of < 2% for a significant degree of fetal oxygen deprivation.

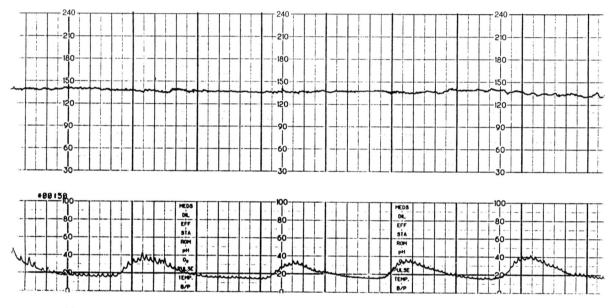

Figure 2   Fetal heart-rate (FHR) tracing reveals a baseline of 140 beats per minute and minimal FHR variability

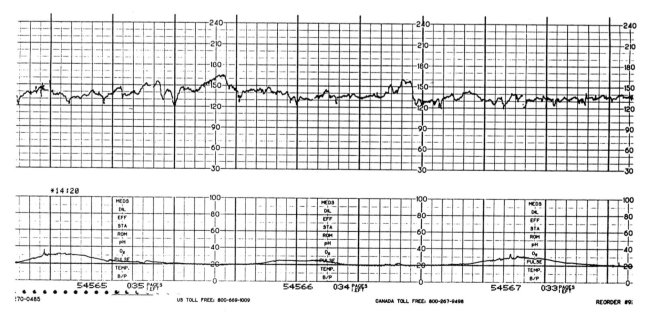

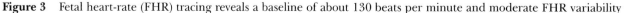

Figure 3   Fetal heart-rate (FHR) tracing reveals a baseline of about 130 beats per minute and moderate FHR variability

Fetal arrhythmias may manifest as regular and irregular irregularities of the fetal heart rate (Figure 4). When these occur, a continuous tracing of the electrocardiographic signals that the fetal monitor is using may be traced via an electrocardiographic monitor. In this manner, the obstetrician may evaluate the presence of P, QRS, and T waves of the fetal cardiac signals. Although most fetal cardiac arrhythmias are transient and of little clinical significance, some have been associated with potential fetal compromise. Fetal supraventricular tachycardia may evoke heart failure and hydrops. A persistent rate of 50–70 beats per minute may represent a complete heart block. Approximately 40% of fetuses with a rate between 50 and 70 beats per minute have congenital heart disease; ventricular septal defects especially are noted. Fetal heart failure and hydrops have been associated with congenital heart block. A persistent fetal rate between 40 and 80 beats per minute can be evaluated by fetal capillary blood sampling or stimulatory test for accelerations to gain commentary regarding acid–base status. A number of fetuses with a persistent bradycardia secondary to an arteriovenous block in this range will have a normal acid–base status and can tolerate labor well.

Periodic heart rate or fetal heart-rate patterns

These are transient alterations in the fetal heart rate associated with uterine contractions. They may be transient increases or transient decreases in heart rate, which are referred to as accelerations or decelerations. Generally, these transient changes are temporally related to the onset of a contraction and return to baseline heart rate prior to the onset of the next contraction.

Fetal heart-rate acceleration

Fetal heart rate acceleration is defined as a visually abrupt increase in FHR at least 15 beats per minute above the baseline with duration between 15 s and 2 min[7]. The onset of acceleration to the peak must be < 30 s. Prior to 32 weeks, accelerations exist if the increase in FHR is ⩾ 10 beats per minute above the baseline and the duration is ⩾ 10 s. Acceleration is prolonged if the duration is ⩾ 2 min but < 10 min[7].

An acceleration in the fetal heart rate may occur at any time, but is frequently associated with a contraction (Figure 3). Generally, the acceleration is thought to represent early or mild cord compression and is a sympathetic nervous system response. The fetal heart-rate acceleration perhaps represents adequate fetal oxygenation.

Fetal heart decelerations

There are four forms of fetal heart decelerations that may be noted during the course of labor.

Early deceleration

This is generally thought to be secondary to fetal head compression as the head moves through the dilating

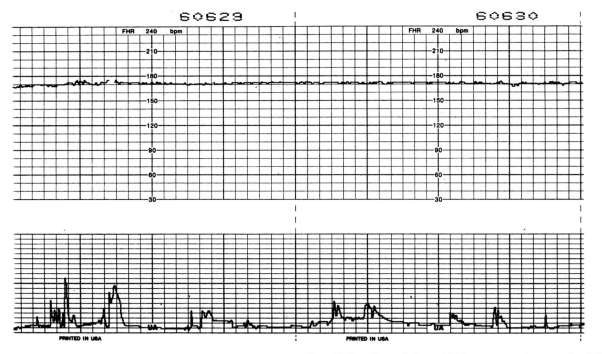

Figure 4 Fetal heart-rate (FHR) tracing reveals fetal tachycardia with baseline of about 170 beats per minute and minimal FHR variability. Fetal arrhythmia is demonstrated by the frequent and very short pause of the fetal heart rate

cervix and the bony pelvis. Early deceleration is defined as a visually apparent gradual decrease and return of FHR to the baseline associated with a uterine contraction. The duration from the onset of the decrease to the nadir of FHR must be ≥ 30 s[7]. Early deceleration is termed such in as much as deceleration begins as the contraction begins, and it represents an inverted mirror image of the uterine contraction, reaching its greatest point of deceleration as the acme of the contraction is reached and returning to baseline as the contraction is terminated (Figure 5). Early deceleration is mediated by the vagus nerve with the release of acetylcholine at the sinoatrial node. It does not fall below 110–100 beats per minute. Classical early deceleration has been demonstrated by a number of studies to be completely innocuous and does not represent any degree of fetal oxygen deprivation or acidosis[12–15] (Tables 1 and 2).

Variable deceleration

Variable deceleration of FHR is defined as a visually apparent abrupt decrease in FHR associated with a uterine contraction. The duration from the onset of the decrease to the nadir of FHR must be < 30 s. The amplitude of the decrease in FHR must be ⩾ 15 beats per minute and the duration of the decrease is ⩾ 15 s

but < 2 min[7]. This may begin before, at the onset of, or following the onset of a uterine contraction. On occasion, it may be seen independent of a uterine contraction. Variable deceleration usually drops many beats per minute in absolute rate within a few fetal heart beats. It is occasionally referred to as the V- or W-shape deceleration because of this sudden drop and often a sudden return to baseline (Figure 5). It is somewhat jagged, irregular, or saw-toothed in nature. The criteria for grading the severity of variable deceleration have been developed[12] (Table 3). Mild variable deceleration is usually innocuous. Repetitive and severe variable deceleration, particularly if it is prolonged, when associated with rising baseline heart rate, loss of FHR variability, and loss of acceleration prior to the deceleration, may herald the onset of significant fetal oxygen deprivation. This pattern is thought to be mediated by the vagus nerve through the barochemoreceptors when the umbilical cord is compressed, causing decreased fetal peripheral vascular resistance with a fall in fetal Po_2, and a rise in Pco_2. To be significant, the fetal heart rate usually falls to < 90 beats per minute. Variable deceleration is the most common periodic pattern noted during the course of labor. As the umbilical cord is compressed, via the vagus nerve, acetylcholine is released at the

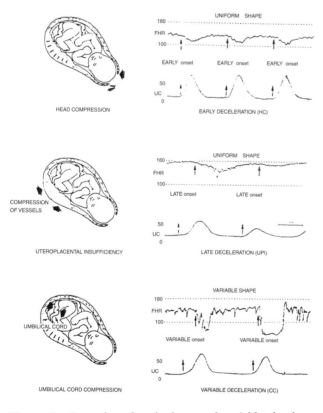

Figure 5 Examples of early, late, and variable decelerations. (From RH Petrie, in *Medicine of the Fetus and Mother*, EA Reece *et al.* eds., JB Lippincott, reprinted with permission.)

Table 1 Relationship between qualitative periodic fetal heart-rate changes and mean fetal pH

Pattern	Kubli et al.[12]	Tejani et al.[13,14]
Normal accelerations	7.30 ± 0.04	7.33 ± 0.01 7.34 ± 0.01
Early decelerations	7.30 ± 0.04	7.33 ± 0.01 7.30 ± 0.01
Variable decelerations (all)		
Moderate	7.26 ± 0.04	
Severe	7.15 ± 0.07	
Late decelerations (all)		7.29 ± 0.01
Moderate	7.21 ± 0.05	
Severe	7.12 ± 0.07	

Table 2 Relationship of fetal heart-rate patterns, fetal acid–base, 5-minute Apgar score, and umbilical acid–base

Pattern	5-min fetal scalp blood pH	Apgar scores ⩾ 7	Umbilical pH ⩾ 7.25
Normal tracing	7.33 ± 0.01	92%	91%
Accelerations	7.34 ± 0.01	91%	97%
Early accelerations	7.33 ± 0.01	92%	93%
Variable decelerations	7.30 ± 0.01	78%	77%
Late decelerations	7.29 ± 0.01	63%	66%

From references 13 and 14, with permission

sinoatrial node, causing a parasympathetic response or fall in fetal heart rate commensurate with the degree of cord compression, as long as the fetal heart rate does not fall to < 80 beats per minute or the duration of the deceleration is not too long. It is uncommon for cord compression, even when repetitive, to be of major clinical significance; however, with moderate and severe variable decelerations, significant reduction in umbilical blood flow may occur, resulting in the accumulation of significant amounts of carbon dioxide in the fetal compartment, thus causing a respiratory acidosis[12–15] (Tables 1, 2 and 4). When the decelerations become severe, repetitive, or prolonged in duration, fetal oxygen deprivation, resulting in a metabolic acidosis, may occur. When this occurs, and there is potential for significant fetal oxygen deprivation, a delay in recovery of the fetal heart rate to the baseline level may be noticed. When this is seen, steps should be taken to correct this pattern by alteration of maternal position, amnioinfusion, or use of a tocolytic agent to remove the stress of uterine activity.

At < 60 beats per minute, nodal control of the fetal heart may be lost. Management should follow the standard management for severe variable deceleration.

Table 3 Grading variable and late decelerations

Criteria of grading	Mild	Moderate	Severe
Variable deceleration; level to which FHR drops and duration of deceleration	< 30-s duration, regardless of level > 80 bpm, regardless of duration 70–80 bpm, < 60 s	< 70 bpm, > 30 to < 60 s 70–80 bpm, > 60 s	< 70 bpm, > 60 s
Late deceleration; amplitude of drop in FHR	< 15 bpm	15–45 bpm	> 45 bpm

bpm, beats per minute; FHR, fetal heart rate. From reference 12, with permission

Table 4 Fetal scalp capillary blood base deficit correlation (collected within 30 minutes prior to delivery) with fetal heart-rate patterns

Fetal heart-rate pattern	Mean (mEq/l) ± SE	Range (mEq/l)
Normal	6.98 ± 0.16	0.3–15.5
Early decelerations	6.97 ± 0.44	1.0–13.4
Mild variable decelerations	7.84 ± 0.19	2.0–13.4
Moderate variable decelerations	8.98 ± 0.44	2.5–21
Severe variable decelerations	10.44 ± 0.93	2.5–15.7
Mild late decelerations	9.29 ± 0.49	2.0–15.5
Moderate late decelerations	10.79 ± 0.43	4.8–16.8
Severe late decelerations	12.88 ± 0.77	10.1–18.8

Adapted from reference 15, with permission

Late deceleration

Late deceleration of FHR is defined as a visually apparent gradual decrease in FHR and return to the baseline associated with a uterine contraction. The duration from the onset of decrease to the nadir of FHR must be ≥ 30 s. The onset, nadir and recovery of the FHR deceleration follow the onset, peak and termination of the uterine contraction, respectively[7] (Figure 5). In many instances, the late deceleration will appear very much as an early deceleration that is delayed in onset. For this pattern to become clinically significant, it must be repetitive in nature. Most investigators believe that there is no such entity as a single late deceleration and that this pattern must be seen following three or more contractions to be called a late deceleration pattern. When the late deceleration is first noted, the deceleration may represent a reflex vagally mediated response, which is associated with normal heart-rate variability. It has been noted that late decelerations develop from fetal myocardial hypoxia, trigger a chemoreceptor response, and cause transient fetal hypotension, thereby stimulating fetal baroreceptors. The degree of potential fetal oxygenation deprivation for a deceleration pattern is related to the duration and depth of the deceleration, as well as the interval from the onset of the contraction to the onset of the deceleration. The shorter the interval from onset of contractions to onset of the deceleration, the greater is the likelihood of a greater degree of oxygenation deprivation. The same is true for the deceleration's duration and depth. The longer a deceleration pattern persists, the greater the likelihood is of significant fetal oxygenation deprivation[16].

Late decelerations may indicate that uteroplacental insufficiency with decreased intervillous exchange between the mother and the fetus may exist, with persistent or intermittent fetal oxygen deprivation. The criteria for grading the severity of late deceleration are given in Table 3. Fetal oxygenation may be impaired as the uterine contraction peaks, thus limiting intervillous-space blood flow. Poorly oxygenated blood ultimately reaches the fetus, thus the late timing of the fetal heart-rate deceleration[12–15] (Tables 1, 2 and 4). Late decelerations are noted with placental abruption, excessive uterine activity of either a spontaneous or oxytocin-induced nature, maternal hypotension, anemia, or ketoacidosis. Mild, repetitive late decelerations of only 5–10 beats per minute may indicate a significant potential for fetal oxygen deprivation such that metabolic acidosis may result. When the clinician notes the pattern of recurrent repetitive late deceleration, the pattern may be corrected by the usual common steps, in as much as up to 35–40% of these fetuses may have significant fetal oxygen deprivation The temporal interval between the onset of fetal heart-rate pattern that may indicate the potential for significant fetal oxygen deprivation and actual damage is unknown, but the interval probably ranges from approximately 0.5 to 2.0 h[16]. The customary correction plan consists of improvement of maternal hypotension, appropriate repositioning of the patient, administration of maternal oxygen, or reduction of the intensity and duration of uterine contractions with a tocolytic agent. For labor to continue with the presence of repetitive late decelerations, normal acid–base values must be obtained at a regular interval of every 15–20 min or commentary from fetal stimulation for evaluation of fetal wellbeing with the presence of fetal accelerations. The continuation of labor in the presence of repetitive late deceleration and reassuring acid–base or fetal stimulatory test is most commonly carried out in the active phase of labor, when a delivery process is not too distant. This situation is most often applicable to a multipara whose delivery is expected quite shortly. It has been demonstrated that the Cesarean section rate in this situation can be significantly lowered with the use of dual fetal surveillance with fetal heart rate and acid–base status.

Prolonged deceleration

Prolonged deceleration of FHR is defined as a visually apparent decrease in FHR below the baseline associated with uterine contractions. The amplitude of the decrease in FHR must be $\geq$ 15 beats per minute below the baseline and the duration from the onset of decrease in FHR to the return of FHR to the baseline is $\geq$ 2 min but < 10 min[7]. This occurs infrequently and unexpectedly. Usually, the fetal heart rate will fall to < 80 beats per minute and the deceleration can last for several minutes, in the manner of a prolonged variable or reflex deceleration. These sudden, prolonged decelerations can be related to uterine activity, fetal manipulation, conduction anesthesia with hypotension, supine hypotension, and a maternal respiratory arrest secondary to intravenous narcotic use. Although the mechanism for the deceleration is usually a reflex mechanism, as with a variable deceleration pattern, if there is no demonstrable, readily apparent, and correctable cause for the sudden prolonged deceleration, the fetal heart rate following recovery should be observed carefully. When a second or third sudden prolonged deceleration occurs, the patient may be moved to an operating room for corrective measures such as would be performed with a severe variable deceleration pattern, including evaluation of maternal

blood pressure, repositioning and oxygenation[17]. The possibility of a prolapsed cord should be investigated. Intravenous fluid may be increased and oxygen may be given to the mother. If delivery is not too far distant, substantiation of a satisfactory fetal acid–base may allow the labor to continue. If this pattern repeats with evidence of fetal oxygen deprivation by acid–base determinations, particularly when associated with the rising fetal base excess and a falling pH, an early vaginal delivery or an operative delivery may be prudent.

Combined (mixed) deceleration

On occasion, fetal heart-rate decelerations appear to be a combination or mixture of two or more decelerations in point of timing, cause, or a visual nature of the pattern. This is referred to as combination or mixed deceleration. Often this is a combination of late and variable decelerations, but on occasion there may be combinations of early and late or early and variable decelerations. In some instances, there may be combinations of accelerations and decelerations. When this mixed-pattern deceleration is noted to be repetitive in nature, the labor should be managed according to the most ominous aspect of the mixed or combined pattern of deceleration. Frequently, this will occur in the active phase of labor or in the second stage of labor. If there is any doubt regarding the potential for fetal oxygen deprivation, additional fetal surveillance regarding the fetal acid–base status will enable the obstetrician to make a logical decision regarding the continuation of labor or the potential need for an early, instrument-assisted vaginal delivery or a Cesarean section.

FETAL ACID–BASE EVALUATION

Acid–base evaluation by fetal scalp capillary blood sampling for fetal acidosis was used to monitor the wellbeing of the known high-risk fetus before continuous fetal cardiotocography was introduced in the late 1960s and early 1970s[18,19]. Fetal acid–base monitoring represents an intermittent commentary regarding the acid–base status or wellbeing of the fetus[20]. Generally, to collect fetal capillary blood from the presenting part, the cervix will need to be dilated approximately 2 cm with an engaged presenting part. The chorioamnion will have to be ruptured, and the patient will need to cooperate. The technique involves positioning the patient in the lateral Sims' or dorsolithotomy position or with hips elevated on an object such as an inverted bedpan so that an elongated cone can be placed into the vagina to rest against the fetal presenting part. The mucus, blood, and fluid is cleared from the scalp or buttocks, and a 2-mm scalpel is used to make a single 'stab-like' incision into the scalp or skin. Free-flowing fetal capillary blood is collected by gravity into a long (355-μl volume), preheparinized capillary tube. Approximately 20 μl of blood (about 1 inch in the capillary tube) is needed to obtain a complete set of respiratory blood gases, including pH, P_{O_2}, P_{CO_2}, bicarbonate, and base excess. Following the collection, the incisional site is inspected and pressure from a forceps-held swab is applied through three contractions. The site is subsequently inspected through a contraction, and if there is no bleeding, the cone is removed.

When the technique was first introduced, fetal scalp capillary blood samples were used for pH determination; later P_{CO_2}, P_{O_2}, bicarbonate, and base excess (base deficit) were added. Because most obstetricians are comfortable with the diagnostic accuracy of normal fetal heart-rate data, intermittent acid–base determinations are used only when fetal heart-rate monitoring is unclear or confusing. Currently, determinations of the fetal acid–base status represent the most precise information that the obstetrician has available for the diagnosis of the loss of fetal health or significant likelihood of clinically pertinent fetal oxygen deprivation. The intrapartum use of fetal capillary respiratory blood gas values with the presence of a maternal temperature greater than 103°F to 104°F (39.4°C to 40°C) should not be relied on as the sole indicator to continue labor, especially if a long labor is anticipated. False values may result from alterations in fetal metabolism with a temperature of this level. Fetal temperatures usually exceed the maternal level by 0.5°C. After the introduction of fetal capillary blood for the determination of respiratory gases, its use became an integral aspect of intrauterine surveillance in many institutions. A number of investigators have demonstrated that fetal stimulation and an evoked heart-rate acceleration may be correlated to a reassuring fetal acid–base status.

Both human and animal work regarding fetal capillary blood sampling during labor for the determination of acid-base status has revealed that there is a correlation between the fetal heart-rate pattern, the severity of that pattern, and the fetal/newborn outcome[12–15] (Tables 1, 2 and 4). During labor, fetal acidosis may result from fetal oxygen deprivation secondary to impaired maternal–fetal exchange in the intervillous space. A transient fall in fetal pH may be secondary to acute umbilical cord compression, leading to the accumulation of carbon dioxide with a resultant fetal respiratory acidosis. Of greater importance is fetal oxygen deprivation, which is due to impaired fetal oxygen–carbon dioxide exchange in the intervillous space. When there is fetal oxygen deprivation sufficient to cause use of the anaerobic (Embden–Meyerhof) pathway for energy production, lactic acid will be accumulated and the fetal pH level will fall. If sufficient fetal oxygen deprivation and acidosis develop, neurological damage or death may result. There is a close relationship between fetal capillary blood gas values that are collected just prior to birth and umbilical cord arterial values collected at birth[21].

Data collection regarding fetal blood pH and respiratory gas evaluation performed at the appropriate time may enable the obstetrician to recognize potential fetal oxygen deprivation prior to damage and allow fetal oxygen deprivation correction from the underlying problem or even a delivery by a route considered to be the safest for both mother and fetus. A number of investigators have considered pH values of ≥ 7.25 to be normal. They consider that a pH range of 7.20 to 7.24 is pre-acidotic. A fetal capillary pH value of ≤ 7.19 has been believed to represent potential fetal acidosis and, if sustained on two collections 10–15 minutes apart, may represent sufficient acidosis to warrant termination of labor. Recent studies have demonstrated that it is uncommon to find significant fetal neurological damage until a pH range of < 7.10 is noted[22], and it is possible that the value may be as low as 7.00[1]. Normal umbilical cord blood and fetal capillary pH and respiratory gas values are given in Tables 5, 6 and 7. Fetal capillary scalp pH values will normally fall in early labor, from approximately 7.35 to 7.25 at delivery. In clinical practice, it has been determined that serial pH determinations correlate best with the clinical setting and are probably of greater significance than an absolute value of one or two determinations of pH. Fetal heart-rate variability provides important commentary on the severity of periodic patterns that may herald potential fetal oxygen deprivation.

A maternal acidosis can cause an apparent fetal acidosis secondary to the equilibration of hydrogen ions (H^+) across the placenta. The presence of a maternal and fetal acidotic state may indicate one of two things. Both the mother and fetus may be producing H^+, or the fetus may be a recipient of H^+ but not truly have

Table 5 Normal umbilical cord acid–base values

	pH	*Po$_2$ (mmHg)*	*Pco$_2$ (mmHg)*	*Base excess (mEq/l)*
Umbilical arterial	7.242	16.6	49.9	−6.8
	(7.10–7.37)	(6.8–33.4)	(37.2–59.5)	[(−3.2)–(−13.6)]
Umbilical venous	7.312	28.9	39.1	−5.5
	(7.20–7.42)	(16.5–42.0)	(33–49.8)	[(2.7)–(−8.6)]

Adapted from reference 22, with permission

Table 6   Fetal capillary blood respiratory gas values

Normal	Respiratory acidosis	Metabolic acidosis
pH 7.25–7.40	Decreased	Decreased
Po_2	Usually stable	Decreased
Pco_2	Increased	Usually stable
Base deficit 0–12	Usually stable	Increased

Table 7   Base deficit (excess)* in fetal capillary blood

Normal	0–9 mEq/l
Borderline	9–11 mEq/l
Potential metabolic acidosis	> 12 mEq/l

*Base deficit and base excess have the same numerical value; however, a positive value is used for base deficit and negative value for base excess, i.e. a base deficit of 6 is the same as a base excess of –6

fetal oxygen deprivation. Maternal and fetal base excess can be compared to distinguish between the fetus with true fetal oxygen deprivation and the fetus who receives H^+ from the mother. Maternal venous blood that is freely flowing without the use of a tourniquet can be collected for determinations of maternal respiratory blood gas values. The fetal pH is usually about 0.1 pH unit below the maternal value. When a maternal acidosis is found, efforts should be made to determine the cause, such as ketoacidosis, sepsis, or hypovolemia. Appropriate corrective therapy then may be initiated. When there is maternal respiratory alkalosis associated with hyperventilation, falsely elevated fetal pH values have been reported.

Base excess

A base excess (deficit) value is an indicator of fetal buffer reserves that are present to neutralize H^+ or fixed acids. The base excess/deficit value can be clinically useful as an indicator of impending loss of fetal wellbeing when fetal pH values are satisfactory but the fetal heart-rate pattern is the cause for concern[22] (Tables 4 and 7). The longer the fetus is exposed to recurrent stress, the more likely it is that its acid–base status will suddenly deteriorate. With recurrent stress, evidenced by fetal heart-rate deceleration, stable pH values, and a rising base excess/deficit status, the temporal interval before deterioration of the fetal status becomes progressively shorter. As with intermittent and continuous fetal heart-rate and pH surveillance, base excess also has an indistinct border between normal and abnormal. Oxygen deprivation-induced fetal/newborn neurologic damage is not observed if a base excess is less than –12 to –14 mEq/l; nevertheless, even at a base excess level of –25 mEq/l or greater, only approximately 40% of newborns will have neurological damage. When fetal base excess/deficit values are

compared with fetal pH determinations and fetal heart-rate patterns, there is a more reliable association of base excess/deficit with the severity of fetal heart-rate patterns than with pH alone. Thus, judicious clinical use of base excess/deficit as an indicator of fetal wellbeing, especially when there are confusing fetal heart-rate patterns, is of significant potential benefit. Now that instrumentation is available that can determine pH and base excess/deficit of fetal capillary blood samples as small as 25–40 μl, this is especially important. On some occasions, before the cervix is sufficiently dilated to collect fetal capillary blood, it may be important to obtain commentary regarding acid–base status or other laboratory information. It is now possible with the use of ultrasound to do a funicentesis (funipuncture, cordocentesis, percutaneous umbilical blood sampling) to collect fetal blood. The use of funicentesis for this purpose is limited, but may have real potential value in situations in which placental blood-flow problems are likely, such as post-term gestation, intrauterine growth restriction, pre-eclampsia, and perhaps severe diabetes mellitus.

Fetal stimulation for evoking a fetal heart-rate acceleration or comparison to pH/buffer evaluation has become more widely used as commentary regarding fetal acid–base status. This allows use of fetal acid–base status without the actual collection of fetal blood for determinations of pH and respiratory gases by a machine. A number of stimuli, including injections of cold sterile water through an intrauterine pressure catheter, pain from the pinching of the fetal scalp, physical movement of the fetus, or a noise as in a vibroacoustic stimulation of the fetal auditory system, have gained popularity in recent years.

Fetal stimulation in some form has been used on a limited basis for three to four decades. Recent investigators have studied the use of an evoked fetal heart-rate acceleration during fetal scalp sampling as a stimulation at the time of the collection of fetal capillary blood. It was observed that, during the fetal capillary blood-collecting process, when the scalp was stimulated, an acceleration of 15 beats per minute with an excursion away from baseline for ⩾ 15 s was almost always indicative of a pH value of ⩾ 7.22[18]. Conversely, the absence of a fetal heart-rate acceleration when the fetus was stimulated is not absolutely predictive of a fetus who is acidotic; although some of the fetuses will be acidotic, the remainder will have a normal acid–base status. An acceleration in response to fetal scalp stimulation generally is accepted as a sufficient acid–base commentary to allow labor to continue. As long as an abnormal fetal heart rate is noted, normal acid–base commentary or acid–base determinations performed at intervals of every 15–20 minutes have been reliable to safely continue labor. When this intermittent form of acid–base commentary is to be used over a prolonged period of time, it is probably prudent to collect a sample of fetal capillary blood, as well as a sample of free-flowing maternal venous blood, occasionally to substantiate a satisfactory acid–base status.

Some investigators have used vibroacoustic stimulation during labor to bring about a fetal heart-rate acceleration[23]. An artificial larynx (AT&T, Parsippany, NJ, USA) that generates 81 decibels of mixed noise and vibration can be placed on the maternal abdomen, approximately one-third the distance from the symphysis pubis to the xiphoid process, to stimulate the fetus. Stimulation intervals of from 2 to 5 s are commonly used. Such a stimulation may evoke a fetal heart-rate acceleration. With such fetal heart-rate accelerations, generally, the fetus is in good condition from the physiological and acid–base status. When using the internal form of fetal heart-rate monitoring, a 5-s vibroacoustic stimulation to the fetus that results in either a 10 beats per minute acceleration with a 10-s excursion away from baseline or a 15 beats per minute acceleration with a 15-s excursion away from baseline as correlated with a mean pH of 7.29 ± 0.07[24]. Again, some healthy fetuses as well as some fetuses with loss of fetal health will not respond with an acceleration. Accordingly, if an acceleration is not achieved through a vibroacoustic stimulation, then it is prudent to collect fetal capillary blood for pH and base excess determination to clarify the picture.

Umbilical cord pH and respiratory blood gas values are frequently used at birth to compare intrapartum fetal heart-rate data with acid–base status and newborn condition[25] (Table 6). These values frequently help identify the degree of fetal/newborn oxygenation at delivery. Following the delivery, 10–30 cm of a doubly clamped segment of the umbilical cord is obtained, and, using two preheparinized small syringes, samples of umbilical cord blood from the artery and vein are collected separately. The blood samples are analyzed for pH and respiratory gases and correlated to both newborn conditions and fetal heart-rate data during labor. By placing the umbilical cord segment or the blood samples on ice, the actual determination may be delayed by a half hour or more while still obtaining reliable determinations. Many obstetricians obtain umbilical artery and vein, pH and respiratory gases as an integral part of the delivery process in selected cases.

For almost 20 years, the potential of continuous fetal pH and respiratory gases from the fetal presenting part has been the aspiration of many obstetricians. A number of electrodes have been evaluated, and continuous pH, P_{CO_2}, P_{O_2}, and base excess/deficit has been available in a few laboratories. In Europe, continuous fetal P_{CO_2}, is becoming more common. Unfortunately, continuous pH and respiratory gases are still under investigation, and it does not appear that they will be available for several years.

AMNIOTIC FLUID

The evaluation of amniotic fluid as a surveillance technique for potential fetal oxygen deprivation represents a small role of primary consideration but a very valuable complementary role of fetal surveillance. The contribution of evaluation of amniotic fluid lies in two aspects: evaluation of volume and evaluation for the presence of meconium.

Amniotic fluid volume

At present, perhaps the most reliable technique for evaluating amniotic fluid is ultrasonography; although used mostly in the antepartum period, intrapartum evaluation may also be valuable, particularly when conditions such as intrauterine growth restriction, pregnancy-induced hypertension, prolonged gestation, and diabetes mellitus are concerned. Amniotic fluid volume can be evaluated by many techniques. One of the most common is the amniotic fluid index[26]. The abdomen is divided into four quadrants and, with the transducer perpendicular to the plane of the table, the greatest depth of amniotic fluid found in each quadrant is obtained. The quadrants are summed and represent the relative amniotic fluid volume. Values of < 5 cm may portend problems associated with cord compression.

Meconium

Meconium evaluation is a reasonably soft marker for potential fetal oxygen deprivation. Two groups of investigators have evaluated the significance of meconium in the amniotic fluid and its relationship to fetal heart rate. Fenton and Steer correlated meconium, fetal heart rate, and newborn outcome using intermittent fetal heart-rate monitoring prior to fetal cardiotocography[27]. Some investigators[28,29] have looked at the significance of meconium, fetal heart rate, and newborn outcomes using continuous fetal heart-rate monitoring. In both instances, the conclusions have been similar. Generally, it is thought that meconium alone, in an otherwise normal fetus, is not a significant marker for the potential of fetal oxygen deprivation. When meconium is present with other markers of potential fetal oxygen deprivation, meconium then becomes an additional marker. The presence of meconium early in a labor, particularly when placental dysfunction may be suspect, such as in prolonged gestation, fetal growth restriction, maternal hypertension or maternal diabetes, may cause a number of clinicians to be concerned about the overall acid–base status of the fetus. The evaluation of acid–base by either direct capillary blood sampling or fetal stimulation may be performed quite early in the labor to establish acid–base status and to identify those fetuses already exposed to chronic fetal oxygen deprivation. It is easy to evaluate meconium from amniotic fluid when the membranes are ruptured. Prior to rupture of the membranes, the use of an amniocentesis or transcervical amnioscopy to evaluate the presence of meconium have been used.

UTERINE ACTIVITY

Both the evaluation of fetal breathing[30,31], and the evaluation of fetal movement or fetal kicking have been established by investigators[32] to have significant potential for the detection of possible fetal oxygen deprivation during the antepartum interval. Although the evaluation of both fetal breathing and fetal movement or kicking during labor can be carried out to a limited degree, their use is usually limited to the early latent period of labor and becomes more difficult as uterine contractions become more frequent, because the fetus tends to move less and it is more difficult to differentiate fetal movement from uterine activity.

Uterine activity evaluation is an important part of intrapartum fetal surveillance. Many clinicians believe that manual palpation of the uterus for contractions or tocodynametric or external uterine monitoring is sufficient to carry out a successful intrapartum fetal surveillance protocol. The early detection of dysfunctional labor secondary to inadequate uterine activity, while not totally dependent on internal quantitated monitoring of uterine activity, certainly is benefited by it. The early detection of a placental abruption can be very rewarding in some instances, and the evaluation of uterine activity for the establishment of the effects of drugs on labor and uterine activity, or progress in labor is equally rewarding. It is the use of uterine activity data for the proper identification of periodic patterns that is critically important. In many instances, the fetal heart-rate data may be good and clear, but uterine activity surveillance, using an external form of fetal monitoring, is of such poor quality that the true identity of fetal heart-rate changes cannot be easily appreciated. For this reason, the use of an intrauterine pressure catheter to evaluate uterine activity is recommended. Although many people believe that the presence of a foreign body such as an intrauterine pressure catheter is a cause of infection, the data do not support this[33–35]. In fact, the presence of an intrauterine pressure catheter frequently decreases the number of cervical examinations that are required during labor, and a reduction in the number of vaginal examinations may lead to reduced incidence of postpartum endomyometritis. Quantitation of uterine activity for the identification of dysfunctional labor requiring oxytocin or the presence of fetal heart-rate abnormalities relating to uterine activity can best be evaluated with the use of an intrauterine pressure catheter. Rising baseline tone, frequent, strong contractions developing into a tachysystole or tetanic contraction may be seen with spontaneous excessive uterine activity, and in drug-induced excessive uterine activity especially in the presence of certain pathophysiological states such as abruptio placentae. Oxygenation of the fetus is obviously proportionate in some of these disorders to the amount of uterine activity. Thus, it may be prudent when evaluating fetal heart-rate and acid–base data for interpretation of the fetal oxygenation status to always be mindful of the potential stress that the fetus is encountering in the form of uterine activity.

FETAL INTRAPARTUM MANAGEMENT

Management options used to avoid the potential of significant fetal oxygen deprivation include control of maternal hypotension, control of uterine activity–hyperactivity, control or alleviation of umbilical cord compression, and appropriate intravenous fluid administration.

Fetal surveillance during labor is principally surveillance with fetal heart-rate monitoring. As long as fetal heart-rate monitoring data are normal, the patient needs no additional monitoring. When heart-rate changes are noted, such as significant tachycardia, bradycardia, late, variable or prolonged decelerations, or significant loss of fetal heart-rate variability, particularly when it had been present previously or following significant fetal stress such as significant uterine hyperactivity, the patient usually responds to correction measures such as maternal supine hypotension, position change, maternal administration of oxygen or fluid, or reduction in oxytocin administration. When these simple measures do not correct the problem, and long-term (> 30 min) or repetitive late or variable decelerations are present, accelerations as a marker of wellbeing may be looked for. Stimulation of the fetus to provoke accelerations or the actual collection for capillary blood acid–base determinations should also be considered. It should be kept in mind that with increasing temporal duration, repetitive fetal heart-rate decelerations are more likely to result in significant fetal oxygen deprivation, although the acid–base status at the time may be satisfactory[17]. Accordingly, dual surveillance that allows the continuation of labor in the presence of questionable or abnormal fetal heart-rate data should be carried out only when the delivery process can be expected within 1–2 h and intermittent acid–base commentary can be obtained at an interval of every 15–20 min. On occasion, when uterine activity is excessive, causing an immediate fetal heart rate abnormality, such as with significant variable decelerations, the temporary us of a tocolytic agent such as intravenous magnesium sulfate by an intravenous injection of 4–6 g over a 15- to 20-min interval or 0.25–0.5 mg of terbutaline subcutaneously may reduce uterine activity sufficiently to allow the fetus to recover and then return to a productive labor[36]. When such a technique is used, careful attention to fetal wellbeing must be utmost in the clinician's mind.

Amnioinfusion

If oligohydramnios is present, the use of an amnioinfusion to buffer the umbilical cord can be of considerable help, especially with a significant cord compression in a premature fetus[37,38]. The use of amnioinfusion in gestations complicated by meconium has been demonstrated to be of benefit. Sadovsky and co-workers have found that amnioinfusion for the elimination of meconium was safe, simple, and effective[39]. Amnioinfusion has been demonstrated to significantly reduce the thickness of meconium, the incidence of neonatal acidemia, and the incidence of significant meconium below the vocal cords at delivery. A number of protocols are used for amnioinfusion. Miyazaki and Taylor[37] and Nageotte and co-workers[38] have advocated the use of amnioinfusion for cord compression, and they use 0.5–1 l of normal saline infused at 150–200 ml/h as long as the decelerative pattern persists. Once the pattern has been ameliorated, a maintenance infusion of 10–20 ml/h is used. Until recently, amnioinfusion required warming of the saline solution to body temperature prior to infusion; recently, however, it has been reported that saline at room temperature has been found to be as effective as fluid warmed to body temperature.

POTENTIAL PROBLEMS OF FETAL SURVEILLANCE

The critics of continuous fetal heart-rate monitoring point out that this technique has caused the Cesarean section rate to soar for obstetrically unwarranted reasons. Although the presence of repetitive late FHR decelerations and decreased FHR beat-to-beat variability have been associated with an increased risk of cerebral palsy, the false-positive rate of detecting cerebral palsy from these abnormal FHR changes is 99.8%. This may partly explain the fact that the rate of cerebral palsy (about 2 per 1000 term infants) remains unchanged, despite an increasing rate of Cesarean section delivery during the last twenty-five years[40,41]. In programs where dual surveillance systems are used, the incidence of Cesarean sections for fetal distress has actually declined[42].

Regarding acid–base monitoring, the problems of infection and bleeding following the collection of fetal scalp blood are real but small. When the scalp puncture site is viewed through three contractions following the collection of capillary blood, significant bleeding thereafter is quite uncommon. In fact, significant bleeding is quite uncommon outside of a pharmacologically induced coagulopathy[43]. The most common of these is with the use of phenobarbital and diphenylhydantoin[44].

Once continued fetal bleeding is identified, usually a small clip placed across the incision site to add pressure to the scalp will take care of the problem. Occasionally, an early instrument-assisted vaginal delivery or a Cesarean section may be required. A small pustule or local infection may be noted at the incision site. Beard gives the incidence of this as approximately 1 in 1000 cases[45]. In most instances, simple drainage will take care of the problem; however, on occasion, antibiotics may be needed for more serious infections.

The use of fetal stimulation to obtain a fetal heart-rate acceleration as a marker of fetal acid–base status without collecting fetal capillary blood is being used with increasing frequency. This form of fetal surveillance is safe, except for the possibility of not being able to identify the fetus with good acid–base status not responding with an acceleration. Nevertheless, some investigators have raised concern about the potential damage to the fetal auditory system[46].

On occasion, a uterine perforation will occur when the uterine pressure catheter is inserted. Almost uniformly, this occurs when the stiff catheter guide is inserted beyond the operator's fingertip. Case reports indicate that complications may occur from time to time, including problems with attachment of the fetal scalp electrode; however, these complications are exceedingly rare.

Intrauterine infection following the use of internal fetal heart-rate monitoring is a concern; however, the infection rate as evidenced by incidence of endometritis is not outside the normal range[34,35]. Gassner and Ledger confirmed these findings, but included the fact that in cases in which internal fetal heart-rate monitoring was used for several hours and the patient underwent Cesarean section, there was an increased incidence of intrauterine infections[33]. A cause-and-effect relationship has not been established.

Some obstetricians are somewhat uncomfortable following a patient with repetitive heart rate indicators of potential fetal oxygen deprivation in the presence of normal fetal acid–base evaluation. In an obstetrical unit that routinely uses acid–base determinations as a secondary surveillance system, especially when base excess is used, dual fetal surveillance is rarely found to be a problem. The 1- and 5-min Apgar score date by Bowe and Hutson and co-workers demonstrate that this is a reasonably safe protocol[1,21]. From the work of Fleisher and associates, it is known that, with repetitive stress, a normal acid–base status can deteriorate over a period of time; thus, it is important that as long as the fetal heart-rate pattern is suggestive of potential fetal oxygen deprivation, commentary regarding acid–base status is necessary every 15–20 min[16]. In this particular instance, the use of fetal capillary blood pH and base excess will be more reassuring than pH alone. Base excess will enable the obstetrician to determine when the fetal buffer reserves are being exhausted, to be shortly followed by a deterioration in the pH values.

Some patients believe that both continuous electronic fetal heart-rate and acid–base surveillance are too technical and too restrictive, and these techniques interfere with the natural birth process. The patients believe that they are not in control, and that monitoring in any form is unwarranted[47,48]. Generally, when the patient expresses this form of doubt, a careful and complete explanation of the means and benefits of this form of monitoring will make her more comfortable. In spite of appropriate antepartum screening, some patients arrive on a delivery service refusing any form of fetal surveillance. When this happens, a careful explanation of the procedure and what is expected of her should be given to the patient, and if the patient continues to refuse appropriate fetal surveillance, in the presence of witnesses, it should be verified in the chart that the patient was offered fetal monitoring and the reasons for needing fetal monitoring were explained to her. Fetal heart-rate data should then be collected when maternal vital signs are collected. Fortunately, the incidence of intrapartum fetal oxygen deprivation is quite small, and it is hoped that neither the patient nor her fetus will adversely be affected by her decision not to use intrapartum fetal surveillance on the frequent basis that current protocols suggest are important.

On occasion, the obstetrician will be required to monitor a multiple gestation in labor. Many commercial monitors now have the ability to monitor two fetuses on one unit. It is possible, by using two monitors, to evaluate up to three fetuses concomitantly. If internal monitoring is being used for the first fetus, a sterile tubing can be run from the dome of the strain gauge of the first monitor to the dome of the strain gauge on the second monitor. With appropriate filling of the tube connecting the two domes, intrauterine pressure can be available on both monitors for the proper evaluation of heart-rate data in relation to uterine contractions.

REFERENCES

1. Gilstrap LC, Leveno KJ, Burris J, *et al.* Diagnosis of birth asphyxia on the basis of fetal pH, Apgar score, and newborn cerebral dysfunction. *Am J Obstet Gynecol* 1989; 161:825–30
2. American College of Obstetricians and Gynecologists. Intrapartum fetal heart rate monitoring. *ACOG Technical Bull* 207, July 1995
3. Hon EH, Quilligan EJ. The classification of fetal heart rate. II. A revised working classification. *Conn Med* 1967; 31:779–84
4. Hon EH. The electronic evaluation of the fetal heart rate. *Am J Obstet Gynecol* 1958;75:1215–30
5. Vintzileos AM, Nochimson DJ, Guzman ER, *et al.* Intrapartum electronic fetal heart rate monitoring versus intermittent auscultation: a meta-analysis. *Obstet Gynecol* 1995;85:149–55
6. Vintzileos AM, Nochimson DJ, Antsaklis A, *et al.* Comparison of intrapartum electronic fetal heart rate monitoring versus intermittent auscultation in detecting fetal acidemia at birth. *Am J Obstet Gynecol* 1995;173:1021–4
7. The National Institute of Child Health and Human Development Research Planning Workshop. Electronic fetal heart rate monitoring: research guidelines for interpretation. *Am J Obstet Gynecol* 1997;177:1385–90
8. Burrus DR, O'Shea M, Veille J-C, Mueller-Heubach E. The predictive value of intrapartum fetal heart rate abnormalities in the extremely premature infant. *Am J Obstet Gynecol* 1994;171:1128–32
9. Catanzarite VA, Schrimmer DB, Maida C, Mendoza A. Prenatal sonographic diagnosis of intracranial haemorrhage: report of a case with a sinusoidal fetal heart rate tracing, and a review of the literature. *Prenat Diagn* 1995;15:229–35
10. Tanaka M, Ikeda T, Suzuki T, *et al.* A case of fetal bradycardia and sinusoidal-like fetal heart rate pattern associated with maternal hypothermia. *Fetal Diagn Ther* 1995;10:207–9
11. Atkinson MW, Belfort MA, Saade GR, Moise KJ. The relation between magnesium sulfate therapy and fetal heart rate variability. *Obstet Gynecol* 1994;83:967–70
12. Kubli FW, Hon EH, Khazin AF, Takemura H. Observations on heart rate and pH in the human fetus during labor. *Am J Obstet Gynecol* 1969;104:1190–206
13. Tejani N, Mann LI, Bhakthavathsalan A, Weiss RR. Correlation of fetal heart rate–uterine contraction patterns with fetal scalp blood pH. *Obstet Gynecol* 1975; 46:392–6
14. Tejani N, Mann LI, Bhakthavathsalan A. Correlation of fetal heart rate with neonatal outcome. *Obstet Gynecol* 1976;48:460–3
15. Hon EH, Khazin A. Observation of fetal heart rate and fetal biochemistry. I. Base deficit. *Am J Obstet Gynecol* 1969;105:721–9
16. Fleischer A, Schulman H, Jagani N, *et al.* The development of fetal acidosis in the presence of an abnormal fetal heart rate tracing. I. The average for gestational age fetus. *Am J Obstet Gynecol* 1982;144:55–60
17. Hutson JM, Mueller-Heubach E. Diagnosis and management of intrapartum reflex fetal heart rate changes. *Clin Perinatol* 1982;9:325–37
18. Clark SL, Gimovsky ML, Miller FC. Fetal heart rate response to scalp blood sampling. *Am J Obstet Gynecol* 1982;144:706–8
19. Zalar RW Jr, Quilligan EJ. The influence of scalp sampling on the Cesarean section rate for fetal distress. *Am J Obstet Gynecol* 1979;135:239–46
20. American College of Obstetricians and Gynecologists. Umbilical artery blood acid–base analysis. *ACOG Technical Bull.* 216, November 1995
21. Bowe ET, Beard RW, Finster M, *et al.* Reliability of fetal blood sampling. Maternal–fetal relationships. *Am J Obstet Gynecol* 1970;107:279–87
22. Wible JL, Petrie RH, Koons A, *et al.* The clinical use of umbilical cord acid–base determinations in perinatal surveillance and management. *Clin Perinatol* 1982;9: 387–97

23. Edersheim TG, Hutson JM, Druzin MD, *et al.* Fetal heart rate response to vibratory acoustic stimulation predicts fetal pH in labor. *Am J Obstet Gynecol* 1987; 157:1557–60

24. Polzin GB, Blakemore KJ, Petrie RH, Amon E. Fetal vibroacoustic stimulation: magnitude and duration of fetal heart rate accelerations as a marker of fetal health. *Obstet Gynecol* 1988;72:621–6

25. Thorp JA, Sampson JE, Parisi VM, Creasy RK. Routine umbilical cord blood gas determinations? *Am J Obstet Gynecol* 1989;161:600–5

26. Moore TR, Cayle JE. The amniotic fluid index in normal human pregnancy. *Am J Obstet Gynecol* 1990; 162:1168–73

27. Fenton AN, Steer CM. Fetal distress. *Am J Obstet Gynecol* 1962;83:354–62

28. Miller FC, Sacks DA, Yeh S-Y. Significance of meconium during labor. *Am J Obstet Gynecol* 1975;122:573–80

29. Miller FC, Read JA. Intrapartum assessment of the postdate fetus. *Am J Obstet Gynecol* 1981;141:516–20

30. Patrick J, Challis J. Measurement of human fetal breathing movements in healthy pregnancies using a real-time scanner. *Semin Perinatol* 1980;4:275–86

31. Patrick J, Campbell LK, Carmichael L, *et al.* Patterns of human fetal breathing during the last 10 weeks of pregnancy. *Obstet Gynecol* 1980;56:24–30

32. Rayburn WF. Clinical significance of maternal perceptible fetal motion. *Am J Obstet Gynecol* 1980;138:210–12

33. Gassner CB, Ledger WJ. The relationship of hospital-acquired infection to invasive intrapartum monitoring techniques. *Am J Obstet Gynecol* 1976;126:33–7

34. Gibbs RS, Listwa HI, Read JA. The effect of internal fetal monitoring on maternal infection following Cesarean section. *Obstet Gynecol* 1976;48:653–8

35. Ledger WJ. Complications associated with invasive monitoring. *Semin Perinatol* 1978;2:187–94

36. Reece EA, Chervenak AF, Romero R, Hobbins JC. Magnesium sulfate in the management of acute intrapartum fetal distress. *Am J Obstet Gynecol* 1984;148:104–6

37. Miyazaki FS, Taylor NA. Saline amnioinfusion for relief of variable or prolonged decelerations. A preliminary report. *Am J Obstet Gynecol* 1983;146:670–8

38. Nageotte MP, Freemen RK, Garite TI, Dorchester W. Prophylactic intrapartum amnioinfusion in patients with preterm premature rupture of membranes. *Am J Obstet Gynecol* 1985;153:557–62

39. Sadovsky Y, Amon E, Bade M, Petrie RH. Prophylactic amnioinfusion during labor complicated by meconium: a preliminary report. *Am J Obstet Gynecol* 1989; 161:613–17

40. Nelson KB, Dambrosia JM, Ting TY, Grether JK. Uncertain value of electronic fetal monitoring in predicting cerebral palsy. *N Engl J Med* 1996;334:613–18

41. MacDonald D. Cerebral palsy and intrapartum fetal monitoring. *N Engl J Med* 1996;334:659–60

42. Shamsi HH, Petrie RH, Steer CM. Changing obstetrical practices and amelioration of perinatal outcome in a university hospital. *Am J Obstet Gynecol* 1979;133:855–8

43. Wood C, Lumbley J, Renou P. A clinical assessment of foetal diagnostic methods. *J Obstet Gynaecol Br Commonw* 1967;74:823–5

44. Mountain KR, Hirsh J, Gallus AS. Neonatal coagulation defect due to anticonvulsant drug treatment in pregnancy. *Lancet* 1970;1:265–8

45. Beard RW. Fetal blood sampling. *Br J Hosp Med* 1970; 3:523–34

46. Richards DS. The fetal vibroacoustic stimulation test: an update. *Semin Perinatol* 1990;14:305–10

47. Molfese V, Sunshine P, Bennett A. Reactions of women to intrapartum fetal monitoring. *Obstet Gynecol* 1982; 59:706

48. Starkman MN. Psychological responses to the use of the fetal monitor during labor. *Psychosom Med* 1976; 38:269

63
Nonimmune fetal hydrops

H.N. Winn

Fetal hydrops denotes a condition of excessive accumulation of extracellular fluid in the form of skin edema, ascites, pleural effusion and/or pericardial effusion which can be diagnosed by ultrasonography (Figures 1 and 2). In the early second trimester (< 20 weeks of gestation) increased nuchal translucency may represent the earliest sign of fetal hydrops[1] (Figure 3). When the excessive fluid is limited to one of the body compartments, the condition may be classified as an isolated finding, such as isolated ascites[2]. Commonly associated ultrasonographic findings include polyhydramnios and increased placental thickness.

Fetal hydrops may be secondary to maternal alloimmunization against fetal red blood cell (RBC) antigens. Nonimmune fetal hydrops (NIH) is distinguished by the absence of maternal IgG antibodies against fetal RBC antigens. The incidence of NIH is about one in 3000 deliveries[3]. The main categories of fetal disorders which are associated with NIH are infection, chromosomal abnormalities, structural anomalies, hematological diseases, metabolic diseases and tumors. The list of conditions associated with NIH is extensive[4], but the following discussion will focus on the common ones.

INFECTION

Common infectious agents associated with NIH include *Toxoplasma gondii*, *Treponema pallidum*, parvovirus (B19), cytomegalovirus (CMV) and adenovirus[4,5]. Adenovirus is probably the most common viral infection in NIH[5]. Maternal infection with these agents tends to be asymptomatic. Diagnosis of maternal infection with *T. gondii*, parvovirus or CMV is made by the presence of organism-specific IgG and IgM in the maternal serum. The presence of *T. gondii*-specific IgG in maternal serum prior to pregnancy confers protection to the fetus. Maternal infection with syphilis is screened by serum venereal disease research laboratory (VDRL) or rapid plasma reagin (RPR) tests and confirmed by the microhemagglutination assay *T. pallidum* (MHA-TP) or fluorescent treponemal antibody absorption (FTA-ABS) test. Fetal infection with parvovirus, *T. gondii*, CMV or adenovirus can be diagnosed by demonstrating the presence of: (i) the organism in the amniotic fluid using polymerase chain

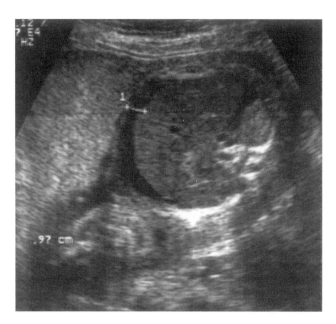

Figure 1 Axial view of the fetal abdomen reveals fetal ascites as a sonolucent area between the anterior abdominal wall and the intestines as marked

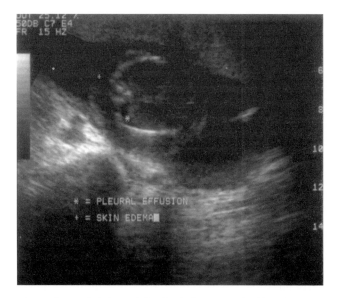

Figure 2 Axial view of the fetal chest reveals skin edema as reflected by the increased skin thickness, and pleural effusion as reflected by the sonolucent area between the posterior chest wall and the lungs

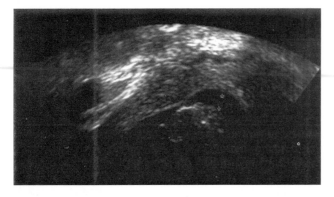

Figure 3 Longitudinal view of the embryo at 11 weeks of gestation reveals increased nuchal translucency in the posterior area of the neck

reaction (PCR)[5–7]; (ii) detection of B19 capsid antigens (VP1 and VP2) using monoclonal antibodies for parvovirus[8]; (iii) the organism-specific IgM antibody in the fetal blood; or (iv) positive culture of the virus from the fetal blood.

The pathogenesis of fetal hydrops in fetal infection includes severe fetal anemia from destruction of fetal erythroid precursors in the case of parvovirus infection and possible hepatic failure and excessive extramedullary hematopoiesis in other cases. Fetal transfusion of red blood cells for severe fetal anemia may resolve fetal hydrops and improve fetal survival. Maternal syphilis infection should be appropriately treated to prevent or reduce the severity of neonatal syphilis. Maternal administration of pyrimethamine and sulfadiazine for *T. gondii* fetal infection may reduce the severity of the neonatal sequelae.

CHROMOSOMAL ABNORMALITIES

Chromosomal abnormalities constitute a major cause of NIH and include Turner syndrome (45X), trisomy 21, trisomy 18, trisomy 16, trisomy 13, triploidy and unbalanced translocations. Turner syndrome is one of the most common chromosomal abnormalities associated with NIH. Cystic hygroma is characterized by the presence of a septated cyst in the paracervical area (Figure 4) and is commonly accompanied by other features of fetal hydrops. Cystic hygroma presumably develops from the lack or maldevelopment of the communication between the vascular and lymphatic systems[9]. The incidence of abnormal chromosomes in patients with first-trimester nuchal cystic hygroma in larger series, each containing at least 29 patients, ranges from 35–60%[10]. Cystic hygroma may also be transmitted as an autosomal recessive disorder[11]. Perinatal mortality is at least 90% in patients with cystic hygroma, and other signs of fetal hydrops or abnormal chromosomes[9], but drops to about 10% in patients with first-trimester nuchal cystic hygroma and normal chromosomes[10].

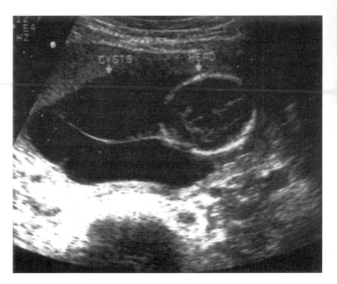

Figure 4 Cystic hygroma. Axial view of the fetal head reveals a septated multiloculated cyst in the paracervical area

FETAL STRUCTURAL ANOMALIES

Fetal anomalies which are commonly associated with NIH include: (i) skeletal dysplasia with a very narrow chest such as thanatophoric skeletal dysplasia and osteogenenesis imperfecta; (ii) pulmonary abnormalities such congenital cystic adenomatoid malformation (CCAM) and diaphragmatic hernia; (iii) cardiovascular abnormalities and cardiac arrhythmia, and (iv) gastrointestinal disorders such as meconium peritonitis and intestinal obstruction.

NEOPLASM

Fetal tumors such as neuroblastomas, teratomas and tuberous sclerosis and placental chorioangiomas have been associated with fetal hydrops. Tuberous sclerosis is an autosomal dominant disorder which manifests as fibroangiomatous tumors affecting many organs. Tuberous sclerosis may cause fetal heart failure or portal hypertension and hepatic failure if the tumors affect the fetal heart or liver respectively. Placental chorioangioma functions as high volume arteriovenous shunts which predisposes the fetus to heart failure and/or anemia[12].

HEMATOLOGICAL DISORDERS

Fetal hemorrhage, hemoglobinopathies and hemolysis are the most common fetal hematological disorders which produce fetal hydrops from severe fetal anemia and fetal hypoxia. Fetal hemorrhage can occur spontaneously or in the setting of abruptio placenta, placenta previa, trauma, or twin transfusion. The amount of fetomaternal hemorrhage can be estimated from the Kleihauer-Betke test. Fetal anemia can be confirmed by funicentesis and severe fetal anemia can be treated with fetal transfusion of red blood cells.

Alpha-thalassemia is an autosomal recessive hemoglobinopathy which occurs mainly in Southeast Asia and Mediterranean descendants. Normal fetal hemoglobin (HbF) has a tetramer consisting of 2 α-chains and 2 γ-chains. A patient with α-thalassemia has reduced or absent synthesis of the α-chains due to deletion of one or more genes. In homozygous α-thalassemia, the affected fetus does not have any α-chains but produces tetramers of γ-chains, also known as Bart's hemoglobins, which do not release oxygen to the tissue effectively because of their high affinity to oxygen. Fetal hydrops develops secondary to fetal hypoxia. The adult carriers of hemoglobinopathy such as α-thalassemia or β-thalassemia have red blood cell mean corpuscular volume (MCV) of less than 80. Diagnosis of fetal α-thalassemia can be made with either DNA analysis of fetal chromosomes for the gene deletion or the presence of Bart's hemoglobin in the fetal blood.

Glucose-6-phosphate dehydrogenase (G6P-D) deficiency may subject the fetus to hemolysis of red blood cells upon exposure to oxidative agents such as fovea beans, sulfasoxazole and methylene blue. This disorder is transmitted as an X-linked recessive pattern and occurs more commonly among African and Greek descendants. Fetal hydrops develops from severe fetal anemia which could be corrected by fetal transfusion of red blood cells.

CLINICAL MANAGEMENT

Perinatal morbidity and mortality are high and depend on the etiology and severity of the fetal hydrops. Isolated fetal conditions such as chylous ascites without an identifiable cause have better outcomes[2]. A detailed ultrasound examination of the fetal anatomy, amniotic fluid, and placenta is essential to rule out coexisting major structural anomalies and signs of fetal infection such as calcifications and hepatosplenomegaly. Initial maternal screening tests include: (i) indirect Coomb's test for red blood cell (RBC) isoimmunization; (ii) a complete blood count (CBC) with differential and indices for infection and thalassemia; (iii) Kleihauer-Betke test for fetomaternal hemorrhage; (iv) serum IgG and IgM antibody titers to *T. gondii*, parvovirus (B19), and cytomegalovirus; and (v) RPR or VDRL titers for *T. pallidum*. Amniocentesis may be performed to analyze fetal chromosomes, to identify antigens of the involved organisms using PCR or monoclonal antibodies, and to determine fetal lung maturity as indicated. Funicentesis may be performed to determine the fetal hemoglobin, CBC, organism-specific antibodies, infectious organisms' antigens, and cultures depending on the potential causes. Fetal therapy may include maternal administration of medications for selected fetal infectious diseases and fetal arrhythmia and fetal administration of red blood cells either by intravascular or intraperitoneal routes for fetal anemia. Close fetal monitoring of fetal well-being is indicated since there is a high incidence of perinatal mortality. The timing of delivery depends on the associated condition, gestational age, fetal growth, the potential success of intrauterine therapies and the status of fetal well-being and fetal lung maturity. The mode of delivery depends on the fetal size and fetal tolerance to labor. Paracentesis may be performed prior to labor and delivery to reduce the risk of abdominal dystocia if fetal ascites are excessive. Presence of an attending neonatologist at the time of delivery for neonatal resuscitation and evaluation is recommended. Fetuses with NIH may benefit from a multidisciplinary approach consisting of maternal-fetal medicine physicians, neonatologists, geneticists, and appropriate pediatric medical or surgical subspecialists.

REFERENCES

1. Jauniaux E. Diagnosis and management of early nonimmune hydrops fetalis. *Prenat Diagn* 1997;17:1261–8
2. Winn HN, Stiller R, Grannum PAT, *et al.* Isolated fetal ascites: prenatal diagnosis and management. *Am J Perinatol* 1990;7:370–3
3. Machin GA. Hydrops revisited: literature review of 1414 cases published in the 1980s. *Am J Med Genet* 1989;34:366–90
4. Norton MA. Nonimmune hydrops fetalis. *Semin Perinatol* 1994;18:321–32
5. Van den Veyver IB, Ni J, Bowles N, *et al.* Detection of intrauterine infection using the polymerase chain reaction. *Mol Genet Metab* 1998;63:85–95
6. Kovacs BW, Carlson DE, Shahbahrami B, *et al.* Prenatal diagnosis of human parvovirus B19 in nonimmune hydrops fetalis by polymerase chain reaction. *Am J Obstet Gynecol* 1992;167:461–6
7. Towbin JA, Griffin LD, Martin AB, *et al.* Intrauterine adenoviral myocarditis presenting as nonimmune hydrops fetalis: diagnosis by polymerase chain reaction. *Pediatr Infect Dis J* 1994;13:144–50
8. Gentilomi G, Zerbini M, Gallinella G, *et al.* B19 parvovirus induced fetal hydrops: Rapid and simple diagnosis by detection of B19 antigens in amniotic fluids. *Prenat Diagn* 1998;18:363–8
9. Chervenak FA, Isaacson MD, Blakemore KJ, *et al.* Fetal cystic hygroma. *N Engl J Med* 1983;309:822–5
10. Trauffer PML, Anderson CE, Johnson A, *et al.* The natural history of euploid pregnancies with first-trimester cystic hygromas. *Am J Obstet Gynecol* 1994;170:1279–84
11. Tricoire J, Sarramon MF, Rolland M, *et al.* Familial cystic hygroma. Report of eight cases in three families. *Genet Counsel* 1993;4:265–9
12. Hirata GI, Masaki DI, O'Toole M, *et al.* Color flow mapping and Doppler velocimetry in the diagnosis and management of a placental chorioangioma associated with nonimmune fetal hydrops. *Obstet Gynecol* 1993;81:850–2

Section VII

Perinatal genetics

64
Basic genetics and patterns of inheritance

D.K. Grange

INTRODUCTION

The field of medical genetics is rapidly expanding. Genetics is becoming increasingly important in the general practice of medicine. Thus, the primary care physician has a responsibility to acquire adequate knowledge of genetics to provide his or her patients with the most up-to-date medical care. In addition to advances in the understanding of the genetic basis for many of the more frequent chromosomal, single-gene and multiple anomaly syndromes, there is greater knowledge of the role of genetics in common disorders such as hypertension, diabetes, heart disease, cancer, psychiatric disorders, and other medical problems. Medical genetics has a particularly great impact in the practice of obstetrics, in the evaluation and the management of fetal abnormalities, resulting in a need for close working relationships between clinical geneticists and specialists in maternal–fetal medicine. As the growth of information and technology continues, it is anticipated that new forms of genetic therapy, at the somatic cell level and possibly at the germ cell level, will be developed[1]. Some of these treatments may be employed preconceptually and during pregnancy, requiring the involvement of obstetricians and gynecologists.

The human genome contains three billion base pairs of DNA, packaged into units known as chromosomes and encoding an estimated 50 000 to 100 000 genes[2]. At the present time, over 10 000 single-gene traits or disorders have been identified[3]. The Human Genome Project, a government-funded research program, was begun in the 1980s and will continue for 15–20 years[4]. Its goal is to completely sequence the human genome. In the process, new genes and new information about the genetic basis for many disorders will be discovered. This has already begun to have a huge impact on the practice of medical genetics and medicine in general.

CYTOGENETICS

Cytogenetics is the study of chromosomes and their abnormalities[5]. The field of cytogenetics is a relative newcomer in clinical laboratory medicine. It was not until the mid-1950s that chromosome analysis could be done. Soon after it was determined that the normal number of chromosomes in humans is 46, rapid discoveries in the area of human cytogenetics were made. In 1959, LeJeune identified the cytogenetic basis of Down syndrome, and around the same time, sex chromosome abnormalities were found in patients with anomalies of sexual development. Techniques for analysis of chromosomes have continued to be improved and refined, allowing more subtle abnormalities to be identified. Newer molecular cytogenetic methods have revolutionized the identification and confirmation of microdeletions and cryptic translocations.

Humans have a total of 46 chromosomes, including 22 pairs of numbered chromosomes, or autosomes, and one pair of sex chromosomes. Females have two X chromosomes, while males have one X and one Y chromosome. Each chromosome is comprised of a single length of double stranded DNA, ranging in size from 50 million to 250 million basepairs. This genetic information is tightly compressed and packaged in the formation of the chromosomes. The DNA molecules are complexed with proteins called histones. The histones are packaged into nucleosomes, which are further compacted into a helical structure known as a solenoid. Finally, the solenoids are wound in a helical fashion and compressed to form the chromatin loops. Chromatin is packaged into chromosomes, which can be viewed microscopically during the metaphase stage of cell division.

Performing karyotype analyses has become an integral part of many areas of medical practice, including obstetrics, pediatrics and oncology. Chromosome analysis first involves obtaining a sample of living tissue. This can be blood, skin, amniotic fluid, products of conception, bone marrow, or any viable solid tissue. Blood is the most frequently obtained sample for routine chromosome analysis. For blood, the lymphocytes are isolated. For amniotic fluid, the amniocytes are obtained by spinning down the fluid and removing the cell pellet. For solid tissues, the tissue is minced and/or sonicated. For all tissue types, the cells are cultured in tissue culture for 48–72 hours. Cell division is arrested at metaphase by the addition of colcemid. The cells are then harvested and placed on a microscope slide. The cell nuclei are ruptured by adding a hypotonic solution, then stained to show the bands, and the metaphase spreads are photographed. Chromosome

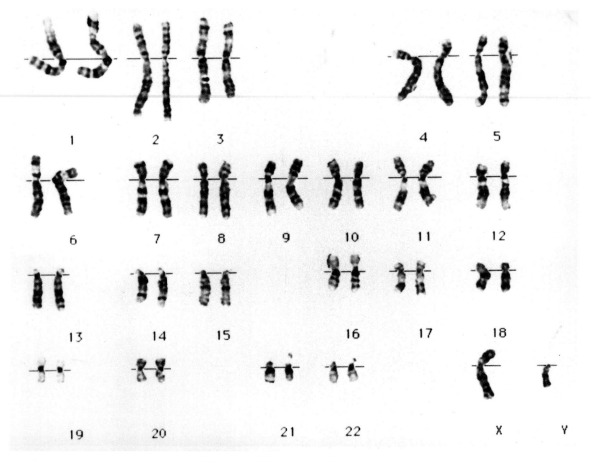

Figure 1   Normal male karyotype

pictures can then be cut manually from the photographs, organized by number and pasted in order for analysis. Each chromosome is studied by looking at the banding pattern to identify not only numerical abnormalities, but also structural problems. Newer computer technology allows karyotype analysis by computer imaging methods which reduces technologist work time. By convention, the 22 autosome pairs are arranged by size, from the largest to the smallest, in four rows, with the pair of sex chromosomes in the lower right corner (Figure 1). Ideograms are schematic representations of banding patterns used by cytogeneticists to standardize numbering of specific bands (Figure 2)[6].

Chromosomes have distinctive structural appearances when viewed microscopically. There are two arms with a central narrowing called the centromere. The shorter arm is termed p for 'petit,' while the longer arm is denoted q, because q comes after p alphabetically. The p arm is always shown at the top on karyotypes. There are three types of chromosomes structurally. Metacentric chromosomes have p and q arms that are almost equal in length, with the centromere located in the middle. Submetacentric

chromosomes have a shorter p arm with the centromere placed closer to the top of the chromosome and acrocentric chromosomes have small p arms called satellites with the centromere located near the top of the chromosome. The ends of chromosomes are called the telomeres (Figure 3).

Various banding techniques are used to visualize the chromosomes. The most frequently used method is Giemsa-banding or G-banding, which results in a specific pattern of dark and light bands on each chromosome. The older method, quinacrine-banding, or Q-banding, produces the same dark and light patterns, but requires the use of a fluorescence microscope and is not used routinely. Reverse-banding, or R-banding, results in the opposite of the dark and light pattern seen with G-banding; this may be used to better see the ends of the chromosomes. C-banding stains the constitutive heterochromatin which is near the centromeres and NOR stain visualizes the nucleolar organizing regions of the satellites and stalks of acrocentric chromosomes. For routine karyotype analysis, G-banding is typically used by most laboratories. Additional stains can be employed if necessary to clarify abnormalities.

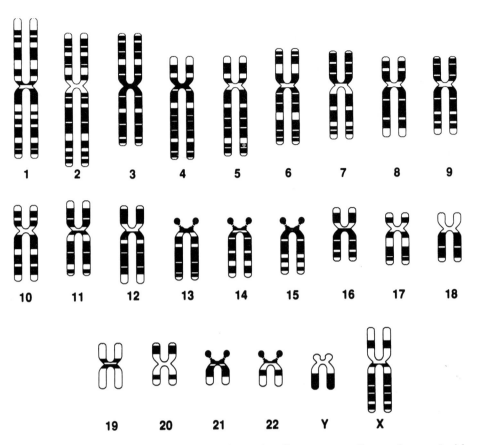

Figure 2   Ideogram of human chromosome showing Giemsa banding patterns. From reference 6 with permission

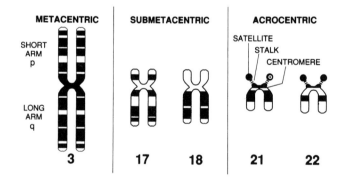

Figure 3   Human chromosome morphology as classified by variation in chromosome size and centromere position. From reference 6 with permission

CHROMOSOMAL ABNORMALITIES

Chromosome abnormalities are seen in 1 in 150 to 1 in 170 livebirths and thus, as a group, contribute significantly to morbidity and mortality among neonates and infants[7]. Any baby that has two or more congenital anomalies should have a karyotype performed (Table 1). Some of the more frequent chromosome anomalies will be reviewed, as well as the categories of chromosome abnormalities.

Table 1   Indications for chromosome analysis

- Suspected recognizable chromosome abnormality
- Infant with two or more malformations
- Mental retardation or developmental delay of unknown etiology, with or without malformations
- Relatives of people with known translocation, deletions, or duplications
- Stillborn infants with malformations or no known reason for fetal demise
- Females with short stature
- Males with infertility, small testes or gynecomastia
- Males with suspected Fragile X syndrome

Aneuploidy

The term 'aneuploidy' refers to an abnormal total number of chromosomes[6]. For example, an individual who has either a missing or extra copy of one of the chromosomes is said to have aneuploidy. Aneuploidy is the most common type of chromosome aberration found in humans and arises by a process known as 'non-disjunction'. Non-disjunction occurs when there is a failure of proper distribution of chromosome pairs into daughter cells during meiosis, leading to gametes that have either an extra copy of a given chromosome or a missing copy of that chromosome. Meiosis is the

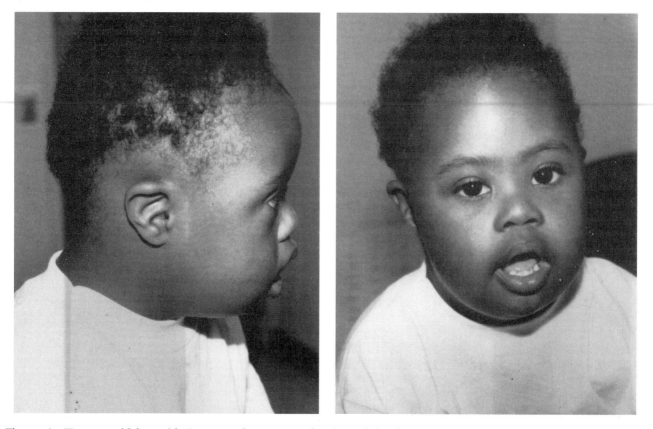

Figure 4 Two-year-old boy with Down syndrome. Note brachycephaly, dysplastic ears, epicanthal folds and upslanting palpebral fissures

process by which the chromosomes in the gamete are reduced from the diploid state (46 chromosomes) to the haploid state (23 chromosomes). There are two cell divisions in meiosis, called meiosis I and meiosis II. In meiosis I cell division, which is also known as the reduction division stage, two haploid cells are formed from one diploid cell. Meiosis II division results in replication of each haploid cell. Non-disjunction can occur in either meiosis I or meiosis II, although 80% of the time it is during meiosis I[8]. There is a clear association between advancing maternal age and an increased risk for non-disjunctional events[9]. However, regardless of parental ages, it has been shown that the extra number 21 in children with trisomy 21 is of maternal origin in 95% of cases and of paternal origin in only 5% of cases[10]. In general, if a zygote has monosomy for an autosome, early embryogenesis will fail and a spontaneous pregnancy loss will occur, sometimes even before the first missed menstrual period. On the other hand, trisomy for an autosome may result in a longer surviving embryo or fetus, or even a liveborn infant. Trisomy 13, trisomy 18 and trisomy 21 (Down syndrome) are the only autosomal trisomies that can result in viable infants in the non-mosaic state. However, mosaicism for many different autosomal

trisomies, that is, the presence of both normal and trisomic cells in one individual, has been described in viable infants. Sex chromosome aneuploidy has, in general, less deleterious effects on the affected individual.

Down syndrome

Down syndrome, or trisomy 21, is the most common autosomal chromosome abnormality seen in liveborn infants (Figure 4). It occurs in approximately 1 in 700 newborns. As mentioned above, the risk of non-disjunction increases with advancing maternal age, and prenatal testing for Down syndrome and other trisomies should be offered to all women who will be over age 35 at the time of delivery[11]. Down syndrome is caused by the presence of three copies of chromosome 21 (Figure 5). In 95% of cases, there is straightforward trisomy 21 (denoted 47,XX,+21 in a female and 47,XY,+21 in a male), with an extra 21 in every cell of the body, arising by non-disjunction. About 2–3% of patients have mosaicism, with some portion of cells having a normal chromosome complement; mosaicism is caused by postzygotic non-disjunction. The features of Down syndrome may be milder in the mosaic form, depending on what percentage of cells are normal.

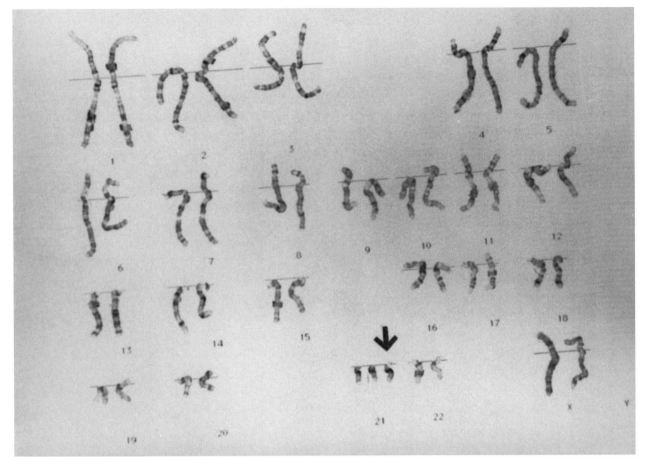

Figure 5   Karyotype of trisomy 21. Arrow indicates extra chromosome 21

About 2% of Down syndrome cases are caused by a translocation, usually a Robertsonian translocation involving another acrocentric chromosome, such as the number 14 (14;21) or the number 21 (21;21). Karyotyping on all newborns with clinical features of Down syndrome will identify those who have the translocation form. Approximately 25% of translocation cases are inherited from a parent, with a high risk of recurrence in future pregnancies[12,13]. Therefore, chromosome analysis should be done on the parents of all cases of translocation type Down syndrome. If a woman is a 14;21 Robertsonian translocation carrier, there is a 15% risk of Down syndrome in each pregnancy, as well as a high risk of recurrent spontaneous abortions due to the other possible unbalanced chromosome complements in the offspring. If a man is a carrier, the risk of a liveborn baby with trisomy 21 is only about 5%[14,15].

Individuals with Down syndrome usually have a moderate degree of mental retardation, with IQ in the 50–60 range. Some have milder mental retardation, while others fall into the severe range. The degree of mental retardation cannot be determined at birth. Early intervention, with involvement in infant stimulation and parent training programs can improve the developmental outcome. Most people with Down syndrome are educable and many can be mainstreamed in regular classrooms in school. Increasing numbers of individuals with Down syndrome are able to live semi-independently and hold jobs in supervised settings.

There are a number of associated birth defects and medical problems in Down syndrome. Approximately 40–50% of babies with trisomy 21 have a congenital heart defect, frequently an atrioventricular canal or septal defect[16]. About 12% of these babies have a malformation of the gastrointestinal tract, most often duodenal atresia, but occasionally Hirschsprung's disease, imperforate anus or tracheoesophageal fistula. Other birth defects include congenital cataracts (3%), syndactyly, eleven pairs of ribs and urinary tract anomalies (2–3%)[16]. Anomalies can be detected by prenatal ultrasound, particularly the heart defects and duodenal atresia. If either of these types of anomalies are seen, prenatal testing for Down syndrome should be considered.

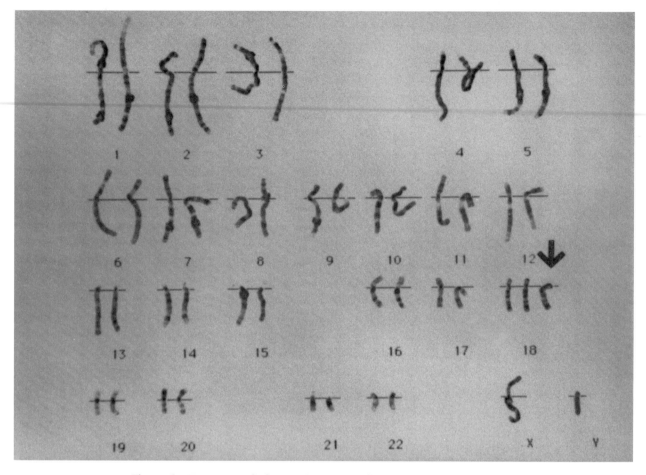

Figure 6 Karyotype of trisomy 18. Arrow indicates extra chromosome 18

Postnatal medical problems, in addition to developmental delay and mental retardation, include poor feeding and hypotonia in infancy, obesity later in life, visual impairment (myopia in 70%), recurrent otitis media and hearing loss, hypothyroidism (20%), atlantoaxial or atlanto-occipital instability (10–30%), and childhood leukemia (1%)[17].

Trisomy 18

Trisomy 18 (Edward syndrome) is a much less common autosomal trisomy, seen in approximately 1 in 7000 liveborn infants[18]. It has been estimated that at least two-thirds of trisomy 18 conceptions are lost by spontaneous abortion. Trisomy 18 is caused by the presence of three copies of the number 18 chromosome, again arising by non-disjunction in meiosis I or meiosis II (Figure 6).

The prognosis for trisomy 18 is extremely poor and the majority of infants die within the first three months of life. There are, however, a few individuals who have survived to their teens and twenties. The associated mental retardation is in the severe to profound range. In general, the birth defects seen in trisomy 18 are more frequent and much more severe than in trisomy 21 (Figure 7). Most infants have significant intrauterine growth restriction, which may be identified by prenatal ultrasound. Approximately 85% of infants have a congenital heart defect, including septal defects, multivalvular dysplasia, and complex anomalies. Other anomalies are dysmorphic facial features, short sternum, joint contractures, overlapping digits, rocker bottom feet, renal abnormalities, and occasionally gastrointestinal tract anomalies and neural tube defects.

Trisomy 13

Trisomy 13 (Patau syndrome) is the third autosomal trisomy which can be seen in liveborn infants (Figure 8). It is less common than trisomy 18 and occurs in about 1 in 12 000 livebirths[18]. As in trisomy

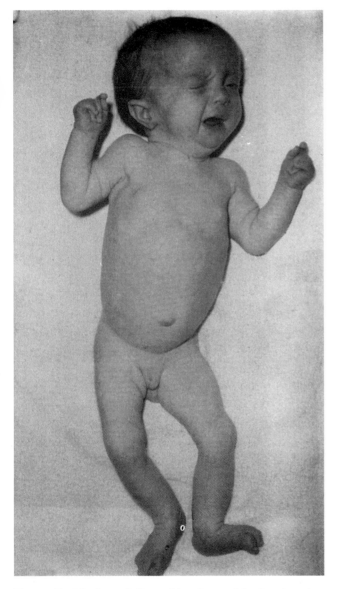

Figure 7 Newborn infant with trisomy 18, showing dysmorphic facies, flexion contracture of fingers and rocker bottom feet

18, the prognosis for trisomy 13 is very poor, with most infants dying in the first three months. Depending on the severity of the associated birth defects, longer-term survival is possible. Infants with trisomy 13 tend to be better grown than those with trisomy 18 (Figure 9). However, they are more likely to have microcephaly, which can be seen by prenatal ultrasound. Congenital heart defects are present in 80–85%, again often of a complex nature. Those with less significant heart defects may survive longer. Holoprosencephaly, cleft lip and palate, renal anomalies and omphalocele are frequent abnormalities in trisomy 13 which may be detected by prenatal ultrasound.

Sex chromosome abnormalities

Sex chromosome abnormalities as a group are very common. Approximately 1 in 500 individuals has a sex chromosome abnormality, although it has been suggested that the true incidence may be higher. Some cases may never be ascertained due to the relatively mild signs and symptoms associated with most of the common sex chromosome problems. Many patients are not diagnosed until adulthood when they may undergo evaluation for infertility or other reproductive problems.

Turner syndrome

Turner syndrome is one of the most familiar sex chromosome abnormalities. It is caused by the presence of only one X chromosome (45,X) in phenotypic females. This classic Turner karyotype is seen in 50% of cases; other cases may be mosaic (45,X/46,XX), or may be caused by an abnormal X chromosome, such as an isochromosome or ring X[6]. Rarely, there may be portions of a Y chromosome present in some cases. Turner syndrome is seen in 1 in 2500 to 1 in 5000 newborn girls. However, it is well known that the incidence is much higher in early pregnancy, with 95% of 45,X embryos and fetuses being lost by spontaneous miscarriage. This would suggest that the incidence among conceptuses could be as high as 1.5%, an extraordinarily high frequency[2].

Features of Turner syndrome detectable by prenatal ultrasound include cystic hygroma, lymphedema or hydrops fetalis; when these abnormalities are seen, the prognosis for survival of the pregnancy is poor[19]. Smaller cystic hygromas may resolve during pregnancy, leaving a webbed neck or excess nuchal skin. Other anomalies seen in Turner syndrome include congenital heart defects, frequently coarctation of the aorta, and renal anomalies, often horseshoe kidney. Lymphedema may be seen at birth, often involving the dorsum of the hands and feet, as well as a shield-shaped chest and wide-spaced nipples. For surviving girls with Turner syndrome, the prognosis for good health and a normal lifespan is excellent. Intelligence is normal, although there may be some specific learning disabilities. However, due to the 'streak' ovaries, puberty and the onset of menses will not occur without hormone therapy and the average adult height without treatment is 57 inches (145 cm). The long-term outcome with estrogen/progesterone replacement and growth hormone therapy is very good. Recently, a number of successful pregnancies in women with Turner syndrome have been reported, with the use of ovum donation and *in vitro* fertilization techniques[20].

Klinefelter syndrome

Klinefelter syndrome is caused by the presence of an extra X chromosome in a phenotypic male (47,XXY)

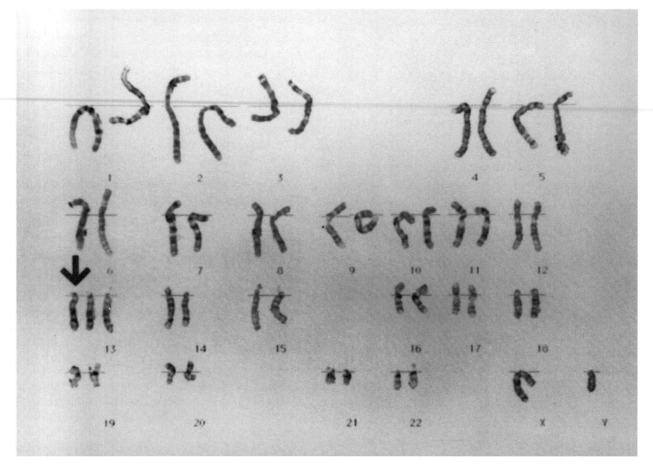

Figure 8   Karyotype of trisomy 13. Arrow indicates extra chromosome 13

and occurs in approximately 1 in 500 to 1 in 1000 males. If Klinefelter syndrome is detected prenatally, it is usually by chance, when an amniocentesis is being done for other reasons. There are no expected fetal anomalies in Klinefelter syndrome and most cases are not diagnosed in infancy. The diagnosis may be suspected in a boy with tall thin body habitus and mild learning disabilities. Testicular size is usually normal in prepubertal boys. However, boys with Klinefelter syndrome fail to go through puberty normally and eventually have small, firm testes and relatively hypoplastic external genitalia. They are sterile, and the diagnosis is sometimes made in an adult infertility or urology clinic.

47,XXX syndrome

This chromosome abnormality is thought to occur in 1 in 1000 women, although the true incidence may be higher. Many cases are probably never ascertained because of the mild nature of the associated signs and symptoms. There is no recognizable phenotype, except perhaps tall stature and mild learning problems. Fertility is normal and the risk of sex chromosome aneuploidy in the offspring of an affected woman appears to be low.

47,XYY syndrome

This chromosome abnormality is also fairly common, occurring in about 1 in 800 men. Again, there is no definite phenotype except taller than expected stature, slightly long facies and long digits. Most individuals have normal intelligence, but there have been reports of personality disorders and antisocial behavior. The incidence may be underestimated due to the nonspecific phenotype. This condition is most often diagnosed serendipitously.

Structural alterations

In addition to aneuploidy, in which there is loss or gain of an entire chromosome, rearrangements, deletions or duplications of portions of chromosomes can occur.

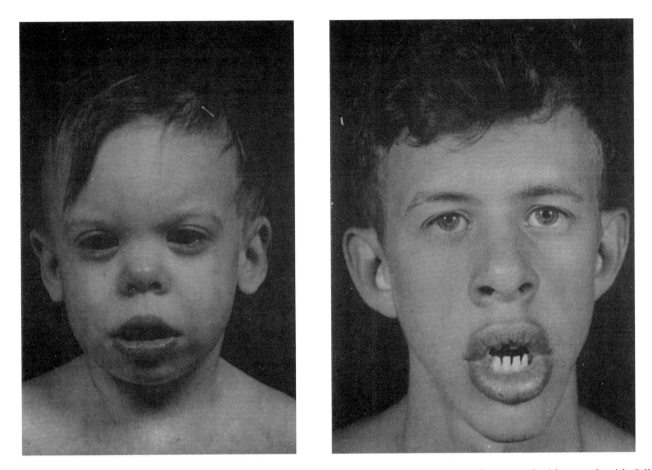

Figure 13   Two unrelated boys with Williams syndrome. Note epicanthal folds, upturned nose and wide mouth with full lips. From reference 22 with permission

the more likely it is that abnormal offspring can be produced, since the duplicated or deleted segments are smaller. The overall risk that a pericentric inversion carrier will have karyotypically abnormal children is estimated to be between 1% and 10%[21].

Finally, isochromosomes result from loss of either the p arm or q arm of a metacentric or submetacentric chromosome, with duplication of the remaining arm, thus causing trisomy for the p or q arm of a pair of chromosomes and monosomy for the opposite arm. This is seen most commonly in some cases of Turner syndrome, when the X chromosome is involved. Isochromosomes for the autosomes would be expected to cause very severe and likely lethal abnormalities in most cases.

Chromosome abnormalities in spontaneous abortions

Chromosomes examined from products of conception from pregnancy losses at various stages of gestation show an exceptionally high rate of chromosomal abnormalities. In fact, as many as 10–15% of early

embryos have a chromosome abnormality, usually leading to spontaneous pregnancy loss[24]. Approximately 50–60% of spontaneous abortions are caused by a chromosome anomaly in the embryo or fetus[25]. At the time of livebirth, approximately 1 in 150 newborns is chromosomally abnormal. Thus, as stated by John Opitz, 'it seems established that most of "humanity" dies before, rather than after birth, and that perhaps only a third survive from the earliest beginnings till [sic] birth…'[26]. The most frequent abnormalities seen are autosomal trisomies (52%), especially trisomy 16 (15%), trisomy 13, 18 and 21. 45,X accounts for 18% of abnormalities and triploidy 17%[27]. There is a steady loss of these abnormal pregnancies throughout the first trimester. By 20 weeks, the incidence has fallen to 27 in 1000 or 2.7% and by full term, the incidence is 6 in 1000 or 0.6%[25].

In the vast majority of cases, the occurrence of a chromosomally abnormal pregnancy with spontaneous abortion does not increase the risk of recurrence in a future pregnancy. A general rule of thumb is that products of conception should be evaluated by karyotype analysis after the third pregnancy loss. Parental

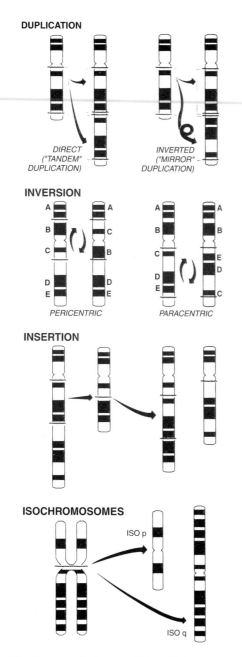

Figure 14   Structural abnormalities of chromosomes. See text for details. From reference 6 with permission

Table 3   Common single-gene disorders

Disease	Incidence
Autosomal dominant	
Adenomatous polyposis coli	1 in 6000
Adult polyoptic kidney disease	1 in 1000
Familial hyper-cholesterolemia	1 in 500
Hereditary nonpolyposis colorectal cancer	up to 1 in 200
Huntington disease	1 in 20 000
Marfan syndrome	1 in 10 000 to 1 in 20 000
Myotonic dystrophy	1 in 7000 to 1 in 20 000
Neurofibromatosis Type I	1 in 3000 to 1 in 5000
Osteogenesis imperfecta	1 in 10 000 to 1 in 15 000
Autosomal recessive	
α_1-Antitrypsin deficiency	1 in 2500–1 in 10 000 Caucasian
Cystic fibrosis	1 in 2000 Caucasian
Hemochromatosis	1 in 5000
Phenylketonuria	1 in 10 000–1 in 20 000
Sickle cell disease	1 in 400 African–Americans
Tay–Sachs disease	1/3000 Ashkenasi Jews
Thalassemia	1 in 50–1 in 100 Asian and Mediterranean population
X-linked	
Duchenne muscular dystrophy	1 in 3500 males
Fragile X syndrome	1 in 1200 males; 1 in 2500 females
Hemophilia A	1 in 10 000 males
Color blindness	8% of males
Glucose-6-phosphate dehydrogenase deficiency	10–15% of African–American males

blood chromosomes should also be analyzed at this point, looking for a balanced translocation in one of the partners. A translocation is found in approximately 5–10% of couples with recurrent miscarriages[28].

MENDELIAN INHERITANCE

In 1865, an Austrian monk named Gregor Mendel published his now famous treatise on the inheritance of characteristics in garden peas, leading eventually to the modern study of genes and inheritance, including human genetic disorders. However, Mendel's original work was largely ignored during his lifetime. In fact, his contemporary, Charles Darwin, apparently never knew of Mendel's research and hypotheses. Mendel's work was 'rediscovered' at the beginning of the 20th century. In 1902, Archibald Garrod reported the first known human Mendelian disorder, alkaptonuria. Over the last century, thousands of human single-gene traits and disorders have been described (Table 3). These conditions have been catalogued by Victor McKusick in his *Mendelian Inheritance in Man*[3].

Since there are two copies of each chromosome, we also have two copies of each gene. Alternative forms of the same gene are called 'alleles'. Each chromosome contains several hundred to several thousand different genes. At the time of conception, one of each pair of genes is inherited from the mother and the other of each pair from the father. Thus, an equal amount of genetic information is received from each parent.

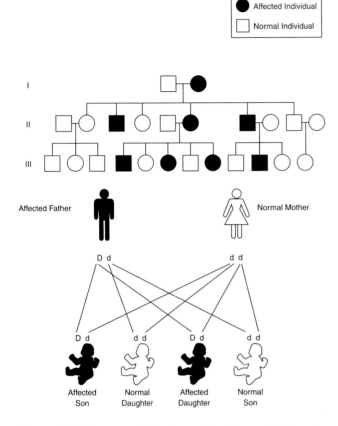

Figure 15 Autosomal dominant inheritance. Both males and females are affected and there is male-to-male transmission of the disorder. From reference 22 with permission

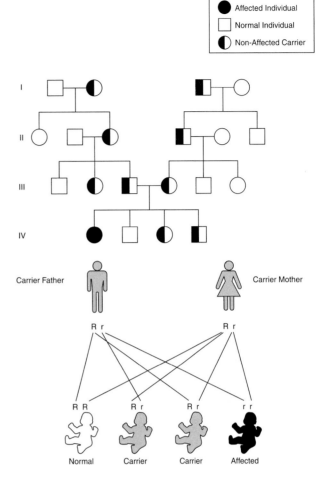

Figure 16 Autosomal recessive inheritance. Note that both parents must be carriers and the affected offspring may be male or female. From reference 22 with permission

There are four basic inheritance patterns of human single gene disorders. These include autosomal dominant and autosomal recessive inheritance, in which the mutant gene is on an autosome, and X-linked dominant and X-linked recessive inheritance, in which the mutant gene is on the X chromosome. Individuals can be heterozygous for a given gene, meaning that they have two different forms, or alleles, of the gene at the same locus on each of the two different chromosomes. Individuals can also be homozygous for a gene, in which the two alleles are identical. Males are said to be hemizygous with respect to genes on the X chromosome, since they have only one copy of the X.

In autosomal dominant genetic disorders, only one copy of a mutant allele is necessary for expression of the disease (Figure 15). Thus, heterozygotes will be affected. The risk of passing on the mutation to an offspring is 50% for each pregnancy. Vertical transmission of the disorder is seen on pedigree analysis, and the condition can often be traced back many generations. However, there are certain caveats to keep in mind when evaluating autosomal dominant disorders. First, there is a high degree of variability of expression of dominant conditions. Even within the same family,

some individuals may be severely affected while others may have very mild and medically insignificant features. Thus, thorough review of medical histories and physical examinations on multiple family members are often parts of a genetic evaluation. Second, there may be reduced penetrance of a dominant disorder. Thus, a heterozygote may not show any manifestations of the mutant gene after a complete medical evaluation. Finally, many autosomal dominant disorders have a high new spontaneous mutation rate and a dominant condition may appear *de novo* in an isolated individual in a pedigree. However, once present, it can be passed on to subsequent generations. Abnormal genes in autosomal dominant disorders often encode structural proteins, such as collagen, which is abnormal in osteogenesis imperfecta, or fibrillin, which is mutant in Marfan syndrome.

In autosomal recessive conditions, two copies of a mutant allele are necessary for expression, and only homozygotes will be affected (Figure 16). Heterozygotes for recessive genes are usually normal and do not have any manifestations of the disease, but they are carriers. Autosomal recessive disorders manifest only if both parents are carriers of the same mutant gene and the offspring receives one mutant allele from each parent. Some individuals with autosomal recessive disorders may be compound heterozygotes, meaning that they have two different mutant alleles of the same gene, resulting in expression of the disorder. Recurrence risk for a recessive disorder is 25% for each pregnancy. There is a 25% chance of having a normal non-carrier child and a 50% chance of having a carrier child. Pedigree analysis usually does not reveal other affected family members outside of the nuclear family group, unless there is consanguinity. The incidence of an autosomal recessive disorder in a population is related to the frequency of heterozygotes. The carrier rate for some conditions is high, while it is very low for others. Recessive conditions have a higher incidence in isolated or inbred populations. Recessive disorders show little variation in expression among affected members within a pedigree, although there may be interfamilial variation due to different mutant alleles. In general, recessive disorders more likely involve genes that encode enzymes or molecules important in cellular functions. Examples include inborn errors of metabolism caused by enzyme deficiencies, hemoglobinopathies, and cellular membrane transport mechanisms, as in cystic fibrosis.

X-linked recessive conditions are caused by mutations in genes on the X chromosome. Since males are hemizygous for X-linked genes, they will express such mutations, while females with a mutant recessive gene on one X chromosome will be carriers with a normal phenotype (Figure 17). There are exceptions to these rules. For example, if the X inactivation process results in a larger proportion of active X chromosomes carrying the mutant allele, a female may have expression or partial expression of the disorder. In X-linked dominant conditions, only one copy of the mutant allele is needed for full expression of the disorder (Figure 18). In this situation, males and females are both affected, but males will generally have more severe manifestations than females, or the mutation may even be lethal in males.

There are very few known Y-linked genes at this time. The most recent edition of *Mendelian Inheritance in Man* lists 18 genes identified on the Y chromosome, including the *SRY* gene, which is involved in male sex determination[3]. Y-linked, or holandric, conditions, such as maleness itself, are passed exclusively from father to son.

MULTIFACTORIAL INHERITANCE

In multifactorial inheritance, it is postulated that genetic influences from both parents, in combination with environmental factors, lead to a specific birth defect or disorder. Examples of birth defects with

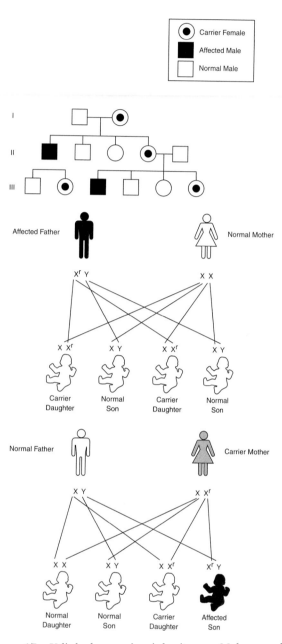

Figure 17   X-linked recessive inheritance. Males can be affected in multiple generations and they inherit the trait from their mothers. From reference 22 with permission

multifactorial inheritance include isolated congenital heart defects, cleft lip with or without cleft palate, cleft palate, neural tube defects, pyloric stenosis, and congenital dislocation of the hips (Table 4). In multifactorial disorders, there is no evidence to suggest simple Mendelian inheritance. For example, the defect does not necessarily appear in sequential generations of a family, as would an autosomal dominant condition due to a single gene mutation. However, there may be clustering of the defect in more than one member of a pedigree. The appearance of multifactorial disorders has been explained by a threshold model in which

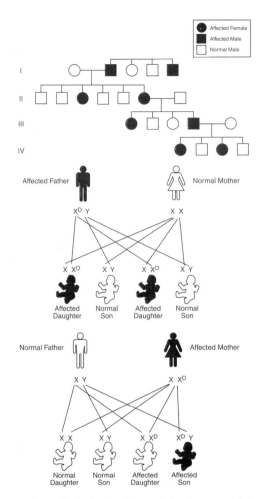

Figure 18 X-linked dominant inheritance. Males and females are affected, but male-to-male transmission does not occur. From reference 22 with permission

Table 4   Multifactorial disorders

Disorder	Incidence
Congenital malformations	
Cleft lip with/without cleft palate	1 in 500–1 in 1000
Cleft palate	1 in 1000
Club foot	1 in 1000
Congenital heart defects	1 in 200–1 in 500
Neural tube defects	1 in 500–1 in 1000
Pyloric stenosis	1 in 300
Adult diseases	
Alcoholism	1 in 10–1 in 20
Alzheimer's disease	1 in 10
Bipolar affective disorder	1 in 100–1 in 200
Cancer	1 in 3
Diabetes (Types I and II)	1 in 10
Coronary artery disease	1 in 3–1 in 5
Schizophrenia	1 in 100

certain genes present in an individual, along with prenatal environmental factors, accumulate towards a threshold. If an individual has enough of these genes and factors, a threshold will be crossed and the defect will appear[29].

Multifactorial disorders often show an increased incidence in one sex or the other. Pyloric stenosis is much more common in males, while dislocation of the hips is more common in females.

Once a couple has had a child with a multifactorial condition, the risk of having a second child with the same disorder is increased over the background population risk. Recurrence risk figures can be estimated for a given defect based on population studies. For example, the incidence of cleft lip with or without cleft palate is 1 in 700 to 1 in 1000 newborns. This risk increases to approximately 4% or 1 in 25 after a family has had one child with cleft lip, representing a forty-fold increased risk. However, the risk is still relatively small, with a 96% chance of having a normal child.

The exact environmental factors contributing to multifactorial conditions remain unknown in almost all cases. Regional factors must play a role, since it is well known that some areas of the world have a markedly increased incidence of certain defects. For example, the incidence of neural tube defects is approximately 1 in 1000 in the general population, but in parts of Great Britain, especially Ireland and Wales, the rate is as high as 7–9 in 1000 births[2]. Genetic influences must also play a role, since immigrants from these areas to other parts of the world still have a somewhat higher rate of neural tube defects[2]. However, other environmental variables such as diet must also be important. It has been shown that folic acid consumption in the diet of pregnant women can significantly reduce the recurrence risk of neural tube defects in subsequent pregnancies. The current recommendation by the Centers for Disease Control (CDC) states that all women of childbearing age who are capable of becoming pregnant should consume 400 μg of folic acid per day[30]. All women who have had a previous child with a neural tube defect should take 4 mg of folic acid per day, beginning two to three months prior to conception and continuing for the first three months of gestation[31]. The CDC is currently planning to supplement flour with folic acid to ensure proper intake for all women, since it is difficult to obtain more than 200 μg of folic acid a day from a typical American diet.

MITOCHONDRIAL INHERITANCE

There are a number of human genetic disorders caused by mutations of mitochondrial DNA (Table 5). Within the cytoplasm of each cell are several hundred mitochondria, which are involved in energy production for

Table 5   Mitochondrial diseases

- Kearns–Sayre disease
- Leber hereditary opticoneuropathy (LHON)
- Mitochondrial encephalopathy, lactic acidosis, and stroke-like episodes (MELAS)
- Myoclonic epilepsy and ragged-red fiber disease (MERFF)

the cell. Each mitochondrion has several copies of its own circular DNA (mtDNA), encoding some enzymes of oxidative phosphorylation, tRNA and rRNA. Because mtDNA is cytoplasmic in location, inheritance is exclusively maternal. Sperm contain very few mitochondria and therefore, both males and females inherit essentially all of their mtDNA from their mothers. There is variable expression of mitochondrial disorders due to heteroplasmy; this term refers to the variability of the proportion of mutant mtDNA within each cell. The proportion of abnormal mtDNA at the somatic level may change over time due to replicative segregation. This can account for the apparent degenerative nature of these disorders noted clinically, which corresponds to an increase in the percentage of abnormal mitochondria[32]. A woman who has a mitochondrial DNA disorder will pass it on to all of her offspring. However, because of the highly variable expression of these conditions, not all offspring would be expected to be affected to the same degree. Offspring of men with mitochondrial DNA disorders cannot inherit the condition because all mitochondria originate from the mother. It is important to remember that there are also many disorders associated with mitochondrial dysfunction that are inherited in a Mendelian fashion, since most proteins active within the mitochondria are encoded by nuclear DNA genes.

COMMON METABOLIC DISORDERS

Inborn errors of metabolism are due to enzyme deficiencies that cause abnormal elevations of intermediary compounds of biochemical pathways in tissues and body fluids, with resultant medical problems. Most have an autosomal recessive inheritance pattern, but a few are X-linked recessive disorders. There are several hundred known inborn errors of metabolism, most of which are very rare[33]. However, they are collectively common and affect about 1 in 1000 newborns.

One of the most common metabolic disorders is the autosomal recessive aminoacidopathy phenylketonuria (PKU), which has an incidence of 1 in 10 000 to 1 in 15 000 newborns[33]. It is caused by a deficiency of the enzyme phenylalanine hydroxylase, which normally converts phenylalanine to tyrosine. Patients with PKU have elevated blood levels of phenylalanine and excretion of phenylketones in the urine. If left untreated, affected individuals will develop

microcephaly and profound mental retardation due to toxic effects of the elevated compounds. However, if diagnosed within the first few weeks of life, with institution of a low phenylalanine diet, mental retardation can be prevented. PKU is the first genetic disorder for which there has been generalized population screening. Since the 1960s all newborns in the USA have been tested for the disorder. This has nearly eliminated PKU as a cause for mental retardation. However, a new problem has emerged; women who were allowed to stop the dietary restriction of phenylalanine after age 6 years are now of childbearing age. The elevated blood level of phenylalanine in a pregnant PKU woman has deleterious effects on the developing fetus, with increased risk for spontaneous pregnancy loss, congenital heart defects, severe microcephaly and mental retardation. Therefore, the PKU diet must be reinstituted prior to conception and continued throughout pregnancy. New guidelines state that all people with PKU should remain on the diet for life.

The USA and most developed countries of the world perform newborn screening for at least two diseases, phenylketonuria and congenital hypothyroidism. Many states have added additional metabolic disorders in their screening programs, such as galactosemia (45 of 50 states), homocystinuria, maple syrup urine disease (MSUD) and biotinidase deficiency, as well as other genetic conditions, including cystic fibrosis and hemoglobinopathies. For each of these disorders it has been shown that early diagnosis in the newborn period can significantly reduce morbidity and mortality. As mentioned above for phenylketonuria, institution of dietary restriction of phenylalanine before one month of age can prevent mental retardation. For other inborn errors of metabolism, such as MSUD and galactosemia, illness, mental retardation and even death can be prevented by early detection and treatment.

POPULATION SCREENING FOR GENETIC DISEASE

Screening tests are a routine part of medical care, with the goal of early identification and treatment of specific and common diseases. For genetic diseases, population screening involves not only affected individuals, but also additional family members. Screening for genetic disease has been defined as the 'search in a population for persons possessing certain genotypes that: (1) are already associated with disease or predisposition to disease or (2) may lead to disease in their descendants'[34]. As outlined in the previous section, newborn screening for metabolic diseases exemplifies the first type of screening, which will result in proper identification of infants with these disorders and institution of treatment. Other examples include presymptomatic genetic testing for Huntington disease, breast cancer or colon cancer.

The second type of screening includes testing of targeted ethnic or racial populations to identify carriers of genetic disease. Examples are cystic fibrosis in Caucasians, Tay–Sachs disease in Ashkenazi Jews and hemoglobinopathies in African–Americans[2]. On a smaller scale, genetic screening can involve karyotype analysis on family members at risk for having a chromosome translocation. Carrier testing is also available for women who are at risk to be carriers for X-linked disorders such as Duchenne muscular dystrophy or Fragile X syndrome. This type of population screening will not affect the health of the carrier, but will have a significant impact on reproductive choices for the family. It is essential that appropriate genetic counseling accompanies the information given regarding carrier status.

GENETIC COUNSELING

Genetic counseling is an important part of the practice of medical genetics. The field of genetics is unique in that a diagnosis of a genetic disorder in an individual has an impact on his or her entire family. Multiple family members and their present or future offspring may be at risk for the genetic disorder as well. Genetic counseling involves the explanation of the manifestations of the disorder, the natural history and treatment, the inheritance pattern, the risks of recurrence and the methods of prenatal and postnatal diagnosis. The genetic counselor also helps the family make the best possible adjustment to the disorder and the risks of recurrence. This often involves referral to a support organization through which the family can make contact with other affected individuals. The vast majority of genetic counselors and clinical geneticists seek to provide non-directive counseling, whereby information about the disorder and the recurrence risk is given in an unbiased and neutral way and the family makes decisions about reproductive options in accordance with their own beliefs and values.

Reasons for referral for genetic counseling include a family history of a known or suspected single gene disorder, chromosomal disorder, or multifactorial condition, carrier status for a genetic disease, consanguinity, advanced maternal age during pregnancy, abnormal screening tests during pregnancy, repeated pregnancy loss or infertility, or teratogen exposure during pregnancy.

In the prenatal clinic setting, the genetic counseling session often precedes any diagnostic testing. During the session, the family history is reviewed in detail, as well as the reasons for referral, the information obtainable by the prenatal testing and the risks of the procedure. If fetal abnormalities are detected, then additional counseling sessions may be required to explain the findings to the family and to discuss options for pregnancy management. If special care or

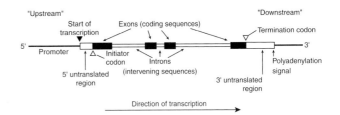

Figure 19 General structure of a typical human gene. From reference 7 with permission

surgery will be needed for the baby immediately after birth, the genetic counselor and the obstetrician may help arrange meetings with the appropriate surgeons or pediatric specialists so that the family is optimally prepared. For cases that are likely to be lethal, it is best to introduce the idea of a postmortem examination before the birth of the baby. In the event of death, a complete autopsy is recommended to search for additional anomalies and to confirm the diagnosis. This helps ensure that accurate genetic counseling, especially with respect to recurrence risk, can be provided in subsequent pregnancies.

MOLECULAR GENETICS

Genes are the basic units of inheritance. As mentioned previously, there are over 10 000 known single-gene traits or diseases, representing only a fraction of the estimated total 50 000–100 000 genes in the human genome. However, over the past five to ten years, there has been a dramatic increase in the number of identified, cloned and sequenced genes associated with human disease. With this new knowledge has come increased availability and demand for both prenatal and postnatal molecular genetic testing. Molecular genetic testing is done for diagnostic purposes to confirm the presence of a disorder, as well as to identify conditions presymptomatically.

Genes are composed of deoxyribonucleic acid (DNA) and are contained on the chromosomes. Each strand of DNA has a specific sequence of four nucleotides, each containing a different base, adenine, thymine, cytosine or guanine. Adenine pairs with thymine and cytosine pairs with guanine as two complementary strands of DNA are wound together to form a double helix. Genes have a common basic structure (Figure 19). First, there are upstream sequences that regulate transcription, known as promoters and enhancers. Then, there is a transcription initiation site, followed by a series of alternating exons and introns. The DNA sequence serves as a template from which messenger RNA (mRNA) is made; this process is known as transcription. As transcription proceeds, a primary mRNA is made from the DNA sequence of the gene, which includes the introns. The intron sequences are then spliced out and the exons are linked together to form the mature mRNA molecule. The function of

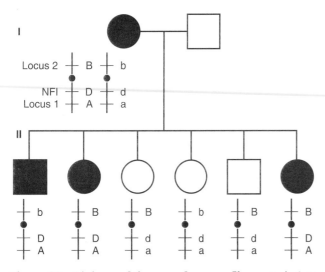

Figure 20 Linkage of the gene for neurofibromatosis 1 to a marker locus. The mother (I–1) is affected with this dominant disease and is heterozygous at the NF1 locus (*Dd*), as well as at two other loci, 1 and 2, on chromosome 17. She carries the *A* and *B* alleles on the same chromosome as the mutant NF1 allele (*D*). The unaffected father is homozygous normal (*dd*) at the NF1 locus, as well as at the two marker loci (*AA* and *BB*). All three affected offspring have inherited the *A* allele at marker 1, whereas the three unaffected offspring have inherited the *a* allele. Thus all six offspring are non-recombinant for NF1 and marker locus 1. However, individuals II-1, II-3, and II-5 are recombinant for NF1 and marker locus 2, indicating that meiotic crossing over has occurred between these two loci. From reference 7 with permission

introns is still not fully understood. Thus, the exons are the only portions of the gene that specify the final protein product. The mature mRNA molecule is used to make the protein product by the process of translation. Groups of three nucleotides, called codons, code for specific amino acids. Transfer RNA (tRNA) and ribosomal RNA (rRNA) interact with the mRNA to assemble the amino acids into a polypeptide chain to form the final protein molecule.

Errors in the sequence of nucleic acids of the DNA produce mutations in genes and often lead to genetic diseases. There are a variety of different kinds of mutations that can occur in genes. Some result in genetic disorders, while others may have no detrimental effect. The most common types of mutations include missense (single amino acid change), nonsense (insertion of stop codon with premature termination of translation), frameshift (insertion or deletion of nucleotides that alters downstream codons), splice site (incorrect splicing of introns) and promoter mutations (decreased transcription of mRNA). A newly identified type of mutation is the expansion mutation, in which there is insertion of many extra copies of a trinucleotide repeat.

Diagnosis is now possible for many genetic disorders using molecular genetic techniques. Testing can be accomplished by either direct mutation analysis or by linkage analysis (Figure 20). In linkage analysis, information about non-disease producing variations, or polymorphisms, such as RFLPs (restriction fragment-length polymorphisms), VNTRs (variable number of tandem repeats) or microsatellite repeat polymorphisms, can trace inheritance of a chromosome containing a disease-producing gene through a family. This method of testing has some disadvantages. First, multiple family members are needed to establish the phase of linkage. Second, some families may not be informative for some linked markers. Third, recombination between the marker and the disease gene may occur, causing inaccuracies in the test results.

In direct DNA testing, the gene must have been isolated and disease-producing mutations identified. Specific mutations can then be sought by a variety of methods. Direct testing is advantageous, since it is likely to be more accurate than linkage analysis and a single individual can be tested without requiring family information. For example, molecular genetic testing for sickle cell disease is highly accurate, since all affected individuals have the same missense mutation at position six of the β-globin chain, which results in a substitution of valine for glutamic acid. This point mutation results in a loss of one MstII restriction enzyme site in the mutant gene, making direct DNA diagnosis by RFLP analysis very straightforward. For other genetic disorders characterized by a relatively small number of common mutations, such as cystic fibrosis, allele-specific oligonucleotide probes (ASOs) of 18–20 nucleotides in length complementary to known normal and mutant DNA sequences can be devised. ASOs are then hybridized to patient DNA samples to identify homozygotes or heterozygotes for specific mutations. Thus, a panel of ASOs for the most common mutations seen in a disorder can be used to rapidly screen patient DNA samples.

GENE THERAPY

With the isolation of disease-producing genes, it has now become feasible to consider cures for genetic disease through various forms of gene therapy[35]. Gene therapy involves insertion of normal copies of genes into individuals who have genetic diseases. This can be potentially be accomplished by either somatic cell or germ cell gene therapy. Most work thus far has focused on somatic cell gene therapy.

There are two ways to approach somatic cell gene therapy. *Ex vivo* gene therapy involves removing a patient's cells from the body, inserting the normal gene copy into the cells and then returning the cells to the body. In *in vivo* gene therapy, cells are treated while in the patient's body. For successful gene therapy, the cell requiring treatment must be easily accessible and relatively long-lived. Some of the earliest human gene therapy trials were performed for severe combined immune deficiency due to adenosine deaminase deficiency, using bone marrow stem cells[36,37]. Other cells under consideration for therapy have included lymphocytes, hepatocytes, muscle cells, and respiratory epithelial cells.

There are a variety of methods available to insert genes into cells. Some are DNA-mediated, such as electroporation, calcium phosphate precipitation, microinjection and liposome fusion. However, viral-mediated methods have received the most attention thus far in human trials of gene therapy. All viruses used for gene therapy are rendered defective (i.e. unable to replicate) by removing their own genes involved in replication and packaging. Then, the desired human gene, along with its own regulatory elements, is inserted into the viral genome. Packaging cell lines are needed to prepare the recombinant virus for use as a treatment vector.

Retroviral vectors are useful because they incorporate their genome into the host genome very efficiently, potentially resulting in long-term correction. These vectors have been used in many of the *ex vivo* gene therapy trials, including treatment of adenosine deaminase deficiency. However, there are certain disadvantages to using retroviruses. They require actively dividing cells for infection. There is also the potential for oncogenesis, since the viral genome is randomly inserted into the host genome. Adenovirus vectors are also being used in human gene therapy, for example, in some of the *in vivo* gene therapy protocols for treatment of cystic fibrosis. Adenovirus can infect non-dividing cells and remains extrachromosomal in the host, which provides some advantages over retrovirus. However, gene expression is transient, decreasing the length of time that the therapeutic effect lasts and requiring repeated treatments. Other viruses being considered for use in gene therapy include adeno-associated virus and herpes simplex virus.

Types of genetic diseases that are amenable to somatic cell gene therapy are primarily autosomal recessive or X-linked disorders that result in almost total lack of normal protein. Reconstitution of even 5–10% of normal protein levels appears to be sufficient to treat these diseases. Dominant disorders that are caused by heterozygosity for mutant and normal genes (dominant-negative mutations) are not likely to be treatable by gene replacement; methods to block production of the mutant protein will be required to treat these conditions.

REFERENCES

1. Jorde LB, Carey JC, White RL. *Medical Genetics*. St. Louis, MO: Mosby, 1995
2. Emery AEH, Rimoin DL. *Principles and Practice of Medical Genetics*, 2nd edn. Vols. 1 and 2, New York: Churchill Livingstone, 1990
3. McKusick VA. *Mendelian Inheritance in Man: Catalog of Autosomal Dominant, Autosomal Recessive, and X-linked Phenotypes*, 11th edn. Baltimore, MD: The Johns Hopkins University Press, 1994, and online Mendelian Inheritance in Man (OMIM) web site (http://www.ncbi.nlm.nih.gov/Omim/)
4. Stephens JC, Cavanaugh ML, Gradie MI, *et al.* Mapping the human genome: current status. *Science* 1990;250:237
5. Therman E. *Human Chromosomes: Structure, Behavior and Effects*, 2nd edn. New York: Springer-Verlag, 1986
6. Gelehrter TD, Collins FS. *Principles of Medical Genetics*. Baltimore, MD: Williams & Wilkins, 1990
7. Thompson MW, McInnes RR, Willard HF. *Genetics in Medicine*, 5th edn. Philadelphia: WB Saunders, 1991
8. Magenis RE. On the origin of chromosome anomaly. *Am J Med Genet* 1988;42:529–33
9. Patterson D. The causes of Down syndrome. *Sci Am* 1987;257:52–60
10. Antonarakis SE and The Down Syndrome Collaborative Group. Parental origin of the extra chromosome in trisomy 21 as indicated by analysis of DNA polymorphisms. *New Engl J Med* 1991;324:872–6
11. D'Alton ME, DeCherney AH. Prenatal diagnosis. *New Engl J Med* 1991;328:114–19
12. Gardner RJM, Veale AMO. *De novo* translocation Down's syndrome: risk of recurrence of Down's syndrome. *Clin Genet* 1974;6:160–4
13. Harper PS. *Practical Genetic Counseling*, 3rd edn. London: Wright, 1988
14. Lister TJ, Frota-Pessoa O. Recurrence risk for Down syndrome. *Human Genet* 1980;55:203
15. Cooley WC, Graham JM. Down syndrome: an update and review for the primary pediatrician. *Clin Pediatr* 1991;30:233–53
16. Jones KL. *Smith's Recognizable Patterns of Human Malformation*, 4th edn. Philadelphia: WB Saunders, 1988
17. Pueschel SM. Clinical aspects of Down syndrome from infancy to adulthood. *Am J Med Genet (Suppl)* 1990;7:52–6
18. Gorlin RJ, Cohen MM, Levin LS. *Syndromes of the Head and Neck*, 3rd edn. New York: Oxford University Press, 1990
19. Bernstein HS, Filly RA, Goldberg JD, Golbus MS. Prognosis of fetuses with a cystic hygroma. *Prenat Diagn* 1991;11:349–55
20. Leclercq G, Buvat-Herbaut M, Monnier JC, *et al.* Syndrome de Turner et grossesse par dans d'ovocytes et fecondation *in vitro*. *J Gynecol Obstet Biol Reprod* 1992;21:635
21. Gardner RJM, Sutherland GR. *Chromosome Abnormalities and Genetic Counseling*. New York: Oxford University Press, 1989
22. Stevenson RE, Goodman R, Hall JG. *Human Malformations and Related Anomalies*. New York: Oxford University Press, 1993
23. Ewart AK, Morris CA, Atkinson D, *et al.* Hemizygosity at the elastin locus in a developmental disorder; Williams syndrome. *Nature Genet* 1993;5:11–16
24. Kalousek DK. Anatomic and chromosome anomalies in specimens of early spontaneous abortion: seven year

experience. *Birth Defects Original Article Series* 1987;23: 153–68

25. Craver RD, Kalousek DK. Cytogenetic abnormalities among spontaneously aborted previable fetuses. *Am J Med Genet (Suppl)* 1987;3:113–19

26. Opitz JM, FitzGerald JM, Reynolds JF, *et al*. The Montana fetal genetic pathology program and a review of prenatal death in humans. *Am J Med Genet (Suppl)* 1987;3:83–112

27. Hassold TJ. Chromosome abnormalities in human reproductive wastage. *Trends Genet* 1986;2:105–10

28. DeWald GW, Michels VV. Recurrent miscarriages: cytogenetic causes and genetic counseling of affected families. *Clin Obstet Gynecol* 1986;29:865–85

29. Bell JI. Polygenic disease. *Curr Opin Genet Dev* 1993;3: 466–9

30. U.S. Department of Health and Human Services, Centers for Disease Control. Recommendations for the use of folic acid to reduce the number of cases of spina bifida and other neural tube defects. *Morbidity Mortality Weekly Rep* 1992;41(RR-14):1–7

31. Centers for Disease Control. Use of folic acid for prevention of spina bifida and other neural tube defects – 1983–1991. *Morbidity Mortality Weekly Rep* 1991;40(30):513–16

32. Luft R. The development of mitochondrial medicine. *Proc Natl Acad Sci USA* 1994;91:8731–8

33. Scriver CR, Beaudet AL, Sly WS, Valle D. *The Metabolic and Molecular Bases of Inherited Disease*, 7th edn. New York: McGraw-Hill, 1994

34. National Academy of Sciences. *Genetic Screening: Programs, Principles and Research*. Washington, DC: National Academy of Sciences, 1975

35. Anderson WF. Human gene therapy. *Science* 1992;256: 808–13

36. Blaese RM. Development of gene therapy for immunodeficiency: adenosine deaminase deficiency. *Pediatr Res* 1992;33(Suppl):49–55

37. Wolff JA. Gene therapy: a primer. *Pediatr Ann* 1993;22: 312–21

65

Fetal genetic disorders

J. Pratt Rossiter and K.J. Blakemore

INTRODUCTION

Since the first clinical use of fetal sex determination by amniocentesis in 1967, there has been a virtual explosion in both the availability and the application of prenatal diagnosis in the management of pregnancy. The rapid expansion of this field has been a result of numerous advances. The quality of ultrasonography has vastly improved, allowing detection of both gross and increasingly more subtle congenital anomalies, and providing accurate guidance for diagnostic procedures including amniocentesis, chorionic villus sampling, fetal blood sampling and fetal biopsy. In turn, the safety of these invasive methods has improved due to higher resolution ultrasonography as well as progress in the development of the techniques themselves. Meanwhile, the 'revolution' in molecular genetics has resulted in the identification of the genes and mutations responsible for many inherited disorders. This knowledge can, in many cases, be applied directly to prenatal diagnosis for pregnancies at risk for specific genetic diseases. All of these factors have contributed to the need for maternal–fetal medicine specialists to become experts in the field of prenatal diagnosis.

This chapter reviews the most common indications for prenatal diagnosis and the invasive methods currently used. The status of preimplantation diagnosis and of prenatal diagnosis using fetal cells isolated from the maternal circulation are considered.

INDICATIONS FOR PRENATAL DIAGNOSIS

The most common reasons for referral for genetic counseling and prenatal diagnosis are summarized in Table 1. Currently, invasive prenatal testing is offered when the likelihood of detecting an abnormality exceeds the statistical risk of pregnancy loss related to the diagnostic procedure. Ethical issues regarding the somewhat arbitrary determination of when to offer prenatal diagnosis must also be considered and universal access to genetic diagnosis has been proposed[1]; however, this practice is presently far from being adopted.

Maternal age

The relationship between advancing maternal age and increasing incidence of chromosomal abnormalities

Table 1 Indications for prenatal diagnosis

Maternal age 33 or more at delivery
Family history of chromosomal abnormality
Parental translocation carrier
Abnormal MSAFP or multiple marker screen
Family history of neural tube defect
Single-gene disorder – family history or carrier detected
   by population screening
Congenital malformation detected by ultrasonography
Anxiety

MSAFP; maternal serum alpha-fetoprotein

due to meiotic non-disjunction is well established[2]. The steadily rising risk with age applies not only to trisomy 21 (Down syndrome), but to any autosomal aneuploidy. The chance of a 35-year-old woman having a liveborn infant with a chromosomal abnormality is 1 in 192[3]. This risk approximates the stated 1 in 200 risk of procedure-related loss with second trimester amniocentesis; thus, women are offered prenatal diagnosis for chromosome abnormalities when they will be 35 years of age or older at the time of delivery. Many chromosomally abnormal fetuses are lost during the course of pregnancy; therefore, the likelihood of having an aneuploid fetus at the time of amniocentesis (usually 16–20 weeks' gestation) is greater than the risk at term[4]. For example, women who will be 33 years old at the time of delivery have a risk of 1 in 200 of having a chromosomally abnormal fetus at the time of amniocentesis[4]. For this reason, some practitioners advocate offering prenatal diagnosis to women who are 33 years of age or older, but no consensus has yet been reached.

Chromosomal abnormalities

Couples with a previous trisomic child are thought to have approximately a 1% risk of recurrence[5], and are thus offered prenatal diagnosis. Siblings and second-degree relatives to an individual with Down syndrome may have a slightly increased risk for having a similarly affected child[6], though most studies have not demonstrated an increased incidence of Down syndrome in second- or third-degree relatives[7,8]. Many people with an affected relative have a high degree of anxiety, which may justify prenatal testing.

Translocations and other chromosomal structural rearrangements can predispose to chromosomally abnormal progeny (see Chapter 64 for a description of translocations). Couples in whom one partner carries a balanced reciprocal translocation are at high risk for recurrent pregnancy loss. At the time of prenatal diagnosis, approximately 10–12% of progeny have an unbalanced chromosome complement[9,10], while this risk declines to 6% of liveborn offspring because of spontaneous abortion[11]. Progeny of Robertsonian translocation carriers are at risk for trisomy or monosomy of the involved chromosomes, with the risk dependent on the specific chromosomes participating in the translocation[9,10]. An extreme example is that of a Robertsonian 21/21 translocation carrier, whose progeny would all be predicted to be either trisomic (Down syndrome) or monosomic (lethal) for chromosome 21. An additional consideration for Robertsonian translocation carriers is that of uniparental disomy (UPD) in the fetus. UPD results from both copies of a chromosome pair being inherited from a single parent. This phenomenon can cause a clinically significant phenotype on the specific chromosomes involved. For example, maternal UPD for chromosome 15 (where both copies of chromosome 15 are derived from the mother) causes Prader–Willi syndrome, which includes among its symptoms mental retardation, hyperphagia, obesity and dysmorphic features. Couples with a history of multiple pregnancy losses should be offered karyotypes to determine if one member is a translocation carrier. Individuals known to be translocation carriers should be offered prenatal cytogenetic testing, as the fetal karyotype result may be normal, balanced, or unbalanced, with the proportion of each karyotype result varying, dependent on the specific translocation[10].

Multiple-marker screening

In 1972, Brock and Sutcliffe described the association of fetal anencephaly and spina bifida with elevations in maternal serum alpha-fetoprotein (MSAFP) levels[12]. Subsequently, studies in the USA[13] and the UK[14] proposed the establishment of screening programs to detect pregnancies complicated by fetal open neural tube defects. During the 1980s, such screening programs became widespread in the USA, where the incidence of neural tube defects is 1–2 per 1000 live births[15]. Elevated MSAFP values are associated not only with open neural tube defects, but also with other fetal abnormalities involving a break in skin integrity such as ventral wall defects (omphalocele, gastroschisis), teratoma, bladder exstrophy, or aplasia cutis. Numerous other fetal and placental abnormalities have been reported in association with elevated MSAFP levels[16,17]. In addition, elevations in MSAFP unexplained by sonographic findings are associated with an increased risk of pregnancy complications,

fetal growth retardation and fetal death[17-19]. The American College of Obstetricians and Gynecologists has proposed an algorithm for the evaluation of pregnancies with elevated MSAFP levels including ultrasonography, amniocentesis for amniotic fluid AFP, and acetylcholinesterase if the amniotic fluid AFP is elevated[15]. Since MSAFP screening became the standard of care in the USA, elevated MSAFP has become a common indication for referral for prenatal diagnosis.

The clinical utility of MSAFP screening expanded substantially when an association was found between low MSAFP values and fetal chromosomal abnormalities[20,21]. Using a combination of maternal age and MSAFP to identify pregnancies at high risk, approximately 20% of Down syndrome pregnancies in women younger than 35 years were detected in prospective trials[22,23]. Subsequently, Down syndrome pregnancies were found to be associated with elevated maternal serum concentrations of human chorionic gonadotropin (hCG)[24] and decreased unconjugated estriol (uE$_3$)[25] as compared with normal controls. In a large, prospective trial using maternal age in combination with maternal serum levels of AFP, hCG and uE$_3$ to assign a risk of fetal Down syndrome of $\geqslant 1:190$, 58% of Down syndrome pregnancies were identified, and 38 amniocenteses were performed for each confirmed case of Down syndrome[26]. This trial included women ranging in age from 16 to 41 years. Since this publication in 1992, multiple marker or 'triple' screening has come into more widespread use. Further applications of the triple screen have followed, with the recognition of a characteristic pattern of low values for AFP, hCG and uE$_3$ in association with trisomy 18[27,28], and a pattern similar to that for an increased risk for Down syndrome (low AFP, low uE$_3$, high hCG) in association with Turner syndrome (45,X)[29,30].

Multiple-marker screening allows the detection of pregnancies which would otherwise not be considered at increased risk for either neural tube defects or chromosomal aneuploidy. One of its main disadvantages is its timing in the second trimester. An abnormal screen, typically obtained at 16–18 weeks' gestation, sets into motion a series of events including: repeat screening in some cases (if AFP is high, *not* for increased risk of aneuploidy), ultrasonography to confirm dating, genetic counseling, and the offer to have amniocentesis for chromosomal analysis and amniotic fluid AFP measurement. At the completion of this evaluation, most patients are beyond 18 weeks' and many are beyond 20 weeks' gestation. By this time, most pregnant women have begun to feel fetal movement and are readily recognized as pregnant by casual observers. In addition, the options for termination are induction methods (prostaglandin and/or urea instillation, prostaglandin suppositories) or dilatation and evacuation at an advanced gestational age. Either method is associated with significantly greater morbidity than first trimester dilatation and curettage, as well as increased medical costs. For these reasons, a current focus of research is to determine whether first trimester maternal serum screening will detect pregnancies at risk for chromosomal abnormalities.

Numerous fetal and placental products are currently being evaluated as possible markers for fetal aneuploidy in the first trimester. These include AFP[31-37], human chorionic gonadotropin and its subunits (free αhCG, free βhCG)[33-40], uE$_3$[33,36,37], pregnancy-specific β$_1$-glycoprotein (SP$_1$)[33,35,41], progesterone[35,38], pregnancy-associated plasma protein A (PAPP-A)[35,39,40,42,43], and immunoreactive inhibin[44]. The published data relating first trimester levels of many of these markers to the risk of Down syndrome were recently analyzed[45]. To date, the most promising first trimester marker appears to be PAPP-A, with median values in Down syndrome pregnancies ranging from 0.31 to 0.50 multiples of the median[39,40,42,43], and low median values also seen in association with trisomies 13 and 18[35,40,43]. Other potentially valuable markers include AFP[31-37], uE$_3$[33,36,37], and SP$_1$[33,35,41]. While free βhCG appears to be markedly decreased in association with trisomies 13 and 18[36,40], its utility as a marker for trisomy 21 is less clear. Though two studies demonstrated a significant rise to 1.96 to 2.1 multiples of the median[36,39], another study showed no significant difference from controls[40]. The combination of multiple maternal serum biochemical markers with an ultrasonographic assessment of nuchal translucency of the posterior fetal neck shows great promise as a first trimester screen for aneuploidy. Nuchal translucency measurements should be performed according to strict criteria, however[46,47]. A screen combining maternal age with first trimester serum analytes and properly performed nuchal translucency measurements would theoretically expect to yield a detection rate of 87% for Down syndrome, at a 5% false positive rate[48]. At this time, further investigation is required prior to widespread application of first trimester serum screening. One concern is the potential loss of information regarding open neural tube defect risk assessment if serum screening is moved into the first trimester.

Family history of single-gene disorders

A family history of a single-gene disorder is another common indication for referral. The need for prenatal diagnosis is dependent on many factors, such as the distance of the relationship between the affected family member and the individual seeking counseling, as well as the frequency of the disease gene in the population. Couples with a previously affected child are obviously at high risk for recurrence, while the risk declines with increased distance from the affected relative (1° > 2° > 3°). For example, parents of a child with an autosomal recessive disorder have a 25% risk

of recurrence with each pregnancy. In contrast, the offspring to the siblings of an affected individual have a risk calculated as follows: the risk of the unaffected sibling being a carrier (2/3) times the risk that the partner is a carrier (the population carrier frequency if the family history is negative), times the risk of having an affected offspring given that both parents are carriers (1/4). Thus, for cystic fibrosis, with a carrier frequency of 1 in 25 caucasian Americans, the risk for an unaffected sibling of an affected individual to have an offspring with cystic fibrosis is $2/3 \times 1/25 \times 1/4 = 1/150$. Carrier testing, when available, can change these odds.

Carrier screening is currently widely available for some recessive conditions, including sickle cell anemia, Tay–Sachs disease, and most recently Canavan disease[49]. In the near future, carrier screening may become available for other relatively common genetic conditions, creating another group of candidates for prenatal diagnosis. Cystic fibrosis-carrier screening is currently available at some sites and is under consideration at others, though the advisability of widespread screening remains controversial[50]. The most recent formal statements from the American Society of Human Genetics[51] and the American College of Obstetricians and Gynecologists (ACOG)[52] both recommend against population-based carrier screening for cystic fibrosis due to limitations in mutation detection, which may result in false reassurance or heightened anxiety. Numerous studies have been published on patient acceptance of screening, responses to test results, application of information to prenatal testing and provider attitudes toward screening[53-58]. In general, most patients accept carrier screening when offered, while medical personnel have more reservations about offering screening. Nevertheless, widespread carrier screening for cystic fibrosis may soon become a reality, and other recessive conditions are sure to follow.

Sonographic findings

As the resolution and therefore the sensitivity of ultrasonography improves, an increasing number of referrals for prenatal diagnosis are generated because of sonographic fetal abnormalities. Some of the more frequent findings include fetal heart defects, ventral wall defects, central nervous system abnormalities, gastrointestinal anomalies, renal anomalies, and, more recently, choroid plexus cysts and nuchal fold thickening. These abnormalities may be found in isolation, in conjunction with chromosomal abnormalities or as part of Mendelian syndromes. As our knowledge of the associated incidence of karyotypic or single-gene abnormalities unfolds, assessment of the need for further prenatal diagnostic evaluation for a given sonographic finding becomes better defined.

INVASIVE PRENATAL DIAGNOSTIC METHODS

While indications for referral for prenatal diagnosis continue to expand, the methods available to prenatally detect genetic disorders are also rapidly improving. In addition to amniocentesis, invasive diagnostic methods currently include chorionic villus sampling, fetal blood sampling, and fetal biopsy for specific indications. Samples obtained by these techniques are used for cytogenetic analysis (karyotype, fluorescence *in situ* hybridization), molecular DNA diagnosis (direct mutation detection, linkage analysis) and/or biochemical evaluation, dependent on the specific diagnosis under consideration. Each invasive procedure has risks and benefits to be considered when offering diagnostic testing.

Midtrimester amniocentesis

The use of amniocentesis to prenatally detect chromosomal abnormalities was first reported in 1967[59]. Since that time, amniocentesis has become a widely accepted method for prenatal diagnosis of chromosomal abnormalities, inherited diseases and some congenital infections. Despite about three decades' experience with midtrimester amniocentesis, determination of the risk of procedure-related pregnancy loss has been difficult. Risk estimates have ranged from 0.5% to 1% in large, prospective, multicenter trials[60-62]. The most recent ACOG Technical Bulletin to consider the question states 'most centers now counsel that the risk of abortion secondary to amniocentesis is 1 in 200 or less'[3].

While fetal loss resulting from amniocentesis is considered the most serious risk of the procedure, other fetal and maternal risks must also be considered. Fetal-needle puncture resulting in scars at birth has been reported[63], but is quite rare. Amniocentesis performed under continuous ultrasound guidance allows sampling of fluid while avoiding fetal parts, thus minimizing the risk of such an injury. Two large prospective trials found an association between midtrimester amniocentesis and neonatal respiratory difficulty[61,62], while a study from the National Institute of Child Health and Human Development (NICHD) of the US National Institutes of Health[60] did not corroborate this finding. An increased incidence of orthopedic postural deformities in association with amniocentesis was reported in the initial UK Medical Research Council (MRC) study[61], but was not found in two other large trials[60,62].

Other complications from midtrimester amniocentesis include chorioamnionitis, leakage of amniotic fluid, and vaginal bleeding. The incidence of chorioamnionitis is < 1 per 1000 procedures[64]. Amniotic fluid leakage occurs in 1–2% of patients[60,62], but is usually self-limited, with reaccumulation of fluid and a normal pregnancy outcome in most cases[65]. The incidence of vaginal bleeding after second trimester amniocentesis is also approximately 1% and is positively correlated with the number of needle insertions required[60].

Early amniocentesis

Traditionally, amniocentesis has been offered at 15–20 weeks' gestation. The timing of the procedure has been based on the ability to reliably obtain diagnostic results with an acceptable complication rate. However, in the late 1980s, in an effort to provide an alternative to chorionic villus sampling for early prenatal diagnosis, several groups began trials to test the safety and accuracy of amniocentesis prior to 15 weeks' gestation. 'Early amniocentesis' at 11–14 weeks became possible due to advances in ultrasonography and tissue culture methods. (Chorionic villus sampling (CVS), a technique available between 10 and 12 weeks' gestation, will be discussed later in this chapter.) The technique for early amniocentesis is quite similar to that for midtrimester amniocentesis, with the following caveats: the target is smaller; the uterus may not abut the maternal abdominal wall, thereby increasing the risk of maternal bowel injury or introduction of intestinal organisms into the uterus; and the amnion and chorion may not be well fused at this gestational age, making entry into the amniotic cavity more difficult. Aids to improve success include continuous ultrasound guidance throughout the procedure, use of a small gauge needle (e.g. 22 gauge), and insertion of the needle perpendicular to the membranes. Approximately 1 ml of amniotic fluid per week of gestational age has been shown to be adequate for culture and analysis, with a minimum of 98% of samples successfully cultured in published reports[66-68].

Numerous papers have described the time interval to diagnosis and the diagnostic accuracy of early amniocentesis, which compare favorably to midtrimester amniocentesis and chorionic villus sampling[69-71]. Some have reported cases of pseudomosaicism, requiring repeat amniocentesis or fetal blood sampling to rule out true mosaicism[72-74]. While many features of early amniocentesis suggested its potential utility as a method for early prenatal diagnosis, studies to evaluate its safety were initially limited. Though many papers were published, they included only descriptions of pregnancy outcome, and were not randomized clinical trials. Reports cited pregnancy loss rates ranging from 0.4% within one week[75] to 2.3% within two weeks of a procedure performed at 11–14 weeks' gestation[73], with many studies showing an intermediate early loss rate[70,74,76-78]. The total loss rate of chromosomally normal pregnancies after early amniocentesis, including early and late spontaneous abortion, fetal death and stillbirth, ranges from 2.3% to 4.2%[69,70,74,76-78]. Because these studies did not include control groups to assess background rates of pregnancy loss at given gestational ages in a matched cohort, the procedure-related pregnancy loss rate was unknown, and therefore unavailable for counseling patients.

Risks other than pregnancy loss which have been described in association with early amniocentesis include amniotic fluid leakage and vaginal bleeding. Mild vaginal bleeding follows approximately 5% of early amniocentesis procedures[69,74] and appears to be unassociated with adverse pregnancy outcome. Fluid leakage occurs in 1.1–4.4% of cases[69,74,76,79,80]. In most instances, the leakage spontaneously resolves with a normal pregnancy outcome. However, most of the published series describe a proportion of patients who experienced pregnancy loss after amniotic fluid leakage related to early amniocentesis. In addition, one paper[74] reported three orthopedic postural deformities (one case each of congenital hip dislocation, scoliosis, and clubfeet) out of a total of 10 cases in which early amniocentesis was complicated by fluid leakage. Two large randomized clinical trials have subsequently shown an association between 11–12 week amniocentesis and club foot. The first, from Denmark, describes a 1.7% frequency of talipes equinovarus following randomization to early amniocentesis vs. no cases of talipes equinovarus following CVS ($p < 0.01$)[80]. Of the nine cases of club foot in the early amniocentesis group, six had had their procedures at 12 weeks, and no cases were seen after procedures later than 12 weeks and 5 days. The second study, from Canada, describes a 1.3% frequency of talipes equinovarus following randomization to early amniocentesis vs. 0.1% following mid-trimester amniocentesis ($p = 0.0001$)[81]. Amniotic fluid leakage was also noted to be significantly higher after early amniocentesis (3.5% compared with 1.7% after midtrimester amniocentesis). Both reports suggest an etiologic mechanism of amniotic fluid leakage with oligohydramnios in the development of club foot following early amniocentesis[80,81].

One advantage of midtrimester amniocentesis over chorionic villus sampling is the ability to measure amniotic fluid levels of AFP, a sensitive marker for open neural tube defects and ventral wall defects. The majority of publications describing pregnancy outcomes after early amniocentesis do not mention AFP. One study that does mention the measurement of amniotic fluid AFP levels found no abnormal results in their series of 130 patients undergoing amniocentesis at 14.0 to 14.9 weeks' gestation[69]. Normal values for amniotic fluid AFP levels in the first trimester have not yet been clearly established. Crandall and co-workers[82] and Drugan and co-workers[83], independently showed a rise in amniotic fluid AFP levels from 11 to 13 weeks' gestation, with a peak at 13 weeks. The peak is then followed by a linear decline until about 20 weeks.

The rise in AFP levels between 11 and 13 weeks is important, because extrapolation from declining values between 14 and 20 weeks would result in failure to detect elevations in AFP at the time of early amniocentesis. In 1993, Wathen and co-workers[78] further corroborated the pattern of rising amniotic fluid AFP levels from 11 to 13 weeks' gestation with a subsequent fall in values. In addition, this group described very high levels of amniotic fluid AFP at eight weeks gestation with a rapid decline until 11 weeks. It appears that more data to establish the range of normal AFP levels in early amniocentesis specimens would be required before this assay could be reliably interpreted and clinically applied.

Detection of acetylcholinesterase in the amniotic fluid is a useful adjunct to amniotic fluid AFP measurement in the second trimester to identify fetuses with an open neural tube defect or a ventral wall defect[85–87]. Several studies have attempted to correlate the presence of acetylcholinesterase in early amniocentesis specimens with fetal anomalies. Burton and colleagues[88] described nine cases in which acetylcholinesterase was detected in amniotic fluid obtained at 11–14 weeks' gestation. (Acetylcholinesterase was measured in cases with an elevated amniotic fluid AFP concentration or a history of neural tube defect in a prior pregnancy.) In four cases, a fetal open neural tube defect was identified. However, in four cases, no explanation for the presence of acetylcholinesterase was found, and repeat amniocentesis at 15–17 weeks revealed normal amniotic fluid AFP and the absence of acetylcholinesterase in each case. The remaining fetus had trisomy 21, though no reason for the positive acetylcholinesterase was found. Evans and co-workers[75] measured acetylcholinesterase in 227 early amniocentesis cases. Results were positive in three cases (1.3%), in association with one case each of ectopia cordis, anencephaly and trisomy 13. Each also had elevated amniotic fluid AFP values. 'Inconclusive' results were obtained in 18 cases (7.9%), three of which had fetal abnormalities (ectopia cordis and encephalocele, posterior urethral valves with obstructive uropathy, and trisomy 13). Thus, equivocal or false-positive acetylcholinesterase results appear to occur much more frequently in early amniocentesis samples than in the midtrimester.

In summary, midtrimester amniocentesis has become the most widely used method for prenatal diagnosis of chromosomal abnormalities and inherited conditions, and plays an important role in the investigation of elevated MSAFP levels. The desire for earlier prenatal diagnosis led to an increase in the availability of amniocentesis at 11–14 weeks' gestation. This technique appears to provide accurate cytogenetic and molecular diagnostic information, although the reliability of this method in the detection of pregnancies complicated by fetal neural tube or ventral wall defects was unproven. The relatively high risk of club foot associated with amniocentesis at 11–12 weeks has, appropriately, curtailed the performance of amniocentesis this early. The risk of club foot following amniocentesis at 13–14 weeks, if any, is still under investigation.

Chorionic villus sampling

The technique of chorionic villus sampling (CVS) was spurred by the desire for prenatal diagnosis in time to allow safer termination options, increased patient privacy and decreased emotional stress. Though methods to obtain trophoblastic tissue were described in the 1960s and 1970s, they were fraught with high failure and complication rates[89,90]. The availability of ultrasound guidance[91] and the development of a thin, malleable catheter for transcervical sampling[92] led to a resurgence of interest in the 1980s. Since the publication of these ground-breaking articles, numerous investigations, including large prospective trials to determine the risks and benefits of CVS, have been undertaken.

CVS is usually performed between 10 and 12.5 weeks of gestation. Cytogenetic, molecular (DNA analysis) and/or biochemical methods can be applied to villus tissue. These assays can detect chromosomal abnormalities, specific gene defects or linkage to at-risk loci, and/or evidence of enzymatic activity abnormalities in pregnancies at known risk for particular inherited conditions. In all of these respects, CVS generally provides the same type of information available through amniocentesis. There are several instances in which the methods are not equivalent in their ability to provide diagnostic information. Notably, CVS is not useful in detecting a fetus with an open neural tube or ventral wall defect. In some cases, the sonogram performed at the time of CVS might identify such a fetus; however, no information regarding AFP level or the presence of acetylcholinesterase can be obtained through CVS. On the other hand, some assays which require tissue samples can be performed on villus tissue but not amniocytes. For example, the prenatal diagnosis of osteogenesis imperfecta is usually based on collagen studies, which cannot be completed on amniotic fluid samples[93]. Thus, in contemplating the preferred method for prenatal diagnosis in a given pregnancy, both the couple's wishes and the ideal means to obtain the desired information must be considered.

The same issues which faced early laboratory investigations of cultured second trimester amniocytes were confronted by early investigators of chorionic villus cells, including maternal contamination and chromosomal mosaicism. Maternal contamination from decidual cells poses a threat to long-term chorionic villus cell cultures. Careful dissection of the villi using a microscope with 40 × magnification will minimize this risk.

Chromosomal mosaicism refers to two (or more) cell lines in the same tissue, organ, or individual. An example would be a villus sample with both a normal (e.g. 46,XX) cell line and a trisomic (47,XX,+21) cell line. Because the placenta arises from different late progenitor cells than the embryo, mitotic errors which result in chromosomal non-disjunction can be limited to cells destined to become chorionic villi[94]. This circumstance is identified as mosaicism by the laboratory at the time of CVS, and is found in about 1% of chorionic villus samples[95]. In contrast, mosaicism is seen in 0.25% of midtrimester amniotic fluid samples[96].

In most cases when mosaicism is found by CVS, the fetus is chromosomally normal[97]. If a mitotic error occurred in a very early progenitor cell, both the villus and the embryonic descendants of this progenitor could contain an abnormality. In such a case, a chromosomal abnormality would often be revealed both at CVS and at follow-up amniocentesis. More often, follow-up amniocentesis in the midtrimester usually has normal cytogenetic results[95]. Though a normal karyotype on amniocytes provides presumptive evidence for a chromosomally normal fetus, it is not a guarantee, as mosaicism can be limited to some fetal tissues.

As is true for any prenatal diagnostic method, patients are most concerned about the risk of procedure-related pregnancy loss. Initial studies to assess the safety of first trimester CVS were descriptions of clinical experience, which described total fetal loss rates from 2 to 7%[98,99]. However, these studies did not address the procedure-related loss rate. A large proportion of the total loss rate represents the naturally occurring spontaneous abortions characteristic of the first trimester. In addition, chromosomally abnormal fetuses are viable in greater proportions at 10–12 weeks than at 16–20 weeks, and would thus be included in the overall CVS loss rate, but not that of midtrimester amniocentesis. These and other issues were subsequently addressed in several multicenter trials of CVS.

A prospective, non-randomized trial, published by the NICHD Collaborative Group[100], compared pregnancy outcomes in patients undergoing first trimester transcervical CVS with a relatively small group of patients undergoing midtrimester amniocentesis. This study showed total loss rates of desired pregnancies of 7.2% in the CVS group and 5.7% in the amniocentesis group. These rates included elective terminations for chromosomal and sonographic abnormalities, as well as spontaneous losses. After correction for differences in gestational age and maternal age between the groups, the total excess loss rate in the CVS group was 0.8% when compared to the amniocentesis group. While this difference was not statistically significant, most centers currently quote a slightly higher procedure-related loss rate for CVS than for second trimester amniocentesis. Many patients, nonetheless, would consider the benefits of early diagnosis to exceed this risk, particularly the greater safety of pregnancy termination at an earlier gestational age. Similar rates of pregnancy loss were found in a large randomized Canadian trial[101], in which the observed difference in loss rates between eligible women with a sonographically viable fetus at 9–12 weeks in the CVS and midtrimester amniocentesis groups was 0.5% (95% confidence interval – 1.57% to +2.57%), which was not statistically significant.

The MRC European trial of CVS[102] was less optimistic about the safety of the procedure. This multicenter, prospective study compared pregnancy outcomes after randomization to either first trimester CVS or midtrimester amniocentesis. The study concluded that CVS 'reduces the chances of a successful pregnancy outcome by 4.6% in comparison with second trimester amniocentesis'. One explanation for the increased loss rate in the MRC trial as compared to the NICHD trial may be related to operator experience; the European study included a larger number of centers, with individual centers contributing fewer patients.

In addition to the pregnancy loss rate, another source of controversy is the question of an increased risk of fetal limb abnormalities in association with CVS. Firth and co-workers[103] reported an unusually high incidence of oromandibular–limb hypogenesis syndromes in pregnancies undergoing CVS at 56–66 days' gestation (8–9 weeks). The authors proposed that a disruption of normal morphogenesis may result from CVS. None of the three large trials[100-102], in which CVS was usually performed at 10–12 weeks' gestation, found such an association. This led Firth to hypothesize that an early gestational age at the time of CVS may predispose to limb reduction defects.

Subsequently, Burton and colleagues[104] reported their experience in which four transverse limb-reduction defects were identified during follow-up after CVS in 436 pregnancies, an incidence far greater than the reported incidence of limb malformations of one in 1500 to 2000 live births[105]. The procedures were performed at 9.6–11.3 weeks' gestation, thus the limb abnormalities cannot be explained by early timing of the CVS. This report has prompted speculation regarding the technique used in the single center involved, particularly since their spontaneous loss rate was considerably higher than that of other centers[106]. A survey conducted in Taiwan[107] also found an association between CVS and limb defects, with a 100-fold increased incidence of severe limb defects after CVS exposure as compared with the general population. However, in this series, 87% of the cases involving limb defects in which the timing of CVS was known were performed prior to 63 days' (9 weeks') gestation. Interestingly, in an effort to objectively evaluate the potential etiologic role of CVS in the development of

limb reduction defects she first described, Firth and colleagues recently reported a series of 75 infants who were exposed to CVS *in utero* and had limb-reduction defects at birth[108]. The authors found a strong correlation between increasing severity of the defects and earlier gestational age at the time of CVS, with the most severe defects following CVS at 9 weeks' gestation or less. These studies and others support postponement of CVS until nine completed weeks of gestation to minimize the risk of fetal injury.

Operator experience may explain the lack of an association with fetal limb defects reported by the majority of US centers. In a recent publication, the World Health Organization reported an incidence of approximately six limb-reduction defects per 10 000 CVS cases[109], which is consistent with the background rate of this congenital anomaly[105]. At this time, many centers feel that patients should be informed of the possible association, made aware of their options, and allowed to select a method of prenatal diagnosis most consistent with their medical and psychosocial needs.

Chorionic villus tissue may be obtained by one of three approaches: transcervical, transabdominal[110,111], or transvaginal[112]. The transcervical method is currently the most widely used, although some claim that transabdominal sampling has a lower risk of infection and is easier to perform due to the technique's similarity with amniocentesis. Several recent prospective, randomized trials compared transabdominal and transcervical methods. Two of these studies, a collaborative study through the NICHD[113] and a single-center study by Brambati and colleagues[114], found no difference in success of sampling, fetal loss, delivery, or neonatal outcome between groups. A third randomized trial[115] showed a significantly greater total fetal loss rate after transcervical CVS (10.9%) when compared with transabdominal CVS (6.3%) and midtrimester amniocentesis (6.4%). The reasons for the differences in fetal loss rates are unclear. In all three studies, an increased incidence of minor symptoms were found in the groups undergoing transcervical CVS.

Common symptoms following CVS include cramping, spotting, and vaginal bleeding. Cramping is reported by 16–22% of women after transabdominal or transcervical CVS[100,113]; 19–32% reported spotting after transcervical procedures, which declined to 4% after transabdominal CVS[100,113]; vaginal bleeding as heavy as a menstrual period was reported by up to 6–7% of patients after transcervical CVS and only 1–2% of women undergoing transabdominal CVS[100,113]. Amniotic fluid leakage is uncommon after CVS, occurring transiently in 1.1% and for several weeks in 0.7% of cases in the initial NICHD study[100], and less frequently in other reports. Of those women who continued to leak fluid, 20% (3 of 14 patients) went on to lose the pregnancy.

Table 2 Indications for fetal blood sampling

Chromosomal
  Karyotype
  Mosaicism
Intrauterine infection
  Toxoplasmosis
  Rubella
  Varicella
  Cytomegalovirus
  Human parvovirus B19
Red cell isoimmunization
Platelet isoimmunization
Hemophilia
Hemoglobinopathies
Immunodeficiency syndromes
Assessment of fetal acid–base status

A significant concern is the risk of infection. For this reason, transcervical CVS is contraindicated in the presence of a genital tract infection, including active herpes genitalis. Case reports of septic abortion and septic shock following CVS have been published[116,117]; however, this complication was not reported in any of the large CVS trials.

Fetal blood sampling

Though amniocentesis or CVS is usually sufficient for prenatal diagnosis, fetal blood sampling can provide rapid and accurate analysis for a multitude of disorders (Table 2). For prenatal cytogenetic analysis, amniocentesis and CVS are the most widely used methods. However, patients occasionally present at late gestational ages with compeling indications for rapid fetal karyotype, such as severe intrauterine growth retardation, oligohydramnios, hydrops fetalis or fetal anomalies. Though CVS or amniocentesis may provide diagnostic information, the quality of a rapid cytogenetic analysis from direct preparations of villus tissue may be poor, and the time required for culture of amniocytes or villi may significantly alter obstetric management. Under such circumstances, fetal blood sampling to obtain a fetal lymphocyte karyotype, which is usually available in two to three days, may be indicated. A clinical example would be a patient in the mid-third trimester of pregnancy presenting with preterm labor, severe fetal growth retardation and a fetal cardiac defect detected by ultrasound. A rapid diagnosis of trisomy 18 would allow that patient to undergo counseling and afford her the option of foregoing tocolysis, antepartum surveillance, Cesarean section for fetal indications and neonatal intervention after birth. Patients may also be offered fetal blood sampling to provide rapid diagnosis at the limits of legal pregnancy termination.

An ever-increasing number of inherited conditions can be diagnosed through molecular and/or biochemical

techniques, as the gene defects, chromosomal locations (for linkage analysis), and/or enzymatic derangements relevant to specific disorders are identified. As a result, fetal blood has become infrequently required for the prenatal diagnosis of coagulopathies, hemoglobinopathies, and other heritable diseases. Historically, some of the first applications of prenatal diagnosis were to detect hemoglobinopathies. This was done initially using fetoscopically-obtained fetal blood, a procedure associated with relatively high rates of morbidity and fetal mortality[118,119]. Later, knowledge of specific gene defects and advancements in molecular technology allowed diagnosis using DNA extracted from amniocytes[120], and subsequently chorionic villi, methods which are now applied for the detection of numerous inherited conditions.

Other specific applications of fetal blood sampling for diagnostic and treatment purposes are considered throughout this text. Examples include fetal evaluation for viral infections, erythroblastosis fetalis, alloimmune thrombocytopenia and assessment of fetal acid–base status. In addition, the techniques and complications of fetal blood sampling are discussed at length in Chapter 56, and therefore will not be considered here.

Fetal biopsy

As is true with fetal blood sampling, the indications for fetal tissue sampling are evolving. These invasive techniques are reserved for highly morbid disorders whose diagnosis is not amenable to analysis of amniocytes, chorionic villi or fetal blood. Fetal tissues that have been biopsied for prenatal diagnosis include skin[121–127], muscle[128,129], liver[130–132], kidney[133] and brain[134].

The most common indications for fetal skin sampling are the diagnoses of genodermatoses, severe hereditary skin disorders with high rates of morbidity and mortality[121,122]. Skin biopsy was initially obtained by fetoscopy, a procedure carrying a fetal loss rate of 4–7%[123,124]. More recently, ultrasound-guided procedures were introduced[125], and are now the method of choice[121,122,126]. The procedure is performed at 17–20 weeks' gestation with a biopsy forceps introduced through a 14-gauge angiocath[126]. Though no study large enough to accurately assess safety has been published, a recent series of 17 cases showed five terminations for affected fetuses and no adverse outcomes in the remaining 12 pregnancies, except for minor skin blemishes in three infants[126].

Fetal skin biopsy analysis is reserved for those genodermatoses whose diagnosis can only be made on skin samples. As clues to the gene location and/or specific molecular defects causing these genetic disorders are found, the need for skin biopsy will diminish, as CVS or amniocentesis will provide diagnostic information in most cases. Table 3 lists some genodermatoses which have been prenatally diagnosed via skin biopsy.

Table 3   Selected genodermatoses diagnosed by fetal skin biopsy

Disorder	Inheritance	Comment
Junctional epidermolysis bullosa	Autosomal recessive	Most commonly prenatally diagnosed genetic skin disease by skin biopsy[127]. Mutations in the gene (*LAMC2*) recently described[176]
Recessive dystrophic epidermolysis bullosa	Autosomal recessive	Mutations in *COL7A1* have been identified[177] and prenatal diagnosis by DNA linkage has been described[178]
Dominant dystrophic epidermolysis bullosa	Autosomal dominant	Mutation in type VII collagen recently described[179]
Non-bullous congenital ichthyosiform erythroderma (lamellar ichthyosis)	Autosomal recessive	
Harlequin ichthyosis	Autosomal recessive	Prenatal diagnosis by morphological abnormality in amniotic fluid cell pellets has been suggested[180]
Bullous congenital ichthyosiform erythroderma (epidermolytic hyperkeratosis)	Autosomal dominant	Mutations in keratins 1 and 10 have been identified in patients[181], prenatal diagnosis by gene sequencing has been reported[182]
Tyrosinase-negative oculocutaneous albinism	Autosomal recessive	
X-linked hypohidrotic ectodermal dysplasia	X-linked recessive	Localized to Xq12–q13.1, mutations described[183] and prenatal diagnosis by linkage available for many families[184]
Anhidrotic ectodermal dysplasia	Autosomal recessive	
Sjögren–Larsson syndrome	Autosomal recessive	Diagnosis by enzymatic analysis of amniocytes has been described[185]

Evaluation of biopsy specimens is specific to the disorder for which the fetus is at risk. Methods include morphological, immunohistochemical and biochemical techniques. The prenatal diagnosis of genodermatoses using fetal skin biopsy has been reviewed recently by Holbrook and colleagues[127].

Fetal skin biopsy, as well as fetal blood sampling, have infrequently been performed for the work-up of chromosomal mosaicism seen in cultured amniocytes[135]. Procedure-related loss rates and knowledge that a skin or blood analysis which is negative for the abnormal cell line cannot entirely rule out fetal mosaicism, have made this an uncommon indication for either procedure.

Fetal muscle biopsy is rarely performed, but has been performed for prenatal diagnosis of muscular dystrophy[128]. Duchenne and Becker muscular dystrophies are caused by mutations in a very large gene on the X chromosome, the gene for dystrophin[136]. Since the dystrophin gene was characterized, prenatal diagnosis has been possible for most fetuses at risk using a variety of molecular methods (polymerase chain reaction, Southern blot and/or restriction fragment length polymorphism linkage analysis) performed on DNA extracted from amniotic fluid or chorionic villi[137]. However, in a few families, the DNA results are uninformative. In such cases, fetal muscle biopsy may provide the sole opportunity for prenatal diagnosis, using immunohistochemical assays for dystrophin. Since very few fetal muscle biopsies have been reported to date[128,129], the safety of the procedure is difficult to assess.

As is the case with fetal muscle biopsy, fetal liver biopsy is reserved for devastating inherited disorders which cannot be diagnosed by analysis of amniocytes and/or chorionic villi. A small number of inborn errors of metabolism are in this category, as they are diagnosed by assay of the activity of enzymes which are primarily expressed in the liver. Examples include ornithine transcarbamylase (OTC) deficiency[130], carbamoyl-phosphate synthetase (CPS) deficiency[131], and glucose-6-phosphatase deficiency[132] (glycogen storage disease, Type 1A). Recent genetic advances have led to the ability to prenatally diagnose OTC deficiency using molecular methods in many cases[138,139], and the promise of similar diagnostic capabilities for CPS deficiency in the near future[140]. As researchers continue to identify the gene mutations responsible for inherited disorders, the rare need for invasive techniques such as fetal skin, muscle and liver biopsy will further diminish.

NON-INVASIVE METHODS FOR PRENATAL DIAGNOSIS

Preimplantation diagnosis

Development of the polymerase chain reaction (PCR)[141] has revolutionized molecular genetics. This technique permits millions of copies of a targeted DNA segment to be amplified from a small DNA sample in a matter of hours. In recent years, this technology has been combined with *in vitro* fertilization in an effort to provide still earlier prenatal diagnosis. For couples at risk for an inherited disorder, results obtained from amniocytes or chorionic villi may present them with a difficult decision of whether or not to continue the pregnancy. Many women would prefer to completely avoid carrying affected fetuses[142], and some would prefer a technology which allows screening embryos prior to implantation.

The technology involved in preimplantation diagnosis includes *in vitro* fertilization, embryo or polar body biopsy, PCR amplification of the DNA sequences of interest, and molecular genetic techniques using the amplified DNA to determine the presence or absence of a specific allele(s) in the embryo. Only those embryos with genetic material predictive of an unaffected fetus are implanted, thus avoiding the need for pregnancy termination.

Methods to obtain the cell(s) required for analysis include biopsy of one to several cells of the two- to three-day embryo, biopsy of the trophectoderm of the five- to six-day blastocyst, and polar body biopsy (removal of the non-functioning haploid product of meiosis I)[143]. Each of these methods has benefits and drawbacks, ranging from the degree of technical difficulty, to variations in pregnancy rates, to errors in diagnosis due to the hazards of single cell analysis. Various embryo biopsy techniques have recently been analyzed[144]. The authors concluded that biopsy of a quarter of the embryo on day three after fertilization (approximately the 12-cell stage) may be the 'most feasible' for preimplantation diagnosis. Accurate diagnoses from polar body biopsy have been described; however, subsequent implantation did not result in successful pregnancies[145].

An important technical consideration is the accuracy of diagnosis. When basing a diagnosis on DNA amplified from a single cell, problems such as contamination, PCR failure and PCR error are of paramount importance. Navidi and Arnheim[146] considered these sources of error mathematically and suggested that blastomere analysis is preferred over polar body analysis, while a combination of the two results in a significantly lower risk of misdiagnosis.

The clinical use of preimplantation diagnosis was first described in 1990 by Handyside and colleagues[147] for sex selection in pregnancies at risk for X-linked diseases. Since that time, this technology has been applied for the specific diagnosis of several disorders, including cystic fibrosis[148], Duchenne muscular dystrophy[149] and alloimmune thrombocytopenia[150].

The potential for preimplantation diagnosis has recently been enhanced by application of single-cell whole-genome preamplification[151]. This method allows analysis of multiple exons and introns within a gene for those diagnoses dependent on evaluation at more than one locus. It also provides sufficient DNA for sex determination as well as specific mutation detection at a sex-linked locus, all amplified from a single cell. Another technique applied to preimplantation diagnosis is fluorescence *in situ* hybridization (FISH), a method using chromosome-specific probes to rapidly determine the copy number of a certain chromosome. This has been done with X and Y chromosome-specific probes for sex determination[152], and probes for the chromosomes most commonly involved in aneuploidy (X, Y, 18, 13 and 21)[153].

As these and other molecular methods and biopsy techniques are further developed, preimplantation diagnosis may become more readily available. However, all of this technology is quite expensive, a factor which must be considered, particularly at a time when the resources available for health care are becoming increasingly limited.

Fetal cells in the maternal circulation

The same molecular techniques (PCR, FISH) which have allowed the development of preimplantation genetic diagnosis have played a major role in efforts to provide prenatal diagnosis based on the analysis of fetal cells obtained from maternal peripheral blood. If this type of non-invasive testing were developed to the point of cost-effective and accurate clinical application, the risks associated with invasive prenatal diagnostic techniques (amniocentesis, CVS) could be avoided. In addition, prenatal diagnosis could potentially be offered to every pregnant woman, rather than limiting testing to those at increased risk.

Though earlier studies suggested that fetal cells exist in the maternal circulation[154,155], more recent work based on PCR technology has proved this with certainty[156]. Requirements to achieve a diagnosis based on fetal cells isolated from maternal blood would include a sensitive and specific method to identify fetal cells, a process to enrich for the infrequent fetal cells, and techniques to analyze the fetal genetic material for prenatal diagnosis. Each of these aspects are currently in the process of development, and a variety of methods have been attempted with varying success.

In order to identify fetal cells, monoclonal antibodies against various fetal cell antigens have been developed. These include antibodies to trophoblasts[157,158], fetal erythrocyte cell surface antigens[159–161], and paternally derived HLA antigens[166,167]. To enrich for fetal cells, the monoclonal antibodies have been fluorescently tagged and used in combination with flow cytometry, a method to sort individual cells based on their specific physical and chemical properties. Characteristics selected for include cell size, cell granularity and the presence of a fluorescent tag[160,161]. By report, multiparameter flow cytometry applied to first-trimester maternal peripheral blood enriches from one fetal nucleated erythrocyte in approximately 10^7 to 10^8 maternal cells to approximately four fetal cells per 1000 maternal cells[160]. The proportion of fetal cells after sorting second-trimester samples was approximately 20 fetal cells per 1000 maternal cells in this study, though other investigators have not described such high yields of fetal cells[164,165]. Alternatives to fluorescence-activated flow cytometry include immunospecific magnetic-activated cell sorting[166], immunomagnetic beads[167], avidin–biotin columns[168], and discontinuous density-gradient centrifugation[169]. The various methods have been reviewed recently and their advantages and disadvantages analyzed by Holzgreve and colleagues[170].

Techniques for genetic analysis that have been applied to fetal cells isolated from the maternal circulation include PCR and *in situ* hybridization. PCR has been used to detect Y chromosome-specific DNA sequences to identify male fetuses in both unsorted[171] and sorted[160,161] maternal peripheral blood. More recently, this technology has been applied to determine fetal rhesus antigen status[172,173]. Fluorescence *in situ* hybridization to detect fetal aneuploidies has also been described using fetal cells derived from the maternal circulation[160,174,175].

The multitude of recent abstracts and papers related to further development of identification, enrichment and diagnostic methods for application to fetal cells in the maternal circulation reflect the ongoing interest in this field. While many of the technical issues remain unresolved, the potential for noninvasive prenatal diagnosis provides a strong motivating force for research efforts.

REFERENCES

1. Druzin ML, Chervenak F, McCullough LB, *et al*. Should all pregnant patients be offered prenatal diagnosis regardless of age? *Obstet Gynecol* 1993;81:615–18
2. Hook EB. Rates of chromosome abnormalities at different maternal ages. *Obstet Gynecol* 1981;58:282–5
3. ACOG Technical Bulletin. Antenatal Diagnosis of Genetic Disorders (number 108). Washington, DC: American College of Obstetricians and Gynecologists, 1987
4. Hook EB, Cross PK, Schreinemachers DM. Chromosomal abnormality rates at amniocentesis and in liveborn infants. *J Am Med Assoc* 1983;249:2034–8
5. Daniel A, Stewart L, Saville T, *et al*. Prenatal diagnosis in 3000 women for chromosome, X-linked, and metabolic disorders. *Am J Med Genet* 1982;11:61–75
6. Tamaren J, Spuhler K, Sujansky E. Risk of Down syndrome among second- and third-degree relatives of a proband with trisomy 21. *Am J Med Genet* 1983;15:393–403
7. Eunpu DL, McDonald DM, Zackai EH. Trisomy 21: rate in second-degree relatives. *Am J Med Genet* 1986;25:361–3
8. Berr C, Borghi E, Rethoré MO, *et al*. Risk of Down syndrome in relatives of trisomy 21 children: a case–control study. *Ann Génét* 1990;33:137–40
9. Boué A, Gallano P. A collaborative study of the segregation of inherited chromosome structural rearrangements in 1356 prenatal diagnoses. *Prenat Diagn* 1984;4:45–67
10. Daniel A, Hook EB, Wulf G. Risks of unbalanced progeny at amniocentesis to carriers of chromosome rearrangements: data from United States and Canadian laboratories. *Am J Med Genet* 1989;31:14–53
11. Neri G, Serra A, Campana M, Tedeschi B. Reproductive risks for translocation carriers: cytogenetic study and analysis of pregnancy outcome in 58 families. *Am J Med Genet* 1983;16:535–61
12. Brock DJH, Sutcliffe RG. Alpha-fetoprotein in the antenatal diagnosis of anencephaly and spina bifida. *Lancet* 1972;2:197–9
13. Macri JN, Weiss RR, Tillitt R, *et al*. Prenatal diagnosis of neural tube defects. *J Am Med Assoc* 1976;236:1251–4
14. U.K. Collaborative Study on Alpha-fetoprotein in Relation to Neural Tube Defects. Maternal serum-alpha-fetoprotein measurement in antenatal screening for anencephaly and spina bifida in early pregnancy. *Lancet* 1977;1:1323–32
15. ACOG Technical Bulletin. Alpha-fetoprotein (number 154). Washington, DC: American College of Obstetricians and Gynecologists, 1991
16. Thomas RL, Blakemore KJ. Evaluation of elevations in maternal serum alpha-fetoprotein: a review. *Obstet Gynecol Surv* 1990;45:269–83
17. Burton BK. Outcome of pregnancy in patients with unexplained elevated or low levels of maternal serum alpha-fetoprotein. *Obstet Gynecol* 1988;72:709–13
18. Waller DK, Lustig LS, Cunningham GC, *et al*. Second-trimester maternal serum alpha-fetoprotein levels and the risk of subsequent fetal death. *N Engl J Med* 1991;325:6–10
19. Evans J, Stokes IM. Outcome of pregnancies associated with raised serum and normal amniotic fluid α-fetoprotein concentrations. *Br Med J* 1984;288:1494
20. Merkatz IR, Nitowsky HM, Macri JN, Johnson WE. An association between low maternal serum α-fetoprotein and fetal chromosomal abnormalities. *Am J Obstet Gynecol* 1984;148:886–94
21. Cuckle HS, Wald NJ, Lindenbaum RH. Maternal serum alpha-fetoprotein measurement: a screening test for Down syndrome. *Lancet* 1984;1:926–9
22. DiMaio MS, Baumgarten A, Greenstein RM, *et al*. Screening for fetal Down's syndrome in pregnancy by measuring maternal serum alpha-fetoprotein levels. *N Engl J Med* 1987;317:342–6
23. New England Regional Genetics Group Prenatal Collaborative Study of Down Syndrome Screening.

Combining maternal serum α-fetoprotein measurements and age to screen for Down syndrome in pregnant women under age 35. *Am J Obstet Gynecol* 1989; 160:575–81

24. Bogart MH, Pandian MR, Jones OW. Abnormal maternal serum chorionic gonadotropin levels in pregnancies with fetal chromosome abnormalities. *Prenat Diagn* 1987;7:623–30

25. Canick JA, Knight GJ, Palomaki GE, *et al*. Low second trimester maternal serum unconjugated oestriol in pregnancies with Down's syndrome. *Br J Obstet Gynaecol* 1988;95:330–3

26. Haddow JE, Palomaki GE, Knight GJ, *et al*. Prenatal screening for Down's syndrome with use of maternal serum markers. *N Engl J Med* 1992;327:588–93

27. Canick JA, Palomaki GE, Osathanondh R. Prenatal screening for trisomy 18 in the second trimester. *Prenat Diagn* 1990;10:546–8

28. Palomaki GE, Knight GJ, Haddow JE, *et al*. Prospective intervention trial of a screening protocol to identify fetal trisomy 18 using maternal serum alpha-fetoprotein, unconjugated oestriol, and human chorionic gonadotropin. *Prenat Diagn* 1992;12:925–30

29. Saller DN, Canick JA, Schwartz S, Blitzer MG. Multiple-marker screening in pregnancies with hydropic and nonhydropic Turner syndrome. *Am J Obstet Gynecol* 1992;167:1021–4

30. Wenstrom KD, Williamson RA, Grant SS. Detection of fetal Turner syndrome with multiple-marker screening. *Am J Obstet Gynecol* 1994;170:570–3

31. Brambati B, Simoni G, Bonacchi I, Piceni L. Fetal chromosomal aneuploidies and maternal serum alpha-fetoprotein levels in first trimester. *Lancet* 1986;2:165–6

32. Milunsky A, Wands J, Brambati B, *et al*. First-trimester maternal serum α-fetoprotein screening for chromosome defects. *Am J Obstet Gynecol* 1988;159:1209–13

33. Brock DJH, Barron L, Holloway S, *et al*. First-trimester maternal serum biochemical indicators in Down syndrome. *Prenat Diagn* 1990;10:245–51

34. Johnson A, Cowchock FS, Darby M, *et al*. First-trimester maternal serum alpha-fetoprotein and chorionic gonadotropin in aneuploid pregnancies. *Prenat Diagn* 1991;11:443–50

35. Brambati B, Chard T, Grudzinkas JC, *et al*. Potential first trimester biochemical screening tests for chromosome anomalies. *Prenat Diagn* 1992;12S:S4

36. Aitken DA, McCaw G, Crossley JA, *et al*. First-trimester biochemical screening for fetal chromosome abnormalities and neural tube defects. *Prenat Diagn* 1993; 13:681–9

37. Cuckle HS, Wald NJ, Barkai G, *et al*. First-trimester biochemical screening for Down syndrome. *Lancet* 1988;1:851–2

38. Kratzer PG, Golbus MS, Monroe SE, *et al*. First-trimester aneuploidy screening using serum human chorionic gonadotropin (hCG), free α-hCG, and progesterone. *Prenat Diagn* 1991;11:751–65

39. Macintosh MCM, Iles R, Teisner B, *et al*. Maternal serum human chorionic gonadotropin and pregnancy-associated plasma protein A, markers for fetal Down syndrome at 8–14 weeks. *Prenat Diagn* 1994; 14:203–8

40. Brambati B, Tului L, Bonacchi I, *et al*. Biochemical screening for Down's syndrome in the first trimester. Personal communication, 1995.

41. Macintosh MCM, Brambati B, Chard T, Grudzinskas JG. First-trimester maternal serum Schwangerschaftsprotein 1 (SP1) in pregnancies associated with chromosomal anomalies. *Prenat Diagn* 1993;13:563–8

42. Hurely PA, Ward RHT, Teisner B, *et al*. Serum PAPP-A measurements in first-trimester screening for Down syndrome. *Prenat Diagn* 1993;13:903–8

43. Brizot ML, Snijders RJM, Bersinger NA, *et al*. Maternal serum pregnancy-associated plasma protein A and fetal nuchal translucency thickness for the prediction of fetal trisomies in early pregnancy. *Obstet Gynecol* 1994;84:918–22

44. Van Lith JMM, Mantingh A, Pratt JJ, for the Dutch Working Party on Prenatal Diagnosis. First-trimester maternal serum immunoreactive inhibin in chromosomally normal and abnormal pregnancies. *Obstet Gynecol* 1994;83:661–4

45. Wald NJ, Kennard A, Smith D. First trimester biochemical screening for Down's syndrome. *Ann Med* 1994;26:23–9

46. Nicolaides KH, Azar G, Byrne D, *et al*. Fetal nuchal translucency: ultrasound screening for chromosomal defects in the first trimester of pregnancy. *Br Med J* 1992;304:867–9

47. Pandya PP, Altman DG, Brizot MI, *et al*. Repeatability of measurement of fetal nuchal translucency thickness. *Ultrasound Obstet Gynecol* 1995;5:334–7

48. Orlandi F, Darmiani G, Hallahan TW, *et al*. First trimester screening for fetal aneuploidy: biochemistry and nuchal translucency. *Ultrasound Obstet Gynecol* 1997;10:381–6

49. ACOG Committee Opinion. Screening for Canavan Disease (no. 212). Washington, DC: American College of Obstetricians and Gynecologists, 1998

50. Gilbert F. Cystic fibrosis carrier screening: comparability of data and uniformity of testing. *Am J Hum Genet* 1994;54:925–7

51. Statement of the American Society of Human Genetics on cystic fibrosis carrier screening. *Am J Hum Genet* 1992;51:1443–4

52. ACOG Committee Opinion. Current Status of Cystic Fibrosis Carrier Screening (number 101). Washington, DC: American College of Obstetricians and Gynecologists, 1991

53. Bekker H, Denniss G, Modell M, *et al*. The impact of population based screening for carriers of cystic fibrosis. *J Med Genet* 1994;31:364–8

54. Schwartz M, Brandt NJ, Skovby F. Screening for carriers of cystic fibrosis among pregnant women: a pilot study. *Eur J Hum Genet* 1993;1:239–44

55. Jung U, Urner U, Grade K, Coutelle C. Acceptability of carrier screening for cystic fibrosis during pregnancy in a German population. *Hum Genet* 1994; 94:19–24

56. Livingstone J, Axton RA, Gilfillan A, *et al*. Antenatal screening for cystic fibrosis: a trial of the couple model. *Br Med J* 1994;308:1459–62

57. Faden RR, Tambor ES, Chase GA, *et al*. Attitudes of physicians and genetics professionals toward cystic

fibrosis carrier screening. *Am J Med Genet* 1994; 50:1–11

58. Rowley PT, Loader S, Levenkron JC, Phelps CE. Cystic fibrosis carrier screening: knowledge and attitudes of prenatal care providers. *Am J Prev Med* 1993;9:261–6

59. Jacobson CB, Barter RH. Intrauterine diagnosis and management of genetic defects. *Am J Obstet Gynecol* 1967;99:796–807

60. The NICHD National Registry for Amniocentesis Study Group. Midtrimester amniocentesis for prenatal diagnosis: safety and accuracy. *J Am Med Assoc* 1976; 236:1471–6

61. Medical Research Council Working Party on Amniocentesis. An assessment of the hazards of amniocentesis. *Br J Obstet Gynaecol* 1978;85:1–41

62. Tabor A, Madsen M, Obel EB, *et al*. Randomised controlled trial of genetic amniocentesis in 4606 low-risk women. *Lancet* 1986;1:1287–92

63. Broome DL, Wilson MG, Weiss B, Kellogg B. Needle puncture of fetus: a complication of second-trimester amniocentesis. *Am J Obstet Gynecol* 1976;126:247–52

64. Porreco RP, Young PE, Resnik R, *et al*. Reproductive outcome following amniocentesis for genetic indications. *Am J Obstet Gynecol* 1982;143:653–60

65. Gold RB, Goyert GL, Schwartz DB, *et al*. Conservative management of second-trimester post-amniocentesis fluid leakage. *Obstet Gynecol* 1989;74:745–7

66. Kwong F, May ND, Rosol HE, *et al*. Cytogenetic prenatal diagnosis in the late first and early second trimester using amniocentesis. *Karyogram* 1988;6:112–4

67. Nicolaides K, Brizot ML, Patel F, Snijders R. Comparison of chorionic villus sampling and amniocentesis for fetal karyotyping at 10–13 weeks' gestation. *Lancet* 1994;344:435–9

68. Lockwood DH, Neu RL. Cytogenetic analysis of 1375 amniotic fluid specimens from pregnancies with gestational age less than 14 weeks. *Prenat Diagn* 1993;13:801–5

69. Shulman LP, Elias S, Phillips OP, *et al*. Amniocentesis performed at 14 weeks' gestation or earlier: comparison with first-trimester transabdominal chorionic villus sampling. *Obstet Gynecol* 1994;83:543–8

70. Shalev E, Weiner E, Yanai N, *et al*. Comparison of first-trimester transvaginal amniocentesis with chorionic villus sampling and mid-trimester amniocentesis. *Prenat Diagn* 1994;14:279–83

71. Kerber S, Held KR. Early genetic amniocentesis – 4 years' experience. *Prenat Diagn* 1993;13:21–7

72. Hackett GA, Smith JH, Rebello MT, *et al*. Early amniocentesis at 11–14 weeks' gestation for the diagnosis of fetal chromosomal abnormality – a clinical evaluation. *Prenat Diagn* 1991;11:311–5

73. Stripparo L, Buscaglia M, Longatti L, *et al*. Genetic amniocentesis: 505 cases performed before the sixteenth week of gestation. *Prenat Diagn* 1990;10: 359–64

74. Penso CA, Sandstrom MM, Garber MF, *et al*. Early amniocentesis: report of 407 cases with neonatal follow-up. *Obstet Gynecol* 1990;76:1032–6

75. Evans MI, Drugan A, Koppitch FC, *et al*. Genetic diagnosis in the first trimester: the norm for the 1990s. *Am J Obstet Gynecol* 1989;160:1332–9

76. Hanson FW, Happ RL, Tennant FR, *et al*. Ultrasonography-guided early amniocentesis in singleton pregnancies. *Am J Obstet Gynecol* 1990;162:1376–83

77. Hanson FW, Zorn EM, Tennant FR, *et al*. Amniocentesis before 15 weeks' gestation: outcome, risks, and technical problems. *Am J Obstet Gynecol* 1987; 156:1524–31

78. Assel BG, Lewis SM, Dickerman LH, *et al*. Single-operator comparison of early and mid-second-trimester amniocentesis. *Obstet Gynecol* 1992;79:940–4

79. Hanson FW, Tennant F, Hune S, Brookhyser K. Early amniocentesis: outcome, risks, and technical problems at ≤ 12.8 weeks. *Am J Obstet Gynecol* 1992;166:1707–11

80. Sundberg K, Bang J, Smidt-Jensen S, *et al*. Randomised study of risk of fetal loss related to early amniocentesis versus chorionic villus sampling. *Lancet* 1997;350:697–703

81. The Canadian Early and Mid-Trimester Amniocentesis Trial Group. Randomised trial to assess safety and fetal outcome of early and mid-trimester amniocentesis. *Lancet* 1998;351:242–7

82. Crandall BF, Hanson FW, Tennant F, Perdue ST. α-Fetoprotein levels in amniotic fluid between 11 and 15 weeks. *Am J Obstet Gynecol* 1989;160:1204–6

83. Drugan A, Syner FN, Greb A, Evans MI. Amniotic fluid alpha-fetoprotein and acetylcholinesterase in early genetic amniocentesis. *Obstet Gynecol* 1988;72:35–8

84. Wathen NC, Campbell DJ, Kitau MJ, Chard T. Alphafetoprotein levels in amniotic fluid from 8 to 18 weeks of pregnancy. *Br J Obstet Gynaecol* 1993;100:380–2

85. Smith AD, Wald NJ, Cuckle HS, *et al*. Amniotic-fluid acetylcholinesterase as a possible diagnostic test for neural-tube defects in early pregnancy. *Lancet* 1979;1:685–8

86. Milunsky A, Sapirstein VS. Prenatal diagnosis of open neural tube defects using the amniotic fluid acetylcholinesterase assay. *Obstet Gynecol* 1982;59:1–5

87. Wald NJ, Barlow RD, Cuckle HS, *et al*. Ratio of amniotic fluid acetylcholinesterase to pseudocholinesterase as an antenatal diagnostic test for exomphalos and gastroschisis. *Br J Obstet Gynaecol* 1984;91:882–4

88. Burton BK, Nelson LH, Pettenati MJ. False-positive acetylcholinesterase with early amniocentesis. *Obstet Gynecol* 1989;74:607–10

89. Mohr J. Foetal genetic diagnosis: development of techniques for early sampling of foetal cells. *Acta Pathol Microbiol Scand* 1968;73:73–7

90. Hahnemann N. Early prenatal diagnosis: a study of biopsy techniques and cell culturing from extraembryonic membranes. *Clin Genet* 1974;6:294–306

91. Kazy Z, Rozovsky IS, Bakharev VA. Chorion biopsy in early pregnancy: a method of early prenatal diagnosis for inherited disorders. *Prenat Diagn* 1982;2:39

92. Ward RHT, Modell B, Petrou M, *et al*. Method of sampling chorionic villi in first trimester of pregnancy under guidance of real time ultrasound. *Br Med J* 1983;286:1542–4

93. Cohn DH, Byers PH. Clinical screening for collagen defects in connective tissue diseases. *Clin Perinatol* 1990;17:793–809

94. Crane JP, Cheung SW. Am embryogenic model to explain cytogenetic inconsistencies observed in

chorionic villus versus fetal tissue. *Prenat Diagn* 1988;8:119–29

95. Vejerslev LO, Mikkelsen M. The European collaborative study on mosaicism in chorionic villus sampling data from 1986 to 1987. *Prenat Diagn* 1989;9:575–88

96. Hsu LYF, Perlis TE. United States survey on chromosome mosaicism and pseudomosaicism in prenatal diagnosis. *Prenat Diagn* 1984;4:97–130

97. Johnson A, Wapner RJ, Davis GH, Jackson LG. Mosaicism in chorionic villus sampling: an association with poor perinatal outcome. *Obstet Gynecol* 1990; 75:573–7

98. Jackson LG, Wapner RA, Barr MA. Safety of chorionic villus biopsy. *Lancet* 1986;1:674–5

99. Hogge WA, Schoenberg SA, Golbus MS. Chorionic villus sampling: experience of the first 1000 cases. *Am J Obstet Gynecol* 1986;154:1249–52

100. Rhoads GG, Jackson LG, Schlesselman SE, *et al*. The safety and efficacy of chorionic villus sampling for early prenatal diagnosis of cytogenetic abnormalities. *N Engl J Med* 1989;320:609–17

101. Canadian Collaborative CVS–Amniocentesis Clinical Trial Group. Multicentre randomised clinical trial of chorion villus sampling and amniocentesis: first report. *Lancet* 1989;1:1–6

102. MRC Working Party on the Evaluation of Chorion Villus Sampling. Medical Research Council European Trial of chorion villus sampling. *Lancet* 1991;337: 1491–9

103. Firth HV, Boyd PA, Chamberlain P, *et al*. Severe limb abnormalities after chorion villus sampling at 56–66 days gestation. *Lancet* 1991;337:762–3

104. Burton BK, Schulz CJ, Burd LI. Limb anomalies associated with chorionic villus sampling. *Obstet Gynecol* 1992;79:726–30

105. Froster-Iskenius UG, Baird PA. Limb reduction defects in over one million consecutive live births. *Teratology* 1989;39:127–35

106. Wapner R. Is chorionic villus sampling a safe procedure? *The Female Patient* 1993;18:59–62

107. Hsieh F-J, Shyu M-K, Shen B-C, *et al*. Limb defects after chorionic villus sampling. *Obstet Gynecol* 1995; 85:84–8

108. Firth HV, Boyd PA, Chamberlain PF, *et al*. Analysis of limb reduction defects in babies exposed to chorionic villus sampling. *Lancet* 1994;343:1069–71

109. World Health Organization/European Regional Office. *Risk of Evaluation of CVS*. Copenhagen: WHO/EURO, 1992

110. Smidt-Jensen S, Hahnemann N. Transabdominal fine needle biopsy from chorionic villi in the first trimester. *Prenat Diagn* 1984;4:163–9

111. Elias S, Simpson JL, Shulman LP, *et al*. Transabdominal chorionic villus sampling for first-trimester prenatal diagnosis. *Am J Obstet Gynecol* 1989;160: 879–86

112. Shulman LP, Simpson JL, Elias S, *et al*. Transvaginal chorionic villus sampling using transabdominal ultrasound guidance: a new technique for first-trimester prenatal diagnosis. *Fetal Diagn Ther* 1993;8:144–8

113. Jackson LG, Zachary JM, Fowler SE, *et al*. A randomized comparison of transcervical and transabdominal

114. Brambati B, Terzian E, Tognoni G. Randomized clinical trial of transabdominal versus transcervical chorionic villus sampling methods. *Prenat Diagn* 1991; 11:285–93

115. Smidt-Jensen S, Permin M, Philip J, *et al*. Randomised comparison of amniocentesis and transabdominal and transcervical chorionic villus sampling. *Lancet* 1992;340:1237–44

116. Blakemore KJ, Mahoney MJ, Hobbins JC. Infection and chorionic villus sampling. *Lancet* 1985;2:339

117. Barela AI, Kleinman GE, Golditch IM, *et al*. Septic shock with renal failure after chorionic villus sampling. *Am J Obstet Gynecol* 1986;154:1100–2

118. Alter BP, Modell CB, Fairweather D, *et al*. Prenatal diagnosis of hemoglobinopathies: a review of 15 cases. *N Engl J Med* 1976;295:1437–43

119. Kan YW, Trecartin RF, Golbus MS, Filly RA. Prenatal diagnosis of β-thalassemia and sickle-cell anaemia: experience with 24 cases. *Lancet* 1977;1:269–71

120. Chang JC, Kan YW. A sensitive new prenatal test for sickle-cell anemia. *N Engl J Med* 1982;307:30–2

121. Cadrin C, Golbus MS. Fetal tissue sampling: indications, techniques, complications, and experience with sampling of fetal skin, liver, and muscle. *West J Med* 1993;159:269–72

122. Shulman LP, Elias S. Percutaneous umbilical blood sampling, fetal skin sampling, and fetal liver biopsy. *Semin Perinatol* 1990;14:456–64

123. Elias S, Esterly NB. Prenatal diagnosis of hereditary skin disorders. *Clin Obstet Gynecol* 1981;24:1069–87

124. Elias S. Use of fetoscopy for the prenatal diagnosis of hereditary skin disorders. In Gedde-Dahl T, Wuepper KD (eds). Prenatal Diagnosis of Heritable Skin Diseases. In *Current Problems in Dermatology*, vol 16. Hönigsmann H ed. Basel: Karger, 1987:1–13

125. Kurjak A, Alfirevic Z, Jurkovic D. Ultrasonically guided fetal tissue biopsy. *Acta Obstet Gynecol Scand* 1987;66:523–7

126. Elias S, Emerson DS, Simpson JL, *et al*. Ultrasound-guided fetal skin sampling for prenatal diagnosis of genodermatoses. *Obstet Gynecol* 1994;83:337–41

127. Holbrook KA, Smith LT, Elias S. Prenatal diagnosis of genetic skin disease using fetal skin biopsy samples. *Arch Dermatol* 1993;129:1437–54

128. Evans MI, Hoffman EP, Cadrin C, *et al*. Fetal muscle biopsy: collaborative experience with varied indications. *Obstet Gynecol* 1994;84:913–17

129. Benzie RJ, Ray P, Thompson D, *et al*. Prenatal exclusion of Duchenne muscular dystrophy by fetal muscle biopsy. *Prenat Diagn* 1994;14:235–8

130. Holzgreve W, Golbus MS. Prenatal diagnosis of ornithine transcarbamylase deficiency utilizing fetal liver biopsy. *Am J Hum Genet* 1984;36:320–8

131. Murotsuki J, Uehara S, Okamura K, *et al*. Fetal liver biopsy for prenatal diagnosis of carbamoyl phosphate synthetase deficiency. *Am J Perinatol* 1994; 11:160–2

132. Golbus MS, Simpson TJ, Koresawa M, *et al*. The prenatal determination of glucose-6-phosphatase activity by fetal liver biopsy. *Prenat Diagn* 1988;8:401–4

133. Greco P, Loverro G, Caruso G, *et al*. The diagnostic potential of fetal renal biopsy. *Prenat Diagn* 1993; 13:551–6

134. Suresh S, Indrani S, Vijayalakshmi S, *et al*. Prenatal diagnosis of cerebral neuroblastoma by fetal brain biopsy. *J Ultrasound Med* 1993;5:303–6

135. Cartolano R, Guerneri S, Fogliani R, *et al*. Prenatal confirmation of trisomy 12 mosaicism by fetal skin biopsy: *Prenat Diagn* 1993;13:1057–9

136. Koenig M, Hoffman EP, Bertelson CJ, *et al*. Complete cloning of the Duchenne muscular dystrophy (DMD) cDNA and preliminary genomic organization of the DMD gene in normal and affected individuals. *Cell* 1987;50:509–17

137. Kazazian HH. Current status of prenatal diagnosis by DNA analysis. *Birth Defects* 1990;26:210–16

138. Grompe M, Caskey CT, Fenwick RG. Improved molecular diagnostics for ornithine transcarbamylase deficiency. *Am J Hum Genet* 1991;48:212–22

139. Liechti-Gallati S, Dionisi C, Bachmann C, *et al*. Direct and indirect mutation analyses in patients with ornithine transcarbamylase deficiency. *Enzyme* 1991; 45:81–91

140. Haraguchi Y, Uchino T, Takiguchi M, *et al*. Cloning and sequence of a cDNA encoding human carbamyl phsophate synthetase I: molecular analysis of hyperammionemia. *Gene* 1991;107:335–40

141. Saiki RK, Gelfand DH, Stoffel S, *et al*. Primer-directed enzymatic amplification of DNA with a thermostable DNA polymerase. *Science* 1988;239:487–91

142. Pergament E. Preimplantation diagnosis: a patient perspective. *Prenat Diagn* 1991;11:493–500

143. Simpson JL, Carson SA. Preimplantation genetic diagnosis. *N Engl J Med* 1992;327:951–3

144. Tarin JJ, Handyside AH. Embryo biopsy strategies for preimplantation diagnosis. *Fertil Steril* 1993; 59:943–53

145. Verlinsky Y, Rechitsky S, Evsikov S, *et al*. Preconception and preimplantation diagnosis for cystic fibrosis. *Prenat Diagn* 1992;12:103–10

146. Navidi W, Arnheim N. Using PCR in preimplantation genetic disease diagnosis. *Hum Reprod* 1991;6:836–49

147. Handyside AH, Kontogianni EH, Hardy K, Winston RM. Pregnancies from biopsied human preimplantation embryos sexed by Y-specific DNA amplification. *Nature* 1990;344:768–70

148. Handyside AH, Lesko JG, Tarín JJ, *et al*. Birth of a normal girl after *in vitro* fertilization and preimplantation diagnostic testing for cystic fibrosis. *N Engl J Med* 1992;327:905–9

149. Kristjansson K, Chong SS, Van den Veyver IB, *et al*. Preimplantation single cell analyses of dystrophin gene deletions using whole genome amplification. *Nat Genet* 1994;6:19–23

150. Van den Veyver IB, Chong SS, Kristjansson K, *et al*. Molecular analysis of human platelet antigen system 1 antigen on single cells can be applied to preimplantation genetic diagnosis for prevention of alloimmune thrombocytopenia. *Am J Obstet Gynecol* 1994; 170:807–12

151. Snabes MC, Chong SS, Subramanian SB, *et al*. Preimplantation single-cell analysis of multiple genetic loci by whole-genome amplification. *Proc Natl Acad Sci USA* 1994;91:6181–5

152. Harper JC, Coonen E, Ramaekers FC, *et al*. Identification of the sex of human preimplantation embryos in two hours using an improved spreading method and fluorescent *in situ* hybridization (FISH) using directly labelled probes. *Hum Reprod* 1994;9:721–4

153. Munne S, Lee A, Rosenwaks Z, *et al*. Diagnosis of major chromosome aneuploidies in human preimplantation embryos. *Hum Reprod* 1993;8:2185–91

154. Walknowska J, Conte FA, Grumback MM. Practical and theoretical implication of fetal/maternal lymphocyte transfer. *Lancet* 1969;1:1119–22

155. Schroder J, de la Chapelle A. Fetal lymphocytes in the maternal blood. *Blood* 1972;39:153–62

156. Lo YM, Wainscoat JS, Gillmer MDG, *et al*. Prenatal sex determination by DNA amplification from maternal peripheral blood. *Lancet* 1989;2:1363–5

157. Covone AE, Mutton D, Johnson PM, Adinolfi M. Trophoblast cells in peripheral blood from pregnant women. *Lancet* 1984;536:841–3

158. Mueller UW, Hawes CS, Wright AE, *et al*. Isolation of fetal trophoblast cells from peripheral blood of pregnant women. *Lancet* 1990;336:197–200

159. Bianchi DW, Flint AF, Pizzimenti MF, *et al*. Isolation of fetal DNA from nucleated erythrocytes in maternal blood. *Proc Natl Acad Sci USA* 1990;87:3279–83

160. Price JO, Elias S, Wachtel SS, *et al*. Prenatal diagnosis with fetal cells isolated from maternal blood by multiparameter flow cytometry. *Am J Obstet Gynecol* 1991; 165:1731–7

161. Wachtel S, Elias S, Price J, *et al*. Fetal cells in the maternal circulation: isolation by multiparameter flow cytometry and confirmation by polymerase chain reaction. *Hum Reprod* 1991;6:1466–9

162. Herzenberg LA, Bianchi DW, Schroder J, *et al*. Fetal cells in the blood of pregnant women: detection and enrichment by fluorescence-activated cell sorting. *Proc Natl Acad Sci USA* 1979;76:1453–5

163. Iverson GM, Bianchi DW, Cann HM, Herzenberg LA. Detection and isolation of fetal cells from maternal blood using the fluorescence-activated cell sorter (FACS). *Prenat Diagn* 1981;1:61–73

164. Bianchi DW, Shuber AP, DeMaria MA, *et al*. Fetal cells in maternal blood: determination of purity and yield by quantitative polymerase chain reaction. *Am J Obstet Gynecol* 1994;171:922–6

165. Hamada H, Arinami T, Kubo T, *et al*. Fetal nucleated cells in maternal peripheral blood: frequency and relationship to gestational age. *Hum Genet* 1993; 91:427–32

166. Gänshirt-Ahlert D, Burschyk M, Garritsen HS, *et al*. Magnetic cell sorting and the transferrin receptor as potential means of prenatal diagnosis from maternal blood. *Am J Obstet Gynecol* 1992;166:1350–5

167. Bertero MT, Camaschella C, Serra A, *et al*. Circulating trophoblast cells in pregnancy have maternal genetic markers. *Prenat Diagn* 1988;8:585–90

168. Berenson RJ, Bensinger WI, Kalamasz D. Positive selection of viable cell populations using avidin–biotin immunoadsorption. *J Immunol Methods* 1986; 91:11–19

169. Bhat NM, Bieber MM, Teng NN. One step separation of human fetal lymphocytes from nucleated red blood cells. *J Immunol Methods* 1990;131:147–9

170. Holzgreve W, Garritsen HSP, Gänshirt-Ahlert D. Fetal cells in the maternal circulation. *J Reprod Med* 1992; 37:410–18

171. Lo YMD, Patel P, Baigent CN, *et al*. Prenatal sex determination from maternal peripheral blood using the polymerase chain reaction. *Hum Genet* 1993;90:483–8

172. Geifman-Holtzman O, Bernstein IM, Berry SM, Bianchi DW. Prenatal diagnosis of fetal Rhesus (Rh) C, D, E type by polymerase chain reaction (PCR). *Am J Obstet Gynecol* 1995;172:265(Abstract 30)

173. Lo YMD, Bowell PJ, Selinger, M, *et al*. Prenatal determination of fetal RhD status by analysis of peripheral blood of rhesus negative mothers. *Lancet* 1993; 341:1147–8

174. Bianchi DW, Mahr A, Zickwolf GK, *et al*. Detection of fetal cells with 47,XY,+21 karyotype in maternal peripheral blood. *Hum Genet* 1992;90:368–70

175. Gänshirt-Ahlert D, Borjesson-Stoll R, Burschyk M, *et al*. Detection of fetal trisomies 21 and 18 from maternal blood using triple gradient and magnetic cell sorting. *Am J Reprod Immunol* 1993;30:194–201

176. Pulkkinen L, Christiano AM, Airenne T, *et al*. Mutations in the gamma 2 chain gene (*LAMC2*) of kalinin/laminin 5 in the junctional forms of epidermolysis bullosa. *Nat Genet* 1994;6:293–7

177. Hovnanian A, Hilal L, Blanchet-Bardon C, *et al*. Recurrent nonsense mutations within the type VII collagen gene in patients with severe recessive dystrophic epidermolysis bullosa. *Am J Hum Genet* 1994; 55:289–96

178. Christiano AM, Uitto J. DNA-based prenatal diagnosis of heritable skin diseases. *Arch Dermatol* 1993;129: 1455–9

179. Christiano AM, Ryynanen M, Uitto J. Dominant dystrophic epidermolysis bullosa: identification of a Gly→Ser substitution in the triple-helical domain of type VII collagen. *Proc Natl Acad Sci USA* 1994; 91:3549–53

180. Akiyama M, Kim DK, Main DM, *et al*. Characteristic morphologic abnormality of harlequin ichthyosis detected in amniotic fluid cells. *J Invest Dermatol* 1994;102:210–3

181. Rothnagel JA, Fisher MP, Axtell SM, *et al*. A mutational hot spot in keratin 10 (KRT 10) in patients with epidermolytic hyperkeratosis. *Hum Mol Genet* 1993;2:2147–50

182. Rothnagel JA, Longley MA, Holder RA, *et al*. Prenatal diagnosis of epidermolytic hyperkeratosis by direct gene sequencing. *J Invest Dermatol* 1994;102:13–6

183. Zonana J, Jones M, Clarke A, *et al*. Detection of *de novo* mutations and analysis of their origin in families with X-linked hypohidrotic ectodermal dysplasia. *J Med Genet* 1994;31:287–92

184. Zonana J. Hypohidrotic (anhidrotic) ectodermal dysplasia: molecular genetic research and its clinical applications. *Semin Dermatol* 1993;12:241–6

185. Tabsh K, Rizzo WB, Holbrook K, Theroux N. Sjögren–Larsson syndrome: technique and timing of prenatal diagnosis. *Obstet Gynecol* 1993;82:700–3

66

Maternal serum α-fetoprotein screening

B.K. Burton

Developments over the past several decades in the field of prenatal diagnosis have had a dramatic impact on selected families at increased risk for birth defects or genetic disorders. Perhaps the most exciting development in recent years, however, has been the emergence of maternal serum α-fetoprotein (MSAFP) screening as a tool for detecting open neural tube defects and chromosomal abnormalities in pregnancy. Maternal serum α-fetoprotein screening is unique among laboratory-based methods of antenatal diagnosis in that it can be reasonably applied to all pregnancies. Although considered experimental little more than a decade ago, it is now part of the standard of care for obstetric patients. Through widespread application of this technology, 80–85% of all open neural tube defects can be detected early in pregnancy, allowing parents the option of pregnancy termination. Because neural tube defects are among the most common and most devastating of all congenital malformations, the potential of MSAFP screening for reducing neonatal morbidity and mortality is substantial. Even beyond its potential for detecting neural tube defects, however, MSAFP screening is also useful in detecting a number of other birth defects and pregnancy complications. Of particular importance was the initial observation that 20–25% of cases of Down syndrome and an undetermined percentage of other chromosomal abnormalities could be detected in women under 35 years of age through follow-up of low MSAFP levels. More recently, the emergence of other serum markers, measured in conjunction with MSAFP, has greatly expanded our ability to identify pregnancies at highest risk for chromosome anomalies.

This chapter focuses on the significance of elevated MSAFP values and of increased risk for Down syndrome identified through low MSAFP and multiple-marker screening. A discussion of the appropriate follow-up of abnormal MSAFP values is provided.

NEURAL TUBE DEFECTS

Neural tube defects are among the most common congenital anomalies, occurring with a frequency of one to two per 1000 births in the USA. Anencephaly and spina bifida occur with approximately equal frequency. All infants with anencephaly, and approximately 80%

of those with spina bifida, have open lesions in which neural tissue is completely exposed or covered only by a thin membrane. Patients with 'closed' lesions have defects that are completely covered by skin or a thick membrane. Open lesions are associated with a poorer prognosis for survival and with a greater incidence of severe handicap. Closed neural tube defects are not typically detected by MSAFP screening.

The cause of neural tube defects is not well understood, but it is important to note that 95% of all affected infants are born to mothers with no previous family history of similar anomalies. The evidence suggests that both genetic and environmental factors play a role in the etiology of most neural tube defects. Couples who have had an affected child have a recurrence risk in future pregnancies of 2–3%; close relatives are at some increased risk as well. A few specific environmental agents, such as valproic acid and perhaps alcohol, have been linked to an increased frequency of neural tube defects. Maternal hyperthermia may also be a factor. Insulin-dependent diabetic mothers are at significantly increased risk and the magnitude of risk appears to be related to diabetic control in early gestation. Perhaps the most important avenue of investigation of environmental causes of neural tube defects, and one that has led to a promising method of prevention, began with several studies in the UK in which mothers of infants with neural tube defects were given periconceptional multivitamins or folic acid supplementation in subsequent pregnancies, with an apparent dramatic reduction in the incidence of recurrence[1–4]. More recently, several studies in the USA attempted to examine the question of whether or not periconceptional vitamin supplementation reduces the incidence of neural tube defects in the general obstetric population[5–7]. Although the results were not uniformly positive, two large studies[5,6] demonstrated a protective effect of multivitamins against the occurrence of neural tube defects. In 1992, Czeizel and Dudas[8] reported the results of a landmark randomized study in Hungary which demonstrated a highly significant decrease in the incidence of neural tube defects among women receiving periconceptional multivitamin supplementation. As a result of the mounting evidence that a large percentage of neural tube defects can be prevented, The Centers for Disease Control issued a recommendation in 1992 that 'all women of childbearing age who are capable of becoming pregnant should consume 0.4 mg of folic acid per day for the purpose of reducing their risk of having a pregnancy affected with spina bifida or other NTDs (neural tube defects)'[9,10]. This amount of folic acid can be obtained from the diet through careful selection of food or from commercial multivitamin preparations. It should be consumed on a continuing basis throughout the childbearing years, since more than 50% of pregnancies in the USA are unplanned[11] and neural tube defects occur within the first month following conception, prior to the initiation of prenatal supplements. At present, the guidelines continue to call for treatment of high-risk women who have previously had a neural tube defect-affected pregnancy with 4.0 mg folic acid daily, although it is not clear that this higher dose is necessary. Treatment of the high-risk patient should be initiated at least 1 month before conception is attempted and continued through the first 3 months of pregnancy. It has been estimated that this strategy, if adopted uniformly, would reduce the incidence of neural tube defects by 70%.

α-FETOPROTEIN IN NORMAL PREGNANCY

α-Fetoprotein (AFP) is a normal fetal protein found in high concentrations in the fetal serum throughout gestation. Its biological function is unknown. α-Fetoprotein disappears rapidly from the circulation during the first few months after birth and is not normally detected in greater than trace amounts in the serum of healthy adult men or non-pregnant women. α-Fetoprotein is present in amniotic fluid in normal pregnancies, presumably reaching the fluid primarily through excretion in the fetal urine. The concentration of AFP normally measured in the amniotic fluid peaks in early pregnancy between 10 and 14 weeks' gestation and decreases steadily thereafter. From the amniotic fluid, AFP diffuses across the fetal membranes and, using standard assay methods, is normally detected in increased quantities in the serum of the pregnant woman beginning at approximately 12 weeks' gestation. Some AFP may also be transported directly across the placenta from the fetal circulation to the maternal circulation, although, under normal circumstances, the transmembranous route predominates. In contrast to amniotic fluid, the normal levels of maternal serum AFP increase steadily throughout pregnancy up to at least 30–32 weeks' gestation. There is a significant concentration gradient from fetal serum to amniotic fluid to maternal serum. Therefore, contamination of either amniotic fluid or maternal serum with even a small quantity of fetal blood can produce AFP levels considerably above normal.

Table 1   Findings associated with elevated amniotic fluid α-fetoprotein

With positive acetylcholinesterase
Open neural tube defects
Ventral wall defects
Fetal demise, including demise of a co-twin
Massive fetal blood contamination

With negative acetylcholinesterase
Ventral wall defects
Fetal blood contamination
Intestinal atresias
Congenital nephrosis
Skin or scalp defects
Fetal demise
Normal fetus

ELEVATED α-FETOPROTEIN AND NEURAL TUBE DEFECTS

An association between open neural tube defects and elevated levels of amniotic fluid AFP has been known since 1972. However, this association is non-specific. In anencephaly or open spina bifida, increased levels of AFP reach the amniotic fluid by diffusion from fetal serum or cerebrospinal fluid across open or leaking membranes. Other 'open' fetal malformations, such as omphalocele or gastroschisis, can therefore also produce elevated levels of amniotic fluid AFP. In addition, elevated levels of amniotic fluid AFP may occasionally be observed in the presence of intestinal atresias, presumably because of decreased swallowing and AFP digestion by the fetus. Congenital nephrosis, and rarely other renal lesions, may lead to increased levels of amniotic fluid AFP through increased excretion in the fetal urine. Elevated amniotic fluid AFP has also been noted in association with Turner's syndrome, particularly when large cystic hygromas are present, and in association with a number of miscellaneous fetal malformations (Table 1).

Elevated levels of amniotic fluid AFP may occasionally be observed when the fetus is completely normal. The most common explanation for this is contamination of the amniotic fluid by fetal blood. Even in the absence of blood contamination, however, rare 'false-positive' elevations of amniotic fluid AFP occur. In the early years of antenatal diagnosis of neural tube defects, these false-positive elevations occasionally resulted in the elective abortion of a normal fetus. The development of a second confirmatory laboratory test has now made such an event extraordinarily unlikely. In most laboratories, gel electrophoresis for detection of the presence of acetylcholinesterase is now routinely carried out on amniotic fluid samples with borderline or elevated AFP.

Acetylcholinesterase, unlike AFP, is not normally present in amniotic fluid. In contrast, it is virtually always present in the face of a significant open neural tube defect. It is variably present in the case of fetal ventral wall defects and in cases of significant fetal blood contamination. If fetal blood contamination is excluded, however, an elevated amniotic fluid AFP finding in association with a positive acetyl-cholinesterase virtually always indicates the presence of a fetal defect. Statistically, the defect is most likely to be an open neural tube defect. On the other hand, negative acetylcholinesterase, even in association with elevated amniotic fluid AFP, strongly suggests that the fetus does not have a neural tube defect.

Shortly after the association between elevated amniotic fluid AFP and fetal neural tube defects was noted, an association between elevated levels of MSAFP and open neural tube defects was also reported. In 1977, the report of the UK Collaborative Study on α-Fetoprotein in Relation to Neural Tube Defects documented the effectiveness of MSAFP screening in selecting pregnant women from the general obstetric population for whom prenatal diagnosis was warranted[12]. Subsequently, several pilot projects were established to determine the efficacy of routine MSAFP screening in the USA. Data from these projects clearly indicated that MSAFP screening is a powerful and effective screening tool that can be successfully integrated into routine obstetric practice[13–15]. A favorable cost–benefit ratio has also been demonstrated[16].

It is essential to bear in mind that, although amniotic fluid AFP determination is a diagnostic test, MSAFP determination is a screening tool only. Much in the same way that patients are identified as candidates for prenatal diagnosis by virtue of their age or family history, MSAFP screening provides another effective means for selecting patients who are at increased risk for neural tube defects and are therefore candidates for the more definitive procedures of ultrasound and amniocentesis. An elevated MSAFP level by no means indicates the presence of a fetal neural tube defect; there are many potential explanations for such a finding (Table 2). Elevated MSAFP does, however, indicate the need for further evaluation.

It is also important to recognize that considerable overlap exists between MSAFP levels observed in pregnancies affected with a fetal neural tube defect and in normal pregnancies. In screening routine pregnancies, a 'cut-off' level defining normal results must be selected such that an acceptable rate of detection of neural tube defects is achieved while the percentage of normal pregnancies subjected to further testing is limited. Practically speaking, it would never be possible to detect all open neural tube defects through MSAFP screening alone. Using cut-off levels commonly employed in the USA, 80–85% of open defects will be identified. Patients and physicians must be aware that defects will be missed through screening and not assume that the birth of an infant with a neural tube

Table 2   Findings associated with elevated maternal serum α-fetoprotein

Common 'benign' findings
More advanced gestational age
Multiple gestation
Normal pregnancy

Fetal abnormalities
Fetal demise
Open neural tube defects
Ventral wall defects
Intestinal atresias
Skin or scalp defects
Congenital nephrosis
Cystic hygroma
Chromosome anomalies, including triploidy, sex
   chromosome anomalies and others

Obstetric complications
Placental abnormalities or insufficiency
Severe oligohydramnios with or without fetal anomalies
Abdominal pregnancy
Partial mole
Late pregnancy complications such as low birth weight
   and stillbirth

Other findings
Maternal liver disease or AFP-producing tumor
Fetal parvovirus infection; possibly other intrauterine
   viral infections
Previous amniocentesis (within 1 week prior to the
   MSAFP determination)
Spontaneous fetomaternal transfusion
Hereditary persistence of α-fetoprotein

AFP, α-fetoprotein; MSAFP, maternal serum α-fetoprotein

defect to a mother with normal results reflects an error in the screening process.

FOLLOW-UP OF ELEVATED MSAFP LEVELS

A rather complex series of follow-up procedures may be triggered by abnormal MSAFP results and it is essential that these proceed in a timely and co-ordinated fashion. Specialized expertise is required in genetic counseling, interpretation of laboratory results and follow-up obstetric services, so the obstetrician must ensure that the patient has ready access to these services and that they are of high quality.

The first step in MSAFP screening is to obtain a blood sample from the patient at approximately 16 weeks' gestation. It is generally agreed that screening should be voluntary, because difficult decisions may follow from abnormal test results. MSAFP screening can be carried out with reasonable reliability any time between 15 and 24 weeks' gestation. Prior to 15 weeks, it is unreliable and the detection rate for neural tube defects is low. Sixteen to 17 weeks' gestation represents the ideal time, because the detection rate for both spina bifida and anencephaly is high and adequate time is available to allow for follow-up testing and the subsequent possibility of pregnancy termination. Fortunately, this coincides with the optimal time for screening for chromosome anomalies using multiple markers.

Once the patient's MSAFP level is determined, it is compared with normal values established within each laboratory for each week of gestation. Each laboratory defines its own normal range, usually using the cut-off of 2.0 or 2.5 multiples of the normal median to define the upper limits of normal. In addition to the patient's gestational age, a number of other factors should be taken into consideration by the laboratory in interpreting an individual MSAFP level. These include maternal weight, race and the presence of insulin-dependent diabetes. Under selected circumstances when the initial MSAFP level is elevated, repeat testing may be considered 1 week later. Approximately 45% of women with an initial MSAFP level between 2.5 and 3.0 multiples of the median will have a normal result on repeat testing. These patients are not at increased risk for neural tube defects or other adverse outcomes of pregnancy and further evaluation is not necessary in this group. In patients with an initial MSAFP level greater than 3.0 multiples of the median, it is very unlikely that a second determination will yield a normal result. Therefore, a repeat test in not recommended in this group prior to proceeding with genetic counseling and further evaluation.

When further testing is indicated because of an MSAFP elevation, it is essential that the patient be counseled regarding the significance of the findings, the nature of neural tube defects and options for further testing. Most individuals with MSAFP elevations do not have a fetus with a neural tube defect. On the other hand, such patients as a group have an overall risk of approximately one in 30 of having an affected fetus, clearly making them candidates for more definitive diagnostic testing.

The specific risk faced by an individual patient of having a fetus with a neural tube defect will depend on a number of factors, including her specific MSAFP level, her race and the background frequency of neural tube defects in the population. The patient whose value is just at the cut-off level will obviously have a risk substantially lower than that of the patient with a more dramatic elevation.

The next step in the testing process is ultrasonography, through which several of the most common causes of MSAFP elevations can be readily identified. The most common 'benign' explanation for MSAFP elevations is more advanced gestational age than originally anticipated. Because MSAFP levels normally rise approximately 15% per week in the mid-trimester, a value interpreted as being elevated at 16 weeks' gestation may be normal for 20 weeks' gestation. Another common explanation for MSAFP elevations is multiple pregnancy. Twins, on average, produce twice as much AFP as the single fetus and, therefore, higher levels of MSAFP are not unanticipated. Although an MSAFP elevation in the range of 2.5–4.0 multiples of the median may be adequately explained by a twin gestation, the presence of twins does not preclude the presence of an open defect in one or both fetuses. Both twins should be carefully examined by ultrasonography. MSAFP levels greater than 4.0 multiples of the median are not adequately explained by twins alone. Patients carrying twins with levels in this range should not only be offered amniocentesis for detection of open fetal defects, but should be followed carefully through the remainder of pregnancy because there is a high incidence of later complications.

In addition to more advanced gestational age and multiple pregnancy, unrecognized fetal demise may be identified by ultrasonography as another explanation for MSAFP elevations. A small percentage of patients with MSAFP elevations will be found at the time of ultrasonography to have severe oligohydramnios. The prognosis in such cases is extremely poor, regardless of whether or not fetal anomalies are present. Less than 10% of patients with severe oligohydramnios and an elevated MSAFP in the mid-trimester will go on to deliver a viable infant.

On rare occasions, elevated levels of AFP measured in the maternal circulation may be of maternal rather than fetal origin. α-Fetoprotein production may occur in adults in association with the acute phase of hepatitis and some other forms of liver disease and in the face of certain malignancies, such as hepatocellular carcinoma and germ-cell tumors. In the otherwise asymptomatic pregnant woman, however, such underlying pathological conditions are extraordinarily rare. Unless other findings are present, evaluation for the possibility of maternal disease is not warranted.

In the course of follow-up of MSAFP elevations, anencephaly should virtually always be diagnosed by ultrasonography alone. Spina bifida is less reliably diagnosed in this fashion and the likelihood of detecting this malformation is clearly related to the expertise of the examiner. Although a number of studies conducted by highly skilled fetal ultrasonographers under optimal conditions have demonstrated a high rate of detection of open spina bifida by ultrasound alone[17,18], leading some to suggest that amniocentesis is not necessary for these patients, the results of these studies cannot be generalized to all centers. Therefore, patients who have elevated MSAFP levels and are found on ultrasonography to have a single viable fetus at the anticipated gestational age, with or without any findings suggestive of open spina bifida, should be offered amniocentesis. The patient can be counseled that normal findings on careful ultrasound examination have reduced her risks of having an affected fetus, but she should be informed that such a malformation cannot be definitively ruled out without amniocentesis. If amniocentesis is performed and the amniotic fluid AFP is elevated or borderline, an acetylcholinesterase determination should be performed. An amniotic fluid AFP with positive acetylcholinesterase, in the absence of fetal blood contamination, is powerful evidence for the presence of a fetal defect. Further evidence that the defect is, in fact, open spina bifida, in contrast to a ventral wall defect, can be obtained by performing scanning densitometry on the electrophoretic gel and calculating the ratio of acetylcholinesterase to pseudo-cholinesterase. In cases of open spina bifida, the ratio is typically greater than 0.15, whereas it is typically below 0.10 in the presence of a ventral wall defect.

If a defect has not been previously visualized, every effort should be made to identify the site and nature of the lesion, as this may be critical to the decision-making process that will follow. Visualization of the defect is most likely to be accomplished by high-resolution ultrasonography in the hands of an examiner skilled in the diagnosis of fetal anomalies. Fetoscopy and amniography have occasionally been used in the past for visualization of fetal defects, but, with the increasing capabilities of ultrasonography, these techniques are currently of little value. Magnetic resonance imaging has recently been utilized in selected circumstances.

The finding of elevated amniotic fluid AFP in association with a negative acetylcholinesterase makes a fetal neural tube defect highly unlikely. Ventral wall defects and fetal blood contamination are the most likely explanations for such findings. Other open fetal defects, such as the scalp defects associated with trisomy 13 or other skin disorders, may also give rise on occasion to elevated amniotic fluid AFP. If high-resolution ultrasonography fails to reveal any abnormality, the amniotic fluid AFP is not extremely high and chromosome analysis of the amniotic cells is normal, the patient can be told that the fetus most probably is normal. The only serious fetal abnormality that consistently produces such biochemical abnormalities with normal findings on high-resolution ultrasonography and chromosome analysis is congenital nephrosis. While common in some parts of Finland, this autosomal recessive disorder is fortunately quite rare in the USA. It should be considered, however, in cases in which both the maternal serum and amniotic fluid AFP levels are exceptionally high. Although placentomegaly and enlarged kidneys may be detected by ultrasonography, these findings are often not present until the third trimester.

Patients undergoing amniocentesis because of elevated MSAFP levels should also be offered chromosome analysis on the amniotic fluid cells. Although patients with MSAFP elevations are at decreased risk of having a fetus with Down syndrome when compared with women of comparable age who have lower MSAFP levels, several large series have demonstrated that they are at increased risk for a variety of other chromosomal abnormalities, even when the amniotic fluid AFP is normal[19–21]. The overall risk to such patients of having a fetus with any chromosomal abnormality may be as high as 1%, which is comparable to the risk faced by the average 36-year-old woman. Sex chromosome anomalies are the most common abnormalities detected in this group. Even if the risk were not greater than the general population risk, women who have already elected to have amniocentesis for AFP testing might choose to have karyotyping, since the added information can be obtained with no added risk. Chromosomal analysis is particularly important when the amniotic fluid AFP turns out to be elevated, because a significant percentage of infants with trisomy 18 or trisomy 13 have open fetal defects, such as spina bifida or omphalocele, which will lead to the amniotic fluid AFP elevation. The presence of such open defects will usually be confirmed by acetylcholinesterase testing or high-resolution ultrasonography. In the face of an open fetal defect, however, the patient's decision with regard to pregnancy termination may be affected by the presence of a major chromosomal abnormality.

Following the identification of a neural tube defect or other fetal malformation *in utero*, it is essential that the parents receive extensive counseling regarding the nature of the defect and options available to them. Continuing support must be available regardless of the parents' decision. In the case of pregnancy termination, follow-up counseling should be arranged to review the findings in the fetus, discuss recurrence risks for future pregnancies and address the emotional issues surrounding such an experience. In the case of parents who choose to continue a pregnancy in the face of a known fetal defect, ongoing counseling and support should be provided. The circumstances of delivery should be planned so as to provide an optimal setting for the care of the mother and infant. Consultation with appropriate specialists, such as neonatologists, pediatric surgeons and geneticists, may be very helpful to the family in advance of the delivery. Whether the presence of open spina bifida or a ventral wall defect alone is an indication for Cesarean section is a subject of debate. One study has suggested that infants with open spina bifida delivered by Cesarean section prior to the onset of labor may exhibit better motor function than those delivered either vaginally or abdominally after the onset of labor[22].

UNEXPLAINED MSAFP ELEVATIONS

If amniocentesis in a patient with elevated MSAFP reveals a normal level of amniotic fluid AFP, the patient can be reassured that there is no evidence for a fetal neural tube defect. It has become increasingly clear, however, that patients in this category constitute a high-risk group for suboptimal outcomes of pregnancy and should be followed for the duration of pregnancy with this in mind (Table 3). There is no consensus at present on the advisability of follow-up testing, such as repeat ultrasonography, non-stress testing or other tests of fetal well being, since there are currently no data available to indicate whether or not such intervention alters outcome. Unexplained elevations of MSAFP have been associated with an increased risk of spontaneous abortion, stillbirth, prematurity, intrauterine growth retardation and neonatal death[23]. Available data also indicate an increased risk of non-neural tube malformations in infants born to mothers with elevated MSAFP but normal amniotic fluid AFP. Other central nervous system malformations, such as isolated hydrocephalus, seem to occur with increased frequency in this group, but the other malformations observed are generally non-specific and variable in nature. The MSAFP elevations observed in patients who later have an adverse pregnancy outcome may reflect placental abnormalities that allow increased transport of AFP directly from the fetal circulation to the maternal circulation. Examination of the placenta at term in such patients has revealed an increased incidence of histological abnormalities, such as chronic villitis, which may correlate with the earlier MSAFP elevation[24].

LOW MSAFP IN CHROMOSOMAL ABNORMALITIES

In 1984, an association between low MSAFP levels and fetal chromosomal abnormalities was first described[25]. This discovery has since been confirmed in many centers in the USA and Europe. Although the initial data focused primarily on Down syndrome, a relationship between low MSAFP levels and other chromosomal abnormalities, such as trisomy 18 and monosomy X (Turner syndrome), has since become apparent. The reason for the association is unclear. The relationship between AFP levels and fetal chromosome anomalies is independent of maternal age, however, so the identification of this relationship made it possible to use two separate variables, namely age and MSAFP level, to calculate a risk of Down syndrome in the fetus for a particular pregnancy. This strategy was subsequently incorporated into most MSAFP screening programs and allowed the detection of approximately 20–25% of cases of Down syndrome in pregnant women under 35 years of age. Since only 25% of cases of Down syndrome can be detected by offering prenatal diagnosis to women aged 35 years or older, the use of MSAFP screening for detecting pregnancies at increased risk effectively doubled the percentage of cases of Down syndrome detected antenatally.

In most centers, definitive diagnostic testing by amniocentesis is offered to pregnant women under the age of 35 if their projected risk of having a fetus with Down syndrome is greater than or equal to that of the average 35-year-old woman (one in 270). Use of this approach identifies approximately 3–4% of women undergoing MSAFP screening as candidates for further testing. Although the potential for detecting some fetuses with chromosomal abnormalities is an additional benefit of MSAFP screening that accrues with little incremental cost, it is important to stress that the majority of fetal chromosome anomalies are not detected using AFP alone. The overlap between MSAFP levels in normal and chromosomally abnormal pregnancies is much greater than is the case with neural tube defect pregnancies. As with elevated MSAFP levels, there are a number of other explanations for low MSAFP levels. These are listed in Table 4.

Methods for projecting risks for Down syndrome based on age and MSAFP levels have been published[26] and the laboratory should provide a projected risk as part of the interpretation of a patient's MSAFP level. The effect of using a projected risk cut-off level for offering further testing, as opposed to a specific definition of a low MSAFP level (such as 0.4 or 0.5 multiples of the median), is to select a different percentage of women for further testing depending on maternal age. A 34-year-old woman will have a Down syndrome risk of one in 250 and will be offered testing at an MSAFP level of 0.7 multiples of the median, whereas a 23-year-old woman will not have a projected Down syndrome risk greater than one in 270 unless her MSAFP level is 0.3 multiples of the median or less.

Table 3 Adverse outcomes of pregnancy associated with maternal serum α-fetoprotein elevations unexplained in the mid-trimester

Spontaneous abortion
Stillbirth
Prematurity
Intrauterine growth restriction
Congenital anomalies
Pre-eclampsia

Table 4 Findings associated with low maternal serum α-fetoprotein

Common 'benign' findings
Less advanced gestational age
Normal pregnancy
Non-pregnancy

Abnormal findings
Missed abortion
Hydatidiform mole
Down syndrome
Other chromosome anomalies

FOLLOW-UP OF LOW MSAFP

The first step in evaluating a patient identified as being at increased risk for Down syndrome based on a 'low' MSAFP level is ultrasonography. The most common explanation for an apparently low value is a gestational age less advanced than previously anticipated. When such a finding is noted and the patient was initially screened prior to 15 weeks' gestation, it is important that another sample be obtained at 16–18 weeks' gestation. Although the less-advanced gestational age may be an adequate explanation for the low value previously obtained, a patient in such circumstances has not been appropriately screened for neural tube defects. Other explanations for a low MSAFP level, such as missed abortion or a molar pregnancy, will also be detected by ultrasonography. If ultrasound examination reveals a viable fetus at the anticipated gestational age, then the patient should be offered amniocentesis. Of all patients undergoing amniocentesis because of low MSAFP, approximately 1% will be found to have a fetus with a chromosomal abnormality. The risk to each individual patient will vary, depending on her specific MSAFP level and age. Patients with normal results on amniocentesis can be reassured that there is no need for further concern. The data suggest that low MSAFP values, except perhaps for those at the very lowest end of the spectrum, differ from unexplained high values in that they do not appear to be associated with an increased risk for other adverse outcomes of pregnancy. Very low MSAFP values (below 0.25 multiples of the median) may be associated with an increased risk of subsequent fetal loss[23], but this observation requires further confirmation.

SCREENING FOR CHROMOSOME ANOMALIES WITH MULTIPLE SERUM MARKERS

Down syndrome

The identification of a link between low MSAFP values and Down syndrome has stimulated efforts to identify other serum markers for this disorder. The best marker yet identified is human chorionic gonadotropin (hCG), which is 2.0–2.5 times higher than normal in pregnancies affected with Down syndrome[27]. Unconjugated estriol, like AFP, is lower than normal in maternal serum when the fetus is affected with Down syndrome[28]. A promising new marker, inhibin-A, is elevated in Down syndrome pregnancies in the mid-trimester[29]. The free α-[30] and β-subunits of hCG[31] have also been found to correlate with Down syndrome and other markers are being investigated as well.

In 1988, it was first proposed that MSAFP, hCG and unconjugated estriol be combined with maternal age to screen all pregnancies for Down syndrome[32]. Using a statistical model for predicting Down syndrome risk based on all four variables and a risk cut-off level of one in 250 in a retrospective study of stored serum samples, 67% of Down syndrome pregnancies were detected with a false-positive rate of 5%. The same model was subsequently applied prospectively in a clinical trial in London and 48% of Down syndrome cases were detected[33]. The results of the first trials in the USA were subsequently published in 1992[34,35] and 1993[36,37] and yielded initial positive rates of 6.6–10.4% with detection rates of 57–83%, depending on the cut-off levels used and the nature of the screened population. Both the initial positive rate and the detection rate increase as a function of maternal age, so studies confined to women under 35 years of age typically yield a lower detection rate than those including women of all ages.

Since the publication of these studies, the combination of AFP, hCG and unconjugated estriol, often referred to as 'triple screening', has come into more widespread utilization in prenatal care. Nonetheless, a number of questions remain unanswered. The contribution of unconjugated estriol to Down syndrome screening in increasing either the sensitivity or specificity of screening and the cost-effectiveness of its utilization has not yet been clearly established. In one series, there was a 6% reduction in the rate of Down syndrome detection when unconjugated estriol was eliminated from the protocol[34], while in another there was improved specificity of screening with no decrease in detection rate when unconjugated estriol was excluded[38]. Therefore, it is not possible at present to conclude that 'triple screening' for Down syndrome is superior to screening using AFP and hCG alone. The use of some form of multiple marker screening, however, has become the standard of care.

When reporting the results of screening using multiple markers, the laboratory must report a projected risk for Down syndrome. The calculation of risk is a very complex one which is typically performed by computer. It is not possible to look at the multiples of the median values on an individual patient's report and determine whether or not the patient's risk for Down syndrome exceeds a given risk cut-off level (most commonly one in 270). If a patient's risk as predicted by multiple-marker screening is below the cut-off used to trigger further testing, no further evaluation is necessary, even if the AFP value is 'low'. It is very clear that the combination of age and multiple markers provides a much more accurate prediction of risk than the use of AFP and age alone. For the same reason, it is inappropriate to adopt a strategy in which patients are initially screened with AFP alone, with multiple-marker screening obtained only on those patients identified as being at increased risk. The benefit of multiple-marker screening in substantially increasing the detection rate for chromosome anomalies is lost in this scenario, since only 20–25% of Down syndrome cases would be found among the patients initially identified as being at risk; subsequently the detection rate for Down syndrome would be reduced even further by the performance of a second test.

Trisomy 18

The pattern of serum markers observed in pregnancies affected by trisomy 18 is clearly different than that associated with Down syndrome, so a different screening strategy must be adopted to allow detection of this disorder[39]. Maternal serum AFP and unconjugated estriol are low in this disorder, as in Down syndrome, but hCG is typically very low as well. Using cut-off values that identify only 0.4% of the screened population as being 'at risk' for trisomy 18, it appears that 60–80% of affected pregnancies can be detected.

Other chromosome anomalies

Although additional data are needed, it appears that a number of other chromosome anomalies may be detected through multiple-marker screening (Table 5). Many 45, XO cases have been detected among patients identified as being at increased risk for Down syndrome[36,40]. Triploidy may be detected through the finding of very low levels of all three markers[41] or through elevated MSAFP[42]. Most trisomy 13-affected pregnancies reported thus far have been associated with normal levels of all three markers, unless there was an open fetal defect present such as an omphalocele.

Protocol for follow-up of patients with positive screening results

Like MSAFP alone, multiple-marker screening should ideally be performed at 15 weeks' gestation or beyond. Patients who have positive screening results indicative of either an increased risk for Down syndrome or an increased risk for trisomy 18 should have an ultrasound examination to confirm gestational age and fetal viability. Many patients with an increased risk for Down syndrome will be shown to have a less advanced gestational age than previously anticipated. If ultrasound findings alter gestational age by more than

10 days, the screening test results should be reinterpreted. If it turns out that the blood sample was drawn prior to 14 weeks' gestation, it should be redrawn at the appropriate time. Samples drawn at 14 weeks can be reliably used for Down syndrome screening, but not for detection of neural tube defects. Therefore, if a multiple-marker screen is inadvertently obtained at 14 weeks, an AFP level only should be repeated at 15 weeks or beyond for screening of neural tube defects. Otherwise the screening test should not be repeated. Patients with a viable singleton pregnancy should be counseled regarding their estimated risk for Down syndrome or trisomy 18 and offered amniocentesis. In the case of twin gestations, an 'average' risk for Down syndrome can be estimated for each fetus, but the detection rate is expected to be considerably lower than in singletons.

Unexplained high or low hCG or unconjugated estriol levels

Since unexplained elevations of MSAFP have been linked to an increased risk of adverse pregnancy outcome, efforts have focused on determining whether or not low or high levels of other markers are predictive of any pregnancy complications. Data are inadequate at present to draw any firm conclusions. Several studies have suggested that elevated hCG may be associated with an increased risk of pregnancy-induced hypertension and intrauterine growth retardation[43–45], while low unconjugated estriol may be associated with an increased risk of pregnancy loss[46].

Screening in women aged 35 years or older

At present, definitive diagnostic testing for chromosome anomalies by either chorionic villus sampling or amniocentesis should be offered to all women who will be aged 35 years or older at the time of delivery. If chorionic villus sampling is performed, an MSAFP determination should be obtained at 16–18 weeks' gestation to screen for open neural tube defects. For patients who choose mid-trimester amniocentesis, no serum screening is necessary, since amniotic fluid AFP determinations are routinely performed.

Despite the promising performance of multiple markers in screening for chromosome anomalies, serum screening should not currently replace the offer of definitive diagnostic testing in patients of advanced maternal age. Most of the data gathered thus far on serum markers relate specifically to Down syndrome, while other chromosome anomalies also occur with increased frequency with advancing maternal age. Some of these, such as trisomy 13, may not be detectable through serum screening. Furthermore, it will never be possible with the serum markers currently

Table 5   Serum markers in various chromosome anomalies

	AFP	*hCG*	*uE₃*
Trisomy 21	low	high	low
Trisomy 18	low*	low	low
Trisomy 13	normal*	normal	normal
Monosomy X	?low†	high	low
Triploidy	low or high	low	low

*Both trisomy 18 and 13 may be associated with an open fetal defect, such as an omphalocele or open spina bifida. In such cases, AFP may be normal or elevated. †AFP may be elevated when large cystic hygromas are present. AFP, α-fetoprotein; hCG, human chorionic gonadotropin; uE₃, unconjugated estriol

available to achieve the almost 100% detection rate for chromosome anomalies which patients over 35 years of age have to come to expect. Nonetheless, it is now quite reasonable to offer patients over 35 years of age the option of serum screening as long as they have the clear understanding that 'normal' test results do not rule out the presence of a chromosomal abnormality in the fetus. At least for Down syndrome, it is clear that serum screening provides a far more accurate method of determining risk than does maternal age alone. This further definition of risk may be particularly helpful to women in the 35–39-year age group who may be undecided about undergoing invasive testing, with an associated risk of fetal loss, when confronted with a risk of chromosome anomalies based on age alone that is 1% or less.

FIRST-TRIMESTER SCREENING

Although maternal serum screening for chromosome anomalies and open neural tube defects is currently conducted only during the second trimester, there are efforts underway to identify screening tools that could be used earlier in gestation. Although MSAFP[47] and unconjugated estriol[48] may be lower than normal in the first trimester when the fetus is affected with Down syndrome, hCG levels appear to be normal[49]. The free β-subunit of hCG is slightly elevated and may be a useful marker when combined with other analytes[50]. The most promising first-trimester marker currently under investigation is pregnancy-associated plasma protein A (PAPP-A), which is significantly reduced at 6–11 weeks' gestation in pregnancies affected with Down syndrome and other chromosome anomalies[50–53]. Although prospective studies are needed, it has been estimated that first-trimester PAPP-A screening could lead to the detection of 60% of Down syndrome pregnancies with a false-positive rate of 5%[50].

PSYCHOLOGICAL EFFECTS OF MSAFP SCREENING

A great deal of concern has been voiced in the past relating to the possibility that the benefits of MSAFP screening might be negated by adverse psychological effects on the women screened. Studies have demonstrated that abnormal MSAFP results are accompanied by significantly heightened anxiety in the pregnant woman and her husband or partner that persists until normal results are ultimately obtained[54,55]. When screening is conducted in an appropriate setting with adequate genetic counseling, however, heightened anxiety does not appear to persist throughout the remainder of the pregnancy. Rather than negating the benefits of MSAFP screening, the heightened anxiety observed in association with abnormal MSAFP results underscores the need to proceed in a timely fashion throughout the screening process and to minimize the time elapsed between the initial serum sample and final diagnosis.

SUMMARY

Maternal serum α-fetoprotein screening should be offered to all patients as a routine component of prenatal care. This technology provides an efficient and cost-effective method of screening for neural tube defects and also provides the physician with important information relevant to a number of other birth defects and complications of pregnancy. As prenatal screening using multiple markers replaces the use of MSAFP alone, the majority of fetal chromosome anomalies will also be detected.

REFERENCES

1. Laurence KM, James N, Miller MH, *et al.* Double blind randomized controlled trial of folate treatment before conception to prevent recurrence of neural tube defects. *Br Med J* 1981;282:1509–11
2. Smithells RW, Seller MJ, Harris R, *et al.* Further experience of vitamin supplementation for prevention of neural tube defect recurrences. *Lancet* 1983;1:1027–31
3. Smithells RW, Sheppard S, Wild J, Schorah CJ. Prevention of neural tube defect recurrences in Yorkshire: final report. *Lancet* 1989;2:498–9
4. MRC Vitamin Study Research Group. Prevention of neural tube defects: results of the Medical Research Council Vitamin Study. *Lancet* 1991;338:131–7
5. Mulinare J, Cordero JF, Erickson JD, Berry RJ. Periconceptional use of multivitamins and the occurrence of neural tube defects. *J Am Med Assoc* 1988;260:3141–5
6. Milunsky A, Jick H, Jick SS, *et al.* Multivitamin/folic acid supplementation in early pregnancy reduces the prevalence of neural tube defects. *J Am Med Assoc* 1989; 262:2847–52
7. Mills JL, Rhoads GG, Simpson JL, *et al.* The absence of a relation between the periconceptional use of vitamins and neural tube defects. *N Engl J Med* 1989;321: 430–5
8. Czeizel AE, Dudas I. Prevention of the first occurrence of neural tube defects by periconceptional vitamin supplementation. *New Engl J Med* 1992;327:1832–5
9. Centers for Disease Control and Prevention. Recommendations for the use of folic acid to reduce number of spina bifida cases and other neural tube defects. *J Am Med Assoc* 1993;269:1233–8
10. Oakley GP Jr. Folic acid-preventable spina bifida and anencephaly (Editorial). *J Am Med Assoc* 1993;269: 1292–3
11. Grimes DA. Unplanned pregnancies in the US. *Obstet Gynecol* 1986;67:438–42
12. United Kingdom Collaborative Study on α-Fetoprotein in Relation to Neural Tube Defects. Maternal serum α-fetoprotein measurement in antenatal screening for anencephaly and spina bifida in early pregnancy. *Lancet* 1977;1:1323–32

13. Macri JN, Weiss RR. Prenatal serum α-fetoprotein screening for neural tube defects. *Obstet Gynecol* 1982; 59:633–9

14. Burton BK, Sowers SG, Nelson LH. Maternal serum α-fetoprotein screening in North Carolina: experience with more than 12,000 pregnancies. *Am J Obstet Gynecol* 1983;146:439–44

15. Haddow JH, Kloza EM, Smith DE, Knight GJ. Data from an α-fetoprotein screening program in Maine. *Obstet Gynecol* 1983;62:556–60

16. Hagard S, Carter F, Milne RG. Screening for spina bifida cystica. A cost–benefit analysis. *Br J Prev Soc Med* 1976;30:40–53

17. Richards DS, Seeds JW, Katz VL, *et al.* Elevated maternal serum alpha-fetoprotein with normal ultrasound: is amniocentesis always appropriate? A review of 26,069 screened patients. *Obstet Gynecol* 1988;71:203–7

18. Nadel AS, Green JK, Holmes JB, *et al.* Absence of need for amniocentesis in patients with elevated levels of maternal serum alpha-fetoprotein and normal ultrasonographic examinations. *New Engl J Med* 1990; 323:557–61

19. Warner AA, Pettenati M, Burton BK. Risk of fetal chromosome anomalies in patients with elevated maternal serum α-fetoprotein. *Obstet Gynecol* 1990;75:64–6

20. Gosden C, Buckton K, Fotheringham Z, Brock DJH. Prenatal fetal karyotyping and maternal serum alpha-fetoprotein screening. *Br Med J* 1981;282:255–8

21. Bobrow M, Lindenbaum RH, Seabright M, Gregson N. Karyotyping amniotic fluids from patients with high serum alpha-fetoprotein. *Lancet* 1981;1:606–7

22. Luthy DA, Wardinsky T, Shurtleff DB, *et al.* Cesarean section before the onset of labor and subsequent motor function in infants with meningomyelocele diagnosed antenatally. *New Engl J Med* 1991;324:662–6

23. Burton BK. Outcome of pregnancy in patients with unexplained elevated or low maternal serum α-fetoprotein. *Obstet Gynecol* 1988;72:709–13

24. Salafia CM, Silberman L, Herrera NE, Mahoney MJ. Placental pathology at term associated with elevated maternal serum α-fetoprotein concentration. *Am J Obstet Gynecol* 1988;158:1064–6

25. Merkatz IR, Nitwosky HM, Macri JN, Johnson WE. An association between low maternal serum α-fetoprotein and fetal chromosomal abnormalities. *Am J Obstet Gynecol* 1984;148:886–94

26. Palomaki GE, Haddow JE. Maternal serum α-fetoprotein, age and Down syndrome risk. *Am J Obstet Gynecol* 1987;156:460–3

27. Bogart MH, Pandian MR, Jones OW. Abnormal maternal serum chorionic gonadotropin levels in pregnancies with fetal chromosome abnormalities. *Prenat Diagn* 1987;7:623–30

28. Canick JA, Knight GJ, Palomaki GE, *et al.* Low second trimester maternal serum unconjugated oestriol in pregnancies with Down syndrome. *Br J Obstet Gynaecol* 1988;95:330–3

29. Wald NJ, Densem JW, George L, *et al.* Prenatal screening for Down syndrome using inhibin-A as a serum marker. *Prenat Diagn* 1996;16:143–53

30. Wald NJ, Densem JW, Smith D, Klee GG. Four-marker serum screening for Down syndrome. *Prenat Diagn* 1994;14:707–16

31. Macri JN, Kasturi RV, Krantz DA, *et al.* Maternal serum Down syndrome screening: free B-protein is a more effective marker than human chorionic gonadotropin. *Am J Obstet Gynecol* 1990;163:1248–53

32. Wald NJ, Cuckle HS, Densem JW. Maternal serum screening for Down syndrome. *Br Med J* 1988; 297:883–7

33. Wald NJ, Kennard A, Densem JW, *et al.* Antenatal maternal serum screening for Down syndrome: results of a demonstration project. *Br Med J* 1992;305: 391–4

34. Haddow JE, Palomaki GE, Knight GJ, *et al.* Prenatal screening for Down syndrome with use of maternal serum markers. *N Engl J Med* 1992;327:588–93

35. Phillips OP, Elias S, Shulman LP, *et al.* Maternal serum screening for fetal Down syndrome in women less than 35 years of age using alpha-fetoprotein, hCG, and unconjugated estriol: a prospective 2-year study. *Obstet Gynecol* 1992;80:353–8

36. Burton BK, Prins GS, Verp MS. A prospective trial of prenatal screening for Down syndrome using maternal serum alpha-fetoprotein, hCG and unconjugated estriol. *Am J Obstet Gynecol* 1993;169:526–30

37. Cheng EY, Leethy DA, Zebelman AM, *et al.* A prospective evaluation of a second-trimester screening test for fetal Down syndrome using maternal serum alpha-fetoprotein, hCG, and unconjugated estriol. *Obstet Gynecol* 1993;81:72–7

38. Dungan JS, Phillip OP, Shulman LP, *et al.* Improved specificity of maternal serum screening for fetal Down syndrome by excluding uE$_3$ level. *Am J Hum Genet* 1993;53:1402A

39. Canick JA, Palomaki GE, Osathanondh R. Prenatal screening for trisomy 18 in the second trimester. *Prenat Diagn* 1990;10:546–8

40. Saller DN Jr, Canick JA, Schwartz S, Blitzer MG. Multiple-marker screening in pregnancies with hydropic and nonhydropic Turner syndrome. *Am J Obstet Gynecol* 1992;167:1021–4

41. Feigin M, Amiel A, Goldberger S, *et al.* Placental insufficiency as a possible cause of low maternal serum human chorionic gonadotropin and low maternal serum unconjugated estriol levels in triploidy. *Am J Obstet Gynecol* 1992;167:766–77

42. Pircon RA, Towers CV, Porto M, *et al.* Maternal serum alpha-fetoprotein and fetal triploidy. *Prenat Diagn* 1989;9:701–7

43. Sorenson TK, Williams MA, Zingheim RW, *et al.* Elevated second-trimester human chorionic gonadotropin and subsequent pregnancy-induced hypertension. *Am J Obstet Gynecol* 1993;169:834–8

44. Gonen R, Perez R, David M, *et al.* The association between unexplained second-trimester maternal serum hCG elevation and pregnancy complications. *Obstet Gynecol* 1992;80:83–6

45. Gravett CP, Buckmaster JG, Watson PT, Gravett MG. Elevated second trimester maternal serum B-hCG concentrations and subsequent adverse pregnancy outcome. *Am J Med Genet* 1992;44:485–6

46. Santolaya-Forgas J, Jessup J, Burd LI, *et al.* Pregnancy outcome in women with low midtrimester maternal serum unconjugated estriol. *J Reprod Med* 1996;41: 87–90

47. Milunsky A, Wands J, Brambati B, *et al*. First trimester maternal serum alpha-fetoprotein screening for chromosome defects. *Am J Obstet Gynecol* 1988;159:1209–13

48. Brock DJ, Barron L, Holloway S, *et al*. First trimester maternal serum biochemical indicators in Down syndrome. *Prenat Diagn* 1990;10:245–51

49. Cuckle HS, Wald NJ, Barkai G, *et al*. First trimester biochemical screening for Down syndrome. *Lancet* 1988;2:851–2

50. Casals E, Fortuny A, Grudzinskas JG, *et al*. First-trimester biochemical screening for Down syndrome with the use of PAPP-A, AFP, and B-hCG. *Prenat Diagn* 1996;16:405–10

51. Hurley PA, Ward RHT, Teisner B, *et al*. Serum PAPP-A measurements in first-trimester screening for Down syndrome. *Prenat Diagn* 1993;13:903–8

52. Brambati B, MacIntosh MCM, Teisner B, *et al*. Low maternal serum levels of pregnancy associated placental antigen (PAPP-A) associated with abnormal fetal karyotype. *Br J Obstet Gynaecol* 1992;100:323–6

53. Muller F, Cuckle H, Teisner B, Grudzinskas JG. Serum PAPP-A levels are depressed in women with fetal Down syndrome in early pregnancy. *Prenat Diagn* 1993;13:633–6

54. Burton BK, Dillard RG, Clark EN. The psychological impact of false positive elevations of maternal serum alpha-fetoprotein. *Am J Obstet Gynecol* 1985;151:77–82

55. Evans MI, Bottoms SF, Carlucci T, *et al*. Determinants of altered anxiety after abnormal maternal serum alpha-fetoprotein screening. *Am J Obstet Gynecol* 1988;159:1501–4

Section VIII

Drug abuse

67

Principles of teratology of drugs and radiation

F.R. Witter

Teratology is the study of birth defects. In this chapter the potential of drugs and radiation to produce birth defects in humans will be explored. Wilson[1] has estimated that of all human malformations less than one percent are due to radiations and four to six percent are due to drugs and environmental chemicals.

Whether an agent produces a teratogenic effect is dependent on the timing of the insult. The conceptus is relatively resistant in the first two weeks following conception (menstrual weeks three and four) when either no effect or loss of the pregnancy are the major outcomes of exposure to teratogenic agents. During this time period the embryo has sufficient reparative powers, if not destroyed, to recover and few malformations occur. The most likely times for chemical teratogenesis are menstrual weeks five to twelve inclusive which corresponds to the time of major organ differentiation. For radiation injury the most likely times for exposure are menstrual weeks 10 to 17 inclusive[2] which correspond to the time of maximum neuronal cell proliferation and migration to the cerebral cortex. No gross malformations due to radiation have been seen in humans without the child exhibiting growth retardation, microcephaly, or gross eye malformations. After the time of gestation of maximal sensitivity, the effects of teratogens in general are to produce growth retardation[3–6].

The criteria for a human teratogen are listed in Table 1[7]. In addition to these criteria the existence of a dose response relationship supports the contention that an agent is a teratogen. Thus for a teratogen with increasing dose of the exposure, there should be an increase in the number or severity of defects produced. Also, it should produce similar defects in experimental animal systems.

DRUGS AS TERATOGENS

Drugs which fulfill the criteria for a human teratogen may produce their effect directly, indirectly or through a toxic intermediate. Direct acting teratogens cause damage in their native form and require only access to the conceptus to do harm. An example of direct acting teratogens are cytotoxic antineoplastic agents, which cause direct cell damage leading to cell death which may result in malformation or pregnancy loss.

Indirect acting teratogens act by perturbing maternal homeostasis to produce damage. Narcotic analgesics are not themselves teratogens; however, they can act as indirect teratogens when taken in sufficient doses to produce maternal hypoxia from respiratory depression. Hypoxia then acts directly to produce malformations by causing cell death in the developing conceptus. Therefore by acting to compromise maternal respiration, narcotics may act as indirect teratogens.

Unlike the first two methods by which a drug can act as a teratogen, those drugs whose teratogenic potential is expressed through a toxic intermediate are not as readily predicted by animal experiments. This is because there are many pathways by which drugs may be metabolized and these may vary between species or even between individuals of the same species. Because of this variation the toxic intermediate may not be produced in all individuals or species. A teratogen acting through a toxic intermediate may be a human teratogen and not one in animal species usually tested, or vice versa. An example of a human teratogen which would fit into this class is thalidomide, which is not a teratogen in the guinea pig.

In addition to the difficulty in extrapolating from animal experiments to man, there are other difficulties with fulfilling the criteria of Table 1. The drug in question might prevent the loss of an already malformed fetus. The condition for which the drug is used might

Table 1 Criteria for recognizing a human teratogenic agent[7]

1. An abrupt increase in the frequency for a particular defect or group of defects.
2. Coincidence of this increase with a known environmental change, such as widespread use of a new drug or sudden exposure to a chemical or a source of radiation.
3. Known exposure to the environmental change early in pregnancies yielding the characteristically defective infants.
4. Absence of other factors common to all yielding infants with the characteristic defect or defects.

produce the malformation. The fetal malformation might cause maternal symptoms for which the drug is taken. Finally, the drug may be commonly used in combination with other drugs that produce the malformation or only a combination of agents, not the individual agents by themselves, might produce the malformation.

Because of these difficulties and the sometimes poor quality of data, differences exist between experts on the teratogenic potential of many agents in humans. An additional reason for conflict in expert opinion on human teratogens is the reason for which the assessment was made. If one wishes to counsel a pregnant woman already exposed to an agent as to its teratogenic potential, then it is appropriate to ignore the potential therapeutic benefit of the agent and use only the information on birth defects available on it[8]. If on the other hand one wishes to prescribe a medication for a condition during pregnancy it is appropriate to use an assessment which balances the therapeutic benefit to the teratogenic risk. The FDA pregnancy categories[9] are an attempt at such an assessment (Table 2).

Table 2   FDA pregnancy categories for drugs[9]

Category A: Controlled studies in women fail to demonstrate a risk to the fetus in the first trimester, there is no evidence of a risk in later trimesters, and the possibility of fetal harm appears remote.

Category B: Either animal reproductive studies have not demonstrated a fetal risk, but there are no controlled studies in pregnant women, or animal reproductive studies that have shown an adverse effect, other than a decrease in fertility, that was not confirmed in controlled studies in women in the first trimester and there is no evidence of a risk in later trimesters.

Category C: Either studies in animals have revealed adverse effects on the fetus, teratogenic or embryocidal or other, and there are no controlled studies in women, or studies in women, or studies in women and animals are not available. Drugs of this class should be given only if the potential benefit justifies the potential risk to the fetus.

Category D: There is positive evidence of human fetal risk, but the benefits from use in pregnant women may be acceptable despite the risk as when the drug is needed in a life-threatening situation or for a serious disease for which safer drugs cannot be used or are ineffective.

Category X: Studies in animals or human beings have demonstrated fetal abnormalities or there is evidence of fetal risk based on human experience or both, and the risk of the use of the drug in pregnant women clearly outweighs any possible benefit. The drug is contraindicated in women who are or may become pregnant.

There are several excellent compendiums of data on teratogenic risk[10–12] to which the reader is referred for details on specific agents. The most common human teratogens used today are listed in Table 3. These agents should be avoided in women who are pregnant or potentially pregnant. The most common agents which have teratogenic potential but whose therapeutic benefit outweighs its risk are listed in Table 4. When assessing maternal drug therapy in pregnancy the first consideration is whether the drug is necessary for maternal survival or well being. Once it is established that this is the case, the most effective agent with the least toxicity and the lowest teratogenic potential should be used in the appropriate dose. Vital therapy should not be withheld from a pregnant woman because of teratogenic risk.

RADIATION AS A TERATOGEN

Unlike drugs, radiation always acts directly on the conceptus to produce birth defects or pregnancy loss. For this reason, it is easier to extrapolate from animal experiments to the human condition for radiation defects. Ionizing radiation produces gross congenital malformations, intrauterine growth retardation and embryonic death. All of radiation's effects have a dose response relationship and a threshold of exposure below which there is no difference between irradiated and nonirradiated populations. Only ionizing radiation has a clearly established teratogenic potential.

Growth retardation and central nervous system effects including microcephaly, mental retardation and eye malformations are the most prominent manifestations of intrauterine radiation exposure in humans. Severe mental retardation has not been observed in

Table 3   Common agents that are teratogens

Anabolic steroids
Androgens
Anticancer agents
Diethylstilbestrol
Isotretinoin
Oral anticoagulants
Oral hypoglycemics
Vitamin A in large doses
Vitamin D in large doses

Table 4   Agents that have teratogenic potential but are used in pregnancy because the benefit of their use outweighs the risk of teratogenesis

Phenytoin
Antimalarials
Propylthiouracil
Aminoglycosides
Antituberculins

patients who received less than 50 rads *in utero*, and there has been no report of radiation induced limb or other gross anomalies in humans where growth retardation or central nervous system anomalies were not also present[13]. Mental retardation has never been seen with radiation exposure prior to ten menstrual weeks gestation in humans[2], in spite of the fact that major organ differentiation occurs from five to twelve menstrual weeks gestation. Radiation exposure prior to ten menstrual weeks results in a high rate of loss and therefore a wide range of malformations are not seen[8].

The gestational ages 10 to 17 menstrual weeks represent the time when the maximum number of infants with mental retardation and central nervous system or eye defects are produced[2]. At 18 menstrual weeks, or greater, few cases of mental retardation are seen[2], however growth retardation continues to be produced. In humans, although malformations are not seen at doses of less than 50 rads, some disturbances of growth can occur with as little as 25 rads[13]. However, at exposures in the range of 20 mrads to 5000 mrads, which is the range of most diagnostic radiology studies, there is an extremely low risk of malformations when compared to the spontaneous rate for humans[13]. The association of prenatal radiation exposure and childhood leukemia or other cancers remains to be determined. However, an increased incidence, 1.5 to 2.4 over the background rate, as a result of *in utero* exposure to radiation at the dosage ranging from 1–4 rads, has been reported[14,15]. X-ray studies with 5 rads or less exposure to the conceptus carry a very low risk and if medically indicated, should be performed with the patient's informed consent.

Special mention should be made of radioiodine during pregnancy. Iodine-131 if given in millicurie doses can damage or ablate the developing fetal thyroid resulting in congenital hypothyroidism of late onset[13]. This can occur after the onset of the iodine concentrating ability of the fetal thyroid at around menstrual week 12 of gestation. Radioiodine is therefore contraindicated in pregnancy.

REFERENCES

1. Wilson JG. Teratogenic effects of environmental chemicals. *Fed Proc* 1977;36:1690–1703
2. Otke M, Schull WJ. In utero exposure to A-bomb radiation and mental retardation; a reassessment. *Br J Radiol* 1984;57:409–14
3. Stewart A. The carcinogenic effects of low level radiation: a re-appraisal of epidemiologists methods and observations. *Health Phys* 1973;24:223
4. Stewart A, Kneale GW. Radiation dose effects in relation to obstetric X-rays and childhood cancers. *Lancet* 1970;1:1185
5. Ford D, Patterson T. Fetal exposure to diagnostic X-rays and leukemia and other malignant disease in childhood. *J Natl Cancer Inst* 1959;22:1093
6. Diamond EL, Schmerler H, Lilienfield AM. The relationship of intrauterine radiation to subsequent mortality and development of leukemia in children: a prospective study. *Am J Epidemiol* 1973;97:283
7. Wilson JG: *Environment and Birth Defects*. New York: New York Academic Press, 1973
8. Friedman JM, Little BB, Brent RL, *et al*. Potential human teratogenicity of frequently prescribed drugs. *Obstet Gynecol* 1990;75:594–9
9. Millstein LG. FDA's "pregnancy categories". *N Engl J Med* 1980;303:706
10. Shepard TH. *Catalog of Teratogenic Agents 8th Ed*. Baltimore, Maryland: Johns Hopkins Press, 1995
11. Brigg GG, Friedman RK, Yaffe JJ. *Drugs in Pregnancy and Lactation: A Reference Guide to Fetal and Neonatal Risk 4th Ed*. Baltimore, Maryland: Williams and Wilkins, 1994
12. Schardein JL. *Chemically Induced Birth Defects 2nd Ed*. New York: Marcel Dekker, 1993
13. Brent RL. Radiation teratogenesis. *Teratology* 1980;21:281–98
14. Harvey EB, Boice JD, Honeyman M, *et al*. Prenatal X-ray exposure and childhood cancer in twins. *N Engl J Med* 1985;312:541–5
15. Swartz HM, Reichling BA. Hazards to radiation exposure for pregnant women. *J Am Med Assoc* 1978;239:1907–8

68

Drug abuse in pregnancy: hallucinogens, stimulants, alcohol and opiates

J.C. Howitt

INTRODUCTION

Substance abuse during pregnancy continues to be a problem of monumental proportions, one that virtually every health professional faces. The drug-abusing population includes women from every portion of society—every ethnic group, every socio-economic stratum[1]. Because the majority of drug-abusing women are in their reproductive years, illicit drug use has become increasingly common in pregnancy. Therefore, it is essential that medical caretakers recognize the hallmarks and subtleties of drug abuse and be prepared to deal with the resulting problems in mother, fetus and neonate.

Relatively little is known about the direct effects of illicit drug use on human pregnancy. Since most women who abuse drugs use more than one drug, studies on effects of drugs in pregnancy are rarely 'pure'. As polydrug use complicates even the best of human studies, and as malnutrition, anemia, and infection are frequently confounding factors, most authors caution against too narrow an interpretation of data regarding the effects of a single drug. Nevertheless, inferences can be drawn from human studies and data extrapolated from animal studies. The following pages contain a contemporary review of the available literature on common drugs of abuse in pregnancy. Caffeine, tobacco, and barbiturates have been excluded from this review.

MARIJUANA

Marijuana use is quite common. Conservative estimates suggest that 51% of 12–17 year olds and 68% of 18–25 year olds have used marijuana at least once; 16.7% and 35% of the respective age groups are current users[2]. Pregnant marijuana abusers are likely to be in a lower socio-economic bracket, to have had less formal education, and are frequently cigarette smokers[3]. Concurrent use of other drugs, especially alcohol, is common[2].

Delta-9-tetrahydrocannabinol (Δ9THC) is the main pharmacologically active component of marijuana. Cannabidiol and cannabinol, other components of marijuana that can affect the metabolism and activity of Δ9THC, do not possess significant pharmacological

activity of their own[4]. The primary site of marijuana metabolism is the liver; the lung also affords some metabolic action. The primary metabolite of Δ9THC (11-hydroxy Δ9THC), which may also be pharmacologically active, is in turn converted to more polar metabolites which are excreted through bile, feces[4] and urine. Two weeks after marijuana use, Δ9THC may still be detected in urine[5]. Smoking marijuana leads to rapid onset of drug action (seconds to minutes), yielding effects which usually last less than 2 hours. Effects of oral ingestion of marijuana initially occur within 30 to 120 minutes and last for 5 to 7 hours[6]. Marijuana is lipophilic and readily distributed to organs with relatively high blood flow (liver, lung, kidney, spleen). However, the brain, which also has a good blood supply, receives comparatively small amounts of marijuana[4], which accumulates mainly in the gray matter. Physiologic effects of marijuana use include: tachycardia, slight decrease in blood pressure, reddening of the conjunctiva, fine hand tremors, and a modest reduction in muscle strength. Marijuana also possesses analgesic activity, has anti-emetic properties, and causes hallucinations in high doses[6]. Following marijuana administration, users experience a brief stimulatory phase in which they may become anxious and restless or euphoric. They typically report enhanced perception of the five senses. A period of sedation follows, in which users seem to move in and out of a 'dream-like' state, during which they have a shortened attention span, an altered sense of time and distance, and impairment of short-term memory. There are no withdrawal symptoms. Moreover, there have been no reports of human lethality from overdose of marijuana[6]. Marijuana smoke contains more carcinogens than tobacco smoke, and tumors can be produced by the application of tars from marijuana smoke to animal skin[2]. Marijuana can also cause extensive pulmonary inflammation and inhibit pulmonary macrophage production. *In vitro* studies have linked marijuana use to changes in cell-mediated immunity[2].

The placenta can accumulate significant amounts of Δ9THC. Placental transfer has been documented in monkeys[7], sheep, and mice and rats[4]. Maternal administration of Δ9THC in these animals yields lower concentrations of marijuana in the fetus than in the mother[4,7–9].

The actual effect of marijuana use on human pregnancy outcome and on the fetus is controversial. Suggested effects include a shortened gestation[10,11] (by 0.8 weeks, the effect reportedly being dose-dependent), a higher occurrence of preterm labor[12] and abruptio placentae[12] (possibly dose-dependent), an increased risk of precipitous labor[5], an increased risk of abnormal antenatal tests[5], a higher likelihood of meconium-staining of amniotic fluid at time of delivery[5], and an increased risk of prolonged, protracted, or arrested labor[5]. Few authors have confirmed the findings of an increased risk of preterm labor or precipitous labor, nor is the increased incidence of meconium a universal finding[3]. Poor maternal weight gain in association with marijuana use has been reported[13], but most investigators have found it impossible to adequately control for effects of malnutrition and cigarette smoking. The incidences of miscarriage, obstetric complications, or major fetal physical anomalies in human pregnancies complicated by marijuana use are the same as those of controls[3]. Pregnant monkeys injected with Δ9THC have an increased risk of spontaneous abortion or delivery of a stillborn, especially when given Δ9THC early in gestation[7]. Hypoxia or anoxia may play a specific role in these occurrences, as Δ9THC given to sheep in late gestation can limit fetal oxygen availability[8].

Two unique minor abnormalities reported among offspring of 'heavy' users (> 6 marijuana cigarettes per week) are the presence of severe epicanthal folds and ocular hypertelorism (unusually wide separation of the eyes). Purported neurobehavioral effects following prenatal exposure to marijuana include an increase in fine tremors and exaggerated and prolonged startle responses in newborn infants. These infants may have a poorer habituation response to visual stimuli[13], but they show a normal response to auditory stimuli[3]. By 12 and 24 months of age, infants exposed prenatally to marijuana are similar to controls when assessed for visual, mental, motor or language capabilities.

Decreased birth weight has been reported in newborn infants of marijuana users, usually as a reflection of intrauterine growth retardation. This decrease fails to achieve statistical significance when data is controlled for the confounding variables of alcohol and nicotine abuse[10,12]. Fried *et al.*[13] found no effect of maternal marijuana use on infant weight, length, head circumference, or Apgar scores. Furthermore, a consistent relationship between marijuana use and the incidences of premature rupture of membranes, fetal distress, and fetal malposition has not been demonstrated[12].

Although controversy remains about certain aspects of the effects of perinatal marijuana use, the frequency of concomitant use of other illicit drugs warrants increased vigilance in the pregnant marijuana user.

LYSERGIC ACID DIETHYLAMIDE (LSD)

The hallucinogen LSD reached its popularity peak in the late 1960s. Since that time, the overall use of LSD has declined dramatically[14,15]. Users in the late 1960s were most often white, above average socio-economically, and college-educated[16].

After oral administration, LSD is rapidly absorbed into the blood. The brain does not selectively concentrate LSD, but is extremely susceptible to its effects[17]. Physiologic effects in humans are generally sympathomimetic in character: pupillary dilation, an increase in blood pressure, tachycardia, hyperreflexia, tremor, nausea, piloerection and increased temperature. LSD induces states of altered perception. Users of LSD claim enhanced awareness and understanding of sensory input[13]. Initial symptoms, which occur within minutes following LSD ingestion, include dizziness, weakness, nausea, and paresthesias. Within 2–3 hours, the user begins to experience visual illusions and affective symptoms. Differences in drug effects apparently exist between users and between episodes of use. Within 4–5 hours, users may experience major panic attacks or merely feel detached. The half-life of LSD is approximately 3 hours; the symptoms begin to abate after approximately 12 hours. There is no withdrawal syndrome, and no deaths have been attributed to the direct effects of LSD.

In 1968 and 1969, three case reports suggested human teratogenicity from prenatal LSD exposure. These involved limb defects, specifically finger abnormalities, and occasionally toe abnormalities of either or both feet[18,19]. Figure 1 depicts one such limb defect on the right hand of an infant. In all three reports,

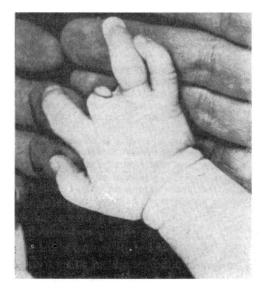

Figure 1 Fetal lysergide exposure resulting in right hand deformities in a 2 month old child. Figure reproduced with permission from reference 18

each fetus had also been exposed to marijuana. In one of the cases, the mother of the affected child had also ingested 3 other drugs (anti-nausea medications) during the early portion of her pregnancy[19]. McGlothlin *et al.*[16] studied the effects of parental LSD exposure and observed an increased risk of spontaneous abortion among women exposed to LSD. In addition, they reported 14 infants of 120 live births with 'congenital anomalies'. However, of these 14 infants, five had a parent with the same problem as the infant, and two had a first cousin with the same problem. Four infants had 'turned-in' feet, one had cystic fibrosis, one had pyloric stenosis, and two were premature but without structural anomaly. In this report, LSD use took place prior to conception. It is unlikely that these anomalies resulted from the reported LSD exposure. Several authors have suggested a causative association between LSD intake and chromosomal damage; others have disputed this correlation[19,20].

Results from animal studies are also controversial. Rats given subcutaneous LSD injections in early gestation (the first 7 days) experienced increased rates of spontaneous abortion, resorption, runting and stillbirth[21]. Later exposure did not appear to have an effect[22]; implantation occurs on day 7, and organogenesis is complete by day 14. Subcutaneous LSD injections in hamsters on day 8 of gestation resulted in neural tube defects, omphalocele, edema in various body parts, parietal and frontal lobe hemorrhages, and sublingual area hemorrhages. Implantation occurs on day 6, and organogenesis is complete by day 13[23]. Other investigators gave LSD subcutaneously to rats, mice, and hamsters during implantation and organogenesis, but were unable to confirm abortifacient or teratogenic effects of LSD[24,25]. Whether or not these animal studies can be extrapolated to human populations is, as always, uncertain.

COCAINE

Cocaine use in pregnancy, especially in conjunction with abuse of other drugs, has become increasingly prevalent[26,27]. Cocaine enjoys its popularity across the spectrum of socio-economic status and ethnic background. The pregnant cocaine abusing population in many studies includes black women in disproportionate numbers[1,27,28]. It appears that black drug abusers and impoverished drug abusers are reported to health authorities more frequently than white or wealthy drug abusers[1].

Polydrug abuse is quite common among women who use cocaine[29,30]. In a retrospective study of 139 cocaine abusing women presenting at greater than 20 weeks gestational age, concomitant use of other drugs such as alcohol, tobacco, marijuana, diazepam, heroin, and methadone occurred in 92.8% of users[29]. Cocaine's routes of entry include sniffing and injecting, along with smoking the freebase form. Cocaine

and its major metabolites are metabolized by the liver and plasma esterases and the cytochrome P450 enzymes[31,32]. Cocaine exhibits some of its peripheral effects by its actions as a local anesthetic. As such, it blocks the impulse in nerve cells by blocking the sodium channel, thereby preventing the rise of membrane potential during depolarization[33,34]. Cocaine also blocks the presynaptic re-uptake of catecholamines at neuron terminals, resulting in accumulation of norepinephrine, dopamine, and epinephrine at postsynaptic sites and in the bloodstream[31,34]. This accumulation causes an increase in sympathetic tone, and thereby vasoconstriction. The major physiologic effects of cocaine use are therefore hypertension, an increase in heart rate, hyperglycemia, hyperpyrexia, and mydriasis. Coronary vasoconstriction can lead to spasm, angina pectoris, acute myocardial infarction, cardiac arrhythmias, and even sudden death. Other potential effects related to acute vasoconstriction include subarachnoid hemorrhage in the presence of an underlying aneurysm or an A-V malformation, occlusive or hemorrhagic stroke[35], and intestinal necrosis[31]. Sniffing or snorting of cocaine can result in anosmia, chronic rhinitis, septal degeneration, necrosis and perforation[32]. Smoking cocaine can cause direct lung damage, and has resulted in pulmonary edema, spontaneous pneumomediastinum and pneumopericardium[32]. Psychiatric problems that can occur following cocaine use include disinhibition, disturbances in judgment, grandiosity, impulsive behavior, hypersexuality, and paranoid psychosis. Abstention symptoms can occur as well. A 'crash' occurs first, consisting of depression, agitation, and anxiety. This is often followed by somnolence and hyperphagia. Then a 'withdrawal' occurs, in which anergia and anhedonia predominate. The extinction phase involves an episodic craving for the drug, which gradually decreases in frequency and severity, but which may last months or years after last drug use[32]. The plasma half-life of cocaine is approximately 40 minutes. The euphoria produced following injection lasts up to 20 minutes following smoking, and between 1 hour and 90 minutes following intranasal use[32].

The placenta possesses cocaine binding sites specific for cocaine[36]. Transplacental passage of cocaine and its metabolites may also involve simple diffusion. Plasma cholinesterase action decreases during pregnancy and is low in the fetus. As fetal glucoronidation and oxidation systems are immature, and as fetal kidneys may provide inadequate clearance, metabolism and clearance of cocaine in the fetus may be insufficient[32].

A multitude of perinatal effects have been associated with gestational cocaine use. However, coexisting risk factors such as multiple drug abuse, malnutrition and lifestyle impede specific relational findings. Burkett *et al.*[29] reported inadequate weight gain (< 19 lbs or 8.6 kg) in 27 of 82 pregnancies, 15 of which were complicated by abuse of multiple substances. Cocaine-related perinatal complications which have not attained statistical significance include a higher rate of stillbirths[26,39], and an increased incidence of fetal distress following cocaine intake[27,39–41]. Controversial findings include increased incidences of spontaneous abortions[37,38], preterm premature rupture of membranes (PROM)[26,30,39,42], chorioamnionitis[30], meconium-stained amniotic fluid[29,30], and precipitous labor[27,30,39,41].

Controversy also surrounds the association between gestational cocaine use and abruptio placentae. In 1983 Acker *et al.*[43] reported 2 cases of abruptio placentae: one patient presented at 21 gestational weeks with vaginal bleeding, back pain and hypertension following intravenous cocaine use; the second presented at 33–34 weeks' gestation with vaginal bleeding and contractions a 'few hours' after snorting cocaine. While other investigators have indicated similar associations[27,37,38], several reports either dispute these findings or indicate low statistical significance[26,41,42,44].

Investigators have attempted to correlate the incidence of abruptio placentae with the time of cocaine exposure. Infants whose urine tested cocaine-positive (suggesting cocaine exposure shortly before delivery) had a similar rate of abruptio placentae to infants whose urine was cocaine-negative (suggestive of past but not recent exposure)[30]. However the rate of both groups was above that of the general population. Chasnoff *et al.*[45] found a similar lack of difference in the placental abruption rate in a group who had used cocaine through only the first trimester compared to a group who used cocaine throughout the pregnancy. These studies suggest that acute cocaine ingestion may not predispose towards an abruption more than chronic or past use of cocaine. Further, in a comparison between 'cocaine only' and 'polydrug' users, there was no significant difference in the occurrences of placental abruptions[41].

As chronic use vs. recent use of cocaine is an issue which complicates clinical studies, and as toxic effects of recent cocaine exposure are important in both the adult and the neonate, improved methods of testing for the presence of cocaine are surfacing. For example, determination of gestational cocaine exposure by hair analysis has been used[46]. This method will help distinguish between occasional and frequent use, but it will not detect very recent use. Since cocaine metabolites can be detected in adult urine 24–36 hours after usage, and because cocaine metabolites can be detected in neonatal urine up to 48 hours after birth, assessment of very recent use is possible. Neonatal meconium assessments are also proving useful for the determination of recent cocaine exposure[47].

Most authors agree that cocaine use increases the likelihood of preterm labor[27,30,41] and of preterm birth[26,28,41,42]. However, in one study, when cocaine use was stratified by the additional substance combinations frequently used[41], 'cocaine only' vs. 'polydrug' comparisons revealed no significant differences in preterm labor or preterm delivery.

Investigators consistently report no cocaine-related effects upon 5 minute Apgar scores[28,41], or umbilical artery pH values[41]. Cherukuri *et al.*[39] assessed the newborn infants of 55 cocaine users and 55 drug-free controls at birth. The cocaine-abusing group and the control groups had similar distributions in race, sex, mean maternal age and parity, a similar lack of prenatal care (40% in each group), a similar rate of concomitant alcohol use (11%), but an uneven rate of tobacco usage (82% cocaine abusers vs. 60% controls). Infants of cocaine-abusing mothers had a clinically insignificant lower mean gestation age (37.4 vs. 39.2 weeks), but more than 50% of the cocaine-using mothers delivered at 37 weeks or earlier. There were no significant differences in mean birthweight, in mean head circumference, or in birth length. No gross congenital anomalies were identified among these infants, though there was one fetal death. Of the cocaine-exposed infants, 38% demonstrated neonatal neurobehavioral abnormalities such as tremulousness, irritability and muscular rigidity. Others reported neonatal disturbances, observed in relation to either independent cocaine use or of cocaine and methamphetamine use, have included sleeping problems, feeding difficulties, vomiting, diarrhea, fever, hypotonia, a highpitched cry, tachypnea, hyper-reflexia[27], tachycardia, seizures, and hyper-responsiveness[28]. A poor sucking response and neurologic deficits are frequently prominent features in these infants[29]. The persistence of an increase in withdrawal signs such as tremulousness, irritability, poor feeding, and diarrhea, when a 'cocaine only' group is compared to a 'polydrug' group, suggests a correlation between prenatal cocaine exposure and neonatal withdrawal symptoms[26]. Apneic spells and/or abnormal pneumograms have been noted by some authors[26,29]. Along these same lines, some authors have commented upon an increased incidence of Sudden Infant Death Syndrome (SIDS) in this population[37], though this association has been disputed by others[48].

Intrauterine growth restriction (IUGR) following gestational cocaine abuse is a common finding[33]. Instances of decreased birthweight[27,41] and of low birthweight (LBW) infants (< 2500 grams)[41,42], including a significant proportion of small for gestational age (SGA) infants, commonly occur following prenatal cocaine exposure[26,28,30,41]. Of the 'cocaine only' vs. 'polydrug' groups studied by MacGregor *et al.*[41], the differences in IUGR between groups were not statistically significant. Though Zuckerman *et al.*[49] have reported that cocaine use is independently associated with a smaller neonatal head circumference (0.43 cm smaller), others have observed that effects of prenatal cocaine exposure on head circumference and birth length are small and not clinically relevant[27,28].

In a retrospective analysis, Chouteau et al.[42] showed that cocaine use is quite predictive of LBW even when other variables such as age, race, gravidity, socio-economic status, and lack of prenatal care are controlled; their analyses were not controlled for alcohol and cigarette use. Burkett et al.[29] noted that the combination of cocaine with tobacco, and of cocaine with other drugs, with the exclusion of alcohol, had larger effects on the incidence of SGA and LBW infants than cocaine alone. Zuckerman et al.[49] have suggested that the effects of marijuana and of cocaine use are additive and nonsynergistic. They were able to show that use of marijuana and of cocaine were independently associated with impaired fetal growth.

Controversy surrounds the subject of cocaine teratogenesis. Suggested congenital anomalies associated with cocaine abuse include skull defects[38], urogenital anomalies[50], urinary anomalies without genital defects[51], and congenital cardiovascular defects such as atrial septal defects (ASD), ventricular septal defects (VSD), cardiomegaly[28], transposition of the great vessels, hypoplastic right heart[38], polydactyly[29], ileal atresia[45], and intracerebral infarctions[45]. Many investigators have found no statistical increase in cocaine-induced congenital anomalies[26,39,41,44], although certain anomalies appear to have occurred with increased frequency (prune-belly with urethral obstruction; amniotic bands with distal limb reduction; jejunal atresia and bowel infarction; multiple anomalies including imperforate anus, horseshoe kidneys, and clubfoot[41]; and VSD, ASD, and complete heart block)[26].

Animal studies of cocaine's effects in pregnancy have assisted investigators with regards to perinatal pathology and potential teratogenic effects related to cocaine use. Woods et al.[52,53] were able to demonstrate in sheep a dose-dependent increase in maternal blood pressure (BP) following intravenous injection of cocaine. The increase in systolic BP, diastolic BP, mean arterial pressure (MAP), and pulse pressure was twice those seen in nonpregnant ewes given an identical dose of cocaine. Following maternal cocaine administration, a decreased fetal arterial PO_2 and an increased fetal MAP and fetal heart rate (FHR) were noted. Direct fetal injection of cocaine resulted in a rapid increase in fetal MAP, and a decrease in FHR (the first 2 minutes after injection) followed by a slow increase of FHR to a peak at 15 minutes. The magnitude of the fetal blood pressure and FHR changes seen with direct fetal administration was less than that seen with maternal drug injection, although the trend was similar. This suggests that cocaine given to the pregnant ewe may produce fetal hypoxemia via uterine artery vasoconstriction, and may produce direct fetal cardiovascular effects via transplacental passage of cocaine into the fetal circulation. It also appears that cocaine-induced uterine artery vasoconstriction, while restricting oxygen transfer to the fetus in a dose-dependent manner, does not limit placental transfer of cocaine to any significant degree.

The animal model has been particularly helpful in exploring potential cocaine teratogenicity. In mice receiving cocaine at specific gestational ages, Mahalik and others[54] reported an increased incidence of cryptorchidism and hydronephrosis, exencephaly, eye defects such as malformed lenses and anophthalmia, bony defects of skull, paws, and sternum. These authors postulate that cocaine may cause these anomalies by decreasing the placental transfer of oxygen. Webster and Brown-Woodman[55] administered cocaine to pregnant rats as single or multiple doses, during specified gestational periods, and examined the fetuses at various times for evidence of hemorrhage or malformation. They found no evidence of teratogenicity when cocaine was given during the main organogenic period, even at toxic maternal doses. However, when given at later specific gestational ages, cocaine exposure was associated with damage to fetal limbs and tail, and hemorrhage in the genital tubercle. In general, cocaine administration was followed by the occurrence of edema and hemorrhage at certain sites. When involved fetuses were reinspected at a later date, reduction anomalies were identified at these sites. It appears, then, that the malformations are a direct result of hemorrhage and edema, followed by necrosis, and subsequent disruption and/or amputation (Figure 2). The authors postulate that the fetal vasculature must attain a certain degree of maturation prior to being able to respond to hypoxia, thereby protecting developing tissues during organogenesis.

Other investigators have been particularly interested in neurobehavioral effects of prenatal cocaine exposure. The cocaine metabolite benzoylecgonine is able to attain high concentrations in fetal, but not maternal brain. This may be linked to neurobehavioral abnormalities that seem to be peculiar to cocaine-exposed offspring. Spear et al.[56] were able to show that cocaine-exposed rat offspring had cognitive defects in some, but not all, conditioning situations. These authors have offered the suggestion, based on their work in the animal model, that chronic exposure to cocaine during gestation may result in down-regulation of dopaminergic systems, relating to subsequent hyperactivity and attention deficit disorders. Other investigators, using the rat model, have provided data which suggests that fetal cocaine exposure during synaptogenesis may result in long-term changes in the neurochemistry of dopaminergic systems, adding that brain effects in the offspring seem to occur at a dose which causes little maternal toxicity[57]. Though controversy is widespread, and lack of knowledge about perinatal effects of cocaine abundant, awareness of its use during gestation is important.

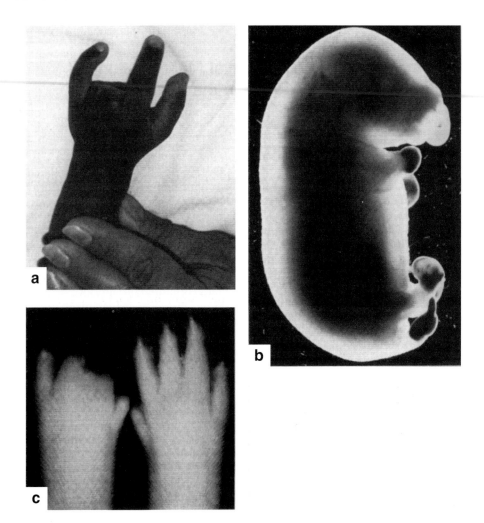

Figure 2   (a) Left hand of an infant born to a mother described as a heavy cocaine user (Chasnoff *et al.* 1988). Note the absence of the 3rd and 4th digits. (Photo courtesy of Dr. I. Chasnoff, Department of Pediatrics, Northwestern Memorial Hospital, Chicago, Illinois 60611). (b) Rat fetus from a dam given a single dose of cocaine (60 mg/kg) 48 hours earlier. Note the severe hemorrhage affecting the footplates and tail and the large fluid-filled blister on the nose and upper lip. (c) Right and left hindlimbs of 5-week rat from a dam given cocaine (60 mg/kg) on day 16 of gestation. Note the reduction of digits 2–4 of the left limb. Figures reproduced with permission from reference 55

AMPHETAMINES

The sympathomimetic amines, of which the most common examples are amphetamine and methamphetamine, have been used to combat obesity and fatigue. Though unorthodox in approach, fanatics among both patient and physician populations have been known to employ this drug of abuse to 'treat' these unpleasant side-effects of pregnancy. Amphetamines work by stimulating the release of catecholamines from sympathetic nerve receptors, preventing their re-uptake, and inhibiting monoamine oxidase, which is responsible for catecholamine breakdown. All these actions serve to increase the availability of norepinephrine and dopamine at the nerve terminal[58,59]. It is this catecholamine 'excess' that accounts for amphetamine's peripheral alpha and beta actions and

central nervous system (CNS) stimulant effects. Vascular effects following amphetamine intake include vasoconstriction and bronchodilation, resulting in increased systolic and diastolic blood pressures, reflex bradycardia, and increased respiratory rate. An enhanced perception of environmental stimuli, mood elevation, and a decrease in hunger and fatigue, are thought to result from amphetamine's ability to stimulate the reticular activating system[60]. Overdose can therefore lead to nervousness, insomnia, hallucinations, confusion, anxiety, headache, pallor or flushing, palpitations, blood pressure instability, cardiac arrhythmias[58], and myocardial infarction[61]. The increasingly popular 'street' drug, methamphetamine, the N-methylated derivative of amphetamine, has CNS effects similar to dextroamphetamine, but with fewer peripheral effects[58]. Also of concern are the so-called 'designer drugs', synthetic analogs of various prescription drugs. Among the stimulants are increasingly popular amphetamine derivatives, which include methylene dioxyamphetamine (MDMA). These drugs share many of the problems of the parent drugs, and they frequently have more unpredictable side-effects[62]. Illegal manufacturing of these derivative drugs may also involve the inclusion of contaminants, which may pose further dangers.

Most investigators who have studied antenatal amphetamine abuse have encountered coexistent abuse of other drugs[63,64]. Because of frequent polydrug abuse, the possibility of drug impurities, and malnutrition, it is difficult to attribute adverse perinatal effects exclusively to amphetamine abuse during pregnancy.

A dearth of information exists about the ability of amphetamines to cross the placenta. In a case reported by Briggs *et al.*[65], neonatal urine was reportedly negative for amphetamines following a 40 mg maternal dose of dextroamphetamine 6–10 hours prior to delivery. This report casts doubt upon the prevailing theory that transplacental passage of amphetamine is a likely occurrence. Nevertheless, amphetamines may have perinatal effects via other mechanisms, and some conclusions can be drawn from available work. Amongst 52 amphetamine abusers[63], differences from controls were noted in infants' birthweights and birth lengths, along with minimal differences in head circumferences. There were no significant differences in pregnancy or neonatal complications in these patients. However, when methamphetamine exposure was coupled with cocaine exposure, increased rates of premature delivery, intrauterine growth retardation, placental abruption, and fetal distress were identified. Multiple regression analysis of these data revealed that methamphetamine and cocaine exposure were independently associated with premature delivery, and decreases in growth parameters[27]. An increase in congenital anomalies following prenatal amphetamine exposure has not been consistently identified[63,65], although an association between prenatal amphetamine use and the occurrence of congenital heart disease has been suggested[66]. The children of amphetamine addicts exhibit normal physical health parameters, (including growth), and normal IQs, but a statistically significant increase in aggressive behavior and peer-related problems has been noted[64].

PHENCYCLIDINE (PCP)

Phencyclidine is usually smoked with tobacco or marijuana. Some of its metabolites are active, but most of the pharmacologic effects result from PCP itself. The half-life of PCP is approximately 3 days. A typical 'high' lasts 4–6 hours, followed by an extended 'coming down' period. Actions of PCP are primarily attributed to its ability to inhibit the reuptake of dopamine, 5-hydroxytryptamine, and norepinephrine at nerve terminals, but distinct saturable and stereospecific binding sites for PCP have also been identified in the CNS[67]. PCP can act as both a stimulant and a depressant. Effects may include hallucinations, euphoria, a subjective state of intoxication, staggering gait, slurred speech, nystagmus, numbness of the extremities, sweating, catatonic muscular rigidity, a blank stare, disorganized thought, drowsiness, apathy, feelings of paranoia or impending death, bizarre behavior, hostility, amnesia, tachycardia, hypertension, hypersalivation, fever, repetitive movements, mood elevation[67,68].

Since PCP crosses the placenta in pigs, rabbits, mice, and humans[68], and as PCP and its monohydroxylated metabolites rapidly cross the blood–brain barrier in mice[68], potential fetal effects are of concern. Case studies have cited neurobehavioral abnormalities in neonates born to women who abused PCP during pregnancy. Although polydrug use complicated the majority of these pregnancies, gestational PCP exposure was specifically associated with jittery and hyperactive neonatal behavior, with bouts of lethargy and blank staring[68]. Increases in neonatal neurobehavioral abnormalities, following prenatal exposure to PCP, have been reported[69]. At ages 3, 6, 12, and 24 months of age, mental and psychomotor exams on these infants have not differed from those of infants with other drug exposure. Growth parameters are similar to those of drug-free controls at birth, and at later assessment times[69]. No congenital structural defects in humans exposed to gestational PCP exposure have been identified[68].

Data from animal studies are proving helpful in the elucidation of neurobehavioral abnormalities following intrauterine PCP exposure. When PCP is given to pregnant rats throughout gestation, changes in concentrations of 5-hydroxytryptamine, which is structurally and functionally related to dopamine and serotonin, are identifiable in discrete brain areas of male offspring[70]. The changes were still present 9 months post-exposure. Other investigators have identified gross structural malformations in the offspring of mice only when dams were given PCP at doses which produced significant maternal toxicity. However, fetal weight was significantly affected at all doses[71]. It is clear that further information is needed about the potential effects of this drug.

ALCOHOL

In the not so distant past, intravenous alcohol was an accepted method of tocolysis for the treatment of preterm labor. Clearly there remain extremes, from no alcohol consumption to frequent heavy imbibing. Not surprisingly, there is a large range of possible pregnancy outcomes within these extremes, varying from no demonstrable effect to specific serious congenital defects[72].

It has been estimated that 44–89% of women drink alcohol at some time during their pregnancies[73]. Heavy drinking (> 10 drinks per week) is thought to occur among 5–10% of obstetric patients[72]. Alcohol use, and alcoholism, involves patients of every ethnic group, of all socio-economic strata, of every age group. It has been suggested that white women are more likely to experiment with drugs and alcohol, and that black women are more likely to have continued use[74]. In a prevalence study of alcohol use in pregnant women, those in the highest consumption category tended to be older, single, heavier smokers, and of higher gravidity[75]. The majority of women involved in this study were white and married.

Alcohol is a small molecule which is readily absorbed from the gastrointestinal tract, and is rapidly distributed throughout the body. Of the alcohol that enters the body, 90–98% is completely oxidized, mainly in the liver by alcohol dehydrogenase[76]. Alcohol is initially metabolized to acetaldehyde, and in turn to acetate and then to acetyl coenzyme A, which is further oxidized via the citric acid cycle or is utilized in various anaerobic reactions. Metabolism of alcohol therefore results in increased production of lactate and fatty acids. Excretion of the unoxidized ethanol occurs via the renal and pulmonary systems[76]. The consumption of excessive alcohol can result in: hypertension, slurred speech, staggering gait, ketoacidosis, myopathy, hepatomegaly, pancreatitis, other upper gastrointestinal disorders, mood swings, memory lapses, blackouts, other neurobehavioral disorders, hematological disorders, and cardiac dysfunction[77]. Ethanol readily crosses the placenta[78], and can interfere with active transport of amino acids across the placenta[72]. Acetaldehyde is a mutagen and is also capable of altering placental transport of nutrients[77]. Unfortunately, the placenta does little in the way of ethanol and acetaldehyde detoxification[79]. Finally, malnutrition and/or specific vitamin deficiencies due to malabsorption from alcohol abuse may play important parts.

Fetal alcohol syndrome (FAS), which may occur secondary to heavy alcohol exposure, has received increasing attention. This syndrome occurs in the offspring of 2.5% to 10% of alcohol-dependent women[72]. FAS is characterized by prenatal and/or postnatal growth retardation (weight, length, and/or head circumference less than the 10th percentile), CNS involvement (signs of neurologic abnormality, developmental delay, or intellectual delay), and characteristic facial dysmorphology (features may include microcephaly, microophthalmia and/or short palpebral fissures, poorly developed philtrum, thin upper lip, or flattening of the maxillary area). The occurrence of FAS is apparently restricted to the offspring of heavy drinkers[80]. Interestingly, progesterone levels are lower than normal in alcoholic women whose offspring develop features of FAS[81].

Fetal alcohol effects (FAE) is the term used when some, but not all, of the criteria for FAS are fulfilled. It occurs more frequently than FAS. Neonatal features which may be associated with heavy prenatal alcohol exposure include: cardiac abnormalities, neonatal irritability and hypotonia, hyperactivity, genitourinary abnormalities, skeletal and muscular abnormalities, ocular problems, or hemangiomas[77]. In children with FAS and FAE, there are large ranges of mental capabilities, in both IQ values and in the extent of mental retardation[82].

Perinatal effects which have been associated with alcohol consumption include an increased risk of: spontaneous abortion[83], stillbirth[75], lower birthweight[80,84], and IUGR[85]. Decreased birthweight does not always remain statistically significant when results are controlled for smoking[75]. Further, the victims of IUGR are exclusively among the offspring of those classified as heavy drinkers[72]. An association between drinking approximately 10 drinks per week at the time of conception and decreased infant size has been identified, suggesting that this effect may actually be periconceptual[86]. A statistically significant association with decreased head circumference has been noted[84], but the reported difference (0.64 mm) is clearly within the range of measurement error. An increased risk of minor physical anomalies following alcohol consumption in the first month of pregnancy has been suggested[84], and disputed[72]. A statistically weak association with fetal distress exists, and links between alcohol abuse of greater than 14 drinks per week and placental abruption, and 5 minute Apgar scores less than 6, have been demonstrated[75]. The consumption of alcohol may also affect antenatal testing, as maternal alcohol consumption may have a transient effect on FHR reactivity[87]. Following maternal ingestion of 0.25 gm/kg of ethanol in healthy pregnant women at term, McLeod et al.[88] noted cessation of fetal breathing movements for up to three hours. The alcohol was not associated with any changes in fetal movement or fetal heart rate.

Structural defects in animals which mimic those seen in humans with FAS or FAE have been created. For example, pregnant mice given alcohol during specific gestational days had fewer pups per litter, with decreased birthweight of the surviving pups[89]. The increase in resorptions and malformations in mice pups exposed to prenatal alcohol is dose-related[90]. A high incidence of hydronephrosis in the offspring was identified, and skeletal, neural, ophthalmic, and cardiac defects were noted[89,90]. According to Sulik et al.[91], craniofacial malformations may be caused by abnormal development of the neural plate and its derivatives, suggesting that the

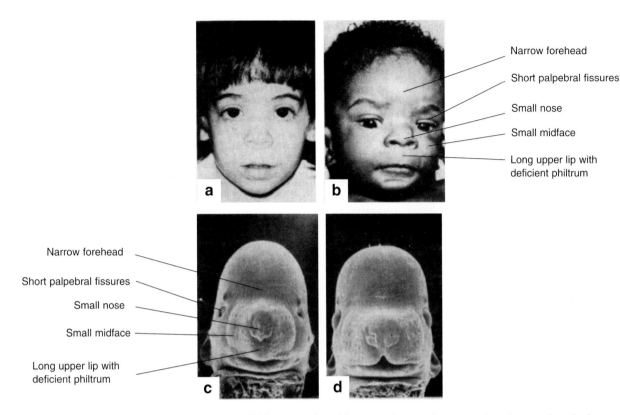

Figure 3   (a and b) Fetal alcohol syndrome in children. 14 day-old mouse fetuses from (c) ethanol-treated and (d) control mothers. Reproduced with permission from reference 91

time of critical exposure is at approximately the third week of human gestation (Figure 3). In another series of experiments[79], the offspring of multiparous alcohol-fed rats exposed to alcohol for a full year had an increased frequency and severity of prenatal effects (resorptions, immature fetuses, decreased fetal weight), as compared to rats with short-term alcohol exposure. The pups of alcoholic dams with the highest serum liver enzyme values were the most affected.

As the reduction of heavy drinking during pregnancy may improve neonatal outcome[72], this is certainly recommended. Unfortunately, withdrawal symptoms can be life-threatening for mother and fetus, so inpatient detoxification may be necessary. Though it must be used judiciously, especially near term, benzodiazepam is a useful agent for the treatment of withdrawal symptoms seen with delirium tremens ('DTs'). Alcoholic acidosis may also be aggravated by pregnancy. Therapy should involve rehydration and reversal of fatty acid mobilization with glucose-containing intravenous fluid, and administration of insulin when necessary to reverse ketogenesis[77].

OPIATES

The warnings of Hippocrates yet pertain: opium during pregnancy may result in 'uterine suffocation'[92]. It

has been estimated that 3 of every 1000 newborns are victims of opiate addiction[93]. Heroin addicts are disproportionately black, while opiate addicts maintained on methadone are disproportionately white[94,95]. Intravenous drug abuse significantly increases risks of infection, and more than 12% of present and former heroin users are known to be chronic carriers of hepatitis B[96]. The need for continued concern about the pregnant opiate addict is heightened by the availability of designer opiates. Designer opiates include 1-methyl 4-phenyl 4-propiooxypiperidine (MPPP) and fentanyl derivatives such as alpha methyl fentanyl ('China White'). These derivatives produce longer-lasting effects with greater potency than fentanyl[97].

Opiates work by binding to various constellations of opioid receptors[98], normally utilized by endogenous opioid peptides. Physiologic effects following exogenous opiate administration include decreased heart rate, decreased respiratory rate, decreased rate of digestion, and constricted pupils. In women of reproductive age, opiate use may cause prolonged amenorrhea. Coma, convulsions, and cardiorespiratory arrest can occur following opiate overdose. Withdrawal signs and symptoms include tachycardia, hypotension or hypertension, increased respiratory rate, nausea, vomiting, stomach and extremities cramps, muscular twitching, 'gooseflesh', chills, tearing, rhinorrhea, yawning, insomnia, irritability, panic, and anorexia[96,98–100]. In the pregnant abuser, withdrawal may be marked by uterine irritability and increased fetal activity, which may precede other maternal withdrawal symptoms[99]. Withdrawal, though distinctly uncomfortable, usually is not life-threatening to the adult[98]. Opiates are likely to affect the fetus, as transplacental passage does occur. Perinatal risks following opiate abuse include spontaneous abortion[96], stillbirth[100,101], preterm birth[95,96,100,101], IUGR[96,101], low birthweight[95,99,102,103], smaller head circumference[102,103], and low birth length[95,102,103]. Approximately 50% of infants born to mothers addicted to heroin had birthweights less than 2500g, as a result of preterm delivery and IUGR[101]. However, birth lengths are similar when controlled for smoking and maternal weight gain, according to at least one author[102]. At the ages of 12, 18, 24, and 36 months, short stature was not more prevalent among the infants of opiate addicts[102,103]. Likewise, infant weights at 12 through 24 months of age did not differ from those of controls[103]. Teratogenic effects following opiate abuse have not been reported[94,100,101]. Dispute remains in regards to respiratory distress syndrome (RDS) occurring less frequently in the opiate-addicted neonate[100]. An increased incidence of sudden infant death syndrome (SIDS) in this population has been reported[104,105].

Strict methadone maintenance has traditionally been the mainstay in prenatal care of the opiate addict. Methadone is a synthetic opiate which blocks the euphoric effects of heroin, thereby decreasing desire for heroin, while preventing the symptoms of withdrawal. Methadone is widely distributed following oral ingestion. It has a long duration of action and extensive nonspecific tissue binding. Peak plasma levels occur between 2 and 6 hours after ingestion of a maintenance dose[96,98,106]. Metabolism occurs primarily in the liver, and methadone is excreted in feces and urine. Methadone readily crosses the placenta, and has been identified in amniotic fluid, umbilical cord blood, and neonatal urine[96]. Both placenta and fetus can further metabolize methadone[107].

Unfortunately, most addicts on methadone maintenance also abuse other drugs[94,96,108,109], the most common of which is concurrent use of heroin. Nevertheless, methadone programs do offer several advantages, for instance methadone-maintained women have more prenatal visits and less anemia than other drug abusers[94,108]. Several studies have confirmed a rate of prenatal care among methadone users which is comparable to that of drug-free controls, and significantly higher than 'untreated' heroin addicts[94,108]. In a study by Edelin *et al.*[108] rates of occurrence of birthweights less than 2500 g were similar in the methadone group and the polydrug group (29.6% and 34% respectively), but they differed significantly from rates in drug-free controls (16.7%). This finding has been confirmed by others[94]. Methadone use is not associated with the occurrence of IUGR[101]. Body weight/gestational age ratios are often low but generally not less than the 10th percentile[109]. Another advantage of methadone therapy is the relative decrease in premature births[101]. In the data from Edelin *et al.*, occurrence of meconium-stained amniotic fluid was similar in drug-abusing groups (46% in methadone-maintained group; 50% in polydrug group), but differed markedly from the drug-free population rate of 12%[108].

It has been suggested by some investigators that fetal opiate withdrawal may be causally related to hypoxia, and to meconium passage *in utero*. Substantiating this idea is the increased incidence of meconium-stained fluid[100] and fetal distress[96] during labor. An increased likelihood of shortened gestation has been reported[100], though the clinical significance of 0.6 weeks[95] is questionable. A decrease in frequency of fetal movements and FHR accelerations after methadone ingestion has been reported[106]. In a retrospective study of 30 infants of drug-abusing mothers with birthweights < 1500 g, (of which 15 were infants of methadone addicts), and matched drug-free controls, a lesser probability of intraventricular hemorrhage (IVH) was noted in infants having had prenatal opiate exposure as compared to infants of drug-free women with similar risk factors. This suggests that gestational opiate exposure may actually offer protection against IVH in these very small infants[110].

There is a 60–90% chance of withdrawal after birth in the neonate whose mother is addicted to opiates. Unless treated, 3–5% of these infants will die[98]. The signs and symptoms of neonatal heroin withdrawal, which typically appear 24–48 hours after birth, consist of hyperactivity, irritability, tremors, convulsions, persistent high-pitched crying, hypertonia alternating with periods of hypotonia, gastrointestinal dysfunction, respiratory distress, sneezing, sweating, tearing, mottling and fever[99,101,111]. Neonatal withdrawal from methadone may be more severe than from other opiates[101,109], may be prolonged[94,101], and may not occur until 2–4 weeks after birth[111]. This is in part due to neonatal storage and prolonged metabolism and excretion of methadone[111].

Newborn infants of opiate addicts often exhibit neurobehavioral abnormalities[103], and methadone-exposed infants are more likely than infants without opiate exposure to have affected motor behaviors at 1 day and 1 month of age, demonstrating hypertonia, tremulousness, and jerky movements[112]. These abnormalities may persist. At 1 year of age, fine motor coordination of methadone-exposed infants is significantly less than that of drug-free controls[94]. As young children, those exposed to prenatal methadone may be hyperactive, with difficulty in fine motor coordination, and with difficulties relating socially[111,112]. Downregulation of opiate receptors in the fetus exposed prenatally to opiates is a likely mechanism of neurobehavioral changes. While plasma levels of β-endorphin in heroin addicts are equal to those of controls at all gestational ages, amniotic fluid levels of β-endorphin from heroin-abusers is less than those of drug-free controls in the second trimester[113].

Data from studies of methadone exposure in the rat tend to support clinical findings. Rat pups perinatally exposed to methadone demonstrate behavioral changes, in that they are abnormally slow to respond to hot-plate stimulation[114]. Prenatal methadone exposure in the rat leads to down-regulation of opioid receptors in the cerebral cortex and hypothalamus, and to a decrease in alpha-adrenergic receptors in the cerebral cortex[115].

GENERAL RECOMMENDATIONS

(1) Inpatient and outpatient counseling of the pregnant substance abuser, when available, should be offered.

(2) In identified substance-users, a screen for the presence of other drugs may be warranted during prenatal care, and/or during labor.

(3) Offer human immunodeficiency virus (HIV) testing, with risk counseling.

(4) A screening sonographic examination for fetal anomalies may prove useful.

(5) Fetal growth surveillance is important.

(6) Antepartum testing such as weekly non-stress testing after 32 weeks' gestation should be considered.

SPECIFIC RECOMMENDATIONS

ALCOHOL: Obtain complete blood count (CBC), red blood cell indices, liver function tests, urine assessment of ketones.

OPIATES:

(1) Ultrasound dating.

(2) Liver function tests on a routine basis.

(3) Hepatitis profiles should be at the first prenatal visit, and at term.

(4) Methadone or other opiates (e.g. oxycodone) should be given when evidence of maternal withdrawal exists.

(5) Usual maintenance doses should be given in labor[96]. For the occurrence of withdrawal signs and symptoms, 10–20 mg of methadone IM should be given. (Methadone is used only to prevent withdrawal; it will not provide adequate analgesia.)

(6) Agonist–antagonist combinations (e.g. Stadol [butorphanol tartrate] and Nubain [nalbuphine hydrochloride]) should not be given, as they will provoke withdrawal[96].

(7) Naloxone should not be given to infants of opiate addicts in the delivery room, as it may provoke neonatal withdrawal[116].

ACKNOWLEDGEMENT

With thanks to Dr James Woods, Jr, for his help in the preparation of this manuscript.

REFERENCES

1. Chasnoff IJ, Landress HJ, Barrett ME. The prevalence of illicit-drug or alcohol use during pregnancy and discrepancies in mandatory reporting in Pinellas County, Florida. *N Engl J Med* 1990;322:1202–6

2. NIDA Research Monograph 31. Petersen RC, ed. Marijuana Research Findings: 1980. Rockville, MD: NIDA, 1980:6–25

3. Fried PA. Postnatal consequences of maternal marijuana use in humans. *Ann NY Acad Sci* 1989;562:123–32

4. Abel EL. Prenatal exposure to cannabis: a critical review of effects on growth, development, and behavior. *Behav Neural Biol* 1980;29:137–56

5. Greenland S, Staisch KJ, Brown N, *et al*. Effects of marijuana on human pregnancy, labor, and delivery. *Neurobehav Toxicol Teratol* 1982;4:447–50

6. Gerald MC. *Pharmacology - An Introduction to Drugs*. Englewood Cliffs, NJ: Prentice-Hall Inc., 1974:335–52

7. Asch RH, Smith CG. Effects of Δ9-THC, the principal psychoactive component of marijuana, during pregnancy in the rhesus monkey. *J Reprod Med* 1986;31:1071–81

8. Clapp JF III, Wesley M, Cooke R, *et al*. The effects of marijuana smoke on gas exchange in ovine pregnancy. *Alcohol Drug Res* 1986;7:85–92

9. Abrams RM, Cook CE, Davis KH, *et al*. Plasma Δ9-tetrahydrocannabinol in pregnant sheep and fetus after inhalation of smoke from a marijuana cigarette. *Alcohol Drug Res* 1985;6:361–9

10. Fried PA, Watkinson B, Willan A. Marijuana use during pregnancy and decreased length of gestation. *Am J Obstet Gynecol* 1984;150:23–7

11. Fried PA, Buckingham M, Von Kulmiz P. Marijuana use during pregnancy and perinatal risk factors. *Am J Obstet Gynecol* 1983;146:992–4

12. Linn S, Schoenbaum SC, Monson RR, *et al*. The association of marijuana use with outcome of pregnancy. *Am J Public Health* 1983;73:1161–4

13. Fried PA. Marijuana use by pregnant women and effects on offspring: an update. *Neurobehav Toxicol Teratol* 1982;4:451–4

14. Jaffe JH. Drug addiction and drug abuse. In Gilman AG, Goodman LS, Rall TW, Murad F, eds. *The Pharmacological Basis of Therapeutics*, 7th edn. New York, NY: MacMillan Publishing Co., 1985:562–5

15. NIDA Research Monograph 35. Richards L, ed. Demographic Trends and Drug Abuse, 1980–1995. Rockville, MD: NIDA, 1981

16. McGlothlin WH, Sparkes RS, Arnold DO. Effect of LSD on human pregnancy. *J Am Med Assoc* 1970;212:1483–7

17. Gerald MC. *Pharmacology - An Introduction to Drugs.* Englewood Cliffs, NJ: Prentice-Hall Inc., 1974:317–34

18. Assemany SR, Neu RL, Gardner LI. Deformities in a child whose mother took L.S.D. *Lancet* 1970;1:1290

19. Titus RJ. Lysergic acid diethylamide: its effects on human chromosomes and the human organism in utero. A review of current findings. *Int J Addict* 1972; 7:701–4

20. Warren RJ, Rimoin DL, Sly WS. LSD exposure in utero. *Pediatrics* 1974;45:466–9

21. Alexander GJ, Miles BE, Gold GM, *et al.* LSD: injection early in pregnancy produces abnormalities in offspring of rats. *Science* 1967;157:459–60

22. Alexander GJ, Gold GM, Miles BE, *et al.* Lysergic acid diethylamide intake in pregnancy: fetal damage in rats. *J Pharmacol Exp Ther* 1970;173:48–59

23. Geber WF. Congenital malformations induced by mescaline, lysergic acid diethylamide, and bromolysergic acid in the hamster. *Science* 1967;158:165–7

24. Roux C, Dupuis R, Aubry M. LSD: no teratogenic action in rats, mice, and hamsters. *Science* 1970;169: 588–9

25. DiPaolo JA, Givelber HM, Erwin H. Evaluation of teratogenicity of lysergic acid diethylamide. *Nature* 1968;220:490–1

26. Neerhof MG, MacGregor SN, Retzky SS, *et al.* Cocaine abuse during pregnancy: peripartum prevalence and perinatal outcome. *Am J Obstet Gynecol* 1989;161:633–8

27. Oro AS, Dixon SD. Perinatal cocaine and methamphetamine exposure: maternal and neonatal correlates. *J Pediatr* 1987;111:571–8

28. Little BB, Snell LA, Klein VR, *et al.* Cocaine abuse during pregnancy: maternal and fetal implications. *Obstet Gynecol* 1989;73:157–60

29. Burkett G, Yasin S, Palow D. Perinatal implications of cocaine exposure. *J Reprod Med* 1990;35:35–42

30. Mastrogiannis DS, Decavalas GO, Verma U, *et al.* Perinatal outcome after recent cocaine usage. *Obstet Gynecol* 1990;76:8–11

31. Plessinger MA, Woods JR Jr. A review of the cardiovascular effects of cocaine use in pregnancy. *Reprod Toxicol* 1991;5:99–113

32. Rosenak D, Diamant YZ, Yaffe H, *et al.* Cocaine: maternal use during pregnancy and its effect on the mother, the fetus, and the infant. *Obstet Gynecol Surv* 1990; 45:348–59

33. Ritchie JM, Greene NM. Local Anesthetics. In Gilman AG, Goodman LS, Rall TW, Murad F, eds. *The Pharmacological Basis of Therapeutics*, 7th edn. New York, NY: MacMillan Publishing Co., 1985:309

34. Gerald MC. *Pharmacology - An Introduction to Drugs.* Englewood Cliffs, NJ: Prentice-Hall, Inc., 1974: 290–1,311

35. Levine SR, Brust JCM, Futrell N, *et al.* Cerebrovascular complications of the use of the "crack" form of alkaloidal cocaine. *N Engl J Med* 1990;323:699–704

36. Ahmed MS, Zhou D-H, Maulik D. Properties of a cocaine binding protein identified in human placental villus tissue. *Placenta* 1989;10A:480

37. Chasnoff IJ, Burns WJ, Schnoll SH, *et al.* Cocaine use in pregnancy. *N Engl J Med* 1985;313:666–9

38. Bingol N, Fuchs M, Diaz V, *et al.* Teratogenicity of cocaine in humans. *J Pediatr* 1987;110:93–6

39. Cherukuri R, Minkoff H, Feldman J, *et al.* A cohort study of alkaloidal cocaine ("crack") in pregnancy. *Obstet Gynecol* 1988;72:147–51

40. Sztulman L, Ducey JJ, Tancer ML. Intrapartum, intranasal cocaine use and acute fetal distress. *J Reprod Med* 1990;35:917–8

41. MacGregor SN, Keith LG, Chasnoff IJ, *et al.* Cocaine use during pregnancy: adverse perinatal outcome. *Am J Obstet Gynecol* 1987;157:686–90

42. Chouteau M, Namerow PB, Leppert P. The effect of cocaine abuse on birth weight and gestational age. *Obstet Gynecol* 1988;72:351–4

43. Acker D, Sachs BP, Tracey KJ, *et al.* Abruptio placentae associated with cocaine use. *Am J Obstet Gynecol* 1983; 146:220–1

44. Lutiger B, Graham K, Einarson, *et al.* Relationship between gestational cocaine use and pregnancy outcome: a meta-analysis. *Teratology* 1991;44:405–14

45. Chasnoff IJ, Griffith DR. Cocaine: clinical studies of pregnancy and the newborn. *Ann NY Acad Sci* 1989; 562:260–6

46. Graham K, Koren G, Klein J, *et al.* Determination of gestational cocaine exposure by hair analysis. *J Am Med Assoc* 1989;262:3328–30

47. Ostrea EM, Parks P, Brady M. The detection of heroin, cocaine and cannabinoid metabolites in meconium of infants of drug dependent mothers: clinical significance. *Pediatr Res* 1989;25:225A

48. Bauchner HJ, Zuckerman B, McClain M. Risk of sudden infant death syndrome among infants with in utero exposure to cocaine. *J Pediatr* 1988; 113:831–4

49. Zuckerman B, Frank DA, Hingson R, *et al.* Effects of maternal marijuana and cocaine use on fetal growth. *N Engl J Med* 1989;320:762–8

50. Chasnoff IJ, Chisum GM, Kaplan WE. Maternal cocaine use and genitourinary tract malformations. *Teratology* 1988;37:201–4

51. Chavez GF, Mulinare J, Cordero JF. Maternal cocaine use during early pregnancy as a risk factor for congenital urogenital anomalies. *J Am Med Assoc* 1989;262:795–8

52. Woods JR Jr, Plessinger MA. Pregnancy increases cardiovascular toxicity to cocaine. *Am J Obstet Gynecol* 1990;162:529–33

53. Woods JR Jr, Plessinger MA, Scott K, *et al.* Prenatal cocaine exposure to the fetus: a sheep model for cardiovascular evaluation. *Ann NY Acad Sci* 1989; 562:267–79

54. Mahalik MP, Gautieri RF, Mann DE. Teratogenic potential of cocaine hydrochloride in CF-1 mice. *J Pharm Sci* 1980;69:703–6

55. Webster WS, Brown-Woodman PDC. Cocaine as a cause of congenital malformations of vascular origin: experimental evidence in the rat. *Teratology* 1990;41: 689–97

56. Spear LP, Kirstein CL, Frambes NA. Cocaine effects on the developing CNS: behavioral, psychopharmacological and neurochemical studies. *Ann NY Acad Sci* 1989;562:290–307

57. Dow-Edwards DL. Long-term neurochemical and neurobehavioral consequences of cocaine during pregnancy. *Ann NY Acad Sci* 1989;562:280–9

58. Gerald MC. *Pharmacology - An Introduction to Drugs*. Englewood Cliffs, NJ: Prentice-Hall Inc., 1974:107–25

59. Middaugh, LD. Prenatal amphetamine effects on behavior: possible mediation by brain monoamines. *Ann NY Acad Sci* 1989;562:308–17

60. Weiner N. Norepinephrine, epinephrine, and the sympathomimetic amines. In Gilman AG, Goodman LS, Rall TW, Murad F, eds. *The Pharmacological Basis of Therapeutics*, 7th edn. New York, NY: MacMillan Publishing Co. 1985:166–9

61. Furst SR, Fallon SP, Reznik GN, *et al*. Myocardial infarction after inhalation of methamphetamine. *N Engl J Med* 1990;323:1147

62. Goodman P, Koz G. *Designer Drugs*. New York, NY: Chelsea House Publishers, 1988

63. Little BB, Snell LM, Gilstrap LC III. Methamphetamine abuse during pregnancy: fetal outcome and fetal effects. *Obstet Gynecol* 1988;72:541–4

64. Eriksson M, Billing L, Steneroth G, *et al*. Health and development of 8-year-old children whose mothers abused amphetamine during pregnancy. *Acta Paediatr Scand* 1989;78:944–9

65. Briggs GG, Samson JH, Crawford DJ. Lack of abnormalities in a newborn exposed to amphetamine during gestation. *Am J Dis Child* 1975;129:249–50

66. Nora JJ, Vargo TA, Nora AH, *et al*. Dexamphetamine: a possible environmental trigger in cardiovascular malformations. *Lancet* 1970;1:1290–1

67. Jaffe JH. Drug addiction and drug abuse. In Gilman AG, Goodman LS, Rall TW, Murad F, eds. *The Pharmacological Basis of Therapeutics*, 7th edn. New York, NY: MacMillan Publishing Co., 1985:565–6

68. Fico TA, VanDerwende C. Phencyclidine during pregnancy: behavioral and neurochemical effects in the offspring. *Ann NY Acad Sci* 1989;562:319–26

69. Chasnoff IJ, Burns KA, Burns WJ, *et al*. Prenatal drug exposure: effects on neonatal and infant growth and development. *Neurobehav Toxicol Teratol* 1986;8:357–62

70. Tonge SR. Neurochemical teratology: 5-hydroxyindole concentrations in discrete areas of rat brain after the pre- and neonatal administration of phencyclidine and imipramine. *Life Sci* 1973;121:481–6

71. Marks TA, Worthy WC, Staples RE. Teratogenic potential of phencyclidine in the mouse. *Teratology* 1980;21:241–6

72. Rosett HL, Weiner L. Alcohol and pregnancy: a clinical perspective. *Annu Rev Med* 1985;36:73–80

73. Rosett HL, Weiner L, Lee A, *et al*. Patterns of alcohol consumption and fetal development. *Obstet Gynecol* 1983;61:539–46

74. Adams EH, Gfroerer JC, Rouse BA. Epidemiology of substance abuse including alcohol and cigarette smoking. *Ann NY Acad Sci* 1989;562:14–20

75. Marbury MC, Linn S, Monson R, *et al*. The association of alcohol consumption with outcome of pregnancy. *Am J Public Health* 1983;73:1165–8

76. Ritchie JM. The aliphatic alcohols. In Gilman AG, Goodman LS, Rall TW, Murad F, eds. *The Pharmacological Basis of Therapeutics*, 7th edn. New York, NY: MacMillan Publishing Co., 1985:372–86

77. Jessup M, Green JR. Treatment of the pregnant alcohol-dependent woman. *J Psychoactive Drugs* 1987;19:193–202

78. Gerald MC. *Pharmacology - An Introduction to Drugs*. Englewood Cliffs, NJ: Prentice-Hall, Inc., 1974: 216–34

79. Sanchis R, Sancho-Tello M, Chirivella M, *et al*. The role of maternal alcohol damage on ethanol teratogenicity in the rat. *Teratology* 1987;36:199–208

80. Hanson JW, Streissguth AP, Smith DW. The effects of moderate alcohol consumption during pregnancy on fetal growth and morphogenesis. *J Pediatr* 1978;92:457–60

81. Smith CG, Asch RH. Drug abuse and reproduction. *Fertil Steril* 1987;48:355–73

82. Streissguth AP, Herman CS, Smith DW. Intelligence, behavior and dysmorphogenesis in the fetal alcohol syndrome: a report on 20 patients. *J Pediatr* 1978;92:363–7

83. Harlap S, Shiono PH. Alcohol, smoking, and incidence of spontaneous abortions in the first and second trimester. *Lancet* 1980;2:173–6

84. Day NL, Jasperse D, Richardson G, *et al*. Prenatal exposure to alcohol: effect on infant growth and morphologic characteristics. *Pediatrics* 1989;84:536–41

85. Russell M. Intrauterine growth in infants born to women with alcohol-related psychiatric diagnoses. *Alcoholism: Clin Exp Res* 1977;1:225–31

86. Wright JT, Toplin PJ. Alcohol in pregnancy. *Br J Obstet Gynaecol* 1986;93:201–2

87. Halmesmaki E, Ylikorkala O. The effect of maternal ethanol intoxication on fetal cardiotocography: a report of four cases. *Br J Obstet Gynaecol* 1986;93:203–5

88. McLeod W, Brien J, Loomis C, *et al*. Effect of maternal ethanol ingestion on fetal breathing movements, gross body movements, and heart rate at 37 to 40 weeks' gestational age. *Am J Obstet Gynecol* 1983;145:251–7

89. Boggan WO, Randall CM. Renal anomalies in mice prenatally exposed to ethanol. *Res Commun Chem Pathol Pharmacol* 1979;23:127–42

90. Randall CM, Taylor WJ. Prenatal ethanol exposure in mice: teratogenic effects. *Teratology* 1979;19:305–12

91. Sulik KK, Johnston MC, Webb MA. Fetal alcohol syndrome: embryogenesis in a mouse model. *Science* 1981;214:936–8

92. Young P. *Drugs in Pregnancy*. New York, NY: Chelsea House Publishers, 1987

93. Farrell M, Dawe S, Strang J. Obstetric liason. *Br J Psychiatry* 1989;155:264–5

94. Wilson GS, Desmond MM, Wait RB. Follow-up of methadone-treated and untreated narcotic-dependent women and their infants: health, developmental, and social implications. *J Pediatr* 1981;98:716–22

95. Little BB, Snell LM, Klein VR, *et al*. Maternal and fetal effects of heroin addiction during pregnancy. *J Reprod Med* 1990;35:159–62

96. Ronkin S, FitzSimmons J, Wapner R, *et al*. Protecting mother and fetus from narcotic abuse. *Contemp Obstet Gynecol* 1988;31:178–87

97. Goodman P, Koz G. *Designer Drugs*. New York, NY: Chelsea House Publishers, 1988

98. Jaffe J, Martin WR. Opiod analgesics and antagonists. In Gilman AG, Goodman LS, Rall TW, Murad F, eds. *The Pharmacological Basis of Therapeutics*, 7th edn. New York, NY: MacMillan Publishing Co., 1985: 491–531

99. Gerada C, Dawe S, Farrell M. Management of the pregnant opiate user. *Br J Hosp Med* 1990;43:138–41

100. Wolman I, Niv D, Yovel I, *et al.* Opiod-addicted parturient, labor, and outcome: a reappraisal. *Obstet Gynecol Surv* 1989;44:592–7

101. Glass L. Effects of narcotics on the fetus. In Morselli PL Garattini S, Sereni F, eds. *Basic and Therapeutic Aspects of Perinatal Pharmacology*. New York, NY: Raven Press, 1975:131–8

102. Lifschitz MH, Wilson GS, O'Brian Smith E, *et al.* Fetal and postnatal growth of children born to narcotic-dependent women. *J Pediatr* 1983;102:686–91

103. Chasnoff IJ, Burns KA, Burns WJ, *et al.* Prenatal drug exposure: effects on neonatal and infant growth and development. *Neurobehav Toxicol Teratol* 1986;8:357–62

104. Chavez CJ, Ostrea EM Jr, Stryker JC, *et al.* Sudden infant death syndrome among infants of drug-dependent mothers. *J Pediatr* 1979;95:407–9

105. Pierson PS, Howard P, Kleber HD. Sudden death in infants born to methadone-maintained addicts. *J Am Med Assoc* 1972;220:1733

106. Archie CL, Lee MI, Sokol RJ, *et al.* The effects of methadone treatment on the reactivity of the non-stress test. *Obstet Gynecol* 1989;74:254–5

107. Pond SM, Kreek MJ, Tong T, *et al.* Altered methadone pharmacokinetics in methadone-maintained pregnant women. *J Pharmacol Exp Ther* 1985;233:1–6

108. Edelin KC, Gurganious L, Golar K, *et al.* Methadone maintenance in pregnancy: consequences to care and outcome. *Obstet Gynecol* 1988;71:399–404

109. Offidani C, Chiarotti M, DeGiovanni N, *et al.* Methadone in pregnancy: clinical-toxicological aspects. *Clin Toxicol* 1986;24:295–303

110. Cepeda EE, Lee MI, Mehdizadeh B. Decreased incidence of intraventricular hemorrhage in infants of opiate dependent mothers. *Acta Paediatr Scand* 1987;76:16–8

111. Caviston P. Pregnancy and opiate addiction. *Br Med J* 1987;295:285

112. Marcus J, Hans SL, Jeremy RJ. Differential motor and state functioning in newborns of women on methadone. *Neurobehav Toxicol Teratol* 1982;4:459–62

113. Volpe A, Facchinetti F, Petraglia F, *et al.* Reduction of B-Endorphin levels in the amniotic fluid of heroin addicts. *Obstet Gynecol* 1986;68:606-9

114. Zagon IS, McLaughlin PJ. Analgesia in young and adult rats perinatally exposed to methadone. *Neurobehav Toxicol Teratol* 1982;4:455–7

115. Wang C, Pasulka P, Perry B, *et al.* Effect of perinatal exposure to methadone on brain opioid and alpha-2-adrenergic receptors. *Neurobehav Toxicol Teratol* 1986;8:399–402

116. Naloxone Use in Newborns. *ACOG Committee Opinion*: 65; February 1989

Section IX

Other maternal/perinatal issues

69

Amnioinfusion

E. Amon, J. Kerns and H.N. Winn

INTRODUCTION

Amnioinfusion is a technique in which a crystalloid solution, usually normal saline, is instilled into the amniotic cavity to replace amniotic fluid which may be absent or low. This technique has been employed with increasing frequency and interest during the past two decades. It is used most often during the intrapartum period to prevent, decrease or eliminate variable decelerations and to dilute meconium in attempts to decrease meconium aspiration syndrome[1-8]. During the antepartum period, amnioinfusion is used less frequently. It is mainly used in this setting to facilitate evaluation of fetal anatomy, less commonly in attempts to reduce fetal complications from prolonged oligohydramnios, and rarely to prevent infectious complications from preterm premature rupture of the membranes (PROM)[9-13].

PATHOGENESIS AND CLINICAL ASPECTS OF OLIGOHYDRAMNIOS

Near the end of the first trimester, the amnion and chorion fuse to create the amniotic cavity, which contains approximately 50 ml of amniotic fluid. In early pregnancy, the amniotic fluid is primarily the product of maternal transudate through the amniotic membranes. By the 16th week of gestation, the amniotic fluid volume is mainly regulated by the processes of fetal urination and fetal swallowing. As the pregnancy progresses, the normal amniotic fluid volume rapidly increases to a maximum (range of 0.5–2.01) at about 34 weeks of gestation. The volume then normally decreases as a natural progression[14].

Oligohydramnios can result from:

(1) Any condition that prevents the formation of urine or prevents the entry of urine into the amniotic sac, including bilateral renal agenesis, bilateral multicystic dysplastic kidneys, infantile polycystic kidney disease and complete lower tract obstructive uropathies;

(2) Uteroplacental insufficiency, particularly in the setting of fetal growth restriction or growth retardation;

(3) Post-term pregnancies;

(4) Rupture of membranes;

(5) Prolonged maternal use of indomethacin or other non-steroidal anti-inflammatory drugs;

(6) Abdominal pregnancy;

(7) Reasons unknown, i.e. idiopathic.

The amniotic fluid environment is necessary for normal fetal growth and development, as evidenced by fetal lung hypoplasia and deformations in the case of Potter's syndrome. Pulmonary hypoplasia may well develop if prolonged oligohydramnios (> 2 weeks) secondary to preterm PROM occurs prior to 24 weeks of gestation. The earlier the gestational age when the premature rupture of membranes occurs, the greater the incidence of lung hypoplasia[15]. Oligohydramnios predisposes to umbilical cord compression, which can lead to fetal hypoxia if resultant interference with blood flow is severe, repetitive and prolonged.

Clinical management involves obtaining a patient history to determine:

(1) If she has had leakage of amniotic fluid;

(2) Risk factors for intrauterine growth retardation (IUGR), such as smoking, drug abuse and hypertensive disorders;

(3) A medication history;

(4) A family history of congenital anomalies, especially urinary tract abnormalities.

Physical examination may reveal the fundal height to be less than expected, leakage of amniotic fluid from the cervical canal and/or positive nitrazine or fern tests. Fetal heart-rate monitoring may reveal variable or prolonged decelerations.

Ultrasound evaluation is essential in assessing the amniotic fluid volume and fetal anatomy. Occasionally, amniocentesis with injection of indigo carmine dye may be necessary to diagnose PROM, especially when there is a history of leakage of fluid in the absence of confirmatory findings.

There are multiple clinical definitions of oligohydramnios. These include a subjective gestalt, or a semi-quantitative measurement scheme. Objective measurements include the one largest vertical pocket and the amniotic fluid index. The latter is a summation of the largest vertical dimensions of the four quadrants of the uterine cavity. If the vertical dimension of the largest pocket of fluid is < 1 cm, severe oligohydramnios is said to exist.

The initial step in the clinical management of oligo-hydramnios is to determine the etiology. Management is then based on gestational age, general maternal health, fetal prognosis and the primary concerns of the patient and family.

INDICATIONS FOR AMNIOINFUSION

General overview

Amnioinfusion is generally classified according to labor status as intrapartum or antepartum. The procedure is performed either transcervically or transab-dominally. Its purpose can be diagnostic, therapeutic or prophylactic (Table 1).

During the antepartum period, amnioinfusion may be used transabdominally to improve sonographic imaging, to obtain fluid for culture and cells for karyo-type, and to restore adequate levels of fluid, possibly to prevent lung hypoplasia and arthrogryposis. In selected cases, amnioinfusion provides a vehicle for antibiotic prophylaxis in preterm PROM.

During the intrapartum period, amnioinfusion may be diagnostic (instilling and aspirating fluid to evalu-ate the microbiology of *in utero* infections), therapeutic (to alleviate cord compression) or prophylactic (to pre-vent meconium aspiration).

Antepartum indications: diagnostic

Oligohydramnios poses a diagnostic challenge for the physician, as the differential diagnosis is broad. Etiologies may include urethral outflow obstruction, absent or diminished renal function, PROM, IUGR, congenital malformations or chromosome anomalies. Conventional sonographic imaging may prove inade-quate to view the fetal anatomy, owing to the absence of a satisfactory acoustic window. Fetal positioning, including crowding of small parts, may also impair visualization. Diagnostic imaging is an important step prior to selecting a course of therapy.

In 1988, Gembruch and Hansmann[16] described transabdominal amnioinfusion to improve ultrasound imaging. Later investigators used amnioinfusion in patients with oligohydramnios and were able to pro-vide an adequate acoustic window and perform a com-prehensive ultrasound evaluation[13]. They confirmed the diagnosis of ruptured membranes by transabdo-minal instillation of indigo carmine and observed the passage of blue dye into the vagina. Fluid could be aspirated during the amnioinfusion procedure and the cells cultured for karyotypic analysis.

Antepartum indications: therapeutic

Fisk and colleagues[11] performed serial amnioinfusion in a few selected cases and found that they could avert lung hypoplasia. Serial infusions were initiated as soon as feasible after the diagnosis of oligohydramnios was made and terminated after the canalicular phase of lung development was complete. Since pulmonary hypoplasia remains the most common cause of neo-natal death following vesicoamniotic shunting for obstructive uropathy, serial amnioinfusion may be a viable option in cases of lower urinary tract obstruction.

Therapeutic amnioinfusion has also been used dur-ing the antepartum period to provide transcervical instillation of prophylactic antibiotics in the setting of PROM[9]. The current management of preterm PROM commonly includes systemic maternal prophylactic antibiotics, rendering the local transcervical approach of the Japanese as inadvisable outside a research set-ting. During complicated and prolonged *in utero* pro-cedures, investigators have used both systemic and transabdominal instillation of antibiotics.

Antepartum amnioinfusion may be a useful aid to improve the success rate of external cephalic version. A group of French investigators instilled about 800 ml of solution transabdominally into patients who had failed standard attempts at external version. In each case, (*n* = 6), a successful follow-up attempt at external version resulted[17].

Intrapartum indications: diagnostic

An indwelling, intrauterine, fluid-filled pressure catheter was initially introduced to monitor uterine tonus and uterine activity. The diagnostic use of this medical device has been expanded. In the clinical set-ting of chorioamnionitis, fluid may be aspirated from a catheter port for Gram-stain evaluation, culture and sensitivity, as indicated. A paucity of amniotic fluid may be detected at the time of amniotomy. This could signify thick meconium. Using the intrauterine fluid-filled catheter, lavage and washings may reveal hidden meconium staining.

Intrapartum indications: therapeutic

Using pregnant monkeys, Gabbe and co-workers[18] demonstrated that removal of amniotic fluid produced variable decelerations, which were subsequently elimi-nated when the fluid volume was restored. Many have reported that a similar mechanism of using fluid as an umbilical cord cushion, via transcervical amnio-infusion in the setting of oligohydramnios, results in a significant improvement in variable and prolonged decelerations which do not otherwise respond to con-ventional methods (intravenous fluids, re-positioning, oxygen administration and manipulation of the pre-senting fetal part).

Accurate measurement of the amount of fluid retained is difficult, because unknown quantities of fluid may leak out during transcervical therapy. Ultrasound is recommended by some to assess the amount of fluid in the four quadrants, with repeat evaluations to measure the change. The change in the amniotic fluid index is used as a guide for further infusion therapy[6,13,19]. After the instillation of a fixed initial amount of 600–800 ml by some investigators, if there is no resolution of the variable decelerations or prolonged decelerations, the amnioinfusion is considered to be a failure[1,19–21]. Still others advocate the initial rate of 10–15 ml/min for the first hour, followed by continuous infusion at a rate of 2–3 ml/min thereafter, or gravity infusion of a fixed amount with periodic evaluation of the amniotic fluid volume index[5]. In all cases of amnioinfusion, the investigators set limits for the amount infused, whether it was by amniotic fluid volume index of 8 cm, total volume infused, total rate infused or the resting tone of the uterus, to define the endpoint of the infusion.

Intrapartum indications: prophylactic

Oligohydramnios in the setting of structurally normal fetuses occurring in the intrapartum period may be caused by membrane rupture, IUGR and postdates. With the loss of the amniotic fluid cushion, there is an increased risk of cord compression, which may lead to variable or prolonged decelerations. These decelerations may be associated with hypoxia and acidosis. Using amnioinfusion, variable decelerations have been eliminated or reduced in frequency or severity during the first and second stages of labor, thereby reducing the associated hypoxia and acidosis and leading to an improved fetal acid–base status at delivery[5,7,8,18].

With prophylactic restoration of amniotic fluid volume at term, Strong and colleagues[6,19] reported a decreased incidence of meconium, severe variable decelerations, end-stage bradycardia, operative delivery for fetal distress and low umbilical artery pH values. The investigators concluded that amnioinfusion prophylaxis at term in patients with membrane rupture and oligohydramnios (amniotic fluid index < 5 cm) resulted in reduced intrapartum morbidity.

The presence of meconium may be the natural response of the gastrointestinal system to maturation. It may also be the response of the fetus to a stressful condition such as hypoxia, acidosis or vagal stimulation. Generally, these etiologies are distinguished by the normality of the fetal heart-rate pattern, with completely normal patterns being indicative of normal maturation.

Meconium has been associated with increased perinatal morbidity and mortality, especially due to aspiration of meconium-stained amniotic fluid. Meconium aspiration syndrome, defined as respiratory distress requiring mechanical ventilation in a neonate with meconium aspiration, carries a mortality rate of approximately 25% and accounts for about 2% of all perinatal deaths[4]. The passage of meconium *in utero* occurs in 8–16% of all deliveries; however, meconium aspiration syndrome occurs in only 1–3% of all cases of meconium-stained fluid. Meconium aspiration may occur before or during labor, or during the process of delivery. When meconium is aspirated into the lower respiratory tract, mechanical obstruction and chemical inflammation occur.

Prior to the use of amnioinfusion, combined obstetric and pediatric suctioning of the neonate's airway during and after delivery was the mainstay of preventing meconium aspiration syndrome. This technique, as described by Carson and colleagues[22], was reported to decrease the frequency of meconium aspiration syndrome, assuming the aspiration occurred during the delivery process.

With the advent of amnioinfusion, investigators have reported its beneficial effects in patients undergoing labor complicated by meconium, or meconium and oligohydramnios. Amnioinfusion resulted in a decreased incidence of:

(1) 1- and 5-min Apgar scores < 7;
(2) Meconium visualized below the cords and in the oropharynx;
(3) The presence of thick meconium;
(4) Umbilical arterial cord pH values < 7.20;
(5) Intrapartum fetal distress;
(6) Operative delivery for fetal distress;
(7) Cesarean delivery rates;

Table 1 Amnioinfusion: classification and indications

	Antepartum	*Intrapartum*

Diagnostic	improve sonographic imaging
	obtain fluid and cells for
	  karyotype and culture
	instillation of indigo carmine to
	  rule out premature rupture of the membranes
		assess for meconium – 'no fluid seen on
		  amniotomy'
		obtain intrauterine cultures

Therapeutic	prevent fetal oligohydramnios sequence
	instillation of antibiotics or other
	  drug therapy
	aid in external cephalic version
		repetitive moderate–severe variable
		  decelerations
		prolonged decelerations
		instillation of antibiotics

Prophylactic		oligohydramnios particulate matter meconium staining

(8) Need for positive pressure ventilation of the newborn[2–4].

The rates of Cesarean delivery for arrest disorders were similar in the infused and control groups.

In summary, the use of amnioinfusion provides an additional therapeutic option in labor to treat patients experiencing variable and prolonged decelerations which are unresponsive to conventional methods. Amnioinfusion also allows for prevention of fetal heart-rate-related complications and meconium-related complications when used prophylactically in the intrapartum setting of oligohydramnios or moderate-to-thick meconium staining. The technique is no longer considered experimental by most. This is evidenced by a recent survey of US obstetrics/gynecology academic training programs, revealing that 96% of responding institutions perform amnioinfusion on a clinical basis[23].

CONTRAINDICATIONS

In general, absolute contraindications to vaginal delivery are also absolute contraindications to intrapartum transcervical amnioinfusion. These include placenta previa and prior ruptured uterus. Other contraindications include conditions in which there would be no fetal benefit, such as lethal fetal anomalies and fetal death. Multiple reports have excluded certain types of patients from entry into their protocols. These exclusions are considered relative contraindications and are listed in Table 2.

Clear evidence of fetal distress generally requires expedient delivery rather than temporization with amnioinfusion. Maternal exclusions include maternal heart disease (New York Heart Association functional classification II or greater), as noted by Sadovsky and colleagues[3]. The exclusion is due to the potential fluid overload from hydration or rapid amnioinfusion. Uterine anomalies, which may result from anatomic size limitation, as in a septate uterus, may be less distensible and less pliable to amnioinfusion and have a less rapid change in the pressure–volume curve. Whether chorioamnionitis is a contraindication is clearly controversial, since some consider this condition to be an indication.

Table 2 Relative contraindications to amnioinfusion

Uterine anomalies
Chorioamnionitis
Maternal heart disease class II, III, IV
Intrauterine growth retardation
Fetal malformations
Fetal distress
Malpresentation
Classical or unknown Cesarean section scar
Abruptio placentae
Multiple gestation

PROTOCOLS

A variety of protocols for amnioinfusion have emerged, all of which have common elements and guidelines. The common elements can be divided into pre-infusion preparation and evaluation, infusion equipment and monitoring, and postinfusion evaluation. The common guidelines are patient education and nursing in-service, evaluation of equipment, defining eligibility for infusion and delineating the limits of the infusion. The ideal protocol defining the recommended infusion technique and rate has not been established. Various protocols are available, with variations defined by different authors for their own purposes. No controlled study has demonstrated the superiority of any given protocol.

In general, an eligible patient during labor has one or more of the following indications:

(1) Variable deceleration with or without oligohydramnios;

(2) Meconium with or without oligohydramnios;

(3) Oligohydramnios either at term or preterm as a result of rupture of the membranes;

(4) Oligohydramnios with intact membranes.

Variable decelerations, as previously discussed, are attributed to cord compression, with multiple studies showing that relieving the cord compression and improving the oxygen delivery to the fetus improve the intrauterine environment and the neonatal outcome.

The recommended protocol may include the following:

(1) Informed consent concerning the clinical setting, risks and benefits, and alternatives. Oral consent is legally sufficient, but is best followed up with written consent for amnioinfusion and Cesarean delivery, if indicated.

(2) A pelvic examination is performed to verify presentation, absence of cord prolapse, cervical dilatation and effacement, and fetal station.

(3) Membrane rupture should be confirmed for transcervical amnioinfusion. An internal fetal heart-rate electrode and an intrauterine pressure catheter ready to perform the infusion should be placed appropriately.

(4) Some authors perform ultrasound for amniotic fluid volume index at the start as well as serially, but this is not necessary. Strong and co-workers[19] showed that 250 ml of infusion into a relatively closed system increases the amniotic fluid volume index by 4–4.3 cm (range 0–7.7 cm).

(5) The intrauterine catheter system chosen should be able monitor intrauterine pressure and instill amniotic fluid.

(6) The fluid chosen for infusion is either normal saline or lactated Ringer's.

(7) Consider warming the infusion to 37 °C for the preterm fetus or rapid infusion.

(8) Infuse normal saline at a rate of 10–14 ml/min. If a faster rate is provided (e.g. 15–25 ml/min by gravity), then warming the fluid to 37 °C is recommended. The initial infusion volume is generally 500–600 ml. Some recommend stopping the infusion after a bolus, while others recommend continuous infusion at a lower rate (2–3 ml/min).

(9) Endpoints for the infusion are individualized, based on experience and the purpose to be achieved. These include:

(a) A predetermined volume of 600–1000 ml;

(b) Resolution of variable decelerations;

(c) An amniotic fluid index $\geq$ 8 or 10;

(d) A slow continuous irrigation and lavage at 2–3 ml/min, as long as fluid is continually draining out of the uterus.

(10) If sonographic monitoring is desirable, the following guidelines are recommended:

(a) If amniotic fluid index > 10 cm, no additional bolus is recommended;

(b) If amniotic fluid index = 5–10 cm, a 250-ml second bolus is added and the patient is re-scanned;

(c) If amniotic fluid index < 5 cm, a 500-ml second bolus is added and the patient is re-scanned.

(11) Periodic re-bolus with 500–600 ml of fluid every 6 h is also appropriate, or a constant low infusion rate of 2–3 ml/min may be used, depending on uterine tone, amniotic fluid index determined by periodic ultrasound evaluation or amniotic fluid index and the estimated amount of fluid loss.

(12) Periodic assessment of the fetal heart-rate pattern, uterine tone and activity, volume infused, vaginal leaking and progress of labor is necessary.

(13) Evaluation for complications.

Meconium staining of the amniotic fluid presents concerns of meconium aspiration and the meconium aspiration syndrome. Amnioinfusion is effective in diluting meconium and reducing the incidence of the sequelae. The recommended protocol is the same as that for variable decelerations, with a preference for continual lavage.

Preterm PROM presents two major concerns. There is potential for cord compression and its sequelae and also for intrauterine infection. There should be a low threshold to initiate therapeutic amnioinfusion and systemic chemoprophylaxis.

Oligohydramnios at term, with membrane rupture occurring during labor, subjects the fetus to the potential of cord compression and its sequelae. The protocol recommended is the same as that for variable decelerations.

COMPLICATIONS

Since the advent of amnioinfusion, the adverse effects and potential complications have been reported by many authors as part of their research protocols or in the form of case reports. Complications are summarized in Table 3.

In a recent survey, 26% of centers reported at least one associated complication. The most frequent complication was uterine hypertonus (14%), followed by fetal heart-rate abnormalities (9%)[23].

Although Posner and colleagues[24] found no change in uterine tone with controlled volumes of amnioinfusion and monitoring, they did report the potential of polyhydramnios with over-infusion. Two cases of polyhydramnios with uterine tenderness, one initially thought to be placental abruption[25] and the other with elevated uterine tone and fetal bradycardia from the amnioinfusion[26], were reported. In both cases, when the excess fluid was removed, the elevated uterine tone and uterine tenderness were relieved. In the case reported by Tabor and Maier, the bradycardia resolved after the excess fluid was removed[26]. Strong and co-workers[27] proposed that, with over-distension and elevated uterine tone, disruption of a previous Cesarean section scar was possible. One case of a disrupted uterine scar was noted during a repeat Cesarean delivery in which there was no resolution of the variable decelerations with amnioinfusion[1]. Strong and colleagues[27] reported no change in the incidence of uterine scar disruption.

One case of cord prolapse was reported, but it was the same case in which the delivery was assisted by mid-forceps. No difference in the incidence of nuchal cords was demonstrated[6].

Miyazaki and Taylor[1] noted one case of fetal bradycardia, which occurred during rapid infusion of room temperature fluid (400 ml over 8 min). The proposed reaction was sudden chilling, leading to vasoconstriction, hypertension and reflex bradycardia in the fetus.

Table 3 Complications of amnioinfusion

Potential neonatal electrolyte imbalance
Potential neonatal hypothermia
Umbilical cord prolapse
Acute polyhydramnios
Fetal bradycardia
Elevated uterine tone
Previous Cesarean section scar disruption
Amnionitis/endometritis
Amniotic fluid embolus

They noted no episodes of bradycardia when the infusate was warmed to 37 °C, regardless of the infusion rate. Thus, warming of the fluid appears unnecessary at rates limited to 10–15 ml/min or less.

The rate of amnionitis as a result of amnioinfusion is variable[13,19]. Patients with a higher rate of amnionitis also had more vaginal examinations. When this element was corrected, the rate was not significantly different from the control (non-infused) group[6]. The majority of investigations reported no significant change in the rates of amnionitis associated with amnioinfusion.

Nageotte and co-workers[7] noted that there were no significant differences in the basic electrolytes (Na, K, Cl) and CO_2 in newborns delivered following amnioinfusion as compared to those not subjected to amnioinfusion. The infusate used in this study was normal saline.

No conclusive evidence of the effect of amnioinfusion on the length of labor is available. The evidence presented by Strong and colleagues[6] suggests that there is a significant increase in the length of labor from 10.1 ± 6.5 to 16.8 ± 12.1 h in their group, whereas Schrimmer and co-workers[8] reported a shorter duration of labor in their group of patients. Macri and colleagues[28] noted no significant change in the lengths of labor between the control group and the amnioinfusion group.

Dibble and Elliott[29] reported possible amniotic fluid embolus in two cases following amnioinfusion. No direct association was made to this rare complication associated with pregnancy. They proposed that these two cases were mild because of the dilutional effect of the infusate on the particulate matter in the amniotic fluid. Other authors have also reported on maternal respiratory distress in association with amnioinfusion[30,31].

CONCLUSIONS

Amnioinfusion is currently useful during the intrapartum period for relief of variable and prolonged decelerations, dilution of meconium, and obtaining fluid for evaluation of meconium staining and microbiology. Some authors propose the use of amnioinfusion to instill antibiotics during the antepartum and intrapartum periods to prevent infection, but this use has been little studied[9,10].

The use of amnioinfusion during the antepartum period is not as well studied. It has been shown to be useful in improving the ultrasound image, obtaining fluid for karyotype or culture, instilling indigo carmine as a test for rupture of the membranes, instilling antibiotics as prophylaxis against or treatment for chorioamnionitis, and restoring fluid volume to decrease the likelihood of lung hypoplasia, arthrogryposis or other fetal compression disorders.

Amnioinfusion is now a firmly established part of the clinical management of complicated obstetric patients.

REFERENCES

1. Miyazaki FS, Taylor NA. Saline amnioinfusion for relief of variable or prolonged decelerations. *Am J Obstet Gynecol* 1983;146:670–8

2. Wenstrom KD, Parsons MT. The prevention of meconium aspiration in labor using amnioinfusion. *Obstet Gynecol* 1989;73:642–51

3. Sadovsky Y, Amon E, Bade ME, Petrie RH. Prophylactic amnioinfusion during labor complicated by meconium: a preliminary report. *Am J Obstet Gynecol* 1989;161:613–17

4. Macri CJ, Schrimmer DB, Leung A, *et al.* Prophylactic amnioinfusion improves outcome of pregnancy complicated by thick meconium and oligohydramnios. *Am J Obstet Gynecol* 1992;167:117–21

5. Nageotte MP, Freeman RK, Garitz TJ, Dorchester W. Prophylactic intrapartum amnioinfusion in patients with preterm premature rupture of membranes. *Am J Obstet Gynecol* 1985;153:557–62

6. Strong TH, Hetzler G, Sarna AP, Paul RH. Prophylactic intrapartum amnioinfusion: a randomized clinical trial. *Am J Obstet Gynecol* 1990;162:1370–5

7. Nageotte MP, Bertucci L, Towers CV, *et al.* Prophylactic amnioinfusion in pregnancies complicated by oligohydramnios: a prospective study. *Obstet Gynecol* 1991;77:677–80

8. Schrimmer DB, Macri CJ, Paul RH. Prophylactic amnioinfusion as a treatment for oligohydramnios in laboring patients: a prospective, randomized trial. *Am J Obstet Gynecol* 1991;165:972–5

9. Ogita S, Imanaka M, Matsumoto M, *et al.* Transcervical amnioinfusion of antibiotics: a basic study for managing premature rupture of membranes. *Am J Obstet Gynecol* 1988;158:23–7

10. Imanaka M, Ogita S, Sugawa T. Saline solution amnioinfusion for oligohydramnios after premature rupture of the membranes. *Am J Obstet Gynecol* 1989;161:102–6

11. Fisk NM, Ronderos-Dumit D, Soliani A, *et al.* Diagnostic and therapeutic transabdominal amnioinfusion in oligohydramnios. *Obstet Gynecol* 1991;78:270–8

12. Sherer DM, McAndrew JA, Liberto L, Woods JR. Recurring bilateral renal agenesis diagnosed by ultrasound with the aid of amnioinfusion at 18 weeks gestation. *Am J Perinatol* 1992;9:49–51

13. Quetel TA, Mejides AA, Salman FA, Torres-Rodriguez MM. Amnioinfusion: an aid in the ultrasonographic evaluation of severe oligohydramnios in pregnancy. *Am J Obstet Gynecol* 1992;167:333–6

14. Brace RA, Wolf EJ. Normal amniotic fluid volume changes throughout pregnancy. *Am J Obstet Gynecol* 1989;161:382

15. Thibeault DW, Beatty EC, Hall RT, *et al.* Neonatal pulmonary hypoplasia with premature rupture of fetal membranes and oligohydramnios. *J Pediatr* 1985;107:273

16. Gembruch U, Hansmann M. Artificial instillation of amniotic fluid as a new technique for the diagnostic evaluation of cases of oligohydramnios. *Prenat Diagn* 1988;8:33–45

17. Benifla JL, Goffinet F, Darai E, *et al.* Antepartum transabdominal amnioinfusion to facilitate external version after initial failure. *Obstet Gynecol* 1994;84:1041

18. Gabbe SG, Ettinger BB, Freeman RK, Martic CB. Umbilical cord compression associated with amniotomy: laboratory observations. *Am J Obstet Gynecol* 1976; 126:353–8

19. Strong TH, Hetzler G, Paul RH. Amniotic fluid volume increase after amnioinfusion of a fixed volume. *Am J Obstet Gynecol* 1990;162:746–8

20. Galvan BJ, VanMullen C, Brookhuizen FF. Using amnioinfusion for the relief of repetitive variable deceleration during labor. *J Obstet Gynecol Neonatal Nurs* 1989;18:222–9

21. Haubrich KL. Amnioinfusion: a technique for the relief of variable decelerations. *J Obstet Gynecol Neonatal Nurs* 1990;19:293–303

22. Carson BS, Losey RW, Bowes WA, Simmons MA. Combined obstetrics and pediatric approach to prevent meconium aspiration syndrome. *Am J Obstet Gynecol* 1976;126:712–15

23. Wenstrom K, Andrews WW, Maher JE. Amnioinfusion survey: prevalence, protocols, and complications. *Obstet Gynecol* 1995;86:572

24. Posner MD, Ballagh SA, Paul RH. The effect of amnioinfusion on uterine pressure and activity: a preliminary report. *Am J Obstet Gynecol* 1990;163:813–18

25. Sorensen T, Subeck J, Benedotte T. Intrauterine pressure in acute iatrogenic hydramnios. *Obstet Gynecol* 1991;78:917–19

26. Tabor BL, Maier JA. Polyhydramnios and elevated intrauterine pressure during amnioinfusion. *Am J Obstet Gynecol* 1987;156:130–1

27. Strong TH, Vage JS, O'Shaughnessy MJ, *et al*. Amnioinfusion among women attempting vaginal birth after Cesarean delivery. *Obstet Gynecol* 1992;79:673–4

28. Macri CJ, Schrimmer DB, Greenspoon JS, *et al*. Amnioinfusion does not affect the length of labor. *Am J Obstet Gynecol* 1992;167:1134–6

29. Dibble LA, Elliott JP. Possible amniotic fluid embolism associated with amnioinfusion. *J Mat Fetal Med* 1992;1:263–6

30. Dragich DA, Ross AF, Chestnut DH, *et al*. Respiratory failure associated with amnioinfusion during labor. *Anesth Analg* 1991;72:549

31. Maher JE, Wenstrom KD, Hauth JC, *et al*. Amniotic fluid embolism after saline amnioinfusion: two cases and review of the literature. *Obstet Gynecol* 1994;83:851

70

Anesthesia and analgesia in pregnancy

G.A. Albright, R.M. Forster and P.J. Bolster

INTRODUCTION

> 'Bring forth men-children only;
> For thy undaunted mettle should compose
> Nothing but males.'
>
> 'Macbeth', Shakespeare

One may suppose that, in this day, the very apotheosis of the hard-driving competent and competitive woman of the 1990s, there may be more than a few to whom Macbeth's admiring statement could be accurately addressed. But now the apron has been dropped, the book of nursery rhymes laid aside and instead the conservative pin-stripped suit is donned, the briefcase hefted; the mother's gaze of compassion overset by the bright-blistered eye of ambition and astute appraisal.

Many Macbeths of both sexes run to and fro the glass-plated market-places of today. Times have changed in most respects. Nevertheless, it remains an immutable fact that the burden of bringing the next generation of intrepid entrepreneurs into being befalls upon 50% or so of the populace and that the final hours of this 9-month manufacturing period still hurt.

There is a resurgent interest in making the experience of giving birth as pleasant and safe as possible. Pecuniary-minded hospital administrators hire interior decorators to redesign their labor suites according to the latest and most fashionable colors of the day. Obstetric monitors address the issue of safeguarding fetal well-being moment-by-moment and many obstetric practitioners are confronted by patients who are no longer interested in labor being a period of self-immolation.

Enter the obstetric anesthesiologist with a wondrous apothecary fairly bristling with new analgesic drugs and techniques to meet the demands of the savvy and sophisticated consumers of today. Within the last decade, several new agents and methods have become relatively commonplace in the vanguard centers of obstetric anesthesia. Consequently as word gets out, more and more hospitals are obligated to duplicate these analgesic measures if for no other reason than to remain competitive. It is our intent then to review some of the fundamentals and to present some of the advances made in the ever-changing field of obstetric anesthesia.

NOCICEPTIVE PATHWAYS OF PARTURITION

The neuronal pathways over which the pain of labor is transmitted have been well delineated. Pain originating from the uterine contractions is carried from the corpus and cervix to Frankenhauser's ganglion by afferent C fibers, then through both the pelvic and the middle and superior hypogastric plexi to ultimately run within the sympathetic chains on each side of the vertebral bodies. These fibers ultimately synapse upon the secondary neurons found in the Rexed laminae of the dorsal horn at spinal segments T10 to L1. Early in the first stage of labor, only the more central segments T11 and T12 are involved. As labor advances, the two outer peripheral dermatones are incorporated as well.

With the onset of the second stage of labor, the focus of pain is shifted from the abdomen to the vagina and perineal floor, which are innervated by the sacral fibers of S2, S3 and S4. These are carried by the pudendal nerve, which travels within the caudae equinae to synapse upon the respective dermatomal segments inside the spinal cord. From the Rexed laminae, the noxious stimuli are transmitted via the secondary neurons to the contralateral spinothalamic tracts, which then ultimately synapse upon the thalamic nuclei, the last interval before reaching the cognitive cortical centers.

During pregnancy, there is an increase in neuronal sensitivity to local anesthetic blockade. Datta and colleagues[1] demonstrated that, when contrasted to its non-pregnant counterpart, pregnancy enhanced the speed of onset of a bupivacaine block upon the vagus nerve of a pregnant rabbit, suggesting either increased local anesthetic penetration through the axonal membrane or an increase in the sensitivity of the receptor site to these compounds. Recently, Butterworth and co-workers[2] demonstrated an increased sensitivity of the median nerve in pregnant women to the local anesthetic effects of lidocaine. They could only speculate that hormonally induced changes in local anesthetic binding sites on the sodium channel, or subtle changes in the myelination of the peripheral nerves, might be the underlying cause(s). They also concluded that the increase in cephalad spread seen during epidural anesthesia resulted primarily from neuronal, not mechanical, causes. Animal studies by Datta and associates[3] and Jayaram and Carp[4] support the theory that progesterone contributes to the increased sensitivity of the parturient to inhalational anesthesia and opiates. This most probably results from a potential ion- or γ-aminobutyric acid-mediated hyperpolarization of neuronal cells[5]. Similar mechanisms are hypothesized for local anesthetics.

Considerable investigative attention has recently been turned towards the goals of identifying the architectural arrangement and composition of the nerve membrane and of the various ionic channels that lie within. Harris and Groh[6] described the phospholipid–protein content of the membrane, finding that phosphatidylcholine predominated in the outer layer, whereas phosphatidylethanolamine and phosphatidylserine were more prevalent within the inner layer. Perhaps more significantly, they reported a large number of gangliosides located in the outer membrane of the axon. These sphingolipid–protein molecules were believed to enhance the ability of local anesthetic molecules to penetrate the lipoprotein membrane and thereby inhibit the influx of sodium through its specific ionic channel. Gangliosides enhance the penetration of the membrane by general anesthetic molecules as well. Therefore, the higher the ganglioside content of a given cell membrane, the greater the sensitivity of that portion of the organ system to the anesthetic effects. A differential in ganglioside content could explain the increased sensitivity of the inhibitory neurons (as compared to the excitatory neurons) to local anesthetic blockade. This could possibly serve to explain the appearance of local anesthetic-induced convulsions prior to the onset of global neuronal depression, as seen clinically when local anesthetics are unintentionally injected intravascularly. It may also conceivably play a role in the increased sensitivity of neurons to the effects of local anesthetics during pregnancy, although this remains as yet to be determined.

The tortoise and the hare

Noxious stimuli are transmitted by both the unmyelinated C fibers and the myelinated A-delta fibers. The C fibers are responsible for carrying the sensation of dull, visceral pain, in contrast to the A-delta fibers, which transmit the sharp, incisional pain. Tourniquet pain is carried by both sets of nerve fibers. Contrary to the earlier teaching concerning the differential sensitivity of these two groups of fibers, it is now believed that the lowly unmyelinated C fibers may actually be more resistant to local anesthetic blockade than their myelinated brethren. This is due to the fact that it takes more 'electrical energy' to make the salutatory leap from one mode to the next in order to perpetuate impulse conduction on the myelinated A-delta fiber.

The C fiber, lacking myelin, simply propagates an impulse to the area of the membrane immediately adjacent to the electrically agitated segment; this requires less electrical energy, allowing the fiber to persist for a longer period of time in the phase of sodium channel blockade induced by ambient local anesthetic agents, despite their lingering presence. Thus, speed of conduction is traded for durability in the C fiber, allowing it to transmit messages in defiance of local anesthetic concentrations which would otherwise prevent such electrical propagation in the faster A-delta fiber. The fact that motor blockade, propagated along A fibers, occurs after sensory blockade is not caused by relative sensitivity, but rather by the architectural arrangement of the various fibers within the dorsal nerve root. The C fibers are located more peripherally and therefore are blocked before the more centrally positioned A fibers.

REGIONAL AND LOCAL ANESTHESIA FOR OBSTETRICS

When local anesthetics are applied in the immediate vicinity of a peripheral nerve, their ability to block the sodium channel is of paramount importance. When applied within the neuraxis, the pharmacodynamic situation becomes far more complex and their action is not limited to a single ionic channel. The local anesthetic molecules are capable of inhibiting a host of membrane-associated proteins, including adenylate cyclase[7], guanylate cylase[8], calmodulin-sensitive proteins[9] and enzymes involved in ion migration, such as the Na^+/K^+-ATPase[10] and Ca^{2+}/Mg^{2+}-ATPase[11]. Enzymes involved in prostaglandin and prostacyclin production are also inhibited[12], along with substance P binding and evoked increases in intracellular Ca^{2+}[13].

Presynaptic calcium channels, which promote neurotransmitter release during depolarization, are blocked by local anesthetics, thereby reducing the amount of transmitter involved[14]. Postsynaptic neuroreceptors are also adversely affected by local anesthetics, such that the chemically gated postjunctional currents are reduced in caliber[15–17].

When local anesthetics are injected into the epidural space, the initial anesthetic effect may indeed evolve as a consequence of sodium channel blockade at the site of the spinal nerve root. Additional mechanisms of anesthesia result from several other effects as the molecules penetrate into the spinal cord itself.

Local infiltration

This technique is simple to perform and it is most commonly used in preparation for the episiotomy incision. Minimal maternal risks are involved when using 5–10 ml of 1% lidocaine, 1% mepivacaine or 2% 2-chloroprocaine. Local infiltration for Cesarean section may be required when anesthesia coverage is unavailable or regional anesthesia is contraindicated and general anesthesia with tracheal intubation impossible. It is not a skill universally shared by all obstetricians, nor is it always simple to execute. When performed satisfactorily it is the least complicated, most direct form of anesthesia, with the least impact upon maternal–fetal physiology. Ranney and Stanage[18] described their technique using 1% procaine in volumes of less than 60 ml. They recommended making three columns, each of four points of infiltration: one midline, the others at points 4 cm laterally. The midline is then infiltrated just under the skin, without deep fascial infiltration. Midline infiltration of the rectus fascia is carried out when the transversalis and peritoneum are exposed. The transversalis and peritoneum are then infiltrated, fanning out from the midline to the more lateral margins. Topical anesthesia of the peritoneum may be performed by splashing 20–30 ml of a sterile, weak local anesthetic solution, such as lidocaine 0.25%, directly onto its surface.

Paracervical block

Paracervical block, a simple technique for labor analgesia, can be performed by the obstetrician when the anesthesiologist is unavailable. However, the injection of 8–20 ml of local anesthetic into the paracervical region has been associated with fetal bradycardia. Although fetal bradycardia is usually transient, experience has demonstrated an increased incidence of intrauterine demise or neonatal morbidity and mortality associated with paracervical block.

The explanation for the fetal bradycardia, which appears between 2–10 min after the injection (although usually transient, may endure for up to 30 min), is controversial. It could be a direct result of local anesthetic-induced fetal myocardial depression; however, animal studies have indicated that relatively large plasma concentrations (40 µg/ml) of lidocaine are well tolerated in the normoxic fetus. Only when hypoxemia and acidosis are concurrent and superimposed will the fetal myocardium fall prey to the depressive effects of the lower plasma concentrations found clinically (6–8 µg/ml) such that a bradycardia may become manifest. It is more likely that fetal bradycardia is a result of systemic fetal hypoxemia resulting from inadequate placental perfusion (owing either to direct uterine arterial vasospasm or to uterine hypertonus) or from umbilical vasoconstriction. Uterine hypertonus has been demonstrated to be an etiological cause of abnormalities in the fetal heart rate[19] and may be secondary to the abrupt sympathetic blockade induced by the local anesthetic. The direct local anesthetic effects upon myometrial tissue include a generalized dose-dependent increase in the resting uterine tone, but a decrease in the strength of contraction. Greiss and

colleagues[20] have suggested that, in addition, there may be a direct vasospastic effect upon the uterine arteries, which may reduce uterine blood flow by as much as 25%. The vasoconstrictive effect is even more pronounced in the vessels of the placenta. It is not mediated by the α-adrenergic receptors, but appears rather to be a result of a direct effect of the local anesthetic upon the vessel wall itself.

Paracervical block should certainly be avoided under conditions of placental insufficiency, prematurity or existent fetal distress. In reality, it has become obsolete in many, if not most, obstetric suites, because of the availability of safer and more effective regional anesthetic techniques. Parturients with fetal bradycardia should be placed in the left lateral decubitus position and given supplemental oxygen to maximize oxygen delivery to the stricken fetus. If present, maternal hypotension should be promptly treated with ephedrine, 5–10 mg intravenously.

Pudendal block

Pudendal block is still an effective and commonly practiced method of providing anesthesia for the second stage of labor, particularly at time of delivery. Perineal anesthesia may be obtained by injecting 10 ml of local anesthetic into the region surrounding the pudendal nerve just below the ischial spine. However, pudendal anesthesia alone is frequently inadequate when forceps are applied or intrauterine manipulations are required. Maternal complications of pudendal anesthesia include infection, hematoma formation and convulsions secondary to unintentional intravascular injection of local anesthetic.

Fetal scalp injection

The unintentional injection of local anesthetic into the fetal scalp is a potential hazard of paracervical and pudendal blocks and of caudal anesthesia. It was initially recognized and documented in 1979 by Hillman and associates[21], who described the clinical consequences of neonatal bradycardia, hypotension, hypoventilation and/or apnea and hypotonia. Seizures were frequently seen within several hours after birth. Treatment consists primarily of promoting adequate urine output and, provided that hypoxia is avoided, the outcome is usually excellent.

Spinal anesthesia and analgesia

Great therapeutic modalities often have rather humble, if not obscure, origins. So it is with spinal anesthesia. Leonard Corning, a neurologist, attempted to inject cocaine into the intrathecal space of his patient in order to cure him of a private sexual malfeasance that was deemed unacceptable by the strict Victorian moral codes of 1885. According to Dr Corning's assessment, no therapeutic benefit was recorded, but this really depends upon the perspective that one chooses. The patient, for his part, may have felt differently.

Fourteen years later, the esteemed August Bier and the hapless Dr Hildebrandt performed spinal anesthetics on each other. Twenty-three minutes later they were able to hammer upon their shins and apply strong pressure to their testicles without experiencing the painful consequences of their peculiar deeds. The large volume of spinal fluid lost by each did cause them to endure the world's first spinal headaches the next morning. Just how much of their subsequent suffering was due to the loss of spinal fluid versus the excessive consumption of wine and cigars enjoyed during their festive celebration of the previous night will never be discerned. Bier could not be sure, but while he languished patiently in bed for a full 9 days, his resident, Dr Hildebrandt, 'feeling very poor but with great physical effort' managed to attend to his professional duties the next morning. Rank has its privileges.

Physiological pharmacology of spinal anesthesia

The cerebrospinal fluid (CSF) is produced by the choroid plexus at a rate of about 500 ml/day. At any one time, there is a total volume of approximately 150 ml, half of which resides intracranially, the other half being found within the spinal cavity. The majority of CSF circulates within the cranial vault; only 10% finds its way into the spinal subarachnoid space. Thus, CSF circulation around the cord is too slow to have any effect upon the distribution of local anesthetic.

Local anesthetics deposited in the subarachnoid space are absorbed into the spinal cord by two processes. One is direct diffusion across the pia mater along a concentration gradient from CSF into the superficial portions of the cord itself. The second mechanism involves penetration through the spaces of Virchow–Robin, which accompany the nutrient arterioles as they enter the cord. By this latter process, molecules of local anesthetic are carried rapidly into deeper areas than by the former mechanism of simple diffusion[22]. Because myelin is predominantly comprised of lipids, the lipid-soluble anesthetic molecules are distributed to the more heavily myelinated tracts of the spinal cord: the posterior and lateral columns and to a lesser extent the anterior corticospinal tracts. Greater concentrations of local anesthetics are reportedly found in the posterior and lateral columns, despite greater vascular access to the anterior portion of the cord. These reports suggest that it is the lipid content of the neurolemma that predominates over tissue blood flow in governing the distribution of lipid-soluble pharmacological agents[23].

Factors which govern the intrathecal spread of local anesthetic solutions (and thus the final dermatomal level achieved) include patient age, spinal column length and position, the site of injection and the position of the needle, the dosage and volume of the agent employed and, finally, the density and baricity of the solution relative to that of the spinal fluid. The chronic increase in intra-abdominal pressure brought about by pregnancy results in an engorgement of the epidural veins, which in turn reduces the volume of CSF in the lower thoracic and lumbar regions of the cord. This results in a greater cephalad spread per given amount of local anesthetic injected[24,25]. A recent study by Pasricha and co-workers[26] found that there was a statistically different height in spinal anesthesia obtained (T2–T3 versus T5–T6) when a standard dose of 8 mg of hyperbaric tetracaine was administered intrathecally to patients in the extremes of morphology: height 1.53 m, weight > 102 kg versus height 1.64 m, weight 73.3 kg, respectively. They concluded that their tall and thin patient population coming to section was better served by larger doses of tetracaine; both spinal cord length and weight will indeed influence dermatomal spread.

Clinical impressions notwithstanding, studies by Marx and colleagues[27], Hopkins and associates[28] and others have demonstrated that neither straining, coughing nor uterine contractions result in an increase in spinal CSF pressure. Increases in skeletal muscle activity arterial pressure, as are found during labor, will cause an increase in CSF pressure. But there is no concomitant intrathecal redistribution of local anesthetics. This is because the transient increase in CSF pressure is instantly transmitted equally and entirely through both the intrathecal and intracranial spaces. Therefore, no pressure differential is ever established and the injected agent is undisturbed[29].

Intrathecal local anesthetics

Tetracaine (8–10 mg) used to be the 'gold standard' in patients undergoing Cesarean section under spinal anesthesia. Lidocaine (60–70 mg) has been employed; bupivacaine (7.5–15 mg) is still the most popular drug currently being utilized. Lidocaine suffers from a relatively brief duration (45–75 min), which conceivably could be out-distanced by the duration of surgery under various clinical circumstances. Intrathecal spread is also less predictable with lidocaine.

Bupivacaine has been found to be well suited for Cesarean section. It is combined with 8.5% dextrose in order to make it hyperbaric and is available as a 0.75% solution, affording 90–120 min of anesthesia when injected into the subarachnoid space. Norris[30] recommends a dose of 12 mg of bupivacaine for patients coming for Cesarean sections who are between 146 cm and 178 cm in height. He found that the average dermatomal level achieved was T3, with a range of T7 to C8. He reasoned that the kyphotic thoracic curvature caused hyperbaric spinal solutions to 'pool' at its nadir, which is at T5–T6. Admittedly, the very obese or very short patients may experience higher levels of dermatomal spread and, conversely, patients whose height exceeds 178 cm may require more than 12 mg of bupivacaine.

Hauch and Hartwell[31] recently published a clinical study in which they found a lower incidence of intraoperative hypotension with bupivacaine compared to equal volumes of 1.0% tetracaine and 10% procaine. They reasoned that bupivacaine may have a less profound sympathetic blockade and/or an induced increase in adrenergic activity (higher plasma catecholamine levels were found with bupivacaine). The tetracaine–procaine combination was also associated with an unnecessarily prolonged motor blockade (260 min versus 133 min with bupivacaine). Higher sensory levels with tetracaine were also demonstrated. Thus, it is tempting to conclude that, when subarachnoid block is selected for Cesarean section anesthesia, bupivacaine is perhaps the most appropriate local anesthetic currently available.

Small amounts of narcotics may be added to intrathecal bupivacaine. Morphine (0.20–0.25 mg) provides extended postoperative analgesia without excessive side-effects. Alternatively, intrathecal fentanyl (25 µg) may be added to enhance operative anesthesia. If an epidural catheter is utilized, epidural morphine may subsequently be administered in the usual doses.

Intrathecal opioids

Intrathecal opioids have added an entirely new dimension to intrathecal analgesia. Early investigative efforts by Wang and co-workers[32] utilized intrathecal morphine in doses of 0.5–1.0 mg. Later investigative efforts have attempted to discern the ideal doses of the newer, more lipid-soluble narcotics, fentanyl and sufentanil, alone or in combination with local anesthetics. Within the field of obstetric anesthesia, narcotics by and large have been used in combination with epidurally administered local anesthetics for analgesia and anesthesia. Intrathecal administration of Duramorph® (0.5–1.0 mg) is less common, in part because of the intensity of the side-effects. Furthermore, the analgesia resulting from narcotics alone is generally inferior to that associated with local anesthetics; the use of narcotics with local anesthetics results in excellent analgesia.

Intrathecal narcotics have recently been recommended for labor analgesia using fentanyl (25 µg) and morphine (0.25 mg) diluted with normal preservative-free saline to 2 ml[33]. An alternative is to use only fentanyl (25 µg) or sufentanil (10 µg) diluted to 2 ml with saline in patients who are not opposed to having an epidural catheter placed. The latter approach gives a shorter duration of analgesia, but dose not have the severity of side-effects associated with morphine or the respiratory monitoring requirements. The use of a new 24–26 gauge Whitacre needle (with a pencil point tip and a side hole) has practically eliminated the risk of spinal headache. This technique is very effective in early labor (the patient rarely feels the second contraction), does not slow labor or interfere with descent or delivery (no autonomic or motor block), but offers no perineal anesthesia. The duration of analgesia is 2–6 h with morphine and 2–3 h with fentanyl and sufentanil. Patients may ambulate and do not require any more monitoring other than that which a patient receives for systemic medication. If the patient agrees, an epidural catheter can be placed immediately after the intrathecal narcotic injection, flushed with several milliliters of saline and activated later, if required. Weaker epidural solutions may be adequate because of the residual analgesic effect of the intrathecal narcotic. Side-effects with intrathecal morphine include a 30% incidence of pruritis as well as nausea and vomiting, especially after delivery. These side-effects may be prevented, or at least minimized, by oral naltrexone (25 mg), given 30 min after delivery. Late respiratory depression is also a potential threat, but is rare in the otherwise young and healthy obstetric population.

Saddle block

Spinal anesthesia has traditionally been utilized in modern obstetrics under two clinical circumstances. The first has been commonly referred to as a 'saddle block' and is of value for an imminent vaginal delivery in a woman who does not have an indwelling epidural catheter. Speed of execution and onset are its main advantages. Rapid anesthesia of the vagina and perineal floor with profound relaxation of the corresponding muscles is provided, yet abdominal muscle tone is maintained. It is ideally suited for an instrumental delivery or the delivery of a premature fetus whose soft calvarium is to be spared compression against a resistant perineal floor. Hyperbaric lidocaine (30–40 mg) or tetracaine (3–4 mg) are the two most commonly used drugs, with the former being the most popular because of its shorter duration. Employing 2 ml of 1.5% hyperbaric lidocaine provides satisfactory anesthesia, yet tends to preserve abdominal muscle tone.

Cesarean section

Another clinical use for spinal anesthesia is during Cesarean section. This technique offers the advantages once again of speed in execution and onset of blockade, which can be of value in the urgent setting of fetal distress. Aspiration and other airway management risks, such as failure to intubate the trachea, which are associated with a general anesthetic, may be obviated. The sensory and motor blockade is profound, more so than with epidural anesthesia. Therefore, supplemental analgesia or sedation is rarely required.

Primary disadvantages of intrathecal anesthesia include maternal hypotension (more profound than epidural anesthesia because of the speed of sympathetic blockade) and the inability to titrate the dose to obtain the dermatomal level desired. The block is fixed at the duration of the specific agent, and it cannot be extended should operative needs lengthen. Continuous spinal anesthesia may avoid this disadvantage, but there have been reports of an association of continuous spinal anesthesia with cauda equina syndrome[34,35] and the potential for local anesthetic-induced neurotoxicity[36,37]. In light of this recent literature, the use of this approach should be judicious.

The most current form of labor analgesia has been termed 'combined spinal–epidural' or CSE. Still popularly referred to as 'paradise analgesia', it is gaining popularity among obstetric anesthesiologists, owing to its rapid onset of analgesia, simplicity of administration and its record of patient safety. To perform CSE, a 17-Tuohy needle is placed in the epidural space and, through it, a 27-Whitacre needle is inserted into the intrathecal space. The Whitacre needle is withdrawn and an epidural catheter is advanced through the epidural needle, which is then removed. The catheter is taped to the patient's back.

Onset of analgesia is within minutes and is quite profound. Motor weakness is minimal, permitting patient ambulation. Although maternal hypotension is rare, 500 ml of preloading with an intravenous crystalloid solution is still recommended. The duration of analgesia is 1–3 h. Side-effects include pruritis, which is common, and, rarely, the experience of difficulty in swallowing caused by the sensation of a 'fullness in the throat'. Both are reversed with small doses of intravenous Narcan (0.2 mg). An additional concern is fetal bradycardia, resistant to changes in maternal position, which may occur within 10–60 min after the administration of CSE. Although the etiology is uncertain, it is hypothesized to be related to a decrease in the circulating epinephrine/norepinephrine ratio, resulting in uterine hypertonus, and/or uterine arterial spasm. Prompt relief has been demonstrated with 50 μg of intravenous nitroglycerin or 0.4 mg of nitroglycerin as a sublingual spray (two puffs per administration). Concerns that the epidural needle may enter the hole made by the Whitacre needle have not proven to be valid.

Subsequent labor analgesia may be instigated with solutions of 0.01% bupivacaine and fentanyl (100 μg/ml). Continuous infusion rates may vary, ranging from 5 to 12 ml/h. Patient-controlled epidural anesthesia (PCEA) may be superimposed upon this background infusion or it may be substituted for the infusion altogether. A popular PCEA regimen is 5 ml incremental doses, which are limited to three per hour and no closer than 5 min apart. As with a conventional epidural anesthetic, labor analgesia may be continued until the birth of the baby.

Combined spinal–epidural techniques

Some investigators and clinicians have combined both epidural catheter insertion and single-shot spinal analgesia into one technique. An epidural Tuohy needle is initially placed into the epidural space and then a spinal needle is directed through it intrathecally. A subarachnoid dose of narcotic and/or local anesthetic is injected through the spinal needle, which is then removed and the catheter passed through the remaining Tuohy needle into the epidural space for maintenance of anesthesia. Finally, the Tuohy needle itself is withdrawn and the epidural catheter left in place until after delivery. The advantages of this technique are that it provides rapid and profound anesthesia, which can easily be extended if the need arises.

Epidural anesthesia and analgesia

Caudal anesthesia pre-dates lumbar epidural analgesia in the history of obstetric analgesia. It does have the advantage of catheter proximity to the sacral segments receiving nociceptive stimuli during the second stage of labor. It otherwise suffers from several disadvantages when compared to the lumbar approach, particularly for analgesia during the first stage of labor. Much more local anesthetic drug (20–25 ml) is required to reach the dermatomal segment of T10, subjecting the mother and fetus to higher plasma concentrations because of greater vascular absorption. Additionally, the catheter is inserted at a location (the sacral hiatus) which is at greater risk for contamination and infection. Therefore, caudal epidural analgesia is generally not preferred in obstetric anesthesia, unless a lumbar approach is contraindicated, as by the presence of a local dermatological infection or a previous laminectomy in that region. Caudal analgesia is occasionally utilized in the 'double-catheter' technique, whereby two catheters are inserted: the lumbar catheter for first stage of analgesia and the caudal catheter for analgesia during the second stage.

Lumbar epidural anesthesia has become, and still remains, the quintessential method of pain relief for labor and delivery. Utilizing the indwelling lumbar epidural catheter, it affords the anesthesiologist the ability to titrate the dosage of analgesic medications both to their desired effect and dermatomal spread, and to maintain analgesia or anesthesia to match the duration required. Finally, it allows for the adjustment of the medications as obstetric needs change. Medications other than the traditional local anesthetics have found their way into the armamentarium of the obstetric anesthesiologist during this last decade.

Absolute perfection continues to elude the questing physician, although he never ceases to continue charging the windmills. Epidural analgesia has its small percentage of failures and its sensory blockade tends to be less profound than that afforded by spinal anesthesia.

Generally speaking, epidural anesthesia is somewhat more time-consuming to perform and the onset of sensory blockade takes slightly longer, although carbonated 2-chloroprocaine comes close to spinal anesthesia in onset time. When compared to spinal anesthesia, in which a small volume of local anesthetic is injected rather precisely over the spinal segment intended to be blocked, epidural anesthesia requires larger volumes. Hence, through vascular absorption, higher plasma levels of local anesthetics are obtained. If local anesthetics are used excessively, these plasma levels could reach toxic levels, resulting in central nervous system and/or cardiovascular toxicity. Similar toxic manifestations may result from unintentional intravascular injection of much smaller quantities of local anesthetics. Unintentional intrathecal injection, resulting in a high spinal block, is an additional concern with epidural analgesia. In either case, airway protection, as well as ventilatory and cardiovascular support, are promptly required; the adverse effect is otherwise self-limiting.

There are a host of physiological benefits afforded to the parturient by epidural analgesia besides the obvious relief of pain. Adequate analgesia reduces maternal catecholamines, whose β_2 effects might instigate or contribute to a dysfunctional pattern of labor[38]. Provided that maternal hypotension is avoided (by adequate hydration and the maintenance of the lateral decubitus position), uterine perfusion generally increases, resulting in less fetal acidosis, particularly at the culmination of the second stage of labor. Maternal hyperventilation in response to the painful uterine contractions, and the consequential hypoventilation during the time between contractions, are both obviated by effective analgesia; the hypocapnia of the former promotes uterine artery vasoconstriction and the hypoventilation of the latter sponsors both maternal and fetal hypoxemia, neither of which are habitually deemed salutary.

Epidural anesthesia is contraindicated under the following circumstances: patient refusal, localized dermatological infection, maternal sepsis with bacteremia, and bleeding diathesis.

Much concern has been generated over the potential deleterious effects of epidural anesthesia upon the course of labor and the well-being of the fetus. The chemical sympathetectomy resulting from epidural blockade is proportional to the number of dermatomal segments involved. In a woman who has been inadequately prehydrated, epidural analgesia for labor may result in maternal hypotension and inadequate uterine perfusion, which may jeopardize fetal oxygenation. Research has demonstrated that a direct relationship exists between decreased uterine blood flow and decreased uterine activity[39]. Progress during the first stage may be impeded if the epidural block is initiated during the latent phase[40]. In addition, epinephrine included in the local anesthetic mixture may be absorbed intravascularly in sufficient quantities to slow labor, according to its β_2 stimulatory properties[41]. Oddly enough, excessive crystalloid prehydration may also retard the progress of labor[42]. Admittedly, most of these desultory effects may be overcome with exogenous oxytocin administration. As a general rule, epidural local anesthetics are usually best withheld until the active phase of labor has commenced.

The actual maelstrom of contention has centered over the effects of epidural analgesia upon the progress of the second stage of labor and the incidence of forceps delivery. Excessive analgesia may separate the parturient from the knowledge that her uterus is currently contracting and that she should therefore bear down and push at this time. Partial motor blockade is not a concern during the first stage of labor, but, during the second stage, it is of paramount importance. The managing obstetrician is concerned not only with the impairment of abdominal muscle tone by the epidural analgesic, but, in addition, the relaxant effect of the epidural analgesic upon the muscles that comprise the vaginal wall, lest malrotation of the presenting fetal head results in the necessity of a low- or mid-forceps delivery[43,44]. These concerns have encouraged many obstetricians to request that the analgesia provided through the epidural catheter be allowed to wear off as the second stage commences, frequently to the dismay and distress of the parturient, who has grown rather fond of the comfort so mercifully provided during the preceding hours of labor.

There are those who maintain that a properly maintained epidural anesthetic will not result in an increase in forceps deliveries, provided that the obstetrician is willing to extend in his mind the limit to which he will allow the second stage to last. Recently, the American College of Obstetrics and Gynecology extended the recommended time over which the second stage of labor may last from 2 h in the unmedicated primipara, to 3 h in the primipara with ongoing epidural analgesia. This recognizes the fact that epidural anesthesia may indeed prolong the second stage, but usually without deleterious effects concerning the mother or neonate. Maresh and Choong[45] noted less neonatal acidemia in those mothers who remained reasonably comfortable during the second stage and that waiting on the part of the obstetrician avoided an increase in forceps deliveries.

Chestnut and colleagues[46] have carried the torch one step further. In 1987 they reported that, although there were indeed modest increases in the duration of the second stage (124 versus 94 min) and in the incidence of forceps deliveries (53% versus 28%) when a constant infusion of 0.125% bupivacaine was maintained, there were also tendencies towards better neonatal acid–base status and Apgar scores. This prompted them to conclude that the prolongation was not deleterious, provided that adequate maternal hydration, analgesia and internal fetal monitoring were maintained. Recently, this same group found that second-stage epidural analgesia maintained by a constant infusion of a lesser concentration of bupivacaine (0.0625%) plus fentanyl (2 µg/ml) not only provided reasonably adequate analgesia, but also avoided both the increase in forceps delivery and the increase in duration of the second stage[47]. This was felt to be the result of reducing yet further the local anesthetic impact on muscle tone, thereby removing any factors which might otherwise have contributed to malrotation of the presenting fetal head. Of greater concern than the incidence of instrumented vaginal delivery is a reported increased incidence of Cesarean section for dystocia in patients receiving epidurals for labor and delivery[48–50]. These reports have been countered by reports which do not show an increase in operative delivery in patients receiving epidural analgesia[46,51,52]. It has proven to be an elusive issue to study secondary to difficulties in randomization and bias elimination, yet proponents and opponents of epidural analgesia continue to try. In most reports, placement of an epidural at 4 cm dilatation or greater did not increase the incidence of Cesarean section; therefore, this has become a guideline on many labor and delivery units.

Epidural local anesthetics

The three local anesthetic agents used most commonly in obstetrics today are bupivacaine, lidocaine, and 2-chloroprocaine. Each is characterized by different speeds of onset and clinical duration. These physical properties are further affected by varying the local anesthetic concentration. The addition of other analgesic agents, such as narcotics, to the local anesthetic mixture affords new dimensions of analgesic flexibility, utilizing different spinal receptor systems to accomplish the traditional goal of relief from pain.

2-Chloroprocaine enjoys the unique advantages of quick onset of action and virtually no accumulation in maternal or fetal plasma, owing to its rapid metabolism by the endogenous esterase enzymes. Its half-life in maternal plasma is only 21 s; the fetal half-life is only slightly longer – 43 s, to be specific. Therefore 2-chloroprocaine is the drug of choice in the setting of fetal prematurity, when avoiding toxic fetal plasma levels of local anesthetics is of primary concern. When carbonated (by adding 2.5 mEq of bicarbonate to a 30-ml volume of 2-chloroprocaine), its speed of onset approaches that of a spinal block. This allows the anesthesiologist to still utilize the indwelling epidural catheter to provide epidural anesthesia for emergency Cesarean section. Insertion of an epidural catheter may be useful in a high-risk patient who may be likely to require an emergency section at any time or in a woman whose upper airway anatomy may render a rapid direct laryngoscopy and tracheal intubation impossible. By employing carbonated 3% 2-chloroprocaine via an indwelling catheter, one may establish epidural anesthesia in a matter of minutes.

As stated above, the 2-chloroprocaine metabolite, 4 amino-2-chlorobenzoic acid, may interfere with local anesthetic binding to the sodium channel receptor. In a similar manner, it may also interfere with and shorten narcotic-induced analgesia[53]. Some investigators, e.g. Hughes and co-workers[54], believe that, in the case of postoperative Duramorph analgesia, the interference is only apparent. They propose that the 2-chloroprocaine wears off before analgesia with Duramorph can begin, thus permitting an undesired 'window' of pain to occur.

Recently, various investigators reported on the neurotoxic effects that 2-chloroprocaine had upon the spinal cord when it was accidentally injected intrathecally[55]. Investigative speculation arose as to whether the toxicity was related to the low pH, the antioxidant sodium bisulfate or to the 2-chloroprocaine itself. Animal results differed, depending on which species were being used. Wang and associates[56] in 1984 concluded that it was the sodium bisulfate that was the causative agent. He found that when sodium bisulfate, adjusted to a pH of 5.3, was applied to the rabbit's subarachnoid space, the characteristic neurological deficits appeared. The application of 2-chloroprocaine alone failed to reproduce the toxic results. Currently, most researchers believe that the bisulfate exists in a state of equilibrium with sulfur dioxide and water with the CSF. Sulfurous acid is formed when the sulfur dioxide crosses the neuronal membrane and it is the former that is the actual neurotoxic agent. Therefore, clinical neurological toxicity is a result of the combination of the bisulfate with the attendant higher acidity. The newer preparations of 2-chloroprocaine have replaced the sodium bisulfate with ethylenediaminetetraacetic acid which lacks neurotoxic potential, even in concentrations ten to 20 times the amount utilized, allowing 2-chloroprocaine to once again be employed with relative impunity.

Lidocaine and mepivacaine are of intermediate onset and duration. They are both employed epidurally for obstetric analgesia or anesthesia. Both lidocaine and mepivacaine are associated with tachyphylaxis upon repeated administration during labor. The underlying mechanisms are incompletely understood, but may to various degrees involve downregulation of the receptors, neuronal edema, decreasing intraneuronal diffusion or altered epidural distribution[57]. Bupivacaine was once held to be the ideal drug for obstetrics. Its ability to block the sensory modalities exceeds the impairment of motor function, thereby satisfying one of the foremost requirements for an obstetric local anesthetic agent. Furthermore, its longer duration reduces the frequency of reinjections through the catheter. Excellent surgical anesthesia is achieved by concentrations of 0.50%, while the dilute concentrations of 0.0625–0.25% satisfy the analgesic requirements for labor.

Epinephrine in concentrations between 1 : 200 000 and 1 : 400 000 potentiates and prolongs the analgesia and anesthesia of lidocaine and bupivacaine when given epidurally[58]. There is also a synergistic effect with local anesthetics when narcotics are added.

Although unintentional intravascular injection of lidocaine may result in seizures, its cardiotoxic effects occur only at much higher plasma concentrations, such that the plasma concentration ratio for cardiovascular to central nervous system toxicity is 3.5 : 1, whereas for the more lipid-soluble agents etidocaine and bupivacaine, the ratio is considerably narrowed, being only 1.5 : 1. Finally, as lidocaine acts to decrease automaticity and depresses phase 4 spontaneous diastolic depolarization, its cardiotoxic effects are manifested essentially as a global depression of myocardial function.

The ability of bupivacaine to effect a blockade of neuronal transmission is enhanced with repeat administration. Indeed, the initial administration of bupivacaine alone may result in a sensory block which is less than completely satisfactory. In some obstetric centers, bupivacaine is often routinely combined with lidocaine to intensify the sensory blockade and to hasten the speed of onset. The overall duration of blockade is still that of bupivacaine; in effect one proverbially obtains 'the best of both worlds'. During the second stage, when impairment of motor function is to be minimized, weak concentrations of bupivacaine (0.0625–0.125%) are combined with fentanyl (50–100 µg) or sufentanil (10–20 µg) for perineal analgesia.

Continuous infusions of bupivacaine (0.04–0.125%) and fentanyl (2.0–5.0 µg/ml) or sufentanil (0.5–1.0 µg/ml) may be employed in lieu of intermittent bolus injections. Rates of infusion may vary from 5 to 15 ml/h. Purported advantages include greater safety, as such a slow infusion rate would only result in the loss of sensory blockade should the catheter migrate intravascularly, and fewer demands upon the anesthesia 'manpower reserve', although, ideally, patients whose analgesia is maintained by continuous infusion should have their levels checked hourly.

A new amide local anesthetic, ropivacaine, has shown promise in the arena of obstetric anesthesia and analgesia. In early testing, this drug has demonstrated similar anesthetic properties to bupivacaine. Advantages of ropivacaine include a less profound motor blockade and decreased cardiotoxicity, both of which could be advantageous in the parturient[59–61].

Bupivacaine cardiotoxicity

Local anesthetic potency and toxicity are both proportionate to their lipid solubility. Bupivacaine and etidocaine, besides being highly protein-bound, are additionally the most lipid soluble of all currently available local anesthetics and, therefore, are the most potent but also the most toxic. All local anesthetics will act to block channel conduction of various ions. At lower concentrations, only the sodium channel, which in the myocardium governs conductance (and therefore heart rate), is affected. Therefore, a decrease in heart rate is one of the earliest signs of local anesthetic myocardial toxicity. The fact that bupivacaine is so lipid soluble confers upon it a 'fast in–slow out' nature with respect to receptor binding properties. This stands in sharp contrast to the less lipid-soluble lidocaine, being typified by a 'fast in–fast out' effect upon the channel receptors. The, 'fast in–slow out' potential of bupivacaine increases its toxic potential in two ways. First, its wash-out time is prolonged, making resuscitation more difficult and, second, it extends the duration of blockade long enough to involve slower action potentials. Lidocaine is limited to affecting the faster action potentials associated with the faster heart rates, but bupivacaine, because of its prolonged dissociation constant, affects the slower action potentials of even the slower heart rates as well.

Bupivacaine decreases myocardial conductivity in a non-homogeneous manner, promoting re-entry dysrhythmias which can lead to malignant dysrhythmias such as ventricular tachycardia or fibrillation. Yet, the toxic effects of bupivacaine are not limited to the myocardial conduction system. As the plasma concentration of bupivacaine rises, it (and the other local anesthetics as well) inhibits the release of calcium from the myocardial sarcoplasmic reticulum, upon which contractility depends. In fact, although bupivacaine is four times as potent a depressor of myocardial conduction as lidocaine, it is up to five times more potent with respect to depression of contractility at slow heart rates.

In summary, bupivacaine pharmacodynamically throws a molecular 'one–two punch' at the hapless myocardium. Initially, it can either lower the heart rate into a state of electromechanical dissociation, in which its depressive effects upon contractility are then maximized[62], or it can incite ventricular tachycardia or fibrillation, in which there is little chance of bupivacaine wash-out unless left ventricular performance can be enhanced by exogenous means. It should additionally be remembered that any local anesthetic effect is heightened if metabolic acidosis and/or hypoxemia are concomitantly present.

Finally, the cardiotoxic effects of bupivacaine are enhanced during pregnancy, which prompted the US Food and Drug Administration in 1983 to no longer recommend the 0.75% formulation for obstetric anesthesia. Pregnancy results in a decrease in the protein binding of bupivacaine and etidocaine (from 95% to 60–70%). This acts to increase the amount of free, unbound bupivacaine available to penetrate the membrane and attach to the channel receptor sites. Additionally, the rapid vertebral–azygos venous blood flow brings higher concentrations of absorbed local anesthetics directly into the sanctuary of the right atrium. Finally, progesterone itself, obviously available in higher concentrations during pregnancy, has the ability to enhance the cardiotoxic potential of bupivacaine and etidocaine, but not lidocaine, by a mechanism not yet completely understood[63].

Test dose

There is a 1% incidence of vascular cannulation by an epidural catheter in the obstetric population[64]. Should such an event go unrecognized, a subsequent injection through the wayward catheter could result in a maternal catastrophe. The quest for the ideal test dose for epidural anesthesia began in 1981 when Moore and Batra[65] recommended the incorporation of 15 µg of epinephrine into a 3-ml bolus of local anesthetic. Should this small dose enter the vascular system, the amount of local anesthetic would be inconsequential and the epinephrine itself would engender a transient increase in maternal heart rate and blood pressure occurring within 20–40 s after injection and lasting 1–3 min.

While this system serves the general non-obstetric population well, the parturient in labor has her own set of endogenous catecholamines rising and falling with the pain of each contraction, making such an 'epinephrine response' extremely difficult to interpret. In addition, concern arose among a number of clinical investigators that epinephrine, even in such a small amount as 15 µg, might cause a reduction in uterine blood flow via its vasoconstrictive α-receptor-stimulating effects. Hood and colleagues[66] reported a 20–40% decrease in uterine blood flow lasting for 3 min in the gravid ewe model in response to the intravascular injection of 10–20 µg of epinephrine. This decrease essentially mimicked the reduction found during a normal uterine contraction and no detrimental effects upon the fetus were observed. Chestnut and Weiner[67] corroborated the results of Hood and associates by demonstrating an epinephrine-induced reduction in uterine artery blood-flow velocity in the gravid guinea pig. Earlier work by Wallis and Shnider[68] had shown that epinephrine injected into the epidural space in the dose range of 60–80 µg (the amount used concomitantly in a normal bolus for establishing labor analgesia) was indeed associated in the gravid ewe with a 14% reduction in uterine blood flow for approximately 15 min. The distribution pattern of blood flow to the placenta versus the myometrium (reduced in favor of the myometrium under conditions of maternal stress) remained, under these circumstances, undisturbed. Finally, no changes in fetal cardiovascular parameters or acid–base status were observed.

It is important to remember that species differences may jeopardize conclusions drawn from observations made in one animal model about the situation that actually exists in another, namely the human being. In 1981, Albright and co-workers[69] examined the impact that 40–50 µg of epinephrine, added to epidurally administered 2-chloroprocaine, had upon the uterine blood flow of women in labor. They found no evidence of a reduction in uterine blood flow, suggesting the hypothesis that unlike the myometrial vascular bed of the lower animals, that of the human undergoes a compensatory vasodilatory response when confronted with a decrease in perfusion pressure.

Although the fears that epinephrine may have a deleterious effect upon the blood supply of the healthy fetus are now considered unfounded, the 15 µg of epinephrine as a test dose has been justifiably criticized with respect to accuracy of interpretation. Chestnut and colleagues[70] found the 15-µg test dose to be of value only when it was used for the non-laboring woman having an epidural catheter inserted for an elective Cesarean section. Both this group and that headed by Leighton[71] reported an unacceptably high instance of false-negative and false-positive interpretations of the epinephrine response in laboring patients. On the other hand, Colonna-Romano and associates[72] found 15 µg of epinephrine to be quite sensitive in laboring patients, but with a less than idealistic specificity. Attempts to devise a more accurate method of interpretation may prove excessively cumbersome for routine bedside employment.

In 1986, Abraham and Harris[73] proposed a simple combination of 3 ml of 1.5% lidocaine (45 mg) made hyperbaric with 7.5% dextrose to which was added Moore and Batral's now classic 15 µg of epinephrine, to serve as a test dose for epidural anesthesia. The hyperbaric lidocaine, if injected intrathecally, would manifest as a spinal block within 2 min; the epinephrine would herald an intravascular injection within 1 min, as described previously. The following year, Grice and Eisenach[74] proposed using a dose of plain local anesthetic. Their initial report recommended 100 mg of 2-chloroprocaine, which was altered in a report published the following year[75] preferring 100 mg of lidocaine, which was equally sensitive and nearly as specific. When compared to the lidocaine test dose, the use of 2-chloroprocaine was found to be associated with a decrease in the duration of the subsequent bupivacaine–fentanyl blockade[76]. This is in accordance with the earlier findings of Hodgkinson and co-workers[77]. Two years after the report of Hodgkinson and colleagues, Corke and associates[78] isolated a metabolite of 2-chloroprocaine, 4-amino-2-chlorobenzoic acid, which, when applied to the sciatic nerve of the animal model, shortened the subsequent bupivacaine-induced blockade. They concluded that 4-amino-2-chlorobenzoic acid interfered with the binding of bupivacaine to the channel receptor.

Alternatives to epinephrine as a test marker have been reported. In 1987, Leighton and Norris[71] reported reasonable success utilizing 5 μg of isoproterenol. This enjoyed the additional advantages of lacking α-receptor-stimulating properties, thereby avoiding any potential component of uterine artery vasoconstriction. Cherala and co-workers[79] recently experimented with 15 mg of ephedrine. Although the resultant increases in blood pressure and heart rate were predictable, their onset time was prolonged and they were therefore easily masked and overwhelmed by the combers of the uterine contractions.

In summary, although some clinicians use epinephrine in obstetrics (with the possible exception of the severe pre-eclamptic), its specificity and sensitivity are lowered unless the patient is not in labor or the contractions are spaced far apart. Slow, incremental injections of local anesthetics, with the attempt to elicit the sensations of tinnitus, circumoral numbness or lightheadedness, is still the safest method in avoiding an unintentional intravascular injection of that which was intended for deposit in the epidural space alone.

Epidural opioids

The epidural administration of narcotics in conjunction with local anesthetics for obstetric analgesia has proved to be valuable in clinical practice. The side-effects of pruritis, urinary retention, nausea and respiratory depression are generally less intense when opioids are administered epidurally. The addition of opioids, whose action upon the μ_1-receptor is that of pure analgesia, produces pain relief without motor and sympathetic blockade. This makes the use of narcotics particularly valuable when retention of motor tone or sympathetic activity is desired.

Pruritis is undoubtedly the most frequent side-effect encountered after intrathecal or epidural narcotic administration. Urinary retention, nausea and delayed respiratory depression have also been documented, but are far less common. Respiratory depression, occurring 12–24 h after the injection of morphine (Duramorph), has been attributed to slow cephalad migration of narcotic, which ultimately reaches the brainstem, or slow diffusion into the μ_2-receptors located near the medullary respiratory control centers. Such respiratory depression is profoundly rare among the young and healthy obstetric population. It is far more frequent in the elderly and among those patients who are concomitantly receiving other central nervous system depressive medications.

The undesirable side-effects are the result of the action of the narcotic upon the μ_2-receptor. Small doses of narcotic antagonists, such as naloxone (Narcan), nalbuphine (Nubain) and orally administered naltrexone[80], are effective in reversing undesirable side-effects yet retaining analgesia to a satisfactory degree. Larger doses of naloxone may also reverse the analgesia

associated with μ_1 activity, along with μ_2-mediated side-effects.

Epidural narcotics are given in doses roughly five to ten times the amount used for intrathecal analgesia. Morphine (Duramorph) set the initial standard against which other narcotics are measured. It has the unique advantage of providing a long duration of analgesic effect, 18–26 h, when used for postoperative analgesia. Being the most water soluble of all the narcotics, its concentration in the CSF remains higher than those concentrations associated with its newer and relatively more lipid-soluble cousins. Lingering on in the CSF, morphine migrates rostral to act upon the medullary μ_2-receptors, producing nausea and potentially respiratory depression. Admittedly, the incidence of respiratory depression is rare (less than one in 10 000 in the otherwise healthy obstetric population), but it has necessitated careful attention to respiratory rates by the nursing staff in centers where it is routinely employed.

Because the long duration of morphine analgesia is so ideal for the initial management of postoperative pain, clinicians have been loathe to give it up. Rather, they have sought to reduce the incidence of side-effects by adding other agents. An interesting report by Lawhorn and associates[81] demonstrated that the addition of 3 mg of butorphanol (Stadol®), a κ-agonist and a μ-antagonist, to 4 mg of morphine, not only maintained excellent postpartum analgesia, but also served to completely eliminate the side-effects of nausea and pruritis associated with the use of epidural morphine alone. Furthermore, the incidence of respiratory depression, as reflected by an oxygen saturation of less than 90% on the pulse oximeter, was found to be less in the butorphanol–morphine group. On the other hand, Naulty and colleagues[82] found that the epidural combination of 2.5 mg of morphine and 20 μg of sufentanil was also effective in providing excellent post-Cesarean analgesia, with significant reductions in side-effects. Again, the incidence of respiratory depression was not increased over that associated with the controls.

The more lipophilic narcotics, fentanyl and sufentanil, are associated with fewer side-effects, being limited primarily to pruritis. Being more lipophilic, they are more rapidly absorbed into the lipid structures of the spinal cord, such as myelin, with far lower concentrations remaining behind in the CSF. DeSousa and Stiller[83] were able to demonstrate that all three agents (fentanyl, alfentanil and sufentanil) were found in the cisterna magna of the ewe within 5 min of epidural injection, with sufentanil being present in the highest amounts and alfentanil in the lowest concentrations.

Epidural administration of fentanyl (50–100 μg) or sufentanil (20–30 μg) has been used in concert with low concentrations of bupivacaine to enhance and increase the duration of analgesia for labor. Both intermittent bolus and continuous epidural infusion techniques have proven to be both safe and effective with regard to both mother and neonate[84,85]. It is interesting parenthetically to observe that sufentanil, when administered systemically, enjoys an analgesic potency nine to 13 times that of its immediate predecessor fentanyl; yet, when it is injected epidurally, the margin of greater potency is reduced to a ratio of only 2–3 : 1, i.e. 20 μg of sufentanil is roughly equivalent to 50 μg of fentanyl.

Earlier reports notwithstanding, alfentanil has now taken its rightful place in obstetric analgesia. Offering a particularly fast speed of onset[86], superior to that of sufentanil and fentanyl, it is most effective when given as a 350–500-μg epidural bolus in concert with 10 ml of 0.125% bupivacaine. This is followed by a continuous infusion of the same concentration of bupivacaine combined with alfentanil (10 μg/kg per hour, at an overall rate of 10 ml/h[87]. Fentanyl (50–100 μg) and/or sufentanil (20–30 μg) have also improved the quality and duration of intraoperative anesthesia when added to surgical concentrations of lidocaine and bupivacaine during Cesarean section, without undue neonatal narcosis[88,89].

Shivering

Intraoperative shivering occurs in 30% of epidural anesthetics, the etiology of which remains enigmatic at this time[90]. Different measures have been instigated in an attempt to reduce this most annoying side-effect, including warming intravenous infusions[91] and even the epidural[92] injection itself. Epidural injections of sufentanil (50–100 μg) or Demerol (25 mg) are sometimes beneficial, as is the intravenous injection of Demerol after general anesthesia.

Tremor is commonly attributed to normal thermoregulatory shivering, occurring apparently independently of changes in core or superficial temperatures or in sensations of cold[93]. Although changes in spinal cord temperature are capable of eliciting thermoregulatory responses in most species, reports are conflicting regarding human beings. The subjective sensation of thermal well-being is mostly controlled by the more superficial skin-surface temperature, as opposed to changes in the core temperature. Furthermore, subjective thermal sensation and the resultant physiological responses, such as vasoconstriction and shivering, are under the control of different thalamic areas and do not necessarily respond in a synchronous fashion[94].

Cold fibers fire tonically and are transmitted via the A-delta fibers, whereas warm receptors transmit their afferent input over the C fibers in an episodic fashion. In those who perceive a sensation of warmth despite decreases in superficial temperatures, local anesthetics may be effecting a block of the more actively firing nerve fibers (phasic block); the slower-firing C fibers carrying the sensation of warmth may be relatively more resistant to the local anesthetic effect. Sessler

and Ponte[95] postulate that tremor during epidural anesthesia is the resultant physiological response to the convergence of several afferent thermal stimuli. Furthermore, pregnancy synergistically adds to the effect of local anesthesia. They discount the notion of heat loss as an inciting cause, observing a balance between the heat lost to the vasodilated legs, as opposed to the heat conserved from the vasoconstricted upper torso, so that the total heat loss to the environment is minimal. Redistribution of body heat may cause a central hypothermia which is not necessarily accompanied by the perception of cold. The shivering that accompanies central hypothermia, while considered a normal thermoregulatory response, is not mediated by epidural thermal receptors. Its etiology remains unknown. Central hypothermia probably has more to do with delayed shivering as seen in the recovery room than with the etiology of the early intraoperative tremors.

Complications of regional anesthetic techniques

Spinal headache

A postdural puncture headache, a potential threat with any intrathecal technique, has been greatly reduced by employing needles of small caliber and a 'pencil-shaped' tip, which spreads the fibers of the subarachnoid membrane rather than cutting them. In particular, Snyder and associates[96] performed 25 spinal anesthetics for Cesarean sections and tubal ligations utilizing a 22-gauge Whitacre needle (with a pencil tip) and compared the incidence of spinal headaches with another group of 25 patients in whom a 26-gauge Quincke needle (with a bevelled tip) was utilized. They reported a 25% incidence of spinal headache in the group of patients for whom the Quincke needle was used, versus an incidence of only 4% when, paradoxically, the larger 22-gauge Whitacre needle was employed. With the increasing popularity of the 25-gauge Whitacre needle, the incidence of postdural puncture headache is less than 1%.

In a recent study by Naulty and colleagues[97], the issue of anesthetic solution potentially promoting a postdural puncture headache was addressed. They found a slightly higher incidence of headache (9.5% and 7.6%) during the first 36 h when solutions of 5% lidocaine with 7.5% glucose and 0.75% bupivacaine with 8.5% glucose were employed. This compares to an incidence of 5.8% when a solution of 1% tetracaine with 10% procaine was used. After 36 h, there were no differences among the three groups in the number of patients requiring epidural blood patches for spinal headaches, the combined incidence being 1.6–1.7%.

They divided the postdural puncture headache conceptually into two phases. The first phase, lasting 24 h or more, was due to reactive vascular hyperemia, a reflexive cerebral vasodilatation that was in response to the short-lived cerebral vasoconstrictive effects of the low concentrations of lidocaine or bupivacaine. Caffeine, a cerebral vasoconstrictor, was effective in treating the reactive vascular hyperemia. Alternatively, since both solutions contained glucose, it was proposed that this agent was potentially capable of causing an osmotic effect on the CSF and/or direct meningeal irritation. That there were fewer headaches in the tetracaine–procaine group may be due to the lack of glucose or to the fact that the esterase enzymes in the CSF may prevent significant concentrations of either ester anesthetic agent from ever reaching the cerebral region.

The second phase conforms to our classical understanding of the 'spinal headache', in that it is due to the meningeal tug in the erect position secondary to CSF leakage. Unresponsive to caffeine, it is successfully treated with the now classic epidural blood patch, which serves to correct the hydraulic deficit.

There is some evidence to suggest that the addition of narcotic to the intrathecally administered local anesthetic may reduce the incidence of spinal headache. Johnson and colleagues[98] reported that mixtures of bupivacaine and fentanyl were retrospectively associated with fewer spinal headaches when compared to those patients who had received bupivacaine alone. They believed that fentanyl altered the cerebral vascular dynamics or perhaps affected the production or release of intermediary substances. Abboud and co-workers[99] were unable to find a similar mitigating effect when intrathecal morphine was combined with bupivacaine. Further clinical investigation will be necessary before this controversial topic can be satisfactorily resolved.

If an inadvertent dural puncture occurs with a Tuohy needle during epidural catheter placement, a severe postdural puncture headache is likely. In 1987, Denny and colleagues[100] suggested that the insertion of a spinal catheter may serve to lessen the incidence of postdural puncture headache. They intimated that the prolonged presence of the foreign-body catheter incited an inflammatory reaction and promoted closure of the hole. Other investigators have been unable to corroborate their fortuitous results[101]. In any case, a majority of these patients will require epidural blood patches.

Maternal hypotension

Maternal hypotension has always been a primary concern of obstetricians, lest regional anesthesia, administered for the mother's benefit, compromises uteroplacental blood flow and jeopardizes fetal well-being. Although epidural anesthesia may also cause maternal hypotension, it is usually less precipitous in

onset and degree than spinal anesthesia, owing to the slower onset of sympathetic blockade.

Resting sympathetic tone maintains a level of arterial and arteriolar vasoconstriction at about 50%. Sympathetic blockade resulting from spinal anesthesia does not completely obliterate arterial vasomotor tone; it is reduced overall by about 12–14%. However, the venous capacitance vessels, in which 70% of the blood volume normally resides, do not possess the ability to retain even a fraction of their resting tone when subjected to a chemical sympathectomy. In sympathetic blockade, virtually 90% of the circulating blood volume essentially stagnates in the venous side, preload is reduced drastically and cardiac output consequently decreases. Furthermore, the atrial stretch receptors remain silent and an exacerbating sinus bradycardia ensues. If the patient is initially hypovolemic, vagal tone is currently enhanced by surgical manipulation of the mesentery, or sympathetic blockade is high enough to incorporate all the cardioaccelerator nerves (T1–T4), then a profound bradycardia or rarely cardiac arrest may result. Subsequent ischemia of the brain stem medullary centers may then result in a respiratory arrest as well.

Therefore, the treatment of hypotension under either regional anesthetic technique must be prompt and aggressive, including oxygen, intravenous fluids, left uterine displacement, instituting Trendelenburg position or raising the legs to increase central blood volumes and venous return thereby restoring cardiac preload. Finally, a vasopressor, such as ephedrine, is frequently necessary. Ephedrine enhances venous and arterial tone, but also exerts a positive inotropic and chronotropic effect upon the myocardium, which increases cardiac output and uterine blood flow.

Cardiac effects

A study by Palmer and associates[102] highlighted the disconcerting fact that ischemic electrocardiogram changes occurred in 35 out of 93 healthy parturients undergoing Cesarean section under either spinal or epidural anesthesia. The changes were indicative of subendocardial ischemia and were sometimes accompanied by complaints of substernal chest pain and dyspnea. The authors concluded that bonafide subendocardial ischemia in young healthy women had indeed occurred for several reasons. First, with a concomitant sympathectomy into the upper thoracic dermatomes, rapid intravenous infusions, the uterine autotransfusion and the expanded intravascular volume associated with pregnancy all resulted in the limited compensatory response of left ventricular expansion. This, in turn, caused an increased myocardial workload and oxygen consumption. Second, decreased diastolic pressure associated with the decreased systemic vascular resistance reduced the coronary perfusion pressure. Thus, increased oxygen demand superimposed upon a decreased oxygen supply caused transient ischemia of the subendocardium, the region associated with the highest intramural pressures during systole. In the light of these findings, the authors recommend less aggressive utilization of prehydration and greater reliance upon vasopressors, such as ephedrine, to maintain adequate blood pressure and ostensibly tissue perfusion. Further investigation by Matthew and colleagues[103] did not correlate ST segment changes with wall motion abnormalities by transthoracic echocardiogram. They, as well as others[104], have concluded that no significant myocardial dysfunction occurs with these electrocardiogram findings. However, the etiology and significance of this finding remain unclear.

Neurological complications associated with epidural anesthesia

It is one of our less redeeming facets that we tend to look for convenient, if not spurious, places upon which to place blame when circumstances go awry or well-laid plans miscarry. So it is with regional anesthesia. The whiteness of our 10-gallon hat that once we so proudly sported not hours before, when all was well and analgesic, now somehow takes on a more tarnished appearance when a neurological complaint arises in the postpartum period. It therefore behoves both the anesthesiologist and the obstetrician to understand the limitations of the potential neurological malfeasance that such an otherwise benevolent procedure is capable of.

Backache is common during pregnancy and well into the postpartum period, having an occurrence rate of 25–45%, regardless of whether or not regional anesthesia was employed[105]. Much of it may be due to ligamentous strain, although moderate-to-severe back pain of a persistent nature may be a true harbinger of serious pathology beneath. For example, the hormonal and postural changes associated with gestation may alter the microscopic structure of the longitudinal ligaments which support the spinal column. Not only may the ligamentous strain account for gestational back pain, but it may also contribute to intervertebral laxity, subjecting the disk to an increased risk of herniation, particularly during the mechanical stresses associated with labor[106]. Protrusion of a lumbar disk would present symptomatically with sciatica, segmental paresthesia, decreased deep tendon reflexes and motor weakness. Low back pain is also commonly due to sacroiliac disk dysfunction. Thoracic disk herniation has also been reported, presenting initially in the immediate postpartum period[107].

The important aspect in treating gestation-related backache is to appreciate the complete differential diagnosis. The occurrence of disk herniation is

unrelated to the concomitant administration of epidural anesthesia, having an overall incidence of one in 10 000 pregnant patients.

Epidural anesthesia may, however, lead to epidural abscess or hematoma. Epidural hematomas present as back pain with motor–sensory loss, usually within the first 24 h after the administration of the epidural block. They are understandably more common in patients who are on anticoagulant therapy, but may also occur in the absence of such therapy[108]. Low-dose 'mini-heparinization' is no longer considered a contraindication to epidural anesthesia[109]. The hazards of initiating anticoagulant therapy in patients who have indwelling epidural catheters have not been well studied, but it is probably unwise to allow the catheter to remain in the epidural space for any significant length of time after anticoagulation has been established.

The persistence of a pharmacologically induced motor–sensory blockade could easily mask the signs and symptoms of a cord compression syndrome. In an unblocked patient, localized back pain, which may be sudden in onset and lacerating in nature, is the most common initial complaint[110], followed by a loss of both motor and sensory function, which may acutely present in a nerve root distribution pattern. Bowel and bladder function may be compromised. As the hematological mass expands, cord or nerve root compression may be joined by vascular compression as well, potentially resulting in further neurological damage because of ischemia and/or necrosis. If a diagnosis of a potentially permanent spinal cord destructive lesion is suspected, a neurosurgical consultation should be promptly obtained. Magnetic resonance imaging of the involved area can document the existence of an intraspinal or epidural mass. An emergency decompressive laminectomy is curative. Recovery is proportional to the speed of diagnosis and therapeutic intervention[111].

Epidural abscess is happily a rare complication of epidural anesthesia (13 in 750 000 epidural anesthetics). Epidural anesthesia is understandably contraindicated when dermatological infection exists directly over the intended site of needle penetration. However, most epidural abscesses occur as a secondary 'seeding' site; the primary nidus of infection exists elsewhere. Unlike an epidural hematoma, the size of this compressive lesion grows slowly over several days to 1 week. The signs and symptoms of an epidural abscess, which include progressive, localized back pain and tenderness exacerbated by movement or coughing, fever, nuchal rigidity, along with leukocytosis and an elevated sedimentation rate, may appear as late as 6 or 7 days after the epidural anesthetic was administered[110]. Treatment is straightforward: intravenous antibiotics and neurosurgical decompression.

The anterior artery spinal cord syndrome may occur as a result of an epidural anesthetic. The anterior spinal artery supplies the ventral two-thirds of the spinal cord, which includes the anterior and lateral spinothalamic tracts, the anterior horn cells and the pyramidal tracts. The posterior dorsal columns are uninvolved. Signs and symptoms include loss of pain and temperature sensations, flaccid paralysis, followed later by spastic rigidity and retention of urine and feces. Motor loss is usually the predominant symptom. The motor–sensory distribution may be bilateral or it may be asymmetrically unilateral[112]. The symptoms are usually transient; complete recovery is the rule. Richardson and Bedder[113] recently reported an occurrence of the anterior spinal artery syndrome in a patient with an indwelling epidural catheter. The symptoms were transient and unilateral; it was postulated that they were the result of temporary arteriolar spasm in response to vascular irritation by the epidural catheter, which was reversed by its removal. Meningeal irritation and radiculitis related to an indwelling epidural catheter have also been described[114].

The blood vessels supplying the spinal cord are relatively unresponsive to the vasomotor effects of catecholamines. It is not felt that the addition of epinephrine, in weak concentrations, to local anesthetics poses a significant risk with respect to promoting vasoconstriction and compromising spinal cord blood supply. The syndrome arises under such clinical circumstances when venous congestion is concomitantly present with systemic arterial hypotension. Neurological ischemia occurs, since the perfusion pressure cannot overcome the resistance it encounters.

GENERAL ANESTHESIA FOR CESAREAN SECTION

Although regional anesthesia is generally held to be the ideal anesthetic for Cesarean section, there are occasions in which a general anesthetic is necessary. In mothers who have had a laminectomy or other surgical procedure over the lumbar and thoracic segments of the vertebral column, regional anesthesia may either be technically impossible or the distribution of local anesthetic may be uneven, leaving some nerve roots totally unblocked. In the setting of fetal distress, there may be insufficient time to instigate an epidural or spinal block. Mothers who have been taking anticoagulants may be at an unacceptably high risk for epidural hematoma should a blood vessel be unintentionally 'nicked'. There is an increased risk of maternal hypotension in the dehydrated or hemorrhaging patient who undergoes regional as opposed to general anesthesia. Of course, there are always the patients who, for one reason or another, have significant fears concerning the insertion of a needle in their backs and refuse regional techniques. Arguing with these patients, shy of an absolute contraindication to general anesthesia, is usually fruitless and ill-advised.

The pregnant patient must always be thought of as having a full stomach. Gastric motility is retarded during pregnancy and uterine encroachment into the upper abdomen presses the stomach against the diaphragm, altering the angle of the gastroesophageal sphincter and lessening its competency. Indeed, many women experience heartburn for the first time during their third trimester. Pain, anxiety and the frequent use of parenteral narcotics are also associated with retardation of gastric emptying. Gastric secretions and, therefore, acidity are also increased with pregnancy.

Although it is not routine to premedicate all laboring patients with antacids and H_2-blockers, these drugs are appropriate for those women in whom a high index of suspicion exists that a Cesarean section is both likely and imminent, as well as for those coming for an elective Cesarean section. A non-particulate antacid, such as Bicitra ®(Alza Pharmaceuticals), has been found to mix more effectively with the stomach contents and poses less of a pulmonary insult than its particulate brethen, such as Maalox ®(Rhône-Poulenc Rorer) and Mylanta ®(Johnson and Johnson), should antacid aspiration occur. It may be given orally literally en route to the operating room in amounts of 30 ml. Ranitidine is an H_2-receptor blocker given to reduce gastric acid secretion. It may be given orally the evening before, and by intravenous route 1 h or less preoperatively. The duration of effect is approximately 6 h. Metoclopramide increases the tone of the gastroesophageal sphincter and increases gastric motility and emptying. It also has mild antiemetic properties and is given as a 10-mg dose intravenously, but slowly, lest mental confusion and anxiety occur.

The induction of general anesthesia is performed after maternal pre-oxygenation and with cricoid pressure, which prevents passive regurgitation once consciousness and the protective pharyngeal and laryngeal reflexes have been ablated by induction agents.

Careful preoperative airway evaluation is absolutely essential when general anesthesia is anticipated for Cesarean section. Maternal oxygen consumption is increased by 20%; at the same time, functional residual capacity is decreased by the same percentage. As a result, maternal hemoglobin desaturation and hypoxemia may occur with frightening rapidity once general anesthesia and skeletal muscle paralysis have been induced. If there is a failed endotracheal intubation during emergency procedures, some patients may be ventilated via the mask throughout surgery, with continuous cricoid pressure. This is not always possible; inability to adequately ventilate the mother at this point may require emergency tracheostomy. Maternal morbidity and mortality are high under these dire circumstances. Failed intubation is currently the greatest cause of anesthetic-related maternal death. Glassenberg and colleagues[115] estimated the failure rate to be between one in 200 to one in 500 general anesthetics.

If a difficult intubation is anticipated preoperatively, an awake fiberoptic intubation with topicalization of the upper airway is a safe, humane and effective alternative to the rigid laryngoscope. The patient remains awake and spontaneously ventilating during the brief period of laryngoscopy and intubation; thus, maternal oxygenation is never in jeopardy. Gentle lifting of the mandible in an anterior direction by an assistant is often helpful. Preoperative administration of an antisialagogue is imperative; glycopyrrolate 0.2 mg intravenously is the agent of choice. Fiberoptic intubation is difficult if copious amounts of blood and secretions are present in the upper airway. Thus, an awake fiberoptic intubation should be attempted prior to laryngoscopic instrumentation of the airway to avoid the almost always inevitable irritation and trauma following the use of a rigid laryngoscope. In the gravida with an anticipated difficult airway, an awake fiberoptic intubation should be opted for initially.

Fiberoptic laryngoscopy is not always successful, however, and it does take a brief, but fixed, amount of time to carry out. If fetal distress dictates that an emergency Cesarean section be performed, in the presence of an anticipated difficult intubation, the anesthesiologist must weigh the risks of an inhalation induction with cricoid pressure versus proceeding with local infiltration until awake intubation can be accomplished. Small amounts of intravenous ketamine (12.5–25 mg) may be employed to supplement anesthesia.

Sodium pentothal (4 mg/kg) has been the classic hypnotic induction agent. Neonatal depression is prevented by not exceeding this dose, as well as by redistribution, dilution and metabolism of the barbiturate in fetal circulation. Half of this dose may be combined with intravenous ketamine (0.5–0.7 mg/kg) if maternal hypotension is a concern or ketamine alone (1.0–1.5 mg/kg intravenously) may be used. Baker and co-workers[116] recently reported favorably on the trial use of propofol (Diprivan), given in doses of 1.5–2.0 mg/kg intravenously as an induction agent for Cesarean section. Propofol was associated with a more rapid maternal recovery profile and no neonatal depression, suggesting that it may prove to be a valuable tool in the induction armamentarium of this decade. Succinylcholine is routinely used to facilitate endotracheal intubation.

Once the trachea is intubated and the airway secured, anesthesia is maintained by combinations of 50% nitrous oxide, 50% oxygen and an inhalational agent in sub-minimum alveolar concentrations. Pregnancy, through mechanisms yet unknown, decreases minimum alveolar concentrations by 20–40%. Since these agents also relax the myometrium, their concentrations are reduced after delivery of the neonate to avoid undue uterine relaxation. Uterine tone postdelivery is routinely augmented with oxytocin. It has been commonplace, should rapid uterine relaxation be mandated at any time intraoperatively, to increase the concentration of the inhalational agents up to 5% for as long as the relaxation is required. Recently, intravenous administration of 50 µg of nitroglycerin, a smooth muscle relaxant, has proved to be equally efficacious. It may be used in lieu of an inhalation agent during Cesarean section, but also has particular value in a routine vaginal delivery in situations which require rapid uterine relaxation (such as a nuchal arm, transverse lie, retained placenta or a breech extraction). This allows the obstetric–anesthetic team to avoid exposing the mother to the hazards of deep general anesthesia.

After the birth of the neonate, intravenous narcotics, such as fentanyl, may be administered as needed. The concentration of nitrous oxide may be increased, but the concentration of the major volatile agent should be reduced to amnesic levels (0.1–0.3%) to avoid uterine relaxation.

Embolization of amniotic fluid or air is an ever-potential threat under general or regional anesthesia, particularly if the uterus is removed from the intra-abdominal cavity. Intramyometrial injections of prostaglandins given in some situations may cause maternal tachycardia, hypotension and elevations in temperature, mimicking sepsis.

The stretching of the abdominal wall by the products of conception may reduce the need for intraoperative muscle relaxants, as will the preoperative use of magnesium. The mother should be able to sustain a head lift for a full 5 s, demonstrating adequate return of consciousness and muscle strength and hence documenting that the airway reflexes are intact, before the trachea is extubated. It is still thought best to administer supplemental oxygen in the delivery room for at least 1 h postoperatively.

EMERGENCY DELIVERY

Emergency delivery may be accomplished by Cesarean section or by vaginal delivery utilizing forceps, vacuum extraction or internal version and extraction, depending on maternal and fetal status, fetal presentation and position, and cervical dilatation.

Vaginal delivery

A previously established lumbar epidural or caudal epidural block provides ideal conditions for emergency vaginal delivery. Otherwise, a low spinal anesthesia may be quickly instituted, depending on the urgency of the situation. Spinal anesthesia with hyperbaric 1.5% lidocaine provides rapid perineal and uterine pain relief to inhibit involuntary bearing down before the cervix is fully dilated in the premature or footling breech. Once the cervix is fully dilated, there is minimal interference with parturient co-operation in expulsion of the fetus. Pudendal block may be used, but generally it is less satisfactory. If necessary, general endotracheal anesthesia should be instituted, using ketamine or pentothal, succinylcholine, cricoid pressure and adding a low concentration of a volatile agent after intubation. The technique is similar to maintenance of Cesarean section anesthesia.

Cesarean section

True emergency Cesarean sections are ideally performed within minutes after recognition of a complication that threatens the life of the mother and/or fetus. General anesthesia should be administered for emergency Cesarean section using 'full aspiration precautions'. This should include an appropriate dose of sodium pentothal or ketamine, a rapid-acting muscle relaxant and a high-inspired oxygen concentration (70%) supplemented with a volatile agent (0.5% halothane, 0.75% isoflurane, 1.0% enflurane). Anesthesiologists should not wait until the surgeons have completed their set-up to initiate general anesthesia, but should time the induction so that surgery can proceed as soon as the surgeons are ready. Furthermore, if 3 min of preoxygenation is not appropriate, four deep vital capacity breaths of a very high flow of oxygen will increase oxygen reserve to some degree. If the patient's trachea cannot be intubated, she should be oxygenated and surgery can be instituted under mask general anesthesia with continuous cricoid pressure. Limited options do exist if this technique is considered too dangerous, including local anesthetic infiltration and waking the patient.

The use of regional block for emergency Cesarean section is either contraindicated or inadvisable, because, first, severe maternal hemorrhage may be present or strongly threatening, or, second, severe or impending fetal distress (prolapsed cord) dictates urgency. Furthermore spinal anesthesia, although fast, may result in rapid and profound maternal hypotension, which will decrease placental blood flow. However, provided that the patient is neither in septic nor hemorrhagic shock, the risks of instituting spinal anesthesia or rapidly augmenting an existing epidural block with 3% 2-chloroprocaine may be less than those associated with general mask anesthesia for the parturient presenting with anatomy that suggests difficult endotracheal intubation. Surgical concentrations of epidural 2-chloroprocaine with sodium bicarbonate require approximately 5 min to strengthen and expand an existing epidural block to a dermatome level of T4–T6. Supplementation with local anesthetic infiltration, and possibly low-dose ketamine, may permit adequate conditions for the start of surgery until the regional block has been augmented.

REFERENCES

1. Datta S, Lambert DH, *et al.* Differential sensitivities of mammalian nerve fibers during pregnancy. *Anesth Analg* 1983;62:1070
2. Butterworth JF, Walker FO, *et al.* Pregnancy increases median nerve susceptibility to lidocaine. *Anesthesiology* 1990;72:962
3. Datta S, Migliozzi RP, Flanagan HL, Krieger NR. Chronically administered progesterone decreases halothane requirements in rabbits. *Anesth Analg* 1989;68:46
4. Jayaram A, Carp H. Progesterone-mediated potentiation of spinal sufentanil in rats. *Anesth Analg* 1993;76:745
5. Majewska MD, Harrison NL, Schwartz RD, *et al.* Steroid hormone metabolites are barbiturate-like modulators of the GABA receptor. *Science* 1986;232:1004
6. Harris RA, Groh GI. Membrane disordering effects of anesthetics are enhanced by gangliosides. *Anesthesiology* 1985;62:115
7. Gordon LM, Dipple D, *et al.* The selective effects of charged local anesthetics on the glucagon- and fluoride-stimulated adenylate-cyclase activity of rat liver plasma membranes. *J Supramol Structure* 1980;14:21
8. Richelson E, Prendergast FG. Muscarinic receptor-mediated cyclic GMP formation in cultured nerve cells – ionic dependence and effects of local anesthetics. *Biochem Pharmacol* 1978;27:2039
9. Butterworth JF, Strichartz GR. Molecular mechanisms of local anesthesia. A review. *Anesthesiology* 1990;72:711
10. Henn FA, Sperelakis N. Stimulative and protective action of Sr^{++} and Ba^{++} on $(Na^+–K^+)$-ATP from cultured heart cells. *Biochem Biophys Acta* 1968;163:415
11. Roufogalis BD. Properties of a $(Mg^{++}–Ca^{++})$-dependent ATPase of bovine brain cortex. Effects of detergents, freezing, cautions and local anesthetics. *Biochem Biophys Acta* 1973;318:360
12. Irvine RF, Hemington N, *et al.* The hydrolysis of phosphatidylinositol by lysosomal enzymes of rat liver and brain. *Biochem J* 1978;176:475
13. Li YM, Wingrove DE, *et al.* Local anesthetics inhibit substance P binding and evoked increases in intracellular Ca^{2+}. *Anesthesiology* 1995;82:166
14. Rana SG, Holz GG, *et al.* Dihydropyridine inhibition of neuronal calcium current and substance P release. *Pflugers Arch* 1987;409:361
15. Steinbach AB. Alteration by Xylocaine (lidocaine) and its derivatives on the time course of the endplate potential. *J Gen Physiol* 1978;277:153
16. Naher E, Steinbach JH. Local anesthetics transiently block currents through single acetylcholine-receptor channels. *J Physiol* 1978;277:153
17. Ruff RL. The kinetics of local anesthetic blockade of endplate channels. *Biophys J* 1982;37:625
18. Ranney B, Stanage WF. Advantages of local anesthesia for Cesarean section. *Obstet Gynecol* 1975;45:163
19. Vasicka A, Robertazzi R, Raji M, *et al.* Fetal bradycardia and paracervical block. *Obstet Gynecol* 1971;38:500

20. Greiss FC, Still JG, Anderson SG. Effects of local anesthetic agents on the uterine vasculature and myometrium. *Am J Obstet Gynecol* 1976;124:889

21. Hillman LS, Hillman RE, *et al.* Diagnosis, treatment and follow up of neonatal mepivacaine intoxication secondary to paracervical and pudendal block during labor. *J Pediatr* 1979;95:472

22. Greene NM. Uptake and elimination of local anesthetics during spinal anesthesia. *Anesth Analg* 1983; 62:1013

23. Cohen EN. Distribution of local anesthetic agents in the neuraxis of the dog. *Anesthesiology* 1968;29:1002

24. Assali NS, Prystowsky H. Studies on autonomic blockade. I. Comparison between the effects of tetraethyl-ammonium chloride (TEAC) and high selective spinal anesthesia on the blood pressure of normal and toxemic pregnancy. *J Clin Invest* 1950;29:1954

25. Barclay DL, Renegar OJ, *et al.* The influence of inferior vena cava compression on the level of spinal anesthesia. *Am J Obstet Gynecol* 1968;101:792

26. Pasricha S, Camillas E, *et al.* Influence of height and weight on spinal analgesia in the term patient. Presented at the *Society for Obstetrical Anesthesia and Perinatology Meeting*, Madison, WI, 1990:abstr

27. Marx GF, Zematis MT, *et al.* Cerebrospinal fluid pressures during labor and obstetric anesthesia. *Anesthesiology* 1961;26:348

28. Hopkins EL, Hendricks CM, *et al.* Cerebrospinal fluid pressure in labor. *Am J Obstet Gynecol* 1965;93:907

29. Greene N. Distribution of local anesthetic solutions within the subarachnoid space. *Anesth Analg* 1985;64: 715

30. Norris MC. Height, weight and the spread of subarachnoid hyperbaric bupivacaine in the term parturient. *Anesth Analg* 1988;67:555

31. Hauch MA, Hartwell BL. Comparative effects of subarachnoid bupivacaine and tetracaine–procaine for Cesarean delivery. *Reg Anesth* 1990;15:81

32. Wang KC, Nauss LA, *et al.* Pain relief by intrathecally-applied morphine in man. *Anesthesiology* 1979;50:149

33. Leighton BL, DeSimone C, *et al.* Intrathecal narcotics for labor revisited. The combination of fentanyl and morphine intrathecally provides rapid onset of profound analgesia. *Anesth Analg* 1989;69:122

34. Rigler ML, Drasner K, *et al.* Cauda equina syndrome after continuous spinal anesthesia. *Anesth Analg* 1991; 72:275

35. Lambert DH, Hurley RJ. Cauda equina syndrome and continuous spinal anesthesia. *Anesthesiology* 1994; 80:1082

36. Drasner K, Sakura S, *et al.* Persistent sacral sensory deficit induced by intrathecal local anesthetic infusion in the rat. *Anesthesiology* 1994;80:847

37. Lambert LA, Lambert HL, *et al.* Irreversible conduction block in isolated nerve by high concentrations of local anesthetics. *Anesthesiology* 1994;80:1082

38. Studd JWW, Crawford JS. The effect of lumbar epidural analgesia on the rate of cervical dilation and the outcome of labor of spontaneous onset. *Br J Obstet Gynaecol* 1980;87:1015

39. Schellenberg JC. Uterine activity during lumbar epidural analgesia with bupivacaine. *Am J Obstet Gynecol* 1977;127:26

40. Friedman EA. Effects of drugs on uterine contractility. *Anesthesiology* 1965;26:409

41. Gunther RE, Bauman J. Obstetrical caudal anesthesia. I. A randomized study comparing 1% mepivacaine with 1% lidocaine plus epinephrine. *Anesthesiology* 1969;31:5

42. Gutsche BB, Cheek TG, *et al.* Rapid intravenous saline infusion decreases uterine activity in labor. Epidural does not (abstr). *Anaesthesiology* 1989;71:A884

43. Walton P, Reynolds F. Epidural analgesia and instrumental delivery. *Anaesthesia* 1984;39:218

44. Hoult IJ, MacLennan AH. Lumbar epidural in labor: relation of fetal malposition and instrumental delivery. *Br Med J* 1977;1:14

45. Maresh M, Choong KM. Delayed pushing with lumbar analgesia in labor. *Br J Obstet Gynaecol* 1983;90:623

46. Chestnut DH, Vanderwalker N, *et al.* The influence of continuous bupivacaine analgesia on the second stage of labor and the method of delivery in nulliparous women. *Anesthesiology* 1987;66:774

47. Chestnut DH, Laszewski L, *et al.* Continuous epidural infusion of 0.0625% bupivacaine–0.002% fentanyl during the second stage of labor. *Anesthesiology* 1990;72:613

48. Thorp JA, Eckert LO, *et al.* Epidural analgesia and Cesarean section for dystocia: risk factors in nulliparas. *Am J Perinatol* 1991;8:402

49. Thorp JA, Hu DH, *et al.* The effect of intrapartum epidural analgesia on nulliparous labor: a randomized, controlled, prospective trial. *Am J Obstet Gynecol* 1993;169:851

50. Ramin SM, Gambling DR, *et al.* Randomized trial of epidural versus intravenous analgesia during labor. *Obstet Gynecol* 1995;86:783

51. Chestnut DH, McGrath JM, *et al.* Does early administration of epidural analgesia affect obstetric outcome in nulliparous women who are receiving intravenous oxytocin? *Anesthesiology* 1994;80:1193

52. Chestnut DH, McGrath JM, *et al.* Does early administration of epidural analgesia affect obstetric outcome in nulliparous women who are in spontaneous labor? *Anesthesiology* 1994;80:1201

53. Naulty JS, Hertwig L, *et al.* Duration of analgesia of epidural fentanyl following Cesarean delivery – effects of local anesthetic drug selection (abstr). *Anesthesiology* 986;65:A18O

54. Hughes SC, Wright RG, *et al.* The effect of pH adjusting 3% 2-chloroprocaine on the quality of post-Cesarean section analgesia with epidural morphine (abstr). *Anesthesiology* 1988;69:A689

55. Reisner LS, Hochman BN. Persistent neurologic deficit and adhesive arachnoiditis following intrathecal 2-chloroprocaine injection. *Anesth Analg* 1980;59:452

56. Wang BC, Hillman DE, *et al.* Chronic neurologic deficits and Nesacaine – an effect of the anesthetic 2-chloroprocaine, or the antioxidant sodium bisulfate? *Anesth Analg* 1984;63:445

57. Morgenson T, Simonson L, *et al.* Tachyphylaxis associated with repeated injections of epidural lidocaine is not related to change in distribution or rate of elimination from the epidural space. *Anesth Analg* 1989; 69:180

58. Eisenach JC, Grice SG, *et al.* Epinephrine enhances analgesia produced by bupivacaine during labor. *Anesth Analg* 1987;66:447

59. Brown DL, Carpenter RL, Thompson GE. Comparison of 0.5% ropivacaine and 0.5% bupivacaine for epidural anesthesia in patients undergoing lower-extremity surgery. *Anesthesiology* 1990;72:633–6

60. Brockway MS, Bannister J, *et al.* Comparison of extradural ropivacaine and bupivacaine. *Br J Anaesth* 1991;66:31–7

61. Scott DB, Lee A, *et al.* Acute toxicity of ropivacaine compared with that of bupivacaine. *Anesth Analg* 1989;69:563–9

62. Lynch C III. Depression of myocardial contractility *in vitro* by bupivacaine, etidocaine, and lidocaine. *Anesth Analg* 1986;65:551

63. Moller RA, Datta S, *et al.* Progesterone-induced increase in cardiac sensitivity to bupivacaine (abstr). *Anesthesiology* 1988;69:A675

64. Verniquet AJW. Vessel puncture with epidural catheters. Experience in obstetric patients. *Anesthesia* 1980;35:660

65. Moore DC, Batra MS. The components of an effective test dose prior to an epidural block. *Anesthesiology* 1981;55:693

66. Hood DD, Dewan DM, *et al.* Maternal and fetal effects of epinephrine in gravid ewes. *Anesthesiology* 1986;64:610

67. Chestnut DH, Weiner CP. Effects of intravenous epinephrine on uterine artery blood flow velocity in the pregnant guinea pig. *Anesthesiology* 1986;65:633

68. Wallis KL, Shnider SM, *et al.* Epidural anesthesia in the normotensive pregnant ewe: effects of uterine blood flow and fetal acid–base status. *Anesthesiology* 1976;44:481

69. Albright GA, Joupilla R, *et al.* Epinephrine; does not alter human intervillous blood flow during epidural anesthesia. *Anesthesiology* 1981;54:131

70. Chestnut DH, Owen CI, *et al.* Does labor affect the variability of maternal heart rate during induction of epidural anesthesia? *Anesthesiology* 1988;68:622

71. Leighton BL, Norris MC, *et al.* Limitations of epinephrine as a test marker of intravascular injection of laboring women. *Anesthesiology* 1987;66:688

72. Colonna-Romano P, Lingaraju N, *et al.* Epidural test dose and intravascular injection in obstetrics: sensitivity, specificity, and lowest effective dose. *Anesth Analg* 993;76:1174

73. Abraham RA, Harris RP. The efficacy of 1.5% lidocaine with 7.5% dextrose and epinephrine as an epidural test dose for obstetrics. *Anesthesiology* 1986;64:116

74. Grice SC, Eisenach JC. Evaluation of 2-chloroprocaine as an effective intravascular test dose for epidural analgesia (abstr). *Anesthesiology* 1987;67:A627

75. Roetman KJ, Eisenach JC. Evaluation of lidocaine as an intravenous test dose for epidural analgesia (abstr). *Anesthesiology* 1988;69:A669

76. Grice SC, Eisenach JC. Effect of 2-chloroprocaine test dosing on the subsequent duration of labor analgesia with epidural bupivacaine–fentanyl–epinehprine (abstr). *Anesthesiology* 1988;69:A668

77. Hodgkinson R, Husain FJ, *et al.* Reduced effectiveness of bupivacaine 0.5% to relieve labor pain after prior injection of 2-chloroprocaine 2% (abstr). *Anesthesiology* 1982;57:A201

78. Corke BC, Carlson CG, Dettbarn WD. The influence of 2-chloroprocaine on the subsequent analgesic potency of bupivacaine. *Anesthesiology* 1984;40:25–7

79. Cherala SR, Mehta D, *et al.* Ephedrine as a marker of intravenous injection in laboring parturients. *Reg Anesth* 1990;15:15

80. Mok MS, Shuai SP, *et al.* Naltrexone pretreatment attenuates side effects of epidural morphine (abstr). *Anesthesiology* 1986;65:A200

81. Lawhorn CD, McNitt J, *et al.* Epidural morphine with butorphanol for postoperative analgesia following Cesarean delivery. Presented at the *Society for Obstetrical Anesthesia and Perinatology Meeting*, Madison, WI, 1990:abstr

82. Naulty JS, Parmet J, *et al.* Epidural sufentanil and morphine for post Cesarean delivery analgesia. Presented at the *Society for Obstetrical Anesthesia and Perinatology Meeting*, Madison, WI, 1990:abstr

83. DeSousa H, Stiller R. Cisternal CSF and arterial plasma levels of fentanyl, alfentanil, and sufentanil after lumber epidural injection. *Anesthesiology* 1989;71:839

84. Capogna G, Celleno D, *et al.* Neonatal neurobehavioral effects following maternal administration of epidural fentanyl during labor (abstr). *Anesthesiology* 1987;67:A461

85. Phillip GH. Epidural sufentanil/bupivacaine combinations of analgesia during labor: effect of varying sufentanil doses. *Anesthesiology* 1987;67:835

86. Kavuri S, Janardham Y. A comparison study of epidural alfentanil and fentanyl for labor pain relief (abstr). *Anesthesiology* 1989;71:A902

87. Heytens L, Cammu H, *et al.* Extradural analgesia during labor using alfentanil. *Br J Anaesth* 1987;59:331

88. Preston PG, Rosen MA, *et al.* Epidural anesthesia with fentanyl and lidocaine for Cesarean section: maternal effects and neonatal outcome. *Anesthesiology* 1988;68:938

89. Vertommen J, Vandmeulen E, *et al.* The effect of adding epidural sufentanil to bupivacaine 0.5% for elective Cesarean section. Presented at the *Society for Obstetrical Anesthesia and Perinatology Meeting*, 1989:abstr

90. Ponte J, Colett BJ, *et al.* Anesthetic temperature and shivering in epidural anesthesia. *Acta Anaesthesiol Scand* 1986;30:584

91. Vincent WS, Chan BS, *et al.* Temperature changes and shivering after epidural anesthesia for Cesarean section. *Reg Anesth* 1989;14:48

92. Webb PJ, James FM III, *et al.* Shivering during epidural anesthesia in women in labor. *Anesthesiology* 1981;55:706

93. Glosten B, Sessler DI, *et al.* Core temperature changes are not perceived during epidural anesthesia during Cesarean section (abstr). *Anesthesiology* 1987;71:A838

94. Satinoff E. Neural organization and evolution of thermal regulation in mammals. *Science* 1978;201:16

95. Sessler DI, Ponte J. Shivering during epidural anesthesia. *Anesthesiology* 1990;72:816

96. Snyder GE, Person DL, *et al.* Headache in obstetrical patients; comparison of Whitacre versus Quincke needles (abstr). *Anesthesiology* 1989;71:A860

97. Naulty JS, Hertwig L, *et al.* Influence of local anesthetic solutions on postdural puncture headache. *Anesthesiology* 1990;72:450

98. Johnson MD, Hertwig L, *et al.* Intrathecal fentanyl may reduce the incidence of spinal headaches (abstr). *Anesthesiology* 1989;71:A911

99. Abboud TK, Zhu J, *et al.* Effect of intrathecal morphine on the incidence of spinal headache. Presented at the *Society for Obstetrical Anesthesia and Perinatology Meeting,* Madison, WI, 1990:abstr

100. Denny N, Masters R, Pearson D, *et al.* Postdural puncture headache after continuous spinal anesthesia. *Anesth Analg* 1987;66:791–4

101. Norris MC, Leighton BL. Continuous spinal analgesia after accidental dural puncture in parturients. Presented at the *Society for Obstetrical Anesthesia and Perinatology Meeting,* Madison, WI, 1990:abstr

102. Palmer CM, Norris MC, *et al.* Incidence of ECG changes during Cesarean delivery under regional anesthesia. *Anesth Analg* 1990;70:36

103. Matthew JP, Fleisher LA, *et al.* ST segment depression during labor and delivery. *Anesthesiology* 1992;77:635

104. Zakowski MI, Ramanathan S, *et al.* Electrocardiographic changes during Cesarean section: a cause for concern? *Anesth Analg* 1993;76:162

105. Groves LH. Backache, headache and bladder dysfunction after delivery. *Br J Anaesth* 1973;45:1147

106. O'Connell JEA. Lumbar disc protrusions in pregnancy. *J Neurol Neurosurg Psychiatry* 1960;23:138

107. Simon JN, Martz DG, *et al.* Spinal cord compression following labor and delivery with epidural analgesia. *Reg Anesth* 1990;19:256

108. Stephanov S, Depreux J, *et al.* Lumbar epidural hematoma following epidural anesthesia. *Surg Neurol* 1982;18:351

109. Allemann BH, Gerber H, *et al.* Rucken marksrahe anaesthesic und subkutan verabreichtes low-dose heparin dihydergot zur thromboembolicprophylaxe. *Anesthetist* 1983;32:80

110. Usubiaga SE. Neurological complications following epidural anesthesia. *Int Anesthesiol Clin* 1975;13:1

111. Laursen J, Fode K, *et al.* Spinal epidural hematomas. *Clin Neurol Neurosurg* 1987;89:247

112. Walton JN. *Brain, Diseases of the Nervous System,* 7th edn. New York: Oxford University Press, 1969:680–2

113. Richardson J, Bedder M. Transient anterior spinal cord syndrome with continuous postoperative epidural analgesia. *Anesthesiology* 1990;72:764

114. Philip K. Complications of regional anesthesia for obstetrics. *Reg Anesth* 1983;7:17

115. Glassenberg R, Vaisrub N, *et al.* The incidence of failed intubation in an obstetrical population during the past decade. Presented at the *Society for Obstetrical Anesthesia and Perinatology Meeting,* Madison, WI, 1990:abstr

116. Baker BW, Longmire S, *et al.* Diprivan (propofol) versus thiopental/isoflurane: a comparison of general anesthetic techniques for Cesarean delivery. Presented at the *Society for Obstetrical Anesthesia and Perinatology Meeting,* abstr

71

Exercise and pregnancy

R. Artal

The health related benefits of exercise are well documented in the general population[1-4]. Pregnancy is a unique period in a woman's life, health awareness increases and women are particularly inclined to continue and conduct an active lifestyle. During their pregnancies, even previously sedentary women may seek to modify their lifestyle and initiate exercise activities. The potential health benefits, safety and feasibility of different amounts and intensities of physical activity in pregnancy are still being investigated. Despite numerous shortcomings in study designs, recent published studies and reviews evaluating the effects of physical activity on pregnancy outcome have identified certain beneficial trends and very few complications[5-7]. Although there are no definite published studies which conclude whether active women have a better pregnancy outcome than their sedentary counterparts, it is logical to assume that maintaining cardiovascular and muscular fitness can benefit women in the long run. Conversely, in the absence of obesity or other related complications, a sedentary lifestyle has not been shown to have deleterious effects on pregnancy outcome either.

In the past, exercise in pregnancy has been scrutinized primarily because of the potential fetal risks. Being aware and cognizant of the potential maternal and fetal risks is essential for exercise guidelines and prescription[8]. Dissemination of such information could only lead to safe conduct of an active lifestyle.

Previous and future guidelines for exercise in pregnancy as formulated by the American College of Obstetricians and Gynecologists (ACOG)[9] have to be primarily geared towards the general population. The vast majority of the population exercises to derive health benefits, while only 10% or less exercises to improve performance. It has been demonstrated in the non-pregnant adult population that the level of exertion required to derive health benefits is relatively moderate[4]. However, guidelines for exercise should in the future include the very active pregnant woman or the elite athlete. Excerpts from the current ACOG guidelines[8] for pregnant women are summarized in Table 1. They are for pregnant women who do not have any additional risk factors for adverse maternal or perinatal outcome.

In this chapter we will review the anatomical and physiological background that provides the basis for

Table 1 Excerpts from ACOG recommendations for exercise in pregnancy

1. During pregnancy, women can continue to exercise and derive health benefits even from mild-to-moderate exercise routines. Regular exercise (at least three times per week) is preferable to intermittent activity.
2. Exercise in the supine position after the first trimester should be avoided. Prolonged periods of motionless standing should be avoided.
3. Women should be encouraged to modify the intensity of their exercise according to symptoms. Pregnant women should stop exercising when fatigued and not exercise to exhaustion. Non-weight-bearing exercise inherently minimizes the risk of injury and facilitates the continuation of exercise during pregnancy.
4. Morphologic changes in pregnancy should serve as relative contraindications to certain types of exercise. Activities which have the potential for abdominal trauma should be avoided.
5. Caloric intake should be ensured.
6. Fluid intake should be adequate to ensure heat dissipation and hydration.
7. Pre-pregnancy exercise should be gradually resumed post partum.

Table 2 Risks of exercise in pregnancy

Maternal	Fetal
Premature labor*	Prematurity*
Musculoskeletal injuries*	Fetal distress or injury*
Hypoglycemia	Fetal growth restriction
Hyperthermia	Fetal malformations

*documented complication

exercise guidelines and prescription in pregnancy, including the maternal and fetal responses to exercise and their potential risks.

Some of the often cited risks have been documented while other remain strictly theoretical (Table 2). Some of the risks are difficult to prove or disprove because of the obvious ethical aspects that such research might involve.

The anatomical and physiological changes which form the basis to the mechanisms potentially leading to injuries during exercise in pregnancy are illustrated in Figure 1[8].

The physicians' role is to advise patients on limitations, contraindications, warning signs and special

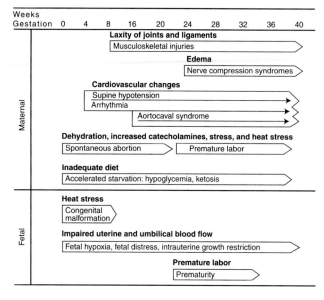

Figure 1   Potential mechanisms leading to injuries during exercise in pregnancy. The top of each box lists the etiology for potential injuries included in each box. The spacing of the boxes reflects the gestational age during which the injury is most likely to occur. Reproduced with permission from Artal R, Wiswell R, Drinkwater B, eds. *Exercise in Pregnancy*. Williams and Wilkins, 1991

concerns. Exercise programs for pregnant women should be conducted by qualified specialists (such as physical therapists, or exercise physiologists) who also have a basic knowledge in obstetrics. The role of obstetricians in this endeavor is essential.

BIOMECHANICAL AND ANATOMICAL CONSIDERATIONS FOR EXERCISE GUIDELINES IN PREGNANCY

Several changes in pregnancy affect the biomechanics of movement. Under the influence of estrogen, progesterone and elastin there is a generalized connective tissue relaxation leading to ligamentous laxity and joint instability[9]. The increase in weight gain increases the load on the musculoskeletal system, producing higher reaction forces. Additional strain on the musculoskeletal system comes from the continuous change in the body center of mass, or point of gravity. The immediate consequence is a combination of progressive lordosis and a limiting in the range of hip joint motion[10]. The change in point of gravity will require greater muscular effort with certain movements, e.g. raising from squatting or sitting positions. One way to reduce the muscular effort of the lower extremity muscles is to utilize the upper extremity muscles when rising from the above mentioned positions. The progressive lordosis in pregnancy frequently results in lower back pain. This potential complication could be prevented or reduced by improved muscular strength, preferably

prior to pregnancy[11]. Most significant, as it relates to exercise guidelines and prescription, is that the biomechanical changes of pregnancy could create balance problems and orthopedic injuries. In addition to back and hip pain, common orthopedic injuries in pregnancy are a consequence of accumulation of interstitial fluid that could result in nerve compression syndromes such as carpal tunnel syndrome.

CARDIOVASCULAR RESPONSES TO EXERCISE IN PREGNANCY

The major hemodynamic response to exercise is redistribution of blood flow away from the visceral organs and towards the working muscles. During exercise the cardiac output to the brain and heart remains unchanged, while the uterine blood flow is significantly restricted depending on the intensity of the exercise. Animal studies suggest that this reduction in uterine blood flow when in excess of 50% may result in abnormal fetal heart rate responses.

Pregnancy is characterized by a significant increase in blood volume, compensated in part by increased venous capacitance and reduced peripheral vascular resistance[12]. Early in pregnancy, the cardiac output increases in excess of the increment in uterine blood flow. Cardiac output reaches maximum values by mid-pregnancy and becomes highly variable in the third trimester. Increases in heart rate, stroke volume and cardiac output are observed not only at rest, but also during submaximal exercise until the third trimester of pregnancy[13].

During cycle ergometry in pregnancy, different kinetic adjustments to the increased maternal mass have been demonstrated[14,15]. The relative increases in cardiac output and stroke volume during exercise are similar in pregnant and non-pregnant subjects[16].

However, during strenuous exercise, the cardiac output response appears to be blunted in pregnancy, a possible reflection of impaired cardiac mechanical functions[15]. These findings are significant from the clinical point of view as the preferential redistribution of blood flow during strenuous exercise does not meet the expected requirements, limiting physical performance. However, unpublished observations indicate that such responses may differ and some elite athletes are capable of overcoming such limitations[17]. At lower exercise intensity, the increase in cardiac output is primarily due to higher heart rate, whereas at higher exercise intensities the contribution is primarily due to increased stroke volume. Hemodynamic changes during rest or exercise in the upright position in pregnancy are influenced significantly by the venous return. Venous return can be significantly impaired in the supine position in pregnancy, even at rest, and can cause symptomatic reduction in cardiac output in 5% or more of pregnant women[18].

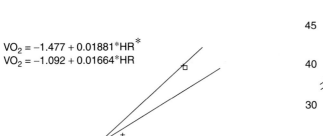
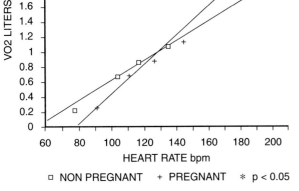

Figure 2 Correlation between oxygen consumption (VO$_2$) and heart rate (HR) during exercise to predict VO$_2$ from submaximal HR. Reproduced with permission from Wiswell RA, Artal R, Romem Y, Kammula R, Dorey F. Hormonal and metabolic response to exercise in pregnancy. *Med Sci Sports Exerc* 1985;17:206

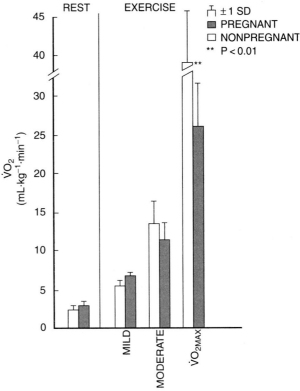

Figure 3 Oxygen consumption during mild, moderate, and VO$_{2max}$ exercise. Reproduced with permission from reference 23

In one invasive study conducted in pregnant women, uterine blood flow during mild cycle exercise was reduced by 25% in healthy women, in their third trimester of pregnancy[19]. A further progressive reduction in blood flow and cardiac output occurs as the intensity of exercise increases. Confirmation for such hemodynamic changes can be found in studies conducted in non-pregnant adults[20]. It is plausible that most of the hemodynamic responses to exercise in pregnancy are a reflection of the hemodynamic changes of pregnancy combined with progressive detraining. The correlation between oxygen consumption (VO$_2$) and heart rate (HR) during exercise is illustrated in Figure 2. Note that the correlations differ in pregnancy compared to the non-pregnant state.

Health benefits could be derived from mild to moderate exercise routines at an intensity of training of 12–14 on the 20 point Borg Scale of Rating of Perceived Exertion (RPE). The RPE scale was first introduced by Borg[21]. A RPE of 12–14 will correspond to a physical activity that will be perceived 'somewhat hard' at the most by the exercising subject and could be more easily monitored than target heart rates.

PULMONARY RESPONSES TO EXERCISE IN PREGNANCY

Significant changes in pulmonary functions parallel the other anatomical and physiological changes of pregnancy. The increase in inspiratory capacity of 300 ml (inspiratory volume + tidal volume) is paralleled by an increased chest circumference and an increase in the resting oxygen consumption by 10–20%. The physiological purpose of the pregnancy state of hyperventilation appears to be aimed at reducing the P_{CO_2} and maintaining pH at 7.44. The increases in tidal volume result in an increase in ventilation, which is the cause of a common subjective feeling of dyspnea. The resulting mild maternal alkalosis facilitates placental gas exchange and prevents fetal acidosis[22]. Many conditions such as strenuous exercise may alter these interactions and affect fetal oxygenation.

Comparison of pulmonary responses during mild, moderate and VO$_{2max}$ exercise (Figure 3) indicates that only a modest increase in VO$_{2max}$ is achieved in pregnancy[23]. This limitation appears to be primarily related to the progressive increase in weight. It does appear that both pregnancy and exercise increase the respiratory demands in the presence of reduced maternal ventilatory reserve. Ventilatory responses and aerobic conditioning have been studied in longitudinal studies in pregnancy and it appears that during submaximal exercise the differences are reflected predominantly in a significant increase in tidal volume during exercise in pregnancy[24].

Another study[25] found that in recreational athletes who maintain a moderate to high level of exercise performance during and after pregnancy, pregnancy is followed by a small increase in VO$_{2max}$.

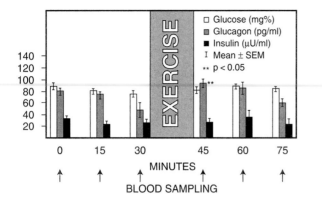

Figure 4 Effect of exercise on maternal glucose, glucagon, and insulin concentrations. The *asterisks* indicate a significant difference for that value when compared to the pre-exercise value. Reproduced with permission from reference 26

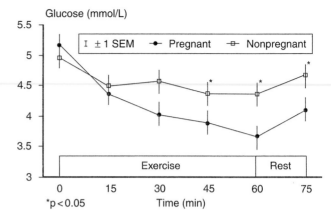

Figure 6 Glucose concentrations during prolonged exercise: pregnant versus non-pregnant. (From Soultanakis HN: Glucose homeostasis during pregnancy in response to prolonged exercise. Postdoctoral thesis, University of Southern California, 1989; with permission.)

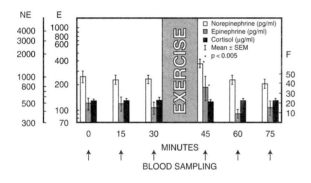

Figure 5 Comparison of preexercise and postexercise concentrations of norepinephrine, epinephrine, and cortisol. The data for norepinephrine (*NE*) and epinephrine (*E*) are illustrated on a logarithmic scale to the *left* of the figure and those for cortisol (*F*) are on a separate scale to the *right* of the figure. The *asterisks* indicate a significant statistical difference for that value when compared to the preexercise value. Reproduced with permission from reference 26

FUEL UTILIZATION DURING EXERCISE IN PREGNANCY

The combined needs of pregnancy and exercise evoke complex hormonal interactions. Stress hormones play an essential role in this process and notably catecholamines, glucagon and cortisol release increase while insulin secretion is suppressed (Figures 4, 5)[26]. Changes in fuel metabolism are modulated to satisfy the requirements of pregnancy (Figures 4, 5). The heavier the workload, the higher the sympathoadrenal activity. Catecholamines promote both glycogenolysis and lipolysis. Epinephrine is recognized to play an essential role in maintaining normoglycemia. Normoglycemia is one of the most guarded physiological functions in pregnancy.

Assessing fuel utilization during exercise in pregnancy is essential because of the possible effects of exercise-induced maternal hypoglycemia. Such events are unlikely to occur during mild–moderate exercise, but very likely to occur during prolonged exercise (Figure 6)[27].

Measurements by indirect calorimetry indicate preferential use of carbohydrates during exercise in pregnancy[28]. Studies have demonstrated that there is a tendency for higher respiratory exchange ratios during pregnancy and during exercise in pregnancy, which suggests a preferential utilization of carbohydrates[28,29] (Figure 7).

The respiratory exchange ratio (RER) is a variable that reflects the ratio between carbon dioxide output (CO_2) and oxygen uptake (VO_2). The RER will provide information on the proportion of substrate derived from various food stuffs. For carbohydrates to be completely oxidized to CO_2 and H_2O, one volume of CO_2 is produced for each volume of O_2 consumed. An RER value of 1.0 would indicate that only carbohydrates are being utilized.

The increases in norepinephrine that parallel the exercise intensity have clinical relevance since norepinephrine has restrictive effects on the splanchnic, renal and uterine blood flow and could precipitate uterine activity[30].

On occasions, uterine activity has been demonstrated to occur during and after physical activity in pregnancy[26]; however, it could potentially have clinical significance only in patients who are at risk for premature labor. And indeed, patients at risk for premature labor are advised to refrain from exercise during pregnancy. (See Table 3 for additional contraindications for exercise in pregnancy).

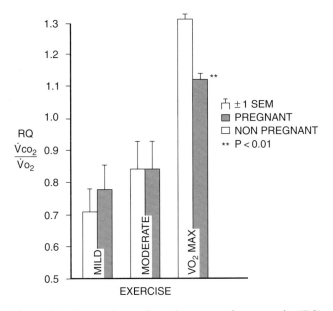

Figure 7 Comparison of respiratory exchange ratio (*RQ*) during mild, moderate, and $\dot{V}O_{2max}$ exercise. Reproduced with permission from reference 23

Table 3 Contraindications to exercise in pregnancy

Absolute contraindications

1. Active myocardial disease
2. Congestive heart failure
3. Rheumatic heart disease (Class II and above)
4. Thrombophlebitis
5. Recent pulmonary embolism
6. Acute infectious disease
7. At risk for premature labor, incompetent cervix, multiple gestations, ruptured membranes
8. Uterine bleeding
9. Intrauterine growth restriction or macrosomia
10. Severe isoimmunization
11. Severe hypertensive disease
12. No prenatal care
13. Suspected fetal distress

Relative contraindications (patients may be engaged in medically supervised programs)

1. Essential hypertension
2. Anemia or other blood disorders
3. Thyroid disease
4. Diabetes mellitus (white class C and above)
5. Breech presentation in the last trimester
6. Excessive obesity or extreme underweight
7. History of sedentary lifestyle

Additional contraindications should be left for the physicians to evaluate

NUTRITION FOR THE ACTIVE PREGNANT WOMAN

The nutritional needs of active pregnant women are not currently defined; however, the recommended dietary intake for pregnant women at large has been well researched. It has been estimated that the caloric cost of pregnancy is approximately 85 000 calories, approximately 300 extra calories per day above prepregnancy requirements. The average weight gain during pregnancy is approximately 12.5 kg, a 20% increase in body weight for most women, with most of the weight gain occurring during the second half of pregnancy.

About 40% of the total gain is represented by the products of conception – fetus, placenta and amniotic fluid[31]. Due to methodology difficulties it has not yet been determined what the true change in body composition during pregnancy is. However, it appears that there is a modest (less than 5%) increase in the percentage of body fat while the remainder is interstitial accumulation of fluids[32]. It is well recognized that individual weight gain in pregnancy can affect the outcome of pregnancy. Obese women (20% above standard weight for height) more frequently deliver large infants (greater than 4.0 kg); conversely, women who begin pregnancy 15% below standard weight for height frequently deliver low birth weight infants. Exertion could further reduce the birth weights of these neonates.

Many active women will begin pregnancy underweight. Among these women there is an increased awareness of body image, and many of them will continue to consume inadequate low calorie diets during their pregnancies. To compensate for these low calorie diets, they will frequently turn to excessive use of vitamins. Excessive intake of vitamins can result in an increased incidence of congenital malformations. Excessive ingestion of vitamin D could result in a neonatal syndrome consisting of supra-valvular aortic stenosis, elfin facies and mental retardation[33]. Hypervitaminosis A may cause urogenital anomalies, ear malformations, cleft palate and neural tube defects[34]. The iron status should be assessed since many of these women may have pre-existing depleted iron stores.

The daily nutritional requirements should include an additional 300 cal/day that are required to provide for the increased basal metabolic needs of pregnancy. Additional calories will be needed depending on the activities conducted. Furthermore, in the postpartum period, lactating women will require an additional 400–600 cal/day to meet the metabolic needs.

FETAL RESPONSES TO MATERNAL EXERCISE

The main concerns related to exercise in pregnancy are focused on the fetus and any potential maternal benefits that could be offset by fetal injuries. In the uncomplicated pregnancy such events are highly unlikely. Most of the potential risks are hypothetical; however, the medical literature lacks the definitive reassuring answers, although it appears that with mild–moderate exercise the risks are minimal.

The principal question that remains to be answered is: To what extent does the selective redistribution of blood flow during exercise offset the transplacental transport of oxygen, CO_2 and nutrients; and if it does, what are the lasting effects, if any?

It is well-recognized that during other obstetrical events transient hypoxia could result initially in fetal tachycardia and an increase in fetal blood pressure. These fetal responses are protective mechanisms for the fetus to facilitate transfer of oxygen and decrease the CO_2 tension across the placenta. Any acute alterations could result in fetal heart rate changes, causing possible fetal distress, whereas chronic effects may result in intrauterine growth retardation. Though fetal demise may be associated with either of the above events, there has never been a report in literature to link them with maternal exercise.

The crux of the theoretical risk is related to the selective redistribution of blood flow during exercise to the exercising muscles, and away from the visceral organs. Studies conducted in non-pregnant[19] and pregnant[35] subjects confirm that blood flow selectively redistributes during exercise. In experimental animal studies, a reduction in uterine blood flow by 50% or more could lead to fetal respiratory acidosis[36]. Theoretically, such events could occur during either strenuous or prolonged exercise. Most of the studies addressing fetal responses to exercise have examined fetal heart rate (FHR) changes during or after exercise[37]. The summary and results of these studies is listed in Table 4[38–59]. Most of the studies demonstrate a minimum or moderate increase in FHR by 10–30 beats/min over baseline during or following maternal exercise. Fetal bradycardia has been reported to occur with a frequency of 8–9%[60]. The mechanism leading to fetal bradycardia during maternal exercise can only be speculated upon; most likely it is either vagal reflex, cord compression, or fetal head malposition. It is unknown whether these transient events have any lasting effects on the fetus, because no long-term studies have been conducted to address this specific question.

Due to the inaccessibility of the fetus, validation of events of fetal bradycardia could ultimately be obtained only with direct internal fetal heart rate monitoring[59] or two dimensional ultrasound[56,57]. In unpublished observations[59], we have demonstrated that in healthy infants of healthy mothers, despite the combined effects of uterine activity during labor with maternal exertion, the uterine perfusion and placental reserve appear not to be affected, and that these fetuses could tolerate such events without obvious signs of fetal distress.

Several studies[61–63] have attempted to assess umbilical blood flow during maternal exercise with Doppler velocimetry, demonstrating various or no changes. Doppler velocimetry studies are technically difficult to conduct during exercise so most measurements are taken before and after exercise, by which time any changes could have returned to normal.

The presence of fetal activity has often been interpreted as a reflection of well-being. The same is true for fetal breathing, which is related to the stage in gestation, diurnal variations, maternal plasma glucose and catecholamine concentrations. And, indeed, a direct relationship has been demonstrated between the sympathetic activity of the mother and the frequency of occurrence of both fetal breathing movements and fetal body movements[64] (Figure 8).

Epidemiological studies have suggested for a long time that a link exists between strenuous physical activities and the development of intrauterine growth retardation. This association appears to be particularly true for mothers engaged in physical work. Working mothers have a tendency to deliver earlier and smaller gestational age infants[65–67]. Corroborating data have been obtained in experimental animals that were forced into strenuous physical activities throughout gestation, and then delivered smaller offspring[68,69]. One study conducted in pregnant women arrived at similar conclusions[70]. Uncontrolled studies done in elite athletes indicate conflicting evidence[71,72]. Most of the studies conducted in pregnant athletes report a very low incidence of complications, but at least one study[72] found that the number of newborn babies of Olympian mothers weighing 2600–3000 g (potentially growth retarded or born prematurely) was greater in their investigations than those weighing in excess of 3500 g. The information available in the literature is too limited to allow risk assignment for either premature labor or fetal growth retardation for exercising mothers. However, clinical observations indicate that patients at risk for premature labor may have labor triggered by exercise. Furthermore, women who are diet-conscious often do not receive the minimum required nutrients. The combined energy requirements of pregnancy and exercise coupled with poor weight gain may lead to fetal retardation.

Exercise, hyperthermia and risk for malformations

During exercise the working muscles generate heat, which could increase the body core temperature to levels which are considered teratogenic. Data obtained in studies conducted in research animals indicate that hyperthermia in excess of 39°C could be teratogenic and frequently results in neurotube defects[73–75].

Human data implicating hyperthermia as teratogenic include primarily case reports[76–79] which may

Table 4 Fetal heart rate responses to maternal exercise

Author	Sample size	Population	GA	Monitoring device	Type of exercise	Intensity of exercise	FHR during exercise	FHR after exercise
Hon & Wohlgemuth[38]	26	Mixed	34–41	Abdominal ECG	Master step test	Moderate	NA	=↑↓
Soiva et al.[39]	24	Mixed	28–40	Phonocardiograph	Bicycle ergometer	Mild, moderate–strenuous	NA	=↑↓
Hodr & Brotanek[40]	56	Mixed	29–36	Phonocardiograph	Master step test	Moderate	NA	=↑↓
Stembera & Hodr[41]	67	Mixed	38–40	Phonocardiograph	Master step test	Moderate	NA	=↑↓
Pokorny & Rous[42]	14	Mixed	36–40	Phonocardiograph	Bicycle ergometer	Mild	=↑	=↓
Pomerance et al.[43]	54	Normal	35–37	Auscultation	Bicycle ergometer	Moderate	NA	↓↑
Eisenberg de Smoler et al.[44]	22	Mixed	28–40	Abdominal ECG	Master step test; treadmill	Moderate	NA	=↓
Pernoll et al.[45]	16	Mixed	24–40	Doppler U/S	Bicycle ergometer	Mild	NA	↑↓
Sibley et al.[46]	7	Normal	17–40	Doppler U/S	Swimming	Strenuous	↑	=
Dale et al.[47]	4	Normal	31–37.5	Doppler U/S	Treadmill	Strenuous	↓	=
Hauth et al.[48]	7	Normal	28–38	Doppler U/S	Jogging	Moderate	NA	↑
Collings et al.[49]	20	Normal	22–34	Doppler U/S	Bicycle ergometer	Strenuous	↑	↑
Artal et al.[50]	15	Normal	35.1 ± 5.65	Doppler U/S	Treadmill	Mild	↑	↑
Artal et al.[50]	15	Normal	34.7 ± 4.31	Doppler U/S	Treadmill	Moderate	↑↓	↑↓
Artal et al.[50]	15	Normal	34.1 ± 6.85	Doppler U/S	Treadmill	VO_{2max}	↑↓	↑↓
Pijpers et al.[51]	28	Normal	35.6	Doppler U/S	Semirecumbent cycling	Moderate	NA	=
Clapp[52]	6	Normal	20 & 32	Doppler U/S	Treadmill	Moderate–strenuous	NA	↑
Jovanovic et al.[53]	6	Normal	36–38.5	Doppler U/S	Cycling	Moderate	↓	↑
Veille et al.[54]	10	Normal	33 ± 3	Doppler U/S	Walking	Moderate–strenuous	NA	↑
Veille et al.[54]	10	Normal	37 ± 1	Doppler U/S	Cycling	Mild–moderate	=	=
Rauramo[55]	61	Mixed	32–40	Doppler U/S	Bicycle ergometer	Mild	NA	↓
Paolone et al.[56]	4	Normal	28–34	M-Mode echocardiograph	Bicycle ergometer and treadmill	Mild–moderate	=	=
Carpenter et al.[57]	45	Normal	20–34	Linear array 2-dimension U/S	Bicycle ergometer	Mild, moderate–strenuous	=	↓ =
Wolfe et al.[58]	12	Normal	37.8 ± 0.6	Doppler U/S	Isometric hand grip	Mild–moderate	=	=
Artal et al.[59]	12	Normal	40 (labor)	Direct fetal scalp monitoring	Bicycle ergometer	Moderate	=	=

GA, gestational age; FHR, fetal heart rate; ECG, electrocardiogram; NA, not available; U/S, ultrasound. Reproduced with permission from Artal R, Posner M. Fetal responses to maternal exercise. In Artal R, Wiswill R, Drinkwater B, eds. *Exercise in Pregnancy*. Williams and Wilkins 1991

suggest an association, but cannot prove causality. The only prospective study, which was conducted with 165 women exposed to first trimester hyperthermia, has failed to confirm its teratogenic effects[80]. Nevertheless, this theoretical risk cannot be dismissed easily, and pregnant women should be advised to avoid hyperthermia during the first weeks of gestation. The malformations implicated are the result of a failure of closure of the neural tube in the phase of embryogenesis that occurs 25 to 27 days after conception, or 50 days from the last menstrual period.

CLINICAL APPLICATIONS FOR EXERCISE IN PREGNANCY

Gestational diabetes occurs in 4–7% of the obstetrical population. Insulin therapy and diet may not be the optimal treatment to attain euglycemia. The hormonal changes of pregnancy reduce insulin peripheral sensitivity, and are further amplified in patients affected by gestational diabetes. Reduced insulin sensitivity may be reversed most efficiently with exercise. Exercise has been recognized for a long time as an adjunct or alternative

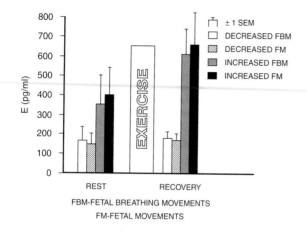

Figure 8 Fetal breathing movements and fetal movements in relation to maternal plasma epinephrine (E) prior to and after exercise. Adapted with permission from Platt LD, Artal R, Semel J, Sipos L, Kammula RK. Exercise in pregnancy II. Fetal responses. *Am J Obstet Gynecol* 1983;147:48

therapeutic modality for Type II diabetic patients. Pregnant diabetics have been denied this option in the past, primarily because of the potential fetal risks. Recent published studies on fetal responses to exercise have removed some of the initial concerns[64].

Exercise training results in sustained insulin sensitivity and improved glucose clearance. Because these functions are altered in gestational diabetes, exercise should be considered not only optional, but preferable, because it obviates insulin therapy. During exercise plasma concentrations of glucose counter-regulatory hormones play an important role in maintaining glucose homeostasis.

Pilot exercise studies conducted in pregnant diabetics indicate that these patients' physiological and metabolic responses are similar to healthy non-diabetics[81–84]. No maternal or fetal adverse responses have been reported to date in pregnant diabetics engaging in mild to moderate physical activities. Nor has there been reported significant complications in non-diabetic, physically active pregnant women.

To date, several studies have tested several exercise prescription regimens for pregnant diabetics. These studies have assessed maternal and fetal safety, and the efficacy of exercise prescription to improve carbohydrate tolerance and obviate insulin therapy.

The prescribed exercise regimens include the following:

1. Artal R *et al.*[82] – 20 min of bicycle ergometry (18 subjects) at 50% VO_{2max} after each meal (3 times/day) for at least 5 days/week for 6 weeks prior to expected day of delivery.

2. Jovanovic-Peterson *et al.*[83] – 20 min arm ergometry (10 subjects) at less than 50% VO_{2max} (daily) for 6 weeks prior to expected day of delivery.

3. Bung P *et al.*[84] – 45 min of bicycle ergometry (21 subjects) at 50% of VO_{2max} 3–4 times/week for at least 6 weeks prior to expected day of delivery.

All the above studies have demonstrated that exercise prescription is feasible in pregnant diabetics and may be utilized as an optional therapeutic approach even in previously sedentary gestational diabetics. The rate of complications observed were similar in the study and control groups. In one study, 2 patients experienced premature labor of which one was successfully tocolyzed[84]. The type, frequency and intensity of exercise utilized in the above studies was sufficient to attain and maintain euglycemia. Non-weight bearing exercise appears to be particularly suited for these type of patients.

It appears that in the absence of either medical or obstetrical complications, exercise prescription can be an optional adjunct therapy for gestational diabetes. This concept has been endorsed by the second[85] and third[86] International Workshops on Gestational Diabetes.

SUMMARY

Women seek to continue an active lifestyle in pregnancy and despite the theoretical risks to both mother and fetus listed in this review, exercise in pregnancy conducted in moderation appears to be, by and large, safe. Questions remain as to the safety and potential benefits for strenuous exercise.

The current published literature includes the following consistent findings[3]:

(1) Women who exercised before pregnancy and continued to do so during pregnancy tended to weigh less, gain less weight, and deliver smaller babies than controls.

(2) All women, regardless of initial level of physical activity, decrease their activity as pregnancy progresses.

(3) No information is available to assess whether active women have better pregnancy outcome than their sedentary counterparts. No information is available on sedentary women.

(4) Physically active women appear to tolerate labor pain better.

(5) Exercise can be utilized as an alternative and safe therapeutic approach for gestational diabetes.

Pregnancy should not be a state of confinement, and cardiovascular and muscular fitness can be reasonably maintained. Restriction of physical activity should be dictated by obstetrical and medical indications only.

REFERENCES

1. Blair SN, Kohl HW, Paffenberges RS, *et al.* Physical fitness and all-cause mortality: a prospective study of healthy men and women. *J Am Med Assoc* 1989;262: 2395–401

2. Bouchard C, Shephard RL, Stephens T, eds. Physical activity fitness and health: international proceedings and consensus statement. Champaign, Ill. Human Kinetics, 1994

3. American College of Sports Medicine - Position stand: The recommended quantity and quality of exercise for developing and maintaining cardiorespiratory and muscular fitness in healthy adults, 1990

4. Pate RR, Pratt M, Blair SN, *et al.* Physical activity and public health: a recommendation from the Centers for Disease Control and Prevention and the American College of Sports Medicine. *J Am Med Assoc* 1995;273: 402–7

5. Artal RM, Dorey FJ, Kirschbaum TH. Effect of maternal exercise on pregnancy outcome. In Artal RM, Wiswell RA, Drinkwater BL, eds. *Exercise in Pregnancy*, 2nd edn. Baltimore: Williams and Wilkins, 1991:225–9

6. Lotgering FK, Gilbert RD, Longo LD. Maternal and fetal responses to exercise during pregnancy. *Physiol Rev* 1985;65:1–36

7. Wolfe LA, Ohtake PJ, Mottola MF, *et al.* Physiological interactions between pregnancy and aerobic exercise. *Exerc Sports Sci Rev* 1989;17:295–351

8. Artal RM, Wiswell RA, Drinkwater BL, *et al.* Exercise guidelines in pregnancy. In Artal RM, Wiswell RA, Drinkwater BL, eds. *Exercise in pregnancy*. Baltimore: Williams & Wilkins, 1991:303

9. ACOG - Technical Bulletin, Number 189 - February 1994

10. Calganeri M, Bird HA, Wright V. Changes in joint laxity occurring during pregnancy. *Ann Rheum Dis* 1982; 41:126–8

11. Gleeson PB, Panol JA. Obstetrical physical therapy. *Phys Ther* 1988;68:1699–702

12. Clapp JF. The effects of exercise on uterine blood flow. In Rosenfeld CR, ed. *The Uterine Circulation.* Ithaca: Perinatology Press, 1989:300–10

13. Wolfe LA, Ohtake PJ, Mottola MF, *et al.* Physiological interactions between pregnancy and aerobic exercise. *Exerc Sport Sci Rev* 1989;17:295–351

14. Guzman CA, Caplan R. Cardiorespiratory response to exercise during pregnancy. *Am J Obstet Gynecol* 1970; 108:600–5

15. Khodignian N, Jacque-Fortunato S, Wiswell RA, *et al.* A comparison of cross-sections and longitudinal methods of assessing the influence of pregnancy on cardiac function during exercise. *Semin Perinatol* 1996;20: 232–41

16. Artal R, Khodignian N, Kammula R, *et al.* Cardiopulmonary adaptations to graded exercise in pregnancy. Proceedings: Society for Gynecologic Investigation, 1986:66

17. Jacque-Fortunateo S, Wiswell RA, Khodignian N, *et al.* A comparison of the ventilatory responses to exercise in pregnant, postpartum and non-pregnant women. *Semin Perinatol* 1996;20:263–76

18. Kerr MG. The mechanical effects of the gravid uterus in late pregnancy. *J Obstet Gynaecol Br Commonw* 1965; 72:513–29

19. Morris N, Osborn SB, Wright HP, *et al.* Effective uterine blood flow during exercise in normal and pre-eclamptic pregnancies. *Lancet* 1956;2:481

20. Rowell LB. Human circulation. In *Regulation During Physical Stress.* New York: Oxford University Press, 1986:232

21. Borg G. *Physical Performance and Perceived Exertion.* Lund, Sweden: Gleenup, 1962;1–63

22. Liboratore SM, Pistelli R, Patalano F, *et al.* Respiratory function during pregnancy. *Respiration* 1984;46:145–50

23. Artal R, Wiswell R, Romem Y, *et al.* Pulmonary responses to exercise in pregnancy. *Am J Obstet Gynecol* 1986;154:378–83

24. South-Paul JE, Rajagopal KR, Tenholder KB. The effect of participation in a regular exercise program upon aerobic capacity during pregnancy. *Obstet Gynecol* 1988;71:175–9

25. Clapp JF III, Capeless E. The VO_2 max of recreational athletes before and after pregnancy. *Med Sci Sports Exerc* 1991;23:1128–31

26. Artal R, Platt LD, Sperling M, *et al.* Exercise in pregnancy: maternal cardiovascular and metabolic responses in normal pregnancy. *Am J Obstet Gynecol* 1981; 140:123–28

27. Soultanakis H, Artal R, Wiswell R. Prolonged exercise in pregnancy: glucose homeostasis ventilatory and cardiovascular responses. *Semin Perinatol* 1996;20:315–24

28. Artal R, Masaki D, Khodignian N, *et al.* Exercise prescription in pregnancy: weightbearing exercise. *Am J Obstet Gynecol* 1989;161:1464–9

29. Clapp JF III, Wesley M, Slcamaker RH. Thermoregulatory and metabolic responses prior to and during pregnancy. *Med Sci Sports Exerc* 1987;29:124–9

30. Zuspan FP, Cibil LA, Pose S. Myometrial and cardiovascular responses to alteration in plasma epinephrine and norepinephrine. *Am J Obstet Gynecol* 1962;84:841–

31. Forbes GB. Methods for determining composition of the human body. *Pediatrics* 1962;29:477–94

32. Jacque-Fortunato S, Khodiginian N, Artal R, *et al.* Body composition in pregnancy. *Semin Perinatol* 1996;20: 340–2

33. Garcia RE, Friedman WF, Koback MM. Idiopathic hypercalcemia and supravalvular stenosis: documentation of a new syndrome. *N Engl J Med* 1964;271: 117–20

34. Bernhardt IB, Dorsey DJ. Hypervitaminosis A and congenital renal anomalies in a human infant. *Obstet Gynecol* 1974;43:750–5

35. Artal R. Unpublished observations

36. Wilkening RB, Meschia G. Fetal oxygen uptake, oxygenation and acid–base balance as a function of uterine blood flow. *Am J Physiol* 1983;244:H749–55

37. Artal R, Romem Y, Wiswell R. Fetal heart responses to maternal exercise. *Am J Obstet Gynecol* 1986;155:729–33

38. Hon EH, Wohlgemuth R. The electronic evaluation of fetal heart rate. *Am J Obstet Gynecol* 1961;81:362–

39. Soiva K, Salmi A, Gronroos M, *et al.* Physical working capacity during pregnancy and effect of physical tests on fetal heart rate. *Ann Chir Gynaecol* 1963;53:187–

40. Hodr J, Brotanek Y. Changes of actography and fetal heart rates in premature deliveries. In Horsky J, Stembera ZK, eds. *Intra-Uterine Dangers to the Fetus*. Amsterdam: Excerpta Medica Foundation, 1967:343

41. Stembera ZK, Hodr J. The exercise test as an early diagnostic aid for fetal distress. In Horsky J, Stembera ZK, eds. *Intra-Uterine Dangers to the Fetus*. Amsterdam: Excerpta Medica Foundation, 1967:349

42. Pokorny J, Rous J. The effect of mother's work on fetal heart sounds. In Horsky J, Stembera ZK, eds. *Intra-Uterine Dangers to the Fetus*. Amsterdam: Excerpta Medica Foundation, 1967:359

43. Pomerance JJ, Gluck L, Lynch VA. Maternal exercise as a screening test for uteroplacental insufficiency. *Obstet Gynecol* 1974;44:383–7

44. Eisenberg de Smoler P, Krachmer SK, Ayala LC, *et al*. El electrocardiogram fetal durante el ejercicio materno. *Ginecol Obstet Mex* 1974;35:521

45. Pernoll ML, Metcalf J, Paul M. Fetal cardiac response to maternal exercise. In Longo LD, Reneau DD, eds. *Fetal and Newborn Cardiovascular Physiology*, vol. 2. New York: Garland Press, 1978:389

46. Sibley L, Ruhling RO, Cameron-Foster J, *et al*. Swimming and physical fitness during pregnancy. *J Nurse-Midwifery* 1981;26:3–12

47. Dale E, Mullinax KM, Bryan DH. Exercise during pregnancy: effects on the fetus. *Can J Appl Sport Sci* 1982;7:98–103

48. Hauth JC, Gilstrap LC, Widmer K. Fetal heart rate reactivity before and after maternal jogging during the third trimester. *Am J Obstet Gynecol* 1983;142:545–52

49. Collings CA, Curet LB, Mullin JP. Maternal and fetal responses to a maternal aerobic exercise program. *Am J Obstet Gynecol* 1983;145:702–7

50. Artal R, Romem Y, Wiswell R. Fetal heart responses to maternal exercise. *Am J Obstet Gynecol* 1986;155:729–33

51. Pijpers L, Wladimiroff W, McGhie Y. Effect of short-term maternal exercise on maternal and fetal cardiovascular dynamics. *Br J Obstet Gynaecol* 1984;91:1081–6

52. Clapp JF III. Fetal heart rate response to running in mid-pregnancy and late pregnancy. *Am J Obstet Gynecol* 1985;153:251–2

53. Jovanic L, Kessler A, Peterson CM. Human maternal and fetal responses to graded exercise. *J Appl Physiol* 1985;58:1719–22

54. Veille JC, Hohimer AR, Burry K, *et al*. The effect of exercise on uterine activity in the last eight weeks of pregnancy. *Am J Obstet Gynecol* 1985;151:727–30

55. Rauramo I. Effect of short-term physical exercise on fetal heart rate and uterine activity in normal and abnormal pregnancies. *Ann Chir Gynaecol* 1987;76:1–6

56. Paolone AM, Shangold M, Paul D, *et al*. Fetal heart rate measurements during maternal exercise – avoidance of artifact. *Med Sci Sports Exerc* 1987;19:605–9

57. Carpenter MW, Sady SS, Hoegsberg B, *et al*. Fetal heart rate response to maternal exertion. *J Am Med Assoc* 1988;259:3006–9

58. Wolfe LA, Lowe-Wylde SJ, Tranmer JE. Fetal heart rate during maternal static exercise. *Can J Sport Sci* 1988; 13:95–6P

59. Artal R, Khodughian N, Paul RH. Intrapartum fetal heart rate responses to maternal exercise. Unpublished

60. Artal R, Romem Y, Paul RH, *et al*. Fetal bradycardia induced by maternal exercise. *Lancet* 1984;2:258–60

61. Moore DH, Jarrett JC, Bendick PJ. Exercise induced changes in uterine artery blood flow, as measured by Doppler ultrasound, in pregnant subjects. *Am J Perinatol* 1989;5:94

62. Morrow RJ, Ritchie WK, Bull SB. Fetal and maternal hemodynamic responses to exercise in pregnancy assessed by Doppler ultrasonography. *Am J Obstet Gynecol* 1989;160:138–40

63. Veille JC, Bacevice AE, Wilson B. Umbilical artery waveform during bicycle exercise in normal pregnancy. *Obstet Gynecol* 1989;73:957–60

64. Artal R, Posner M. Fetal responses to maternal exercise. In Artal R, Wiswell RA, Drinkwater B, eds. *Exercise in Pregnancy*, 2nd edn. Baltimore: Williams & Wilkins, 1991

65. Fox ME, Harris RE, Brekken AL. The active-duty military pregnancy: a new high-risk category. *Am J Obstet Gynecol* 1977;129:705–7

66. Taferi N, Naeye RL, Gobzie A. Effects of maternal undernutrition and heavy physical work during pregnancy on birth weight. *Br J Obstet Gynaecol* 1980; 87:222–6

67. Naeye RL, Peters E. Working during pregnancy; effects on the fetus. *Pediatrics* 1982;69:721

68. Terada M. Effect of physical activity before pregnancy on fetuses of mice exercised forcibly during pregnancy. *Teratology* 1974;10:141–4

69. Nelson PS, Gilbert RD, Longo L. Fetal growth and placental diffusing capacity in guinea pigs following long-term maternal exercise. *J Dev Physiol* 1983; 5:1–10

70. Clapp JF, Dickstein S. Endurance exercise and pregnancy outcome. *Med Sci Sports Exerc* 1984;16:556–62

71. Erdelyi GJ. Gynecological survey of female athletes. *J Sports Med Phys Fit* 1962;2:174–5

72. Zaharieva E. Olympic participation by women; effects on pregnancy and childbirth. *J Am Med Assoc* 1972; 221:992–5

73. Edwards MJ. Congenital defects in guinea pigs: fetal resorptions, abortions and malformations following induced hyperthermia during early gestation. *Teratology* 1969;2:313–28

74. Skreb N, Frank Z. Developmental abnormalities in the rat induced by heat shock. *J Embryol Exp Morphol* 1983; 11:445

75. Kelham L, Ferm VH. Exencephaly in fetal hamsters exposed to hyperthermia. *Teratology* 1976;14:323–6

76. Miller P, Smith DW, Shepard TH. Maternal hyperthermia as a possible cause of anencephaly. *Lancet* 1978;1: 519–21

77. Shiota K. Neural tube defects and maternal hyperthermia in early pregnancy. Epidemiology in a human embryonic population. *Am J Med Genet* 1982;12:281–8

78. Edwards MJ. Hyperthermia as a teratogen. *Teratol Carcinog Mutagen* 1986;6:563–82

79. Harvey MAS, McRorie, Smith DW. Suggested limits to the use of hot tubs and saunas by pregnant women. *Can Med Assoc J* 1981;125:50–4

80. Clarren SK, Smith DW, Harvey MAS. Hyperthermia – a prospective evaluation of a possible teratogenic agent in man. *J Pediatr* 1979;95:81–3

81. Artal R, Wiswell R, Romem Y. Hormonal responses to exercise in diabetic and nondiabetic pregnant patients. *Diabetes* 1985;34(suppl 3):80–86

82. Artal R, Masaki D. Exercise in gestational diabetes. *Pract Diabetol* 1989;8:7–14

83. Jovanovic-Peterson L, Durak EP, Peterson CM. Randomized trial of diet versus diet plus cardiovascular conditioning on glucose levels in gestational diabetes. *Am J Obstet Gynecol* 1989;161:415–9

84. Bung P, Artal R, Khodignian N, *et al*. Exercise in gestational diabetes: an optional therapeutic approach? *Diabetes* 1991;40(suppl 2):182–5

85. Summary and recommendations of the Second International Conference on Gestational Diabetes Mellitus. *Diabetes* 1985;34:123–6

86. Metzger BE. Summary and recommendations of the Third International Workshop–Conference on Gestational Diabetes Mellitus. *Diabetes* 1991;40(suppl 2): 197–201

72

Mature gravidas

C.C. Egley

OVERVIEW

The total number of patients becoming pregnant in the United States after the age of 35 is at an all-time high. Most of this increase has been caused simply by the large cohort of women born during the 'baby boom' years reaching their 35th birthdays during the 1990s. Other reasons for delaying fertility include late (or second) marriage, delayed fertility, and pursuit of career[1]. Of the women who become pregnant after age 35, 85% do so before the age of 40. Pregnancy beyond the age of 50 is exceedingly rare[2].

There is evidence from both nature[3] (studies of the Hutterite population) and science[4] (results from artificial insemination of women of various ages whose husbands were azoospermic) that fertility gradually decreases after the age of 29.

FETAL AND NEONATAL RISKS

The risk of trisomy 21 and other nondisjunction gradually increases from the age of 20 (1:1923) till 30 (1:885); then it begins to sharply increase after the age of 30 with even sharper increases in risk during subsequent 5-year intervals[5]. The risk of carrying a fetus with trisomy 21 is 1:365 at the maternal age of 35 and increases to 1:12 at the age of 49. It is thus clear that patients over the age of 35 [and younger patients with a positive family history, low maternal serum alpha-fetoprotein (MSAFP), abnormal triple marker, ultrasound evidence] should be offered prenatal diagnosis. Ultrasound or MSAFP (alone or in combination) are neither sensitive nor specific enough in this age group, so these patients need to be offered chorionic villus sampling, genetic amniocentesis, or in certain cases

Table 1 Regression-derived estimated rates per 1000 of cytogenetic abnormalities by maternal age at time of amniocentesis

Maternal age (years)	47, + 21*	47, + 18	47, + 13**	47,XXX	47,XXY	Other clinically significant abnormalities†	All abnormalities‡
33††	2.4	0.6	0.4	0.4	0.4	1.1	4.6 – 5.4
34††	3.1	0.8	0.4	0.5	0.5	1.2	5.8 – 6.5
35	4.0	1.0	0.5	0.6	0.6	1.3	7.4 – 8.0
36	5.2	1.3	0.6	0.7	0.8	1.3	9.5 – 9.9
37	6.7	1.6	0.6	0.8	1.0	1.4	12.1 – 12.2
38	8.7	2.1	0.7	1.0	1.2	1.5	15.4 – 15.2
39	11.2	2.6	0.9	1.2	1.5	1.6	19.6 – 19.0
40	14.5	3.3	1.0	1.4	1.9	1.7	25.0 – 23.8
41	18.7	4.2	1.1	1.7	2.4	1.8	31.9 – 29.9
42	24.1	5.2	1.3	2.0	3.0	1.9	40.7 – 37.6
43	31.1	6.6	1.5	2.4	3.8	2.0	51.9 – 47.5
44	40.1	8.4	1.8	2.9	4.7	2.2	66.1 – 60.0
45	51.8	10.6	2.0	3.4	5.9	2.3	84.3 – 76.0
46	66.8	13.3	2.4	4.1	7.4	2.4	107.5 – 96.5
47	86.2	16.9	2.7	4.9	9.3	2.6	137.1 – 122.6
48	111.2	21.3	3.1	5.9	11.7	2.7	174.8 – 155.9
49	143.5	26.9	3.6	7.0	14.6	2.9	222.9 – 198.6

* A value of 0.08 per 1000 should be added to this figure to allow for structural rearrangements associated with Down's syndrome
** A value of 0.06 per 1000 should be added to this figure to adjust for structural rearrangements associated with Patau's syndrome
† Includes structural rearrangements associated with Patau's and Down's syndromes
‡ The first value of the range given is derived from a regression equation analysis on all abnormalities, the second by adding values for all abnormalities. Including abnormalities of more questionable significance would result in addition of about 2.7 per 1000 at the lower ages (around 35 years) and about 2.1 per 1000 at the older ages to the second values given in the range
†† Values extrapolated from regression equation derived for ages 35 to 39 years. (Reference 22)

Table 2 Estimated rates per 1000 of cytogenetic abnormalities at time of expected live birth

Maternal age (years)	47, + 21*	47, + 18	47, + 13**	47,XXX	47,XXY	Other clinically significant abnormalities[†]	All abnormalities[‡]
33	1.6	0.2	0.2	0.4	0.4	0.8	2.9 – 3.5
34	2.0	0.2	0.2	0.5	0.4	0.8	3.7 – 4.2
35	2.6	0.3	0.3	0.5	0.6	0.9	4.7 – 5.2
36	3.4	0.4	0.3	0.6	0.7	0.9	5.9 – 6.4
37	4.4	0.5	0.4	0.8	0.9	1.0	7.6 – 7.9
38	5.7	0.6	0.4	0.9	1.1	1.0	9.7 – 9.8
39	7.3	0.8	0.5	1.1	1.4	1.1	12.3 – 12.1
40	9.4	1.0	0.5	1.3	1.7	1.2	15.7 – 15.2
41	12.2	1.2	0.6	1.6	2.2	1.2	20.1 – 19.0
42	15.7	1.6	0.7	1.9	2.7	1.3	25.6 – 23.9
43	20.2	2.0	0.8	2.2	3.4	1.4	32.6 – 30.2
44	26.1	2.5	1.0	2.7	4.3	1.5	41.6 – 38.1
45	33.7	3.2	1.1	3.2	5.4	1.6	53.0 – 48.2
46	43.4	4.0	1.3	3.8	6.8	1.7	67.6 – 61.0
47	56.0	5.1	1.5	4.6	8.5	1.8	86.2 – 77.5
48	72.3	6.4	1.8	5.5	10.7	1.9	109.9 – 98.5
49	93.3	8.1	2.0	6.5	13.4	2.0	140.1 – 125.3

* A value of 0.06 per 1000 should be added to this figure to allow for structural rearrangements associated with Down's syndrome
** A value of 0.03 per 1000 should be added to this figure to adjust for structural rearrangements associated with Patau's syndrome
[†] Includes structural rearrangements associated with Patau's and Down's syndromes
[‡] First value of range given is derived from regression analysis on all abnormalities; second, by adding values for all abnormalities. Including abnormalities of more questionable significance would result in addition of about 2.7 per 1,000 at the lower ages (around 35 years) and about 2.1 per 1000 at the oldest ages to the second values in the range. (Reference 22)

percutaneous umbilical blood sampling. Triple marker testing and ultrasound, however, may be useful in preventing more invasive procedures in such patients[6–8]. Experimentally, fetal cells may be recovered from maternal blood. These cells can then be analyzed for fetal karyotype. After the age of 40, there is an increased risk of other major fetal malformations that would not be diagnosed with routine karyotype analysis[9]. In this age group, detailed ultrasonographic examination (Level II) should also be offered in addition to karyotype analysis. It is also important to remember that up to 40% of women referred for genetic amniocentesis because of increased maternal age also have family histories suggestive of other fetal genetic abnormalities that would not be picked up on routine karyotype analysis[10]. Therefore, the mature gravida may profit from expert genetic counseling.

There is a gradual increase in the incidence of stillbirths (but not neonatal deaths) as women age[10–13]. Only 14% of the increase in stillbirths is accounted for by congenital anomalies; half the increase in stillbirths is accounted for by an increase in the incidence of (1) abruptio placenta, (2) large placental infarcts, and (3) placental growth retardation. These three diseases are the result of uteroplacental underperfusion. While medical diseases that are a function of increasing age (diabetes, hypertension) may account for some of this uteroplacental underperfusion, there is good evidence that as women age, the branches of the uterine arteries that pass through the myometrium develop specific

sclerotic lesions and it is these lesions that account for most of the underperfusion of the placenta, thus predisposing to fetal death (Tables 1 and 2).

MATERNAL RISKS

The risk of maternal mortality increases with increasing maternal age starting at about the age of 40 in white patients and about 30 in black patients. After the age of 35, the overall relative risk of maternal death is 4.3 compared with women age 20 through 34 years[14,15]. However, the maternal mortality has decreased significantly over the past 15 years in each age group so that it is probably safer for a 35 year old to go through a pregnancy today than it would have been for her 15 years ago at the age of 20.

During pregnancy, older women are more likely to have placenta previa[16], diabetes mellitus, leiomyomata, rhesus sensitization, dizygotic twinning, malpresentation, malposition, and gestational trophoblastic neoplasia (GTN)[17]. Special surveillance must be in place for GTN, especially in the gravida who is beyond the age of 40. Patients over the age of 35 are also significantly more likely to have chronic hypertension or pregnancy induced hypertension, with more than 30% of women over the age of 40 developing hypertensive complications. The incidence of cervical incompetence is higher in the older gravida.

During labor, the older parturient is more likely to develop protraction disorders[18] and her fetus is more likely to develop late decelerations[19]. It is important for the clinician to be aware that there is a marked increase in the Cesarean rate for the older patient. The reason for the increased Cesarean section rate is not clear, but it may be that the older patient gets labeled as 'high-risk' and therefore the obstetrician has a lower threshold for performing a Cesarean section[20]. Induction of labor is also more common among older patients.

THE GOOD NEWS

In many respects, the older patient fares as well as, or better than her younger counterpart[19,21]. The incidence of preterm labor, neonatal intensive care unit admissions, and birth weight less than 2500 g is actually less common in the older patient. The fetus is no more likely to suffer bradycardia, tachycardia, or prolonged decelerations during labor. The incidence of spontaneous abortion, urinary tract infections and chorioamnionitis is no higher in the older patient. Maternal anemia is less frequent in the older patient.

MANAGEMENT POINTS

(1) If the maternal age is greater than 35, prenatal diagnosis should be offered to rule out fetal chromosomal abnormalities. Good quality genetic counseling should also be available to obtain a good family history and ethnology.

(2) If maternal age is greater than 40, there are additional risks: (a) GTN must be ruled out by early ultrasound and quantitative human chorionic gonadotropin assays and (b) the fetus is at higher risk for anomalies that may be missed by karyotype analysis but may be diagnosed with ultrasonography.

(3) The fetus has a five-fold increased risk of stillbirth and may benefit from close surveillance during the third trimester.

(4) While the 35-year-old gravida's risk is increased compared to her 20-year-old sister, her risk today, at the age of 35, is no greater than it would have been 15 years ago if she had become pregnant at the age of 20.

REFERENCES

1. Friede A, Baldwin W, Rhodes PH, *et al.* Older maternal age and infant mortality in the United States. *Obstet Gynecol* 1988;72:152

2. Natter CE. Pregnancy after fifty. *Obstet Gynecol* 1964;24:641

3. Guttmacher AF. Factors affecting normal expectancy of conception. *J Am Med Assoc* 1956;161:855

4. Schwartz D, Mayaux MJ. Female fecundity as a function of age. Results of artificial insemination in 2193 nulliparous women with azoospermic husbands. Federation CECOS. *New Engl J Med* 1982;306:404

5. Hook EB. Rates of chromosome abnormalities at different maternal ages. *Obstet Gynecol* 1981;58:282

6. Donnenfield AE, Carlson DE, Librizzi RT, *et al.* Prospective multicenter study of second-trimester nuchal skinfold thickness in unaffected and Down syndrome pregnancies. *Obstet Gynecol* 1994;814a:8144

7. Bahado-Singh RO, Goldstein I, Uerpairojit B, *et al.* Normal nuchal thickness in the midtrimester indicates reduced risk of Down syndrome in pregnancies with abnormal triple-screen results. *Am J Obstet Gynecol* 1995;173:1106

8. Munne S, Alikani M, Tomkin G, *et al.* Embryo morphology, developmental rates, and maternal age are correlated with chromosome abnormalities. *Fertil Steril* 1995;64:382–91

9. Goldberg MF, Edmonds LD, Oakley GP. Reducing birth defect risk in advanced maternal age. *J Am Med Assoc* 1979;242:2292

10. Rubin MS, Malin J, Maidman J. Genetic counseling before prenatal diagnosis for advanced maternal age: an important medical safeguard. *Obstet Gynecol* 1983;62:155

11. Naeye RL. Maternal age, obstetric complications, and the outcome of pregnancy. *Obstet Gynecol* 1983;61:210

12. Cnattingius S, Berendes HW, Forman MR. Do delayed childbearers face increased risks of adverse pregnancy outcomes after the first birth? *Obstet Gynecol* 1993;81:512

13. Raymond EG, Cnattingius S, Kiely JL. Effects of maternal age, parity, and smoking on the risk of stillbirth. *Br J Obstet Gynaecol* 1994;101:301–6

14. Buehler JW, Kaunitz AM, Hogue CJ, *et al.* Maternal mortality in women aged 35 years or older: United States. *J Am Med Assoc* 1986;255:53

15. Sachs BP, Layde PM, Rubin GL, *et al.* Reproductive mortality in the United States. *J Am Med Assoc* 1982;247:2789

16. Zhang J, Savitz DA. Maternal-age and placenta previa: a population-based, case-control study. *Am J Obstet Gynecol* 1993;168:641–5

17. Spellacy WFN, Miller SJ, Winegar A. Pregnancy after 40 years of age. *Obstet Gynecol* 1986;68:452

18. Cohen WR, Newman L, Friedman EA. Risk of labor abnormalities with advancing maternal age. *Obstet Gynecol* 1980;55:414

19. Kirz DS, Dorchester W, Freeman RK. Advanced maternal age: the mature gravida. *Am J Obstet Gynecol* 1985;152:7

20. Gordon D, Milberg J, Daling J, *et al.* Advanced maternal age as a risk factor for Cesarean delivery. *Obstet Gynecol* 1991;77:493

21. Kessler J, Lancet M, Borenstein R, *et al.* The problem of the older primipara. *Obstet Gynecol* 1980;56:165

22. Hook EB, Cross PK, Schreinemachers MS. Chromosomal abnormality rates at amniocentesis and in live born infants. *J Am Med Assoc* 1983;249:2034–8

73

Neonatal diseases I

W.J. Keenan and S.S. Toce

NUTRITION

The transition from fetal to extra-fetal life is significantly challenging even for the child born at term. Nutritional needs must be met by rapid adaptation of the relatively untried gastrointestinal system and the child must master the complex neurologic task of successful feeding behavior. The premature infant faces even more nutritional challenges as nutrient stores at birth are low and there are higher requirements for rapid growth[1,2]. Mechanisms for feeding, digestion, and absorption are immature. Concomitant illnesses may interfere with growth potential, add to organ dysfunction, and further increase the demand for energy and nutrients.

A goal of neonatal nutrition is to meet the metabolic requirements of the developing organ systems, satisfy normal growth requirements and avoid deficiency or excess states without imposing detrimental stress on developing metabolic or excretory systems. Optimal neonatal growth rates are difficult to determine but attempting to follow the intrauterine growth curve and accretion rates of the third trimester fetus appears to be a reasonable starting point. The fetus gains approximately 10 g/day at 21 weeks, 20 g/day at 29 weeks and 35 g/day at 37 weeks.

Energy requirements

The energy balance describes the relationship between intake, expenditure and storage or growth. Table 1 gives the approximate intakes and expenditures one might expect for a term and a preterm infant.

Energy expenditure is highly dependent upon the extent of ongoing illness, the thermal environment and the amount of rest allowed from nursing and

Neonatal nutritional balance

	Preterm	Term
Body weight, kg	1.3	4.0
Resting energy expenditure, kcal/kg/day	47.0	40.0
Rate of weight gain g/kg/day	15.0	7.5
Minimum intake, kcal/kg/day	130.0	120.0

medical care procedures. Excreted calories, mostly a small portion of the ingested fat, are about 15 kcal/kg/day. An expected intake would allow for these losses and expenditures while making sufficient energy available to provide for at least 15 g/kg/day of growth. The caloric distribution probably should be that of human milk: 10–15% protein, 40–50% carbohydrate and 40–50% fat. A protein intake of 2–4 g/kg/day appears to provide adequate protein nutrition without the undesirable effects of excess protein.

Human milk

For the human infant no other food appears to be superior to human milk. For term infants human milk is nutritionally adequate for the first six months. The protein content of human milk is quantitatively low, 2.3 g/100 ml in colostrum and 1.0 g/100 ml after the second week postpartum. The protein is primarily lactalbumin (and whey) with high concentrations of taurine and cysteine. The fat portion contains cholesterol and 10–12% of total lipid is easily digested median chain triglyceride. The major carbohydrate of human milk is lactose which enhances the absorption of calcium and magnesium and promotes the intestinal growth of lactobacilli. The anti-infective properties of human milk include the high content of IgM, IgG, IgA and secretory IgA. Human milk also contains lysozymes, leukocytes, and lactoferrin and transferrin which bind iron necessary for the growth of some Gram-negative organisms. Human milk from the premature infant's own mother appears to be uniquely adapted towards the nutritional needs of the premature infant. For the first two weeks postpartum, the milk has a higher protein and sodium chloride content than mature 'term' human milk. Many very low birth weight infants receiving human milk require additional protein, sodium chloride, calcium and/or phosphorus[3]. Enfamil Human Milk Fortifier and Similac Natural Care are available to meet some of these needs.

In the absence of human milk, there are a number of cow milk based and soy proprietary formulas that meet the needs of most term infants. Iron supplemented formulas are recommended to avoid the morbidity associated with iron deficiency. Because these formulas do not meet the nutritional needs of the premature infant, special formulas have been developed which are whey predominant, have higher caloric, mineral and vitamin content and are more easily digestible. Growth of the premature infant while on these formulas matches that of the fetus *in utero*. Because of inadequate calcium and phosphorus absorption with soy formulas fed to premature infants, long term feeding with these formulas is not recommended for infants born preterm.

Initiation of feedings

The term infant may ideally suckle at the breast immediately after delivery or be formula fed in the first few hours after delivery. Repeat feedings are then offered on an *ad lib* every 2–4 hour schedule. The usual term infant begins to approach 150 ml/kg/day and 120 calories/kg/day by the end of the third day.

The initiation of enteral feedings for the extremely low birth weight infant is an important and vexing challenge. The very early initiation of hypocaloric enteral feedings occupies considerable current clinical interest. Half strength or full strength feedings at 0.5–1.0 ml/kg/h are advocated by many. Some data indicate that early hypocaloric feedings reduce the time required to achieve full enteral feedings and promotes feeding tolerance without increasing the risk for necrotizing enterocolitis (NEC)[4–6]. Most extremely low birth weight infants will require parenteral nutrition as discussed in a subsequent section. The pace of advancing enteral feedings is governed by the tolerance to volume and calories and by the concern for necrotizing enterocolitis. Several studies have indicated that the pace of advancing enteral feedings in the high risk low birth weight infant ought to be limited to a daily increase of about approximately 20 ml/kg to minimize the risk of necrotizing enterocolitis.

Route of feeding

Nipple feeding is appropriate for the infant with coordinated suck and swallow and active gag reflex. Coordination generally does not occur before 32 weeks post conceptual age. Gavage feedings are indicated in newborns who cannot safely be nippled, who have poorly coordinated suck–swallow or little feeding vigor. The importance of non-nutritive sucking at the time of gavage feedings has recently been emphasized. Intermittent gavage feedings can be given every 1–4 h, generally every 3 h. Gastric distention may stimulate the vagus and gastrocolic reflex with resultant rapid transit of nutrients through the gut. This method is generally well tolerated. Continuous gavage infusion via infusion pump for very low birth weight (VLBW) infants (< 1500 g) has been suggested because of the small gastric capacity in the premature, the prolonged transit time with resultant improved absorption,

improved pulmonary mechanics and reduced energy requirements. Infants below 1250 g may benefit the most by this method. Transpyloric feedings are felt to have less risk of aspiration and may be appropriate for the infant with demonstrated aspiration or certain infants with major gastrointestinal problems. The position of a silicone or polyurethane catheter in the duodenum or jejunum is confirmed radiographically. Isosmolar feedings are recommended to prevent 'dumping' syndrome. We feel that all duodenal and jejunal feedings should be given by continuous infusion. Because of the increased risk of bowel perforation, transpyloric feedings are not indicated for routine use. Gastrostomy tube feedings are generally reserved for infants with selected surgical conditions or those infants in whom adequate nipple feedings will never be a reasonable expectation. Parenteral nutrition is indicated only when enteral feedings are inadequate or contraindicated. If the gut works, use it!

Parenteral nutrition

Parenteral nutrition is an important adjunct in the nutritional management of the high risk newborn. Prevention of catabolism and provision of adequate nutrients are critical to the reduction of morbidity and mortality. Parenteral nutrition is often used as a 'nutritional bridge' to protect the nutritional status during the days and weeks necessary to establish adequate enteral nutrition. Parenteral nutrition is usually considered when enteral feeding is contraindicated or inadequate. While no clearly documented benefit of short term total parenteral nutrition (TPN) has been demonstrated, other lines of evidence indicate that the very low birth weight infant can be nutritionally compromised by the second day of inadequate nutrition. Institution of TPN in the first days of life in the high risk newborn in whom early feeding is not anticipated is indicated to enhance protein anabolism and promote growth.

Glucose is the main energy source of parenteral nutritional solutions but the glucose tolerance of the high risk infant may be very limited. Hyperglycemia is a common problem, emphasizing the vulnerability of the VLBW or extremely low birth weight infant to carbohydrate disequilibrium. Generalized stress state, altered secretion of glucoregulatory hormones and diminished tissue responsiveness to these regulatory hormones are often problematic for the VLBW or extremely low birth weight infant. In addition, the extremely low birth weight (birth weight $\leqslant 1000$ g) does not limit hepatic glucose output even when external glucose availability is adequate. Usually dextrose concentrations of 5 g/dl are begun initially, delivering 6–8 mg/kg/min. Early detection of hyperglycemia is achieved by frequent glucose monitoring. Plasma glucose levels greater than

150–200 mg/dl may require intervention. Hypotonic solutions in general are to be avoided but the delivery of glucose may need to be altered. Early institution of intravenous protein may stimulate insulin release and reduce the incidence of hyperglycemia.

There is no general agreement whether the infusion of exogenous insulin is indicated in the hyperglycemia of the VLBW infant. Continuous infusion of insulin does allow for a higher caloric intake with lower blood glucose values and less glucosuria in these low birth weight infants. Suggested initial doses of insulin are between 0.05 and 0.1 units/kg/h. Dosing is adjusted on the basis of frequent monitoring of plasma glucose.

Lipid

The premature infant rapidly becomes deficient in essential fatty acids in the absence of enteral or parenteral fat[7]. The requirement for essential free fatty acids in premature babies can be met by the administration of 1 g/kg/day linoleic acid or 2 g/kg/day of commercially available intravenous lipid[7]. Lipid infusion is usually begun at 0.5–1 g/kg/day and advanced in 0.5–1 g/kg/day increments as tolerated. Lipid dose is gradually increased to a maximum dose of 2–3 g/kg/day or 40–50% of the calories. Lipid is usually infused over a 24-h period to maximize tolerance. Lipid intolerance is demonstrated by triglyceride levels greater than 150–180 mg/dl. Extreme prematurity, intrauterine growth restriction, liver dysfunction and infection are associated with lipid intolerance.

Protein

Intravenous protein in the very low birth weight/extremely low birth weight infant is usually begun at approximately 1–1.5 g/kg/day. To match *in utero* protein accretion, protein administration is increased incrementally until the child is receiving 2.7–3.5 g/kg/day[8]. Metabolic acidosis and increased blood urea nitrogen (BUN) are often seen in protein loads in excess of 3.5–4.0 g/kg/day. Metabolic acidosis seen with lower protein loads is poorly understood and may be related to factors other than dietary protein. When the underlying cause of acidosis cannot be corrected, lactate may be added to parenteral nutritional solutions to correct acidosis and is compatible with the calcium/phosphorus content of the TPN solutions. Since lactate is substituted for chloride, long term use of lactate may lead to hypochloremic alkalosis and is not recommended. The newborn infants are at an increased risk of TPN associated cholestasis and cholestasis of other etiologies. Starvation, sepsis (particularly Gram-negative), high protein loads, caloric excess, circulatory congestion and liver dysfunction are among many factors that appear to predispose to cholestasis. Newer pediatric TPN formulations (Trophamine and Aminosyn PF) may be associated with a lower incidence of TPN associated cholestasis. TPN associated cholestasis can best be avoided by aggressive promotion of enteral feedings. If cholestasis develops (i.e. conjugated bilirubin > 0.6 mg/dl) institute enteral feedings if at all possible, avoid caloric excesses, reduce or eliminate copper and manganese supplements and consider the use of taurine-containing pediatric amino acid solutions.

Complications

Metabolic bone disease can be seen in premature infants on long term TPN. Calcium and phosphorus intake is limited because of poor solubility in the parenteral nutritional solutions. Osteopenia, fractures and poor linear growth may result. Hypophosphatemia and elevated alkaline phosphatase may help identify this bone disease of nutritional deficiency. The most serious TPN associated complications are those associated with central catheters. The incidence of catheter related sepsis is increased with decreased gestational age. Perforation of a vessel or viscus and thrombus formation are less frequently seen, but potentially serious complications. A high index of suspicion for catheter related morbidity will allow early detection and treatment of complications.

Assessment of nutrition status

Weight and weight change should be checked daily and plotted on an appropriate weight grid. The premature infant should be plotted according to corrected gestastional age until 24 months of age. Length and head circumference are usually measured and plotted weekly. Total serum protein, albumin and prealbumin measurements may assist in the assessment of protein nutritional status. Serum electrolytes should be followed as clinically indicated. Growth is affected by birth weight, gestational age, severity of illness and ongoing illnesses as well as nutritional intake.

Failure to grow

The major cause of the failure to grow is the unavailability of adequate calories. If adequate calories, 120–180 kcal/kg/day, are being provided to the child who fails to grow further evaluation is indicated. Frequent causes of failure to grow include infection (especially urinary tract infection), late metabolic acidosis, increased energy requirements (i.e. bronchopulmonary dysplasia; BPD), prematurity, subclinical hypoxemia and failure to provide thermal protection. Examinations to detect malabsorption, congenital heart disease, renal disease, metabolic disease, congenital infections, or a chromosomal problem may be indicated.

Summary

Nutrition plays a particularly important role in the developing newborn. Because of the vulnerability of growth and maturation to nutritional insults, there exists a potential for permanent sequelae. Many questions remain to be resolved: Is it reasonable to attempt to match intrauterine growth? Can the newborn compensate for suboptimal postnatal growth? How well does 'normal' somatic growth protect the nutritional promotion of motor and cognitive development? Is more necessarily better? Provision of adequate micro- and macronutrition to support growth and development while minimizing morbidity associated with enteral or parenteral feeding is one of the most rapidly evolving aspects of neonatal care today.

PATENT DUCTUS ARTERIOSUS

The ductus arteriosus, an important fetal circulatory pathway, is normally open in all infants at the time of birth. In the term and near term infant the ductus arteriosus begins to close immediately after birth and is anatomically closed in almost all infants by 48–96 hours. However this closure is delayed in the preterm infant and an incidence of persistently patent ductus arteriosus (PDA) is inversely proportional to gestational age and time after birth.

Incidence

A national collaborative study documented symptomatic patent ductus arteriosus (sPDA) in 42% of infants with birth weights less than 1000 g, 20.6% of infants with birth weights 1000–1499 g and 7.8% in infants with birth weights 1500–1700 g. The range of the incidence of sPDA among the thirteen participating centers in that study was 11–36%[9]. The onset of symptoms associated with a PDA is usually by 10 days, often by 2–5 days. Data from several studies are compatible with an effect of clinical phototherapy in maintaining ductal patency.

Pathophysiology

The early postnatal constriction of the ductus arteriosus is a functional interaction between local oxygen levels, neurohormonal factors and the smooth muscle of the ductus arteriosus[10]. Ductal constriction in response to oxygen shows a developmental progression with the least vasoconstrictive response to high oxygen levels. The duct also responds to the prostaglandins and thromboxane. Prostaglandin E_2 (PGE_2) appears to have the most potent vasodilatory effects. Many other clinical events that affect the ductal opening and closure may work through a prostaglandin mechanism. Besides immaturity, clinical risk factors for the development of a sPDA include the degree of respiratory distress, postnatal artificial surfactant use,

episodes of hypoxemia, administration of excess fluids, and anemia.

As pulmonary vascular resistance falls, the shunt through the PDA shifts from a right to left pattern to a left to right pattern, with an increasing volume pumped by the left ventricle. Effective systemic blood flow may be reduced, pulmonary edema develops and the left ventricle and atrium dilate[10]. The presence of a large shunt through the PDA is thought to adversely affect the course of respiratory distress syndrome (RDS), increase the requirement for ventilatory assistance, increase the risk of BPD and contribute to intestinal and central nervous system (CNS) ischemia.

Diagnosis

The presence of a PDA with left to right shunting is usually suspected in the presence of an increased pulse pressure and the sometimes inconsistent presence of a systolic murmur in a premature infant. A systolic or less often continuous murmur, hyperdynamic precordium, tachypnea, hepatomegaly and signs of respiratory insufficiency often ensue. Pulmonary congestion and cardiomegaly are seen in about one third of the infants with a sPDA. Echocardiography to confirm a PDA and to exclude complicating congenital heart disease is indicated when therapeutic intervention is being planned.

Treatment

A sPDA in a preterm infant will close spontaneously in approximately 80% of cases. Part of the decision to treat rests on the balance of consequences of an untreated PDA in that particular patient, the possibility of spontaneous closure and the morbidity associated with specific therapies. Several aspects of non-specific or supportive treatment deserve particular attention.

Enteral feedings

An increase in the incidence of necrotizing enterocolitis has been seen in children with large left right ductal shunts. The PDA may act as a 'mesenteric steal' rendering the bowel relatively ischemic. The patient's vulnerability to the development of necrotizing enterocolitis should be an important consideration. It is unclear whether or not withholding enteral feeding in the presence of a symptomatic PDA will result in a reduced incidence of necrotizing enterocolitis.

Fluid restriction

Fluid overload may be a feature of a patient with a sPDA. Fluid restriction appears to lessen pulmonary congestion but prolonged fluid restriction will place the patient at significant risk for undernutrition and renal dysfunction. Studies of the administration of low and high volume fluids to preterm infants and clinical experience are compatible with the notion that excess fluid administration will increase the risk of developing a sPDA. Two randomized prospective studies have examined the role of high fluid and low fluid volume infusions on the development of the sPDA[11,12]. In one study the high fluid group (169 ml/kg/day) had a lower maximum weight loss, higher caloric intake and 12.9% sPDA versus 2.3% incidence of sPDA in the low fluid group (122 ml/ kg/day). The other study design compared very low birth weight infants allowed to lose a maximum of 8–10% of the body weight versus those allowed to lose 13–15%. The incidence of sPDA of 29.5% versus 20.4%, respectively, was not significantly different. These results lend support to the use of an individualized fluid management plan for the VLBW infant.

Diuretics

Induction of diuresis may reduce the cardiac congestion and pulmonary edema. Furosemide has an action on renal tissue mediated by prostaglandins. Furosemide treatment of very low birth weight infants has been associated with increased presence of prostaglandin metabolites in the urine and some potential for dilatation of the ductus arteriosus by furosemide seems to exist. Various studies utilizing furosemide in preterm infants have not shown a consistent effect on increasing the incidence of PDA. Longer term use of diuretics is associated with a variety of electrolyte imbalances and is not a good choice for long term treatment of the patient with a sPDA.

Digoxin

This drug has been used in children with sPDA but appears to offer little help to the maximally contracting generally healthy myocardium. Digoxin toxicity is frequent in the preterm infant. Digoxin is no longer used widely.

Catecholamines

While having no specific effect upon the ductus arteriosus, inotropic catecholamines offer short-term assistance to an overloaded myocardium but administration of inotropic agents does not address the primary problem of persistently patent arteriosus with a large left to right shunt.

Specific treatment for PDA

A large number of trials have documented the efficacy of intravenous or oral administration of indomethacin in promoting ductal closure. Indomethacin probably exerts its effect through inhibiting the dilatory effect of prostaglandin at the smooth muscle of the duct[13]. The most common dose given is 0.2 mg/kg given intravenously or orally for three doses every 12–24 h. Relative contraindications for the administration of indomethacin include an elevated serum creatinine greater than 1.2 mg/dl, platelet count less than 50 000/μl, coagulopathy, necrotizing enterocolitis and possibly the presence of a CNS hemorrhage. Approximately 20% of infants will fail to close the sPDA in response to indomethacin. Another 20% will reopen the duct after an initial constrictive response. Babies < 1000g, > 10 days old at time of treatment or > 36 weeks corrected post-conceptual age have higher relapse rates. A second course of indomethacin is probably a reasonable approach for many of these children. Longer courses of treatment, continuous infusions and indomethacin dosing based on pharmacologic data have all been reported as successful. Since indo-methacin inhibits the prostaglandin effect upon regional perfusion in the kidney, caution should be used in the child with a low blood volume (fluid restriction and diuretics), reduced systemic flow (left to right shunt), congestive heart failure, and renal insufficiency (elevated serum creatinine). Indomethacin has been anecdotally reported to be associated with ileal perforation. Surgical ligation appears to be safe and effective. The surgical related mortality and morbidity are very low. Two studies that included early ligation of the PDA reported a significantly lower incidence of necrotizing enterocolitis in surgically treated infants versus those treated with general medical support[14,15]. Mortality and other major morbidities were not significantly different between the groups.

Prevention

A large number of randomized clinical trials have examined the effectiveness of prophylactic indomethacin administration on the PDA in the preterm infant. Prophylactic administration of indomethacin does decrease the incidence of sPDA but does not affect neonatal mortality or major morbidities except for a slight reduction in the incidence of intraventricular hemorrhage. Prophylactic diuretic therapy, vitamin E administration and inositol supplementation have not been shown to affect mortality. The incidence of sPDA is reported to be approximately 3-fold lower in the group of infants whose mothers received prenatal steroids. Whether the prenatal steroid had a specific effect upon the ductal tissue or whether steroids acted through a reduction in the severity of hyaline membrane disease is speculative.

PERIVENTRICULAR– INTRAVENTRICULAR HEMORRHAGE

The most common neuropathic finding in the preterm infant and one of the most common causes of acute perinatal CNS dysfunction is periventricular–intraventricular hemorrhage (PIVH). It is the second leading cause of neonatal death after RDS. The development of non-invasive CNS imaging techniques such as neuroultrasonography has helped describe a broad spectrum of lesions from small hemorrhages in the subependymal germinal matrix with no discernable sequelae to intraparenchymal hemorrhage with infarction and serious sequelae. Wide spread use of ultrasonography has allowed the use of grading schemes that have some prognostic usefulness (Table 2).

Table 2 Grading system for periventricular–intraventricular hemorrhage (from reference 16)

Grade	Ultrasonographic findings
I	Hemorrhage confined to the germinal matrix
II	Some blood seen in normal sized ventricle
III	Blood seen in enlarged ventricle
IV	Blood seen in ventricle plus intraparenchymal hemorrhage

Incidence

PIVH occurs predominantly in very low birth weight infants but can occur even in infants born at full term. Most hemorrhages are evident using non-invasive imaging by two days after birth, but some occur up to about seven days after birth. Several studies have documented that about 14% of all PIVH is evident at birth. The prevalence of any form of PIVH in preterm infants less than 1500 g birth weight in tertiary centers is approximately 40–50%. In our recent series of 71 consecutively admitted VLBW infants the incidence of any PIVH was 25.9%. Grades III or IV were seen in 11.8%. Mortality rate in children with Grade IV PIVH was 47.8%. The incidence of PIVH was inversely proportional to gestational age.

Children with severe PIVH often have a mix of severe organ dysfunctions such as RDS and other problems of prematurity. The mortality associated with PIVH is reported to be 25–50%, with a higher mortality seen with more severe lesions[17].

Germinal matrix

The subependymal germinal matrix is a periventricular layer of pluripotential precursors of neurons and glia. This layer is most prominent between 24 and 34 weeks' gestation and then gradually involutes as the neural elements migrate to intended functional sites in the central nervous system. This germinal matrix has a rich but thin and vulnerable vascular supply with almost no supportive stroma.

Hemorrhage in the subependymal germinal matrix hemorrhage may disrupt the migration of critical neurocellular elements in the network near the head of the body of the caudate nucleus. However, no long-term clinical consequences of isolated subependymal germinal matrix hemorrhage have yet been identified.

Intraventricular hemorrhage

Most intraventricular hemorrhage appears to be a consequence of subependymal germinal matrix hemorrhages rupturing into the lateral ventricle. A large hemorrhage may fill the ventricle and result in clot formation.

Arachnoid dysfunction or mechanical blockage caused by the clot may result in the accumulation of abnormal amounts of ventricular fluid causing post-hemorrhagic hydrocephalus. Many infants who show acute ventricular dilatation will have spontaneous resolution. Progressive ventricular dilatation is a major sequela of intraventricular hemorrhage. Clinical hydrocephalus requiring ventricular drainage is seen in about 14% of infants with intraventricular hemorrhage and is more frequent with grades III and IV PIVH.

Parenchymal hemorrhage

Hemorrhage into the periventricular substance of the cerebrum is seen in 10–20% of infants with PIVH (9.3% in our most recent series) and is an important cause of neurodevelopmental handicap. Periventricular hemorrhage may occur because of venous or arterial bleeding and may be the result of infarction. Periventricular venous infarction, usually unilateral, has been linked to the venous obstruction caused by a large ipsilateral intraventricular hemorrhage.

Periventricular leukomalacia

Periventricular leukomalacia in the premature infant appears to occur as a consequence of hemorrhagic infarction or can appear as an ischemic non-hemorrhagic lesion. Ischemia leading to areas of necrosis in the periventricular white matter results in edema, macrophage infiltration and astrocytic proliferation. Glial replacement and sometimes cyst formation may then follow. Destruction of white matter can result in secondary enlargement of the lateral ventricles (hydrocephalus ex vacuo). Large amounts of destruction are associated with periventricular changes apparent on central nervous system imaging. Extensive periventricular leukomalacia usually involves the descending motor tracks with spastic dysfunction most commonly affecting the lower limbs. Spastic quadriplegia and visual defects can also be seen with extensive injury[18].

Etiology

Attempts have been made to define a relationship between any number of perinatal events and occurrence of PIVH. The risk factors that can be defined consistently are prematurity and acute pneumothorax, hypotension, acute expansion of blood volume, acidosis, coagulation problems, abrupt changes in serum osmolality with bicarbonate infusion, hypercarbia, hypocarbia, hyperglycemia, and fluctuations in erebral blood flow or systemic blood pressure. A firm cause and effect with any of these risk factors except prematurity remains to be established.

Diagnosis

Major PIVH may be associated with changes in central nervous system function and disturbance of cardiorespiratory stability. Many infants, however, have no clinical signs attributed to PIVH. The major method of diagnosis is routine screening usually utilizing bedside neuroultrasonography through open fontanelles. The evolution of various lesions of PIVH may be followed with serial imaging. Optimal timing for CNS screening remains to be determined. In our nursery, screening ultrasonography is done at 7–10 days of age.

Evolution/Sequelae

Smaller hemorrhages tend to gradually resolve without evidence of anatomic abnormality. Clinical studies have identified that infants with grade I–II PIVH have the same risk of neurodevelopmental handicap as appropriate control preterm infants. More severe degrees of hemorrhage tend to be associated with post-hemorrhagic hydrocephalus and periventricular leukomalacia. The incidence of major handicap in infants with grade III–IV PIVH appears to be about 11%[16]. Post-hemorrhagic hydrocephalus may in itself not increase neurodevelopmental risk but is often associated with more extensive original and residual injury. As mentioned earlier, periventricular leukomalacia evolving to multicystic formation is associated with a major incidence of motor disability. Hydrocephalus ex vacuo is often associated with extensive neurologic and developmental dysfunction.

Treatment

Management of infants with PIVH is generally supportive, attempting to achieve or maintain clinical homeostasis. No treatment specifically directed to acute PIVH has been shown to be effective. Post-hemorrhagic hydrocephalus is most often communicating. Pharmacologic suppression of cerebral spinal fluid production (e.g. acetazolamide) and hyperosmolar therapy have not been proven very effective. Rapid progressive ventricular dilatation is usually treated with surgical ventricular drainage. If the dilatation is slowly progressive over several weeks, serial lumbar punctures are often used. Although there are few data that definitively support the long-term benefits of such an approach, if ventricular dilatation continues, ventriculoperitoneal shunting of cerebral spinal fluid is usually done. If the ventricular dilatation is arrested, intermittent observations without intervention are probably the best alternative.

Prevention

The most effective prevention of PIVH is the reduction of preterm birth[19]. One note of optimism is that while the incidence of preterm birth has remained unchanged or increased in the last decade, a poorly understood reduction of PIVH incidence has been seen in many prenatal centers around the USA[20].

Obstetric events

Several studies have indicated that very low birth weight infants born at a tertiary perinatal center have a lower incidence of PIVH than those born outside such a center. Non-randomized selection of subjects and multiple confounding variables interfere with any definitive conclusion. A number of obstetric related events have been examined for a relationship with PIVH. No consistent effect has been seen. A study comparing electronic fetal monitoring with intermittent auscultation did not demonstrate an influence on the incidence of PIVH. Several trials have suggested an association of the use of antenatal steroids with the reduction of PIVH. In a randomized controlled study, Morales demonstrated that the group that received antenatal steroids had a lower incidence of all PIVH grades combined[21]. The role of antenatal steroids in the prevention of PIVH is not firmly established.

Phenobarbital

Prophylactic phenobarbital treatment of premature infants was initially reported to be associated with reduction of the incidence of PIVH. Randomized control studies have failed to confirm this observation. Phenobarbital administration to women at acute risk of preterm delivery has not shown a reduction in PIVH severity and incidence.

Indomethacin

Indomethacin dramatically reduces PIVH in the canine model. Several clinical studies have yielded both confirmatory and contradictory results. The potential role of indomethacin in clinical practice is still undefined.

Pancuronium

One prospective trial of paralysis with pancuronium was shown to be associated with less fluctuation of arterial blood pressure and cerebral blood flow velocity. A reduction in the incidence in severity of PIVH was attributed to this increased stability[22]. Other clinical studies have not been supportive of the use of pancuronium.

Ethamsylate

A large multicenter trial concluded that ethamsylate, a non-steroidal anti-inflammatory agent, was effective in reducing both the incidence and severity of PIVH. Definition of effectiveness requires further study.

Vitamin E and vitamin K

Neonatal vitamin E supplementation and antepartum maternal administration of vitamin K have each been suggested to be effective in the prevention of PIVH. The data concerning vitamin E are contradictory and those concerning vitamin K are confounded with important clinical variables.

Summary

Available studies do not yet outline a safe and effective clinical approach to the prevention of PIVH in the premature infant. Further improvements in care and prevention will probably be made through greater understanding of the pathophysiologic mechanisms involved.

APNEA OF PREMATURITY

Most preterm infants exhibit various patterns of respiratory effort including regular respirations, periodic breathing and longer respiratory pauses or apnea. The risk/benefit of diagnostic and therapeutic efforts can be judged better if we understand the pathologic significance of apnea occurring in the preterm infant. Apnea has been defined as being pathologic when there is 'cessation of breathing for twenty seconds or longer; or briefer episodes if associated with bradycardia, cyanosis or pallor'[23]. The significance of apnea of prematurity probably rests more with the primary diagnosis than with the apnea related consequences of prolonged or recurrent hypoxemia and/or hypotension. Although extensive clinical monitoring has been used for a number of years our understanding of which clinical apneic events might be associated with significant cerebral hypoxia is still very poor. Patterns of cessation of respiration without respiratory effort known as central apnea, patterns of respiratory effort without air flow, obstructive apnea, and mixed (both central and obstructive) apnea are seen at various times in large numbers of preterm infants with or without associated hypoxemia. In addition, hypoxemia and/or bradycardia without apnea is sometimes seen in very high risk infants presumably because of hypoventilation, intrapulmonary circulatory disturbances or reflex bradycardia.

Incidence

Martin has reported that more than 50% of all surviving infants < 1500 g, require interventions because of recurrent prolonged apneic spells[24]. Our recent experience in a tertiary referral center indicated that 715 of 1457 (49%) consecutively admitted infants with birth weight less than 1500 g experience apnea requiring treatment.

Etiology

The basic underlying mechanisms that account for apnea of prematurity are unclear. Apnea of prematurity may in part result from decreased carbon dioxide responsiveness, vulnerability to hypoventilation, predilection for upper airway obstruction, hypoxemic depression of carbon dioxide responsiveness and/or decreased responsiveness of respiratory reflexes. While some data exist to support each of these hypotheses no generalizable explanation has yet emerged[24].

Diagnosis

Apnea is diagnosed through the combined use of electronic monitoring and bedside observation. Generally apneas of 15–20 s or shorter respiratory pauses associated with cyanosis, hypotension and/or bradycardia are recorded. The typical preterm infant with apnea will have a mixed pattern of central and obstructive apneas. A major criterion for the diagnosis of idiopathic apnea of prematurity is the absence of major pathology that could itself be related to the apnea. An appropriate search for possible complications should be carried out with each apneic infant and any underlying pathology treated. The apneic preterm infant should be evaluated for major infection including pneumonia, meningitis, and urinary tract infection, early necrotizing enterocolitis, metabolic problems including hypoglycemia, and stressful thermal environment[25]. Most of this is done by a review of the history, clinical examination, a period of observation and relatively few laboratory screening tests. Factors possibly predisposing the infants to apnea such as feeding stress, severe anemia, gastroesophageal reflux, seizures, airway positioning, laryngopharyngeal stimulation and fatigue may require attention[26].

Treatment

Treatment of apnea of prematurity should begin with a search for any underlying pathology and specific treatment instituted. If the apneic spells are not consistently responsive to gentle tactile stimulation additional therapeutic intervention might be indicated.

The most common therapeutic approach to apnea to prematurity is treatment with methylxanthines. Approximately 70% of infants with apnea of prematurity will respond to this approach with major decrease or disappearance of the apnea. Oral theophylline is used as a loading dose of 2.5–6 mg/kg and

2.0–4.0 mg/kg/day divided into two doses. A serum level of 6–10 µg/ml is usually adequate. Side-effects include agitation, jitteriness, vomiting and tachycardia[27]. Alternatively oral caffeine can be given as a loading dose of 10 mg/kg as caffeine base and 2.5–5.0 mg/kg once per day beginning on day two of therapy. A serum level of 8–20 µg/ml is usually achieved. In the dosages cited caffeine is equally as effective as theophylline and seems to be associated with fewer gastrointestinal or central nervous system side-effects[28]. A small increase in FiO_2 may be effective in reducing apnea in some children. Close monitoring to avoid hyperoxia is required.

Kinesthetic stimulation in the form of a rocking bed has been effective in some studies. Correction of anemia occasionally reduces the number and severity of apneic spells. Anemia is common and usually well tolerated in the preterm infant and often is not related to the apnea. Transfusion should not be undertaken routinely as it has a poorly predictable effect on frequency and severity of apnea of prematurity. There are a small number of preterm infants with hypoxemic episodes poorly responsive to any of the above measures.

No generally therapeutic approach can be universally recommended. To repeat a note of caution, the possible underlying pathology should be sought even if the apneic infant is responsive to any of the above measures. The role of home monitoring for the infant with symptomatic apnea of prematurity at the time of discharge is unclear. The treatment plan should be individualized.

Outcome

Severe, recurrent apnea of prematurity is a weak statistical risk factor for the development of cerebral palsy. While apnea with severe bradycardia has been demonstrated to be associated with reduced cerebral blood flow, any cause-effect relationship is obscure. Prognosis appears to be related to clinical conditions other than apnea. Apnea of prematurity improves with time probably as the maturation of the central nervous system and neuroflexive systems improve. Once apnea has resolved, recurrence is rare.

SEIZURES

Seizure activity in the newborn period can represent a primary pathology in the central nervous system or be a manifestation of systemic or metabolic events. The presence of neonatal seizures generally represents a relative medical emergency since interference with the cardiorespiratory status can be life threatening. Additionally, the disorder accounting for the seizures can represent ongoing but treatable injury to the central nervous system and prolonged neuroleptic activity may add an injurious effect to the developing brain.

Some laboratory evidence indicates that seizure activity in an immature animal interferes with myelinization and cell division. Positron emission tomographic studies suggest that ongoing seizures may increase cerebral vulnerability because metabolic requirements may exceed available energy.

Etiology/incidence

Several groups of investigators have reported on the incidence and etiology of neonatal seizures in select populations[29,30]. Potential etiologic mechanisms include:

(1) metabolic;

(2) infections;

(3) toxicity;

(4) hypoxia–ischemia;

(5) anomalies;

(6) CNS trauma/hemorrhage;

(7) benign familial or non-familial.

Metabolic causes for neonatal seizures include hypoglycemia, hypocalcemia, hyponatremia, hypomagnesemia, hypernatremia, and inborn errors of amino acid, carbohydrate or organic acid metabolism. Hypoglycemia is most likely to occur in association with perinatal depression, prematurity, postmaturity, intrauterine growth restriction or in infants who are large for gestational age. Routine screening for early neonatal blood glucose level is a widespread practice but no particular standard for screening is universally recommended. Early nutritive practices in both stressed and non-stressed newborns seems to have reduced the number of symptomatic newborns with hypoglycemia. Hypocalcemia with serum calcium levels less than 7.5 mg/dl is often seen in infants with perinatal stress but hypocalcemia appears to be an uncommon cause of neonatal seizures.

Meningoencephalitis can be associated with neonatal seizures. Approximately 55% of infants with neonatal bacterial meningitis exhibit seizures. Common viral etiologies for encephalitis are herpes simplex and enterovirus. Toxicity from injected local anesthetics intended for the mother have been reported to cause refractory seizures. Neonatal drug withdrawal from narcotics or a variety of sedatives can also result in seizures.

Seizures associated with perinatal hypoxemic ischemic encephalopathy most commonly begin between 6 and 24 h after birth. About 70% of infants with moderate encephalopathy secondary to hypoxemia–ischemia will develop seizures. Seizures associated with perinatal hypoxemic ischemic encephalopathy may be very difficult to control and the refractoriness denotes a very poor neurologic outcome[31]. Major malformations of the central nervous system such as holoprosencephaly, and probably more subtle malformations, can also be associated with high incidence of seizure disorder during the neonatal period.

Small amounts of subarachnoid bleeding (in an otherwise healthy appearing infant) can be associated with one or more seizures usually within the first three days after birth. These seizures do not recur and are associated with a good neurological prognosis. Severe PIVH in the preterm infant can be associated with seizures. When seizures occur in association with PIVH the extent of the seizure disorder appears to correlate with the severity of the PIVH[32]. Cerebral infarction and traumatic intracranial hemorrhage such as subdural hematomas can also be associated with neonatal seizures. One dramatic current association with cerebral infarct and seizures is the use of cocaine in the immediate prepartum period. Benign transient familial neonatal seizures are often seen by the second day after birth and usually are no longer seen by age 2 years. A strong pattern of neonatal seizures is seen in some family members who have normal development and neurologic outcomes. A benign non-familial pattern is also recognized. Seizures most commonly occur around day five. The neonatal seizures in both entities can be quite severe and often require considerable anticonvulsant therapy. However, the disease of both entities appears to be mostly self-limited. The familial pattern seems to be associated with an increased risk of epilepsy later in life[33].

Diagnosis

A variety of autonomic and motor manifestations of neonatal seizures have been identified. Major motor manifestations include focal, non-focal, tonic, clonic, myoclonic, general or non-generalized seizures. Movements of the leg or rowing movements of the arms may be the only major motor abnormalities seen. Repetitive sucking, grimacing, or chewing movements are common facial demonstrations of neonatal seizure activity. These movements may precede more generalized tonic clonic seizures. Nystagmus, horizontal deviation of the eyes, staring or blinking are often the earliest signs of neonatal seizures. Apnea and hyperpnea are common autonomic disturbances in neonatal seizures. Tremors or repetitive myoclonic jerks usually can be distinguished from seizure activity by suppressing the movement with resistance or movement and by the absence of state or autonomic change associated with seizures.

Critical clues to the etiology of seizures are often provided by family or perinatal history. The timing of seizure onset may be helpful. Seizures associated with hypoxemic ischemic encephalopathy, drug withdrawal, benign familial seizure disorder and hypoglycemia are most often seen in the first several days after birth while those associated with infectious disease or inborn error of metabolism are most often seen towards the end of the first week.

Screening for hypoglycemia and hypocalcemia is usually done for every infant with a seizure. Evaluation for bacterial or viral infection, intracranial hemorrhage, or hypoxemic ischemic encephalopathy is pursued as clinically indicated. A lumbar puncture is indicated to rule out meningitis unless the etiology of the seizures is already firmly determined. Hypoglycemia persisting or recurring after 5–7 days suggests that an inborn error of metabolism be pursued. Noninvasive imaging, such as computed tomography scans, is often helpful when the diagnosis has not been identified. Recording of the electroencephalograph may be useful to clarify the relationship between questionable clinical manifestations and possible paradoxical electrical discharge.

Treatment

Treatment of neonatal seizures is begun immediately. Correction of metabolic abnormalities such as hypoglycemia or hypocalcemia may be curative. Monitoring the response to initial and continued therapy is recommended. Prompt diagnosis and treatment deserve emphasis. In addition to specific convulsant therapy, it may be necessary to support oxygenation and ventilation.

Anticonvulsants are usually indicated if seizures persist or are likely to recur. Dosage ranges for commonly used anticonvulsants are seen in Table 3. Phenobarbital is the most likely used first anticonvulsant and is given in 10 mg/kg increments with slow intravenous push up to 40 mg/kg total dosage if seizures persist. Phenytoin (Dilantin) is a commonly used second drug. It is important to recognize the lethal potential of phenytoin (Dilantin) overdose. Fosphenytoin, a phenytoin prodrug, appears to be a safer alternative and is ordered in phenytoin equivalents. Diazepam, lorazepam[34] and midazolan are used as second or third anticonvulsants and some feel that they are a useful primary therapy.

Table 3   Anticonvulsants for neonatal seizures

Phenobarbital	10 mg/kg IV push repeated PRN up to 40 mg/kg total	3–4 mg/kg/day IV or PO
(phenytoin equivalents) Fosphenytoin	10 mg/kg IV push up to 20 mg/kg total	4–8 mg/kg/day IV or PO
Lorazepam	0.05–0.1 mg/kg per dose IV slow push	
Midazolam	0.05–0.15 mg/kg IV slow push	

IV, intravenous; PO, orally; PRN, as needed

One potential effect of the many anticonvulsants used alone or in combination is respiratory depression.

All anticonvulsants except phenobarbital are usually discontinued after improvement in the acute neurologic status. The etiology, if it can be defined, is useful in determining duration of anticonvulsant therapy. A corrected metabolic disorder should be associated with a low potential for recurrence for recurrent seizures. On the other hand, malformations in the central nervous system are associated with a high potential for recurrence for recurrent seizures.

Prognosis

Neurodevelopmental prognosis associated with neonatal seizures is primarily related to the etiology of the seizures themselves and the extent of the primary pathology. Children with hypoxemic ischemic encephalopathy and persistent, difficult-to-treat seizures are at a very high risk of permanent sequelae. Seizures related to subarachnoid hemorrhage, a promptly responsive metabolic disorder or a familial pattern generally are associated with a good prognosis. Outcomes for seizures associated with inborn errors of metabolism, such as maple syrup urine disease, are related to the success in treating the primary disorder. In very general terms seizures with prematurity, with early onset, of long duration or refractiveness to treatment denote a poorer prognosis. Infants with a normal electroencephalogram and neurologic exam at the time of discharge from the hospital are more likely to have a good outcome.

NECROTIZING ENTEROCOLITIS

Necrotizing enterocolitis (NEC) is the most common serious gastrointestinal disorder encountered in the neonatal intensive care unit. The clinical presentation of NEC ranges from insidious dysfunction of the gastrointestinal tract to a catastrophic pattern of shock, sepsis and intestinal perforation. NEC continues to be a major contributor to infant mortality and morbidity[35]. Affected bowel is dusky in appearance and grossly distended with edema and scattered intramural hemorrhage. The bowel has subserosal gas collection (pneumatosis intestinalis), areas of necrosis, and may have areas of perforation. Histologically, coagulation necrosis begins with the mucosa and can extend across the full thickness of the bowel wall. Inflammation is seen but is usually only moderate in degree.

Incidence

Necrotizing enterocolitis is said to constitute approximately 5% of all admissions to the neonatal intensive care unit (NICU) and accounts for the majority of children with severe long term complications of bowel function. Reported mortality is approximately 20–40%[36]. The incidence of NEC increases with decreasing birth weight but this disease can occur in term infants. In the years 1990–1994, NEC was seen in 2.2% of the in-born admissions to our tertiary referral center and 97.7% of affected infants were less than 2500 g birth weight. NEC accounted for 4.7% of the admissions to our out-born NICU and was associated with a 23.9% mortality rate. In this outborn population 9.4% of all infants with NEC were greater than 2500 g birth weight. Prominent risk factors in the term and near term infant are polycythemia and congenital heart disease.

Etiology

The etiology of NEC probably is a multifactorial mix of intestinal ischemia, enteral demand and infection[36]. Enteral alimentation is felt to have a major role in the pathogenesis since almost all children who develop necrotizing enterocolitis have been fed enterally (158 of our last 159 infants with NEC). Enteral feeding could be the major risk factor because formula might furnish the substrate for bacterial overgrowth, cause major changes in interluminal pH and increase the risk for intestinal hypoxemia by promoting a mismatch between oxygen consumption and mesenteric circulation. Stressful perinatal events also appear to be major risk factors.

Necrotizing enterocolitis also appears to be an epidemic event, appearing in clusters, although the presence of possible triggering events such as wide spread rotovirus infection in the nursery has been documented infrequently.

Diagnosis

Necrotizing enterocolitis usually presents during the first week after birth but may present somewhat later especially in the extremely preterm infant. Risk factors for NEC include prematurity, asphyxial episodes, respiratory distress, patent ductus arteriosus, polycythemia, exchange transfusions or previous episodes of shock. The diagnosis of NEC is generally based on a high index of suspicion, evidence of gastrointestinal dysfunction and characteristic changes on the abdominal radiograph. The initial signs and symptoms of necrotizing enterocolitis are quite variable, ranging from slowly developing feeding intolerance to a cataclysmic presentation of peritonitis and shock. Abdominal distention, increased volume of prefeeding gastric aspirates, bilious gastric content and blood in the stool are frequently early signs of NEC. Increasing apnea, decreasing tolerance to handling, lethargy, and pallor are also seen. Findings on the abdominal examination can be minimal or can reveal visable bowel loops, tenderness of the abdominal wall, guarding, or abdominal wall erythma. Serial examinations of the abdomen are helpful.

Laboratory evidence may reflect inflammation, with increased white blood count, left shift and/or thrombocytopenia. Hypoventilation and/or metabolic acidosis are frequently seen. Occasionally a child will have disseminated intravascular coagulation and coagulation studies are performed as clinically indicated.

Radiologic examinations should include a flat plate of the abdomen and a cross table lateral or left lateral decubitus. The decubitus film with the liver in the superior position or the cross table film provide the most sensitive views to discover free intraperitoneal gas. The patient should be in a position at least 20 min prior to an examination to allow for the suspected intraperitoneal gas to collect in a position visible on the film. The earliest radiologic sign of NEC is ileus with distended intestinal loops. A stagnant dilated bowel loop may be seen on serial films. Pneumatosis intestinalis is evidence of abnormal gas accumulation within the bowel wall and provides strong diagnostic evidence of NEC. Gas accumulation within the portal veins probably represents drainage of the pneumatosis intestinalis and may be associated with rapid clinical deterioration. The flat plate may also furnish evidence of edema of the bowel wall or ascites. The occurrence of pneumoperitoneum in the presence of clinical signs of NEC is evidence of intestinal perforation. Some infants will have perforation without demonstrating pneumoperitoneum on radiographic examination. Serial films in the patient with suspect or documented NEC are generally done every 6–8 h to detect evidence supportive of intestinal gangrene and perforation. Diagnostic paracentesis and careful serial clinical exams may both furnish strong independent evidence of gangrene, perforation, and/or advancing peritonitis[37,38].

Treatment
General clinical support

The cardiovascular status of the child with NEC may be compromised by translocation of fluids outside of the vascular space ('third space' accumulation in the bowel, peritoneum and interstitial spaces) and toxic factors decreasing effective circulation. Affected children most often require generous expansion of vascular volume, transfusion with packed red blood cells as necessary, and ionotropic support of the circulation as clinically indicated. Oral feedings are immediately discontinued and gastric drainage provided. Correction of metabolic acidosis with bicarbonate or tris buffers may or may not be helpful. Many children with NEC can show progressive hypoventilation or apnea and prompt support of ventilization and supplemental oxygen therapy may be indicated. Nutrition should be provided by the intravenous route. Associated electrolyte and coagulation abnormalities should be corrected.

Anti-infective

Antibiotic combinations with both Gram-positive and Gram-negative coverage are provided. Many clinicians advocate specific treatment with anaerobic coverage but convincing evidence of clinical effectiveness is lacking. Since a number of currently implicated microorganisms are methicillin-resistant staphylococci, we most commonly include vancomycin in the initial antibiotic regimen. The utility of intravenous immunoglobulin is uncertain. No evidence exists that the administration of fresh frozen plasma for its possible non-specific anti-infective properties might outweigh the definite risk of transmitted infection. Bell and Martin described the use and role of oral aminoglycosides in the treatment of acute NEC[39] but the effectiveness of the strategy was not confirmed in a single small prospective study[40].

Acute follow-up

While the outcome of a patient with acute NEC is still in doubt a careful watch for signs of advancing peritonitis, intestinal perforation or other clinical deterioration must be continued. Clinical and radiologic exams should be repeated at approximately 6–8 h intervals. Serial blood counts may provide evidence of ongoing inflammation or consumption of platelets. Measures of acid–base status are followed carefully.

Indications for laparotomy

There is general agreement that laparotomy is indicated if there is unequivocal evidence of intestinal perforation, gangrene, or clinical signs of progressive peritonitis. Unremitting metabolic acidosis, persistent shock, thrombocytopenia or the presence of fixed dilated intestinal loops suggest intestinal gangrene and provide relative indications for surgical exploration[41]. Specific surgical therapy is dictated by the clinical appearance of the bowel and the patient. Resection of gangrenous bowel and closure of perforations are performed. Primary anastamosis is feasible in occasional infants. An ileostomy or colostomy is often provided. A 'second look' exploratory laparotomy may be useful in the unstable infant 24–36 h after the initial operation. This 'second look' operation may provide the opportunity to remove clearly defined non-viable bowel, exclude the possibility of additional perforation and remove additional purulent material from the peritoneum[42].

Post acute care

Antibiotics are usually continued for 10–14 days. Total parenteral nutrition is aggressively provided to try to establish an anabolic state. Small amounts of lactose free formula are usually initiated after 7–10 days of asymptomatic recovery. Secondary reanastomosis of the intestine may be carried out at any time the patient demonstrates a period of adequate anabolism and growth. The patient who retains only a marginal length of bowel presents a difficult therapeutic challenge for the combined team of pediatricians and surgeons.

Prevention

Several studies provide evidence that the rapid advancement (> 20 ml/kg/day) of enteral feedings to infants with birth weights less than 1500 g presents a significant risk factor for the development of NEC. Neither the early initiation of oral feedings nor its delay are convincingly associated with reduction in the incidence of NEC[43].

The feeding of human milk to prevent NEC has been a major clinical investigative interest for more than twenty years. Laboratory induced NEC in a rat pup model can be prevented by the feeding of fresh mother's milk while the feeding of formula does not prevent the development of NEC-like illness. Although NEC is occasionally seen in infants who were exclusively fed mother's milk, Lucas and Cole[44] have reported a protective effect of human milk in a prospective multicenter study of 926 preterm infants. Preterm infants receiving only human milk had a 1.2% incidence of NEC, those who were receiving partial human milk feedings 2.5% and formula fed infants 7.2%. Statistical correction for other risk factors demonstrated a 3–10-fold risk reduction of NEC related to human milk[44].

Several groups have reported their experience with oral aminoglycosides in the prevention of NEC. Oral kanamycin, gentamicin and colistin have been studied. While these experiences are not universally positive the administration of oral aminoglycosides appears to decrease the incidence of a radiologic and clinical NEC in high risk populations over limited periods of time. The number of NEC related deaths may not be reduced significantly, and aminoglycoside use promotes the development of antibiotic-resistant enteric flora. While the use of oral aminoglycoside might be considered for use during an endemic situation it is not to be recommended routinely. One report showed a reduction in NEC incidence associated with the use of an oral IgA–IgG preparation. Several prospective trials of prenatal steroids have suggested a reduction in the incidence of NEC in the groups whose mothers were treated with steroids. These results appear quite encouraging. Early surgical closure of the patent ductus arteriosus in low birth weight infants has been associated with a significant reduction in the incidence of NEC[14,15]. A significant effect on mortality was not demonstrated and the place of aggressive management of the PDA remains undetermined.

In summary, the most solid current support for preventative strategies in the prevention of NEC in high risk infants appears to be prevention of prematurity, avoidance of rapid advancement of oral feedings and the use of human milk whenever possible.

RETINOPATHY OF PREMATURITY

Vascular retinopathy occurring in the immature and incompletely vascularized retina of preterm infants is known as retinopathy of prematurity (ROP)[45]. The vasculopathy can completely resolve with resulting normal vision, can result in partial scarring and some deformity of the retina, or can result in significant scarring and complete retinal separation and blindness. When first described in the 1940s this vasculopathy was called retrolental fibroplasia (RLF) and virtually disappeared between 1950 and 1970 when the use of supplemental oxygen to preterm infants was curtailed. The resurgence of ROP in modern neonatal care as a result of increased survival of extremely premature infants is a major cause of morbidity in the extremely low birth weight infant. Phelps estimates that 770 infants each year are blinded as a result of ROP and that another 2300 have significant interference with normal vision[46].

Incidence

A very useful classification for staging retinopathy of prematurity is based on the 1984 international classification of acute retinopathy of prematurity (ICROP) which describes the disease by its location in the retina (zone), the amount of circumference involved (clock hours), the appearance of the active edge of vasculopathy or the extent of the scarring (stage), and the presence or absence of accelerated vasculopathy which seems to mark a major risk of aggressive progression (plus disease)[47].

Zone one describes the most posterior or immature retina, zone two the intermediate portion of the retina and zone three the most peripheral and last portion of the retina to vascularize. Stage one describes a clear flat demarcation line between the vascular and avascular retina. Stage two describes a transition line that has formed a pink ridge with or without a small amount of neovascular proliferation behind the ridge. Stage three describes the presence of extra-retinal fibrovascular proliferation which may extend into the vitreous. Stage four represents partial detachment with exudative traction on the retina and stage five describes complete retinal detachment.

Disease presenting in a more posterior or immature zone, with a more advanced stage of disease and a large number of involved clock hours, has a worse prognosis than disease presenting in the peripheral (more mature) retina, with a milder stage and fewer clock hours of involvement.

All investigators have described an inverse relationship of gestational age at birth to the incidence of ROP. The multicenter study of retinopathy of prematurity and cryotherapy showed an incidence of 66% in infants weighing less than 1251 g at birth[48]. Eighteen per cent developed moderate or severe ROP and 6% had extensive disease (3+) which in that study was the threshold for the initiation of cryotherapy. In a multicentered study of 3025 premature infants Purohit *et al.* reported retinal detachment in 9/54 (16.7%) of infants with a birth weight between 500 and 749 g[49].

In our recent 4 year experience with 871 consecutively admitted very low birth weight infants (< 1500 g), stage 4 ROP was seen in 1.38%. Among the infants with birth weights of 500–799 g the stage 4 ROP was seen in 8.9% and stage 5 disease in 2.2%.

Etiology

Retinal growth proceeds at 15–18 weeks' gestation from the optic disc outward. Growth and vascularization is not complete until about 40 weeks' gestation. If the progress of retinal development and vascularization is disrupted for whatever reason retinopathy of prematurity ensues. The results of this disruption of vascular development can be transitory with minimal or no scarring, or may progress to a more permanent injury of the retina.

No single hypothesis has been fully validated but the current theories of the pathogenesis of enciting events of ROP include hypoxia, ischemia triggered by hyperoxia, a failure of vasoconstriction in hyperoxia exposing the developing retina to hyperoxic injury, the hyperoxic stimulation of gap junction formation and the local leak of vascular proliferative factors, hyperoxia and free radical formation, and light induced changes in the immature retina promoting free radical formation and disrupted retinal growth. Very little is understood about factors that either promote the vasculopathy or allow regression.

Diagnosis

Infants at risk of ROP usually undergo regular screening examinations with the aid of an indirect ophthalmoscope. The American Academy of Pediatrics recommends that all infants less than 28 weeks or ⩽ 1500 g at birth undergo retinal examination[50]. The first exam usually takes place at 4–6 weeks after birth, 31–33 weeks corrected age, or before discharge from the hospital, whichever is earlier. The examinations are repeated as an inpatient or outpatient at regular intervals until the retina is fully vascularized. Active ROP is followed carefully to detect disease that may be amenable to intervention or more hopefully until the disease is resolved and the retina fully vascularized.

Disease initiating early in extrauterine life in the posterior part of the retina and with accelerated inflammatory change has the worst prognosis for eventual visual impairment.

Treatment

Advancing ROP of a moderate to severe degree can be treated with retinal ablative therapy using cryotherapy or laser therapy. The collaborative cryotherapy trial demonstrates a reduction of poor visual outcomes from 55.5% to 33.9% with the application of cryotherapy to selected eyes[48]. Near-total retinal detachment can be treated with a fair chance of anatomical correction but with a poor prognosis for useful vision.

Prevention

Partially effective therapy (laser and cryotherapy) for some cases of retinopathy of prematurity has been available for only a relatively short period of time. A variety of attempts have been made to explore more preventative strategies. Clinical trials examining the influence of exogenous surfactant, indomethacin, inositol, and vitamin E have provided no convincing evidence of a role in the prevention of ROP. Initial studies of prophylactic vitamin A and the reduction of ambient light reaching the eye have shown some promise. No specific preventative strategy other than that of reducing preterm births can be recommended at this time.

CEREBRAL PALSY

Cerebral palsy is the term given to a group of disorders marked by abnormalities of muscle tone and signs and symptoms demonstrable in early infancy. While some change occurs with age and maturation the general abnormalities of tone and movement show a static course without progression. Cerebral palsy is generally classified by its clinical manifestations and is better described as a symptom complex rather than a disease. Spastic cerebral palsy is characterized by hyperreflexia and hypertonus with flexor tone usually dominant over extensor tone. Topographic description of the involved limbs further classifies the involvement. Hemiplegia describes the involvement of arm and leg on one side with normal findings of the other limbs. Diplegia, the type most often associated with preterm birth, describes considerably more involvement of the lower than the upper extremities. Quadriplegia describes the involvement of all four limbs with the arms at least as affected as the legs.

Extrapyramidal cerebral palsy is characterized by abnormal posture, ataxia, hypertonus and involuntary movements (athetosis). Mixed cerebral palsy with both spastic and extrapyramidal involvement is seen in about 20% of affected children. The severity of cerebral palsy ranges from very little handicap through severe limitations of daily activities. An increased severity of cerebral palsy is usually associated with an increased risk of associated problems such as mental retardation, seizure disorder, visual motor abnormalities, deafness and bulbar dysfunction.

Incidence

Grether *et al.*[51] have estimated that moderate to severe cerebral palsy occurs in 1.23/1000 three year old children. Despite extensive expansion of perinatal care and electronic fetal monitoring the incidence of cerebral palsy has remained largely unchanged. The increased survival of the very low birth weight infant has been reported to be associated with increased cerebral palsy rate in that population but is balanced by a large portion of survivors without cerebral palsy[52]. Very low birth weight children are disproportionately represented and account for about 25% of all those with cerebral palsy.

Etiology

The etiology of most cases of cerebral palsy remains unknown. Low birth weight and prematurity are probably the most important identifiable risk factors for the development of cerebral palsy. The reasons for the intrauterine growth failure and/or untimely delivery, as well as the high incidence of critical neonatal illness in these populations, probably accounts for a sizeable proportion of increased incidence of cerebral palsy associated with low birth weight and prematurity. The development of cystic periventicular leukomalacia seen on cerebral ultrasound or computerized tomographic scanning is a very high risk marker for the eventual development of cerebral palsy[53].

No more than 3–13% of cases of cerebral palsy are attributable to perinatal events. In the series reported by Ellenberg and Nelson,16% of children with cerebral palsy had serious perinatal depression and neonatal neurologic symptomatology[54]. Conversely most children with cerebral palsy do not have identifiable signs of perinatal asphyxia. The clearest, but not conclusive, cluster of illness possibly identifying an immediate perinatal origin of significant central nervous system dysfunction are prolonged low Apgar scores, severe umbilical cord blood acidemia, abnormalities of respiratory drive, persistent abnormalities of muscle tone, abnormalities of consciousness and responsiveness, early seizures and evidence of asphyxial injury in other organs such as lung, heart, kidney or liver. The mortality of severe neonatal depression is high. It is remarkable that while mortality is high, surviving children with one minute Apgar scores of zero have only a 32% incidence of neurologic morbidity. Children with marked lasting neonatal depression and poorly responsive seizures have a high risk of the eventual development of cerebral palsy. Individual data such as fetal heart rate patterns, Apgar scores, presence of meconium in amniotic fluid and cord blood pH have a poor predictive value for development of cerebral palsy.

Prenatal central nervous system injury, maldevelopment of the central nervous system, maternal illness and genetic association have been implicated in the etiology of some cases of cerebral palsy.

Congenital malformations involving organ systems other than the central nervous system are also associated with an increased risk of development of cerebral palsy and this relationship is especially true among infants with low birth weight. The presence of chorioamnionitis has also found to be associated with a higher risk of cerebral palsy. Twin birth and especially the intrauterine death of one twin is associated with an increased number of malformations of both the central nervous system or other organs, prematurity, and low birth weight. These associations probably account for the five times increased risk of cerebral palsy seen among twins.

Other associations important in cerebral palsy include chemicals toxic to the central nervous system, identifiable trauma, extreme hyperbilirubinemia and encephalitis from a variety of etiologies.

Most children with cerebral palsy do not have a history compatible with any of the above proposed etiologies. In one study, utilizing magnetic resonance imaging of the central nervous system, Volpe suggested that about one third of the cases of cerebral palsy were secondary to abnormalities of neuronal migration[55].

Diagnosis

Diagnosis can be suspected in a child who falls behind in early developmental milestones and has abnormalities of neurologic tone. Serial neurologic examinations and follow up will be necessary to clarify the significance of such findings. Many children with some delay and some early neurologic signs will demonstrate normalization of these abnormal signs over time. Capute and coworkers[56] have proposed that an early diagnosis of cerebral palsy can be approached by the systematic examination of the young infant for the persistence of primitive reflexes. A particularly ominous neurologic pattern is that of hypotonia which progresses to hypertonia. Limitation of the poplitial angle in a former premature infant supports the diagnosis of spastic diplegia.

A careful patient history is extraordinarily helpful. However the presence of neonatal distress is very nonspecific for the development of cerebral palsy. Neurologic disease progression or the loss of tone suggests diagnoses other than cerebral palsy. Because of the above difficulties definitive diagnosis may be difficult prior to 2 years of age.

Treatment

The treatment of cerebral palsy is a difficult, complex and controversial area. The treatment plan for an individual should depend on the child's motor deficits and cognitive difficulties. Specific modalities to avoid contractures, minimize or balance abnormalities of muscle tone, promote ambulation and maximize appropriate learning and self help capabilities are part of an individualized plan of care. A program of selected physical therapy, pharmacologic and surgical alterations of muscle tone, bracing/supporting and splinting, education interventions and psychological support should be directed by a multidisciplinary team experienced in the care of the family and child with cerebral palsy.

Prevention

The most dramatic reduction in cerebral palsy occurred with the modern management of severe neonatal hyperbilirubinemia beginning in the 1950s. Exchange transfusion and other treatments developed later have almost totally eliminated kernicterus as a cause of cerebral palsy. The discovery that benzyl alcohol preservative in parenteral fluids given to small preterm babies was toxic to the central nervous system led to its elimination from use. This was associated with further reduction of the risk of cerebral palsy in very low birth weight children[57]. Extensive investment in acute perinatal care issues such as electronic fetal monitoring does not seem to have any effect on the risk of cerebral palsy. The reduction of the rate of preterm births is a difficult to achieve societal goal but probably would have a large impact on the rate of cerebral palsy.

REFERENCES

1. American Academy of Pediatrics, Committee on Nutrition: Nutritional needs of low-birth-weight infants. *Pediatrics* 1985;75:976
2. Adamkin DH. Nutrition in very, very low birth weight infants. *Clin Perinatol* 1986;13:419–43
3. Gross SJ, Slagle TA. Feeding the low birthweight infant. *Clin Perinatol* 1993;20:193–209
4. La Gamma EF, Brown LE. Feeding practices for infants weighing less than 1500 g at birth and the pathogenesis of necrotizing enterocolitis. *Clin Perinatol* 1994;21:271–306
5. McKeown RE, Marsh TD, Amarnath U, *et al*. Role of delayed feeding and of feeding increments in necrotizing enterocolitis. *J Pediatr* 1992;121:764–70
6. Berseth CL. Effect of early feedings on maturation of the premature infants' small intestine. *J Pediatr* 1992;120:947–53
7. Farrell PM, Gutcher GR, Palta M, *et al*. Essential fatty acid deficiency in premature infants. *Am J Clin Nutr* 1988;48:220–9
8. Zlotkin SH, Stallings VA, Pencharz PB. Total parenteral nutrition in children. *Pediatr Clin North Am* 1985;32:381–400
9. Ellison RC, Peckham GJ, Lang P, *et al*. Evaluation of the preterm infant for patent ductus arteriosus. *Pediatrics* 1983;71:364–72
10. Baylen BG, Meyer RA, Kaplan S, *et al*. The critically ill premature infant with patent ductus arteriosus and pulmonary disease – an echocardiographic assessment. *J Pediatr* 1975;86:423–32
11. Bell EF, Warburton D, Stonestreet BS, Oh W. Effect of fluid administration on the development of symptomatic patent ductus arteriosus and congestive heart failure in premature infants. *New Engl J Med* 1980;302:598–604
12. Lorenz JM, Kleinman LI, Kotagal UR, *et al*. Water balance in very low-birthweight infants: relationship to water and sodium intake and effect on outcome. *J Pediatr* 1982;101:423–32
13. Gersony WM, Peckham GJ, Ellison RC, *et al*. Effects of indomethacin in premature infants with patent ductus arteriosus: results of a national collaborative study. *J Pediatr* 1983;102:895–906
14. Cotton RB, Stahiman MT, Bender HW, *et al*. Randomized trial of early closure of symptomatic patent ductus arteriosus in small preterm infants. *J Pediatr* 1978;93:647–51
15. Cassady G, Crouse DT, Kirklin JW, *et al*. A randomized controlled trial of very early prophylactic ligation of the ductus arteriosus in babies who weighed 1000 g or less at birth. *New Engl J Med* 1989;320:1511–16
16. Papile LA, Munsick-Bruno G, Lowe L. Relationship of cerebral intraventricular hemorrhage and early childhood neurologic handicaps. *J Pediatr* 1983;103:273–7
17. Hawgood S, Spong J, Yu VYH. Intraventricular hemorrhage incidence and outcome of very low birth weight infants. *Am J Dis Child* 1984;138:136–9
18. McMenamin JB, Schackelford GD, Volpe JJ. Outcome of neonatal intraventricular hemorrhage with periventricular echo-dense lesions. *Ann Neurol* 1984;15:285–90
19. Philip AGS, Allan WC, Tito AM, *et al*. Intraventricular hemorrhage in preterm infants: declining incidence in the 1980's. *Pediatrics* 1989;84:797–801
20. Hobar JD. Prevention of periventricular–intraventricular hemorrhage. In Sinclair JC Bracken MB, eds. *Effective Care of the Newborn Infant*. Oxford University Press, 1992
21. Morales WJ, Diebel ND, Lazan AJ, *et al*. The effect of antenatal dexamethasone administration on the prevention of respiratory distress syndrome in preterm gestations with premature rupture of membranes. *Am J Obstet Gynecol* 1986;154:591–5
22. Perlman JM, Goodman S, Kreuser KL, *et al*. Reduction in intraventricular hemorrhage by elimination of fluctuating cerebral blood flow velocity in preterm infants with respiratory distress syndrome. *New Engl J Med* 1985;312:1353–7
23. American Academy of Pediatrics Task force on prolonged apnea. Prolonged apnea. *Pediatrics* 1978;61:651–2
24. Martin RJ, Miller MJ, Carlo WH. Pathogenesis of apnea in preterm infants. *J Pediatr* 1986;109:733–41

25. Perlstein P, Edwards N, Sutherland J. Apnea in premature infants and incubator air temperature changes. *N Engl J Med* 1970;282:461–6

26. Thach BT, Stark AR. Spontaneous neck flexion and airway obstruction during apneic spells in preterm infants. *J Pediatr* 1979;94:275–81

27. Sims ME, Yau G, Rambhatta S, *et al.* Limitations of theophylline in the treatment of apnea of prematurity. *Am J Dis Child* 1985;139:567–70

28. Murat I, Moriette G, Blin D, *et al.* The efficacy of caffeine in the treatment of recurrent idiopathic apnea in premature infants. *J Pediatr* 1981;99:984–9

29. McInerny TK, Schubert WK. Prognosis of neonatal seizures. *Am J Dis Child* 1969;117:261–4

30. Painter MJ, Bergman I, Crumrine P. Neonatal seizures. *Pediatr Clin North Am* 1986;33:91–109

31. Bergman I, Painter MJ, Hirsch RP, *et al.* Outcome in neonates with convulsions treated in an intensive care unit. *Ann Neurol* 1983;14:642–7

32. Volpe JJ. *Neurology of the Newborn,* 3rd Edn. W.B. Saunders Company 1995

33. Miles DK, Hines GL. Benign neonatal seizures. *J Clin Neurophys* 1990;3:369–79

34. Deshmukh A, Witteret W, Schnitzler E, *et al.* Lorazepam in the treatment of refractory neonatal seizures. *Am J Dis Child* 1986;140:1042–4

35. Holzman IR, Brown DR. Necrotizing enterocolitis: a complication of prematurity. *Semin Perinatol* 1986;10:208–16

36. Kliegman RM, Fanaroff AA. Necrotizing enterocolitis. *N Engl J Med* 1984;310:1093–1103

37. Kosloske AM, Goldthorn JF. Paracentesis is an aid to the diagnosis of intestinal gangrene: experience in 50 infants and children. *Arch Surg* 1982;117:571–5

38. Ricketts RR. The role of paracentesis in the management of infants with necrotizing enterocolitis. *Am Surg* 1986;52:61–5

39. Bell MJ, Kosloske AM, Benton C, *et al.* Neonatal necrotizing enterocolitis: prevention of perforation. *J Pediatr Surg* 1973;8:601–5

40. Hasen TN, Ritter DA, Speer ME, *et al.* A randomized controlled study of oral gentamycin in the treatment of necrotizing enterocolitis. *J Pediatr* 1980;97:836–39

41. O'Neill J, Holcomb GW. Surgical experience with neonatal necrotizing enterocolitis. *Ann Surg* 1979;189:612–9

42. Weber TR, Lewis JE. The role of second-look laparotomy in necrotizing enterocolitis. *J Pediatr Surg* 1986;21:323–5

43. Bauer CR. Necrotizing enterocolitis. In Sinclair JC, Bracken MB, eds. *Effective Care of the Newborn Infant.* Oxford University Press, 1992

44. Lucas A, Cole TJ. Breast milk and neonatal necrotizing enterocolitis. *Lancet* 1990;336:1519–23

45. Watts JL. Retinopathy of prematurity. In Sinclair JC, Bracken MB, eds. *Effective Care of the Newborn Infant.* Oxford University Press, 1992

46. Phelps DL. Retinopathy of prematurity: an estimate of cisoin loss in the United States 1979. *Pediatrics* 1981; 67:924–5

47. New international classification of retinopathy of prematurity. *Pediatrics* 1984;74:127

48. Cryotherapy for retinopathy of prematurity cooperative Study Group. Multicenter trial of cryotherapy for retinopathy of prematurity. *Arch Ophthalmol* 1990;108:1408–16

49. Purohit D. Risk factors for retrolental fibroplasia: incidence and treatment. *Arch Dis Child* 1985;60:698

50. Hauth JC, Merenstein GB. (eds). Guidelines for Perinatal Care. *American Academy of Pediatrics* 1997

51. Grether JK, Cummins SK, Nelson KB. The California cerebral palsy project. *Pediatr Perinatal Epidemiol* 1992; 6:339–51

52. McCormick MC. Has the prevalence of handicapped infants increased with the improved survival of the very low birth weight infant? *Clin Perinatol* 1993;20:263–77

53. Leviton A, Pooneth N. White matter damage in preterm newborns – an epidemiologic perspective. *Early Hum Dev* 1990;24:1–22

54. Ellenberg JH, Nelson KB. Cluster of perinatal events identifying infants at high risk for death or disability. *J Pediatr* 1988;113:546–52

55. Volpe JJ. Value of MR in definition of neuropathy of cerebral palsy *in vivo. Am J Neuroradiol* 1992;13:79–83

56. Capute AJ, Palmer FB, Shapiro BK, *et al.* Primitive reflex profile: a quantitation of primitive reflexes in infancy. *Dev Med Child Neurol* 1984;26:375–83

57. Benda GI, Hiller JL, Reynolds JW. Benzyl alcohol toxicity: impact on neurologic handicaps in surviving very low birth weight infants. *Pediatrics* 1986;77:507–12

74

Neonatal diseases II

J.G. Dawson, J.L. Rosenbaum and F. Sessions Cole

HYPOGLYCEMIA

As early as the 1930's, the risk of hypoglycemia associated with specific clinical situations was recognized. However, the scope and even the definition of the problem have remained controversial[1]. The following blood glucose levels have been determined in one study as one standard deviation below the mean[1]:

Preterm infants	< 20 mg%
Term infants < 72° of age	< 30 mg%
Term infant beyond 72° of age	< 40 mg%

The incidence of hypoglycemia in term infants using these criteria has varied from 0.4% to 8.1%. This wide variation reflects the important confounding effects of maternal intrapartum glucose administration, nursery feeding practices, and biologic heterogeneity of affected infants[2]. Newborn infants are hypoglycemic more frequently than older children or adults for several reasons, including their relatively small carbohydrate stores, less efficient mobilization of glycogen stores, and greater glucose utilization particularly in their proportionately larger brains.

Several physiologically distinct groups of infants have been identified as being at particularly high risk for hypoglycemia[1]. Infants who are small for gestational age, born to mothers with chronic uteroplacental insufficiency, have decreased glycogen and adipose stores to mobilize in the immediate newborn period. Infants born to mothers with recurring hyperglycemia, particularly those with diabetes mellitus, may develop compensatory fetal hyperinsulinemia that is slow to adapt to the postnatal state. Rarely, infants may also have primary disorders of pancreatic islet cell function such as adenomas or beta cell hyperplasia that lead to primary hyperinsulinemia. Recognition of the higher risk status of infants in these groups is important in detecting infants with neonatal hypoglycemia but will not identify all infants. Glucose screening protocols are therefore widely used for all newborn infants.

The significance of neonatal hypoglycemia is nearly as controversial as its definition. As early as the 1960's, long-term follow-up of newborns with recurrent and severe hypoglycemia revealed an increased incidence of neurodevelopmental sequelae[1]. More recently, concern for infants with more moderate degrees of hypoglycemia has been raised with the demonstration of increased sequelae in preterm infants with frequently recurring ($\geqslant$ 5 days) hypoglycemia (< 45 mg/dl, plasma)[3]. Other studies have detected subtle evidence of transient neurologic dysfunction in newborn infants with levels as high as 45 mg/dl (blood), most of whom were asymptomatic. The impact of low blood glucose levels on short-term and long-term central nervous system function is likely to be greater in the presence of other conditions that are known to be deleterious to the brain, particularly hypoxia and ischemia.

In light of these considerations, the approach to neonatal hypoglycemia emphasizes the recognition of high risk patients, the prevention of low blood glucose levels particularly in those at risk groups, and prompt recognition and intervention when necessary. Many of these efforts begin early in the pregnancy, with screening for maternal glucose intolerance and for intrauterine growth retardation, and continue in the peripartum period with avoidance of maternal hyperglycemia and with intervention to minimize fetal hypoxia and ischemia[2]. The same principles guide postnatal management: interventions to prevent or treat hypoxia and ischemia, to minimize excess glucose utilization by preventing cold stress, to treat with oral or parenteral glucose, and to provide serial surveillance for response to interventions. Severe and persistent hypoglycemia may require the placement of central vascular access to deliver hyperosmotic, glucose-containing (25–50 mg%) solutions (15–20 mg/kg/min of glucose) or pharmacologic interventions (e.g. glucagon or corticosteroids).

HYPOCALCEMIA

Like hypoglycemia, the definition of hypocalcemia is not absolute, although most studies use values of ionized calcium (Ca^{2+}) of < 3.0–4.0 mg/dl. The proportion of the total calcium that exists as the physiologically active ionized form will vary with several factors including the infant's acid–base status and serum protein concentration. This physiologic variation makes measurement of the ionized Ca^{2+} important. The newborn infant is particularly at risk for development of hypocalcemia at birth, when mechanisms optimized for regulation of intrauterine calcium concentration via high trans-placental Ca^{2+} transport and high fetal calcitonin levels change[4]. The identification of infants at high risk for hypocalcemia facilitates appropriate screening and treatment.

Early neonatal hypocalcemia is the most common type, and it is detected more frequently in specific clinical situations such as prematurity, asphyxia, and in infants of diabetic mothers. Late onset hypocalcemia beyond the first three days of life occurs less frequently and may be associated with increased phosphate loads seen occasionally in the ingestion of cow's milk.

The approach to treatment begins with the identification of infants at greatest risk. In those infants who are asymptomatic, treatment may simply consist of usual enteral feedings and continued surveillance, as calcitonin levels fall postnatally. In infants with symptoms of hypocalcemia, particularly seizures or tetany, parenteral infusions of calcium salts can be administered through a secure peripheral or central venous catheter or through a central arterial catheter but not through a peripheral arterial catheter. These infants should also be screened for hypomagnesemia, correction of which improves the response to calcium.

NEONATAL SCREENING FOR METABOLIC DISORDERS

In the USA, individual states have adopted a variety of approaches to the detection of inherited metabolic disorders. Screening for phenylketonuria (PKU), galactosemia, and hypothyroidism occurs in most, although some states also include screening for such diverse diseases as hemoglobinopathies, homocystinuria, maple syrup urine disease, tyrosinemia, cystic fibrosis and others. Blood samples are collected from heel-stick specimens on filter papers, for processing by a centralized state laboratory. Screening levels for results are set to optimize the sensitivity of the test, and provision is then made for confirmatory testing, along with appropriate counseling and management for those patients who are confirmed to be affected.

The criteria used to select the disorders for which screening will be performed include the availability of a reliable assay on newborn blood, the existence of a therapeutic intervention that will substantially improve outcome, the incidence of the disease in a population, and the cost[5]. Galactosemia, with an incidence of $\sim 1 : 50\,000$ live births, can be treated with a diet excluding the galactose found in milk products. The treatment of phenylketonuria requires a special diet low in phenylalanine. Interestingly, as a result of those early screening programs, many women are now surviving into their child-bearing years. If they are not maintained on their restrictive diets throughout pregnancy, even some of the offspring who do not have the genetic defect of PKU may be born severely affected (microcephaly, mental retardation,

congenital heart disease) secondary to the elevated maternal levels of phenylalanine[6].

PERSISTENT PULMONARY HYPERTENSION

In 1969 Gersony and colleagues[7] described two cyanotic infants who presented with 'persistent physiologic characteristics of the fetal circulation in the absence of recognizable cardiac, pulmonary, hematologic or central nervous system disease.' This condition was termed 'persistent fetal circulation' (PFC). Since that time, however, PFC has become recognized as a syndrome caused by a variety of clinical conditions rather than a single disease and has been termed persistent pulmonary hypertension (PPHN). It is defined by postnatal persistence of right to left shunting at the ductal and/or atrial level. Although in most cases pulmonary pressures are elevated, they may be normal or low[7–9].

The exact incidence of PPHN is unclear. Goetzman and Riemenschneider[10] have estimated that the disease occurs in approximately 1 in 1500 live births. Most commonly the syndrome is related to a wide spectrum of lung diseases, but may also be caused by primary congenital heart disease or other idiopathic etiologies.

Rudolph has identified three anatomic varieties of pulmonary hypertension based on pulmonary vascular anatomy. These include: (1) maladaptation, (2) increased pulmonary vascular smooth muscle development and (3) pulmonary underdevelopment[9].

Maladaptation refers to the failure of the pulmonary vascular resistance to decrease after birth. Common predisposing factors causing pulmonary vasoconstriction include hypoxia, acidosis, sepsis and hyperviscosity[11–14]. Endogenous pulmonary vasoactive substances such as the leukotrienes may also play an active role[15].

Histological evidence of increased muscularization of the small intraacinar arteries have been demonstrated by Murphy and co-workers[16]. These changes are associated with various predisposing factors including chronic intrauterine hypoxemia, meconium aspiration and maternal ingestion of nonsteroid inflammatory drugs such as aspirin and indomethacin[17–20].

Pulmonary hypertension is often associated with pulmonary underdevelopment. These conditions classically include diaphragmatic hernia, oligohydramnios, and neuromuscular diseases. In these cases the number of bronchial generations, the number of alveoli per acinus and arterial caliber may be affected and are generally decreased[18,21].

Structural cardiac abnormalities associated with pulmonary hypertension or cyanosis must be differentiated from primary pulmonary disorders. Long[22] has grouped these into five categories. These include: (1) obstruction to pulmonary venous drainage,

(2) congenital cardiomyopathies, (3) obstruction to left ventricular outflow, (4) obligatory left to right shunts and (5) miscellaneous cardiac disorders.

The pathophysiology of PPHN is directly related to changes in pulmonary vascular resistance. When pulmonary vascular resistance is greater than systemic vascular resistance, blood is shunted right to left through the foramen ovale and/or a patent ductus arteriosus.

Responses of the pulmonary vasculature to changes in oxygen tension and hydrogen ion concentration have also been demonstrated. Rudolph and Yuan[23] observed dramatic increases in pulmonary vascular resistance in newborn calves associated with hypoxia (Pao_2 < 40 torr) and acidosis (pH < 7.2). These observations have been confirmed in clinical studies as well. Moreover, myocardial dysfunction and congestive heart failure are commonly associated with pulmonary hypertension[8,13,24]. Endothelin and nitric oxide, respectively a potent vasoconstrictor and vasodilator of the pulmonary vasculature, may play a role in the pathogenesis of PPHN[25].

The diagnosis of PPHN should be considered in the clinical setting of a cyanotic term or post-date infant who has experienced perinatal hypoxic–ischemic insult and/or acidosis[10,26,27]. Frequently, there is history of meconium aspiration[17]. Less frequently, preterm infants may demonstrate PPHN in association with hyaline membrane disease or sepsis. In all cases, primary congenital heart disease must be rigorously excluded before PPHN is diagnosed.

The bedside diagnosis of PPHN may be made with the use of pre- and post-ductal arterial blood gases, hyperoxia test or hyperoxia-hyperventilation[26,28]. When an infant is placed in a high oxygen environment (FiO_2 1.0), an increase in arterial oxygen concentration to 150 mmHg or greater generally excludes cyanotic heart disease. If the Pao_2 is <150 mmHg, hyperventilation by bag and mask ventilation or mechanical ventilation may result in an increase in Pao_2 to >150 mmHg after a critical pH has been reached.

Definite confirmation of ductal/foramen shunting and absence of congenital heart disease requires evaluation with 2-D echocardiography or, infrequently, cardiac catheterization[29,30].

Management strategies for PPHN have changed dramatically since the first description of the disease. In the early 1970s management was conservative, including use of oxygen, physiologic ventilator support and drugs aimed at improving cardiac function, i.e. digoxin and diuretics[31]. With the observation that pulmonary vascular resistance was related to a critically low pH, hyperventilation to induce a respiratory alkalosis was utilized[32,33]. Pharmacologic agents that directly decrease pulmonary vascular resistance, i.e. tolazoline, sodium nitroprusside[34–36], and isoproterenol have been used[34–36]. Ionotropic agents including dopamine and dobutamine are often employed[37,38]. Despite these multiple therapeutic interventions, there was still 50% mortality[26]. Extracorporeal membrane oxygenation (ECMO) was introduced as a rescue therapy in 1982 for infants in which an 80–90% mortality rate was expected based on historical data[39,40]. With the use of ECMO, published survival rates approach 85%[41]. More recently, a return to more conservative management without hyperventilation and hyperoxia has produced similar outcomes[42–44]. Clearly, further studies are indicated to determine the most appropriate management for infants with this syndrome.

RESPIRATORY DISORDERS

Hyaline membrane disease

In 1959, Avery and Mead[45] noted the lack of surfactant in lungs of newborn infants who died of hyaline membrane disease (HMD) and thereby established the pathophysiologic role of surfactant in this disease. Over the ensuing four decades, further research has helped elucidate an understanding of the biophysical, biochemical, and cellular basis of hyaline membrane disease. Surfactant is synthesized by Type II alveolar epithelial cells and secreted into the alveolar space. It is composed of a mixture of phospholipids, particularly disaturated phosphatidylcholine (lecithin) and phosphatidylglycerol (PG), and lung-specific surfactant associated proteins. The proteins' function is both lowering alveolar surface tension and in the regulation of secretion and uptake of surfactant. The surfactant monolayer which lines the alveolar surface minimizes surface tension, maintains alveolar patency at end expiration, reduces the amount of pressure necessary to expand alveoli, and thus prevents atelectasis. Study of the control of synthesis, secretion and uptake of surfactant components has implicated several important regulatory mechanisms that may modify normal developmental patterns of production and explain the wide gestational age range over which surfactant may first be produced (26–36 weeks). For example, endogenous and exogenous glucocorticoids accelerate surfactant appearance in alveoli both *in vitro* and *in vivo*. In contrast, insulin may retard surfactant production.

Because of the importance of fetal lung maturity for neonatal outcome, extensive investigation has focused on measurements of pulmonary surfactant maturity in amniotic fluid samples. Measurements of amniotic fluid lecithin/sphingomyelin ratio (L/S) and PG are used most frequently. These same measures have also been used postnatally on gastric or tracheal aspirate specimens, to characterize biochemically the cause of respiratory distress in newborn infants. However, differences in the maturation of surfactant production are not the sole determinants of respiratory distress in premature newborns. To varying degrees, structural maturation of the distal airway, the influx of serum proteins that inhibit the surface tension lowering properties of surfactant, the marked lack of compliance of the chest wall, decreased diaphragmatic contractility, or perinatal events may contribute to the development, or severity of HMD[46].

The clinical course of HMD is characterized by the onset of respiratory distress in the first hours of life, worsening compliance and oxygenation for the first 48–72 hours, then improvement during the subsequent 72 hours. As progressive atelectasis occurs, work of breathing and intrapulmonary vascular shunting increase. Grunting by the infant increases end expiratory pressure in the airways and thereby helps to maintain alveolar patency. However, atelectasis is accompanied by hypoxemia, acidosis and hypercarbia. On necropsy, interstitial edema is prominent, and the airways are filled with proteinaceous cellular debris (the 'hyaline membranes'). These changes are reflected radiographically by the appearance of a reticulogranular infiltrate and prominent air bronchograms. Pulmonary function tests reveal a marked decrease in total lung capacity, in functional residual capacity, and in compliance. The typical clinical course may be modified adversely by the development of air leaks, by hypoxic–ischemic injury to the pulmonary endothelium, or to the myocardium, by left to right or bidirectional shunting across a persistently patent ductus arteriosus, or by concomitant infection. In addition, both oxygen therapy and mechanical ventilation with positive pressures can induce epithelial injury in the airways. While some infants recover promptly, others will develop chronic lung disease, or bronchopulmonary dysplasia, a heterogeneous disease whose possible etiologies include developmental immaturity of the premature infant's lung, oxygen toxicity and barotrauma, or other genetic, developmental or nutritional factors not yet well understood.

The therapeutic approaches to this disease center most importantly on its prevention, and secondarily on the use of mechanical and pharmacologic measures. Preventive measures include the timely use of amniotic fluid pulmonary maturation testing, to help guide management of tocolysis in cases of preterm labor. In addition, use of antepartum steroids to help induce pulmonary maturation decreases the incidence of hyaline membrane disease in singleton pregnancies with no evidence of any short- or long-term detrimental effects on the child[47]. Preventive measures are also important in the peripartum period, when the availability of adequately trained personnel to assist in the initial stabilization of the newborn is necessary. These early interventions may decrease the degree or duration of hypoxia or ischemia, and ensure the best possible transition to the extrauterine environment. In addition, by recognizing the signs of respiratory distress, early administration of appropriate amounts of positive airway pressure may prevent worsening atelectasis[48].

A primary development in both the understanding of the pathophysiology of respiratory distress and in its treatment is the recent development of several exogenous surfactant preparations. These have been derived from several sources, including human amniotic fluid, bovine lung extracts and from purely synthetic formulations. All have been shown *in vitro* to lower surface tension like native surfactant, and *in vivo* to ameliorate the clinical course of HMD in some premature infants. Specifically, surfactant replacement therapy has been associated with a significant decrease in the incidence of air leaks, an improvement in oxygenation, and a less consistent decrease in the mean airway pressure needed to maintain adequate gas exchange. In many but not all studies, these acute changes have been accompanied by a decrease in mortality. However, they have not led to a consistent decrease in the incidence of BPD or severe IVH[49].

The patient selection criteria most frequently used have included infants with clinical and radiographic features of at least moderate HMD. In addition, some studies have administered surfactant prophylactically to those infants most at risk of developing HMD, e.g. infants < 1200 g at birth. When these two strategies, rescue vs. prophylactic, have been compared in a prospective, randomized fashion, both have been effective[50,51]. Furthermore, some patients did not respond to either strategy. This lack of response suggested either that their disease was not surfactant deficiency, that the dose administered was inappropriate for their disease, or that exogenous surfactant function was inhibited by factors in the lung, e.g. extravasated serum protein. The administration of these products requires neonatal personnel skilled in their use with appropriate ancillary support, as pulmonary compliance of these infants may change rapidly after treatment[52]. Many controversies remain about the optimal utilization of these products.

Meconium aspiration

Meconium stained amniotic fluid has long been a source of controversy and concern. Occurring in approximately 8–20% of all deliveries, its presence has historically been associated with fetal compromise and fetal hypoxemia[53–55].

Meconium differs from adult stool in many ways. Composed primarily of water, meconium lacks the intestinal bacteria necessary to convert primary bile acids to secondary bile acids. In addition, since most of the fluid in meconium is derived from amniotic fluid, the contents of protein, lipid, and sterols parallel that of amniotic fluid[56,57].

Meconium is seldom passed before 34 weeks' gestation. This delay may be related to immaturity of bowel innervation, as well as prolonged transit time in the preterm fetus[58]. Although meconium is passed more commonly during periods of hypoxemia, the exact relationship to fetal distress remains unclear[54–56]. In baboons, acute sublethal perinatal asphyxia or instillation of meconium into the neonatal lungs via the endotracheal tube at the time of delivery, does not produce persistent pulmonary hypertension, or abnormal pulmonary arteriolar muscularization, as frequently seen in severe meconium aspiration syndrome[59].

Meconium causes chemical inflammation and airways obstruction. Air trapping in the distal airways may result in hyperexpansion of alveoli and atelectasis and lead to uneven ventilation and intrapulmonary shunting. Hypoxemia and acidosis are common[54]. Airleaks occur in as many as 50% of infants with meconium aspiration. Pulmonary hypertension is a frequent complicating factor[60].

The diagnosis of meconium aspiration should be suspected in the clinical setting of meconium stained amniotic fluid and fetal distress. The infant is often post date or shows physical signs of placental insufficiency. Respiratory distress is common with cyanosis, grunting, flaring, and retractions. The diagnosis can be confirmed by chest X-ray which has a typical appearance of irregular pulmonary densities creating a 'snowstorm' appearance[54,61]. In patients having more than trace meconium-stained amniotic fluid, amnioinfusion of saline solution into the maternal uterine cavity during labor reduces the neonatal risk of having meconium below the vocal cords and meconium aspiration syndrome[62].

Carson *et al.*[63] have shown that the obstetrician can clear the airway in approximately 90% of affected infants by suctioning the nasopharynx immediately after the head is delivered. After delivery of the infant and before respirations are established, the vocal cords should be visualized and suctioning of the trachea through an endotracheal tube should be performed when thick or particulate meconium is present[64–68]. These simple procedures have been shown to decrease the neonatal morbidity and mortality associated with meconium stained amniotic fluid.

Treatment is otherwise symptomatic. Attention to adequate oxygenation and ventilation is imperative. Coexisting metabolic acidosis may require correction. In the most severe cases, mechanical ventilation may be helpful with pulmonary toilet and management of pulmonary hypertension[61,69]. Surfactant replacement therapy given within six hours of birth may improve neonatal oxygenation and reduce the incidence of air leaks, thus facilitating ventilation[70].

ERYTHROBLASTOSIS FETALIS

The identification by Landsteiner in 1940 of the rhesus (Rh) factor on human red blood cells (RBC), the subsequent development of improved methods of antenatal diagnosis and prevention by Liley, and development of postnatal treatment by Diamond have radically changed the incidence of Rh hemolytic disease of the newborn. Before these developments, it is estimated that nearly 1% of all pregnancies would result in isoimmunization, with a perinatal mortality of 17.5%. More recent series suggest a perinatal mortality rate of 1.5%[71]. As these measures have succeeded, however, the relative importance of other isoimmunizing antigen groups (e.g. Kell, C) has increased.

Placental transfer of maternal anti-D IgG with resultant hemolysis of fetal RBC causes anemia and hydrops fetalis. Anemia may occur despite compensatory increases in red cell production via extramedullary hematopoiesis which occurs in the liver and spleen in response to increased levels of erythropoietin. If this compensation fails to maintain red cell mass, an increase in plasma volume occurs to sustain normal blood volume. Tissue oxygen delivery may be compromised despite these mechanisms, particularly when oxygen consumption increases, e.g. when the newborn must suddenly take over the roles of respiration and temperature maintenance at birth. The extreme example of failure of these compensatory mechanisms is hydrops fetalis.

With ongoing hemolysis, bilirubin is produced from the degradation of hemoglobin and is bound to albumin. In the fetus, bilirubin is rapidly cleared by the placenta. Postnatally, the infant's own hepatic clearance mechanisms must be utilized but may be too immature to handle the increased bilirubin load. Accumulation of unconjugated bilirubin in plasma, that exceeds the binding capacity of circulating albumin, may cross the blood–brain barrier and injure specific areas in the brain. Displacement of bilirubin from albumin by organic acids (increased in hypoxemic infants), or by exogenous substances like sulfonamides or salicylates may increase the risk of transfer into the brain[72]. The neuropathology of bilirubin encephalopathy is characterized by selective staining and neuronal death particularly in the basal ganglia and brainstem. Clinically, this is accompanied by the development of classic signs of kernicterus, particularly opisthotonus and movement disorders, upward gaze abnormalities, and sensorineural hearing deficits[73,74].

Most jaundiced infants do not develop kernicterus. In isoimmunized infants, the risk of kernicterus may increase with increasing serum bilirubin levels. In one study of infants with Rh hemolytic disease with bilirubin levels of 25–40 mg%, 12 of 23 infants developed kernicterus. Several studies of term infants with lower levels have found little evidence for long-term cognitive deficits although transient effects on brainstem auditory evoked responses have been seen. In the case of sick premature infants, there is greater concern as postmortem findings consistent with kernicterus may be seen in very premature infants at even lower bilirubin concentrations[74].

As noted above, the incidence of kernicterus has greatly decreased since the Rh factor was first described, a fact that is in large measure secondary to effective prevention with administration of Rhogam to Rh negative pregnant patients. However, some infants will still need therapy, particularly if they are premature or if there is significant hemolysis. Phototherapy results in photoisomerization of bilirubin in the most superficial capillaries to a form that is more readily cleared from the body[75]. In those infants at greatest risk of developing kernicterus, double-volume exchange transfusion may be necessary to decrease the amount of circulating and bound anti-D IgG as well as to decrease the amount of circulating bilirubin.

NEONATAL SEPSIS

Neonatal sepsis poses a difficult diagnostic dilemma for physicians who care for infants. In the preantibiotic era, case fatality rates exceeded 90%[76,77]. The incidence of sepsis is low: 1–10/1000 term births and 1–10/250 preterm births are affected[78–80]. Furthermore, symptoms may be absent or nonspecific early in the disease course. Due to the high mortality of untreated infection, many unaffected infants are treated. Thus, sepsis evaluation remains a high cost, low yield diagnostic intervention with evaluation of twenty infants performed for each infection identified[81].

By definition, sepsis may be 'early onset' (first seven days of life) or 'late onset' (seven days to two months of life). Common bacterial pathogens include group B streptococcus, *Listeria monocytogenes*, *Escherichia coli*, and other Gram-negative enterics that colonize the maternal genitourinary tract[82]. Nosocomially acquired infections pose a significant problem in the neonatal intensive care setting. Coagulase negative staphylococcal infections have become the predominant hospital acquired organism, replacing *Staphylococcus aureus* and Gram-negative organisms[83–85].

The fetus and newborn can be exposed to infection by several different mechanisms. The newborn may be infected by transplacental passage of a maternal blood-borne organism. Neonatal sepsis may also be acquired from a localized maternal infection, such as chorioamnionitis where the infant is prone to aspirate infected amniotic fluid. A small group of infants will become infected after colonization with maternal organisms acquired by passage through the birth canal. Health care personnel can also transmit organisms through poor hand washing technique[82].

In an attempt to identify more accurately infants who will develop infection, clinicians have investigated a variety of risk factors[86,87]. Host factors appear to be the most important[82]. Male infants are two to six times more likely to develop infection than female infants. The immune system also plays a major role. The neonate's immune system is immature in many regards. There is decreased ability to localize spread of organisms secondary to decreased response to chemotactic factors and decreased opsonic activity[82]. Impaired phagocytosis and cidal activity have also been reported[82,88]. Prematurity alone increases the risk of acquiring an infection eight to ten-fold[82].

Maternal risk factors have been evaluated in great detail. Premature rupture of membranes, maternal fever +/− chorioamnionitis, and colonization with group B streptococcus have all been implicated[89–91]. These risk factors are additive and must be considered in light of overall clinical risk factors[92,93].

The clinical signs and symptoms of sepsis may be subtle or overt. Feeding difficulties or behavioral changes may precede temperature instability, or respiratory difficulties[82]. Any perturbation of normal may be associated with infection even in the absence of maternal risk factors.

Multiple screening tests have been utilized to aid in determining which infants should be treated. These include such blood tests as C-reactive protein, erythrocyte sedimentation rate, and other acute phase reactants[93–96]. The value of the complete blood count has been debated[97]. Neutropenia (defined as < 1750) has been shown to be a more reliable indicator of sepsis than neutrophilia[98]. An increased immature to total neutrophil count of greater than 0.2 has also been associated with an increased risk of sepsis[98]. However, the wide range of predictive values of both tests limits their usefulness.

Although a positive blood culture is the most commonly used test to document sepsis, blood cultures may not be as reliable as previously thought. Examples of systemic bacterial infection without positive blood cultures include the symptomatic infant with a positive urine latex and negative blood culture[99], symptomatic congenital pneumonia with positive tracheal aspirates, X-ray findings and negative blood cultures[100], as well as autopsy evidence of sepsis in infants whose cultures were negative postmortem[101,102].

The decision to evaluate cerebrospinal fluid (CSF) is controversial. The overall yield of positive CSF cultures in asymptomatic newborns with septic risks is low[103,104]. Routine evaluation of CSF in very low birth weight infants presenting with respiratory distress syndrome produces a low yield of positive CSF cultures[105,106]. However, not all infants with meningitis exhibit symptoms early in the course of the disease. The frequency of infants with negative blood cultures and positive CSF cultures has been reported as high as 15%[107]. Thus the decision to evaluate spinal fluid should be individualized based on clinical findings and associated risk factors.

Management of neonatal sepsis requires prompt treatment with antibiotics once laboratory investigations and the decision to treat have been made. If culture results are not available at the time antibiotic therapy is instituted, broad spectrum antibiotics should be chosen to cover likely etiologic agents. Once an organism has been isolated, therapy should be based upon known antibiotic sensitivities.

Treatment is otherwise largely symptomatic and supportive in nature. When infection is focal, attention may be directed at the affected organ system. Septicemia, however, implies bacteremia with major physiologic changes. All infants should have frequent cardiorespiratory status monitoring. Hypotension or decreased perfusion may require vigorous fluid resuscitation and/or use of ionotropic agents. Frequent blood gas analysis with correction of metabolic acidosis may be needed. Metabolic abnormalities such as hypocalcemia, hyponatremia and glucose imbalance require meticulous attention. Disseminated intravascular coagulation may occur necessitating transfusion of blood products. Multiple immunologic therapies have been investigated[88]. Exchange transfusions have been used with varying success. Theoretical advantages of exchange transfusion include improved oxygen delivery, removal of endotoxins, and provision of immunologically active white blood cells, complement and immunoglobulins. Transfusion of adult neutrophils in septic, neutropenic infants was initially promising therapy[108]. However, consistent benefit has not been documented in follow-up studies. This therapy awaits demonstration of definitive efficacy in a large study. Human immunoglobulin replacement therapy has been used safely, but its benefit prophylactically is questionable[109–111]. Hyperimmune and human-human monoclonal antibodies may be used in the future but ongoing studies are needed to elucidate further their efficacy. Steroid use has had anecdotal success, but not documented in clinical studies.

REFERENCES

1. Cornblath M, Schwartz R. *Disorders of Carbohydrate Metabolism in Infancy*, 2nd edn. New York: WB Saunders, 1976

2. Miedovnik M, Mimouni F, Tsang RC, *et al*. Management of the insulin-dependent diabetic during labor and delivery. Influences on neonatal outcome. *Am J Perinatol* 1987;4:106–14

3. Lucas A, Morley R, Cole TJ. Adverse neurodevelopmental outcome of moderate neonatal hypoglycemia. *Br Med J* 1988;297:1304–8

4. Hillman LS, Rojanasathit S, Slatopolsky E, *et al*. Serial measurements of serum calcium, magnesium, parathyroid hormone, calcitonin, and 25-hydroxy-vitamin D in premature and term infants during the first week of life. *Pediatr Res* 1977;11:739–744

5. Mamunes P. Neonatal screening tests. *Pediatr Clin North Am* 1980;27:733–51

6. Waisbren SE, Levy HL. Effects of untreated maternal hyper-phenylalaninemia on the fetus: further study of families identified by routine cord blood screening. *J Pediatr* 1990;116:926–9

7. Gersony WM, Duc GV, Sinclair JC. "PFC" syndrome (persistence of the fetal circulation) (abstract). *Circulation* 1969;40S:III:87

8. Riemenschneider TA, Nielsen HC, Ruttenberg HD, *et al*. Disturbances of the transitional circulation: Spectrum of pulmonary hypertension and myocardial dysfunction. *J Pediatr* 1976;89:622–5

9. Rudolph AM. High pulmonary vascular resistance after birth. I. Pathophysiologic considerations and etiologic classification. *Clin Pediatr* 1980;19:585–90

10. Goetzman BW, Riemenschneider TA. Persistence of the fetal circulation. *Pediatrics* 1980;2:37–40

11. Fishman A. Hypoxia on the pulmonary circulation: how and where it acts. *Circ Res* 1976;38:221–31

12. Geggel RL, Aronovitz MJ, Reid LM. Effects of chronic *in utero* hypoxemia in rat neonatal pulmonary arterial structure. *J Pediatr* 1986;108:756–9

13. Gersony WM. Persistance of the fetal circulation syndrome: Definition of the problem. In Peckham GS, Heymann MA, eds. *Cardiovascular Sequelae of Asphyxia in the Newborn*. Report of the eighty-third Ross conference on pediatric research. Ross Laboratories, Columbus, Ohio, 1982:70–5

14. Gross GP, Hathoway WE, McGaughey HR. Hyperviscosity in the neonate. *J Pediatr* 1973;82:1004–12

15. Stenmark KR, James SL, Voelkel NF, *et al*. Leukotriene C4 and D4 in neonates with hypoxemia and pulmonary hypertension. *N Engl J Med* 1983;309:77–80

16. Murphy JD, Aronovitz MJ, Reid LM. Effects of chronic *in utero* hypoxia on the pulmonary vasculature of the newborn guinea pig. *Pediatr Res* 1986;20:292–5

17. Fox WW, Gewitz MW, Dinwiddie R. Pulmonary hypertension in perinatal aspiration syndromes. *Pediatrics* 1977;59:205–11

18. Haworth SC, Reid L. Persistent fetal circulation: newly recognized structural features. *J Pediatr* 1976;88:614–20

19. Manchester D, Margolis HS, Sheldon RE. Possible association between maternal indomethacin therapy and primary pulmonary hypertension of the newborn. *Am J Obstet Gynecol* 1976;126:467–9

20. Van Marter LJ, Leviton A, Allred EN. Persistent pulmonary hypertension of the newborn and smoking and aspirin and nonsteroidal antiinflammatory drug consumption during pregnancy. *Pediatrics* 1996;97(5):658–63

21. Goldstein JD, Reid LM. Pulmonary hypoplasia resulting from phrenic nerve agenesis and diaphragmatic amyoplasia. *J Pediatr* 1980;98:282–7

22. Long WA. Structural cardiovascular abnormalities presenting as persistent pulmonary hypertension of the newborn. *Clin Perinatol* 1984;11:601–26

23. Rudolph AM, Yuan S. Responses of the pulmonary vasculature to hypoxia and H+ ion concentration changes. *J Clin Invest* 1966;45:399–411

24. Rowe RD, Hoffman T. Transient myocardial ischemia of the newborn infant: a form of severe cardiorespiratory distress in full-term infants. *J Pediatr* 1972;81:243–50

25. Steinhorn RH, Millard SL, Morin FC. Persistent pulmonary hypertension of the newborn: role of nitric acid and endothelin in pathophysiology and treatment. *Clin Perinatol* 1995;22:405–28

26. Fox WW, Duara S. Persistent pulmonary hypertension in the neonate: diagnosis and management. *J Pediatr* 1983;103:505–14

27. Levin DL, Heymann MA, Kitterman JA, *et al*. Persistent pulmonary hypertension of the newborn infant. *J Pediatr* 1976;89:626–30

28. Jones RWA, Baumer JH, Joseph MC. Arterial oxygen tension and response to oxygen breathing in differential diagnosis of congenital heart disease in infancy. *Arch Dis Child* 1976;51:667–73

29. Hegyi T, Hiatt IM. Tolazoline and dopamine therapy in neonatal hypoxia and pulmonary vasospasm. *Acta Paediatr Scand* 1980;69:101–3

30. Johnson GL, Cunningham MD, Desai NS, *et al*. Echocardiography in hypoxemic neonatal pulmonary disease. *J Pediatr* 1980;96:716–20

31. Brown R, Pickering D. Persistent transitional circulation. *Arch Dis Child* 1974;49:883–5

32. Drummond WH, Gregory GA, Heymann MA, *et al*. The independent effects of hyperventilation, tolazoline, and dopamine on infants with persistent pulmonary hypertension. *J Pediatr* 1981;98:603–11

33. Duara S, Gewitz MH, Fox WW. Use of mechanical ventilation for clinical management of persistent pulmonary hypertension of the newborn. *Clin Perinatol* 1984;11:641–52

34. Benitz WE, Malachowski N, Cohen RS, *et al*. Use of sodium nitroprusside in neonates: efficacy and safety. *J Pediatr* 1985;106:102–10

35. Goetzman BW, Sunshine P, Johnson JD, *et al*. Neonatal hypoxia and pulmonary vasospasm: response to tolazoline. *J Pediatr* 1976;89:617–21

36. Korones SB, Eyal FG. Successful treatment of "persistent fetal circulation" with tolazoline. *Pediatr Res* 1975;9:367

37. Drummond WH. Use of cardiotonic therapy in the management of infants with PPHN. *Clin Perinatol* 1984;11:715–28

38. Fiddler GI, Chatrath R, Williams GJ, *et al*. Dopamine infusion for the treatment of myocardial dysfunction associated with a persistent transitional circulation. *Arch Dis Child* 1980;55:194–8

39. Barlett RH, Roloff DW, Cornell RG, *et al*. Extracorporeal circulation in neonatal respiratory failure: a prospective randomized study. *Pediatrics* 1985;76:479–87

40. Short BL, Miller MK, Anderson KD. Extracorporeal membrane oxygenation in management of respiratory failure of the newborn. *Clin Perinatol* 1987;14:737–48

41. Glass P, Miller M, Short B. Morbidity for survivors of extracorporeal membrane oxygenation. Neurodevelopmental outcome at one year of age. *Pediatrics* 1989;83:72–8

42. Dworetz AR, Moya FR, Sabo B, *et al*. Survival of infants with persistent pulmonary hypertension without extracorporal membrane oxygenation. *Pediatrics* 1989;84:1–6

43. Schapiro D, Soliman A. Is extracorporeal membrane oxygenation necessary to reduce mortality and morbidity in patients with meconium aspiration syndrome (abstr). *Pediatr Res* 1988;23:424A

44. Wung JT, James LS, Kilchevsky EM, *et al*. Management of infants with severe respiratory failure and persistence of the fetal circulation, without hyperventilation. *Pediatrics* 1985;76:488–94

45. Avery ME, Mead J. Surface properties in relation to atelectasis and hyaline membrane disease. *Am J Dis Child* 1959;97:517–23

46. Moya FR, Grass I. Prevention of respiratory distress syndrome. *Semin Perinatol* 1988;12:348–58

47. Crowley PA. Antenatal corticosteroid therapy: a meta-analysis of the randomized trials, 1972 to 1994. *Am J Obstet Gynecol* 1995;173:322–35

48. Bloom RS, Cropley C. *Textbook in Neonatal Resuscitation*. American Academy of Pediatrics, 1987

49. Hennes HM, Lee MB, Rimm AA. Surfactant replacement therapy in respiratory distress syndrome, meta-analysis of clinical trials of single-dose surfactant extracts. *Am J Dis Child* 1991;145:102–4

50. Kendig JW, Notter RH, Cox C, *et al*. A comparison of surfactant as immediate prophylaxis and as rescue therapy in newborns of less than 30 weeks gestation. *N Engl J Med* 1991;324:865–71

51. Dunn MS, Shennan AT, Zayack D. Bovine surfactant replacement therapy in neonates of less than 30 weeks gestation: a randomized controlled trial of prophylaxis versus treatment. *Pediatrics* 1991;87:377–86

52. American Academy of Pediatrics Committee on Fetus and Newborn. Surfactant replacement therapy for respiratory distress syndrome. *Pediatrics* 1991;87:946–7

53. Abramovic A, Brandes JM, Fuchs K, *et al*. Meconium during delivery: a sign of compensated fetal distress. *Am J Obstet Gynecol* 1974;118:251

54. Avery GB, ed. *Neonatology, Pathophysiology, and Management of the Newborn*, 3rd edn. JB Lippincott, 1987:438–9

55. Woods JR, DolKart L, Creasy RK, *et al*. *Maternal Fetal Medicine*, 2nd edn. New York: WB Saunders, 1989:404–13

56. Lackkainen TJ, Lentonen PJ, Hess AE. Fetal sulfate and nonsulfate bile acids in intrahepatic cholestasis of pregnancy. *J Lab Clin Med* 1978;92:185

57. Miettinen TA, Laa Kkainen TJ. Gas liquid chromatographic and mass spectrometric studies on sterols in vernix caseosa, amniotic fluid and meconium. *Acta Chem Scand* 1968;22:2603

58. Becker RF, Windle WF. Fetal swallowing, gastrointestinal activity and defecation *in utero*. *Surg Gynecol Obstet* 1940;70:603

59. Cornish JD, Dreyer GL, Snyder GE, *et al*. Failure of acute perinatal asphyxia or meconium aspiration to produce persistent pulmonary hypertension in a neonatal baboon model. *Am J Obstet Gynecol* 1994;171:43–9

60. Chen CM, Kao HA, Shih SL. Relationship of chest roentgeno-graphic features and outcome in meconium aspiration syndrome. *Acta Padiatr Sin* 1990;31:24–8

61. Co E, Vidyasager D. Meconium aspiration syndrome. *Compr Ther* 1990;16:34–9

62. Dye TD, Aubrey R, Gross S, *et al*. Amnioinfusion and the intrauterine prevention of meconium aspiration. *Am J Obstet Gynecol* 1994;171:1601–5

63. Carson BS, Losey RW, Bowes WA, *et al*. Combined obstetric and pediatric approach to prevent meconium aspiration syndrome. *Am J Obstet Gynecol* 1976;126:712–5

64. Benny PS, Malani S, Hoby MA, *et al.* Meconium aspiration–role of obstetric factors and suction. *Aust NZ J Obstet Gynecol* 1987;27:36–9

65. Cunningham AS, Lawson EE, Martin RJ, *et al.* Tracheal suction and meconium: a proposed standard of care. *J Pediatr* 1990;116:153–4

66. Hageman JR, Conley M, Francis K, *et al.* Delivery room management of meconium staining of the amniotic fluid and the development of meconium aspiration syndrome. *J Perinatol* 1988;8:127–31

67. Holtzman RB, Branzhaf WC, Silver RK, *et al.* Perinatal management of meconium staining of the amniotic fluid. *Clin Perinatol* 1989;16:825–38

68. Linder N, Aranda JV, Tsur M, *et al.* Need for endotracheal intubation and suction in meconium stained neonates. *J Pediatr* 1988;112:613–5

69. Wiswell TE, Tuggle JM, Turner BS. Meconium aspiration syndrome: have we made a difference? *Pediatrics* 1990;85:615–21

70. Findlay RD, Taeusch W, Walther FJ. Surfactant replacement therapy for meconium aspiration syndrome. *Pediatrics* 1996;97:48–52

71. Nathan DG, Oski FA, eds. Isoimmune hemolytic diseases. In *Hematology of Infancy and Childhood*, 3rd edn. New York: WB Saunders Co. 1987:44–66

72. Perlman M, Frank JW. Bilirubin beyond the blood-brain barrier. *Pediatrics* 1988;81:304–15

73. Turkel SB, Miller CA, Guttenberg ME, *et al.* A clinical pathologic reappraisal of kernicterus. *Pediatrics* 1982;69:267–72

74. Volpe JJ. Bilirubin and brain injury. In *Neurology of the Newborn*, 2nd edn. New York: WB Saunders, 1987:386–408

75. Scheidt PC, Bryla DA, Nelson KB, *et al.* Phototherapy for neonatal hyperbilirubinemia: six-year follow-up of the NICHHD clinical trial. *Pediatrics* 1990;85:455–63

76. Dunham EC. Septicemia in the newborn. *Am J Dis Child* 1933;45:229–53

77. Nyhan WL, Fouse K. Septicemia of the newborn. *Pediatrics* 1958;22:268–78

78. Freedman RM, Ingram DL, Gross I, *et al.* A half century of neonatal sepsis at Yale. *Am J Dis Child* 1981;135:140–4

79. Hodgman JE. Sepsis in the neonate. *Perinatal Neonatal* 1981;5:45

80. Placzek MM, Whitelaw A. Early and late neonatal septicemia. *Arch Dis Child* 1983;58:728

81. Boyer KM. Diagnosis of neonatal sepsis and perinatal infections. *Mead Johnson Symp Perinat Dev Med* 1982:40–6

82. Wilson CB. Developmental immunology and role of host defenses in neonatal susceptibility. In Remington JS, Klein JO, eds. *Infectious Diseases of the Fetus and Newborn*. New York: WB Saunders, 1990:17–67

83. Freeman J, Epstein MF, Smith NE, *et al.* Extra-hospital stay and antibiotic usage with nosocomial coagulase-negative staphylococcal bacteremia in two neonatal intensive care unit populations. *Am J Dis Child* 1990;144:324–9

84. St. Geme JW III, Joseph W, Harris MC. Coagulase-negative staphylococcal infection in the neonate. *Clin Perinatol* 1991;18:281–302

85. St. Geme JW III, Bell LM, Baumgart S, *et al.* Distinguishing sepsis from blood culture contamination in young infants with blood cultures growing coagulase-negative staphylococci. *Pediatrics* 1990;86:157–62

86. Tollner V. Early diagnosis of septicemia in the newborn: clinical studies and sepsis score. *Eur J Pediatr* 1982;138:331

87. Philip AGS, Hewitt JR. Early diagnosis of neonatal sepsis. *Pediatrics* 1980;65:1036

88. Yoder MC, Polin RA. Immunotherapy of neonatal septicemia. *Pediatr Clin North Am* 1986;33:481–501

89. St. Geme JW Jr, Murray DL, Carter JA, *et al.* Perinatal infection after prolonged rupture of membranes: an analysis of risk management. *J Pediatr* 1984;104:608–13

90. Varner MW, Galask RP. Conservative management or premature rupture of the membranes. *Am J Obstet Gynecol* 1981;140:39

91. Baker CJ. Summary of the workshop on perinatal infections due to group B streptococcus. *J Infect Dis* 1977;136:137

92. Boyer KM, Gadzala CA, Kelly PD, *et al.* Selective intrapartum chemoprophylaxis of neonatal group B streptococcal early-onset disease: II. Predictive value of prenatal cultures. *J Infect Dis* 1983;148:802–9

93. Boyer KM, Gadzala CA, Burd LI, *et al.* Selective intrapartum chemoprophylaxis of neonatal group B streptococcal early-onset disease: I. Epidemiologic rationale. *J Infect Dis* 1983;148:795–801

94. Adler SM, Denton RL. The erythrocyte sedimentation rate in the newborn period. *J Pediatr* 1975;86:942–8

95. Sann L, Bienvenu F, Bienvenu J, *et al.* Evolution of serum pre-albumin, C-reactive proteins, and orosomucoid in neonates with bacterial infection. *J Pediatr* 1984;105:977–81

96. Mathers NJ, Polhandt F. Diagnostic audit of C-reactive protein in neonatal infection. *Eur J Pediatr* 1987;146:147

97. Weitzman M. Diagnostic utility of white blood cell and different cell counts. *Am J Dis Child* 1985;129:1183

98. Manroe BL, Weinberg AG, Rosenfeld CR, *et al.* The neonatal blood count in health and disease. I. Reference values for neutrophilic cells. *J Pediatr* 1979;95:89–98

99. Nelson SN, Merenstein GB, Pierce JR. Early onset group B streptococcal disease: is it underdiagnosed? *J Perinatol* 1987;6:234

100. Sherman MP, Goetzman BW, Ahlfors CE, *et al.* Tracheal aspiration and its clinical correlates in the diagnosis of congenital pneumonia. *Pediatrics* 1980;65:258–63

101. Pierce JR, Merenstein GB, Stocker JT. Immediate postmortem cultures in an intensive care nursery. *Pediatr Inf Dis J* 1984;3:510

102. Squire E, Favara B, Todd J. Diagnosis of neonatal bacterial infection. Hematologic and pathologic findings in fatal and nonfatal cases. *Pediatrics* 1979;64:60

103. Hendricks-Munoz KD, Shapiro DL. The role of the lumbar puncture in the admission sepsis evaluation of the premature infant. *J Perinatol* 1980;10:60–4

104. MacMahon P, Jewes L, deLouvois J. Routine lumbar punctures in the newborn - are they justified? *Eur J Pediatr* 1990;149:797–9

105. Eldadah M, Frenkel LD, Hiatt IM, *et al*. Evaluation of routine lumbar punctures in newborn infants with respiratory distress syndrome. *Pediatr Infect Dis J* 1987; 6:243–6

106. Schwersenski J, McIntyre L, Bauer CR. Lumbar puncture frequency and cerebrospinal fluid analysis in the neonate. *Am J Dis Child* 1991;145:54–8

107. Visser VE, Hall RT. Lumbar puncture in the evaluation of suspected neonatal sepsis. *J Pediatr* 1980;96:1063

108. Christensen RD, Rothstein G, Anstall HB, *et al*. Granulocyte transfusion in neonates with bacterial infection, neutropenia, and depletion of bone marrow neutrophils. *Pediatrics* 1982;70:1–6

109. Christensen KK, Christensen P. Intravenous gammaglobulin in the treatment of neonatal sepsis with special reference to group B streptococci and pharmacokinetics. *Pediatr Infect Dis* 1986;5(Suppl 3):S189–S192

110. Kliegman RM, Clapp DW. Rational principles for immunoglobulin prophylaxis and therapy of neonatal infection. *Clin Perinatol* 1991;18:303–24

111. Magny JF, Bremard-Oury C, Brault D, *et al*. Intravenous immunoglobulin therapy for prevention of infection in high risk premature infants. Report of a multicenter, double blind study. *Pediatrics* 1991;88:437–43

75

Neoplasia and pregnancy

T.J. Herzog and D.G. Mutch

Cancer complicates approximately one in 1000 pregnancies[1]. The Third National Cancer Survey found that 12. 8% of all cancers in women occur during the reproductive years, and the three most common cancers in decreasing order of frequency are thyroid, cervical and melanoma of the skin[2]. Malignancy in pregnancy is a rare and distressing condition which requires consideration of mother and fetus. Specific issues which complicate medical management of malignancy in pregnancy include the possible benefits of pregnancy termination to allow aggressive treatment, the effect of therapy on the developing fetus, the timing of delivery or termination with ongoing treatment, and the role of altered immune and hormonal status during pregnancy which may affect the prognosis of the coexistent cancer. Most malignancies in females occur outside the reproductive age group; therefore, there are few large studies which adequately examine these issues in detail. However, in reviewing the composite literature, several general guidelines have emerged. First, the anatomical and physiological changes of pregnancy can obscure the signs and symptoms of early malignancy. Patient complaints are often dismissed as simply symptoms of pregnancy, thereby delaying the performance of timely examination and diagnostic studies. Second, although immunosurveillance may be altered in pregnancy, stage-for-stage the prognosis and survival data for malignancy in pregnancy when properly treated are not significantly different than those for the non-pregnant population. Finally, the risk of an anomalous fetus resulting from treatment depends upon the gestational age of the fetus, as well as the mode and intensity of therapy. Many cancers arising during pregnancy can be treated aggressively with surgery, chemotherapy and even radiation, without necessarily requiring therapeutic abortion.

GYNECOLOGICAL MALIGNANCIES

The following section details the gynecological malignancies by disease site. Staging for the major gynecological malignancies is presented in Tables 1–5[3]. Overall, endometrial cancer has the highest incidence among gynecological malignancies for all age groups, followed by cervical and ovarian cancer. The incidence of gynecological malignancies in the reproductive age

Table 1 International Federation of Obstetrics and Gynecology (FIGO) staging of vulvar carcinoma. From reference 3

Stage 0 Tis	carcinoma *in situ*; intraepithelial carcinoma
Stage I T1 N0 M0	tumor confined to the vulva and/or perineum – 2 cm or less in greatest dimension. No nodal metastasis
Stage II T2 N0 M0	tumor confined to the vulva and/or perineum – more than 2 cm in greatest dimension. No nodal metastasis
Stage III T3 N0 M0 T3 N1 M0 T1 N1 M0 T2 N1 M0	tumor of any size with: (1) adjacent spread to the lower urethra and/or the vagina, or the anus; and/or (2) unilateral regional lymph node metastasis
Stage IVA T1 N2 M0 T2 N2 M0 T3 N2 M0 T4 any N M0	tumor invades any of the following: upper urethra, bladder mucosa, rectal mucosa, pelvic bone and/or bilateral regional node metastasis

Table 2 FIGO staging for vaginal carcinoma. From reference 3

Stage 0	carcinoma *in situ*, intraepithelial carcinoma
Stage I	the carcinoma is limited to the vaginal wall
Stage II	the carcinoma has involved the subvaginal tissue, but has not extended to the pelvic wall
Stage III	the carcinoma has extended to the pelvic wall
Stage IV	the carcinoma has extended beyond the true pelvis or has involved the mucosa of the bladder or rectum; bullous edema as such does not permit a case to be allotted to Stage IV *Stage IVa* spread of growth to adjacent organs and/or direct extension beyond the true pelvis *Stage IVb* spread to distant organs

group is altered, as cervical cancer far outranks ovarian cancer while endometrial carcinoma is rarest, unless one considers gestational trophoblastic disease (GTD)

Table 3 FIGO staging for cervical carcinoma. From reference 3

Stage 0	carcinoma *in situ*, intraepithelial carcinoma
Stage I	the carcinoma is strictly confined to the cervix (extension to the corpus should be disregarded)
	Stage Ia preclinical carcinoma of cervix, that is, those diagnosed only by microscopy
	Stage Ia1 minimal microscopically evident stromal invasion
	Stage Ia2 clinical detected microscopically that can be measured; depth ⩽ 5 mm from the base of the epithelium, either surface or glandular, from which it originates and horizontal spread
	Stage Ib clinical lesions confined to the cervix of preclinical lesions greater that Ia
	Stage Ib1 clinical lesions no greater than 4.0 cm in size
	Stage Ib2 clinical lesions greater than 4.0 cm in size
Stage II	carcinoma extends beyond the cervix, but not to pelvic wall. The carcinoma involves the vagina, but not as far as the lower third
	Stage IIa no obvious parametrial involvement
	Stage IIb extension to the pelvic wall and/or hydronephrosis or non-functioning kidney
Stage III	carcinoma has extended to the pelvic wall or tumor involves the lower third of the vagina. Hydronephrosis or non-functioning kidneys are Stage III, unless due to other causes
	Stage IIIa no extension to the pelvic wall
	Stage IIIb extension to the pelvic wall and/or hydronephrosis or non-functioning kidney
Stage IV	*Stage IVa* spread of growth to adjacent organs (i.e. bladder or rectal mucosa)
	Stage IVb spread to distant organs

Table 4 FIGO staging for endometrial carcinoma. From reference 3

Stage IA, G123	tumor limited to endometrium
Stage IB, G123	invasion to less than one-half of the myometrium
Stage IC, G123	invasion to more than one-half of the myometrium
Stage IIA, G123	endocervical glandular involvement only
Stage IIB, G123	cervical stromal invasion
Stage IIIA, G123	tumor invasion of serosa and/or adnexa, and/or positive peritoneal cytology
Stage IIIB, G123	vaginal metastases
Stage IIIC, G123	metastases to pelvic and/or para-aortic lymph nodes
Stage IVA, G123	tumor invasion of bladder and/or bowel mucosa
Stage IVB	distant metastases, including intra-abdominal and/or inguinal lymph nodes

G1: 5% or less of a non-squamous or non-morular solid growth pattern
G2: 6–50% of a non-squamous or non-morular solid growth pattern
G3: > 50% of a non-squamous or non-morular solid growth pattern

Table 5 FIGO staging for ovarian carcinoma. From reference 3

Stage I	growth limited to ovaries
IA	growth limited to one ovary; no ascites present containing malignant cells; no tumor on external surfaces; capsule intact
IB	growth limited to both ovaries; no ascites present containing malignant cells; no tumor on external surfaces, capsule intact
IC	tumor involving one or both ovaries either with tumor on external surfaces, or with capsule ruptured, or with ascites containing malignant cells, or with positive peritoneal washings
Stage II	growth involving one or both ovaries with pelvic extension
IIA	extension and/or metastases to uterus and/or tubes
IIB	extension to other pelvic tissues
IIC	tumor either Stage IIA or IIB, but with tumor on surface of one or both ovaries, or with capsule(s) ruptured, or with ascites present containing malignant cells, or with positive peritoneal washings
Stage III	tumor involving one or both ovaries with peritoneal implants outside the pelvis and/or positive retroperitoneal or inguinal nodes. (Superficial liver metastasis equals Stage III. Tumor is limited to the true pelvis but with histologically proven malignant extension to small bowel or omentum)
IIIA	tumor grossly limited to the true pelvis with negative nodes, but with histologically confirmed microscopic seeding of abdominal peritoneal surfaces
IIIB	tumor of one or both ovaries with histologically confirmed implants of abdominal peritoneal surfaces, none exceeding 2 cm in diameter; negative nodes
IIIC	abdominal implants greater than 2 cm in diameter; negative and/or positive retroperitoneal or inguinal nodes
Stage IV	growth involving one or both ovaries, with distant metastasis. (If pleural effusion is present, there must be positive cytology to allot a case to Stage IV. Parenchymal liver metastasis equals Stage IV)

in this group. A brief outline of etiology, epidemiology, diagnosis and treatment of each disease site is presented, with specific reference to pregnancy.

Vulvar carcinoma

Carcinoma of the vulva represents only about 4% of gynecological malignancies and is quite rare in pregnancy, because the vast majority of vulvar malignancies occur in postmenopausal patients. Approximately 15%

of vulvar cancers are found in women under 40 years of age. Of these, about 90% of the cases are squamous cell cancers. Other cell types include melanoma, adenocarcinoma, basal cell carcinoma and sarcoma. Presenting symptoms are similar to those of the non-pregnant state and include itching, irritation, discharge and occasionally bleeding. The etiology of vulvar cancer is unknown, but common patient characteristics include obesity, diabetes, hypertension and perhaps less-than-optimal vulvar hygiene. Recent evidence suggests that human papillomavirus infection is a causative or associative factor in pre-invasive vulvar intraepithelial neoplasia, as well as in invasive vulvar cancer. Examination of the vulva will demonstrate areas of ulceration, exophytic growth, hyper- or hypopigmentation, or red or white discoloration. The key to early diagnosis is biopsy. All abnormal areas of the vulva, including raised, depressed, discolored or warty lesions, deserve consideration for biopsy. Biopsy may be performed in the office under local anesthesia by simple excision or by utilizing the Keyes punch biopsy instrument. Toluidine blue staining and colposcopy may be used as adjunctive procedures, but should not substitute for biopsies, even in lieu of pregnancy.

A review of pregnancy-associated vulvar cancers in the literature by Barclay[4] revealed only 31 reported cases. Since this review, several other small series have been added. The youngest reported patient was 17 years old, whilst the average age was 27. Such a small number of patients presenting with vulvar carcinoma during pregnancy limits the development of guidelines for prognosis and treatment; nonetheless, certain conclusions can be drawn. Prognostically, these patients appear to do as well stage-for-stage with proper treatment as their non-pregnant counterparts. Treatment for vulvar intraepithelial neoplasia should be conservative with multiple biopsies to rule out invasion and then close follow-up, including colposcopy, until definitive therapy can be carried out postpartum. Invasive disease should be treated as in the non-pregnant state during the first and second trimesters, with radical or modified radical resection and groin node dissection. Lesions less than 2 cm in diameter and with invasion of 1 mm or less which are confined to the vulva with no evidence of nodal involvement may be considered for radical local excision. Bilateral or multiple ipsilateral positive groin nodules require adjunctive radiation to the groin and pelvis. Even if radiation is given after the period of organogenesis, the risk of spontaneous pregnancy loss is great. Thus, depending on the wishes of the patient, radiation treatment may be delayed until after delivery[4,5]. Alternatively, in this unusual circumstance, consideration may be given to a pelvic node dissection which, if negative, might allow omission of pelvic irradiation. Positive or close margins of resection, while also treatable with radiation, may be considered for re-excision during pregnancy to avoid the deleterious effects of radiation.

Invasive lesions presenting late in pregnancy (third trimester) may be widely excised and definitive treatment delayed until after delivery. These patients must be informed that these alternative forms of therapy during pregnancy deviate from the standard of treatment and may carry an increased risk of recurrence. The route of delivery is generally not altered by treatment, including radical vulvectomy and groin node dissection. Marked vaginal constriction and perineal fibrosis rarely necessitate Cesarean section delivery.

Human papillomavirus/warts of lower genital tract

The human papillomavirus (HPV) is the causative agent of genital warts and is related to a variety of skin diseases in humans, including lower genital tract carcinoma. Over 60 types have been identified to date. HPV is of concern during pregnancy for several reasons. First, the virus may be transmitted to the fetus, usually in the form of laryngeal papillomas. Also, the papillary lesions can proliferate and cause soft tissue dystocia or potential hemorrhage upon attempted vaginal delivery. When the lesions are occluding the introitus and vagina or are large and friable, treatment with trichloracetic acid, and rarely laser or cryotherapy, may be attempted. Podophyllin and interferon are contraindicated in pregnancy. Without adequate resolution of obstructive or hemorrhagic papillomas, Cesarean section is indicated. When smaller lesions or subclinical infections are present, the decision as to the route of delivery is problematic. Recent evidence suggests that perinatal transmission of HPV may not be avoided by abdominal delivery, since possible transplacental *in utero* infection may be possible with intact membranes. Further studies are required to elucidate potential benefits of Cesarean section delivery over vaginal delivery to avoid maternal–fetal transmission.

Vaginal carcinoma

The occurrence of vaginal cancer has limited demographic overlaps with the reproductive age group, as the vast majority of cases are diagnosed in patients beyond 50 years of age[6]. Less than 2% of gynecological malignancies are of primary vaginal origin. Metastatic disease from the cervix or vulva is far more common and must always be excluded. Up to 95% of cases are of squamous cell origin, while melanomas, sarcomas and adenocarcinomas, including clear cell histologies, are also found.

The incidence of squamous cell carcinoma of the vagina during pregnancy is very rare, with fewer than 20 reported cases[1]. Symptoms of vaginal cancers are bleeding or discharge. More advanced disease may present with symptoms of bladder or bowel dysfunction, including frequent urinary tract infections, urinary retention, constipation or tenesmus. While a persistently abnormal Papanicolaou's (Pap) smear may rarely provide initial evidence of vaginal cancer, thorough speculum examination with biopsy of suspicious gross lesions provides definitive diagnosis. Pre-invasive disease, vaginal intraepithelial neoplasia, which is far more common than invasive disease in the pregnant population, is best diagnosed with the use of colposcopic-guided biopsies. If biopsy confirms pre-invasive disease, treatment with laser, 5-fluorouracil (FU) or other ablative therapy can be postponed until completion of the pregnancy.

In the exceptional event that invasive cancer of the vagina is discovered during pregnancy, treatment is generally unaltered, except possibly during the late second or third trimester, when postponement of treatment until after delivery may be considered. Therapy is dependent upon the location and stage of disease, but the primary mode of treatment is radiation. Surgery is a viable option when early-stage disease is confined to the upper one-third of the vagina and is thus resectable with radical hysterectomy and upper vaginectomy. Disease localized to the distal portion of the vagina has been reported as resectable with lower vaginectomy. Utilizing radiation or surgery, fetal loss is inevitable.

Surgery allows preservation of ovarian function in this young population. Advanced-stage disease of any histology requires prompt treatment, which may necessitate hysterotomy for removal of products of conception, thus allowing initiation of radiation therapy.

Several histological types of vaginal cancer, although rare, tend to occur more commonly than squamous cell carcinoma in women of reproductive age. Adenocarcinoma, usually of the clear cell variety, may develop after *in utero* exposure to diethylstilbestrol. The link between diethylstilbestrol exposure and clear cell adenocarcinoma of the lower genital tract, including the cervix, was well established by 1971, after which the use of diethylstilbestrol during pregnancy was discontinued. The risk of developing adenocarcinoma of the vagina or cervix is actually less than one in 1000 for those exposed to the transplacental carcinogen diethylstilbestrol. Approximately one-third of diethylstilbestrol-exposed patients develop adenosis, which may be a precursor to clear cell carcinoma. Such diethylstilbestrol-linked malignancies rarely occur before 14 years of age or after 30 years of age. Thus, frequent cervical and vaginal cytology with careful colposcopic evaluation for abnormal findings are indicated beginning at menarche. Most clear cell adenocarcinomas are diagnosed early (Stage I) and thus have a good prognosis with an 80% 5-year survival. In pregnancy, treatment is largely unaltered, as surgery is performed without fetal regard, unless in the final trimester, in which case delay until after delivery may be contemplated.

Melanomas are very rare as primary tumors of the vagina. The lower posterior one-third of the vagina is the most frequent site of origin. Sarcoma botryoides of the vagina generally occurs in infants and children and presents as a group of cystic masses. The occurrence of both vaginal melanomas and sarcomas is exceedingly rare and reportable in pregnancy. Both tumors have a very poor prognosis, and management must be individualized according to the stage of disease, desires of the patient and gestational age.

Cervical neoplasia

The most common gynecological neoplasia, both pre-invasive and invasive, encountered during pregnancy arises from the cervix. Although the mean age of diagnosis for carcinoma of the cervix is 50 years, this disease process has a bimodal peak incidence with age ranges of 35–39 years and 60–64 years[7]. Clearly, this early peak corresponds with the reproductive age group. The incidence of pre-invasive and invasive cancer of the cervix is estimated to be 1.3 and 0.45–1.0 per 1000 pregnancies, respectively[8].

Pre-invasive disease

Cervical intraepithelial neoplasia (CIN) generally arises in the transformation zone between squamous-lined ectocervix and columnar-lined endocervix and has a peak age in the mid- to late twenties. The role of HPV infection is not completely understood, but it appears to play a role in the genesis of CIN. The progression of CIN to invasive disease does not appear to be accelerated by pregnancy, despite the possibility that pregnancy represents an immunocompromised state. As in the non-pregnant state, the screening method of choice for CIN is the Pap smear, which should be performed at the first prenatal visit.

Abnormal Pap smear   Management of the abnormal cervical Pap smear is a clinical dilemma often encountered during pregnancy. One acceptable algorithm for the management of abnormal cervical cytology during pregnancy is presented in Figure 1. In determining which diagnostic and therapeutic interventions to utilize in assessing an abnormal Pap smear in pregnancy, maternal risk in the form of underdiagnosed invasive cancer, and thus inadequate or delayed treatment, must be balanced against fetal risk, in the form of premature rupture of membranes, chorioamnionitis and spontaneous abortion, from conization. Recent evidence indicates that conservative management can be exercised with low-grade cervical lesions without significant maternal risk. LaPolla and colleagues[9] reported a cytological and histological concordancy rate of 84% in 248 pregnant patients with abnormal Pap smears who underwent colposcopically directed biopsies and found no false-negative results after rigorous postpartum follow-up. Patsner[10] used serial evaluation of the Pap test, colposcopy and directed biopsy to rule out occult or new malignancy in a large group of pregnant patients with mild dysplasia; the conclusion of this study was that patients with mild dysplasia require only one antepartum colposcopy prior to thorough postpartum re-evaluation, without significant increased risk of developing invasive cervical cancer. Advocacy of conservative management assumes that colposcopy is performed by an experienced operator, while cytology and histology are reviewed by a reliable laboratory. If these standards are not met, more frequent colposcopy and closer follow-up are required. In general, we recommend more than one antepartum colposcopic evaluation if there is a large time lag between the initial examination and delivery.

Colposcopy during pregnancy The pregnant cervix is actually quite amenable to colposcopy. The transformation zone tends to evert as pregnancy progresses, allowing for optimal colposcopic visualization of the cervix. Colposcopic appearance of the pregnant cervix is highlighted by edamatous and hyperemic changes secondary to increased vascularity and an underlying decidual stromal reaction. Clinically, increased friability with brisk bleeding upon cervical contact may be encountered during pregnancy and, if persistent, is an indication for evaluation. Acetic acid staining is often more intense during pregnancy, causing some minor abnormalities to be interpreted falsely as significant lesions. Nonetheless, aceto-white areas, especially more opaque changes with mosaicism, punctuation or frankly atypical vessels, deserve histological evaluation by biopsy. Any gross lesion and the worst representative abnormal areas by colposcopic visualization should be biopsied regardless of gestational age unless delivery is imminent, whereby biopsy may be delayed up to several weeks. Cervical biopsy during pregnancy may cause increased bleeding, which is generally well controlled by silver nitrate sticks, ferric sulfate solution, or, rarely, suture placement. In a series of 100 pregnant patients, Hacker and associates[8] reported a diagnostic accuracy of 99.5% and a complication rate of 0.6% for colposcopy with biopsies. As noted in Figure 1, no endocervical curettage should be performed on any patient with known or suspected pregnancy. The overall goal of a thorough colposcopic cervical examination in pregnancy is to exclude invasive disease, thus averting unnecessary conizations and allowing safe postponement of ablative therapy for CIN, including carcinoma *in situ*, until after delivery. Thus, the treatment of all forms of CIN in pregnancy is conservative, with requisite follow-up for postpartum therapy.

Cone biopsy during pregnancy Inadequate colposcopic visualization of either the transformation zone or the entire proximal extent of a lesion is generally averted during pregnancy, owing to eversion and slight cervical dilatation. In addition, endocervical curettage is not performed during pregnancy; thus, the primary indications for conization during pregnancy are histological microinvasive disease or marked discordance between a Pap smear suggestive of carcinoma and a histological specimen with minimal abnormalities. Every effort should be made to reconcile such discordance by review of the cytological interpretation and even repeat colposcopic biopsies to avoid unnecessary conization during pregnancy. When conization is required to rule out invasive disease in pregnancy, it is best performed in the first or early second trimester when the risk of spontaneous abortion and bleeding from the increased vascularity of the cervix are reduced. Averette and co-workers[11] collected the largest series of conizations during pregnancy with 180 patients and reported that 9.4% required a blood transfusion and 63% underwent a spontaneous abortion. The rates of spontaneous abortion and preterm delivery were similar to those of the general population. Others have described less frequent but significant complications associated with cone biopsy in pregnancy, including cervical infection, stenosis, chorioamnionitis, preterm labor, thrombophlebitis, pulmonary embolism and cervical laceration during labor. In an attempt to minimize bleeding and violation of the endocervical canal, DiSaia and colleagues[7] and others[6] have advocated excising a shallow 'coin'-shaped biopsy rather than a 'cone'-shaped specimen. Multiple hemostatic sutures can be placed at the vaginal reflection of the cervix and a vasoconstrictive agent can be used to infiltrate the cervical stroma in an attempt to decrease blood loss.

Cone cerclage has been described as a safe method for performing diagnostic conization during pregnancy[12]. The biopsy shape is usually smaller and shallower, resulting in an increased risk of residual disease with positive margins. The compilation of seven studies by Hacker and colleagues[8] showed 43.4% of cones for carcinoma *in situ* have residual disease upon repeat conization or hysterectomy. Cone biopsy performed during pregnancy should therefore be considered a diagnostic rather than a therapeutic procedure.

Invasive cervical carcinoma

Up to 3% of all cases of cervical cancer are diagnosed during pregnancy and the incidence of invasive disease varies from one to 13 cases per 10 000 pregnancies[7,8]. Pregnancy is not thought to play an etiological role in the development of cervical carcinoma, since the age-adjusted incidence is the same in pregnant as in non-pregnant women. Despite increases in estrogen and progesterone levels, the natural history of cervical cancer is likewise unaffected by pregnancy, as the prognosis is the same in pregnant and non-pregnant patients[7,8,13]. Precise survival data by stage for pregnancy complicated

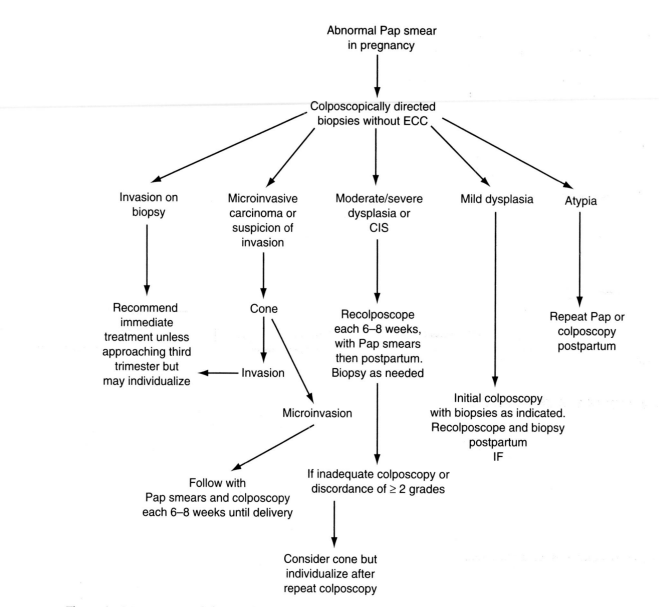

Figure 1   Management of abnormal Pap smears in pregnancy. ECC, endocervical curettage; CIS, carcinoma *in situ*

by invasive cervical carcinoma are difficult to ascertain, because more than 15 series reported a span greater than 30 years and their treatment, as well as staging, vary[14]. Nonetheless, stage-for-stage, 5-year survival rates are the same for pregnant and non-pregnant patients, with rates approaching 100% for Stage IA, 85% for IB and 60–70% for Stage II using aggregate data from more recent studies[5,8,15]. The average age of patients with cervical cancer in pregnancy is 30 years, while the average parity is four, but neither variable has been shown to be of prognostic value[8]. Table 6 shows the breakdown by trimester (stage and 5-year survival) in cases of cervical cancer associated with pregnancy. Highlighted is the trend of decreased survival and increased likelihood of advanced stage at presentation

as pregnancy progresses. Selection bias may influence the data. Patients who defer prenatal care and present later in pregnancy, or even during delivery, are more likely to ignore early symptoms of cervical cancer and not comply with regular cytological screening.

The distribution of histology is similar to the non-pregnant state; 95% or more are squamous cell carcinomas and 3% are adenocarcinomas. The cornerstone of detection remains the Pap smear. Biopsy is the requisite for diagnosis. Vaginal bleeding or abnormal discharge are the most frequent symptoms. Early-stage disease is often asymptomatic, but advanced disease may present with symptoms of urinary retention, pelvic pain, lymphedema or weight loss. Once the diagnosis is made, thorough staging should be performed

Table 6 Cervical carcinoma associated with pregnancy

| | Trimester | | | | | |
	1st	2nd	3rd	Postpartum	Total	Average
Time of diagnosis	19.3	14.2	14.9	51.6	100	N/A
5-year survival	68.6	62.7	51.7	46.3	N/A	51.3
Stage[*]						
IB	64.3	60.6	50.0	46.5	N/A	55.4
II	28.0	30.8	20.7	29.4	N/A	27.2
III/IV	7.7	8.6	29.3	24.1	N/A	17.4

[*]Adapted from reference 8; N/A, not applicable

and may include cytoscopy, proctoscopy and sigmoidoscopy. Imaging studies should be used judiciously; magnetic resonance imaging may be the study of choice, as excellent soft-tissue delineation is obtained without ionizing radiation. Single-exposure intravenous pyelography can be used and renal ultrasound may also be of value. Cervical malignancies tend to be understaged during pregnancy, because proper work-up is not performed and because parametrial induration may be less prominent and more difficult to detect[5].

Treatment for invasive forms of cervical carcinoma depends on stage of pregnancy and disease, as well as upon the wishes of the mother. Figure 2 outlines broad recommendations for treatment during pregnancy, which should be modified to the individual characteristics of the tumor and patient desires.

Microinvasive tumors confirmed by conization to be invading less than 3 mm below the basement membrane with negative margins and without lymph-vascular space involvement may be safely allowed to continue to term if desired. When microinvasion is discovered early in pregnancy, repeat cytology and colposcopy to exclude regrowth of the tumor after conization is indicated[8]. Route of delivery should be based primarily on obstetric indications. If Cesarean section is indicated, a Cesarean extrafascial hysterectomy can be performed at delivery. Close postpartum follow-up without surgery is advocated by some when future childbearing is desired in selected patients with minimal microinvasive disease[7].

Frankly invasive tumors of the cervix demand prompt treatment, although slight delay of up to 6–8 weeks has been shown not to alter prognosis[8,15]. For Stage IB and selected IIA tumors early in pregnancy, radical hysterectomy with ovarian preservation is effective therapy with the fetus *in situ* up to 18–20 weeks; thereafter, hysterotomy and uterine evacuation via fundal incision should be first performed. Radiation is equally efficacious, and no hysterotomy is necessary prior to 20 weeks' gestation with radiation therapy. External beam therapy is initiated and spontaneous abortion ensues. However, if the pregnancy is advanced, hysterotomy is required prior to

intracavitary radiation. Alternatively, a modified radical hysterectomy can be performed in certain cases[7]. For IB and IIA tumors found in the third trimester, classical Cesarean section via a fundal incision can be followed by radical hysterectomy with pelvic and periaortic lymph node dissection. If radiation is planned, lymph node dissection alone can be performed, which may guide subsequent therapy.

With advanced-stage tumors beyond IIA, radiation is the treatment of choice. Commencement of treatment is immediate, with the exception of late-second- or third-trimester pregnancies when treatment may be delayed until after documentation of fetal pulmonary maturity and delivery.

Route of delivery has not been shown to be of prognostic significance. Choice of route should be based on obstetric indications, extent of cervical tumor involvement and therapy planned. In general, early lesions allow for vaginal delivery if otherwise indicated, while advanced disease favors abdominal delivery because of the risk of cervical laceration and hemorrhage or infection.

Endometrial carcinoma

Endometrial carcinoma in pregnancy is extremely rare. There are fewer than ten well-documented cases in the world literature and great care is necessary to exclude misdiagnosis secondary to an intense Arias-Stella phenomenon. Diagnosis is usually made at dilatation and curettage for spontaneous or therapeutic abortion. Treatment is unaltered by pregnancy.

Gestational trophoblastic disease

The term 'gestational trophoblastic disease' comprises a wide variety of pathological entities, from the benign hydatidiform mole to the highly malignant choriocarcinoma. Hydatidiform mole has been observed since the era of Hippocrates. Richardson and Hertig provided the first account of a hydatid mole in 1638, while in 1827 the midwife Bolvin was the first to ascribe moles as products of gestational origin. In 1895, Felix Morchand

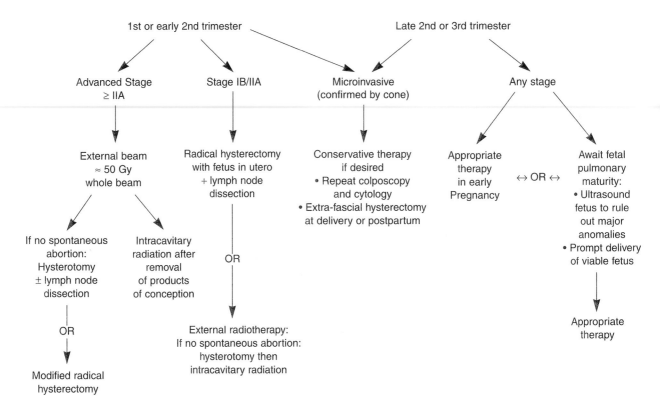

Figure 2   Management of cervical carcinoma in pregnancy

finally demonstrated that hydatidiform moles and their malignant sequelae derived from trophoblast, but his concept was not widely accepted until 1903[16,17].

Trophoblast may be regarded as the first organ of the developing embryo. Normal trophoblast is a unique tissue which bears several characteristics of cancer. Among these are the ability to invade the myometrium and embolize into the maternal circulation. Whether the trophoblast is normal or neoplastic, it contains both syncytiotrophoblast and cytotrophoblast and secretes human chorionic gonadotropin (hCG) in proportion to its volume. This fact allows clinicians to monitor this disease and predict eradication of trophoblastic tissue from the host[18].

Abnormal trophoblastic proliferation is manifested in two entities: partial and complete hydatidiform mole. The complete mole consists of abnormal trophoblast of paternal origin with a karyotype of 46,XX. This entity presents with abnormal bleeding 95% of the time between the 6th and 16th week gestational age. Other manifestations of molar gestation include pre-eclampsia, hyperemesis and hyperthyroidism. Rarely, patients can present with trophoblastic embolization and symptoms of congestive heart failure or pulmonary edema. hCG levels are usually markedly elevated above those appropriate for the gestational age of the pregnancy. The diagnosis is generally made with ultrasound. Histologically, complete hydatid moles are characterized by hydropic villi, proliferation

of both syncytiotrophoblast and cytotrophoblast, absence of fetal vessels and no definitive fetal structures[19,20].

In contrast, the diagnosis of partial mole is usually made at the time of curettage for a presumed missed or incomplete abortion. The clinical features are similar to those of a complete mole, but less severe. In addition, partial moles are usually of polyploid karyotype and associated with fetal structures.

The incidence of complete hydatidiform mole varies throughout the world from a high of one in 450 in Japan to one in 2500 in the USA[21]. These data are based on population base studies. The treatment of choice for a complete mole is suction curettage. Blood products, such as packed red blood cells, should be made available preoperatively, as blood loss can be unexpectedly high. Furthermore, a substantial risk of postevacuation pulmonary edema from trophoblastic deportation or rapid fluid replacement is possible. The incidence of malignant sequelae of complete moles is about 15%. The incidence of malignancy following a partial mole is much less. All moles require careful follow-up with weekly hCG levels. A rising or plateauing level requires immediate attention to staging and initiation of cytotoxic therapy[22,23].

The malignant sequelae of molar gestation ranges from invasive mole to the highly malignant choriocarcinoma. The prognosis for these entities is excellent with proper treatment. Two major staging

Table 7   Prognostic scoring system for staging gestational trophoblastic neoplasia

Score[*]	0	1	2	4
Age	< 39	> 39		
Prior pregnancy	mole	abortion	term	
Interval (months)[†]	4	4–6	7–12	> 12
Pretreatment hCG (log)	< 3	< 4	< 5	> 5
ABO group (female × male)		O × A	B	
		A × O	AB	
Largest tumor (cm)	< 3	3–5	5	
Site of metastases		spleen kidney	gastrointestinal tract, liver	brain
Number of metastases	0	1–4	4–8	> 8
Prior failed chemotherapy agents			single	multiple

[*]Prognosis is determined by summing the scores for each individual factor. Total score < 4 = low risk, 5–8 = middle risk, > 8 = high risk; [†]Interval is the time between termination of prior pregnancy and start of chemotherapy

systems have been proposed for malignant disease: the World Health Organization prognostic scoring system and a clinical staging system proposed by Hammond and colleagues of the South-eastern Regional Trophoblastic Disease Center (Tables 7 and 8)[24,25]. Once malignant trophoblastic disease is diagnosed, staging studies consisting of computed tomography scans of the head, abdomen and pelvis need to be performed. A chest X-ray is mandatory. Computed tomography of the chest may identify low-risk patients who are likely to fail primary single-agent therapy[26]. Cure for the groups with a good prognosis approaches 100% in published studies[25]. The last remaining challenge for cure in this disease lies in those patients with the following poor prognostic factors of brain or liver metastases:

(1)   hCG of greater than 40 000 IU/l;

(2)   Long duration of symptoms (usually greater than 4 months);

(3)   Malignant disease preceded by a term pregnancy.

A survival of 50–85% is reported in this group of patients. Good prognosis, or low-to-medium-risk disease, may be treated with single-agent therapy (methotrexate or actinomycin D), while patients with poor prognostic factors should be treated with multi-agent therapy (Table 9).

Pelvic mass in pregnancy

Pelvic masses in pregnancy present difficult management problems, because one must also consider the fetus as well as the patient. Therefore, the proper treatment of this problem is not always clear and requires clinical judgement. Fortunately, pregnancy

Table 8   Clinical classification of gestational trophoblastic neoplasia (GTN)

I   Non-metastatic GTN
II   Metastatic GTN
   (1) Good prognosis
     (a) Serum hCG < 40 000 mIU/ml (random) or urinary hCG < 100 000 IU (24 h)
     (b) Symptoms present less than 4 months
     (c) No brain or liver metastases
     (d) No prior chemotherapy
     (e) Prior pregnancy a mole or abortion of ectopic pregnancy
   (2) Poor prognosis
     (a) Serum hCG > 40 000 mIU/ml (random) or urinary hCG > 100 000 IU (24 h)
     (b) Symptoms present more than 4 months
     (c) Brain or liver metastases
     (d) Failure of prior chemotherapy
     (e) Antecedent term pregnancy

complicated by a pelvic mass is relatively uncommon, with the reported incidence varying from one in 230 pregnancies to one in 2489; the average of all fourteen reports in the literature is one in 991[27-29]. Prior to the advent of ultrasound, fibroids, ectopic pregnancies, appendicitis and pelvic kidneys were frequently included in the diagnosis of pelvic mass. These entities are now frequently diagnosed accurately with ultrasound, avoiding unnecessary laparotomy[30-32].

Most masses found during pregnancy are benign[33]. The most common masses found during gestation are serous or mucinous cystadenoma or mature teratoma. The most common malignant pelvic mass found during pregnancy is a dysgerminoma followed by tumors of epithelial origin, many of which are of low malignant potential. The incidence of ovarian cancer concomitant with pregnancy is one in 8000 to one in

Table 9   EMA–CO chemotherapy for high-risk patients

	Week 1,3,5, etc.: EMA	*Week 2,4,6, etc.: CO*
Day 1	actinomycin D 0.5-mg intravenous push etoposide 100 mg/m² intravenously in 200 ml normal saline over 30 min methotrexate 100-mg/m² intravenous push methotrexate 200 mg/m² intravenously over 12 h	vincristine 1-mg/m² intravenous push (maximum 2 mg) cyclophosphamide 600 mg/m² intravenously over 20 min
Day 2	actinomycin D 0.5-mg intravenous push etoposide 100 mg/m² intravenously in 200 ml normal saline over 30 min folinic acid 15 mg orally or intramuscularly twice daily for four doses, starting 24 h after initiation of methotrexate	

20 000 pregnancies. Only up to 5% of pelvic masses during pregnancy are malignant, versus 20% in the non-pregnant state[7]. One-third of masses, benign or malignant, found during pregnancy are of germ-cell origin. The remainder consist of a miscellaneous array of simple cysts, fibroids and theca lutean cysts. Masses over 15 cm identified during pregnancy are seldom malignant[34–36].

Masses discovered during pregnancy can be managed expectantly or surgically. Expectant management is frequently complicated by acute rupture, torsion, tumor previa or malignancy. Grimes[21] reported that these complications occurred most commonly when masses were greater than 5 cm. Acute rupture or torsion resulting in an acute abdomen occurred in 34% of patients expectantly managed. Tumor previa occurred about 5% of the time, while malignancy occurred only in about 4.5% of cases. Surgical management seeks to avoid these complications and remove the mass under more controlled and less emergent conditions. If possible, most clinicians postpone surgery until the second trimester, since inadvertent removal of the corpus luteum before this time can result in spontaneous abortion. Tocolysis by magnesium sulfate or β-mimetics during and after surgery may be beneficial.

Extensive preoperative discussion with the patient and family is required prior to laparotomy, because of the possibility of malignancy. If a malignancy is found, the patient should be staged and treated as if she was not pregnant. Pelvic washings should be obtained, extent of disease assessed and appropriate surgery performed. If conservative criteria apply, such as unilateral epithelial tumor of grade I or borderline differentiation or germ-cell origin, then unilateral salpingo-oophorectomy and staging may be performed without hysterectomy. Furthermore, the patient may alter her treatment based on her desire to preserve the fetus. Suggestions for possible management of pelvic masses by trimester can be found in Figures 3–5.

NON-GYNECOLOGICAL MALIGNANCIES

Breast cancer

One in nine women will develop breast cancer during her lifetime, representing one-third of all cancers in women[37]. Approximately 15% of breast cancers occur in women under age 41 years of age; one in 3000 pregnancies is complicated by breast cancer, with 3% of all breast cancer being diagnosed during pregnancy or lactation[1]. The incidence of breast cancer in association with pregnancy is expected to continue to rise, owing to the trend toward delayed childbearing.

Breast engorgement and hypertrophy during pregnancy may delay the detection of breast cancer. Some cases of inflammatory cancer, as well as some masses, can be confused with mastitis or other pregnancy-related changes. Most cases present with a painless lump often noted by the patient upon self-examination. The initial prenatal visit should include a thorough breast examination and detailed instructions on breast self-examination.

Mammography should be limited during pregnancy to minimize radiation exposure. In addition, pregnancy changes, such as elevated water density, increase the rates of false-positive and false-negative mammographic examinations[38]. In short, any palpable mass should be biopsied regardless of circumstances, including pregnancy or lactation. Fine-needle aspiration has a specificity and sensitivity of about 95% and no harmful effects upon the pregnancy have been reported[39]. If fine-needle aspiration is unsuccessful, open biopsy, preferably under local anesthesia, is performed. Radioisotopic bone scan, generally avoided during pregnancy, may be necessary when metastases are clinically suspected. Adequate maternal hydration may increase fetal exposure to radiation. Ultrasound for discriminating solid-form cystic breast lesions may be a valuable diagnostic adjunct in pregnancy.

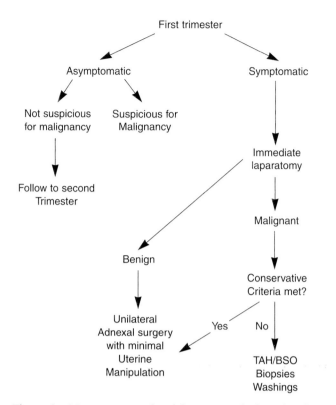

Figure 3 Management of pelvic masses during the first trimester of pregnancy. TAH/BSO, total abdominal hysterectomy with bilateral salpingo-oophorectomy

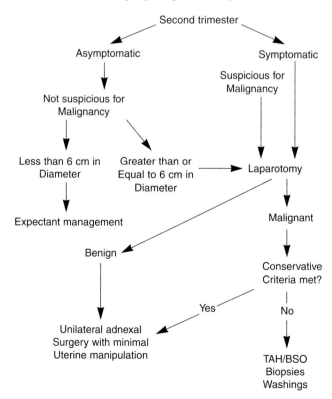

Figure 4 Management of pelvic masses during the second trimester of pregnancy. TAH/BSO, total abdominal hysterectomy with bilateral salpingo-oophorectomy

Although treatment of breast cancer is largely unaltered during pregnancy, certain issues must be considered. Modified radical mastectomy with axillary node dissection is generally the procedure of choice for early-stage disease during pregnancy. In the non-pregnant state, wide local excision with axillary node dissection and radiation is a viable alternative for small unifocal masses. This alternative is less attractive during pregnancy, as radiation with boost doses to the tumor bed would cause internal scatter, resulting in fetal radiation exposure above acceptable levels[39]. Treatment may be modified by delaying radiation until after delivery if the diagnosis is made in the third trimester, while carrying out lumpectomy and axillary dissection during pregnancy. There is a paucity of data for the role of adjuvant chemotherapy in pregnancy for patients with positive or negative nodes. Chemotherapy, if chosen, is best withheld until the second trimester, despite no documentation of overwhelming risk of congenital anomalies, growth retardation or preterm delivery[40]. Advanced disease calls for careful individualization of treatments. Delay of palliative treatment until achievement of fetal viability is a reasonable option when the diagnosis is made late in pregnancy. Otherwise, aggressive palliative treatment should be instituted without delay. Such treatment, which includes radiation, multi-agent chemotherapy and hormonal therapy, separately or in combination, poses a considerable unmeasurable risk to the fetus. If such advanced disease is diagnosed early in pregnancy, termination may be considered. Therapeutic abortion does not appear to enhance maternal remission or survival in early-stage disease; however, it does allow for prompt initiation of therapy in advanced disease.

Prognosis for pregnancy-associated breast cancer has been traditionally deemed dismal based on early reports. More recent studies have shown that the prognosis for breast cancer, stage-for-stage, is unchanged by pregnancy. Prognosis is most influenced by maternal age with 5-year survival rates of 75% for women over 40 years of age, but only 55% for those under 40 years of age[40,41]. Pregnancy-associated breast cancer tends to present at later stages with twice the rate of lymph node involvement (74% versus 37%), even controlled for age[40]. This worse prognosis may be due to delayed diagnosis and treatment of pregnant patients. In addition, pregnancy-induced hormonal changes may alter the behavior of tumors. Over 70% of women with pregnancy-associated breast cancer had estrogen-receptor-negative tumors[40].

Although pregnancy early in the reproductive years is thought to be protective against breast cancer, pregnancy after breast cancer should be delayed several years as pregnancy remains a high-risk period for recurrence of these hormonally responsive tumors. The overall prognosis, both maternal and fetal, appears unaltered by subsequent pregnancy[41].

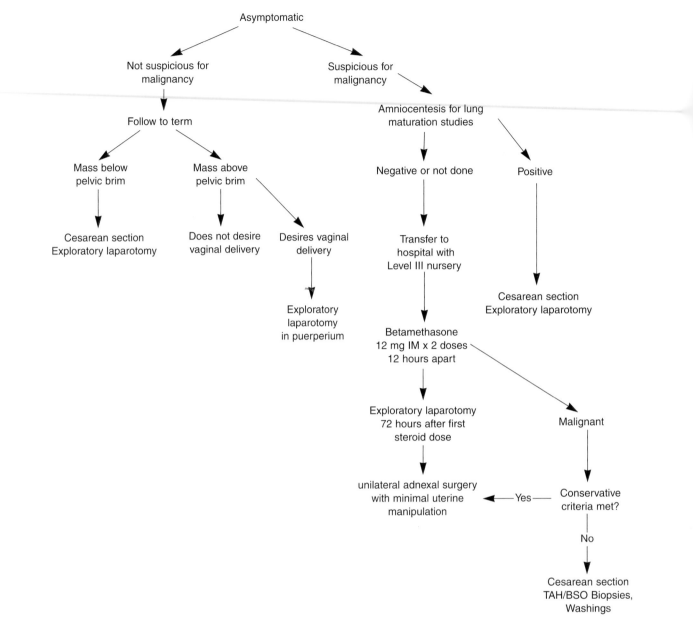

Figure 5   Management of pelvic masses during the third trimester of pregnancy, remote from term. TAH/BSO, total abdominal hysterectomy with bilateral salpingo-oophorectomy

Colorectal carcinoma

Colorectal carcinoma, one of the leading causes of cancer death in females, occurs only in one in 50 000 to one in 100 000 pregnancies, with approximately 200 reported cases; most cases originate distally below the level of the peritoneal reflection[42,43]. The mean age of diagnosis is 32 years[43].

Presenting symptoms include constipation, obstipation, abdominal pain, rectal or abdominal mass, rectal bleeding, nausea and vomiting. Many of these signs and symptoms represent common complaints of normal pregnancy and therefore delayed diagnosis in pregnancy is common. Rectal bleeding of guaiac-positive stool is an alarming symptom which requires full evaluation. Routine digital examination should be performed during prenatal evaluation. Distribution of lesions appears to be similar to that in the non-pregnant population, with 57% arising in the rectum, 20% in the sigmoidcolon and 23% in the remainder[44]. If a colorectal lesion is suspected during pregnancy, sigmoidoscopy and/or colonoscopy with biopsy are the diagnostic procedures of choice. Barium enema should be avoided if possible. Serum tumor markers, such as carcinoembryonic antigen and α-fetoprotein, are difficult to interpret because of their elevation in normal pregnancy[42]. If a markedly elevated serum α-fetoprotein occurs in the setting of normal amnionitic fluid α-fetoprotein, extrauterine origins, including colorectal carcinoma, should be considered. Increased surveillance is recommended for patients with a history of familial polyposis, Gardner's syndrome or villous adenomas.

Treatment during the first two trimesters is generally immediate surgery with limited regard for the pregnancy, although frequently the pregnancy is unharmed if cancer had not metastasized to other pelvic structures. Even distal tumors may be resected with primary re-anastomosis using automatic staplers and abdominoperineal or low anterior resection procedures. If optimal resection is prevented by the gravid uterus, hysterectomy may at times be necessary; such a possibility must be addressed with the mother prior to surgery. If tumor is unresectable, diverting colostomy for decompression and palliation is the treatment of choice to allow the pregnancy to progress towards term. During the third trimester, one can await fetal maturity and perform Cesarean section with subsequent tumor excision or diverting colostomy, depending on the extent of disease. If the tumor is discovered near term, vaginal delivery may be considered, provided that tumor is not obstructing the pelvic outlet. With advanced-stage and surgically unresectable tumor identified at any stage of pregnancy, consideration may be given to awaiting fetal maturity, thus delaying palliative treatment until after delivery[45]. Chemotherapy or irradiation for colorectal cancer during pregnancy has a limited role, with no evidence of prolonging survival.

Pregnancy has not been shown to affect maternal prognosis or the natural source of colorectal cancer. The prognosis of pregnant women with colorectal carcinoma is dismal.

There are no reported 5-year survivors for colon cancer. Few with rectal carcinoma are reported, owing to the advanced stage at presentation. Over one-half of pregnant patients with colorectal carcinoma present with Duke's stage C or a more advanced stage (see Table 10 for staging)[43]. Theoretically, the estrogen-binding capacity of cells derived from colorectal carcinomas may indicate accelerated cancer growth during pregnancy. However, survival data between pregnant and non-pregnant patients are comparable stage-for-stage.

Hematological malignancies

Leukemia

The development of leukemia during pregnancy is rare, with an incidence of one in 75 000 pregnancies[46]. Acute and chronic leukemias occur with equal frequency. Among the acute forms, acute myelogenous leukemia is more common than acute lymphocytic leukemia. Ninety per cent of the cases are chronic myelocytic leukemia, with the remainder being chronic lymphocytic leukemia[47].

The majority of pregnant women found to have leukemia are diagnosed during routine prenatal care.

Table 10 Duke's staging for colorectal carcinoma

A	penetration into, but not beyond, the bowel wall
B	penetration through the bowel wall
C	positive lymph node involvement
D	distant metastasis

Signs and symptoms of acute leukemia include anemia, granulocytopenia, thrombocytopenia, splenomegaly, fatigue, fever, infection and evidence of a bleeding diasthesis. The diagnosis of leukemia can only be confirmed by bone marrow examination.

Acute lymphocytic leukemia in adults is seen in the 30–40-year-old age group. While anemia and splenomegaly are common, only 25% of patients will have a white blood cell count of greater than 50 000/mm[3,48]. In contrast, acute myelogenous leukemia most commonly occurs in 30–60-year-old women and 75% will have white blood cell counts greater than 50 000/mm[3]. The usual age of presentation of acute leukemia during pregnancy ranges from 23 to 28 years[47].

Chronic leukemia usually presents with lymphadenopathy, splenomegaly, leukocytosis and constitutional symptoms. Chronic myelocytic leukemia accounts for the majority of chronic leukemias complicating pregnancies, with a median age of 35 years[49]. Chronic lymphocytic leukemia is generally indolent, with a median age onset of 60 years, which accounts for its relative rarity during gestation.

Experience in the treatment of leukemia during pregnancy is limited. Without treatment, the median survival time for patients with acute leukemia is 2 months. With treatment, 65–75% of adults with acute lymphocytic leukemia will gain complete remission; however, recurrence is common and only one-third of patients with acute lymphocytic leukemia will be long-term survivors. A similar proportion of individuals under 60 years of age treated for acute myelogenous leukemia will achieve complete remission, with 40% of these experiencing eventual cure[49]. Chronic leukemia is more indolent and can be successfully controlled with chemotherapy for a long period of time.

The patient diagnosed with acute leukemia during pregnancy poses a difficult problem. Due to the poor prognosis and rapid progression of this disease, immediate treatment is needed. Since there is no evidence that pregnancy alters the natural course of leukemia, terminating the pregnancy will not improve survival of the patient. Combination chemotherapy has become the therapeutic management of choice in patients with acute leukemia. Children who were exposed to chemotherapeutic agents *in utero* showed normal growth and development from 1 to 17 years of age[50]. Remission rates of pregnant women treated with combination chemotherapy compare favorably with those in comparable non-pregnant women. Standard anti-leukemic agents, such as cytoarabine and anthracyclines, can be safely administered during the second and third trimesters. However, antifolates should be avoided during the first trimester, owing to a 10–20% risk of congenital anomalies[51].

Intrathecal chemotherapy and whole-brain radiation may safely be performed during any trimester of pregnancy[13]. There is an increased risk of infection and spontaneous abortion associated with leukemia treatment[52]. Patients diagnosed with acute leukemia during the first half of pregnancy have only a 50–60% chance of producing a healthy live infant.

Chronic leukemia is generally a more indolent disease and treatment should be withheld until after delivery if possible. As seen with acute leukemia, pregnancy does not appear to alter the natural course of chronic leukemia. The median survival for pregnant women with chronic leukemia is not significantly different from that expected for non-pregnant women.

Lymphoma

Lymphoma is a relatively common malignancy presenting during the reproductive years. It occurs in one in 1000 to one in 6000 pregnancies. Approximately 25–40% of lymphomas are Hodgkin's type, with the average age of onset being 32 years. Hodgkin's disease is the most common type of lymphoma associated with pregnancy[54].

The majority of women with lymphoma are asymptomatic. On physical examination, 80% will have superficial lymphadenopathy. Those with Hodgkin's disease are more likely to have localized lymphadenopathy. A small percentage of patients have fever, night sweats, weight loss or pruritis, which are associated with poor prognosis. Biopsy is the 'gold standard' of diagnosis. The histological pattern of Hodgkin's disease is most commonly nodular sclerosing or lymphocytic, which is associated with a better prognosis compared to patients with mixed cellularity or lymphocyte depletion pattern. Patients with non-Hodgkin's lymphoma commonly present with high- or intermediate-grade diffuse histological patterns and have a poorer prognosis than those with a nodular pattern[53].

After diagnosis, the staging of lymphoma is difficult in the presence of the gravid uterus. The treatment of lymphoma depends on accurate staging, which requires procedures such as lymphangiography, intravenous pyelography, computed tomography scans and staging laparotomy, all of which expose the fetus to radiation. Minimal evaluation requires examination by the physician, chest radiographs, bone marrow biopsy with aspirate, and core and imaging of the abdomen. Abdominal ultrasound examination for retroperitoneal adenopathy or hydronephrosis may be helpful in staging. The value of magnetic resonance imaging for evaluating lymphoma remains unclear.

Once staging is complete, treatment generally should not be compromised because of the pregnancy. In the non-pregnant woman, nodal radiotherapy and combination chemotherapy result in cures for 70% of patients with Hodgkin's disease and 50% of patients with non-Hodgkin's lymphoma[54]. Patients in the third trimester with localized Hodgkin's disease can be allowed to deliver prior to therapy[51]. Treatment during the first and second trimesters and in patients with advanced disease or high-grade tumors is more complex. Localized disease above the diaphragm can be treated with radiotherapy with abdominal shielding. More extensive disease is best treated with combination chemotherapy to reduce the large fetal radiation exposure. The same considerations concerning combination chemotherapy as discussed with leukemia apply to lymphoma.

Melanoma

Melanoma represents 1% of all cancers diagnosed in the USA, with approximately 30% occurring in women of reproductive age[55]. It complicates pregnancy with an estimated incidence of 0.14–2.8 cases per 1000 pregnancies[56].

The majority of patients present with a change in the size and color of a pre-existing nevus. More advanced melanomas may present with ulceration and bleeding. Excisional biopsy of the entire suspicious pigmented lesion is the diagnostic procedure of choice. Microscopic measurement of the actual tumor thickness, as outlined by Breslow, most accurately reflects the prognostic index and is of utmost importance in the clinical management of patients[57]. The Clark level, which describes the anatomical level of invasion, should also be assessed. Following histopathological evaluation of the biopsy, the patient should be clinically staged with a thorough history and complete physical examination. The most common clinical staging system defines Stage I as local disease without clinically palpable regional lymph nodes, Stage II as having suspiciously palpable regional lymph nodes, and Stage III as having distant metastases[58]. Further tests, such as serum liver function studies radionucleotide, or computed tomography scans of the liver, bone or brain, should be performed only for specific signs or symptoms suggesting metastatic disease.

Local excision with wide margins is the only effective cure for melanoma and this approach should not be influenced by pregnancy[59]. Regional lymphadenectomy has not proven to be beneficial when lymph nodes are not palpable, but clinically involved lymph nodes should be excised. Distant metastatic disease may be treatable with systemic chemotherapy with a response rate of 20–25%. Metastatic melanoma is resistant to most forms of therapy. Immunotherapy or radiotherapy are unproven modalities during pregnancy.

Pregnancy-associated increases in pigmentation and melanocyte stimulating hormone, presence of estrogen receptors on 46% of melanomas, reports of rapidly fatal courses in pregnancy and reports of tumor regression postpartum or with hormonal therapy have led to speculation that the course of malignant melanoma may be adversely affected by pregnancy[60]. Melanoma is one of the most unpredictable cancers. Extensive research had failed to provide conclusive evidence for either a beneficial or deleterious effect of pregnancy on its clinical course. Most recent studies which control for prognostic factors have demonstrated similar survival in both pregnant and non-pregnant patients. When controlling of tumor site, age, Breslow thickness and Clark level, an overall mortality of 25% in the pregnancy group was found during a 7-year mean follow-up period[61].

Although Reintgen and colleagues[55] reported no difference in survival for patients who developed melanoma during pregnancy or for those who became pregnant within 5 years of diagnosis, most clinicians advise patients to avoid a subsequent pregnancy for 2–5 years after diagnosis, since 60–86% of melanomas recur during this period[55,59]. In addition, when melanoma complicates pregnancy, both the fetus and placenta should be examined closely after delivery because melanoma is the most common tumor metastasizing to the fetus and placenta. Overall, this phenomenon is exceedingly rare, with fewer than 20 reported cases. Termination of the pregnancy is not warranted, as infant survival, even with metastatic melanoma, is 75%[59,60]. Nonetheless, the fact that melanoma is overwhelmingly the predominant tumor metastasizing to the fetus or placenta suggests that melanoma has important immune and endocrine interactions in pregnancy.

Thyroid cancer

Thyroid cancer is the most frequently encountered cancer in the reproductive age group, with 50% of cases occurring in women 15–44 years of age. In the general population, it is a relatively uncommon cancer, with an estimated incidence in women of 5.5 per 100 000, which is two to three times the incidence in men[62]. Some case–control studies suggest hormonal factors may play an etiological role in the development of thyroid cancer[63]. This theory is supported by isolated studies showing an increased incidence in pregnancy and a decreased incidence, equal to that in males, following menopause. No consensus about the impact of pregnancy on thyroid cancer has been reached, however, as the precise incidence of thyroid cancer in pregnancy is unknown[64].

The most common histological type is papillary, followed by follicular and mixed papillary–follicular. These histologies have a favorable prognosis, whereas the less commonly occurring medullary and anaplastic patterns do not. The usual clinical presentation is that of a single thyroid nodule which has up to a 20% chance of being malignant. Rapid growth, fixation of the nodule to the surrounding structures or cervical lymphadenectomy are common findings for advanced disease. Risk factors for developing thyroid cancer are prior head or neck irradiation and a family history of multiple endocrine neoplasms. Diagnosis is often made by palpation, but must be confirmed by biopsy. Fine-needle aspiration has been shown to be a safe and effective technique in pregnant women, with false-positive results being exceedingly rare and false-negative results occurring in only 5–10% of cases[13]. Radioisotope nuclear scanning is contraindicated in pregnancy, because radioactive isotopes are taken up by the fetus. Other methods, such as ultrasound, can be used to distinguish solid-form cystic nodules. Thyroid function tests may also be helpful. Normally, pregnancy witnesses a hypertrophy of the thyroid gland from follicular cell hyperplasia, and total triiodothyronine and thyroxine levels are elevated while triiodothyronine resin uptake is decreased secondary to increased thyroid-binding globulin. Thyroid stimulating hormone is in the normal to slightly elevated range.

Treatment of choice for all primary carcinomas is surgery. Cancer discovered during the first or second trimester should prompt immediate surgery[64]. In the third trimester, a brief delay to allow fetal pulmonary maturity may be acceptable. Well-differentiated forms of papillary and follicular histology are treated with subtotal thyroidectomy. Extensive neck dissection performed for cervical lymphadenectomy carries an increased incidence of spontaneous abortion. Poor prognostic medullary or anaplastic forms may present at very advanced stages, in which case regard for fetal development may predominate. Treatment with radioactive iodine is contraindicated, since it crosses the placenta and is trapped by the fetal thyroid. Overall, prognosis during pregnancy appears unchanged stage-for-stage and histology-for-histology; thus, abortion or prevention of subsequent pregnancy is unwarranted. When surgery is performed, vigilance for hypothyroidism and hypoparathyroidism should be maintained throughout pregnancy as well as postpartum. Thyroid hormone replacement is safe and effective in pregnancy.

Bone and soft tissue sarcomas

Bone and soft tissue sarcomas are relatively common malignancies in the reproductive age group. Their presence in association with pregnancy, however, is very rare, as there are less than 50 such recorded cases in the literature[65]. The majority of these cases are osteosarcomas, followed by Ewing's sarcomas. Genital sarcomas of the cervix, vagina and vulva include liposarcomas, histiocytomas, myosarcomas and leiomyosarcomas, with and without peritoneal dissemination.

The majority of patients present with symptoms of localized pain or a mass. Diagnostic procedures commonly used to assess sarcomas include radiographs with abdominal shielding during pregnancy. Osteogenic sarcomas may require radioisotopic bone scanning, which is thought to be of low risk to the fetus[66]. Definitive diagnosis of any type of sarcoma requires biopsy. Although pregnancy has no proven deleterious effects on the natural course of sarcomas, delayed diagnosis results in postponed treatment. These tumors present at advanced stages, which may explain isolated reports of worsened prognosis for sarcomas in pregnancy[67]. The aggressive biological behavior of pelvic sarcomas may be enhanced by hypervascularity or hormonal stimulus; however, an impaired prognosis for most sarcomas associated with pregnancy remains unsubstantiated.

Owing to the diversity of histological types, anatomical locations, stages of disease and forms of treatment for different types of sarcomas, it is difficult to generalize treatment options. Since maternal prognosis for all types of sarcomas is poor, a combination of surgery, irradiation and aggressive multi-agent chemotherapy is warranted[68]. Most clinicians recommend that the pregnant woman should be managed without regard for the pregnancy during the first two trimesters of gestation. In cases presenting in the third trimester, the fetus may be delivered by vaginal delivery or Cesarean section for obstetric indications as soon as pulmonary maturity is documented, so that aggressive treatment can be initiated. Although based on limited experience, more recent reports advocate the initiation of multi-agent chemotherapy for control of systemic disease during any stage of gestation. Such therapy is based on the rationale that mortality in sarcomas often results from distant metastases and not local recurrence, and chemotherapy is relatively well tolerated by the fetus with the exception of the first trimester.

Tumors of the central nervous system

The Third National Cancer Study indicates that 21% of brain tumors affect women in the childbearing years[2]; however, only 220 cases of central nervous system (CNS) tumors occurring during pregnancy have been reported in the world's literature over the past 90 years[69]. Intracranial tumors occur in pregnancy with a reported frequency of 3.6 per 10^6 births[70]. Certain CNS tumors, such as meningiomas, pituitary adenomas and vascular neoplasms, have a slightly increased incidence during pregnancy. Although not well established, the fact that meningiomas predominate in women, enlarge rapidly during pregnancy and express estrogen and progesterone receptors suggests a causal relationship between the tumors and pregnancy[71]. Pregnancy normally results in pituitary enlargement secondary to hyperplasia of prolactin-secreting acidophilic cells and it also appears to stimulate the growth of pituitary microadenomas, making them clinically apparent[72]. The relative frequency of CNS vascular tumors is also increased during pregnancy, with hemangioblastomas and spinal hemangiomas predominating. This increased incidence is attributed to retrograde engorgement of vascular channels in the tumor secondary to increased venous pressure from compression of the inferior vena cava in the gravid uterus, as well as an overall increased blood volume[73]. These factors permit occult vascular tumors to become clinically apparent.

Symptoms of brain tumors manifesting during pregnancy, such as nausea and vomiting, can be mistakenly attributed to the pregnancy. In addition, headache and visual disturbances commonly caused by brain tumors may be misinterpreted as signs of pre-eclampsia. Spinal cord tumors cause symptoms of spinal cord compression, depending on the level involved. Early symptoms, such as fatigue, backache and nerve-root irritation, may also be confused with common pregnancy-related complaints.

The diagnosis of CNS tumors can be established by radiographic studies, such as computed tomography scans, magnetic resonance imaging, myelography and angiography. Prolactin levels are useful in assessing pituitary tumors and examination of the cerebrospinal fluid is helpful with spinal cord tumors. Definitive diagnosis of any tumor requires histological examination. The coexistence of a CNS tumor and pregnancy should not preclude diagnostic studies.

The management of CNS tumors must be considered on an individual basis. Immediate treatment is usually not necessary unless symptoms are severe and progressive. Once the diagnosis is established, the patient should be closely observed for sudden increase in intracranial pressure, loss of visual fields or progressive neurological deficits. The treatment of choice for most CNS tumors, including meningiomas and spinal cord tumors, is surgery. Other tumors may respond to radiation therapy, which is not contraindicated during pregnancy provided the tumor is above the thoracic region and the fetus can be appropriately shielded. When symptoms are mild or occur during the third trimester, careful observation with conservative medical treatment aimed at reducing intracranial pressure until fetal maturity is suggested[74]. When symptoms are severe, treatment is mandatory without regard to the pregnancy to prevent further neurological deficits or death. The best mode of delivery in the presence of increased intracranial pressure remains to be determined.

REFERENCES

1. Donegan WL. Cancer and pregnancy. *Cancer* 1983;33: 194–214
2. Third National Cancer Survey. Incidence data. *NCI Monogr* 1975;41:108–11

3. Creasman WT. New gynecologic cancer staging. *Obstet Gynecol* 1990;75:287

4. Barcly DL. Surgery of the vulva, perineum and vagina in pregnancy. In Barber HRK, Graber EA, eds. *Surgical Disease in Pregnancy*. Philadelphia: WB Saunders, 1974

5. Yagizi R, Cunningham FG. Cancer and pregnancy. *Williams Obstet* 1990;4(Suppl):1–15

6. Lutz MH, Underwood PB, Rozier JC, Putney FW. Genital malignancy in pregnancy. *Am J Obstet Gynecol* 1977; 129:536–42

7. DiSaia PJ, Creasman WT. Cancer in pregnancy. In DiSaia PJ, Creasman WT, eds. *Clinical Gynecologic Oncology*. St. Louis, MO: CV Mosby, 1989

8. Hacker NF, Berek JS, Lagasse LD. Carcinoma of the cervix associated with pregnancy. *Obstet Gynecol* 1982; 59:735–46

9. LaPolla JP, O'Neill C, Wetrich D. Colposcopy management of abnormal cervical cytology in pregnancy. *J Reprod Med* 1988;33:301–6

10. Patsner B. Management of low grade cervical dysplasia during pregnancy. *South Med J* 1990;83:1405–12

11. Averette HE, Nasser N, Yankow SL, Little WA. Cervical conization in pregnancy. *Am J Obstet Gynecol* 1970;106: 543–8

12. Goldberg GL, Ataras MM, Block B. Cone cerclage in pregnancy. *Obstet Gynecol* 1991;77:315–17

13. Jacob JH, Stringer CA. Diagnosis and management of cancer during pregnancy. *Semin Perinatol* 1990;14: 79–87

14. Zemlickis D, Lishner M, Degendorfer P, *et al*. Maternal and fetal outcome after invasive cervical cancer in pregnancy. *J Clin Oncol* 1991;9:1956–61

15. Lee RB, Neglia W, Park RC. Cervical carcinoma in pregnancy. *Obstet Gynecol* 1981;58:584–9

16. Obner WB. Choriocarcinoma: historical notes. In Szulman AE, Buschsbaum J, eds. *Gestational Trophoblastic Disease*. New York: Springer Verlag, 1987

17. Dehner LP. Gestational and nongestational trophoblastic disease. *Am J Surg Pathol* 1980;4:43–58

18. Vaitukaitis JL, Braunstein GD, Ross GT. A radioimmunoassay which specifically measures human chorionic gonadotropin in the presence of human luteinizing hormone. *Am J Obstet Gynecol* 1972;113:751–8

19. Voss IP, Riottanm G, Kazii T. Hydatidiform mole: two entities. *Am J Obstet Gynecol* 1977;127:167–70

20. Lawler SD, Fisher RA, Dent J. A prospective genetic study of complete and partial hydatidiform moles. *Am J Obstet Gynecol* 1991;164:1270–7

21. Grimes DA. Epidemiology of gestational trophoblastic disease. *Am J Obstet Gynecol* 1984;150:309–18

22. Kahan EI. Clinical management and the neoplastic sequelae of trophoblastic embolization associated with hydatidiform mole. *Obstet Gynecol Surv* 1987;42: 484–8

23. Berkowitz RJ, Goldstein DP, DuBeshten B, Bernstein MR. Management of complete molar pregnancy. *J Reprod Med* 1987;32:634–9

24. Bageshawe KD. Risk and prognostic factors in trophoblastic neoplasm. *Cancer* 1976;58:1373–85

25. Hammond CB, Berchert LG, Tyrey L, *et al*. Treatment of metastatic trophoblastic disease: good and poor prognosis. *Am J Obstet Gynecol* 1973;115:451–7

26. Mutch DG, Soper JT, Baker ME, *et al*. Role of computer axial tomography of the chest in staging patients with nonmetastatic gestational trophoblastic disease. *Obstet Gynecol* 1986;68:348–52

27. Katsumi T. Ovarian tumors in pregnancy. *Am J Obstet Gynecol* 1964;90:511–16

28. Novak ER, Lombrow C, Woodruff DJ. Ovarian tumors in pregnancy: an ovarian tumor registry review. *Obstet Gynecol* 1975;46:401–6

29. Hamilton HG, Higgins RS. Ovarian tumors in pregnancy. *Int Abstr Surg* 1979;89:525

30. Gustafson GW, Gardener SH, Stout FE. Ovarian tumors complicating pregnancy: a review of 45 surgically proved cases. *Am J Obstet Gynecol* 1954;67:1210–23

31. Levine W, Diamond B. Surgical procedures during pregnancy. *Am J Obstet Gynecol* 1961;81:1046–52

32. Child CG, Douglas RG. Surgical problems arising during pregnancy. *Am J Obstet Gynecol* 1943;47:213–28

33. Beischen HA, Buttery BW, Fortune DW, McCafee CAJ. Growth and malignancy of ovarian tumors in pregnancy. *Aust NZ J Obstet Gynecol* 1971;11:208–20

34. Dougherty CM, Lund CJ. Solid ovarian tumors complicating pregnancy: a clinicopathologic study. *Am J Obstet Gynecol* 1950;60:261–72

35. Chung A, Birnbaum SJ. Ovarian cancer associated with pregnancy. *Obstet Gynecol* 1977;41:211–14

36. Bitson JR, Golden ML. Cancer and pregnancy. *Am J Obstet Gynecol* 1961;85:345–54

37. American College of Obstetricians and Gynecologists. *Carcinoma of the Breast*. Technical bulletin no.158. ACOG, 1991

38. Gallenberg MM, Loprinzi CL. Breast cancer and pregnancy. *Semin Oncol* 1989;16:369–76

39. Hoover HC. Breast cancer during pregnancy and lactation. *Surg Clin North Am* 1990;70:1151–63

40. Nugent P, O'Connell TX. Breast cancer and pregnancy. *Arch Surg* 1985;120:1221–4

41. Petrek JA, Dukoff R, Rogatko A. Prognosis of pregnancy-associated breast cancer. *Cancer* 1991;67:869–72

42. Gonsoulin W, Mason B, Carpenter RJ. Colon cancer in pregnancy with elevated maternal serum α-fetoprotein level at presentation. *Am J Obstet Gynecol* 1990;163: 1172–3

43. Nesbitt JC, Moise KJ, Sawyers JL. Colorectal carcinoma in pregnancy. *Arch Surg* 1985;12:636–40

44. Girard RM, Lamarche J, Bailot R. Carcinoma of the colon associated with pregnancy. *Dis Colon Rectum* 1981;24:465–73

45. Hill JA, Kassam SH, Talledo OE. Colonic cancer in pregnancy. *South Med J* 1984;77:375–8

46. McLain CR. Leukemia in pregnancy. *Clin Obstet Gynecol* 1974;17:185–94

47. Juarez JM, Quarado P, Felia J, *et al*. Association of leukemia and pregnancy: clinical and obstetric aspects. *J Clin Oncol* 1988;11:159–65

48. Wiernek PH. Acute leukemia in adults. In DeVita VT, ed. *Cancer: Principles and Practice of Oncology*, 3rd edn. Philadelphia: JB Lippincott, 1989

49. Koren G, Weiner L, Lishner M, *et al*. Cancer in pregnancy: identification of answered questions on maternal and fetal risks. *Obstet Gynecol Surv* 1990; 45:614

50. Reynoso EE, Shepard FA, Messner HA, *et al*. Acute leukemia during pregnancy. *J Clin Oncol* 1987;5: 1098–106

51. Williams SF, Bitran JD. Cancer and pregnancy. *Clin Perinatol* 1985;12:609–23

52. Caligiuri MA, Mayer RJ. Pregnancy and leukemia. *Semin Oncol* 1989;16:388–96

53. Steiner-Salz D, Yahalom J, Samuelov A, *et al*. Non-Hodgkin's lymphoma associated with pregnancy. *Cancer* 1985;56:2087–91

54. DeVita VT, Hellman S, Rosenberg SA. Hodgkin's disease and the non-Hodgkin's lymphomas. In DeVita VT, ed. *Cancer: Principles and Practice of Oncology*, 3rd edn. Philadelphia: JB Lippincott, 1989

55. Reintgen DS, McCarty KS, Vollmer R, *et al*. Malignant melanoma and pregnancy. *Cancer* 1985;55:1340–4

56. Allen HH, Nisker JA. *Cancer in Pregnancy: Therapeutic Guidelines*. Mt. Kisco, NY: Futura, 1986

57. Balch CM, Murad TM, Soony ST, *et al*. A multifactorial analysis of melanoma. I. Prognostic, histopathologic features, comparing Clark's and Breslow's staging methods. *Ann Surg* 1978;188:732–42

58. Ho VC, Sober AJ. Therapy for cutaneous melanoma: an update. *J Am Acad Dermatol* 1990;22:159–76

59. Wong DJ, Strassner HT. Melanoma in pregnancy. *Clin Obstet Gynecol* 1990;33:782–91

60. Colbourn DS, Nathanson L, Belilos E. Pregnancy and malignant melanoma. *Semin Oncol* 1989;16:377–87

61. Slingluff LL, Reintgen DS, Vollmer RT. Malignant melanoma arising during pregnancy: a study of 100 patients. *Ann Surg* 1990;211:552–9

62. Hod M, Sharony R, Friedman S, Ovadia J. Pregnancy and thyroid carcinoma: a review of the incidence, course and prognosis. *Obstet Gynecol* 1989;44:774–9

63. Preston-Martin S, Bernstein L, Pike MC, *et al*. Thyroid cancer among young women related to prior thyroid disease and pregnancy history. *Cancer* 1987; 55:191–5

64. Rosen IB, Walfish PG. Pregnancy as a predisposing factor in thyroid neoplasia. *Arch Surg* 1986;121: 1287–90

65. Yutaka K, Kenji I, Tadayuki A. Sarcoma associated with pregnancy. *Am J Obstet Gynecol* 1989;161:94–6

66. Simon MA, Phillips WA, Bonfiglio M. Pregnancy and aggressive or malignant bone tumors. *Cancer* 1984;53: 2564–9

67. Huvos AG, Butler A, Bretsky SS. Osteogenic sarcoma in pregnant women. *Cancer* 1985;56:2326–31

68. Haerr RW, Pratt AT. Multiagent chemotherapy for sarcoma diagnosed during pregnancy. *Cancer* 1985; 56:1028–33

69. Roelunk NCA, Kamphorst W, van Alphen H, *et al*. Pregnancy related primary brain and spinal tumors. *Arch Neurol* 1987;44:209–15

70. Haas JF, Janisch W, Staneczed W. Newly diagnosed primary intracranial neoplasms in pregnant women: a population based assessment. *J Neurol Neurosurg Psychiatry* 1986;49:874–80

71. Wan WL, Geller JL, Feldon SF, *et al*. Visual loss caused by rapidly progressive intracranial meningiomas during pregnancy. *Ophthalmology* 1990;97:18–21

72. Magyar DM, Marshall JR. Pituitary tumors and pregnancy. *Am J Obstet Gynecol* 1978;132:739–49

73. Apuzzio J, Pelioso MA, Ganesh VV, *et al*. Spinal cord tumors during pregnancy. *Int J Gynecol Obstet* 1980; 17:608–10

74. Simon RH. Brain tumors in pregnancy. *Semin Neurol* 1988;8:214–21

76

Placental transport, metabolism and perinatal nutrition

J.M. Dicke

PLACENTAL NUTRIENT TRANSPORT

The placenta is a structure of fetal origin which actively participates in nutrient exchange between mother and fetus. Far from being a passive conduit for the transfer of substances from mother to fetus, the placenta is a metabolically and morphologically dynamic organ which adapts to the peculiar demands of the developing conceptus. The following is an overview of placental development and nutrient exchange mechanisms.

There are two placental components: a fetal portion (chorion) and a maternal portion (endometrium). About 3 days after fertilization, the zygote, a ball of 12–16 cells, enters the uterine cavity and develops into the blastocyst. This structure differentiates into an inner cell mass, or embryoblast, and an outer cell layer, or trophoblast. Implantation of the blastocyst and endometrial invasion begin on day 7, at which time the trophoblast differentiates into the cytotrophoblast and syncytiotrophoblast. The syncytiotrophoblast is a large multinucleated mass which develops adjacent to the embryonic pole. The syncytiotrophoblast is a true syncytium with no cell boundaries. Described by Hertig[1] as 'invasive, ingestive and digestive', the syncytiotrophoblast penetrates the endometrial capillaries and glands. Glycogen- and lipid-laden stromal cells (decidual cells) at the implantation site are an early source of nutrition for the embryo. The cytotrophoblast consists of actively dividing cells that migrate into the overlying syncytiotrophoblast. By day 9, isolated spaces, or lacunae, are present in the syncytiotrophoblast. These spaces fill with maternal blood and secretions from eroded endometrial capillaries and glands. The connection of uterine vessels with lacunae in the syncytiotrophoblast represents the beginning of the uteroplacental circulation. As maternal blood flows into the lacunae of the syncytiotrophoblast, nutrients become available to the developing embryo over a relatively large surface area. Early circulation is established as oxygenated blood is delivered into the lacunae from spiral arteries, while deoxygenated blood is removed by the uterine veins. Adjacent lacunae fuse to form lacunar networks, which develop into the intervillous spaces of the placenta.

At 13–14 days following fertilization, the cytotrophoblast proliferates and produces localized clumps that project into the syncytiotrophoblast, forming primary chorionic villi on the outer surface of the chorionic sac. Following development of the primary chorionic villi, implantation is complete. At this point, the conceptus is entirely imbedded in the endometrium, the defect in the surface epithelium disappears and marked decidual reaction occurs. Shortly after the primary chorionic villi develop, they begin to branch and fill with mesenchyme, loosely organized undifferentiated mesodermal cells, denoting progression to secondary villi. Mesenchymal cells within the secondary villi differentiate into blood capillaries, resulting in the arteriocapillary vascular network which distinguishes tertiary chorionic villi. Vessels in the tertiary villi become connected with the embryonic heart through vessels that differentiate in the mesenchyme of the chorion. By about day 21, embryonic blood starts to circulate through the capillaries of the tertiary villi, allowing for exchange of nutrients between the maternal and embryonic circulations.

The placenta in man and most other primates is classified as hemochorial, indicating that, as the chorion penetrates the uterine stroma and destroys the endometrial capillaries, it comes in direct contact with maternal blood. The separation of maternal and fetal circulations by only trophoblastic epithelium places the trophoblast in a unique position to regulate nutrient transport from mother to fetus. Flux across the syncytiotrophoblast is the rate-limiting step in the transfer of most major nutrients. Directional transfer of nutrients and other compounds, with differences in flux rates, is a basic principle of placental exchange. Known mechanisms of cellular transport are present in the microvillous and basal plasma membranes of the trophoblast. The microvillous membrane is in contact with the maternal circulation, while the basal membrane faces the fetal circulation. In other species, multiple tissue layers are interspersed between maternal and fetal blood, all of which may influence maternal–fetal transfer.

Placental maturation is characterized by morphological changes which increase its functional capacity.

These include a marked increase in the number of terminal villi in the intervillous space and a modification of their structure. During the first trimester, villi are composed of well-defined cytotrophoblastic and syncytiotrophoblastic layers, with few capillaries in abundant stroma. In the second trimester, there is marked capillary proliferation such that, by the third trimester, there is a high ratio of capillaries to stroma. In addition, morphometric studies of the placenta in multiple species indicate that, as gestation advances, the surface area of the placental villi increases and placental thickness decreases[2]. In humans, the syncytiotrophoblast thins greatly and the underlying cytotrophoblast becomes less prominent. These observations suggest that growth of the surface across which maternal–fetal exchange occurs correlates with increased fetal metabolic demand. These changes in placental morphology are accompanied by an increase in placental permeability. Studies in sheep indicate a marked increase in urea permeability in the last third of gestation, even after placental growth has ceased. The increase in permeability is accompanied by an increase in fetal and placental blood flows, suggesting a maturation of several aspects of placental function[2]. In humans, as in most species, the ratio of fetal to placental weight increases with advancing gestation[3]. The more rapid growth of the fetus during later gestation places significant demands on placental transport function. The relative lag in placental weight versus fetal weight suggests that enhanced transport capacity results from placental maturational changes, rather than increased placental size.

The notion that a small placenta can restrict fetal growth is supported by a number of observations. Intrauterine growth restriction, induced experimentally by uterine artery ligation, removal of uterine caruncles, severe maternal undernutrition and embolization of uterine vasculature, is characterized by reductions in both fetal and placental growth[4]. In sheep undergoing uterine carunculectomy, there is reduced placental implantation area, decreased placental size and a corresponding decrease in fetal size and placental glucose transfer, which is proportional to the reduction in cotyledonary number and weight[5]. In growth-restricted human fetuses, placental growth may cease after 36 weeks, with earlier slowing of fetal growth. In addition, high fetal : placental weight ratios have been associated with an increased risk of fetal distress and other perinatal problems in appropriately grown, as well as small-for-gestational-age, infants[3]. These findings suggest that, when placental size is small relative to the fetus, there may be an imbalance between placental nutrient supply and fetal demand.

Current understanding of placental transport mechanisms derives primarily from the following experimental approaches:

(1) *Maternal loading with amino acids*   Using a variety of animal models, amino acids have been administered both orally and by direct injection into the maternal circulation via indwelling catheters. Although complicated by concurrent maternal and fetal metabolism, these experiments have demonstrated the capacity of the placenta for rapid, accumulative and stereospecific transport[6].

(2) *Placental slices*   Using whole villous slices, three membrane transport systems for neutral amino acids have been defined. Uptake kinetics, preincubation effects and characterization of the active nature of the transport process have also been described[7]. While relatively simple to perform technically, these studies are compromised by the difficulty of preparing uniform samples, the loss of polarity of the trophoblastic tissue and the large extracellular fluid space which makes determination of tissue uptake imprecise.

(3) *Membrane vesicles*   The development of techniques for the isolation of microvillous and basal plasma membranes from human placenta minimized the problems associated with placental slices. Using membrane vesicle preparations, amino-acid and glucose transport systems were able to be more completely characterized[8,9]. These preparations allow the performance of experiments with both the maternal- and fetal-facing membranes of the trophoblast under well-defined conditions on either side. While useful for the study of transport capacity, this technique does not allow determination of actual transfer, or flux, of nutrients in the placenta. Other limitations include the relative isolation from the maternal–placental–fetal environment present during development and the inability to investigate substrate metabolism within the trophoblast.

(4) *Placental perfusion models*   In the human placenta, anatomical relations of the blood vessels, umbilical cord and the chorionic plate have been utilized for recirculating perfusions of one or more cotyledons. These preparations have been employed to study the production, metabolism and transport of glucose, amino acids, hormones and O_2. Using this technique, active stereospecific placental transport that functions unidirectionally from the maternal to the fetal side has been demonstrated for a variety of amino acids[10]. This methodology permits evaluation of directionality of transport and minimizes the effects of maternal and fetal metabolism. However, such studies are technically complex and subject to hemodynamic and anatomic variables, making interexperimental comparisons problematic.

(5) *Cultured trophoblast*   The application of cultured trophoblast to the investigation of the development

of cellular (membrane) mechanisms of nutrient transport is a relatively recent development made possible by controlling trophoblast differentiation *in vitro* and establishing preparations with bilayer cellular architecture similar to that *in vivo*[11]. Pure trophoblast cell models are useful for delineating mechanisms of transplacental transfer and hormone secretion and their relation to intracellular metabolism. Other potential advantages of this technique include the ability to study inductive or maturational changes in placental function and to maintain cells for study over extended periods of time.

Using these and other techniques, a number of mechanisms of transplacental exchange have been described, including:

(1) Simple diffusion: a passive process of substance movement from an area of high concentration to an area of low concentration which occurs down a chemical or electrical gradient and does not require energy.

(2) Facilitated diffusion: a process in which a carrier molecule in the membrane moves a substance from an area of high concentration to an area of low concentration at a more rapid rate than expected on a physiochemical basis. The carrier enhances transfer rate without energy expenditure.

(3) Active transport: occurs against a concentration gradient when a carrier within the membrane forms a complex with the substance to be transported. This process requires expenditure of metabolic energy and is subject to competitive inhibition.

(4) Bulk transport: refers to the transfer of water molecules, carrying dissolved substances, in response to an osmotic pressure gradient. This results in a faster rate of transfer than simple diffusion.

(5) Organellar transport: occurs primarily by pinocytosis, a process in which the trophoblast surface membrane invaginates to surround a substance. The vesicle so formed crosses the trophoblast and is expelled on the opposite side. Similar transport may also occur via coated vesicles, multivesicular bodies or lysosomes.

Respiratory gas exchange

Oxygen and carbon dioxide

Provision of O_2 to the developing conceptus is thought to result largely from simple diffusion. Measurements of placental diffusing capacity in multiple species, including primates, indicate that O_2 and CO_2 tensions readily achieve equilibrium at the maternal intervillous space and fetal capillary[12]. The difference in partial pressures of O_2 between maternal blood in the intervillous space and fetal blood in the villous capillaries is the driving force for placental O_2 transfer. However, estimates of O_2 transfer are complicated by the relatively high O_2 consumption of the uterus and placenta. In sheep, uteroplacental tissues consume approximately one-half of the uterine O_2 uptake, with the remainder utilized by the fetus. Considered on a weight-specific basis, uteroplacental O_2 consumption is four- to five-fold greater than that of the fetus, whose metabolic rate is double that of the adult. Estimates of uteroplacental metabolism near term suggest that the metabolic rate of trophoblastic tissue is as high as that in brain, liver, kidney and many tumor cells[13]. Transplacental O_2 exchange is also influenced by the characteristics of maternal and fetal hemoglobin. O_2 uptake by fetal hemoglobin is stimulated by the rise in fetal blood pH and fall in maternal blood pH, which occurs secondary to CO_2 transfer (the Bohr effect). In addition, 2,3-diphosphoglycerate releases O_2 from maternal hemoglobin more readily than from fetal hemoglobin. In general, placental O_2 transfer is a very efficient process, with the rate-limiting factor being the provision of O_2 to the placenta via the maternal circulation.

Placental CO_2 transfer also occurs by simple diffusion. The partial pressure gradient between maternal and fetal blood in the placenta is estimated to be between 4 and 30 mmHg. Factors regulating CO_2 transfer are similar to those described for O_2 transfer and there is minimal placental diffusion resistance to CO_2[14]. Fetal red blood cells contain sufficient carbonic anhydrase to maintain adequate CO_2 transfer, and the release of CO_2 from fetal hemoglobin in the placenta is enhanced by concurrent O_2 uptake (the Haldane effect).

Transfer of organic nutrients

Carbohydrates

Glucose is the major source of carbon and energy for the developing fetus, and glucose metabolism accounts for a significant portion of fetal oxygen consumption[15]. Placental glucose transfer varies directly with the maternal plasma glucose concentration, uterine uptake of glucose and the maternal–fetal glucose concentration gradient. Maternal blood glucose levels exceed fetal blood levels by about 20 mg/100 ml, originally suggesting that glucose transfer occurred via simple diffusion. Placental glucose transporters were subsequently characterized in both the microvillous (maternal-facing) and basal (fetal-facing) membranes[16,17]. The microvillous glucose transporter has been identified as a protein of 50 kDa[18]. Studies using microvillous and basal membranes have demonstrated that transplacental glucose transfer is saturable and stereospecific, with characteristics suggesting facilitated diffusion. These transporters are insulin-independent and have a similar molecular structure and regulation to those occurring in the brain and on erythrocytes. They permit bidirectional glucose transport across the placenta and facilitate placental glucose uptake from both maternal and fetal circulations[13]. Placental glucose transport capacity increases substantially as pregnancy advances, owing to increases in both the glucose gradient across the placenta and the number of glucose transport proteins[19].

Glucose supplied via the maternal circulation is primarily consumed by the uterus and placenta, rather than the fetus. At mid-pregnancy, an estimated 80–85% of total uterine glucose consumption is utilized by the uteroplacental unit[20]. Studies using glucose clamp techniques in the maternal and fetal circulations of gravid sheep have demonstrated that uteroplacental glucose consumption limits glucose transport into the umbilical circulation, accounting for the relative fetal hypoglycemia. It is estimated that the arterial glucose concentration in fetal sheep would increase from a normal value of 200 mg/l to approximately 450 mg/l if placental glucose consumption were lacking[21]. Such consumption contributes to the transplacental glucose gradient.

More recent studies indicate uteroplacental glucose consumption is primarily a function of fetal glucose concentration and independent of maternal glucose[22]. It has been demonstrated that, when maternal and fetal glucose concentrations are the same, approximately 80% of uteroplacental glucose consumption is derived from the fetal glucose supply[21]. In addition, the glucose transport capacity of the fetal surface of the placenta exceeds that of the maternal surface. These observations indicate that uteroplacental glucose metabolism is predominantly placental, i.e. by the tissues having direct access to glucose in the umbilical circulation.

Placental glucose consumption is normally substantial, but decreases when the mother becomes hypoglycemic[13]. This is important, because it decreases the demand of the fetus when maternal glucose supplies are limited and encourages the diversion of maternal glucose from placental to fetal metabolism. In addition, the fetal capacity for endogenous glucose production allows the fetus some direct control over glucose utilization by its own tissues, as well as those of the placenta. Under these conditions, the inverse relationship between glucose transfer to the fetus and placental glucose consumption, and its regulation by the fetal glucose concentration, protects both fetus and placenta without further diminishing an already limited maternal glucose supply.

The glucose taken up by placental tissues is not utilized solely for oxidative metabolism. Up to one-third of the glucose consumed may be converted to the three-carbon sugar, lactate[23]. Lactate is second only to glucose as a metabolic fuel and carbon source for growth. The observation that fetal blood concentrations of lactate exceed maternal blood levels was originally attributed to presumed chronic fetal hypoxia, resulting in anaerobic metabolism, increased fetal lactate production and excretion into the placenta via the umbilical circulation. Subsequently, it was demonstrated that, under normal physiological conditions, fetal tissues in humans and other species are adequately oxygenated and that placental lactate production under aerobic conditions is a normal phenomenon[24].

The role of lactate in fetal metabolism was first suggested by studies using fetal lambs. Under steady-state conditions during late gestation, the concentration of lactate in the umbilical vein was higher than that in the umbilical artery, indicating net consumption of lactate by the fetus. Similar arteriovenous differences in lactate concentration were also noted in the uterine circulation, indicating that lactate is normally produced by the uteroplacental tissues in the presence of high oxygen-utilization rates and released into both circulations. Studies of lactate/oxygen quotients in several species other than sheep also indicate that lactate is delivered from uteroplacental tissues into the maternal and umbilical circulations[25] and that such delivery is not regulated by simple concentration differences. Late in gestation, there is more lactate delivered into the fetal circulation than into the maternal circulation, despite higher fetal lactate concentrations[26]. These findings suggest that both the microvillous and basal membranes possess lactate transport mechanisms. Studies using microvillous membrane vesicles have identified a lactate transport system which is sodium-independent and stimulated by an H^+ gradient[27]. Lactate transfer apparently occurs as a lactate–H^+ complex via a transporter which is regulated by the size and direction of the lactate and H^+ gradients across the microvillous membrane. This transport system may represent a mechanism by which endogenously produced placental lactate is removed from the syncytiotrophoblast via the maternal circulation, thereby maintaining intracellular pH and preventing damaging accumulations of lactic acid within the placenta. The mechanism of lactate transport in the basal membrane is currently unknown.

Amino acids

Amino acids are the primary source of nitrogen for fetal growth and are essential for protein synthesis[15]. Lacking a storage form in the body, amino acids are used as fuels and oxidized when not required for accretion into protein. Protein synthesis requires the simultaneous presence of a specific mixture of constituent amino acids in order to proceed[28]. Animal studies suggest that even small decreases in the delivery of particular amino acids may result in inadequate availability and limit fetal growth[29]. In small-for-gestational-age human fetuses, significant reductions in many essential amino acids have been demonstrated many weeks prior to delivery[30].

All essential and most non-essential amino acids are transported by the placenta into the umbilical circulation, from where they are taken up into the fetal liver[31,32]. Many amino acids are supplied to the fetus in excess of the amounts necessary for protein synthesis[33]. Amino acids are taken up into the trophoblast by means of several transport-specific membrane proteins identified via competitive inhibition studies with non-metabolizable analogs. Studies using microvillous and basal plasma membrane vesicles have confirmed the presence of certain transport systems similar to those described in other mammalian cells, as well as special adaptations of these systems unique to the nutritive function of the placenta. The microvillous membrane employs transport systems common to other cell types. Neutral amino-acid transporters identified in the microvillous membrane include:

(1) System A: a ubiquitous sodium-dependent system that strongly supports transport of methylamino-isobutyric acid, alanine, serine and proline;

(2) System N: a sodium-dependent system that interacts with histidine and glutamine;

(3) Several sodium-independent systems, one of which has a high affinity for leucine and other branched-chain amino acids and resembles the L system of other cell types.

Basal-membrane transport systems are similar to those of intestine and include:

(1) A sodium-dependent system with affinity for methylaminoisobutyric acid, similar to the A system of the microvillous membrane;

(2) A sodium-dependent system resistant to inhibition by methylaminoisobutyric acid with characteristics of the ASC system;

(3) A sodium-independent system with an affinity for leucine, phenylalanine and 2-aminobicyclo-[2,2,1]-heptane-2-carboxylic acid (BCH) that resembles the L system.

The appropriate transfer of amino acids from mother to fetus requires the co-ordinated activity of all of the amino-acid transporters present in these membranes[34].

These transport systems require energy to concentrate amino acids within the intracellular matrix of the trophoblast. *In vitro* and *in vivo* studies indicate that inhibition of glycolysis and aerobic metabolism can inhibit activity of these transporters. Accurate measurements of uterine amino acid uptake from maternal plasma are difficult to obtain, although there are positive arteriovenous differences for most amino acids. Studies using labeled amino acids have demonstrated their incorporation into placental proteins and structural tissue. At term, the placenta possesses enzymes capable of utilizing amino acids through a variety of metabolic pathways, including glycogenesis, protein synthesis and gluconeogenesis. A small quantity of amino acids are also used for oxidation, the production of other amino acids by transamination pathways, and synthesis of secreted protein products such as placental lactogen, human chorionic gonadotropin and lipoproteins[13].

Lipids and related compounds

Fetal fat is derived primarily from either transplacentally acquired free fatty acids or from the fetal synthesis of lipid from carbohydrate acetate. Placental transport capacities for fatty acids differ markedly among different species. Fetal fat contents vary likewise in relation to placental lipid transport. The human placenta transports lipids rapidly, resulting in the fattest of all newborns. Lipid stores in human infants at term account for approximately 18% of body fat, with most deposition occurring in the second half of gestation[13,35].

The primary group of naturally occurring lipids transported by the placenta is the free fatty acids. Essential fatty acids (such as linolenic acid, docosahexaenoic acid and arachidonic acid) are derived from fatty acids in the maternal diet and transported to the fetus via the placenta. Studies of concentration gradients from mother to fetus and umbilical vein to artery suggested that placental transport of free fatty acids occurred via simple diffusion[36]. The finding that free fatty acid flux across the placenta correlated with the difference between maternal and fetal free fatty acid concentrations supported this conclusion[37].

The discovery of a plasmalemmal fatty acid-binding protein in the membranes of heart, liver, intestine and other tissues provided evidence that fatty acids are transferred across plasma membranes via a carrier-mediated mechanism[38,39]. A similar protein has been isolated and purified from human placental membrane[40]. While the contribution of the plasmalemmal fatty acid binding protein to the placental transport and metabolism of fatty acids is uncertain, it is thought to be involved in the extraction of fatty acids from the maternal circulation for provision to the fetus. Thus, evidence suggests that the passage of free fatty acids across the human placenta results from both passive diffusion and mediated transport, with the relative contributions of these mechanisms remaining to be clarified.

Following entry into the trophoblast, fatty acids may be used by the placenta for glycerolipid synthesis, membrane biosynthesis, oxidation for energy or transfer to the fetus. Although the factors regulating lipid flux through these pathways are uncertain, the maternal plasma free fatty acid concentration is apparently one determinant[41]. In women who are fasting and in those who have diabetes mellitus, conditions in which plasma free fatty acids are increased, placental triacylglycerol content is also increased.

Vitamins

Data derived from experiments using membrane vesicles and/or placental perfusions suggest that water-soluble vitamins (ascorbate, folate, riboflavin and thiamin) are actively transported across the placenta by means of specific transport proteins capable of concentrating these compounds against a concentration gradient and generating higher fetal than maternal levels[35]. Vitamin C exists in blood as the oxidized (dehydroascorbate) or reduced (ascorbate) form. Dehydroascorbate is more rapidly taken up by the microvillous membrane, where it is metabolized to the more useful ascorbate form and released into the fetal circulation[42]. In perfused guinea-pig placenta, folate uptake occurs via high-affinity transporters which can be inhibited by 5-methyltetrahydrofolate, the major plasma form[43]. A placental folate binding protein, which may be related to those found in other cell types, has also been identified in human placental villous homogenate[44]. In human placental perfusion studies, riboflavin transfer was saturable and occurred via a low-capacity transport system with preferential transfer in the fetal direction. The riboflavin recovered in the fetal perfusate was unmetabolized, while that concentrated in the placenta underwent partial metabolism to flavin adenine dinucleotide and flavin mononucleotide[45,46]. These findings suggest that riboflavin is actively transported across the placenta via a transporter in the microvillous membrane. Perfusion experiments also suggest a similar mechanism for thiamine transfer. Thiamine transport was saturable and occurred against a concentration gradient, with higher levels in the placenta than in either perfusate and with greater transfer in the fetal than in the maternal direction[47]. These data are consistent with the presence of a thiamine transporter in the microvillous membrane.

In general, the concentrations of lipid-soluble vitamins in fetal blood are slightly lower than those in maternal blood. The transplacental flux of vitamin A is not well defined. Vitamin A exists in the blood as a complex of retinol and retinol-binding protein. Two mechanisms of placental transfer have been proposed. The human placenta possesses surface receptors which bind the retinol-binding protein. Transplacental passage of the retinol-binding protein complex may be the primary route of vitamin A transport in early gestation[48]. A second possible mechanism involves binding of the maternal retinol-binding protein to its receptor and release of retinol into the syncytiotrophoblast. A retinol ester is then formed by the placenta and secreted into the circulation as a lipoprotein[49]. There are contradictory data on the placental transfer of vitamin D. In humans, both 25-hydroxyvitamin D_3 and 1,25-dihydroxyvitamin D_3 have been positively correlated in maternal and cord blood, suggesting

diffusion[50]. Others, however, have not observed an association between maternal and fetal blood levels, suggesting little transfer across the placenta and resulting in speculation that vitamin D is produced by the placenta to meet fetal needs[51]. Vitamins E and K are present in higher concentrations in maternal plasma than umbilical cord plasma. α-Tocopherol (vitamin E) does not cross the rabbit placenta[52] and studies with human placenta indicate that it inhibits vitamin-K transport[53].

Growth factors

Growth factors are peptides that stimulate intercellular communication on many levels and affect many aspects of cell behavior[54]. Unlike postnatal growth, which is primarily affected by classical endocrine hormones, embryogenesis is regulated by polypeptide growth factors whose effects are exerted locally in an autocrine or paracrine fashion[55]. Growth factors bind to membrane receptors, after which the receptor complex is internalized and degraded. Biological effects attributed to growth factors include stimulation of glucose uptake, amino-acid transport, synthesis of RNA, DNA and proteins, and cell replication[54]. Individual target-cell response depends upon cell site, growth conditions, state of development and the presence or absence of other growth factors[56]. Peptide growth factors are present early in development, suggesting that the conceptus is sensitive to changes in the uterine milieu[57].

Growth-factor expression is influenced by oxygenation, nutrition and fetal insulin[54]. Insulin is critical for fetal development, its effects a result of its metabolic activity[58]. Insulin-like growth factor-I (IGF-I) and IGF-II are present in many fetal tissues and promote cellular division and differentiation through their local (autocrine and/or paracrine) effects[55,59]. Evidence suggests that IGF-I is a regulator of fetal growth. Levels of IGF-I increase throughout the latter half of pregnancy and maternal IGF-I concentrations correlate with birth weight[60]. In humans, birth weights have been shown to correlate with cord blood IGF-I levels, with lower values being present in preterm than term infants[61,62]. IGF-I also has anabolic and anticatabolic effects. It promotes glucose and amino-acid uptake and inhibits protein breakdown[63,64]. In studies using human first-trimester chorionic villi, IGF-I causes increased uptake of the amino acid analog α-[methyl-H-3]-aminoisobutyric acid and enhances glucose transport[65].

Developmental analysis of growth kinetics in mouse embryos indicates that the prenatal effects of IGF-I stem from its interaction with the type 1 IGF receptor (IGF1R). Unlike IGF-I, which is pre- and postnatally active, the effects of IGF-II are limited to the period of embryogenesis and are only partially mediated by IGF1R. A second receptor, XR, has been characterized and this serves only IGF-II signalling. Distinct from the effects of IGF-II on embryonic growth, the IGF-II–XR complex influences only placental growth[55,66].

Epidermal growth factors (EGF) are another of the group of peptide growth factors which play a role in mammalian growth and development. Members of the human EGF family include EGF, transforming growth factor-α (TGF-α) and amphiregulin. These growth factors are structurally related and bind to a single EGF receptor (EGF-R)[67]. The major effect of EGF in target cells is enhancement of cell proliferation and EGF receptors have been identified in most cell types[67]. Studies in mice have demonstrated EGF receptors in placental, embryonal and fetal tissues and EGF stimulation of protein synthesis during the morula-blastocyst stage and in post-implantation tissue[68]. Receptors for EGF have been identified in human placenta (hEGF)[69]. hEGF is thought to influence fetoplacental growth and development by stimulating cellular proliferation and placental and fetal membrane hormone production[70]. Early in the first trimester (less than 6 weeks' gestation), placental EGF and its receptor are localized primarily to the cytotrophoblast where it induces trophoblast proliferation. At 6–12 weeks' gestation, EGF is localized to the syncytiotrophoblast where it stimulates differentiated trophoblast activity[71].

Transforming growth factor-β (TGF-β) is the prototype of a multifunctional cytokine, in that it can act as both an inhibitor and a stimulator of cell proliferation and differentiation, as well as regulate the synthesis of many of the components of the extracellular matrix[72]. TGF-β isoforms are found on most cell types, and TGF-β mRNA levels confirm that human placenta is a source of TGF-β, suggesting that it also plays a role in the local control of the trophoblast-endometrial unit[73,74].

SUMMARY

The placenta is a complex dynamic organ which undergoes morphological and functional maturational changes allowing it to actively participate in the provision of essential nutrients to the developing conceptus. Placental transport, or flux, is a complex process influenced by a number of factors, including blood flow, placental permeability and area available for exchange, concentration differences and carrier systems capable of concentrating certain substrates against a gradient via relatively specific transport proteins. The use of placental perfusions, isolated preparations of microvillous and basal plasma membranes, and trophoblast culture have allowed the identification and characterization of various transport mechanisms. Current evidence suggests that the placenta actively regulates nutrient transport using mechanisms which are similar to those of other cells, but which are uniquely adapted to the needs of the fetoplacental unit.

REFERENCES

1. Hertig AT. *Human Trophoblast*. Springfield, IL: Charles C. Thomas, 1968
2. Battaglia FC, Meschia G. Fetal and placental growth. In Battaglia FC, Meschia G, eds. *An Introduction to Fetal Physiology*, 1st edn. Orlando: Academic Press, 1986: 1–27
3. Molteni RA, Stys SJ, Battaglia FC. Relationship of fetal and placental weight in human beings: fetal/placental weight ratios at various gestational ages and birth weight distributions. *J Reprod Med* 1978;21:327–34
4. Bassett JM. Current perspectives on placental development and its integration with fetal growth. *Proc Nutr Soc* 1991;50:311–19
5. Owens JA, Falconer J, Robinson JS. Effect of restriction of placental growth on fetal and utero–placental metabolism. *J Dev Physiol* 1987;9:225–38
6. Page EW. Transfer of materials across the human placenta. *Am J Obstet Gynecol* 1957;74:705–15
7. Smith CH, Adcock EW, Teasdale F, *et al*. Placental amino acid uptake: tissue preparation, kinetics and preincubation effect. *Am J Physiol* 1973;224:558–64
8. Smith CH. Mechanisms and regulation of placental amino acid transport. In Kilberg MS, ed. *Report of Nutrient Transport Symposium: Amino Acid Transport in Eukaryotic Cells and Tissues. Fed Proc* 1986;45:2443–5
9. Johnson LW, Smith CH. Monosaccharide transport across microvillous membrane of human placenta. *Am J Physiol* 1980;238:C160–8
10. Schneider H, Mohlen KH, Dancis J. Transfer of amino acids across the *in vitro* perfused human placenta. *Pediatr Res* 1979;13:236–40
11. Kliman HJ, Nestler JE, Sermasie E, *et al*. Purification, characterization, and *in vitro* differentiation of cytotrophoblast from term placentae. *Endocrinology* 1986;118:1567–82
12. Bissonette JM, Longo LD, Novy MJ, *et al*. Placental diffusing capacity and its relation to fetal growth. *J Dev Physiol* 1979;1:351–9
13. Hay WW Jr. Energy and substrate requirements of the placenta and fetus. *Proc Nutr Soc* 1991;50:311–19
14. Longo LD, Power GG. Problems in the placental transfer of carbon dioxide. In Moghissi KS, Hafez ESE, eds. *The Placenta, Biological and Clinical Aspects*. Springfield, IL: Charles C. Thomas, 1974:89–125
15. Battaglia FC, Meschia G. Principal substrates of fetal metabolism. *Physiol Rev* 1978;58:499–527
16. Ingermann RL, Bissonett JM. Effect of temperature on kinetics of hexose uptake by human placental plasma membrane vesicles. *Biochim Biophys Acta* 1983;734:329–35
17. Johnson LW, Smith CH. Glucose transport across the basal plasma membrane of human placental syncytiotrophoblast. *Biochim Biophys Acta* 1985;815:44–50
18. Johnson LW, Smith CH. Identification of the glucose transport protein of the microvillous membrane of human placenta by photoaffinity labelling. *Biochem Biophys Res Commun* 1982;109:408–13
19. Molina RD, Meschia G, Battaglia FC, Hay WW. Gestational maturation of placental glucose transfer capacity in sheep. *Am J Physiol* 1991;261:R697–704

20. Battaglia FC. Metabolic aspects of fetal and neonatal growth. *Early Hum Dev* 1992;29:99–106

21. Simmons MA, Battaglia FC, Meschia G. Placental transfer of glucose. *J Dev Physiol* 1979;1:227–43

22. Hay WW Jr, Molina R, DiGiacomo JE, Meschia G. Model of placental glucose consumption and glucose transfer. *Am J Physiol* 1990;258:R569–77

23. Sparks JW, Hay WW Jr, Bonds D, *et al*. Simultaneous measurements of lactate turnover rate and umbilical lactate uptake in the fetal lamb. *J Clin Invest* 1982;70:179–92

24. Hauguel S, Challier JC, Cedard L, Olive G. Metabolism of the human placenta perfused *in vitro*: glucose transfer and utilization, O$_2$ consumption, lactate and ammonia production. *Pediatr Res* 1983;17:729–32

25. Battaglia FC, Meschia G. Fetal and placental metabolism. Part I. Oxygen and carbohydrates. In Battaglia FC, Meschia G, eds. *An Introduction to Fetal Physiology*, 1st edn. Orlando: Academic Press, 1986:49–99

26. Sparks JW, Hay WW Jr, Bonds D, *et al*. Partition of maternal nutrients to the placenta and fetus in the sheep. *Eur J Obstet Gynecol Reprod Biol* 1983;14:331–40

27. Balkovetz DF, Leibach FH, Mahesh VB, Ganapathy V. A proton gradient is the driving force for uphill transport of lactate in human placental brush border membrane vesicles. *J Biol Chem* 1988;263:13823–30

28. Bessman SP. The justification theory: the essential nature of the non-essential amino acids. *Nutr Rev* 1979;37:209–20

29. Joyce J, Young M. A comparison of the effect of a reduction of maternal blood flow on the placental transfer of glucose and amino nitrogen from mother to foetus. *J Physiol (London)* 1974;239:5–6

30. Cetin I, Corbetta C, Sereni LP, *et al*. Umbilical amino acid concentrations in normal and growth-retarded fetuses sampled *in utero* by cordocentesis. *Am J Obstet Gynecol* 1990;162:253–61

31. Battaglia FC. Metabolic aspects of fetal and neonatal growth. *Early Hum Dev* 1992;29:99–106

32. Hay WW. The role of placental–fetal interaction in fetal nutrition. *Semin Perinatol* 1991;15:424–33

33. Carter BS, Moores RR Jr, Battaglia FC. Placental transport and fetal and placental metabolism of amino acids. *J Nutr Biochem* 1991;2:4–13

34. Smith CH, Moe AJ, Ganapathy V. Nutrient transport pathways across the epithelium of the placenta. *Ann Rev Nutr* 1992;12:183–206

35. Battaglia FC, Meschia G. Fetal and placental metabolism. Part II. Amino acids and lipids. In Battaglia FC, Meschia G, eds. *An Introduction to Fetal Physiology*, 1st edn. Orlando: Academic Press, 1986:100–35

36. Morris FH Jr, Boyd RDH, Mahendran D. Placental transport. In Knobil E, Neill JD, eds. *The Physiology of Reproduction*, 2nd edn. New York: Raven Press, 1994:813–61

37. Stephenson TJ, Stammers JP, Hull D. Effects of altering umbilical flow and umbilical free fatty acid concentration on transport of free fatty acids across the rabbit placenta. *J Dev Physiol* 1991;15:221–7

38. Sorrentino S, Potter DJ, Berk PD. From albumin to the cytoplasm: the hepatic uptake of organic anions. In Popper H, Schaffner F, eds. *Progress in Liver Disease*. Philadelphia: Saunders, 1990:203–24

39. Sorrentino S, Berk PD. Free fatty acids, albumin and the sinusoidal plasma membrane: concepts, trends and controversies. In Tavaloni N, Berk PD, eds. *Hepatic Organic Anion Transport and Bile Secretion*. New York: Raven Press, 1993:197–219

40. Campbell FM, Taffesse F, Gordon MJ, Dutta-Roy AK. Plasma membrane fatty-acid binding protein in human placenta: identification and characterization. *Biochem Biophys Res Commun* 1995;209:1011–17

41. Thomas CR, Locoy C, St Hillaire RJ, Burnzell JD. Studies on the placental hydrolysis and transfer of lipids to the fetal guinea pig. In Miller RK, Thiede HA, eds. *Fetal Nutrition, Metabolism and Immunology: Role of the Placenta*. New York: Plenum Press, 1983:135–48

42. Choi JL, Rose RC. Transport of metabolism of ascorbic acid in human placenta. *Am J Physiol (Cell Physiol)* 1989;257:C110–13

43. Sweiry JH, Yudilevich DL. Characterization of folate uptake in guinea pig placenta. *Am J Physiol (Cell Physiol)* 1988;254:C735–43

44. Antony AC, Utley C, VanHaorne KC, Colhouse JF. Isolation and characterization of a folate receptor from human placenta. *J Biol Chem* 1981;256:9684–92

45. Dancis J, Lehanka J, Levitz M. Transfer of riboflavin by the perfused human placenta. *Pediatr Res* 1985;19:1143–6

46. Dancis J, Lehanka J, Levitz M. Placental transport of riboflavin: differential rates of uptake at the maternal and fetal surfaces of the perfused human placenta. *Am J Obstet Gynecol* 1988;158:204–10

47. Dancis J, Wilson D, Hoskins IA, Levitz M. Placental transfer of thiamine in the human subject: *in vitro* perfusion studies and maternal-cord plasma concentrations. *Am J Obstet Gynecol* 1988;159:1435–9

48. Torma H, Vahlquist A. Uptake of vitamin A and retinol-binding protein by human placenta *in vitro*. *Placenta* 1986;7:295–305

49. Vahlquist A, Nilsson S. Vitamin A transferred to the fetus and to the amniotic fluid in Rhesus monkey (*Macaca mulatta*). *Ann Nutr Metab* 1984;28:321–33

50. Boullion R, VanAssche FA, VanBaelen H, *et al*. Influence of the vitamin D-binding protein on the serum concentration of 1,25-dihydroxyvitamin D$_3$. Significance of the free 1,25-dihydroxyvitamin D$_3$ concentration. *J Clin Invest* 1981;67:589–96

51. Delvin EE, Glorieux FH, Salle BI, *et al*. Control of vitamin D metabolism in preterm infants: feto-maternal relationships. *Arch Dis Child* 1982;57:754–7

52. Bortolotti A, Traina GL, Barzago MM, *et al*. Placental transfer and tissue distribution of vitamin E in pregnant rabbits. *Biopharm Drug Dispos* 1990;11:679–88

53. Kazzi NJ, Ilagan NB, Liang KC, *et al*. Placental transfer of vitamin K$_1$ in preterm pregnancy. *Obstet Gynecol* 1990;75:334–7

54. Hill BJ, Han VKM. Control of cellular multiplication and differentiation. In Sharp F, Fraser RB, Milner RDG, eds. *Fetal Growth*. Heidelberg: Springer Verlag, 1989;84–98

55. Baker J, Liu J-P, Robertson EJ, Efstratiadis A. Role of insulin-like growth factors in embryonic and postnatal growth. *Cell* 1993;75:73–82

56. Sporn MB, Roberts AB. Peptide growth factors are multifunctional. *Nature (London)* 1988;332:217–19

57. Blay J, Hollenberg MD. The nature and function of polypeptide growth factor receptors in the human placenta. *J Dev Physiol* 1989;12:237–48

58. Gluckman P, Harding J. The regulation of fetal growth. In Hernandez M, Argente J, eds. *Human Growth: Basic and Clinical Aspects*. Amsterdam: Elsevier Scientific Publishers, 1992:253–9

59. Hill DJ, Han VKM. Paracrinology of growth regulation. *J Dev Physiol* 1991;15:91–4

60. Hall K, Hansson U, Lundin G, *et al*. Somatomedin levels in pregnancy: longitudinal study in healthy subjects and patients with GH deficiency. *J Clin Endocrinol Metab* 1984;59:587–94

61. Samaan NA, Schultz PN, Johnston DA, *et al*. Growth hormone, somatomedin C, and nonsuppressible insulin-like activity levels compared in premature, small, average birth weight, and large infants. *Am J Obstet Gynecol* 1987;157:1524–8

62. Lassarre C, Hardouin S, Daffos F, *et al*. Serum insulin like growth factors and insulin like growth factor binding proteins in the human fetus. Relationships with growth in normal subjects and subjects with intrauterine growth retardation. *Pediatr Res* 1991;29:219–25

63. Sara VR, Hall K. Insulin-like growth factors and their binding proteins. *Physiol Rev* 1990;70:591–614

64. Clemmons DR, Smith-Banks A, Underwood LE. Reversal of diet-induced catabolism by infusion of recombinant insulin-like growth factor-I in humans. *J Clin Endocrinol Metab* 1992;75:234–8

65. Kniss DA, Shubert PJ, Zimmerman PD, *et al*. Insulin-like growth factors – their regulation of glucose and amino acid transport in placental trophoblasts isolated from first-trimester chorionic villi. *J Reprod Med* 1994;39:249–56

66. Liu J-P, Baker J, Perkins AS, *et al*. Mice carrying null mutations of the gene encoding insulin-like growth factor (IGF-1) and type 1 IGF receptor (IGF 1R). *Cell* 1993;75:59–72

67. Fisher DA, Lakshmanan J. Metabolism and effects of epidermal growth factor and related growth factors in mamals. *Endocr Rev* 1990;11:418–38

68. Garnica AD, Chan W-YC. The role of the placenta in fetal nutrition and growth. *J Am Coll Nutr* 1996;15:206–22

69. Hock RA, Hollenberg MD. Characterization of the receptor for epidermal growth factor urogastrone in human placental membrane. *J Biol Chem* 1980;225:10731–6

70. Thorburn GC, Waters MJ, Young IR, *et al*. Epidermal growth factor: a critical factor in maturation? In Whelan J, ed. *The Fetus and Independent Life, CIBA Foundation Symposium 86*. London: Pittman, 1981:172–91

71. Marvo T, Matsuo H, Murata K, Mochizuki M. Gestational age-dependent dual action of epidermal growth factor on human placenta early in gestation. *Endocrinology* 1992;75:1366–72

72. Sporn MB, Roberts AB. Transforming growth factor-β: recent progress and new challenges. *J Cell Biol* 1992;119:1017–21

73. Vuckovic M, Genbacev O, Kumar S. Immunohistochemical localization of TGF-β in first and third trimester human placenta. *Pathobiology* 1992;60:149–50

74. Meunier H, Rivier C, Evans RM, Bale W. Gonadal and extragonadal expression of inhibin α, β$_A$ and β$_B$ subunits in various tissues predicts diverse functions. *Proc Natl Acad Sci USA* 1988;85:247–51

77

What is obstetric ethics?

F.A. Chervenak and L.B. McCullough

INTRODUCTION

This chapter provides an overview of ethics as an essential tool in clinical maternal–fetal medicine. We first define two basic ethical principles, beneficence and respect for autonomy. On this basis, we then provide an account of the clinical–ethical concept of the fetus as a patient. On the basis of this clinical–ethical concept, we identify its implications for clinical practice, particularly directive versus non-directive counselling for fetal benefit. Finally, we provide the reader with tools for evaluating the literature on the ethics of maternal–fetal medicine[1].

THE LANGUAGE AND CONCEPTS OF ETHICS

For centuries, ethics has been defined as the disciplined study of morality. Morality concerns both right and wrong behavior (i.e. what one ought and ought not to do) and good and bad character (i.e. virtues and vices). Since the goal of ethics is to improve human behavior and character, the fundamental question that ethics addresses is: 'What ought morality to be?' This question involves two further questions: 'What ought our behavior to be?' and 'What virtues ought to be cultivated in our moral lives?' Ethics in maternal–fetal medicine deals with these same questions, focusing on what morality ought to be for physicians caring for pregnant women.

The bedrock for what morality ought to be in clinical practice for centuries has been the obligation to protect and promote the interests of the patient. This general ethical obligation needs to be made more specific if it is to be clinically useful. This can be accomplished by attending to two perspectives in terms of which the patient's interests can be understood: that of the physician and that of the patient[2].

The principle of beneficence

The most ancient of these two perspectives on the interests of patients in the history of medical ethics is the perspective of medicine. On the basis of scientific knowledge, shared clinical experience and a careful, unbiased evaluation of the patient, the physician should identify those clinical strategies that will probably serve the health-related interests of the patient and those that will not do so. The health-related interests of the patient include preventing premature death, and preventing, curing or at least managing disease, injury, handicap, or unnecessary pain and suffering[3]. That these matters are constitutive of any patient's health-related interests is a function of the competencies of medicine as a social institution[2]. We cannot overemphasize the point that the identification of a patient's interests is not a function of the personal or subjective outlook of a particular physician, but rather one of rigorous clinical judgement.

The ethical principle of beneficence structures this rigorous clinical perspective on the interests of the patient, because it obliges the physician to seek the greater balance of goods over harms for the patient as a consequence of clinical care. On the basis of rigorous clinical judgement, physicians should identify those clinical strategies that are reliably expected to result in the greater balance of goods (i.e. the protection and promotion of health-related interests) over harms (i.e. impairments of those interests). The principle of beneficence has an ancient pedigree in Western medical ethics, at least back to the time of Hippocrates[3].

The principle of beneficence in maternal–fetal medicine should be distinguished from the principle of non-maleficence, commonly known as *Primum non nocere* or 'First, do no harm'. It is important to note that *Primum non nocere* does not appear in the Hippocratic Oath or in the texts that accompany the Oath. Instead, the principle of beneficence was the primary consideration of the Hippocratic writers. For example, in *Epidemics*, the text reads: 'As to diseases, make a habit of two things – to help or to at least do no harm'[4]. In fact, the historical origins of *Primum non nocere* remain obscure.

There are more than historical reasons to reject *Primum non nocere* as a principle of clinical ethics, because virtually all medical interventions involve unavoidable risks of harm. If *Primum non nocere* were to be made the primary principle of clinical ethics, virtually all of maternal–fetal medicine would be unethical.

Primum non nocere is therefore superseded in the ethics of maternal–fetal medicine by the principle of beneficence. The latter is sufficient to alert the physician to those circumstances in which a clinical intervention has the potential to harm the patient. When a clinical intervention is on balance harmful to a patient, it should not be employed.

The principle of respect of autonomy

A well-formed clinical perspective on the interests of the patient is not the only authoritative perspective on those interests. The perspective of the patient on the patient's interests is equally worthy of consideration by the physician[2]. This is because the patient has developed a set of values and beliefs according to which she is capable of making judgements about what will and will not protect and promote her interests. It is commonplace that, in other aspects of her life, the patient regularly makes such judgements concerning matters of considerable complexity, e.g. choosing a professional calling, rearing children, entering into contracts and writing a will of property. Despite the complexity of these decisions, she is rightly assumed to be competent to make them, with the burden of proof on anyone who would challenge her competence.

The same is true regarding health-care decisions made by the pregnant patient. She must be assumed by her physician to be competent to determine which clinical strategies are consistent with her interests and which are not. In making such judgements, it is important to note that the patient utilizes values and beliefs that can range far beyond the scope of health-related interests, e.g. religious beliefs or beliefs about how many children she wants to have. Beneficence-based clinical judgement, because it is limited by the competencies of medicine, gives the physician no authority to assess the worth or meaning to the patient of the patient's non-health-related interests. Therefore, these are matters solely for the pregnant patient to determine.

The ethical significance of this perspective is captured by the ethical principle of respect for autonomy. This principle obligates the physician to respect the integrity of the patient's values and beliefs, to respect her perspective on her interests and to implement only those clinical strategies authorized by her as the result of the informed consent process.

Respect for autonomy is put into clinical practice by the informed consent process. This process is understood to have three elements:

(1) Disclosure by the physician to the patient of adequate information about the patient's condition and its management;

(2) Understanding of that information by the patient;

(3) A voluntary decision by the patient to authorize or refuse clinical management[5].

Beneficence and respect for autonomy applied in maternal–fetal medicine

There are obviously beneficence-based and autonomy-based obligations to the pregnant patient[2,6]. The physician's perspective on the pregnant woman's interests provides the basis for beneficence-based obligations owed to her. Her own perspective on those interests provides the basis for autonomy-based obligations owed to her. Because of an insufficiently developed central nervous system, the fetus cannot meaningfully be said to possess values and beliefs. Thus, there is no basis for saying that a fetus has a perspective on its interests. There can, therefore, be no autonomy-based obligations to any fetus[2,6,7]. Hence, the language of fetal rights has no meaning and therefore no application to the fetus in obstetric ethics, despite the popularity of right-to-life talk in public and political discourse in the USA and other countries. Obviously, the physician has a perspective on the fetus's health-related interests and the physician can have beneficence-based obligations to the fetus, but only when the fetus is a patient. Because of its importance for the ethics of maternal–fetal medicine, the topic of the fetus as a patient requires careful consideration, to which we now turn.

THE ETHICAL CONCEPT OF THE FETUS AS A PATIENT

The ethical concept of 'the fetus as a patient' has recently come to prominence, largely because of developments in fetal diagnosis and management strategies to optimize fetal outcome[8–12], and has become widely accepted[13–20]. This concept has considerable clinical significance, because, when the fetus is a patient, directive counselling (i.e. recommending a form of management for fetal benefit) is appropriate and, when the fetus is not a patient, non-directive counselling (i.e. offering but not recommending a form of management) is appropriate. However, these apparently straightforward roles for directive and non-directive counselling are often difficult to apply in actual clinical practice because of uncertainty about when the fetus is a patient.

One approach to resolving this uncertainty would be to argue that the fetus is or is not a patient in virtue of personhood[21–26] or some other form of independent moral[27–30]. This approach fails to resolve the uncertainty and we will therefore defend an alternative approach that does resolve the uncertainty.

The independent moral status of the fetus

One prominent approach for establishing whether or not the fetus is a patient has involved attempts to show whether or not the fetus has independent moral status.

Independent moral status for the fetus means that one or more characteristics that the fetus possesses in and of itself and, therefore, independently of the pregnant woman or any other factor, generate and therefore ground obligations to the fetus on the part of the pregnant woman and her physician.

An impressive variety of characteristics have been nominated for this role, e.g. moment of conception, implantation, central nervous system development, quickening and the moment of birth[31–33]. Given the variability of proposed characteristics, there is marked variation among ethical arguments about when the fetus acquires independent moral status. Some take the view that the fetus has independent moral status from the moment of conception or implantation[34–36]. Others believe that independent moral status is acquired in degrees, thus resulting in 'graded' moral status[27,29]. Still others hold, at least by implication, that the fetus never has independent moral status so long as it is *in utero*[28].

In the enormous literature on this subject, there has been no closure on an authoritative account of the independent moral status of the fetus[37,38]. This is not an unsurprising outcome, because, given the absence of a single methodology that would be intellectually authoritative for all of the markedly diverse theological and philosophical schools of thought involved in this endless debate, closure is impossible. For closure ever to be possible, debates about such a final authority within and between theological and philosophical traditions would have to be resolved in a way satisfactory to all, an inconceivable intellectual and cultural event.

It is best, therefore, to abandon futile attempts to understand the fetus as a patient in terms of independent moral status of the fetus and turn to an alternative approach that makes it possible to identify the ethical concept of the fetus as a patient and its clinical implications for directive and non-directive counselling.

The dependent moral status of the fetus

Our analysis of the ethical concept of the fetus as a patient begins with the recognition that being a patient does not require that one possesses independent moral status[30]. Rather, either before or after birth, being a patient means that one has an interest in the applications of the clinical skills of the physician. Put more precisely, a human being – with or without independent moral status – is properly regarded as a patient when two conditions are met: first, that a human being is presented to the physician and, second, there exist clinical interventions in which that human being is justifiably thought to have an interest. Such an interest exists when these interventions are reliably expected to be efficacious, in that they are reliably expected to result in a greater balance of goods over harms for the human being in question and that

human being already is, or is reliably expected to become, a child or person[39]. We call this the dependent moral status of the fetus.

The authors have argued elsewhere that beneficence-based obligations to the fetus exist when the fetus is reliably expected later to achieve independent moral status (sometime during the second year postpartum)[2]. That is, the fetus is a patient when the fetus is presented to the physician and there exist medical interventions, whether diagnostic or therapeutic, that reasonably can be expected to result in a greater balance of goods over harms for the person or child the fetus can later become after birth. The ethical concept of the fetus as a patient, therefore, depends on links that can be established between the fetus and the child, it later achieving independent moral status. These links establish the present interest of the fetal patient in future outcomes of clinical management and subsequent development. The authors emphasize that this is not an argument from or for the potentiality of the fetus to become a person.

The viable fetal patient

One such link is viability. Viability is not an intrinsic property of the fetus, because viability must be understood in terms of both biological and technological factors[38,40,41]. It is only in virtue of both factors that a viable fetus can exist *ex utero* and thus later achieve independent moral status. Moreover, these two factors do not exist as a function of the autonomy of the pregnant woman. When a fetus is viable, i.e. when it is of sufficient maturity so that it can survive into the neonatal period and later achieve independent moral status given the availability of the requisite technological support, and when it is presented to the physician, the fetus is a patient.

Viability exists as a function of biomedical and technological capacities, which are different in different parts of the world. As a consequence, there is, at the present time, no world-wide, uniform gestational age to define viability. In the USA, the authors believe that viability presently occurs at approximately 24 weeks of gestational age[42,43].

When the fetus is a patient, directive counselling for fetal benefit is ethically appropriate. In clinical practice, directive counselling for fetal benefit involves one or more of the following: recommending against termination of pregnancy; recommending against non-aggressive management; or recommending aggressive management. Aggressive obstetric management includes interventions such as fetal surveillance, tocolysis, Cesarean delivery or delivery in a tertiary-care center when indicated. Non-aggressive obstetric management excludes such interventions. Directive counselling for fetal benefit, however, must take account of the presence and severity of fetal anomalies, extreme prematurity and the physician's obligations to the pregnant woman.

In clinical practice, it is very important to appreciate that the strength of directive counselling for fetal benefit varies according to the presence and severity of anomalies. As a rule, the more severe the fetal anomaly, the less directive counselling should be for fetal benefit[7,44]. In particular, when there is '(1) a very high probability of a correct diagnosis and (2) either (a) a very high probability of death as an outcome of the anomaly diagnosed or (b) a very high probability of severe irreversible deficit of cognitive developmental capacity as a result of the anomaly diagnosed'[45], counselling should be non-directive in recommending between aggressive and non-aggressive management[44,45]. Directive counselling against termination of the viable fetus that meets these criteria is a subset of ongoing clinical ethical investigation[46].

By contrast, when lethal anomalies can be diagnosed with certainty, there are no beneficence-based obligations to provide aggressive management[44,47]. Such fetuses are not patients; they are appropriately regarded as dying fetuses and the counselling should be non-directive in recommending between non-aggressive management and termination of pregnancy, but directive in recommending against aggressive management for the sake of maternal benefit[44].

The strength of directive counselling for fetal benefit in cases of extreme prematurity of viable fetuses does not vary. This is also the case for what we term just-viable fetuses[2], those with a gestational age of 24–26 weeks, for which there are significant rates of survival, but high rates of mortality and morbidity[42,43]. These rates of morbidity and mortality can be increased by non-aggressive obstetric management, while aggressive obstetric management may favorably influence outcome. Thus, it would appear that there are substantial beneficence-based obligations to just-viable fetuses to provide aggressive obstetric management. This is all the more the case in pregnancies beyond 26 weeks' gestational age[42,43]. Therefore, directive counselling for fetal benefit is justified in all cases of extreme prematurity of viable fetuses, considered by itself. Of course, such directive counselling is only appropriate when it is based on documented efficacy of aggressive obstetric management for each fetal indication. For example, such efficacy has not been demonstrated for routine Cesarean delivery to manage extreme prematurity[42].

Any directive counselling for fetal benefit must occur in the context of balancing beneficence-based obligations to the fetus against beneficence-based and autonomy-based obligations to the pregnant woman[2,6]. Any such balancing must recognize that a pregnant woman is obligated only to take reasonable risks of medical interventions that are reliably expected to benefit the viable fetus or child later. The unique feature of ethics in maternal–fetal medicine is that whether, in a particular case, the viable fetus ought to be regarded as presented to the physician is, in part, a function of the pregnant woman's autonomy.

Obviously, any strategy for directive counselling for fetal benefit that takes account of obligations to the pregnant woman must be open to the possibility of conflict between the physician's recommendation and a pregnant woman's autonomous decision to the contrary. Such conflict is best managed preventively through informed consent as an ongoing dialog throughout the pregnancy, augmented as necessary by negotiation and respectful persuasion[2,48].

The pre-viable fetal patient

The only possible link between the pre-viable fetus and the child it can become is the pregnant woman's autonomy, because technological factors cannot result in the pre-viable fetus becoming a child. This is simply what pre-viable means. The link between a fetus and the child it can become, when the fetus is pre-viable, can therefore be established only by the pregnant woman's decision to confer the status of being a patient on her pre-viable fetus. The pre-viable fetus has no claim to the status of being a patient independently of the pregnant woman's autonomy. The pregnant woman is free to withhold, confer or, having once conferred, withdraw the status of being a patient on or from her pre-viable fetus according to her own values and beliefs. The pre-viable fetus is presented to the physician solely as a function of the pregnant woman's autonomy.

Counselling the pregnant woman regarding the management of her pregnancy when the fetus is pre-viable should be non-directive in terms of continuing the pregnancy or having an abortion, if she refuses to confer the status of being a patient on her fetus. If she does confer such status in a settled way, at that point the fetus becomes a patient and beneficence-based obligations to her fetus come into existence; furthermore, directive counselling for fetal benefit becomes appropriate for the pre-viable fetus. Just as for viable fetuses, such counselling must take account of the presence and severity of fetal anomalies, extreme prematurity and obligations owed to the pregnant woman.

For pregnancies in which the woman is uncertain about whether to confer such status, the authors propose that the fetus be provisionally regarded as a patient[2]. This justifies directive counselling against behavior that can harm a fetus or future child in significant and irreversible ways, e.g. substance abuse, until the woman settles on whether to confer the status of being a patient on the fetus.

In particular, non-directive counselling is appropriate in cases of what we term near-viable fetuses[2], i.e. those which are 22–23 weeks' gestational age, for which there are anecdotal reports of survival[42]. In the authors' view, for these fetuses aggressive obstetric and neonatal management should be regarded as clinical investigation, i.e. a form of medical experimentation – not standard of care. There is no obligation on the part of a pregnant woman to confer the status of being a patient on a near-viable fetus, because the efficacy of aggressive obstetric and neonatal management has yet to be proven for this population.

The *in vitro* embryo

A subset of pre-viable fetuses as patient concerns the *in vitro* embryo. It might, at first, seem that the *in vitro* embryo is a patient because such an embryo is presented to the physician. However, for there to be beneficence-based obligations to a human being, it also must be the case that there exist medical interventions in which, as we pointed out above, that human being is justifiably thought to have an interest. This is because, in terms of beneficence, whether the fetus is a patient depends on links that can be established between the fetus and its later achieving independent moral status. Therefore, the reasonableness of medical interventions on the *in vitro* embryo depends on whether that embryo later becomes viable. Otherwise, no benefit of such intervention can meaningfully be said to result. An *in vitro* embryo, therefore, becomes viable only when it survives *in vitro* cell division, transfer, implantation and subsequent gestation to such a time that it becomes viable. This process of achieving viability occurs only *in vivo* and is therefore entirely dependent on the woman's decision regarding the status of the fetus(es) as a patient, should assisted conception successfully result in the gestation of the pre-viable fetus(es). Whether an *in vitro* embryo will become a viable fetus and whether medical intervention on such an embryo will benefit the fetus are both functions of the pregnant woman's autonomous decision to withhold, confer or, having once conferred, withdraw the moral status of being a patient on the pre-viable fetus(es) that might result from assisted conception.

It therefore is appropriate to regard the *in vitro* embryo as a pre-viable fetus rather than as a viable fetus. As a consequence, an *in vitro* embryo should be regarded as a patient only when the woman into whose reproductive tract the embryo will be transferred confers that status. Thus, counselling about how many *in vitro* embryos should be transferred and about pre-implantation diagnosis should be non-directive[49]. As to the former, information should be presented about the prognosis for a successful pregnancy and the possibility of confronting a decision about selective reduction, depending on the number of embryos transferred[50]. However, no definitive recommendation should be made about these matters, because directive counselling for fetal benefit is not appropriate until the woman confers the status of being a patient on the *in vitro* embryo. In short, the woman should have the final say about how many embryos are to be transferred. Pre-implantation diagnostic counselling should be non-directive, because the woman may elect not to implant abnormal embryos. These embryos are not patients and so there is no basis for directive counselling.

HOW TO EVALUATE THE LITERATURE OF ETHICS IN MATERNAL–FETAL MEDICINE

Inquiry into the various issues in ethics in maternal–fetal medicine is sure to continue and expand. We therefore provide the reader with tools appropriate to the task of evaluating this literature.

Descriptive versus normative obstetric ethics

The first tool is a basic distinction between descriptive and normative ethics in maternal–fetal medicine. Descriptive ethics employs the long-established methods of the quantitative and qualitative social sciences to obtain data about actual ethical beliefs and practices regarding the ethical dimensions of obstetrics. Normative ethics, by contrast, is concerned with what ethical beliefs and practices in obstetrics ought to be. Normative ethics employs the qualitative methods of rigorous ethical analysis and argument, as we have above. Descriptive obstetric ethics provides an important reference point for normative ethics, but descriptive ethics can never tell us what the beliefs and practices of obstetricians ought to be, only – and importantly – what they actually are. Articles on descriptive obstetric ethics are becoming increasingly common in the literature[51].

Criteria for rigorous ethical analysis and argument in normative ethics

The main qualitative methods of normative ethics are ethical analysis and argument. Ethical analysis identifies component elements of ethical issues in terms of ethical principles, such as beneficence and respect for autonomy, and virtues, such as compassion and integrity[2]. Ethical argument utilizes ethical principles and virtues as premises from which conclusions can reliably be drawn. Over the centuries, philosophical ethics has developed a number of criteria for intellectually rigorous ethical analysis and argument in normative ethics. Our reading of that history is that six criteria are relevant for evaluating ethical analysis and argument for their intellectual rigor.

The first of these is clarity, which requires that terms and concepts be provided precise meanings. Consider for example the popular phrase, 'right to life'[34]. Clarifying this phrase leads to the recognition that 'right to life' does not refer to a single right, but to at least three. These are:

(1) The right not to be killed unjustly;

(2) The right not to have technological or biological supports discontinued unjustly;

(3) The right to have such supports continued for as long as it is reasonable to do so.

This three-part distinction has clinical significance, because each of these rights makes different demands upon the pregnant woman and the physician. For example, the first version seems limited by very few exceptions, whereas the third version must admit of many exceptions because no human being has an overriding right to the property or body of another human being. Yet another clarification can be made about the 'right to life'. In the first two senses just identified, the right is a negative right, i.e. a right to non-interference. In the third sense identified above, the right to life is a positive right, i.e. a claim to the resources of others, including the physician. There is a temptation to trivialize the criterion of clarity as a definition of terms. As the preceding example illustrates, clarity involves much more than mere definition, e.g. careful explanation and the introduction of relevant distinctions.

A second criterion is consistency. Consistency makes two requirements of ethical analysis and argument. First, once key terms and phrases have been clarified, they should always be used with the same meaning to avoid confusion and clinical errors. Second, consistency requires that arguments be free of contradiction. That is, the conclusion of an argument should logically follow from its premises. For example, an inconsistent argument about abortion might be one in which different senses of the 'right to life' are introduced into the premises and the conclusion of an argument. An example would be asserting the first version of the right to life as the sole premise of an argument and concluding that abortion in the case of rape or incest is permissible because the fetus does not have an overriding right to continue to exist under those circumstances. The problem is that this conclusion does not follow from a premise that asserts the right of the fetus not to be killed unjustly. This is because such a right stands independently of how the fetus is conceived. Hence, the exceptions claimed in the conclusion, rape and incest, are inconsistent with the first sense of a fetal right to life. Hence the argument fails because of a lack of consistency. Unfortunately, this does not prevent this position from being advanced in public debate.

A third criterion is coherence. Coherence requires the premises of an argument to join together into a meaningful whole. For example, simply listing ethical principles without demonstrating their connection to each other fails to satisfy the criterion of coherence. Thus, if one were to say that criminal penalties for drug use during pregnancy were ethically unjustified on the grounds of the principles of autonomy and beneficence, without showing how in clinically meaningful terms the two principles complement each other regarding this topic, such a stringing together of principles would fail the criterion of coherence.

A fourth criterion is clinical applicability. Clinical applicability requires that normative ethics can actually be used to guide and direct clinical judgement and behavior in maternal–fetal medicine. That is, normative ethics worthy of the name is never an 'ivory tower' enterprise, because normative obstetric ethics should be solidly grounded in clinical reality.

A fifth and related criterion is clinical adequacy. Clinical applicability means that normative obstetric ethics applies to present clinical realities. Clinical adequacy means that normative obstetric ethics will be applicable in future, as yet unforeseen, clinical situations.

Finally, all of the preceding criteria presuppose a well-known criterion of scholarship, namely, completeness. Just as in clinical research, so, too, in normative ethics, no ethical analysis and argument in the ethics of maternal–fetal medicine is complete unless it takes account of, and responds to, the existing literature on the subject being addressed.

Readers may conveniently recall these criteria for intellectual rigor in normative obstetric ethics as the 'six C's': clarity, consistency, coherence, clinical applicability, clinical adequacy and completeness[52].

Pitfalls to be avoided

Careful evaluation of the literature in obstetric ethics involves the identification of pitfalls to be avoided. These pitfalls occur when the inherent limitations in the several disciplines that contribute to normative obstetric ethics are ignored. Because of their prominence, we will consider law, religion, professional consensus, uses of authority, and philosophy.

The main limitations of the law – common, statutory, regulatory and administrative – are its incomprehensiveness and possible inconsistency. While the law is surely clinically applicable and clinically adequate to many areas of obstetric practice, it is silent or virtually silent in many other areas. For example, some state courts have issued court orders for Cesarean delivery for fetal distress or placenta previa. However, no court has addressed, or is likely to address, a pregnant woman's disinclination to appear for prenatal care until she is in labor, although there would be justified ethical doubts about such behavior on beneficence-based grounds concerning both the woman's and the fetal patient's interests. Moreover, the law is largely silent on the virtues that physicians in the practice of maternal–fetal medicine ought to cultivate. Yet, attention to virtues such as compassion and integrity is critical for any adequate response to society's concerns about the dehumanization of obstetric practice[2].

The law is also at risk for internal conflict and thus possible inconsistency. On the one hand, statutory and regulatory law governing publicly funded health care seems to obligate physicians to do less for their patients. On the other hand, the common law of malpractice seems to obligate physicians to do more. Ignoring the incomprehensiveness or possible inconsistency of the law involves a pitfall.

The main limitations of religion are its potential lack of clinical applicability and clinical adequacy. This is because obstetric ethics based on religious belief requires all to accept, first, the existence of a deity or some transcendent reality and, second, a particular interpretation within a community of faith of what the deity or transcendent reality deems to be the ultimate good of human beings – two conditions that can never be satisfied in a pluralistic society that includes people of different religions, as well as atheists or agnostics[22]. In addition, because the intellectual warrant of medicine, the biomedical sciences, and because the legal warrant of medicine, licensure by the state, are secular in character, any ethics of maternal–fetal medicine based on religion cannot be presumed to be clinically applicable or clinically adequate. To suggest otherwise involves a serious pitfall.

The main limitation of consensus[53] concerns the distinction drawn earlier between descriptive and normative ethics. The limitation of consensus is that it is a version of descriptive ethics. Taking consensus to be normative obstetric ethics involves a serious pitfall.

Uses of authorities are also subject to limitations[54]. The problem here is that the intellectual authority of any expert view in obstetric ethics depends on the quality and rigor of the analysis and argument that supports the view (i.e. satisfying the six C's) and not on the prestige of an individual, an academic institution, professional association, or government commission or agency. These individuals or institutions may well have produced well-reasoned analysis and argument. The pitfall of inappropriate uses of authorities occurs when one overlooks the need to evaluate the statements of authorities according to the six C's. Such statements, therefore, should not be taken at face value.

The main limitation of philosophical ethics is a function of its subject matter. Aristotle noted centuries ago that a science or area of knowledge can only be as exact as its subject matter[55]. The subject matter of philosophical ethics comprises human beliefs and behaviors, which are notoriously inexact. From this fact, Aristotle correctly concluded that philosophical argument in ethics cannot ever be exact in the sense that geometric proofs are exact. The lesson of Aristotle for our time is that the aims of any endeavor in the normative ethics of maternal–fetal medicine should be intellectually rigorous ethical analysis and argument that acknowledge intellectually rigorous competing ethical analysis and argument. This should not be a disabling shortcoming, provided that the ethical analysis and argument in question satisfy the six C's. The pitfall of philosophical ethics is to treat one's ethical analysis and argument as final and irrefutable and thus above the necessity to acknowledge competing ethical analysis and argument.

Accepting this limitation of philosophical ethics has great value, because doing so obliges one to be willing to receive, and respond in a thoughtful way to, the critical evaluation of others. Every experienced clinician knows that failure to be open to critical evaluation of one's clinical judgement and practice in scientific matters more often than not leads to preventable problems in the care of patients. The same is true for clinical judgement and practice in ethical matters. In other words, the lack of finality that at first appears to be a serious limitation, turns out on closer consideration to be an intellectual and clinical virtue and thus a powerful antidote to narrow-mindedness and inflexibility.

REFERENCES

1. Chervenak FA, McCullough LB. What is obstetric ethics? *J Perinat Med* 1996;23:331–41
2. McCullough LB, Chervenak FA. *Ethics in Obstetrics and Gynecology*. New York: Oxford University Press, 1994
3. Beauchamp TL, Childress JF. *Principles of Biomedical Ethics*, 3rd edn. New York: Oxford University Press, 1989
4. Hippocrates. *Epidemics* i:xi. Jones WHS. Translation. Loeb Classical Library, vol 147. Cambridge: Harvard University Press, 1923
5. Faden RR, Beauchamp TL. *A History and Theory of Informed Consent*. New York: Oxford University Press, 1986
6. Chervenak FA, McCullough LB. Perinatal ethics: a practical method of analysis of obligations to mother and fetus. *Obstet Gynecol* 1985;66:442–6
7. Chervenak FA, McCullough LB. Does obstetric ethics have any role in the obstetrician's response to the abortion controversy? *Am J Obstet Gynecol* 1990;163:1425–9
8. American Academy of Pediatrics Committee on Bioethics. Fetal therapy: ethical considerations. *Pediatrics* 1988;81:898–9
9. American College of Obstetricians and Gynecologists. Committee on Ethics. *Patient Choice: Maternal-Fetal Conflict*. Washington, DC: American College of Obstetricians and Gynecologists, 1987
10. American College of Obstetricians and Gynecologists. *Ethical Decision-making in Obstetrics and Gynecology*. Technical Bulletin. Washington, DC: American College of Obstetricians and Gynecologists, 1989
11. Harrison MR, Golbus MS, Filly RA. *The Unborn Patient*. New York: Grune & Stratton, 1984
12. Liley AW. The foetus as a personality. *Aust NZ J Psychiatr* 1972;6:99–105
13. Fletcher JC. The fetus as patient; ethical issues. *J Am Med Assoc* 1981;246:772–3

14. Mahoney MJ. Fetal–maternal relationship. In Reich WT, ed. *Encyclopedia of Bioethics*. New York: Macmillan, 1978:485–9

15. Mahoney MJ. The fetus as patient. *West J Med* 1989; 150:517–40

16. Murray TH. Moral obligations to the not-yet born: the fetus as patient. *Clin Perinatol* 1987;14:329–44

17. Newton ER. The fetus as patient. *Med Clin North Am* 1989;73:517–40

18. Pritchard JA, MacDonald PC, Gant NF. *Williams' Obstetrics*, 17th edn. Norwalk: Appleton–Century–Crofts, 1985;xi

19. Shinn RL. The fetus as patient: a philosophical and ethical perspective. In Milunsky A, Annas GJ, eds. *Genetics and the Law III*. New York: Plenum Press, 1985

20. Walters L. Ethical issues in intrauterine diagnosis and therapy. *Fetal Ther* 1986;1:32–7

21. Anderson G, Strong C. The premature breech: Cesarean section or trial of labor? *J Med Ethics* 1988; 14:18–24

22. Engelhardt HT, Jr. *The Foundations of Bioethics*. New York: Oxford University Press, 1986

23. Fleming L. The moral status of the fetus: a reappraisal. *Bioethics* 1987;1:15–34

24. Ford NM. *When Did I Begin? Conception of the Human Individual in History, Philosophy and Science*. Cambridge, UK: Cambridge University Press, 1988

25. Strong C. Ethical conflicts between mother and fetus in obstetrics. *Clin Perinatol* 1987;14:313–28

26. Strong C, Anderson G. The moral status of the near-term fetus. *J Med Ethics* 1989;15:25–7

27. Dunstan GR. The moral status of the human embryo. A tradition recalled. *J Med Ethics* 1984;10:38–44

28. Elias S, Annas GJ. Reproductive genetics and the law. Chicago: Year Book Medical Publishers, 1987

29. Evans MI, Fletcher JC, Zador IE, *et al.* Selective first-trimester termination in octuplet and quadruplet pregnancies: clinical and ethical issues. *Obstet Gynecol* 1988; 71:289–96

30. Ruddick W, Wilcox W. Operating on the fetus. *Hastings Cent Rep* 1982;12:10–14

31. Curran CE. Abortion: contemporary debate in philosophical and religious ethics. In Reich WT, ed. *Encyclopedia of Bioethics*. New York: Macmillan, 1978: 17–26

32. Hellegers AE. Fetal development. *Theol Stud* 1970; 31:3–9

33. Noonan JT, ed. *The Morality of Abortion*. Cambridge: Harvard University Press, 1970

34. Bopp J, ed. *Restoring the Right to Life: The Human Life Amendment*. Provo: Brigham Young University, 1984

35. Bopp J, ed. *Human Life and Health Care Ethics*. Frederick, MD: University Publications of America, 1985

36. Noonan JT. *A Private Choice. Abortion in America in the Seventies*. New York: The Free Press, 1979

37. Callahan S, Callahan D, eds. *Abortion: Understanding Differences*. New York: Plenum Press, 1984

38. Roe v. Wade, 410 US 113 (1973)

39. Chervenak FA, McCullough LB. The fetus as patient: implications for directive versus non-directive counselling for fetal benefit. *Fetal Diagn Ther* 1991;6:93–100

40. Fost N, Chudwin D, Wikker D. The limited moral significance of fetal viability. *Hastings Cent Rep* 1980; 10:10–13

41. Mahowald M. Beyond abortion: refusal of Cesarean section. *Bioethics* 1989;3:106–21

42. Hack M, Fanaroff AA. Outcomes of extremely-low-birth-weight infants between 1982 and 1988. *N Engl J Med* 1989;321:1642–7

43. Whyte HE, Fitzhardinge PM, Shennan AT, *et al.* Extreme immaturity: outline of 568 pregnancies of 23–26 weeks' gestation. *Obstet Gynecol* 1993;82:1–7

44. Chervenak FA, McCullough LB. An ethically justified, clinically comprehensive management strategy for third-trimester pregnancies complicated by fetal anomalies. *Obstet Gynecol* 1990;75:311–16

45. Chervenak FA, McCullough LB. Nonaggressive obstetric management: an option for some fetal anomalies during the third trimester. *J Am Med Assoc* 1989; 261:3439–40

46. Chervenak FA, McCullough LB, Campbell S. Is third trimester abortion justified? *Br J Obstet Gynaecol* 1995; 102:434–5

47. Chervenak FA, Farley MA, Walters L, *et al.* When is termination of pregnancy during the third trimester morally justifiable? *N Engl J Med* 1984;310:501–4

48. Chervenak FA, McCullough LB. Clinical guides to preventing ethical conflicts between pregnant women and their physicians. *Am J Obstet Gynecol* 1990;162:303–7

49. Grifo JA, Boyle A, Tang YX, *et al.* Preimplantation genetic diagnosis. *Arch Pathol Lab Med* 1992;116:393–7

50. Wapner RJ, Davis GH, Johnson A, *et al.* Selective termination of multifetal pregnancies. *Lancet* 1991; 335:90–3

51. Wertz DC, Fletcher JC. *Ethics and Human Genetics: A Cross-cultural Perspective*. Heidelberg: Springer-Verlag, 1989

52. Chervenak FA, McCullough LB. How to critically evaluate positions on obstetric ethics. *J Reprod Med* 1993; 38:281–4

53. Moreno J. Ethics by committee: the moral authority of consensus. *J Med Phil* 1988;14:411

54. Rachels J. When philosophers shoot from the hip. *Bioethics* 1991;5:67

55. Aristotle. *Nichomachean Ethics*. Indianapolis: Bobbs–Merrill, 1962

Index